Manipal Manual of
Clinical Methods in
Surgery

Differential Diagnosis and Clinical Discussion

Included

Viva Voce Examination

Manipal Manual of
Clinical Methods in
Surgery

Differential Diagnosis and Clinical Discussion

Included
Viva Voce Examination

Chief editor

K Rajgopal Shenoy MBBS, MS, FRCS (Glasgow)

Professor
Department of Surgery
Ex-Associate Dean–Academics
Kasturba Medical College, and
Consultant Surgeon, Kasturba Hospital, Manipal 576104
Karnataka, India
Manipal Academy of Higher Education (MAHE)
email: kallyarajgopalshenoy@gmail.com

Co-editor

Anitha Shenoy (Nileshwar) MBBS, MD, FRCA

Professor and Head
Department of Anaesthesiology
Kasturba Medical College, and
Consultant Anaesthesiologist, Kasturba Hospital, Manipal 576104
Karnataka, India
Manipal Academy of Higher Education (MAHE)
email: anitharshenoy@gmail.com

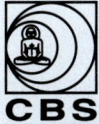

CBS

CBS Publishers & Distributors Pvt Ltd

New Delhi • Bengaluru • Chennai • Kochi • Kolkata • Mumbai
Bhubaneswar • Hyderabad • Jharkhand • Nagpur • Patna • Pune • Uttarakhand

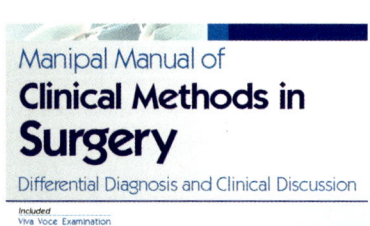

Manipal Manual of
**Clinical Methods in
Surgery**
Differential Diagnosis and Clinical Discussion

Included
Viva Voce Examination

ISBN: 978-93-87964-30-3

Copyright © Editors and Publisher

First Edition: 2019

Published by Satish Kumar Jain and produced by Varun Jain for

CBS Publishers & Distributors Pvt Ltd
4819/XI Prahlad Street, 24 Ansari Road, Daryaganj, New Delhi 110 002
Ph: 23289259, 23266861, 23266867   Fax: 011-23243014   Website: www.cbspd.com
e-mail: delhi@cbspd.com; cbspubs@airtelmail.in

Corporate Office: 204 FIE, Industrial Area, Patparganj, Delhi 110 092
Ph: 4934 4934   Fax: 4934 4935   e-mail: publishing@cbspd.com; publicity@cbspd.com

Branches

- **Bengaluru:** Seema House 2975, 17th Cross, K.R. Road,
  Banasankari 2nd Stage, Bengaluru 560 070, Karnataka
  Ph: +91-80-26771678/79   Fax: +91-80-26771680   e-mail: bangalore@cbspd.com
- **Chennai:** 7, Subbaraya Street, Shenoy Nagar, Chennai 600 030, Tamil Nadu
  Ph: +91-44-26260666, 26208620   Fax: +91-44-42032115   e-mail: chennai@cbspd.com
- **Kochi:** 42/1325, 1326, Power House Road, Opp KSEB Power House, Ernakulam 682 018, Kochi, Kerala
  Ph: +91-484-4059061-65   Fax: +91-484-4059065   e-mail: kochi@cbspd.com
- **Kolkata:** No. 6/B, Ground Floor, Rameswar Shaw Road, Kolkata-700014 (West Bengal), India
  Ph: +91-33-2289-1126, 2289-1127, 2289-1128   e-mail: kolkata@cbspd.com
- **Mumbai:** 83-C, Dr E Moses Road, Worli, Mumbai-400018, Maharashtra
  Ph: +91-22-24902340/41   Fax: +91-22-24902342   e-mail: mumbai@cbspd.com

Representatives

- **Bhubaneswar**   0-9911037372   • **Hyderabad** 0-9885175004   • **Jharkhand**   0-9811541605   • **Nagpur**   0-9021734563
- **Patna**   0-9334159340   • **Pune**   0-9623451994   • **Uttarakhand** 0-9716462459

Printed at Manipal Technologies Limited., Manipal, Karnataka, India

to

All patients who form the central pillar of the book.
All discussions revolve around patients.
They have been generous in their approval in taking photographs
and have given consent for educational purpose in spite of their sufferings
and
KASTURBA HOSPITAL, MANIPAL

Forewords

Medical undergraduate students are often told that patients are their best teachers. The caveat here is in making the patients talk and listening to them. The art of history taking and clinical examination is best learnt from good teachers and good books. *Manipal Manual of Clinical Methods in Surgery* by Dr Rajgopal Shenoy and Dr Anitha Shenoy provides a unique way of introducing surgery to undergraduate students. Syndromic approach in surgical teaching has been practiced for long but this excellent manual takes it beyond the classic approach and enters the exciting realm of differential diagnosis. Here is an example of a good book written by good teachers.

This handy, ready to refer, illustrated manual will be useful resource for medical students. Books like this have to be a necessary part of a medical student's repertoire. I have a suspicion that this Manual will see several reprints and editions.

Prof H Vinod Bhat
Vice-Chancellor
Manipal Academy of Higher Education (MAHE)
Manipal

I have great pleasure in writing the Foreword to this book. The *Manipal Manual of Surgery*, and *Manipal Manual of Instruments* by Dr Rajgopal Shenoy and Dr Anitha Shenoy have been popular among the students of surgery. This book on *Manipal Manual of Clinical Methods in Surgery* is borne out of more than three decades of extensive experience of the authors in teaching and evaluation of the undergraduate and postgraduate surgical students of many Universities of Karnataka and neighbouring states. Dr Rajgopal Shenoy has been a popular resource person in many CMEs and PG teaching programs. All the clinical cases encountered by the students in the general surgery examination have been covered in 29 chapters.

There are some unique features of this book. The 'Clinical Discussion' presented in the form of questions and answers is helpful to prepare the students to face the clinical examination of short and long cases. The common case scenario along with clinical photographs is followed by the analysis of the signs, the logic and reasoning in making the diagnosis. The 'Clinical Wisdom' and 'Clinical Boxes' highlighted in color leave a lasting impression in the minds of the reader and improve retention. The liberal use of colorful clinical photographs and diagrams enhances the learning experience. The language is easy to understand and has a consistent style which is lacking in many books written by multiple authors.

The book is student-friendly and envisages to lay firm foundation to basic principles of clinical methods in surgery in both undergraduate and postgraduate learners of surgical science. I am sure this book will be as popular as the earlier books by the same authors.

Prof Ashok Godhi MS, FRCS (Glasgow)
Prof of Surgery
Former Principal, JNMC, Dean (FoM)
KLE Academy of Higher Education
Belagavi

It gives me immense pleasure to write the Foreword on latest in the series of Manipal Manuals—*Manipal Manual of Clinical Methods in Surgery*. This is a different book altogether with clinical discussion, differential diagnosis, a lot of change in script as well as illustrations in the manual.

I appreciate the efforts of Professor K Rajgopal Shenoy and Dr Anitha Shenoy (Nileshwar) in bringing out this practical manual for day-to-day use in surgical floors. His untiring efforts became fruitful in bringing out this beautiful manual for students and surgical faculty. I definitely say that this book is more useful to develop a competent medical graduate and postgraduate. This book is helpful not only for resident doctors but also for practising surgeons as a rapid reference book. Dr Shenoy is a popular faculty in CME of most of the South Indian medical colleges. He has prepared this book with his vast experience in general surgery and with expert opinions from senior professors and colleagues.

The language he has used in the book is very easy for understanding and the content is more informative. The emphasis is mainly on the practical and routinely used material. Hence, it is more helpful in ward rounds and discussions. The diagrams in this book assist the reader in gaining proper knowledge of the topic and create utmost interest in the minds of readers.

I wish good luck to the readers who are going to use this manual for examination purpose. I congratulate the author and publisher for their untiring efforts in bringing out a new jewel in the hands of practising surgeons.

With best wishes

NV Ramaniah
Principal
(Former Professor and Head, Department of Surgery)
SV Medical College, Tirupathi
Chittoor District
Andhra Pradesh

Preface

One cannot become a competent clinician unless sufficient time is spent with the patients. Clinical knowledge cannot be gained just from reading books but must be obtained from bedside.

This manual is not just another book. It is unique and is taking birth at a time when many books on clinical methods are available in the market. A general feeling exists among students that clinical methods are not all that important because everything can be diagnosed by investigations. This is simply not true. Clinical methods are important. Many clinical illustrations in this manual will help the students learn clinical methods properly. In addition, this manual will help the students to discuss the cases properly in the examinations within the limited time frame.

After examining the students in various universities over the last 25 years or more, I realised that there will always be an element of anxiety or fear among students. Many students who score very high marks in theory have failed in the clinical examination. The reasons can be many: Firstly, they may not have seen a particular case at all and that is the case they get in the university examination, and secondly, different examiners ask different questions and a kind of ambiguity may be present in the exam hall (performing hall).

So, what does Manipal Manual on clinical methods offer? I have tried my level best to provide you with relevant clinical methods, high quality clinical photographs, common and uncommon case discussions with examples. I always tell the students that seeing is believing. One careful look at the clinical photographs will tell you so many aspects about the disease and description of the disease—whether it is a swelling, ulcer, gangrene or abdominal mass. As far as I know, I can say that the details given in the chapter on abdominal mass/skin tumours and many others are not available in any other book on clinical methods. This was possible because of the vast experience gained from patients (bedside) not only after working in KMC, Manipal since 1986 but also after participation in several CMEs all over India. Thus, contributions of various teachers, both senior and junior, have been carefully selected and inserted in the book. The whole idea of this book is to make the clinical methods simple, easy to understand and help students answer the questions in the clinical examination. Some photographs have been included more than once at different places in the book to aid explanation of different clinical aspects and also to help the student by not having to go back and forth to look at those photographs.

A word of caution: There is no end to the questions asked by examiners and no limit for anyone to insert the answers in a book. Questions and answers given in each chapter help the students to get a feel of facing a real examination. I have made a sincere attempt in this *Manipal Manual of Clinical Methods in Surgery* to give most probable questions and answers. It is up to the readers to make use of the book properly so as to sail smoothly through the sea of examination and reach the shore safely. My best wishes to all the students.

Students of many other disciplines such as Ayurveda or homeopathy can also use the manual since it is easy to understand because of many figures, photos, tables, clinical case capsules, clinical wisdom, clinical boxes and flowcharts.

Practising surgeons and even general practitioners can make use of the book because of clinical discussions and quick reference to a few guidelines in the management.

I have added a section of Viva Voce because it is also part of clinical examination. Thus, carrying this one book solves many of your problems and reduces anxiety.

Dear students, please do make use of the clinical facilities in your hospital to the maximum during your clinical postings. Read well, prepare well, study all photographs given in *Manipal Manual of Clinical Methods in Surgery* carefully and achieve success with flying colours. Give me a feedback about the book—good or bad with suggestions.

K Rajgopal Shenoy

Email: kullyarajgopalshenoy@gmail.com

Acknowledgements

Abhay Taranath Kamath
Professor and Head
Department of Oro-Maxillo-Facial Surgery

and

Deepika Kamath
Associate Professor
Department of Pedodontics
Manipal College of Dental Sciences
Manipal
Chapter on Examination of Jaw Swelling

Clinical Photographs, Clinical Methods and Clinical Discussion

This was made possible because of active participation in various conferences, several continuing medical and surgical education (CME and CSE) teaching programs conducted by several medical colleges in India over more than three decades. I am very grateful to all of you. My sincere apologies if I have forgotten to include the names of a few resource persons.

1. Bangalore Surgical Society Annual CMEs since 2007. It is here I had opportunity to meet several senior and junior faculties not only from Bangalore but also from most of Southern states and gain knowledge from them. However, it is my duty to mention the key anchor of the clinical sessions, Dr Anjanappa and others who assisted him. They are Dr MR Srivatsa and Dr CS Rajan to whom I am very much thankful.

2. Sri Venkateshwara Medical College, Tirupathi
   Dr Ramaniah NV, Dr Srihari, Dr Manohar, Dr Haribabu

3. Karnataka Institute of Medical Sciences, Hubballi
   Dr Gurushantappa, Dr Mallikarjuna Desai, Dr Madakatti

4. Government Medical College, Mysore
   Dr Geetha Avadani, Dr MA Balakrishna, Dr Dinesh, Dr Ravikumar

5. Vijayanagar Institute of Medical Sciences, Bellary, Karnataka, India
   Dr Vidyadhar Kinhal, Professor and Head

6. MS Ramaiah Medical College, Bangalore
   Dr MR Srivatsa, Dr Bagali Baba Sab, Dr SV Kulkarni, Dr Bharathi, Dr Sreekar Pai

7. Calicut Medical College, Calicut, Kerala
   Dr P Rajan, Dr KK Rajan, Dr Shashi, Dr Sreejayan

8. Madurai Medical College, Madurai
   Dr Marudhu Pandyan, Dr Amutha, Dr Damodharan, Dr Chitra, Prof. Satyavan and others

9. Sri Ramachandra Medical College, Chennai
   Dr Balaji Singh, Dr Ravi, Dr Vishwanath Pai

10. Christian Medical College, Vellore
    Dr Iniyan Samarasan, Dr Sukriya Nayak, Dr MJ Paul

11. Jawaharlal Nehru Medical College, Belagavi
    Dr Ashok Godhi, Dr V M Uppin, Dr Shashi Uppin, Dr AC Pangi

12. NKP Salve Institute of Medical Sciences, Nagpur
    Dr Murtaza Akhtar, Dr Satish Deshmukh, Dr BS Gedam

13. JSS Medical College, Mysore
    Dr Siddesh G, Dr Madu, Dr (Late) Manjunath Shenoy

14. Goa Medical College, Goa
    Dr Dilip Amonkar

15. Shivamogga Institute of Medical Sciences, Shivamoga
    Dr Sushil Kumar, Dean and Dr SV Mohan

16. Nizam's Institute of Medical Sciences, Hyderabad and ASI Telangana Branch
    Dr N Bheerappa, Dr Sureshchandra Hari, Dr Sridhar

17. Sri Mookambika Institute of Medical Sciences, Kulashekar, Tamil Nadu
    Dr Velayudhan Nair, Dr Sounderrajan, Dr Mukambika, Dr Vinu Gopinath

18. PSG Medical College, Coimbatore, Tamill Nadu
    Dr Premkumar, Dr Vimal Kumar, Dr Rajesh Kumar, Dr Sunay Bhat

19. St. John's Medical College, Bengaluru
    Dr LN Mohan, Dr Arun Kilpadi

20. Gokulam Medical College, Thiruvananthapuram
    Prof. Dayananda Babu

21. Lourde Hospital, Kochi
    Dr Santhosh John Abraham

We wish to acknowledge and thank

Dr Ramdas M Pai, Chancellor, Manipal Academy of Higher Education (MAHE), Mrs Vasanthi Ramdas Pai and Dr Ranjan Pai, CEO, MEMG, for giving us an opportunity to grow in this prestigious institution from postgraduation (1983) till date.

Prof HS Ballal, Pro-Chancellor, Manipal Academy of Higher Education (MAHE) for providing constant encouragement.

Prof H Vinod Bhat, Vice-Chancellor, Manipal Academy of Higher Education (MAHE) for writing the Foreword and giving support to academic activities.

Prof CR Ballal, my guru, my well-wisher and mentor, for all-time support and encouragement.

Prof MG Shenoy, Prof. U. Santosh Pai, Prof. BH Anand Rao, Prof. H. Diwakar Shenoy, Prof. P. Sampath Kumar, Prof. Annappa Kudva, Prof. Ramachandra L, Prof. S.S. Prasad, KMC, Manipal, for their support. My sincere thanks to Late Professors of Surgery—Dr N. Rajan, Dr MN Nayak also, under whom I had worked and gained clinical wisdom.

Dr Ashok Godhi, a very senior teacher, clinician and resource person, my well-wisher and my mentor, shared the stage with me on many occasions during CMEs and contributed to the book and also wrote Foreword.

Dr Ramaniah NV, another well-wisher and guide, who always encouraged me wherever we met—CME halls, workshops and conferences. Sir, your contributions are also included.

Dr Keerthan Upadhya and Dr Krishna Kalyan Reddy have gone through the manuscript with utmost patience, have given suggestions for changes and corrected grammatical errors. I am indebted to them.

Dr Sunil Krishna, Dr Chitra Bhat, Department of Surgery, Dr Joseph Thomas, Assistant Professor, Department of Plastic and Reconstructive Surgery, KMC, Manipal, for timely help in updating the subject.

Dr Muqurab Ali Khan, Dr Kartik, Dr Vishnu, Dr Venkatesh, Dr Kawari Saubhagya, Dr Shruthi Pandith, Dr Aneesh, Dr Akanksha Rajput, Dr Shravya, Dr Pawan Bhat, Postgraduates, Department of Surgery, for correcting the text meticulously and giving suggestions.

Dr Navneeth Kamath, Dr Kausthabh KP, interns have not only corrected but have also given suggestions about the type of questions and usefulness of the text. I am very much thankful to them.

Dr Swathi John, Dr Priya Pai, Dr Sravya, Dr Anshika Gupta, Dr Suhas Dr Samarth, Dr Vani, Dr Jaya, Dr Vijay, Dr Akansha Singh, Dr Sravya, Dr Sonalika, Dr Ateesh Shetty, (interns), Shantanu Gulati, Anwesha Das, Divyanshu Chawla, Shivani Shenoy K, Kanika Arora, Raj Shekar (students) have also done the corrections at the final phase of the book.

Mr YN Arjuna, Sr VP—Publishing, CBSP&D, for his help with the prepress work; Mrs Ritu Chawla, AGM—Production, CBSP&D, for resetting and repagination the text with an attractive page layout and design; Mr Wilfred Lobo, Chetana Printers, Mangalore, a friend of mine who had helped to compose my previous books and also helped me with a few chapters while preparing this manual; Mr SK Jain, Managing Director, for excellent production of this book.

Our apologies if we have omitted anyone who may have contributed to this venture, as it is unintentional.

Medicine must be learnt from patients and so, this book could be written because of the large number of patients who attended Kasturba Hospital, a teaching hospital attached to KMC, who agreed for photographs and students who inspired me from the time I joined this institution in 1986. All of you (students, both undergraduate and postgraduate) are alumni now. This book has taken this shape because of you: Students. We are ever grateful to you. Do enjoy reading *Manipal Manual of Clinical Methods in Surgery*.

K Rajgopal Shenoy

Anitha Shenoy

Contents

1

Introduction to Examination of a Surgical Patient

INTRODUCTION

When I was a student, clinical examination was the only method available to detect a disease and to guide its management in majority of the patients. Radiological investigations were minimal and hence it was very important to do a complete clinical examination with judicial use of clinical methods. It was not uncommon to find a large crowd of faculty members accepting the so-called 'final diagnosis' from a senior professor even though it was proved 'wrong' later by laparotomy or by investigations. Gone are those days of the so-called 'final word'! We now believe in evidence-based science.

Today, after 30 years, because of the availability of a variety of investigations such as CT (computerised tomography) scan, MRI (magnetic resonance imaging) scan, and endoscopies, diagnosis of many conditions has become easy. Consequent to this, students may cut short the history-taking and clinical methods. **In India, clinical methods are still relevant in the clinical examination.** It should be remembered that clinical medicine is the most important and most challenging part of medicine where, students will develop communication skills, interpretation skills and analytical skills. Above all, this communication gives them an opportunity to know what suffering is and teaches them how to conduct themselves with the patients.

STUDENT–PATIENT RELATIONSHIP

The very fact that a person has come to the hospital means that he has some complaints. Complaints can be major or minor. The first thing students

need to do before commencing history-taking and examination is *to make the patient comfortable.* A comfortable patient is more likely to co-operate with eliciting history and permitting clinical examination. This is also the first lesson in establishing doctor–patient rapport (Clinical Box 1.1).

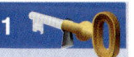

Clinical Box 1.1

Clinical code of conduct
- Dress well, wear proper shoes and look neat.
- Read well and come—do not read in front of the patient.
- Be sensitive to the feelings of the patients.
- Make the patient comfortable.
- Talk to the patient in his own language.
- Allow the patient to express himself.
- Follow up your patient till he is discharged from the hospital.
- Do not discuss patients' problems in public.
- Insist on a female nurse while examining female patient.

Enough time should be spent in the history-taking, and taking the patient into confidence. It is always better to talk to the patient in his own language. Patients can explain the events better in their own language than a language known to the students but not to them. Often, when you ask one question you may get a lengthy answer. In such situations, it is better to listen to the patient than tell him that it is irrelevant or not required, etc. *Allow the patient to express himself. It helps in building of rapport.*

The students should conduct themselves with dignity and be sensitive to the feelings of the patients. *Dress well, wear proper shoes and look neat.* This inspires confidence in them. Students are required to carry the following instruments—stethoscope, knee hammer, pen torch, skin marking pencil and measuring tape.

Name: What is the patient's name?

You get familiarised with the patient by calling him by his name. Don't you feel happy when a teacher calls you by your name?

Age: What is patient's age?

Some diseases are common in certain age groups. Following are a few examples:

- Tuberculous lymphadenitis in young patients
- Cystic hygroma (lymphatic cyst) and haemangioma in children
- Oral cancer in elderly patients
- Secondaries (metastasis) in the neck lymph nodes common in elderly patients
- Thromboangiitis obliterans (TAO) is common in men smokers between 30 and 40 years of age and atherosclerotic disease is common after 50 years.
- Appendicitis is common in young patients
- Branchial cyst, though congenital, appears in second or third decade
- Gallstones are typically seen in fatty female patients around 40 years of age
- Malignancies mostly occur in elderly patients. Examples: Carcinoma stomach in middle-aged men, bronchogenic carcinoma in old-aged men. *However, it should be remembered that testicular tumours occur in young boys.*

Gender: What is the patient's gender?

For reasons less known, certain diseases are more common in women than in men.

Following are a few examples

- Tuberculous lymphadenitis is more common in women
- Postcricoid carcinoma is more common in women
- Apical bronchogenic carcinoma is common in men smokers
- *Haemophilia* is seen *exclusively in male* children even though it is *transmitted by females.*

Occupation: What is the patient's occupation?

Some diseases are related to occupation

- Varicose veins (dilated, tortuous veins) occur in patients who require to stand for a prolonged period of time such as agriculturists, hotel workers, traffic police, etc.
- Truck drivers, sailors in India have increased incidence of HIV.
- Carcinoma lip is common in those with outdoor occupation such as agriculturists. Hence, it is called *country man's lip*. It is due to ultraviolet rays resulting in solar keratosis or actinic cheilitis which can predispose to carcinoma lip.
- Gardeners are susceptible to *thorn prick* injuries which can give rise to *implantation dermoid cyst* (page 72).
- Trumpet blowers may have laryngocoele
- If a patient is a *teacher or a singer,* who may present with *thyroid swelling*—utmost care should be taken during surgery *to avoid injuries to laryngeal nerves.* Possible complications should be clearly explained to the patients.
- Farmers and butchers can get anthrax
- Hydatid disease is common in shepherds and butchers.

Place: Where is he/she from?

Certain regions of the state or country have increased incidence of some diseases.

- Thyroid swellings are more common in low lying areas wherein iodine content of the water is less. Such goitres are called *endemic goitres.*
- Chronic pancreatitis is more common in Kerala state.
- Gall stone disease is more common in patients from North Indian states.
- Peptic ulcer is common in South India.
- Gall bladder cancer is more common in Gangetic river belt.

Socioeconomic status: What is his/her socioeconomic status?

- *Poor socioeconomic status:* Thromboangiitis obliterans, carcinoma penis.
- *Higher socioeconomic status:* Atherosclerotic disease in the form of ischaemia of the limbs and malignant melanoma (cutaneous malignancy).

Date of admission: When did he/she get admitted to the hospital?

This is for record purposes.

- Did he/she get admitted from outpatient department (OPD) which means it is an elective case.
- Did he/she get admitted through casualty which means it must have been an emergency situation.
- Does he/she have any records from referring hospital—if so, please make a note of it and get more details.

SUMMARY

After getting all this information, please summarise and present the case. One example is given below:

Mr Gangadhar, a 35-year-old male patient, a teacher by occupation, coming from Manipal, presented to the outpatient department with the following complaints.

COMPLAINTS

Every complaint is important. All complaints must be listed in the *chronological* order, i.e. every disease starts with certain complaints. Hence, whichever complaint appeared first has to be mentioned first. A few examples are given below.

Example 1: Thyroid swelling (Fig. 1.1)

1. Swelling in front of the neck—5 years
2. Palpitation since 3 months

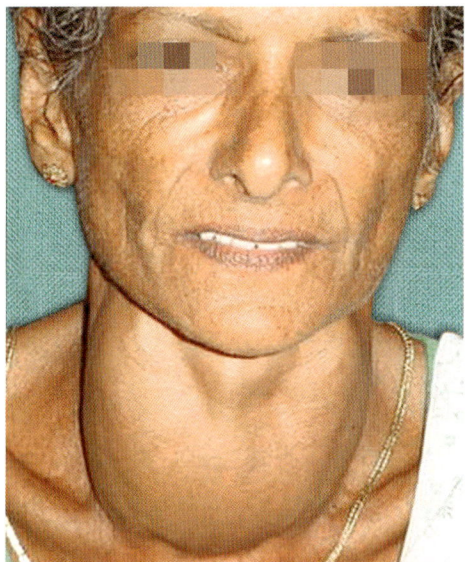

Fig. 1.1: She was a 48-year-old lady who had multinodular goitre of 10 years duration. She also had palpitations

Analysis of the complaints: Swelling is of 5-year duration—it means it is likely to be a benign lesion. It is in front of the neck—so, most probably it is a thyroid swelling.

Patient has developed palpitations since 3 months: It means thyroid gland is producing more hormones. Hence, toxic features have developed in this swelling—hence the case is mostly toxic goitre.

Example 2: Ulcer over leg in a 50-year-old diabetic man

1. Ulceration in the sole of the foot—6 months
2. Swelling in the groin—10–15 days

Analysis of the complaints: Ulcer in the leg started first. This may be malignant as in squamous cell carcinoma or malignant melanoma (skin cancers) and the groin swelling could be metastasis in lymph nodes. In case the ulcer is benign such as trophic ulcer (diabetic foot), the groin swelling may be due to lymph node enlargement due to secondary infection.

Example 3: Case of dysphagia in a 75-year-old man

1. Difficulty in swallowing—3 months
2. Swelling over neck—15 days

Analysis of the complaints: Difficulty in swallowing is dysphagia. This started first and could be due to some lesion in the posterior third of the tongue, oropharynx or oesophagus. This was followed by swelling in the neck, most likely due to metastasis in a lymph node.

Example 4: Case of mass in the epigastrium (upper abdomen) in a 50-year-old man

1. Early satiety, loss of appetite since 2 months
2. Vomiting since 10 days
3. Swelling on the left side of the neck since 3 days.

Analysis of the complaints: With the first complaints, he may be having some malignancy in the upper abdomen mostly carcinoma stomach. Vomiting indicates obstruction, may be in the pylorus. Hence, it may be carcinoma antrum of the stomach. Swelling in the left supraclavicular region is most likely due to lymph node enlargement. (Enlarged supraclavicular lymph node in malignancies is called Virchow's node.) Thus, the case may be advanced carcinoma stomach with lymph node metastasis.

Example 5: Case of lump in the breast in a 40-year-old lady

1. Lump in the breast—6 months
2. Axillary swelling—2 months
3. Abdominal distension—10 days

Analysis of complaints: Lump in the breast can be due to carcinoma of the breast or a benign aetiology such as fibroadenoma. Axillary swelling is due to enlargement of axillary group of lymph nodes. Abdominal distension can be due to ascites (fluid) caused by spread of malignant cells into the peritoneal cavity. Last two symptoms cannot be caused by fibroadenoma but can be caused by carcinoma breast.

Example 6: Case of ulcer in the leg in a 35-year-old male

1. Dilated veins in the leg—2 years duration.
2. Itching—3 months duration.
3. Ulcer—15 days

Here again, dilated veins started first. They are called varicose veins. Itching appeared later. It is due to skin changes caused by dilated veins carrying deoxygenated blood. As it progresses, skin ulceration develops (Fig. 1.2).

- Chronological order of presentation is a must.
- You should not jump to conclusions in the beginning but you should analyse the case right from the beginning. Ask yourself, is this the diagnosis or is it something else?
- Can I explain all symptoms of the patient with this diagnosis?

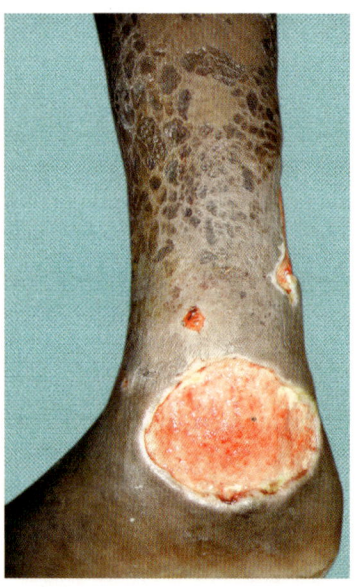

Fig. 1.2: Venous ulcer leg

HISTORY OF PRESENT ILLNESS

- History of present illness includes history from the time complaint started till the time of your presentation of the case. Narrate the sequence of all events in detail. However, any irrelevant history need not be mentioned. In the beginning, you will not be in a position to conclude what is relevant and what is not. Hence, it is better to present all that the patient tells you.

- Take any case and start asking questions about the complaints: How did it start, when did it start, how is the growth, has it been growing slowly, has it grown big within a short period or has it become smaller in size? Any other complains?

- *How and when*: Many thyroid swellings start insidiously or they are noticed by relatives or friends. In such cases, it is better to say swelling is *insidious* in onset. On the other hand, haemorrhage in multinodular goitre appears suddenly. Look at another example. The patient may tell you that he had a small swelling in his back since 3 years and never gave him any problem but suddenly since previous night onwards, he is getting pain. It could be *infection in a sebaceous cyst.* This is described as *sudden onset of pain.*

Progress of the Disease

- *Rapid progress is a feature of malignancies* (Fig. 1.3): Examples—soft tissue sarcoma, poorly differentiated carcinoma, and carcinoma oral cavity. Phyllodes tumour of the breast grows very rapidly. This, however, is often benign (page 295, Fig. 20.12).

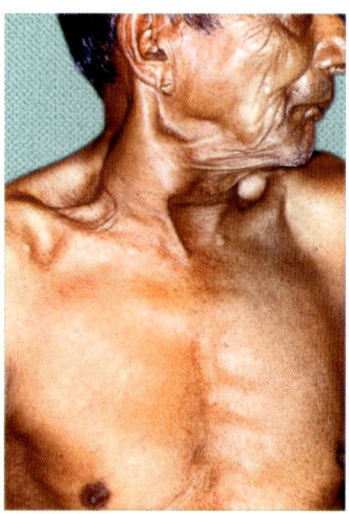

Fig. 1.3: Metastasis in the neck 2 months duration

- *Slow progress is a feature of benign diseases:* Examples—cystic swellings, goitres, etc. Size of the swelling may decrease as in inflammatory diseases or resolving haematoma—patient says he had a fall and then noticed swelling in his thigh. It is becoming smaller in size over the last few days.
- Malignant swellings do not decrease in size.

Pain

- Any ulcer or any swelling which starts with *pain and fever* indicates *inflammatory* condition. Examples are—boil, carbuncle (abscess in diabetic patients usually seen in the nape of the neck). Low grade fever may be a part of inflammation, but high degree fever indicates presence of pus (abscess). Thyroiditis can present as swelling and pain.

  Painful benign swelling can be arising from nerve fibres such as neurofibroma or neurilemmoma.

- However, a swelling which was painless initially but later became painful can be due to various reasons:

  a. Secondary infection, e.g. sebaceous cyst.

  b. Malignant tumour infiltrating bone, e.g. carcinoma buccal mucosa infiltrating mandible. In this situation, pain is constant, dull aching and well localised.

  c. Malignancy infiltrating nerve fibres, e.g. carcinoma tongue involving lingual nerve, sarcoma thigh infiltrating sciatic nerve, etc. In this situation, the pain radiates along the nerve fibres. Some patients describe this as *shooting type of pain.*

Thus, I have given a few complaints and analysis. With each disease, you will find many such complaints and you should try to elicit more details about each one of them.

History-taking is an art. To be more effective, good knowledge of the subject is necessary. To be more successful, more number of patients should be examined. If you achieve this, you will be a successful doctor.

Past History

- Once again, all relevant complaints and the treatment received from the patient have to be recorded in the chronological order. Students may feel some of them may not be relevant but you have to record them. At this stage, what you feel is not relevant may be an important relevant history and later may clinch the diagnosis. Here are a few examples:

1. A patient presented to the hospital with a sinus (blind track with opening) in the chin discharging pus. His past history is that he had been getting recurrent pain in his tooth. Students may feel it is irrelevant but the fact is that the *caries teeth are responsible* for this sinus formation (Fig. 1.4).

2. A patient presented to the hospital with a huge swelling in the groin. She had a lesion in the left fourth toe of the foot which had been amputated 3 years back. What is the relevance of this history? The lesion excised may be a malignant melanoma and groin swelling is due to enlarged lymph nodes (Figs 1.5 and 1.6).

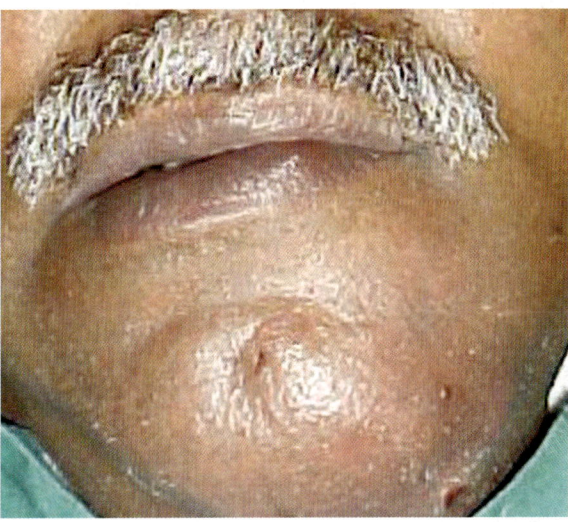

Fig. 1.4: Median mental sinus (*Courtesy:* Dr Dinesh BV, Associate Professor of Surgery, KMC, Manipal)

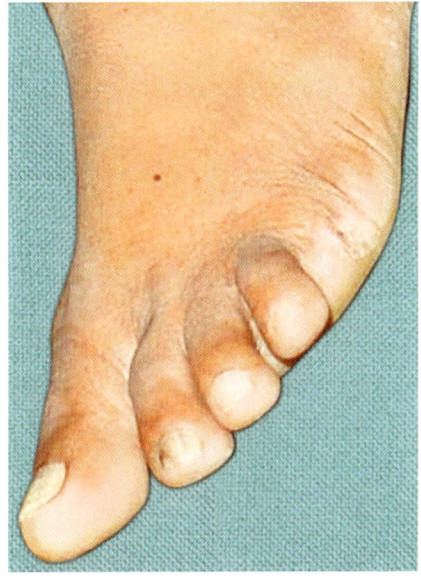

Fig. 1.5: Observe the foot, little toe had been amputated 3 years back for malignant melanoma (*Courtesy:* Prof U Santosh Pai, Ex-Professor of Surgery, KMC, Manipal)

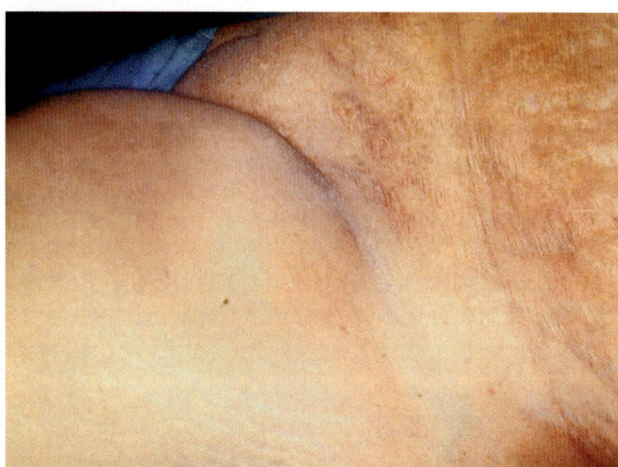

Fig. 1.6: Patient presented 3 years later with enlarged inguinal lymph nodes

3. Patient had undergone abdominal surgery in the past. Please take all the details. Whether the surgery was elective or emergency, what about patient's condition before and after surgery, was any blood transfusion given? What was the patient told after the surgery? What was the histological diagnosis or biopsy report? Getting details about previous surgery will help you in many ways. *Example*: If he was operated for cancer of the stomach by gastrectomy, the present problems can be due to the incision (incisional hernia) or due to recurrence or due to metastasis ascites, palpable nodular liver, etc.

Personal History

• This mainly refers to some of the habits such as smoking, consumption of alcohol, tobacco and betel nut chewing, etc. Detailed history should include number of beedis or cigarettes smoked, amount of alcohol consumed or pan chewed, etc.

– Heavy smoking (refer to page 109 for pack year index—PYI) alcohol and nonvegetarian diet predispose to carcinoma of the upper aerodigestive tract such as oral cancer or carcinoma oesophagus.

– Smoking also causes bronchogenic carcinoma and Buerger's disease (thromboangiitis obliterans).

– Pan chewing with areca causes oral cancer.

• Is the patient married or single, a widow or widower? How is the family—number of children and their health?

• Bachelors and frequent travellers have increased chances of sexual exposure and related diseases including HIV infections. (Syphilis is almost rare nowadays.)

• Frequent travelling, consumption of water and food can also precipitate hepatitis, amoebiasis, etc.

• Altered bowel or bladder habits reflect diseases of the colon/urinary tract.

• Tuberculous infection of the lungs can easily spread from one person to another, if precautions are not taken properly.

• Missed period is most important history which gives a clue in the diagnosis of ruptured ectopic gestation, which presents as acute abdominal pain and shock. Menstrual history in females is very important in cases of carcinoma of the breast and in acute abdomen in females.

• Pre-/postmenopausal status also is important deciding factor while treating cases of carcinoma breast.

Family History

1. Enquire whether any member of the family has suffered from similar diseases.

• Carcinoma colon runs in families

• Carcinoma breast can be familial

• Medullary carcinoma thyroid can also be familial.

2. First degree relatives can also be affected by the genetic diseases.

• Haemophilia

• Polycystic disease of the kidney

• Diabetes

• Piles

3. Undoubtedly, cardiac diseases (myocardial infarction) have strong genetic predisposition.

Treatment History

1. *Drugs*: Often patients are receiving antidiabetic agents (oral hypoglycaemic agents and injection insulin), antitubercular agents, antihypertensive drugs, anticonvulsants, antithyroid, anticoagulants, etc. More patients are receiving *antiplatelet* agents for cardiac/neurologic conditions. Make a note of these.

Each drug has some side effects. Try asking whether any of the symptoms is related to these drugs. *Example:* Hepatitis can be caused by rifampicin—a drug used to treat tuberculosis.

2. Any surgical procedures which are known for recurrences—if inadequate excision has been done for malignant tumours, the lesion can recur, e.g.

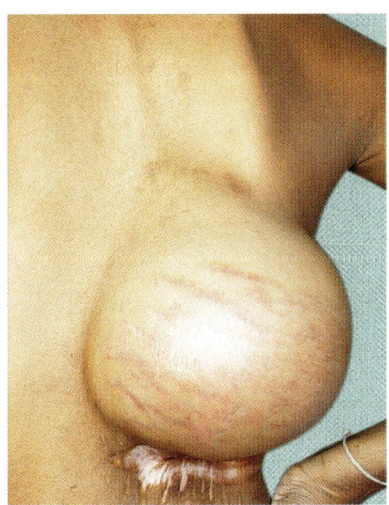

Fig. 1.7: Recurrent soft tissue sarcoma back

sarcoma. Other tumours also can recur in spite of adequate (Fig. 1.7) excision such as desmoid tumours, keloid, fibromatosis.

3 Any hospitalisation for major illness such as for a surgical procedure or for a medical illness.

4. Treatment for any allergic reactions/asthma

5. History of laparotomy/family planning procedures.

GENERAL PHYSICAL EXAMINATION

General survey of the patient from *head to toe* must be done now. The important points and their relevance are given below:

1. *General appearance*: A quiet, co-operative patient indicates that he is not in agony. Patients who are in pain will not cooperate with students and will never be quiet.

   - Comment on mental state: Is he conscious with orientation to time, space and person? Is he drowsy? If these features are not there, say he is normal.

   - An emaciated, cachectic patient is typically having carcinoma oesophagus, tuberculosis, etc.

   - Prominent eyes associated with a thyroid swelling suggest primary thyrotoxicosis (Fig. 1.8).

2. *Attitude*: Occasionally, the diagnosis can be arrived at by looking at the attitude of the patients in the bed. A few examples are given below:

   - An elderly male sitting in the outpatient department with *handkerchief spitting saliva frequently* is almost diagnostic of carcinoma of the posterior third of the tongue.

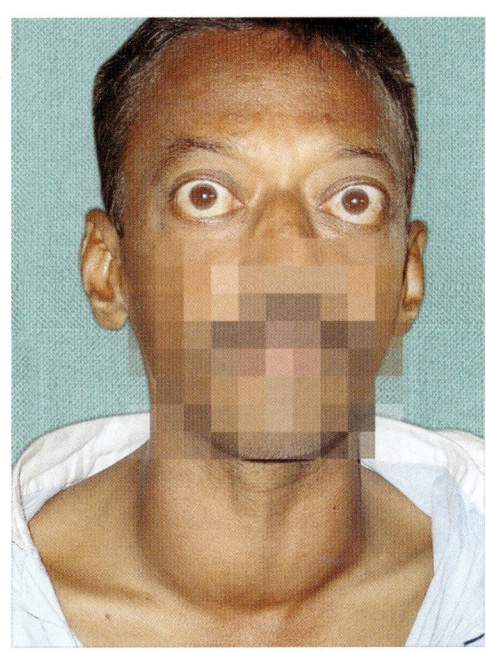

Fig. 1.8: He was 31-year-old with loss of weight of 12 kg in 3 months. There was diffuse enlargement of the gland with exophthalmos. Case of primary thyrotoxicosis

   - *A restless patient* who is sweating even in cold climatic conditions may be having thyrotoxicosis.

   - *A child sitting* with hands pressing the chin up may be having *tuberculosis of the cervical spine* with collapse of vertebrae **(Rust sign)**.

   - *Chronic smoker,* who is unable to sleep in the night—sitting on the bed with his legs *hanging down is probably* having severe *ischaemic rest pain (TAO)* (Fig. 1.9).

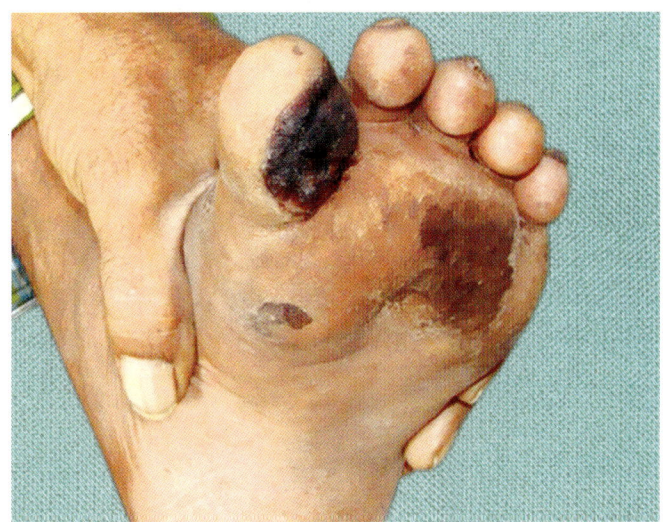

Fig. 1.9: Attitude of TAO patient—foot is tightly held by hand. Observe gangrene, ulcer, skin changes and ridged nails

3. **Build and nourishment**: Average build indicates adequate nutrition. Poor nutrition indicates malnutrition or chronic diseases such as tuberculosis, uncontrolled diabetes or carcinoma.

- A patient with a tall build and marfanoid features may be having medullary carcinoma of the thyroid.
- Interestingly varicose veins of the leg are common in tall and obese patients.
- Short built—dwarfism can be due to various causes specially endocrinal as in hypopituitarism.
- Assessment of the nourishment is done by calculating body mass index (BMI). It is easy, simple and reliable method.

$$\text{BMI} = \frac{\text{Body weight in kilograms}}{\text{Height in square metres}}$$

Accordingly, patients can be classified as:

a. Underweight = Less than 18.5 kg/m²

b. Normal weight = 18.5 to 25 kg/m²

c. Overweight = 25 to 30 kg/m²

d. Obese = Over 30 kg/m²

- Some changes will indirectly reflect on nutritional status. They are wasting of muscles, flat nails, angular cheilitis, skin changes, thinning or loss of hair, dementia, neurological changes, etc.

4. **Anaemia**: Anaemia refers to decreased haemoglobin or circulating red blood cells and manifests as pallor. Look at the conjunctiva and look for anaemia. Anaemia may be because of nutritional cause, blood loss from gastrointestinal tract or due to chronic diseases including tuberculosis or carcinoma. Pallor refers to pale skin and conjunctival discolouration.

- Mucous membrane is the ideal site to look for pallor (oral mucosa and tongue).
- Lower eyelid is turned down to look for conjunctival pallor (Fig. 1.10).

There are many causes of low haemoglobin.

A. **Gastrointestinal tract bleeding**: Common causes are chronic duodenal ulcer, chronic gastric ulcer, portal hypertension, haemorrhoids, etc. Carcinoma stomach and carcinoma caecum are notorious that sometimes they present with anaemia due to occult blood loss and iron deficiency anaemia.

B. **Malignant tumours**: The occurrence of anaemia can be the first diagnostic clue to suggest a malignant disease, and is **present in more than 30% of cancer patients.**

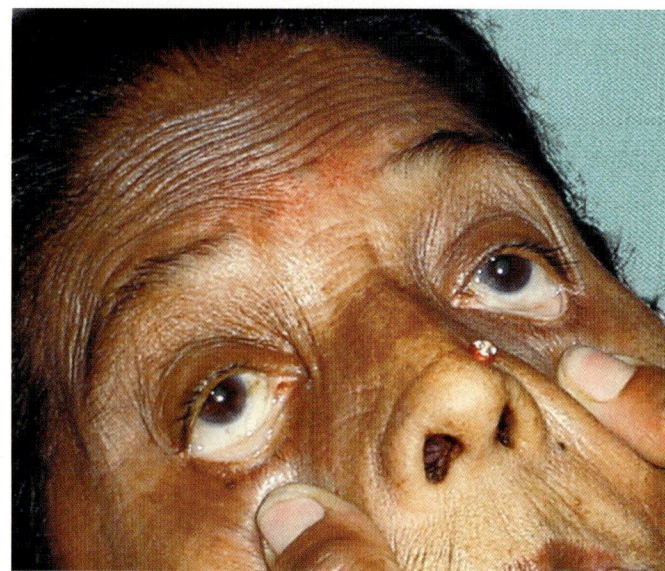

Fig. 1.10: Gross pallor: Patient had carcinoma caecum

- **Invasion of bone marrow**: Certain cancers, such as leukaemias, lymphomas, myeloma, carcinoma breast and prostate, invade the bone marrow. The bone marrow contents decrease or change due to accumulation of abnormal amyloid protein, necrosis (dead tissue) and fibrosis leading to anaemia.
- **Cancer and immune response**: This immune response results in the secretion of proteins called **cytokines** that serve a signaling function between components of the immune system. *These cytokines appear to reduce the production of some haematopoietic growth factors, notably erythropoietin,* and can *impair the bone marrow* response to erythropoietin.
- **Carcinoma and bleeding**: Carcinoma stomach, carcinoma caecum, carcinoma rectum, and renal cell carcinoma also give rise to bleeding resulting in anaemia.
- **Cancer treatment**: Surgery, radiotherapy, chemotherapy with a single drug or in combination will give rise to anaemia.

C. **Nutritional deficiencies**: Iron, B$_{12}$ or folic acid.

D. **Haemolysis**: Haemolytic anaemias, which present as splenomegaly, mild icterus and anaemia, are classical examples encountered in the surgical ward.

5. **Icterus**: Yellowish discolouration of sclera, skin, and mucous membranes indicates jaundice. In obstructive jaundice, sclera can occasionally have deep yellow or even greenish hue due to oxidation

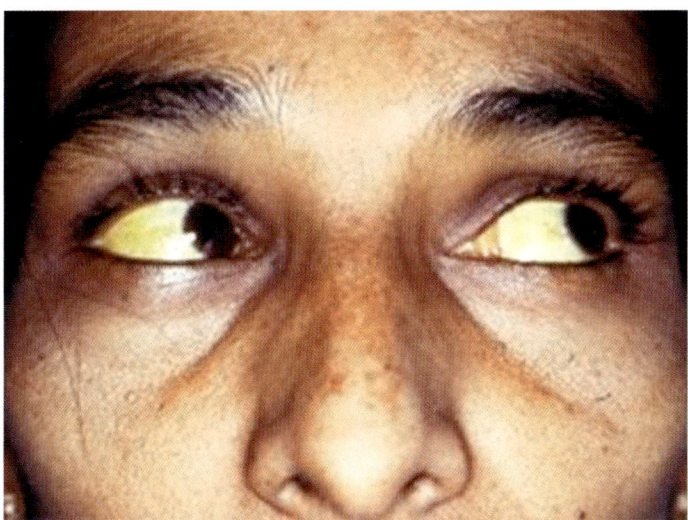

Fig. 1.11: Lemon yellow eyes in hereditary spherocytosis (*Courtesy:* Prof U Santosh Pai, Ex-Professor of Surgery, KMC, Manipal)

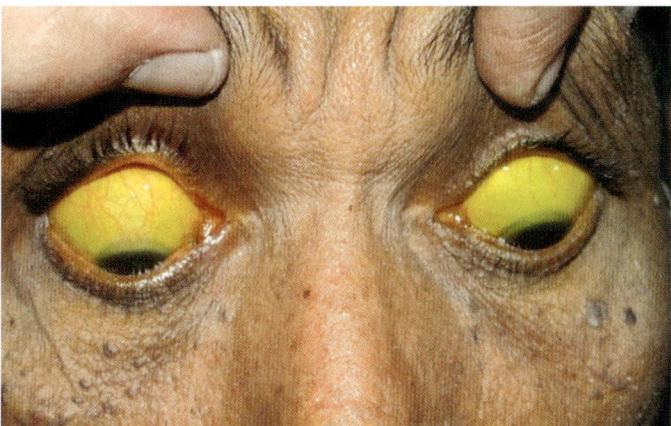

Fig. 1.12: Obstructive jaundice

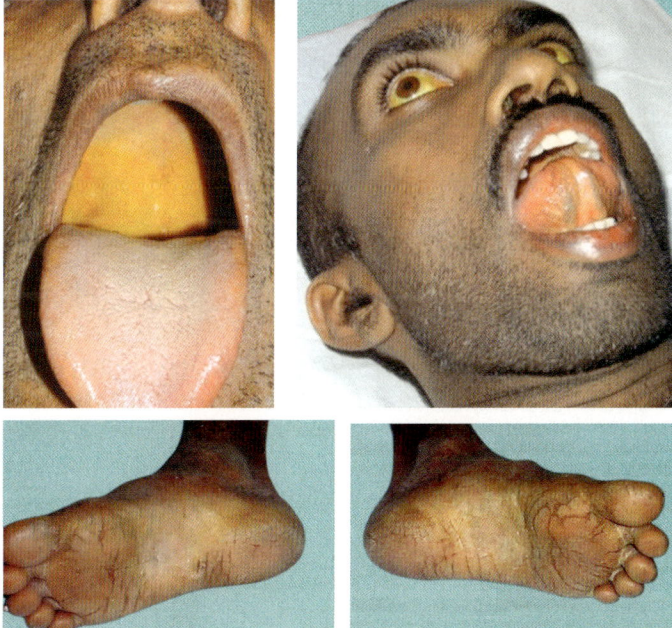

Figs 1.13 to 1.16: Greenish yellow changes in obstructive jaundice. Sites to look for jaundice are sclera palate, undersurface of the tongue and even feet

of bilirubin to biliverdin. *Generalised yellow colour may be present not only in jaundice but also in pernicious anaemia and carotenaemia. However, sclera will not be yellow in carotenaemia.* Depending upon the depth of the jaundice, it can be of following types:

- *Pale yellow colour:* Haemolytic jaundice
- *Orange yellow:* Hepatocellular jaundice
- *Greenish yellow:* Obstructive jaundice (Figs 1.12 to 1.16)

- **Obstructive jaundice (surgical jaundice):** It is diagnosed when patients have dark urine, pale stools, itching with or without abdominal pain. Eyes are deep yellow in colour and sometimes have greenish colour due to biliverdin. Carcinoma head of pancreas, periampullary carcinoma, stones in the common bile duct and stricture are common causes. (For more details refer to page 352). Conjugated hyperbilirubinaemia is a feature. Conjugated bilirubin is water-soluble and stains the urine dark. Unconjugated bilirubin is tightly bound to albumin and not filtered at the glomerulus.

- **Hepatic jaundice:** Common drugs causing hepatic damage are paracetamol, dextropropoxyphene, INH, rifampicin, PAS, phenytoin, propylthiouracil, halothane, etc.

- **Cholestatic jaundice:** Common drugs causing cholestasis are dextropropoxyphene, erythro mycin, sulfasalazine, PAS, chlorpromazine, phenytoin, etc.

6. *Cyanosis:* Bluish or purple discolouration of skin and mucous membrane due to poor oxygenation is called cyanosis. Bluish discolouration of the conjunctiva occurs due to many causes including respiratory and cardiac causes. Thus lips, tongue, and tip of the fingers are the common sites to look for. It is found in medical patients with cardiac illness or respiratory diseases. Severe pneumonia, pulmonary oedema, and chronic obstructive pulmonary diseases are a few examples. Congenital heart diseases, and valvular diseases are the other causes. More details are given in medical books.

7. *Clubbing:* It refers to bulbous enlargement of terminal phalanges. **It occurs due to arteriovenous shunt resulting in increased vascularity of the**

local part. Clubbing is seen in many conditions, the important ones being chronic pulmonary diseases such as bronchiectasis, lung abscess, emphysema, bronchogenic carcinoma, and cardiovascular causes such as congenital and cyanotic heart diseases, subacute bacterial endocarditis, etc. For a surgeon, clubbing can be found in a condition called thyroid acropachy (pretibial myxoedema with clubbing of fingers and toes). Biliary cirrhosis, non-small cell lung carcinoma, and inflammatory bowel disease are a few other causes.

8. *Koilonychia*: It means 'spoon-shaped nails' as seen in anaemia. Pink nails indicate good circulation and pale-ridged nails indicate poor circulation (leukonychia). *Onycholysis*: Destruction of nails is seen in local fungal infections and psoriasis.

9. *Generalised lymphadenopathy*: When two or more anatomical sites of the lymph nodes are palpable, it is called generalised lymphadenopathy.

- Common causes for generalised lymphadenopathy include lymphoma, tuberculosis, infectious mononucleosis, leukaemia, etc. These are all systemic diseases. If they are present, they have to be mentioned. Any localized or regional lymphadenopathy should be mentioned later along with the local examination. *Example*: In a case of carcinoma breast, examination of axillary lymph nodes and supraclavicular group of lymph nodes becomes part of **regional or local examination.**

  - Neck, axilla and groin are the common sites of lymph node enlargement. There are many causes of lymphadenopathy which will be discussed later.

  - When a lymph node is palpable, size is more than 1 cm in the neck or 2 cm in the groin, when the node is hard or when the node is fixed, it is called a 'clinically significant lymph node'. However, supraclavicular lymph node when it is just palpable (shotty) is significant as it very often signifies underlying malignancy.

  - **As per oncology principles, if a node is palpable in the drainage area of the primary cancer, it is considered significant.**

  - It should be remembered that inguinal vertical chain of lymph nodes can be more than 2 cm but may not be significant specially in Indian patients due to bare foot walking or due to recurrent filarial infections.

  - Palpable epitrochlear node may suggest non-Hodgkin's lymphoma.

- When multiple nodes in one group are enlarged, it is called regional lymphadenopathy.

- Multiple, matted, mobile nodes—tuberculosis.

- Tender lymph nodes suggest enlargement following acute infections.

- Large rubbery, non-matted bulky nodes are typical of Hodgkin's lymphoma (Fig. 1.17).

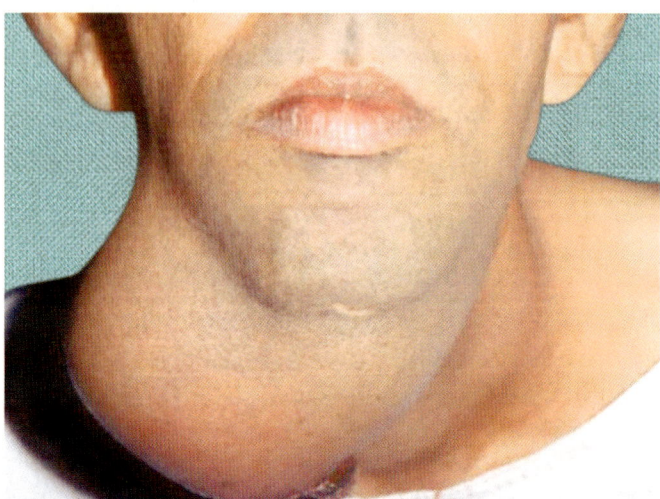

Fig. 1.17: Advanced stage of Hodgkin's lymphoma: Bilateral massive enlargement of nodes

10. *Oral cavity* (details are given in oral cavity chapter)

  - Bad odour of the oral cavity reflects malignancy very often. It is due to putrefying bacterial infection in a malignant lesion.

  - Any ulcer/leukoplakia must be noted.

  - Hygiene can be poor.

  - *Teeth*: Nicotine stains are of smoking. These suggest diseases related to tobacco, e.g. thromboangiitis obliterans and oral cancer (Fig. 1.18).

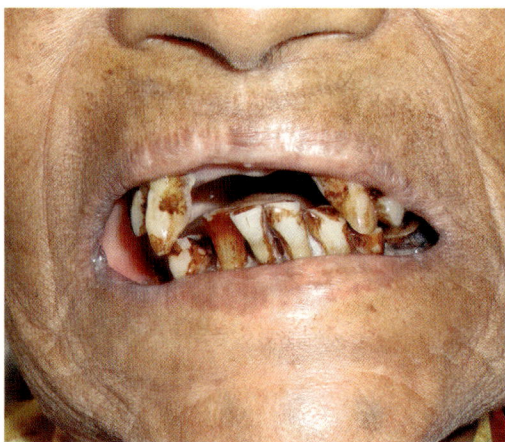

Fig. 1.18: Carcinoma buccal mucosa infiltrating mandible—severe trismus. Also observe tobacco stains

Teeth may fall off spontaneously, if there is expansion of the mandible or destruction of the mandible as in osteomyelitis or malignancies infiltrating the mandible. Dentigerous cyst arises from unerupted permanent tooth.

- Examine the tongue, buccal mucosa and lips especially for any nonhealing ulcers which suggest malignancy.

11. *Pedal oedema*: Pitting refers to depression created by the pressure of the finger over the oedematous part. It is checked in the lower third of the medial side of the leg (Figs 1.19 and 1.20).

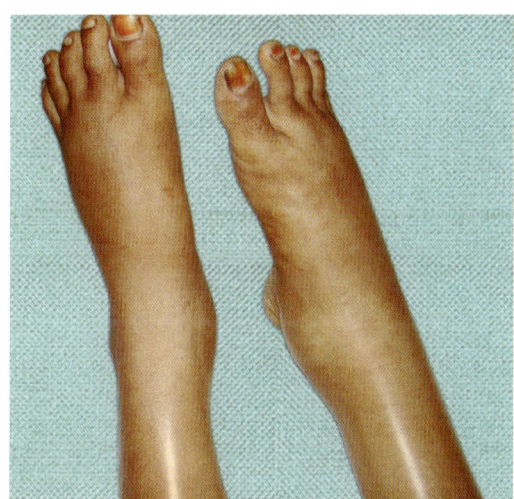

Fig. 1.19: Bilateral pedal oedema—a case of severe hypoproteinaemia in nephrotic syndrome

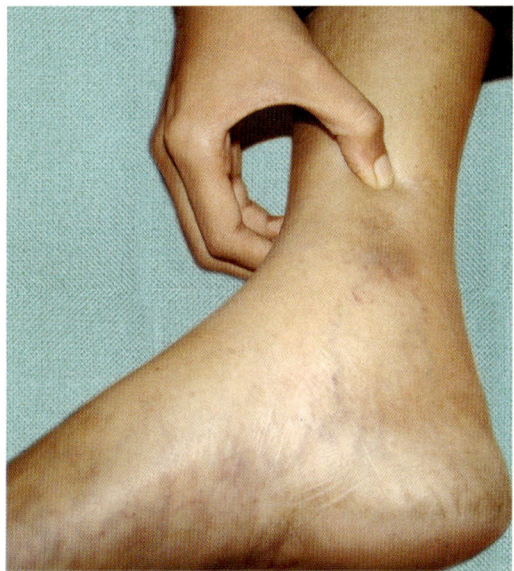

Fig. 1.20: Pitting test to check for oedema of leg

12. *Spinal tenderness*: This is specially highlighted in Indian cases because Pott's spine or tubercular (TB) spine is a common problem. Tenderness over the spine is one of the common signs of the TB spine. It is elicited by exerting firm pressure over the *lateral aspect of the spinous process* of the vertebrae—and rotation of the vertebral body results in pain. *Kyphotic deformity of the 2 or 3 vertebrae* together is called *gibbus*. Deformity of one vertebra is called *knuckle*.

- Tenderness is also a feature in old fracture spine.
- Spine is one of the common sites of metastasis from haematogenous spread. A few examples are—carcinoma breast, carcinoma prostate, renal cell carcinoma, lymphoma, and multiple myeloma (Clinical Box 1.2).

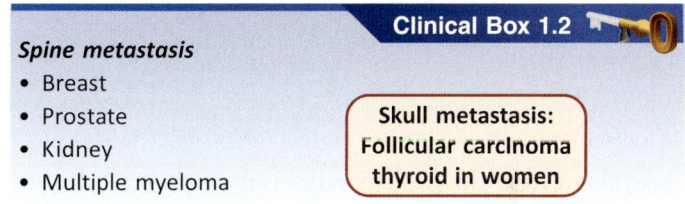

Clinical Box 1.2

Spine metastasis
- Breast
- Prostate
- Kidney
- Multiple myeloma

Skull metastasis: Follicular carcinoma thyroid in women

13. *Pulse*: More details on the pulse are given in medicine books. However, relevant points for students of surgery have been given here.

- Pulse volume is *weak* in peripheral vascular diseases such as TAO or atherosclerotic vascular diseases.
- *High volume* pulse is seen in thyrotoxicosis
- *Low volume* pulse is seen in hypotension, typically in haemorrhagic shock.
- *Tachycardia* is a feature of thyrotoxicosis and many other medical conditions.
- *Bradycardia* is seen in athletes.
- Arterial wall *thickening* is seen in atherosclerotic vascular diseases.
- *Dancing brachialis*: Thickened prominent pulsation of the brachial artery is suggestive of atherosclerotic disease. It is also called **locomotor brachialis** (Fig. 1.21).

14. *Blood pressure*: It should be made as a common practice to measure the blood pressure in all patients. More details are given in medicine books.

- Hypertension should be controlled well before surgery to avoid complications such as cerebral haemorrhage or cardiac failure following the surgical procedure.

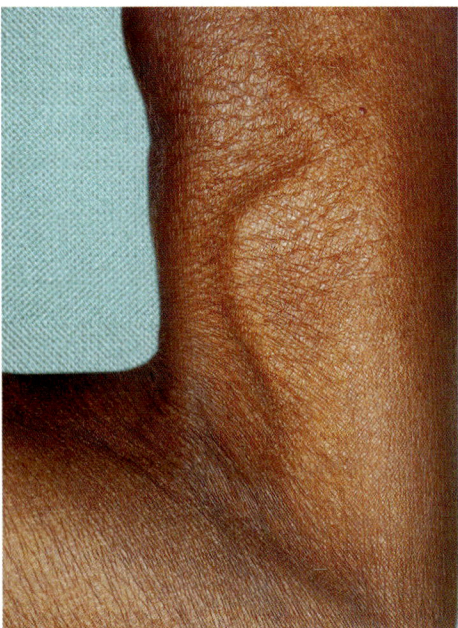

Fig. 1.21: Locomotor brachialis

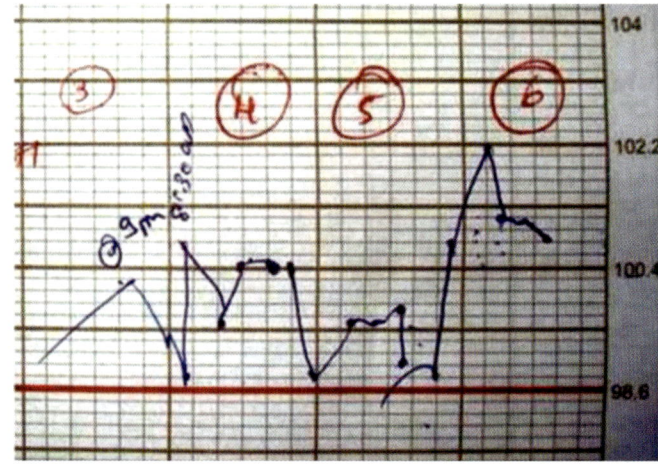

Fig. 1.22: Postoperative fever

- Bilateral renal mass with hypertension should suggest the possibility of polycystic kidneys.

- Renal conditions are very important causes of hypertension—acute glomerulonephritis can result in microscopic haematuria which is a clue to the renal cause of hypertension.

- Malignant hypertension with papilloedema in a young patient can be due to phaeochromo-cytoma—functioning tumour of the adrenals.

- **Pulsatile arteries,** collaterals in the scapular region with hypertension suggest **coarctation of aorta.**

15. *Temperature*: Is the patient normothermic, hypo-thermic or hyperthermic?

- The patient looks sick, not interested in what is happening around or he may be covering himself when he has a high temperature—diagnosis of fever can be done even from a distance when you see him. Fever indicates certain degree of infection—may be bacterial, viral or fungal. There are numerous causes of fever which are of interest to physicians. A few important aspects of surgical fever are given below:

- **High grade fever** with or without chills and rigors suggests following conditions:

  a. **Abscess**—may be intra-abdominal or in the soft tissues—boil or carbuncle in diabetic patients.

  b. Urinary tract infection—quite common in female patients.

  c. Biliary tract infections—cholangitis

  d. Malaria, filaria and pneumonia

- Low grade fever suggests a low grade continuing inflammation or infection as in diabetic cellulitis being treated or postoperative low grade fever due to wound infection.

- Evening rise of temperature with some chills may be due to tuberculous infections (not necessarily seen in all patients).

- **Hyperpyrexia** is a complication of surgery following thyroidectomy for primary thyrotoxi-cosis. It occurs in unprepared patients who are undergoing thyroidectomy. However, it is rarely seen nowadays.

- Fever in a postoperative patient can be due to many reasons (Fig. 1.22). Common causes (6 **Ws**) are given in Clinical Box 1.3.

Clinical Box 1.3

Mnemonic for the causes of fever: Rule of 'W'
1. **W**ater: Urinary tract infection
2. **W**ind: Respiratory tract infection
3. **W**alking: Deep vein thrombosis
4. **W**ound: Surgical site infection
5. **W**onder drug
6. **W**hat did we do? (Anastomosis—it may be leaking)

16. *Respiration*: Normal breathing is abdomino-thoracic.

- In cases of peritonitis, there will be minimal movement of the abdomen. Hence, breathing is mainly thoracic.

- *Tachypnoea* refers to increased respiratory rate and is referred to as number of breaths per minute. *It may be the early sign of sepsis.* More details are given in medicine books.

LOCAL EXAMINATION (REGIONAL EXAMINATION)

Local examination: This term is used widely in clinical surgery books. What it means is examination of the diseased part. However, better terminology is regional examination. This is especially relevant in malignancies. To give an example when you examine a case of carcinoma of the buccal mucosa, you not only examine the cancerous growth but will also examine teeth, mandible, palate, gums, etc. Hence, better term is regional examination.

- Adequate light should be present. Daylight is preferred. Mild jaundice can be missed in artificial lighting conditions.
- Position of the patient:
  1. Supine and lateral positions for abdominal examination
  2. Prone position for examination of the back, checking plane of the abdominal mass, whether intraperitoneal or retroperitoneal
  3. Sitting position for examination of head and neck, oral cavity
  4. Standing position for varicosity of veins, varicocele and inguinoscrotal swelling (hernia).
- **Local examination must be done in the following order:** Inspection, palpation, percussion and auscultation.
- Please do not start palpating as soon as you see a lesion such as swelling or ulcer. Spend some time in inspection which can reveal so much information and clue to the diagnosis in many cases. The importance of each of these examinations has been given below with examples.

Inspection

- This must be done in good daylight with adequate exposure of the patient. Explain to the patient what you are doing and why you are doing?
- Specific examination of swelling or ulcer is given under the respective chapters. A few general principles of each of these methods are given here.
- Some books mention that examination of neck requires exposure from chin to nipple. Just imagine a young lady with a small 2 cm nodule in the thyroid being examined for swelling in the neck is also asked to expose her chest. Is it required? One should be extremely careful while examining a female patient specially breast, groin, and abdomen. A female attendant, preferably a nurse, should always be present with you till you complete examination of a female patient.

- Look at this example: If you suspect follicular carcinoma thyroid, it can spread by blood spread and can metastasise to ribs. This will manifest as swelling. What is the best solution? Just after examination of the neck, ask the patient whether she has any swelling or pain in her rib cage or chest wall. If it is present, then examine the area. Otherwise, it is not required. We should also be aware that the participation of the patient, co-operation and support of the patient during clinical examination differs from a government college hospital to a private medical college hospital.
- Whole body examination (all systems) is more relevant in a situation that necessitates undressing of patient as in malignancies.
- Spend sometime in carefully inspecting the local area or the part. Vital clues can be obtained which can clinch the diagnosis without even touching the patient.
  - *A patient with a swelling in the posterior triangle of the neck has minimal ptosis of the upper eyelid*: It is called pseudoptosis and diagnosis is Horner's syndrome (Fig. 1.23).
  - *Patient with thyroid swelling:* Lower border of the swelling is not seen in case of retrosternal goitre.
  - *Prominent veins are present over the swelling in the thigh:* This suggests increased vascularity, may be a soft tissue sarcoma.
  - Pulsatile swelling may be an aneurysm.
  - Mild deviation of the angle of the mouth can be due to injury or paralysis of the marginal mandibular nerve.
  - Multiple holes discharging pus is a carbuncle (sieve-like appearance) (Fig. 1.24).

Clinical Wisdom

No wonder a surgeon should have Eagle's eyes.

Palpation

- Palpation is done with palmar aspect of the fingers.

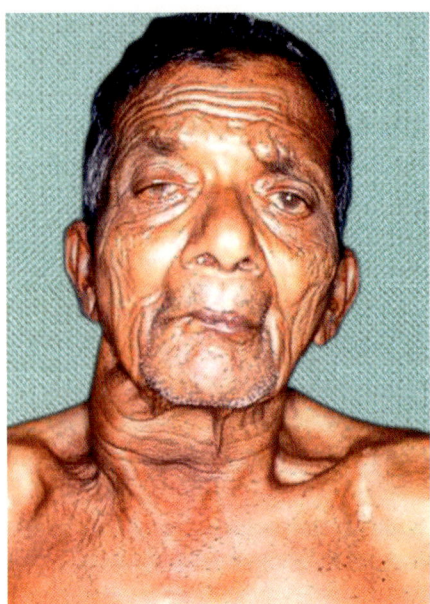

Fig. 1.23: Pseudoptosis due to lymph node metastasis on the right middle and lower cervical lymph nodes (*Courtesy:* Prof BH Ananda Rao, KMC, Manipal)

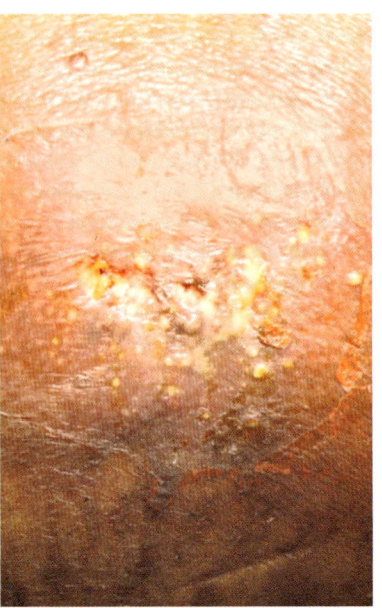

Fig. 1.24: Carbuncle on the back of neck region—common site, sieve-like appearance or cribriform appearance—pathognomonic sign

- Palpation should be gentle. Reassure the patient that you will not hurt them.
- More details about what points are to be noted under palpation are given in the respective chapters.
- Local rise in temperature and tenderness have to be mentioned first under palpation for swellings. Please also check in the chapters on neck and thyroid.
- In the abdomen, start palpation away from the site of the mass or pain.
- Different methods of palpation are available, e.g. *Dipping method* while examining the abdomen in cases of ascites.
- The most important vital clues or signs are elicited with palpation—such as extent of the lesion, consistency, mobility, plane, fixity of the swelling. Details have been given in respective chapters.

Percussion

Organs that are solid, hollow, or those containing air or liquid give different sounds on percussion similar to percussion instruments. This forms the basis of the percussion. A few examples are given below.

- Percussion over the chest is resonant because of the underlying lung which contains air.
- Normally percussion over the sternum is resonant, but if there is retrosternal extension of the thyroid swelling, it may be dull.

- Resonant note all over the abdomen may indicate distended loops of intestine in cases of intestinal obstruction or paralytic ileus.

- It should be remembered that the clinical method of examination such as percussion should be used, only if you feel it is useful. There is no point in percussing over the thyroid swelling, cause inconvenience to the patient and say it is dull.
- Rare case of laryngocoele in the neck may give tympanitic note.
- Percussion over the stomach mass is impaired resonant because of growth and air. However, in advanced cases, it may be dull due to a large stomach tumour which has filled the lumen of the stomach.

Auscultation

This is an important method of clinical examination in medicine for respiratory system and cardiovascular system which will be dealt in detail in medicine. However, a few relevant things to be remembered in surgery are given below.

- A swelling with a **bruit suggests increased vascularity** typically seen in arteriovenous malformations.
- Logically speaking, in a case of swelling in the neck, if on palpation, you find a thrill, then auscultate for a bruit, e.g. carotid artery aneurysm, dilatation of subclavian artery in cases of cervical rib.

- In primary thyrotoxicosis, you may find a bruit at the upper pole of the thyroid gland (due to increased vascularity).

- Auscultation of the trachea can be done to check air entry.

- Auscultation of the abdomen should be done in right iliac fossa for bowel sounds. Bowel sounds that are heard are from the small bowel, which ends in the right iliac fossa. Hence, it is logical to auscultate right iliac fossa (Fig. 1.25).

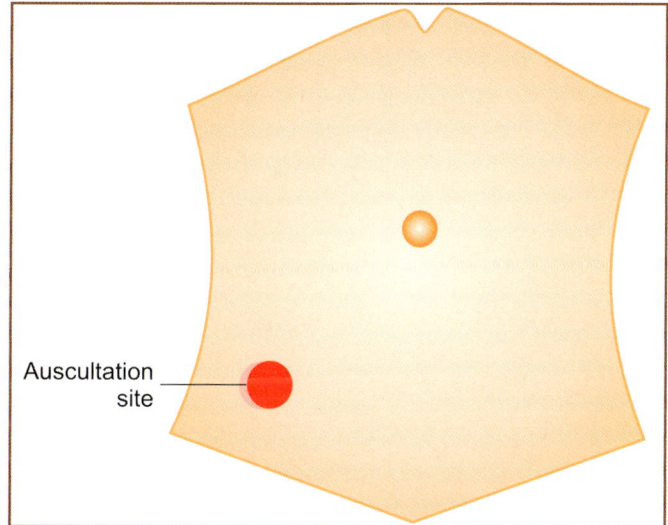

Auscultation site

Fig. 1.25: Sir Henry Hamilton Bailey has called this site as abdominal post

Left Supraclavicular Lymph Node Examination—Virchow's Node (Refer to Page 27)

- Vast majority of intra-abdominal malignancies, testicular tumours spread to left supraclavicular lymph nodes via thoracic duct.

- It felt in the posterior triangle just above clavicle.

- Physician should stand behind the patient, flex the patient's neck and tilt the neck to left side.

- Palpable supraclavicular node in malignancies is called Troisier's sign.

PER RECTAL (PR) AND PER VAGINAL (PV) EXAMINATION

- Details are given in chapter on abdominal mass.

- However, purpose is to feel for growth in the rectum and to feel for rectovesical deposits **(Blummer Shelf)** which occur due to transcoelomic spread in malignancies.

- In women, it has to be checked in the **Douglas pouch** (rectouterine pouch).

SYSTEMIC EXAMINATION

- *Respiratory system:* Examination for normal or abnormal sounds such as rhonchi or crepitations must be done. They reflect status of the lungs. It is necessary to assess the lungs before surgery. Lungs are often the site of metastasis from a primary elsewhere in the body. Common primary sites in cases of metastasis of lungs are: Carcinoma colon, carcinoma breast, malignant melanoma, etc. Metastases in the lungs are usually round, and are called **cannon ball secondaries.** Pleural effusion is quite a common metastatic manifestation of carcinoma breast.

- *Cardiovascular system*: It is examined for heart sounds, any abnormal sounds, etc. Cardiovascular system can give a clue in some cases, e.g. a patient with upper limb acute ischaemia of the fingers is found to have mid-diastolic murmur on auscultation of the heart. It is a case of mitral stenosis with emboli causing ischaemia.

- *Skeletal system*: Skeletal system is examined thoroughly. Firstly, ask the patient about *bony pains* and ask him to point out the site. Accordingly, look for any tenderness. Ask the patient for any *bony swelling* of recent origin, e.g. follicular carcinoma thyroid can have metastasis in skull bones, ribs and other flat bones. Malignant lesions such as sarcoma and carcinoma can infiltrate the bone and give rise to *pathological fractures*. This may result in *abnormal mobility* of the bones. This also should be tested in appropriate cases.

Clinical Wisdom
1. Follicular carcinoma thyroid: Bony swelling
2. Carcinoma breast: Bony pains, tenderness
3. Tuberculosis spine: Tenderness, deformity and cold abscess

CLINICAL DIAGNOSIS/WORKING DIAGNOSIS

- At the end of the clinical examination, students should quickly summarise. Think of possibilities by elimination process and come to a clinical diagnosis. This diagnosis may or may not be right but we start working from there and hence it is also

Clinical Box 1.4

Summary of Clinical Examination
- When you talk to the patient, be well prepared—do it with dignity. Explain what you are doing, why you are doing.
- It is important to realize that examiners expect students to conduct well and behave well with the patient
- Clinical examination should be complete—no short cuts. Even if a few findings are missed, it does not matter. What is important is that you have examined the relevant parts.
- Interpretation of the data should start from the time when you start taking history. It should continue at every level of examination and findings.
- When final diagnosis is given, mentally prepare yourself for possible questions such as—Why? What? How? What else?
- Give a common diagnosis first
- Rare diagnosis are rarely correct.
- Get ready with answers to the questions on investigations and treatment.
- Observe/watch carefully how a senior clinician examines the patient (Fig. 1.26)

called the 'working diagnosis' or simply diagnosis (Clinical Box 1.4).

- While giving the clinical diagnosis, common diagnosis has to be kept in mind. As the old saying goes, *'common things are common'*.
- It is important to realise that while giving a diagnosis you not only use your five senses properly but also use the most important 6th sense—**common sense**.

- While giving a diagnosis, first think of the anatomical diagnosis meaning which anatomical structure this is arising from, e.g. Is it from lymph nodes? thyroid gland? or submandibular salivary gland? stomach? or kidney? etc. Then consider what pathological condition is affecting this structure. Both combined together form the clinical diagnosis, e.g. tuberculous lymphadenitis, carcinoma parotid, carcinoma tongue, metastasis in cervical lymph nodes, carcinoma stomach, hydronephrosis, etc.

- **As far as possible, try to give one diagnosis:** It may not explain all physical signs and symptoms which is difficult in many situations. To give a few examples: A patient may have lymph nodes in the neck which are matted suggesting tuberculosis. He may also have a nonhealing lesion in the tongue which is indurated (hard). The diagnosis will be carcinoma tongue with metastasis in the lymph nodes rather than tuberculosis of the tongue with neck nodes (carcinoma tongue is more common than tuberculosis of the tongue).

- When there are multiple swellings or masses in the neck, lymph node swellings should be offered as the *first diagnosis.*

- A lady has a thyroid swelling with another swelling in the scalp bone. *The complete diagnosis* is not just carcinoma thyroid but also with metastasis in the skull bone.

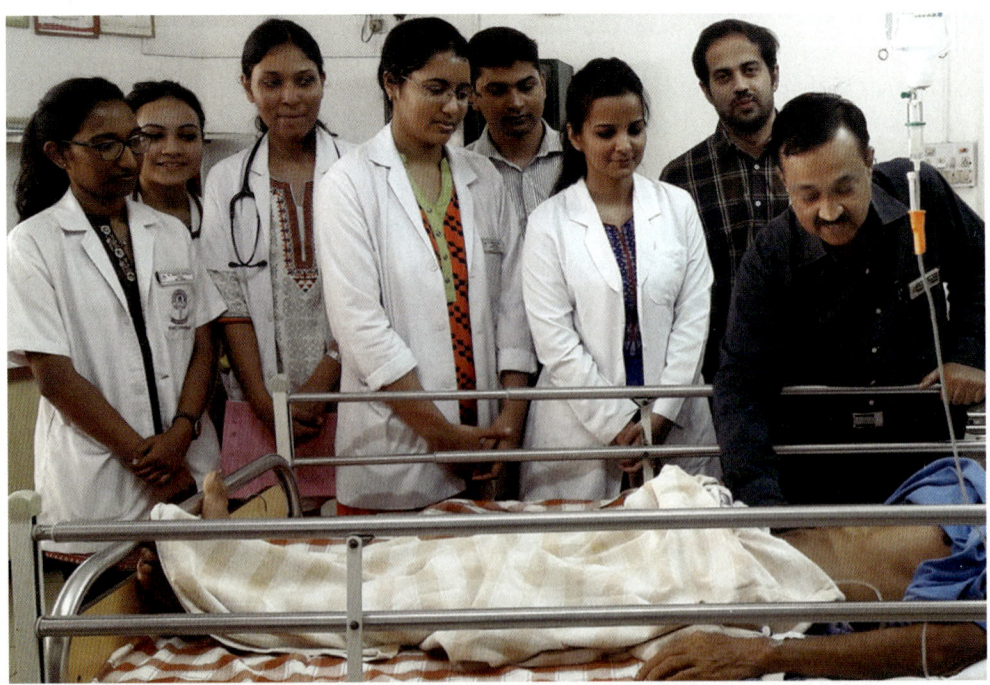

Fig. 1.26: Students can attain many skills by observing a clinician examining the patients

- As you study and present different cases, you will find the appropriate adjectives in the diagnosis. The whole purpose is to *highlight the important aspects* while giving the clinical diagnosis.

DIFFERENTIAL DIAGNOSIS

- In a given case, all findings may not fit with one diagnosis which prompts to give a differential diagnosis.

- Sometimes the physical findings are so typical there is only one diagnosis and there is no differential diagnosis as in a typical case of carcinoma breast or carcinoma cheek (buccal mucosa).

- **The differential diagnosis should be the nearest possible diagnosis:** One example is given here. A nonhealing lesion in the tongue can be malignant, if there is induration. However, nonhealing can also be due to constant irritation caused by dentures. If signs are equivocal, carcinoma of the tongue should be the first diagnosis followed by dental ulcer as second diagnosis. In case of jaw tumours or salivary gland tumours, it is difficult to give a firm diagnosis. First mention it is a jaw tumour, followed by a few differential diagnoses such as adamantinoma, dental cyst, etc.

- Take another example, a sebaceous cyst. If it has a sebaceous punctum, it is diagnostic and no other differential diagnosis needs to be offered. However, if the punctum is absent, you have to consider other swellings such as dermoid cyst, lipoma, etc.

- Swelling in the palmar aspect of the hand was diagnosed as sebaceous cyst. The differential diagnosis was dermoid cyst. The diagnosis was wrong. **Why? There are no sebaceous glands in the palm and sole. Hence, sebaceous cyst cannot occur in these areas.**

The clinical discussion ends here. However, it is good practice to now think of relevant investigations in a given case, their interpretation and planning of treatment. You will be able to understand further only when you have studied the subject well. For now, I will stop the case sheet documentation and clinical diagnosis.

Please note: There is always anxiety and apprehension in the clinical examination for dental, MBBS and MS students. In an attempt to reduce this tension and anxiety, I have given the possible list of cases with their page numbers, which can be allotted to you as long or short cases. This list may differ from place to place. I am confident that this list and clinical methods will benefit you.

Long Cases (Most Probable Cases) and Clinical Methods

1. Multinodular goitre (P 268)
2. Carcinoma thyroid (P 268)
3. Thyrotoxicosis (P 268)
4. Solitary nodule thyroid (P 286)
5. Parotid tumours (P 208)
6. Occlusive arterial diseases (TAO atherosclerosis) (P 106)
7. Varicose veins (P 139)
8. Carcinoma breast (P 293)
9. Groin hernias, incisional hernia (P 441)
10. Hepatoma, secondaries in the liver, hydatid cyst (P 377)
11. Carcinoma stomach (P 384)
12. Pseudocyst of pancreas (P 386)
13. Obstructive jaundice (P 381)
14. Right iliac fossa mass (P 398)
15. Cystic swelling in the abdomen (P 409)
16. Renal swelling (P 393)
17. Splenomegaly (P 390)
18. Lymphoma (P 149)
19. Retroperitoneal tumour (P 404)

Short Cases (Most Probable Cases) and Clinical Methods

1. **Examination of neck swellings:** For example, lymph nodes, branchial cyst, cold abscess, salivary gland enlargement, haemangioma, lymphangioma, etc. (P 245)
2. **Examinatin of cystic and solid swellings:** Sebaceous cyst, dermoid cyst, neurofibroma, lipoma (P 52)
3. Skin tumours (P 188)
4. Jaw swellings: Adamantinoma, dental cyst, dentigerous cyst (P 237)
5. Differential diagnosis of leg ulcer (P 31)
6. Sinus—median mental, osteomyelitis jaw, etc. (P 94)
7. Lymphadenopathy (P 247)
8. Soft tissue sarcoma (P 59)
9. Oral Cancer (P 224)
10. Cervical rib (P 126)
11. Lymphoedema (P 148)
12. Hydrocoele (P 458)
13. Carcinoma penis (P 471)
14. Fibroadenoma, phyllodes (P 293)
15. Epigastric hernia (P 455)

2

Surgical Patient—Symptoms and Signs of Surgical Importance

INTRODUCTION

- Now that you have some idea what to ask the patient and what to examine, let us study some important symptoms and signs in more detail. To give an example, the patient says, 'I have no appetite, I have severe weight loss, I lost 15 kg weight in 3 months'. He also says, 'I have pain abdomen'. In addition to what has already been given in the first chapter, some new important signs have been given in this chapter such as bimanual palpation, ballottement, etc. Students should know these before examination of the patients specially in abdominal cases.

- In the same fashion, when you examine the swelling, a few signs such as fluctuation and transillumination have been given here which will help you in your clinical examination.

LOSS OF APPETITE (ANOREXIA)

Loss of appetite is an important manifestation of intra-abdominal malignancies, especially carcinoma stomach. However, many causes of loss of appetite have been mentioned. A few are given below.

1. *Gastric causes*: Carcinoma stomach is the most important diagnosis to be borne in mind in patients who come with loss of appetite and upper GI (gastrointestinal) symptoms. In gastric ulcer, patients are afraid to take food because food intake aggravates the pain even though appetite may be near normal.

2. *Parasitic causes*: Roundworm infestation may produce loss of appetite but weight loss is not a feature.

3. *Hepatic causes*: Patients who have malignant tumour such as hepatoma and prodromal stage of viral hepatitis can have loss of appetite.

4. *Chronic illness*: Chronic alcoholic disease, cirrhosis, uraemia, chronic pulmonary disease, advanced malignancies are common causes of chronic illness.

5. *Psychiatric illness*: Anxiety, depression, and stress are common causes. **Anorexia nervosa** occurs in young girls with significant weight loss and they refuse to eat due to fear of putting on weight. **Bulimia nervosa** is an eating disorder characterised by recurrent binge eating, followed by compensatory behaviour. The most common form is defensive vomiting, sometimes called purging.

FLUSHING

It occurs due to dilatation of capillaries resulting in spreading erythema of the skin. Generally, more common in women.

1. *Menopausal flushing*: They are called **hot flushes.** They are short attacks lasting for 15 minutes. Sweating is an important feature.

2. *Alcohol*: Flushing is common after consumption of alcohol as certain wines contain histamine. Food and drugs may also contribute.

3. *Carcinoid syndrome*: Flushing is the commonest clinical feature of carcinoid syndrome.

4. *Phaeochromocytoma*: Flushing with fainting is a feature along with other features such as hypertension.

5. *Zollinger-Ellison syndrome*: Flushing and diarrhoea are its features.

HICCUP

- It occurs due to spasmodic contraction of the diaphragm. Hiccup can occasionally be so troublesome that the patient is completely exhausted.
- It can be classified into central and peripheral causes.
- Central causes are given in more detail in medical books. They occur due to cerebral anoxia.
- Peripheral causes are called surgical causes. They are as follows:

  a. **Early postoperative period:** Hiccups occur due to distension of the stomach as a result of paralytic ileus. Incidence of this complication is less in laparoscopic surgeries. Overdistended stomach pushes the diaphragm cephalad resulting in irritation and hiccups. **Treatment is by insertion of nasogastric tube.**

  b. **Peritonitis:** Irritation of undersurface of the diaphragm in peritonitis can result in hiccups. Once peritonitis is treated, symptom may disappear.

  c. **Renal failure:** Patients with advanced renal failure can present with hiccups. Look at the tongue first—**brown dry tongue** clinches the diagnosis.

- Hiccups may also be treated by drawing the attention of the patient away from illness, keeping ice cubes on the tongue, tab chlorpromazine 50 mg oral or a sharp pulling of the tongue outwards.

PAIN

- Many patients come to the hospital because of pain. Pain is very much subjective and cannot be measured unlike temperature, pressure, etc. Presence and extent of fever can be measured using thermometer, say 104°C. Pain cannot be measured like that. Many varieties of pain are present. Understanding the nature of each pain may give vital clue to the diagnosis in many cases.
- Start asking questions such as how long the pain has been present? How is the progress? Has it worsened recently? Or has it been constant since many months? Has it become less any time? Has the pain come down and how is it relieved?
- *Periodicity*: Chronic pain of peptic ulcer will completely disappear for some time. It is called periodicity. **Trigeminal neuralgia** also shows periodicity.
- Location of the pain and movement of the pain.

1. **Radiation:** It means pain which is present at one site extends to another site. Example: In patients with chronic pancreatitis, pain in the epigastrium is radiated to back. When carcinoma stomach infiltrates pancreas, patients complain of pain radiating to the back.

2. **Referred pain:** The pain is felt at a distance from its source and there is no pain at the site of disease. It occurs when central nervous system fails to differentiate between somatic and visceral nerve impulses from the same spinal segment. In acute cholecystitis, inflammatory oedema accumulates in the under surface of the diaphragm. Diaphragm is supplied by phrenic nerve (C3, 4, 5). Cutaneous supply to tip of the shoulder comes from supraclavicular nerves (C4, 5).

3. **Ureteric colic** pain is referred to genitalia and groin due to irritation of genitofemoral nerve (L-1).

4. **Migrating pain:** Classically seen in acute appendicitis wherein initially pain is felt in the umbilical region (visceral pain due to distension of the appendix). Later, it migrates to right iliac fossa when parietal peritoneum is irritated.

Nature of Pain

1. **Dull aching or vague pain:** Usually it is a dull aching pain or discomfort, very nonspecific, often subsides on its own.

2. **Throbbing pain:** It is typical of an abscess especially when it is in a tight space—examples are breast abscess, acute paronychia, etc. Pain is severe, throbbing and it is due to pressure on nerve endings.

3. **Burning pain:** It is typical of peptic ulcer disease and reflux oesophagitis. (More details are given on page 349)

4. **Scalding pain:** When the pathology is in the urinary tract such as stone in the bladder, cystitis, the patient experiences scalding type of pain while urinating.

5. **Sickening feeling:** It occurs with pressure or blow on the testis or in cases of torsion testis. It is felt in the umbilical region.

6. **Shooting pain:** It is a type of radiating pain but classically described for sciatica—pain that shoots down the leg.

7. **Stabbing pain:** It is a sharp, severe, short-lived pain that is classically seen in perforated duodenal ulcer.

8. **Constricting pain:** It means compression or constriction from all around as in **angina pectoris.** Herpes zoster also can produce constrictive type of pain but from one side as in neck or thorax.

9. **Colicky pain** is due to **obstruction** to hollow viscus. It is intermittent. When it comes, it is a severe pain which lasts for a few minutes and subsides slowly. Colicky abdominal pain is associated with frequent vomiting as in intestinal obstruction.

Aggravating factor

- Burning pain of peptic ulcer is aggravated by eating spicy food.
- Pain from lumbar disc prolapse becomes worse on movement of the spine.
- Any pain due to peritonitis, such as acute appendicitis, will cause pain on movement of the abdominal wall as coughing, jumping or jolting.

Relieving factor

- Peptic ulcer pain is relieved to some extent by taking antacids or pantoprazole, etc.
- Pain of pancreatitis is relieved to some extent by sitting and bending forward.

ITCHING: PRURITUS

A number of pathological processes can lead to pruritus: Inflammation, hypersensitivity, degenerative changes, malignant tumours, and even psychological abnormalities. Itching of the skin can be due to local causes such as clothing, parasitic, vaginal and rectal discharge, etc. Urticaria and eczema are other causes. A few causes of surgical interest are given below.

- *Intrahepatic and extrahepatic biliary obstruction* (cholestatic pruritus). Obstructive jaundice is an important disease of surgeon's interest that causes itching. **Scratch marks** on the **body with jaundice** gives the clue to the diagnosis. It is caused by bile acids in the blood (cholemia) or skin, but there is a poor correlation between the skin concentration of bile salts and intensity of pruritus. Another cause is an *elevation of endogenous opioids* in the blood and treatment with the *opiate antagonist naloxone improves pruritus*. The itch in patients with cholemic pruritus can be lessened by treatment with cholestyramine, phototherapy and plasmapheresis which lower or remove the unknown circulating pruritogen; antihistamines can be used as adjuvants. Ursodeoxycholic acid (10–15 mg/kg)

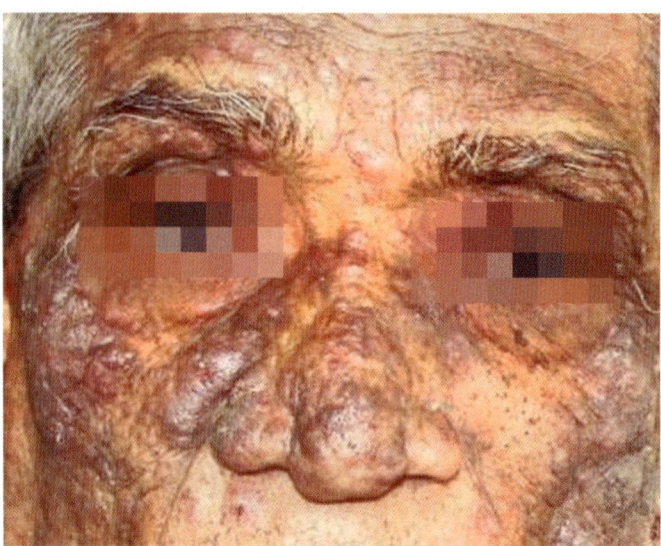

Fig. 2.1: Skin lesions in lymphoma

has been used with good success. Interestingly, some serotonin subtype-3-receptor antagonists such as *ondansetron, given intravenously*, have been *helpful in the treatment of cholestatic pruritus.*

- Patients with mycosis fungiodes, a low grade non-Hodgkin's lymphoma can have skin lesions with itching (Fig. 2.1).

- **Chronic renal failure:** Proliferation of mast cells in the skin, release of histamine, allergic reactions to the material used for dialysis, uremic neuropathy affecting motor, sensory and autonomic nerves, changes in the calcium phosphate product, endogenous opioids and others. Probably the cause is multifactorial. Pruritus is not seen in acute renal failure.

- Hepatic failure, polycythaemia, and thyrotoxicosis are some other causes.

- **Drugs:** Testosterone, chlorpromazine, oral contraceptive pills, erythromycin, allopurinol, rifampicin can also provoke cholestatic jaundice and pruritus.

PEDAL OEDEMA

- Accumulation of fluid in the extravascular space results in oedema.

- In venous obstruction, capillary hydrostatic pressure increases resulting in pedal oedema. In hypoalbuminaemia, fall in the oncotic pressure results in oedema, e.g. nephrotic syndrome.

- In prolonged standing, military and traffic men, air travels, mild oedema is common due to *inadequate lymphatic drainage which is critically dependent* on calf muscle activity.

- Irrespective of the causes, oedema fluid accumulates in the dependent areas in the body due to gravity. Thus, pedal oedema or mild ankle oedema occurs in those who stand or travel for a long time. Sacral oedema is common in recumbent (bedridden) patients. Interestingly, oedema of the eyelids is common in nephrotic syndrome—due to loose connective tissue.
- At least 5 litres of fluid should accumulate for clinically detectable generalised oedema.
- **Pitting on pressure:** Presence of fluid in the subcutaneous plane can be confirmed by eliciting a sign called pitting on pressure. Apply firm pressure over the oedematous part for about 15 seconds. In legs, this should be about 2–3 cm above the medial malleolus. Once pressure is released, one can see pitting in the area. However, once pressure is released, it may fill back (Figs 2.2 and 2.3).
- **Two types**

  A. **Generalised oedema** is due to disorders of heart (congestive cardiac failure), kidney (nephrotic syndrome), liver (cirrhosis), gut (malabsorption syndrome) or nutritional (severe anaemia).

  B. **Local oedema:** It is of surgical importance. Various causes are given below:

  - *Inflammatory:* Any injury, infections such as cellulitis, snake bites or bee stings
  - *Venous disorders:* Varicose veins with perforator incompetence and patients with deep vein thrombosis (Fig. 2.4)
  - *Lymphatic disorders* such as primary lymphoedema, filariasis
  - *Allergic:* It can be generalised or local

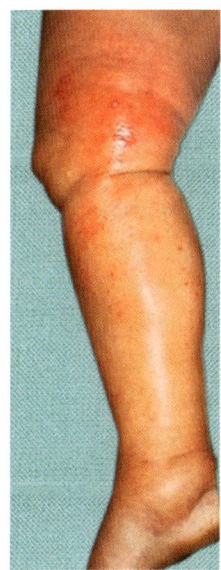

Fig. 2.4: Acute oedema of the proximal and distal limb due to iliac vein thrombosis caused by a tumour in the pelvic cavity

Endocrinal: Myxoedema due to accumulation of mucopolysaccharides. In primary thyrotoxicosis, special variety of nonpitting oedema develops which has been called pretibial myxoedema.

- *Tumours:* Sudden appearance of unilateral limb oedema suggests proximal obstruction. In women, pelvic mass should be ruled out. Soft tissue sarcomas can present with unilateral limb oedema caused by obstruction to common iliac vein.
- *Deep vein thrombosis:* Depending upon the level of obstruction of deep veins, oedema develops. Example: When common iliac vein is thrombosed, entire lower limb will be oedematous. When calf muscle veins are thrombosed, oedema is confined to the lower leg—an appearance which has been described as *inverted beer bottle appearance*.

A FEW SIGNS OF SURGICAL IMPORTANCE

PROMINENT VEINS

Visible veins or prominent veins signify some pathology. Loss of subcutaneous fat is the common cause of prominent veins. However, obstruction to the venous return results in opening of alternate channels which result in prominent venous channels. A few examples are given below.

1. **In caput medusae** (veins around umbilicus in portal hypertension), blood flow is towards the

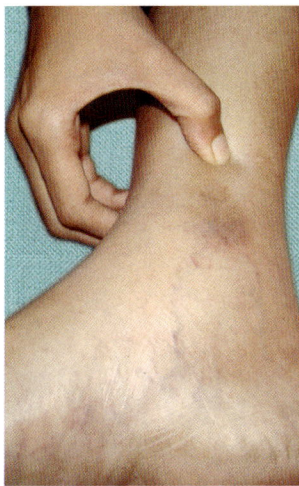

Fig. 2.2: Method of eliciting pitting

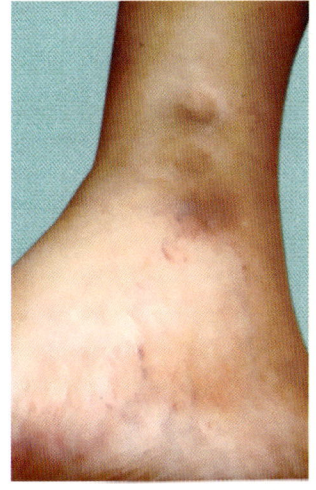

Fig. 2.3: You can see the pitting caused due to oedema

heart from veins above umbilicus, but blood flow is towards groin from veins below the umbilicus (Figs 2.5 to 2.8).

2. **In cases of inferior vena caval obstruction,** prominent veins will develop in the flanks. They are called inguino-axillary veins. Blood flow is from below upwards towards axilla (Figs 2.9 and 2.10).

3. **In superior vena caval obstruction,** prominent veins will develop over the upper chest and in neck. Blood flow is towards the heart. This can happen in cases of retrosternal goitre and mediastinal growths (Fig. 2.11).

4. **External jugular vein:** Engorgement of external vein suggests increased central venous pressure as in circulatory overload which may be dangerous in patients with cardiogenic shock.

5. **Varicose veins:** Dilated tortuous veins in the leg are called varicose veins (Fig. 2.12).

6. **Sarcoma:** Dilated prominent veins over a swelling is usually in cases of sarcoma. It suggests increased vascularity (Fig. 2.13).

7. **AV fistula:** Veins become tortuous and thickened almost like an artery. So, it is called arterialisation of veins (Fig. 2.14).

8. Veins can also be seen in unusual site (Fig. 2.15).

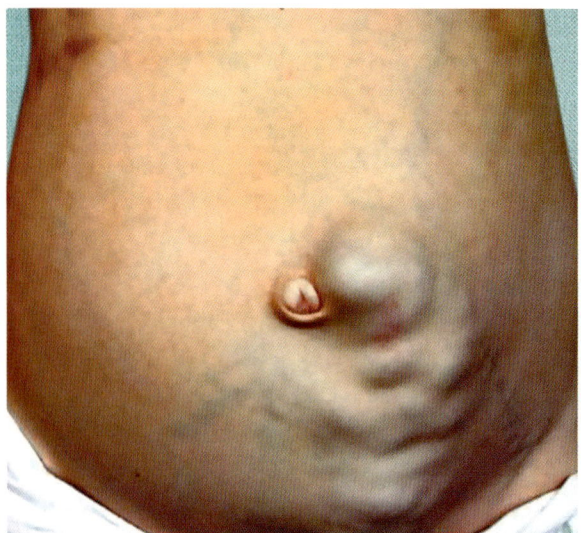

Fig. 2.5: Caput medusae in portal hypertension

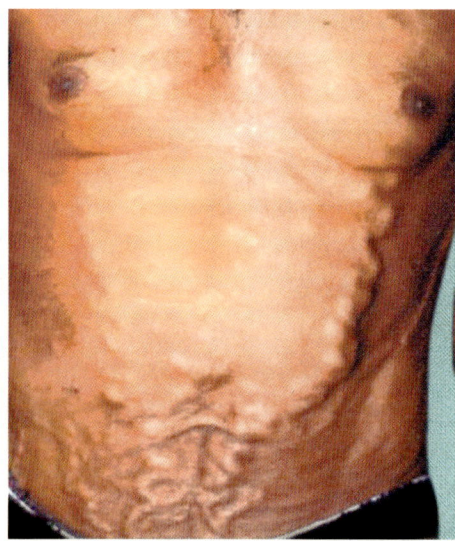

Fig. 2.6: Tortuous veins in the anterior abdominal wall

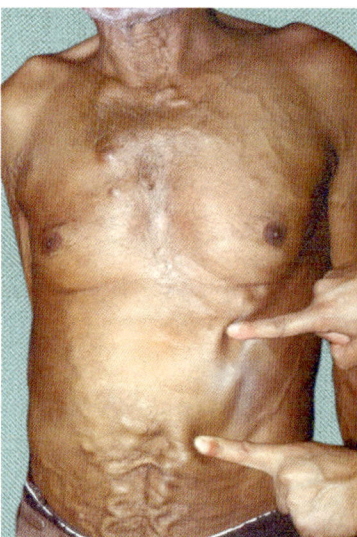

Fig. 2.7: Checking for direction of blood flow

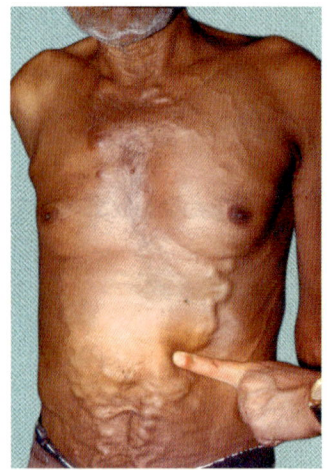

Fig. 2.8: Veins in the anterior abdominal wall—testing for refilling

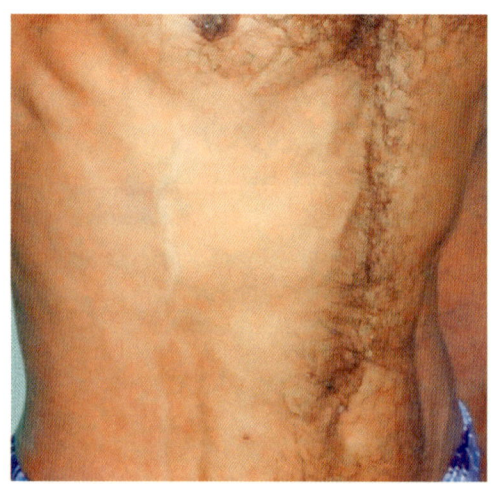

Fig. 2.9: Flank veins—inguinoaxillary veins due to inferior vena caval obstruction caused by hepatoma

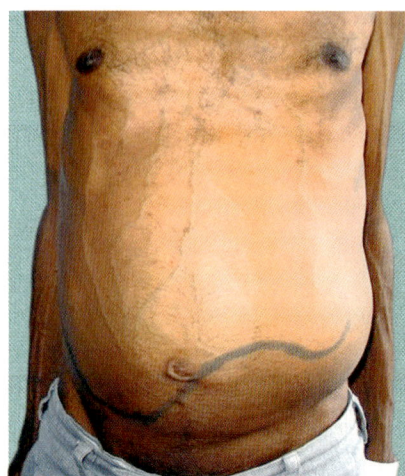

Fig. 2.10: Large liver mass with abdominal wall veins

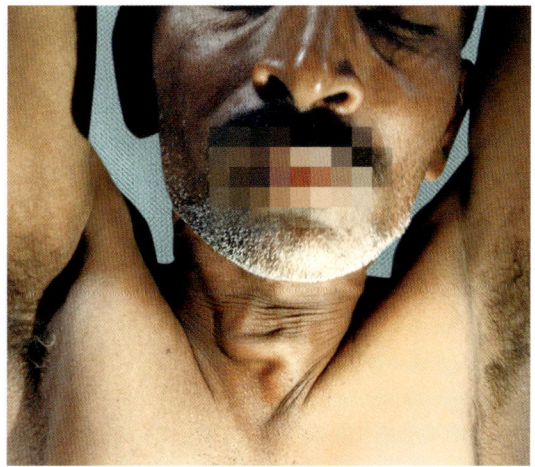

Fig. 2.11: Retrosternal goitre—on raising the hands and touching the ears, veins become more prominent suggesting superior vena caval obstruction (Pemberton test)

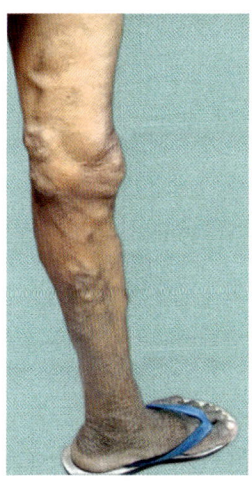

Fig. 2.12: Dilated veins in the leg—varicose veins

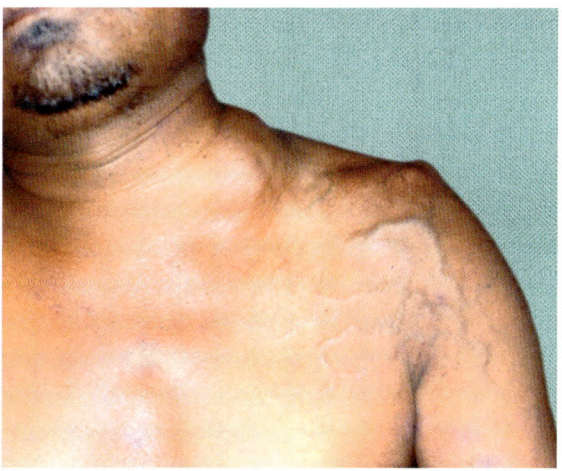

Fig. 2.13: Synovial sarcoma shoulder region—see the secondary vascularity due to pressure effects

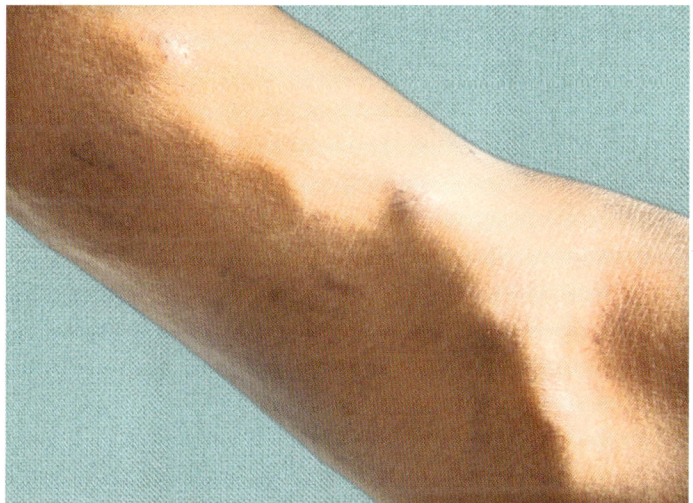

Fig. 2.14: Most common type of AV fistula you see today is in the nephrology ward—created to facilitate haemodialysis

FLUCTUATION (Fig. 2.16)

- It should be done only when swelling is soft to find out whether the swelling contains fluid or not. Detailed method of eliciting fluctuation is given on page 57.
- When cystic swelling is compressed at one spot, other end opposite to it will be raised due to increase in the pressure within the swelling. It is elicited in two directions.
- *Cross-fluctuation test*: When the swelling has two components connected to each other with a narrow channel or different anatomical regions but are adjacent, cystic swellings will exhibit cross-fluctuation test. A few examples are given below.
  1. *Compound palmar ganglion:* Swelling is not only in the lower forearm but also in the palm. Part of the swelling is situated deep to palmar aponeurosis and projects out in the area of least resistance or anatomical barrier.

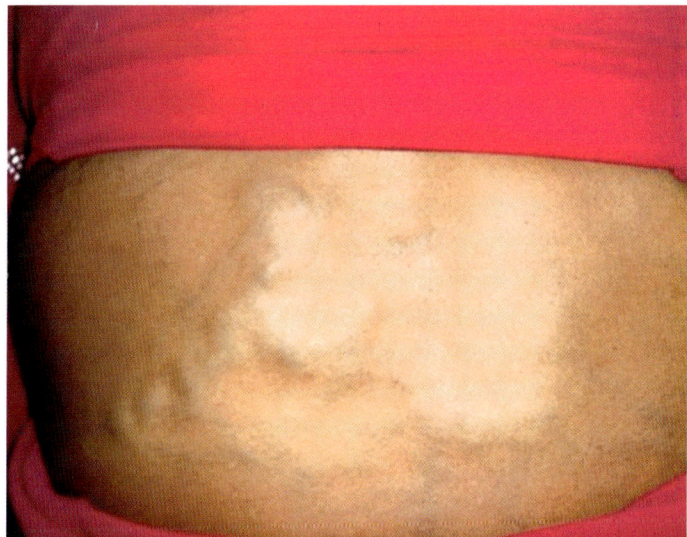

Fig. 2.15: Varices in the back in portal hypertension. Unusual site

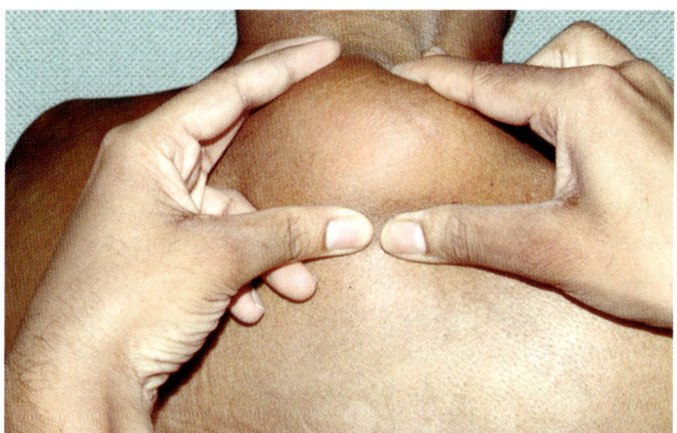

Fig. 2.16: Fluctuation test

2. *Plunging ranula*: Ranula (page 259) insinuates under fibres of mylohyoid and manifests as swelling in the submandibular region.

3. *Hydrocoele en bisac*: Portion of hydrocoele sac is under abdominal wall—deep to internal oblique. (Main sac is in the scrotum and the other sac is deep to internal oblique).

4. *Bubo-(swollen inflamed lymph node in the groin) iliopsoas abscess*: In both situations, pus is both above and below the inguinal ligament. Cross-fluctuation between two swellings—one above and one below the inguinal ligament, indicates the communication between the two swellings—which is the principle behind positive cross-fluctuation test.

TRANSILLUMINATION

- When light is passed through a swelling containing clear fluid, the light can be seen on the other side of the swelling. This is called transillumination positive. It only tells you that the swelling contains clear fluid. An X-ray roll is made like a pipe and used as transilluminoscope (Fig. 2.17).

- Thus you *should not be able to elicit transillumination test*, if the swelling is *hard* or even firm, e.g. metastatic lymph nodes, neurofibromas, etc.

- **Swellings which are transilluminant**
  1. Lymphangioma
  2. Ranula
  3. Meningocoele
  4. Epididymal cyst
  5. Vaginal hydrocoele

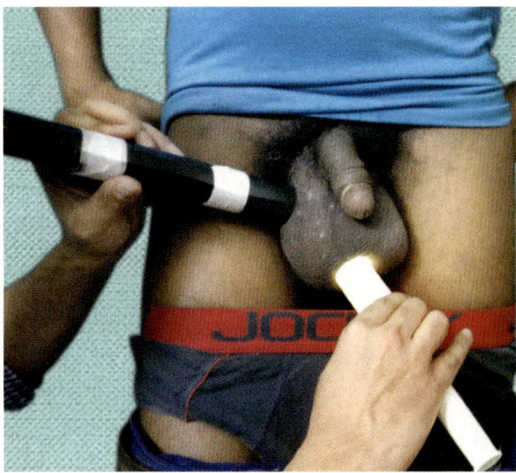

Fig. 2.17: Transillumination

- **Precautions to be taken while eliciting this test are**
  1. Avoid surface transillumination (do not put the torch light very superficial).
  2. Avoid any mass or tissue within the swelling which can obstruct the light—this can happen in scrotal hydrocoele.
  3. This test should be done in a dark room.

MOBILITY

- This test, also called intrinsic mobility test, is an important feature of any benign swelling or lumps. When a tumour arises from a structure, an attempt is made to move the lump. If the tumour moves freely, it is benign.

- All malignant tumours exhibit a property of local infiltration. They also cause a lot of desmoplastic reaction resulting in fibrosis. As a result of this, the lump may not move freely and they have restricted mobility. Students should look for this sign carefully because often this may be the only important sign available for the diagnosis.

- A few examples are given below:
  A. Restricted mobility in a hard breast lump suggests carcinoma breast.
  B. Restricted mobility in a thyroid nodule suggests carcinoma thyroid.
  C. Restricted mobility in a soft tissue swelling suggests soft tissue sarcoma.
  D. Restricted mobility in a hard node in the neck suggests malignancy (*refer* to Clinical Case Capsule).

■ Clinical Case Capsule

A 24-year-old young man was admitted with a swelling in the forearm of 3 months duration. The candidate diagnosed the case as a neurofibroma. It was deep to deep fascia. It was feeling firm. The patient did not have any tingling and numbness on compressing the swelling. Candidate also gave differential diagnosis of fibrolipoma and haematoma. He failed. He had forgotten to look for intrinsic mobility test. Swelling had restricted mobility on movement. It was a case of sarcoma.

Clinical Wisdom

It should be remembered that inflammatory swellings (lymph node) also will have restricted mobility but they will be very tender.

BIMANUAL PALPATION

- It means the swelling can be palpated by both hands simultaneously. Bimanual palpation should be done in every mass in the lumbar region, a few in the hypochondrial regions and pelvic masses.

- Kidney is a **peripherally placed organ**, in the loin. When it enlarges, it enlarges both anteriorly and posteriorly. In such cases, it is palpable with both hands—one hand kept anteriorly and another hand kept posteriorly. This is called bimanual method of palpation.

- Thus enlarged masses arising from kidney, liver, spleen and ascending colon can be bimanually palpable.

- Thus when kidney is enlarged, start palpating with flat of fingers. Anteriorly, it is palpable and posteriorly it is palpable in the renal angle. Apart from kidney, any large mass in the lumbar region such as colonic mass can be bimanually palpable.

- **Bimanual palpation in bladder masses:** Under anaesthesia, the mass is palpated with a finger passed in the rectum in males, the vagina in females while the abdomen is palpated simultaneously with the other hand in the suprapubic region. Thus, bladder neoplasms can be appreciated better, especially to determine staging.

- **Bimanual palpation in pelvic masses:** Under anaesthesia, the mass is palpated with a finger is passed in the rectum in males, the vagina in females while the pelvic mass is palpated simultaneously with the other hand.

BALLOTTEMENT

- **Ballottement means tossing about.**

- Originally, this was described to confirm pregnancy exceeding 3 months or near term to see if the baby's head is engaged. A gentle push is given to the foetus using fingers within one of the cervical fornices. Foetus is displaced up for a while only to comeback and hit fingers. This is also called *internal ballottement*.

- **Pelvic ballottement** is done for a mass arising from the pelvis. Gentle downward push is given to the mass by the abdominal hand and the bouncing sensation is felt by the fingers inside vagina. In males and in virgins, this test can be done by fingers within rectum instead of vagina. This is also called *interno-external ballottement*.

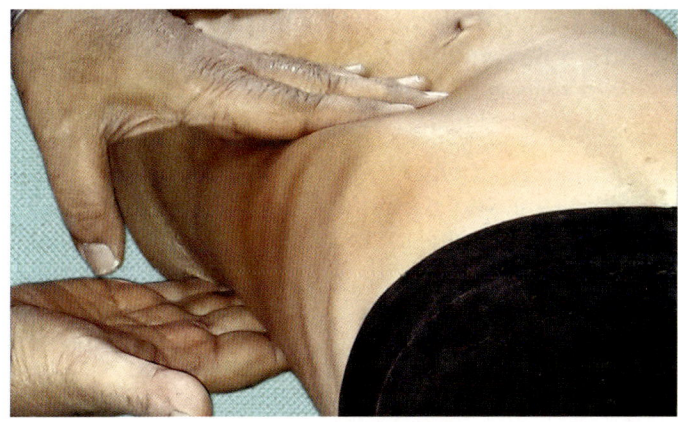

Fig. 2.18: Ballottement

- **Renal ballottement:** Classically kidney is not only bimanually palpable but also ballottable. The patient is asked to lie down on the couch in the supine position. One hand is laid flat on the mass so that flexor surface of the fingers are in contact with the mass. Fingers of the other hand are passed behind the flank so that they are in contact with the back lateral to sacrospinalis muscle (in fact, this is the renal angle). Now toss the mass with gentle, short, quick forward thrusts from behind. This hand is called displacing hand. If these movements are felt by anteriorly placed hand (watching hand), as a bouncing sensation, ballottement is said to be positive. *Renal ballottement is also called external ballottement* (Fig. 2.18).

- **Renal ballottement is possible due to following reasons**

  1. Kidney is covered by pad of fat within fascia of Gerota.

  2. It has a pedicle similar to ovary.

  3. When it enlarges, it can enlarge both anteriorly and posteriorly.

Clinical Wisdom

- It should be remembered that most of the renal masses are bimanually palpable and ballottable. However, in advanced renal malignancies, due to fixity, mass may not exhibit ballottability. Thus, all ballottable swellings are bimanually palpable but bimanual swellings need not be ballottable.
- It is also possible to have bimanual palpability in cases of massive enlargement of liver or spleen or even an ascending colonic mass but they are not ballottable.

CREPITUS

- It is a type of cracking sound which is to be experienced by palpating fingers. It is not a sound which is either audible or heard with stetho-scope.

- Crepitus of the subcutaneous tissue is of importance to surgeons. Various causes are classified as given below.

  1. **Lung injury:** Mostly it is caused by traumatic fractures of ribs. Fractured segment penetrates the lung and results in leakage of air into subcutaneous tissues. It is called surgical emphysema.

  2. **Laryngeal injury:** Injury to larynx, tracheostomy, and ruptured bronchus are the other causes.

  3. **Infective:** Gas gangrene is a classical example which produces crepitus due to gas production in the subcutaneous plane. It should be remembered that even anaerobic organisms will produce crepitus. Severely toxic patient who is ill and has crepitus is likely to be due to gas gangrene than other causes.

  4. **Rupture/perforation of the oesophagus:** One of the important signs to look for when you suspect oesophageal perforation is to look for crepitus in the supraclavicular fossa.

  5. **Other causes:** These are mainly orthopaedic causes. Fractured segments, osteoarthritic joints, tenosynovitis (inflammation of the synovial lining of the joint) as in de Quervain's disease.

  6. **Laryngeal crepitus** refers to the grating feeling elicited while moving the laryngeal cartilages especially the thyroid cartilage sideways against the cervical vertebrae.

> This is due the friction between the posterior border of the thyroid alae and the transverse process of the cervical vertebrae.
>
> Crepitus is *normally present and if it is absent 'Bocca's sign is said to be positive.'*
>
> Laryngeal crepitus is absent in postcricoid malignancy, retropharyngeal abscess or any lesion in the retropharyngeal space pushing the laryngeal cartilages forwards.

TRACHEAL TUG

- Classically described for aortic aneurysm. Left bronchus is crossed by arch of aorta.

- Gently hold the cricoid cartilage and apply upward pressure in an extended neck. So in cases of aortic aneurysm, with each heart beat, trachea is pulled down due to compression effect caused by aneurysm over the bronchus. This is described as *tracheal tug.* This sign is called **Oliver's sign.**

- Thus, tracheal tug can be absent in carcinoma larynx due to fixity.

PIGMENTATION

1. *Acanthosis nigricans*: Bilateral symmetrical pigmentation in the axilla, groin, nipples and umbilicus. It can also be in face and neck. It is not a premalignant lesion, but it is commonly associated with carcinoma stomach, other causes being Cushing's syndrome, acromegaly, etc.

2. *Haemochromatosis*: Bronzing of the skin from melanin deposition occurs in about 90% of patients and about half with haemosiderin deposition.

3. *Addison's disease*: Dark brown pigment of the body along with greyish pigmentation of the mucous membrane is characteristic.

4. *Café au lait spots*: Seen in von Recklinghausen's disease (Fig. 2.19).

5. Melanoma

6. *Drugs*: Busulphan

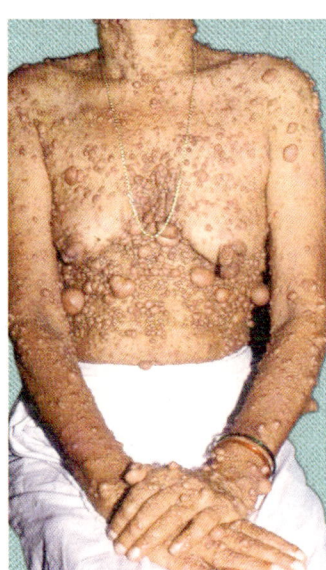

Fig. 2.19: Von Recklinghausen's disease—multiple neuro-fibromatosis with cafe au lait spots

SKIN LESIONS

I. Nonpalpable

- **Macule:** Flat, circumscribed lesion in the skin having a diameter less than 1 cm (Fig. 2.20)

- **Patch:** Flat circumscribed lesion in the skin having a

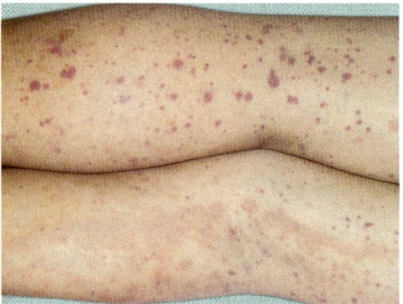

Fig. 2.20: Macule

diameter 1 cm or more—vitiligo patch, hypopigmented patch in leprosy.

II. Palpable

- **Papule** (Fig. 2.21): A solid elevated lesion up to 5 mm in diameter, e.g. wart.

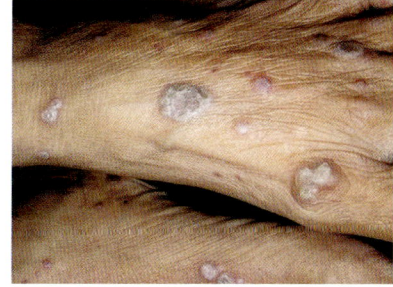

Fig. 2.21: Papule

- **Nodule:** A solid elevated lesion more than 5 mm, usually about 1 cm in diameter. Metastatic deposits in the skin, hard subcutaneous nodule in rheumatoid arthritis, nodule of neurofibromatosis.

- **Plaque** (Fig. 2.22): It is classically seen in psoriasis. It is a confluence of papules or nodules having large, flat topped, raised lesion.

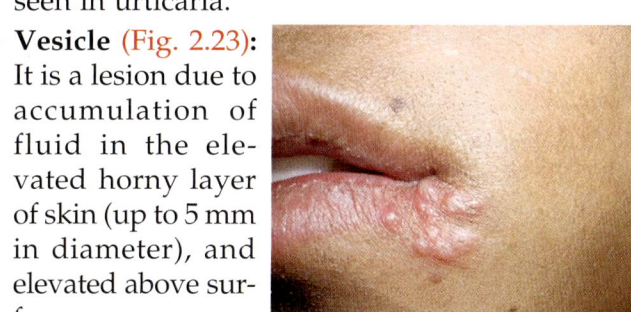

Fig. 2.22: Plaque

- **Wheal:** It is a round elevated lesion due to accumulation of fluid in dermis. It is a primary lesion seen in urticaria.

- **Vesicle** (Fig. 2.23): It is a lesion due to accumulation of fluid in the elevated horny layer of skin (up to 5 mm in diameter), and elevated above surface.

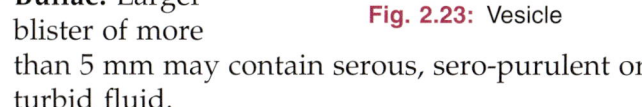

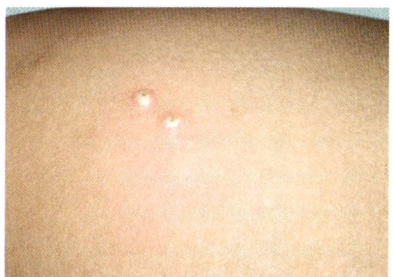

Fig. 2.23: Vesicle

- **Bullae:** Larger blister of more than 5 mm may contain serous, sero-purulent or turbid fluid.

- **Pustule** (Fig. 2.24): Classically described for hair follicle infection. It is a small, yellow, elevated, circumscribed lesion in the skin.

Fig. 2.24: Pustule

VIRCHOW NODE

Enlargement of supraclavicular node by metastasis specially on the left side is called Troisier's sign and this node is called Virchow's node. It indicates intra-abdominal or thoracic disease, including testis.

- It also receives lymphatics from left upper limb, left side of the chest including the breasts.

- It is felt by 2 methods. In the first method, stand behind the patient, tilt his head to the left side and palpate the supraclavicular node on left side.

- When it is grossly enlarged, it can also be felt by palpating above the clavicle in the posterior triangle (Fig. 2.25).

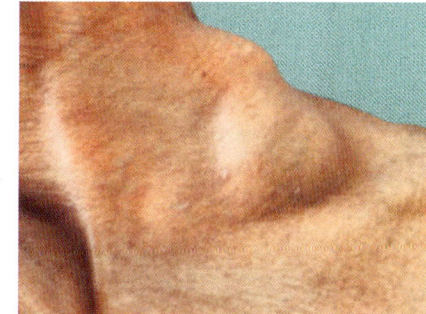

Fig. 2.25: Virchow's node (left supraclavicular node)

- This node is located at the junction of internal jugular vein and left subclavian vein. The thoracic duct drains here.

- Reflux from thoracic duct into this node occurs in intra-abdominal malignancies.

SCALENE NODE (Fig. 2.26)

- This node gets enlarged in bronchogenic carcinoma. It is in between the two heads of the sternocleidomastoid. It is anterior to scalenus anterior muscle.

- These nodes are the first ones to receive lymphatics from bronchogenic carcinoma.

- They are also members of supraclavicular group.

- When the CT scan/PET scan was not available for the diagnosis, it was a common practice to do 'scalene pad of fat' biopsy.

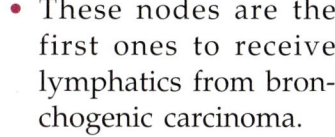
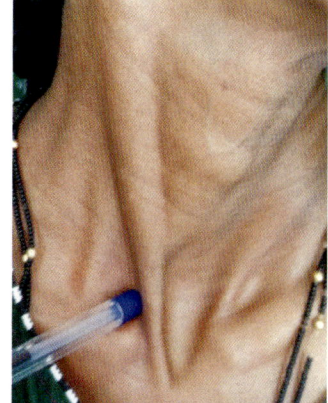

Fig. 2.26: Scalene node

Skin lesions—Figs 2.20 to 2.24 *contributed by* Dr Satish Pai, Head, Department of Skin and VD, KMC, Manipal

- Injury to the thoracic duct, and internal jugular vein can occur.

- Phrenic nerve is deep here. Injury to phrenic nerve due to cautery can occur here.

TONGUE

Normal colour of the tongue is red because of rich vascularity and capillary network close to the surface.

- Discolouration can be due to chewing betel nut, iron-containing medicine or due to moniliasis.

- *Dry tongue* suggests dehydration. Common causes are late intestinal obstruction, renal failure, acute pancreatitis, etc. Coated tongue is seen in debilitating diseases including pancreatitis (Figs 2.27 and 2.28).

- *Geographic tongue* (glossitis migrans) refers to changes that happen in the tongue after surgery for peritonitis and following antibiotics. Epithelial regeneration and denudation occur quickly and thus scallops or rings appear (Fig. 2.29).

- *Fissure*: Congenital fissure (Fig. 2.30) is more common. It appears by 3–4 years of age and fissures are in all directions. In the midline, the fissure is more deep. Fissures are more transverse than horizontal. (In secondary syphilis, fissures are longitudinal.)

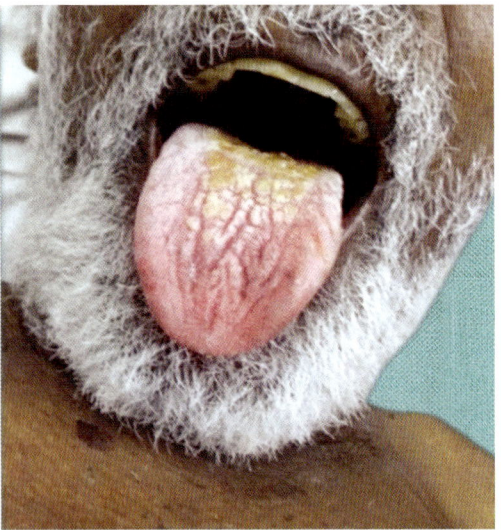

Fig. 2.27: Dry tongue in intestinal obstruction

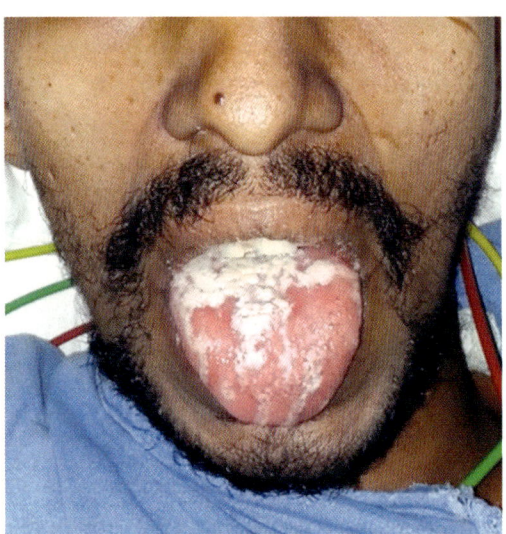

Fig. 2.28: Dry coated tongue in acute pancreatitis

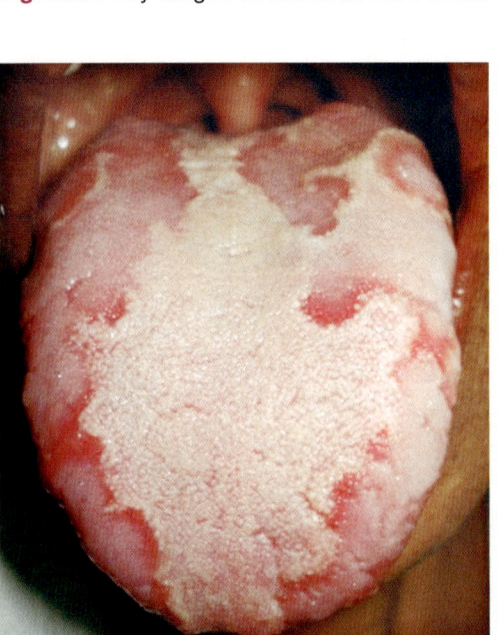

Fig. 2.29: Geographic tongue

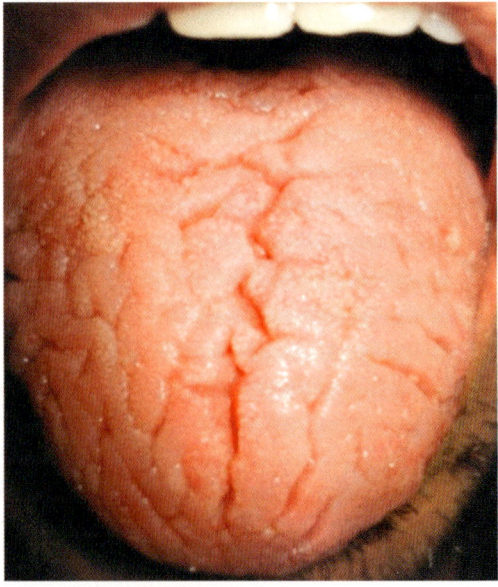

Fig. 2.30: Fissured tongue

- **Tongue tie:** The patient is not able to protrude the tongue outside or move the tongue upwards, if there is a short frenulum—it is due to tongue tie (Fig. 2.31).

- **Glossitis** and **stomatitis:** Very many causes are responsible for red inflamed lesions within oral cavity including lips and tongue. They are nutritional deficiencies, vitamin deficiencies (B_1, B_2, B_6, B_9), bacterial and viral fevers, allergy, etc. The term atrophic glossitis refers to smooth bald tongue without any papilla. Iron deficiency anaemia is one of the causes of bald tongue. Syphilis used to be one of the causes of atrophic gastritis. Now it is rare. Median rhomboid glossitis is caused by fungal infection of the oral cavity. Immuno-suppression and corticosteroid use are commonly blamed for this. Many antibiotics including cephalosporins, clarithromycin, and drugs such as corticosteroids, carbamazapine, methotrexate can cause glossitis (Figs 2.32 and 2.33).

- Carcinoma arising from leukoplakia (Fig. 2.34).

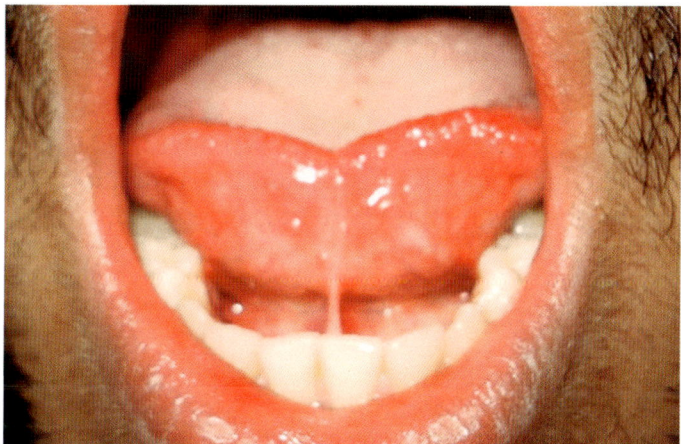

Fig. 2.31: Tongue tie

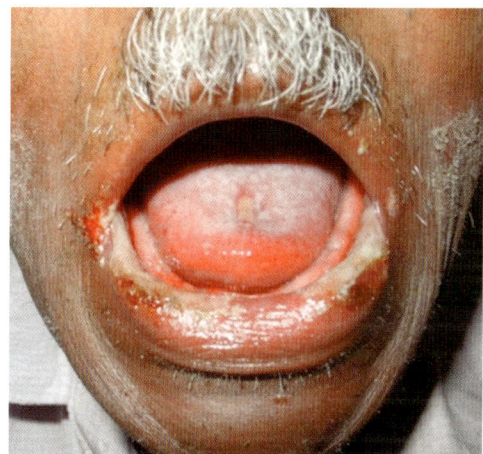

Fig. 2.32: Methotrexate-induced stomatitis and glossitis

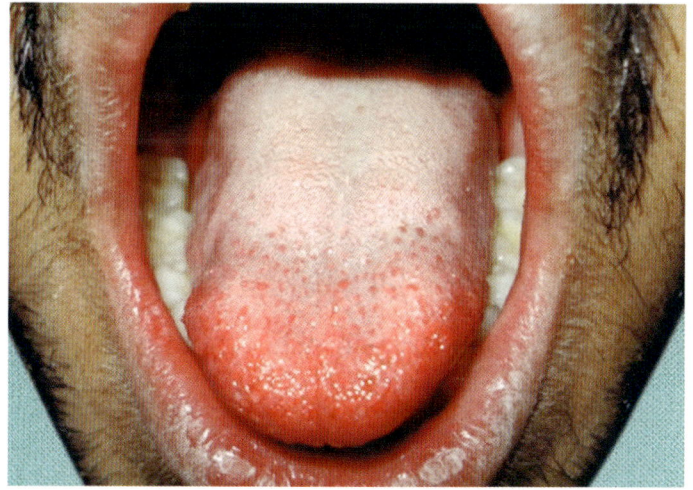

Fig. 2.33: Allergic glossitis

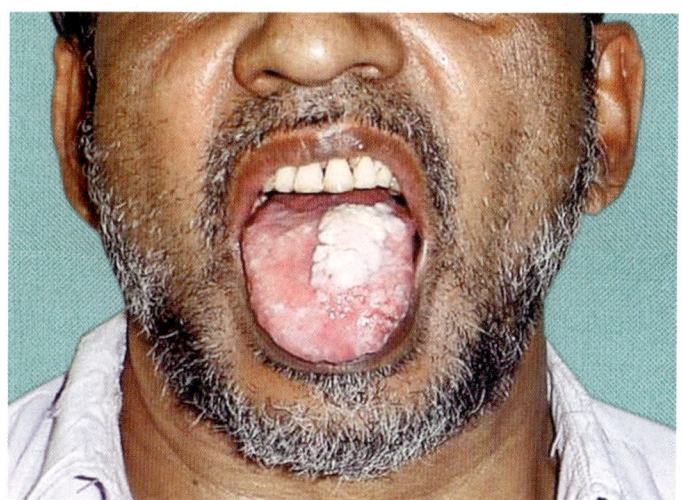

Fig. 2.34: Carcinoma *in situ* in leukoplakia

(*Courtesy:* Dr Keertilatha Pai, Dean, Manipal College of Dental Sciences, Manipal, Figs 2.29 to 2.34)

3

Examination of an Ulcer

DEFINITION

An ulcer is a discontinuity in the skin or mucous membrane. It occurs due to death of cells (surface epithelium) following surgical debridement of tissues or due to trauma.

INTRODUCTION

Ulcer leg is an important cause of morbidity and also a cause of mortality in elderly patients, especially with diabetes. It is an important short case in the clinical examination because it is common. In fact, a few examiners make a statement that if you do not know ulcer properly, you do not deserve to pass MBBS examinations. So, study ulcer in full detail along with proper clinical methods.

It is also important to realise that history and examination for ulcer differ when they occur in different locations. To give an example: Loss of sensation, pain and trauma are important history for ulcers in the leg. However, such history is least important for ulcers in the face or other areas. Students should try to analyse every case in a different way, i.e. site, specific history and examination. An attempt has been made here to give you site-specific history and examination.

Clinical Wisdom—the most common

- Ulcer over face: Basal cell carcinoma
- Ulcer over neck: Tuberculosis
- Ulcer over chest wall: Tuberculosis
- Ulcer over genitalia: Sexually transmitted diseases
- Ulcer over the toes: Ischaemic ulcers
- Ulcer over the sole: Trophic ulcers
- Ulcer over gaiter area: Venous ulcers
- Ulcer on the nape of neck: Carbuncle
- Ulcer on the scrotum: Fournier's gangrene
- Ulcer over shin: Traumatic ulcer

Please remember **these are the most common locations of the ulcers.** First rule out these before you give alternate diagnosis.

CLASSIFICATION

- It is classified into clinical classification and pathological classification

- Clinical classification is given in Table 3.1.

Table 3.1: Clinical classification

Spreading	Callus	Healing
No granulation tissue	Pale granulation tissue	Red granulation tissue
Plenty of discharge	Serous discharge	Minimal serous discharge
Excessive slough	Slough present	Slough absent
Surrounding area inflamed and oedematous	Induration at the base, edge and surrounding area	Signs of inflammation are minimal
Purulent smell present	Smell can be present	Smell is absent

HISTORY OF PRESENT ILLNESS

- *How did it start?* Often leg ulcers start after trauma— ask a question, did you have trauma? It is but natural that agriculturists, field workers, manual labourers are susceptible. Trivial trauma may be the precipitating factor for development of ulcers in diabetic patients and in patients with occlusive arterial disorders like **T**hrombo**A**ngiitis **O**bliterans (TAO).

- *Before the onset of ulcer*, were *you getting any crampy or a catch-like* pain in the legs while walking? If present, it indicates arterial occlusion. TAO and atherosclerotic disease are the two common arterial occlusive disorders affecting the limbs (*refer* to page 106 for more details). Crampy pain late in the evening may also be due to venous disorders such as varicose veins (dilated tortuous veins in the leg). Sudden severe pain in the limbs, followed by change in colour, and then black patches are suggestive of gangrene. Once gangrenous skin is removed, it results in ischaemic ulcers.

- How is the progress ? Is it becoming big, remaining the same or is it healing? An ulcer which is becoming big is a spreading ulcer, e.g. diabetic ulcer. Ulcer which remains same may be a chronic ulcer, e.g. callous ulcer. Ulcer which is becoming small is a healing ulcer, e.g. treated diabetic ulcers or venous ulcers. A nonhealing and spreading ulcer can also be malignant specially malignant melanoma (malignant skin tumour arising from melanin pigment). Leg is one of the common sites of melanoma.

- Do you appreciate sensations in the sole of the foot? Those who have neuropathy may have loss of sensation. Diabetes is the most common cause of neuropathic foot. Totally anaesthetic foot is classical of leprosy. Ulcers developing in neuropathic feet are called trophic ulcers.

- Recurrent ulcerations in the leg with jaundice suggest sickle cell anaemia.

- Sudden appearance of black patches followed by ulcerations are suggestive of fixed drug reactions— once the black patches (gangrenous skin) are removed, it results in ulcer.

- History of chronic smoking should be elicited.

Clinical Wisdom

Site specific history and examination should be done

PAST HISTORY

- Any history suggestive of chronic illness such as diabetes, leprosy, and tuberculosis (rarely cutaneous tuberculosis can present as an ulcer or a wart-like lesion, more so in children).

- In basal cell carcinoma, it is common to get a history of recurrence of a swelling/lesion which is treated as benign lesion.

GENERAL PHYSICAL EXAMINATION

It is done to check for general health of the patient.

- *Chronic anaemia*: Poor wound healing
- *Jaundice*: Sickle cell anaemia
- *Multiple matted nodes in the neck*: Tuberculosis
- *Evidence of atherosclerosis*: Thick arteries, hypertension
- Nicotine stains on the lips, oral cavity.

CLINICAL EXAMINATION OF AN ULCER

Inspection

1. *Location of the ulcer*: Whenever possible, describe the location in relation to a bony landmark. Example: Ulcer is located 4 cm away from medial malleolus.

   - Arterial ulcer: Tip of the toes, dorsum of the foot.
   - Long saphenous varicosity with ulcer: Medial side of the leg.
   - Short saphenous varicosity with ulcer: Lateral side of the leg just above the lateral malleolus.
   - Trophic ulcers or perforating ulcers: Over the sole at pressure points.
   - Nonhealing ulcer: Over the shin and lateral malleolus.

2. *Number, size, shape and extent*
   - Traumatic ulcers, tubercular ulcers or venous ulcers may be multiple. When multiple ulcers are present, find out which one started first.
   - Ischaemic ulcers are small but deep lesions.
   - Describe the vertical and horizontal diameter.
   - Venous ulcers are generally ovoid in shape. Tuberculous ulcers are generally oval in shape.
   - Irregular shape suggests carcinomatous ulceration.
   - Syphilitic chancre is single, but lymph nodes are multiple.

3. *Floor of the ulcer*: This is the part of the ulcer which is exposed or seen.

- Red granulation tissue: Healing ulcer (Fig. 3.1)
- Necrotic tissue, slough: Spreading ulcer (Fig. 3.2)
- Tendons, ligaments and bones may be visible in ischaemic ulcers or in diabetic ulcers after debridement.
- Pale, scanty granulation tissue: Tuberculous ulcer **(apple-jelly granulation)**
- Wash-leather slough: Gummatous ulcer
- Part of the bone: Neuropathic ulcer
- Nodular: Epithelioma
- Black tissue: Malignant melanoma

4. *Discharge from the ulcer*

- Serous discharge: Healing ulcer
- Purulent discharge: Spreading ulcer
- Bloody discharge: Malignant ulcer

- Discharge with bony spicules: Osteomyelitis
- Greenish discharge: Pseudomonas infection

5. *Edge and margin*: Edge is between the floor of the ulcer and the margin. *The margin is the junction between the normal epithelium and the ulcer.* It represents the areas of maximum cellular activity. If destruction dominates as in spreading ulcers, the edge is inflamed, oedematous and angry looking (*stage of extension*). When ulcer shows evidence of healing, the edge will be bluish due to granulation tissue covered with thin epithelium (*stage of transition*). In a healed ulcer, the outermost part of the edge is whitish due to fibrosis (*stage of repair*). Various types of edges of ulcers are given in Fig. 3.3.

- *Sloping edge* is seen in all healing ulcers such as traumatic ulcers, venous ulcers (Fig. 3.4).
- *Punched out edge* is seen when there is loss of sensation to the foot. These ulcers are called trophic ulcers. Diabetic neuropathy, leprosy

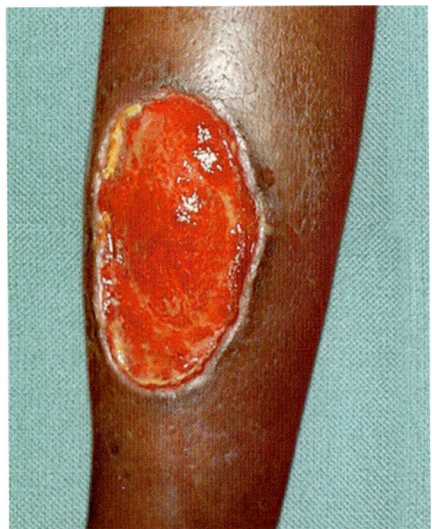

Fig. 3.1: Traumatic ulcer

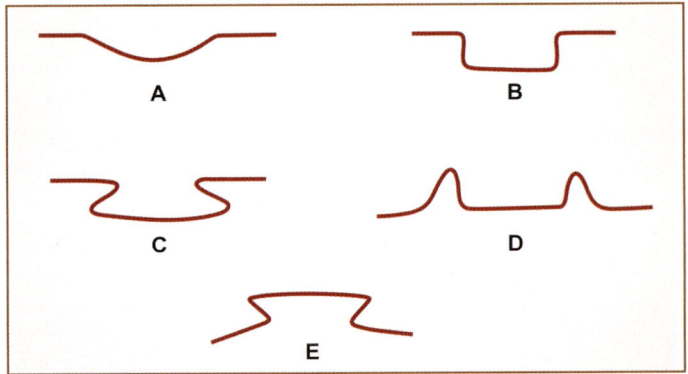

Fig. 3.3: Different types of edges of ulcer

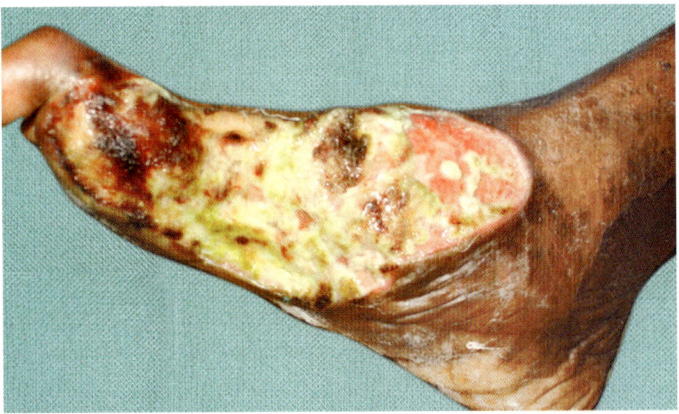

Fig. 3.2: Slough—dead soft tissue—typical spreading ulcer in a diabetic patient

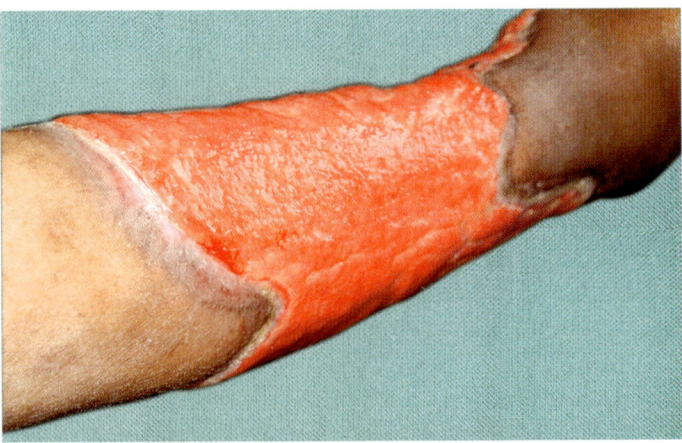

Fig. 3.4: Sloping edge

nerve injuries and myelomeningocoele are a few examples where in trophic ulcers occur. Ischaemic ulcers also may have punched out edge (square cut).

Gummatous ulcers also have punched out edges. Gummatous ulcers occur in tertiary syphilis. They are rare. They have punched out edge due to endarteritis obliterans caused by syphilitic organisms. (Please do not give a diagnosis of gummatous ulcer in the clinics.) Chronic non-healing ulcers also may have punched out edges (Fig. 3.5).

- *Undermined edge* is seen in tuberculous ulcers, probably due to more destruction of sub-cutaneous tissues than the skin. The edge is classically thin and bluish in colour (Fig. 3.6).

- *Raised edge* (beaded edge) is seen in rodent ulcers or basal cell carcinoma (Fig. 3.7).

- *Everted edge* (rolled out) is diagnostic of squamous cell carcinoma. The edge grows very rapidly and it occupies the normal skin and thus gets everted (Fig. 3.8).

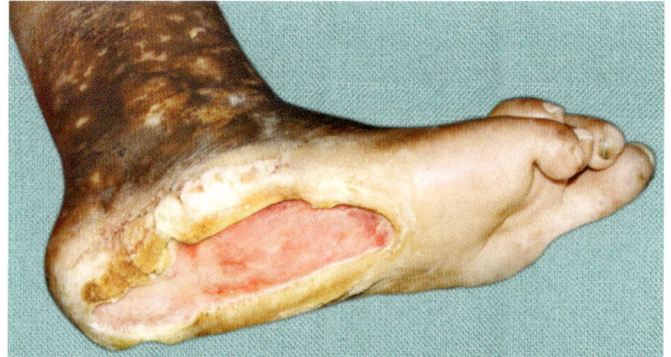

Fig. 3.5: Punched out edge—neuropathic ulcer (classically described for gummatous ulcer)

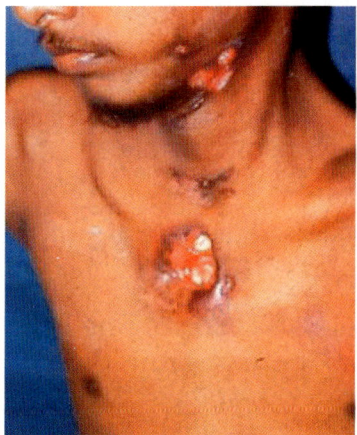

Fig. 3.6: Tubercular ulcers over the sternum and neck

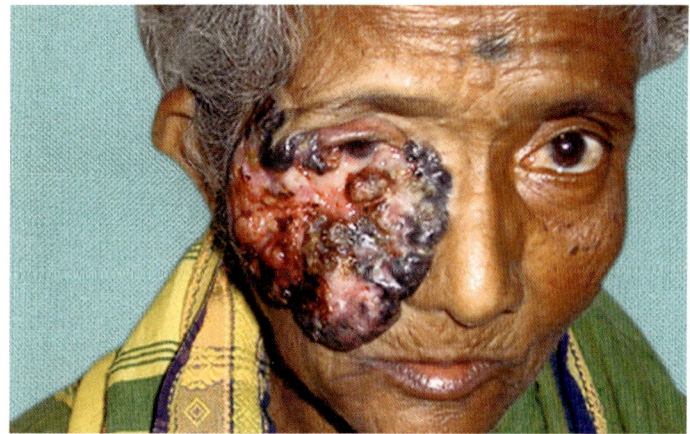

Fig. 3.7: Elevated edge—basal cell carcinoma (*Courtesy:* Prof Vidyadhar Kinhal, HOD, Surgery, VIMS, Bellary, Karnataka)

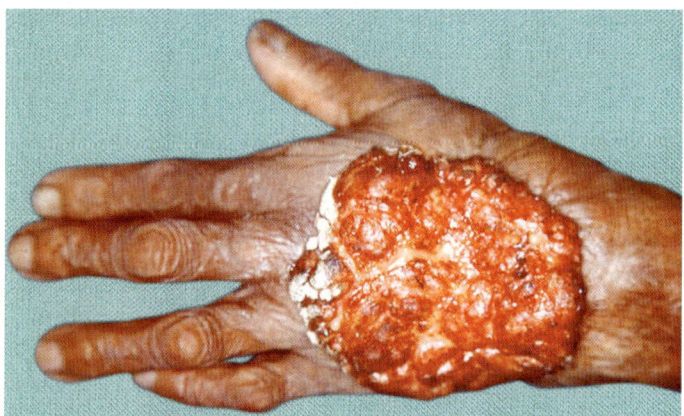

Fig. 3.8: Everted edge—squamous cell carcinoma

6. *Surrounding area*
   - Thick and pigmented—venous ulcer (Figs 3.9 and 3.10).
   - Thin and dark—arterial ulcer.
   - Red and oedematous—spreading ulcers like diabetic ulcer.
   - Scar around the ulcer—Marjolin's ulcer.

7. *Any other obvious findings in the leg*
   - Equinus deformity suggests venous ulcers.
   - Grossly swollen leg may be due to deep vein thrombosis. Such limbs are called postphlebitic limb.
   - A few toes may be absent—due to surgical procedures as in diabetic foot or in ischaemic limbs.
   - Ulcers with multiple sinuses suggest madura foot.
   - Significant wasting of calf muscles indicates ischaemic ulcers (disuse atrophy).

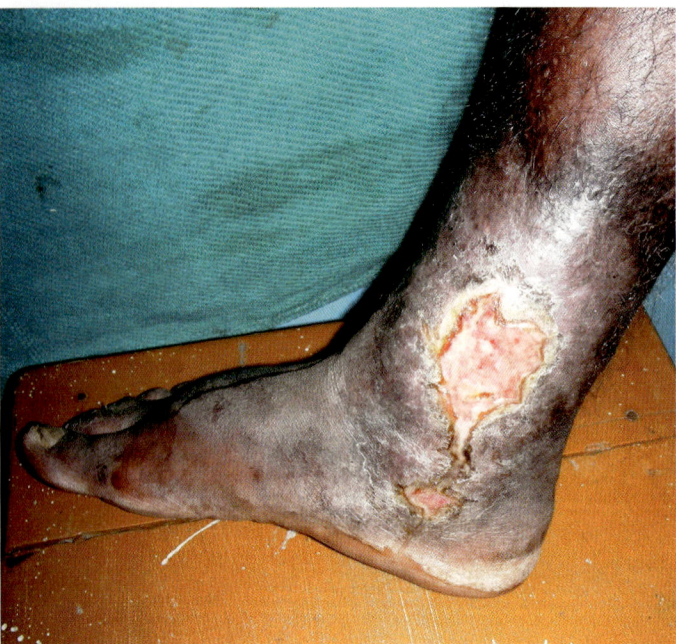

Fig. 3.9: Spreading venous ulcer. You can see unhealthy granulation tissue and discharge

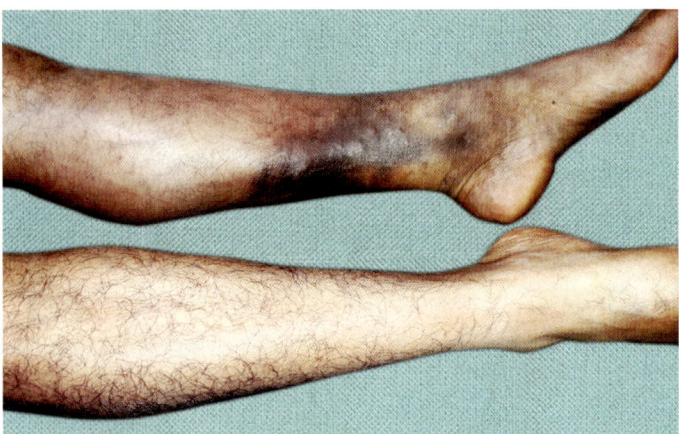

Fig. 3.10: Pigmentation of medial side of the leg

Palpation

1. *Tenderness*: This is the first sign to be elicited. One need not put too much pressure on the ulcer to elicit tenderness. If pain is elicited on gentle palpation, it is said to be positive which means ulcer is tender.

   - Acutely inflamed ulcer—tender
   - Venous ulcer—may or may not be tender
   - Arterial ulcer—tender
   - Tubercular ulcer—nontender
   - Malignant ulcers—nontender

   It is important to realise that even malignant ulcers are painful, if they are infected or when they infiltrate bones

2. *Edge*: Induration (hardness) of the edge is characteristic of squamous cell carcinoma. Some degree of induration can also be seen in chronic ulcers and long-standing varicose ulcers (Fig. 3.11). Induration occurs due to extensive fibrosis. It is said to be a host defense mechanism. *By causing fibrosis, lymphatic spread is delayed.* Tenderness of the edge is characteristic of infected ulcers and arterial ulcers.

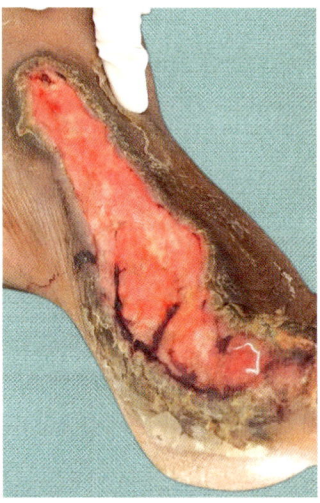

Fig. 3.11: Palpation of the ulcer

3. *Base*: *It is the area on which ulcer rests.* Pick up the ulcer between thumb and index finger and tissues beneath can be appreciated. If the ulcer cannot be lifted up, the base cannot be made out. The base can be tendons, muscles or bone depending upon the site of ulcer. *Marked induration at the base is diagnostic of squamous cell carcinoma.* Hunterian chancre (occurs in primary syphilis) is a benign ulcer and produces significant induration. Hence, it is also called a hard chancre (Clinical Box 3.1).

> **Clinical Box 3.1**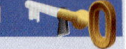
>
> *Induration*
> - It means hardness
> - Maximum induration—squamous cell carcinoma
> - Minimal induration—malignant melanoma
> - Brawny induration—abscess
> - Cyanotic induration—chronic venous congestion as in varicose ulcer
> - The base and the surrounding area should be examined for induration

4. *Depth*: It is not an important sign. However, if possible try to assess the depth of the ulcer. Penetrating or perforating ulcers in the sole of the foot, pressure sores (bedsores) can be very deep and up to the bone.

5. *Mobility:* Gentle attempt is made to move the ulcer to know its fixity to the underlying tissues. Malignant ulcers are usually fixed, benign ulcers are not (Fig. 3.12).

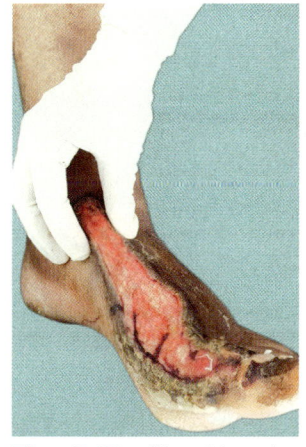

   It is difficult to move a large ulcer on the dorsum of the foot or in sole even when it is benign.

6. *Bleeding:* Malignant ulcer is friable like a cauliflower. On gentle palpation, it bleeds. Granulation tissue as in a healing ulcer also bleeds.

Fig. 3.12: Checking for mobility

   Once again, students should not use force to elicit bleeding. What is important is bleeding on gentle touch—which is a sign of malignancy?

7. *Surrounding area* (Fig. 3.13):
   - Thickening and induration is found in squamous cell carcinoma.
   - Tenderness and pitting on pressure indicates spreading inflammation surrounding the ulcer.
   - Colour changes indicate ischaemia of the foot.
   - If dilated veins are present, the ulcer is due to varicosity.
   - Loss of sensations in the surrounding areas suggests neuropathic ulceration.

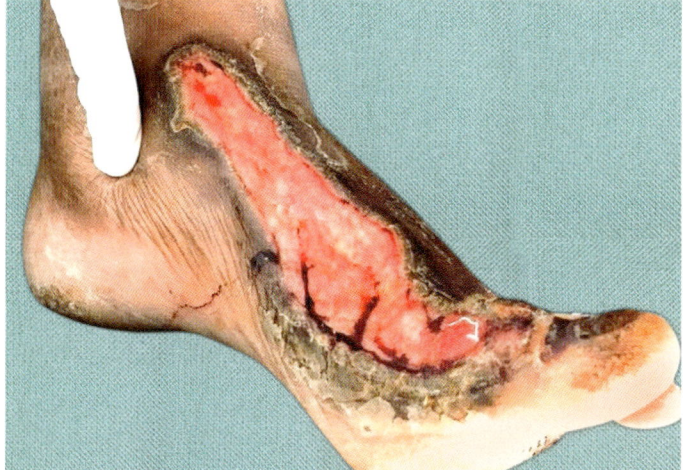

Fig. 3.13: Surrounding area to be checked for induration, oedema or tenderness

8. *Muscle wasting:* Measure the girth of calf muscles from a fixed point (both sides). Wasting of muscles is classically found in occlusive arterial diseases (Fig. 3.14).

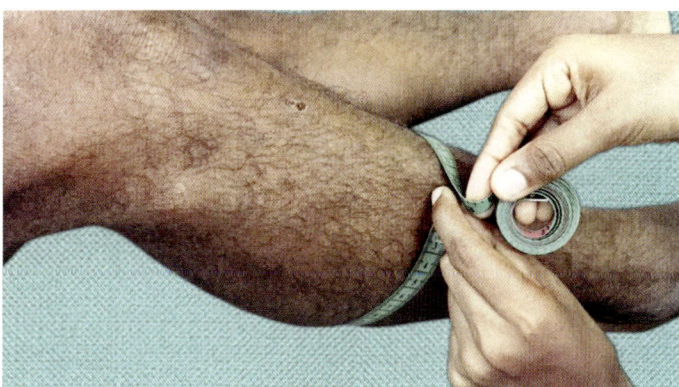

Fig. 3.14: Examination for wasting of the muscles

RELEVANT CLINICAL EXAMINATION

1. *Arterial pulsations:* Detailed examination of peripheral vessels is discussed under peripheral vascular disease. However, dorsalis pedis, posterior tibial, popliteal and femoral arteries should be palpated in cases of lower limb ulcers. Presence of weak pulses or absent pulses indicates occlusive arterial disease (Fig. 3.15).

2. *Varicose veins:* If present, it is most probably a varicose ulcer. However, AV fistula can present as distal ulcers, with arterialisation of veins and a continuous murmur.

3. *Sensations:* Loss of vibration sense and loss of ankle jerk occur early in cases of diabetic neuropathy. Later, touch and pain are lost. *Totally anaesthetic feet are characteristic of leprosy* (Figs 3.16 and 3.17).

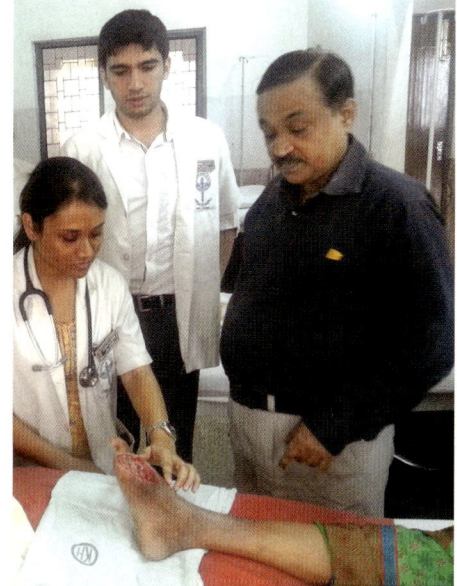

Fig. 3.15: Checking for dorsalis pedis artery pulsations in a case of TAO

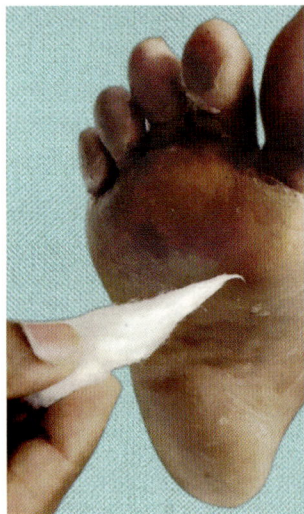

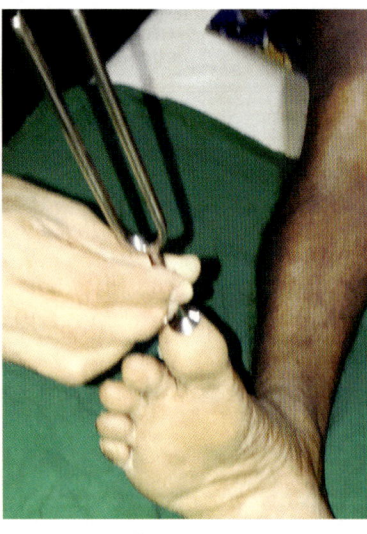

Fig. 3.16: Testing for touch sensation

Fig. 3.17: Checking for vibration sense

In every case of suspected neuropathic ulcer, examine the spine. If you see a scar, it might be due to operation on myelomeningocoele. Suspect spina bifida, if there is tuft of hair or lipoma or skin dimpling in the spine region (Figs 3.18 and 3.19).

4. *Function of the joint*: Movements of the involved joint are restricted either due to pain, involvement of the joint or due to infiltration into the joint by malignant ulcers.

5. *Regional lymph nodes*
   - Tender and enlarged—acute secondary infection
   - Nontender and enlarged—chronic infection
   - Nontender and hard—epithelioma
   - Nontender, large, firm, multiple—malignant melanoma (Figs 3.20A and B).

Remember to examine: Pulsations, sensations, veins, function and lymph nodes.

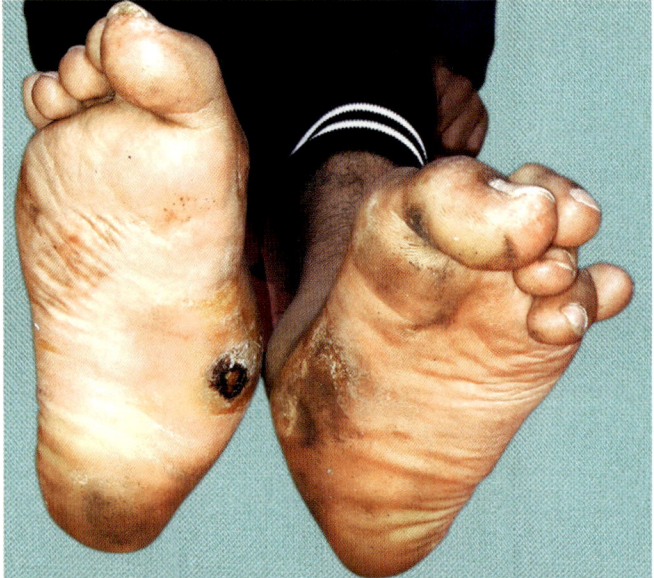

Fig. 3.18: Trophic ulcers in myelomeningocoele

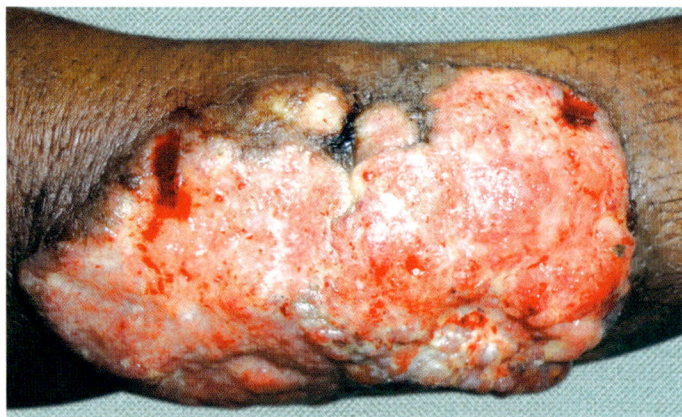

Fig. 3.20A: Epithelioma leg

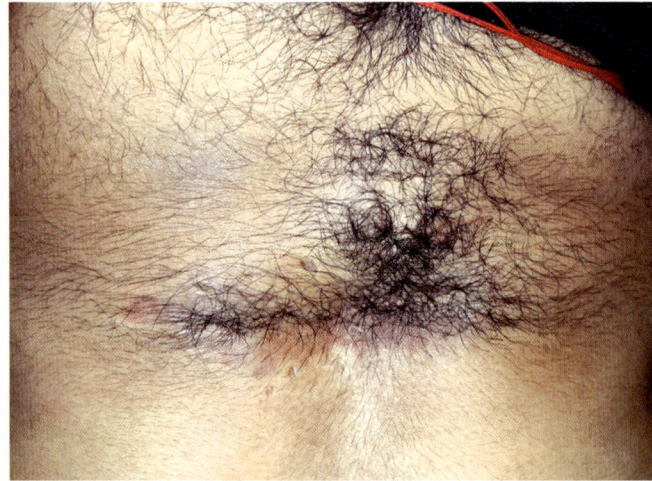

Fig. 3.19: Scar at the back—operated for myelomeningocoele

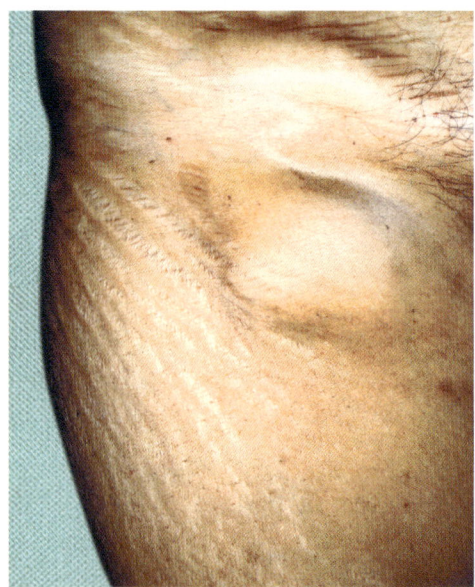

Fig. 3.20B: Lymph nodes in the groin

Systemic Examination

1. Central nervous system (CNS) and spine in neuropathic ulcers. There may be gibbus as in cases of TB spine or operated scar due to myelo-meningocoele, etc. (Figs 3.19 and 3.20).

2. Cardiovascular system (CVS) may reveal murmur as in cases of arteriovenous fistula or features suggestive of cardiac diseases.

3. Splenomegaly in blood dyscrasias such as in early stages of sickle cell anaemia.

A mention of examination of spleen is irrelevant in a case of arterial, venous or neuropathic ulcer. It is important only when patients present with blood dyscrasias. Students should develop this clinical wisdom.

Diagnosis

- When you are asked about the diagnosis, think of pathological diagnosis and clinical diagnosis.

- Examples:

    a. Trophic ulcer due to diabetes—callous ulcer

    b. Diabetic ulcer leg—healing

    c. Venous ulcer leg—healing

    d. Traumatic healing ulcer

INVESTIGATIONS

1. *Complete blood picture:* Hb%, TC, DC, ESR, peripheral smear:

    - Low Hb% is found in chronic ulcer. It is either nutritional or due to frequent blood loss during dressings as in diabetic ulcer.

    - High total count indicates infection.

    - Peripheral smear is done to rule out anaemia and sickle cell disease.

2. Fasting and postprandial blood sugar to rule out diabetes.

3. *Chest X-ray:* PA view to rule out pulmonary diseases such as tuberculosis, chronic obstructive pulmonary disease (COPD).

4. Pus for culture/sensitivity

5. Doppler/duplex scan/lower limb angiography in cases of arterial diseases

6. X-ray of the part to look for:

    - Osteomyelitis—common in diabetic ulcers

    - Periostitis tibia—common in varicose ulcers

7. *Biopsy:* Non-healing/malignant ulcers

Biopsy in a non-healing ulcer is done to rule out malignancy and also for any histological surprises (treatable causes such as tuberculosis). No biopsies are done in traumatic ulcers.

TREATMENT

It can be classified:

- **Local treatment:** It is given in Clinical Box 3.2.

- Control of systemic disease/causative factors/disease.

Clinical Box 3.2

Local treatment of ulcers in the leg (8 Ds)
- **D**ressings
- **D**esloughing agents
- **D**ebridement
- **D**isarticulations
- **D**rugs
- **D**iabetes control (if diabetic)
- **D**isease control (TAO, varicose veins, etc.)
- **D**ermal cover

Damage control—amputations

CLINICAL DISCUSSION

How do you classify ulcers?

Ulcers can be classified based on the pathology or clinical features.

Pathological Classification

A. Nonspecific ulcers

1. *Traumatic ulcer:* Trauma can be mechanical. This is the commonest cause of leg ulcer. It can be physical trauma due to burns or radiation. It can also be due to chemicals such as acids.

2. *Venous ulcers:* These include varicose ulcers and post-thrombotic ulcers which can occur following deep vein thrombosis.

3. *Arterial ulcers:* Following are a few examples of arterial ulcers:
    - Buerger's disease—common
    - Atherosclerotic vascular disease—common
    - Vasospastic disorders such as Raynaud's disease—uncommon
    - Martorell's ulcers or hypertensive ulcers—rare
    - Patients with rheumatoid arthritis can develop leg or foot ulcers due to vasculitis.

4. *Neurogenic ulcer (neuropathic ulcer, trophic ulcers)*
    - Leprosy and diabetes are the common causes.
    - Paraplegia, meningomyelocoele, posterior tibial nerve injury, tabes dorsalis are the other causes.

5. *Tropical ulcer:* It is a rare ulcer due to malnutrition associated with infection caused by Vincent's organisms.

6. *Diabetic ulcer foot or diabetic ulcer leg*

7. *Blood dyscrasias:* Sickle cell anaemia, thalassemia, leukaemia, etc. can produce recurrent ulcerations in the leg.

B. *Specific ulcer*: This is due to specific type of organisms, e.g. tubercular ulcers, syphilitic ulcers, actinomycotic ulcers.

C. *Malignant ulcers*: Malignant ulcers are squamous cell carcinoma, basal cell carcinoma, and malignant melanoma. Malignant ulcers are discussed in Chapter 13.

DIFFERENTIAL DIAGNOSIS

TRAUMATIC ULCERS

- These can occur anywhere in the body. However, these are more common where skin is closely applied to bony prominences, e.g. shin, malleoli, over which there are no muscles (Fig. 3.21).
- These are usually single, very painful ulcers of healing type. With proper dressings and antibiotics, these usually heal within 5–7 days.
- *Footballer's ulcer* is the name given to those nonhealing ulcers which occur in the leg over the shin due to direct trauma caused by the football.
- Sometimes, these ulcers may take a long time to heal. If not treated properly, it gets adhered to the bone.

VENOUS ULCER

- It occurs due to increased venous hydrostatic pressure.
- Located on the medial side of lower one-third of the leg in cases of long saphenous varicosity and on the lateral aspect of the leg in short saphenous varicosity (Fig. 3.22).
- It is shallow and superficial
- Never penetrates deep fascia
- Usually painless unless it is infected or causes periostitis tibia
- Shows evidence of healing
- Usually associated with varicose veins
- Typically lower leg around the ulcer is pigmented.
- Elevation of leg, dressings, compression stockings and treatment of varicose veins is the treatment of choice.

ARTERIAL ULCERS/ISCHAEMIC ULCERS

- Occur in the distal parts of the lower limbs such as toes, dorsum of the foot and over pressure points in the sole of the foot.

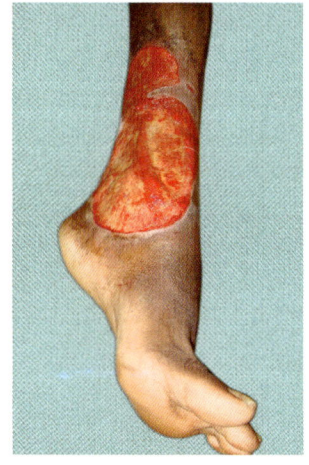

Fig. 3.21: Traumatic ulcer following hot water burns

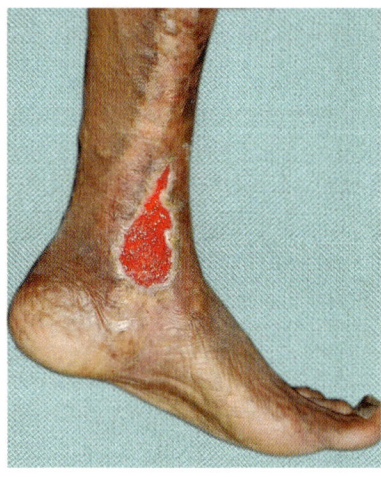

Fig. 3.22: Venous ulcer—left leg

- These are very painful and occur in young patients who have Buerger's disease (thromboangiitis obliterans—TAO) or occur in elderly patients due to atherosclerotic vascular disease.
- TAO commonly occurs in chronic smokers.
- Sudden occurrence of gangrene (Fig. 3.23) followed by ulcerations is typically seen in embolic causes such as atheromatous plaques, cardiac vegetations, etc.
- The ulcer is dry, deep and penetrates deep fascia.
- Evidence of chronic ischaemia in the rest of the foot clinches the diagnosis (see Table 3.2 for differences between arterial and venous ulcers).

Dry ulcers, deep ulcers, distal ulcers, disturbing sleep (severe pain), in a dying or dead limb are ischaemic ulcers.

NEUROPATHIC ULCER/TROPHIC ULCER

This type of ulcer develops in an anaesthetic limb. The causes of neuropathy are (Fig. 3.24):

- Diabetic neuropathy
- Meningomyelocoele
- Leprosy
- Alcoholic neuropathy

Table 3.2: Differences between arterial and venous ulcers

	Arterial ulcer	Venous ulcer
Location	Tips of toes	Medial or lateral side of leg
Pain	Very painful	Absent
Number and shape	Many and irregular	Single and oval
Depth	Deep, penetrates deep fascia	Superficial, does not penetrate deep fascia
Pigmentation	Not a feature	Usually present
Nature of the vessels	Peripheral pulses are weak or absent; veins are not dilated	Peripheral pulses are normal; veins are dilated

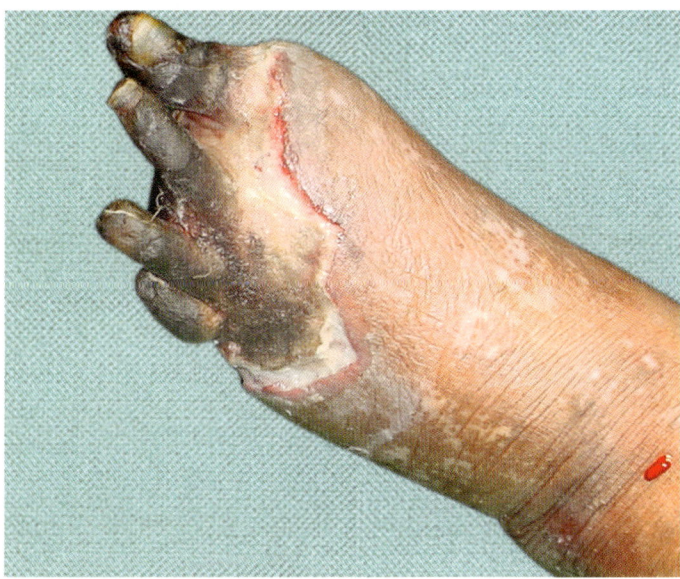

Fig. 3.23: Gangrene of the toes with ulcer in a case of polycythemia

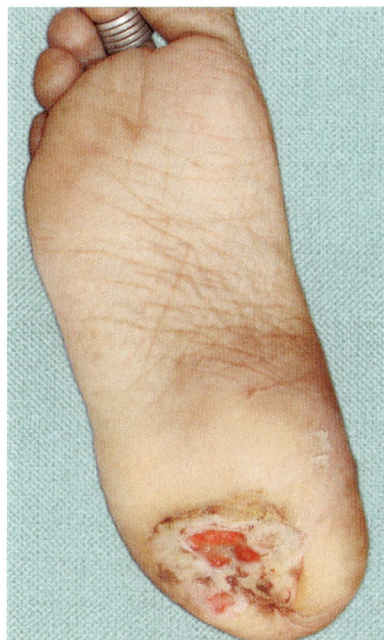

Fig. 3.24: Trophic ulcer due to diabetic neuropathy

- Nerve injuries/spine injuries
- Transverse myelitis
- Ulcer develops on the pressure points such as beneath heel, beneath the first and fifth metatarsals and gluteal region (decubitus ulcer). It develops as a callosity, gets infected, suppurates and leaves a central hole discharging pus. Slowly, it burrows deep inside, may involve bone and cause osteomyelitis. Hence, it is also called perforating ulcer.
- Trophic ulcers are caused by inadequate blood supply, malnutrition and neurological deficit. These are also included in this group.

DIABETIC ULCER LEG

- It is more common in the foot as it is vulnerable for injuries.
- High blood sugars, loss of sensations—neuropathy can be distal and diffuse with a stocking type of distribution. Neuropathy, poor blood supply due to micro- and macroangiopathy, poor resistance (diabetes is an immunocompromised status) predispose to ulcerations in the foot.
- Starts after trivial trauma, starts spreading rapidly, if untreated with features of toxicity. Cellulitis, abscess, spreading fasciitis, gangrene, and osteomyelitis are different stages of diabetic foot (Clinical Box 3.3).
- Ulcers are infected with purulent discharge. Foul odour of wet gangrene is characteristic. Patients look toxic with high blood sugars and ketoacidosis.
- Often, these ulcers may take a long time to heal even after treatment.
- Pus culture and sensitivity is obtained first and appropriate antibiotics are given.
- Different types of diabetic ulcer legs are given in (page 40, Figs 3.25 to 3.30)

Treatment

- If the ulcer is non-healing with slough, initial management should include desloughing agents and surgical removal of the slough.
- Once the ulcer starts healing with red granulation tissue, skin grafting is done.
- When the ulcer and gangrene involve the toe, disarticulation of the toe with removal of distal portion of head of the bone is done so that the healing is faster. Later, skin grafting is required, if the wound is kept open.
- When the infection is spreading, aggressive debridement is done with drainage of the pus, removal of the debris and multiple fasciotomy, if required.
- When the life is in danger, amputation may have to be done.
- Immobilisation of the foot in a plaster of Paris posterior slab with a walking boot almost cures the trophic ulcer within 2–3 weeks, provided the primary disease is controlled.

Clinical Box 3.3

Diabetic ulcer foot
- Distal and diffuse neuropathy
- Decreased blood supply
- Defective immune functions
- Dangerous organisms

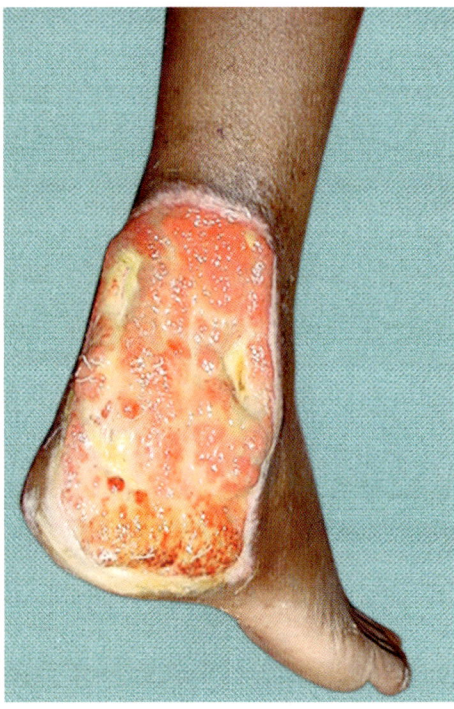

Fig. 3.25: Diabetic ulcer leg with a few areas of healing and a few areas with slough

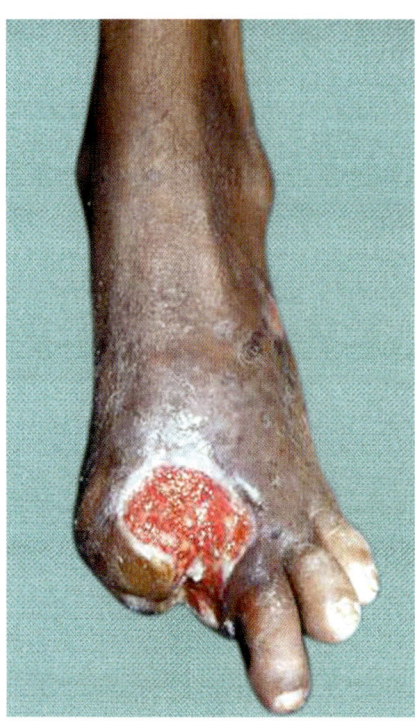

Fig. 3.26: Diabetic ulcer resulted after amputation of great toe and second toe

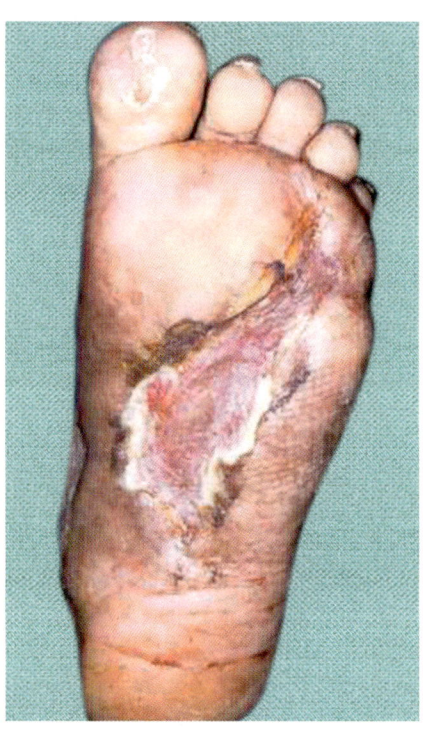

Fig. 3.27: Diabetic ulcer resulted after debridement and now it is healing ulcer

Patient in Fig. 3.28 had sustained trivial injury to the calcaneous region. Diabetic status was uncontrolled. He developed severe infection and sloughing of tendo Achillis tendon and eventually underwent below knee amputation

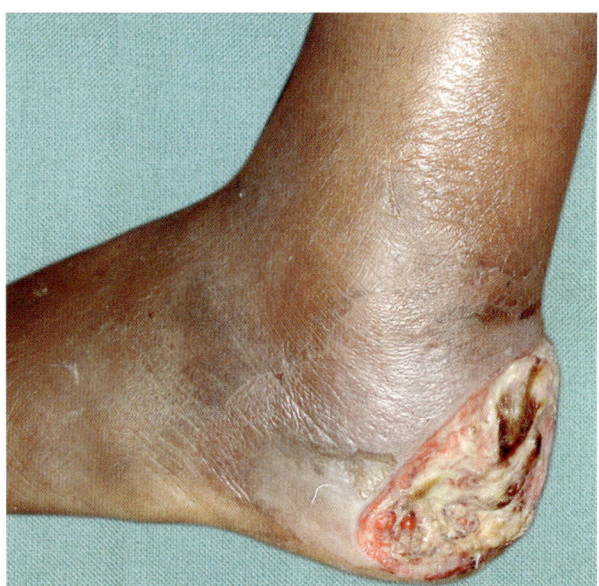

Fig. 3.28: Diabetic ulcer over the calcaneous region with slough

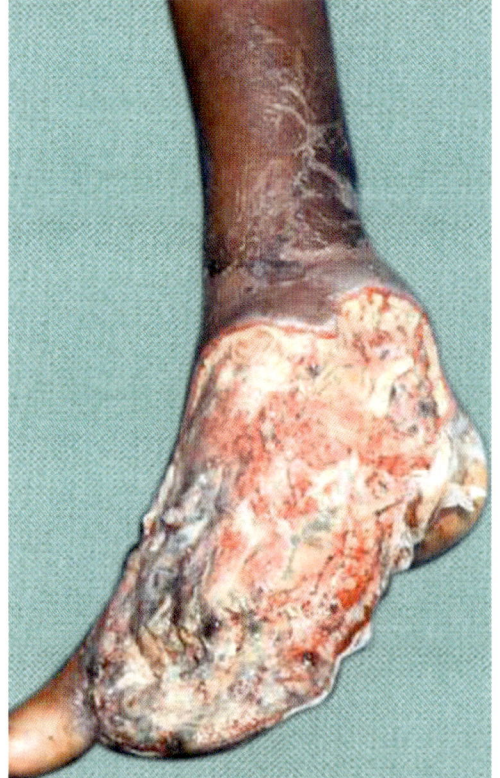
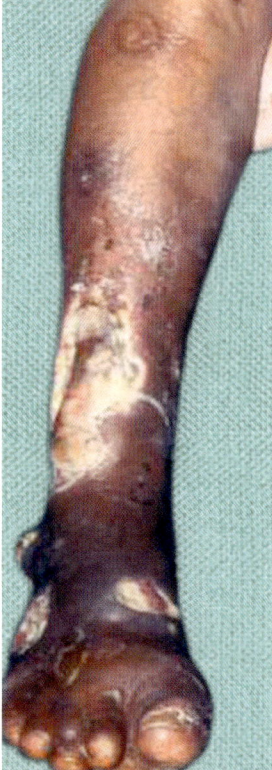

Figs 3.29 and 3.30: Diabetic ulcer with gangrene which is spreading and life-threatening. Such patients will present with ketoacidosis and they require amputation

MALIGNANT ULCER

- Squamous cell carcinoma and malignant melanoma can occur in the limbs.
- Marjolin's ulcer is a type of squamous cell carcinoma arising from scar tissues.
- Melanoma can occur in the sole—acral lentigerous variety *(refer to page 193)* or in the leg as nodule (nodular variety).
- Edges are everted, floor with cancerous tissue (granular tissue).
- May penetrate deeper tissues and thus mobility gets restricted.
- Usually painless unless it is infected or infiltrated.
- Non-healing ulcers.
- Significant lymph nodes in the groin (hard) will clinch the diagnosis.

TROPHIC ULCER

It occurs in tropical countries. The precipitating factors are:

- Malnutrition
- Humid zones
- Poor immunity
- Trauma or insect bite

The infection is caused by Vincent's organisms such as Bacteroides, *B. fusiformis* and *Borrelia vincentii*. It starts as a pustule with extensive inflammation. The pustule bursts and the ulcer spreads rapidly and causes destruction of surrounding tissue. Hence, it is also called **phagedenic ulcer** *(rapidly spreading ulcerative destructive lesion)*. The edges are undermined, floor contains slough, and there is copious seropurulent discharge. Healing is delayed for days to a month. Metronidazole may be quite useful in bringing down the inflammation. Broad spectrum antibiotics may also be required in cases of secondary infections. If healing takes place, it leaves behind a scar.

POST-THROMBOTIC ULCER

It occurs due to deep vein thrombosis (Fig. 3.31). It may affect calf veins or it may be due to femoral vein thrombosis. It is an example of venous ulcer or gravitational ulcer.

Precipitating Factors

- Accidents involving lower leg
- Following childbirth
- After abdominal operation

Clinical Features

- Bursting pain in the limb, extensive induration of the leg or thigh depending upon site of thrombosis.

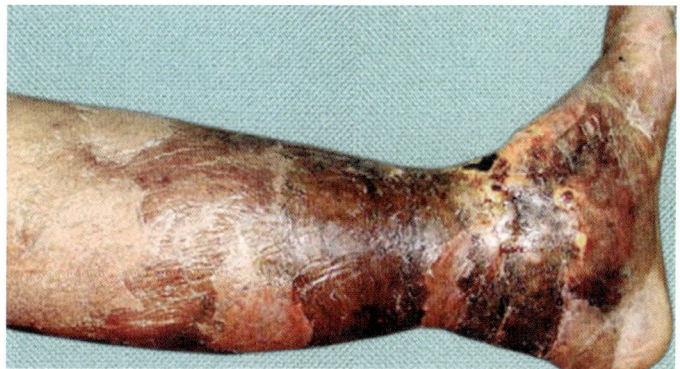

Fig. 3.31: Extensive ulceration of the leg with lipodermato-sclerosis following deep vein thrombosis

- The ulcer is non-healing with scanty granulation tissue.
- The ulcer is deep and always infiltrates deep fascia.
- Due to increased hydrostatic venous pressure, the part is significantly indurated (cyanotic induration) pigmented, thickened with a rise in local temperature.
- The ulcer is not associated with superficial varicosity.
- **Homan's sign** is positive in calf vein thrombosis. It is elicited by forcible dorsiflexion of the foot with the knee extended causing pain in the region of calf.
- **Moses sign:** Squeezing of the calf muscles from side-to-side also produces pain.

  These two signs are positive in acute cases.

Treatment

- Rest and elevation of the leg
- Appropriate antibiotics
- Elastic crepe bandage

With conservative treatment for a few days to a few weeks, veins may get recanalised and the ulcer may heal. The treatment can be very, very difficult *(refer to chapter on varicose veins, page 145).*

MARTORELL'S ULCER

- Affects elderly patients over the age of 50 years.
- Commonly affects hypertensive patients. Hence, the name hypertensive ulcers.
- Atherosclerosis is also a precipitating factor even though all peripheral pulses are usually present.
- It occurs due to sudden obliteration of endarterioles of the skin on the back or outer side of calf region.
- Severe pain, and ischaemic patch of skin which later develops into a deep punched out non-healing ulcer are other clinical features.
- Healing is delayed due to vascular insufficiency.

BAZIN'S ULCERS

- These ulcers exclusively occur in young females and occur in the lower third of leg and ankle region.

- Usually seen in those patients who are obese with thick ankles and abnormal amount of subcutaneous fat.
- These begin with erythematous purplish nodules (hence the name erythrocyanosis frigida) on the calves which later rupture producing non-healing ulcer.
- Aetiology of these ulcers is not clear. It is supposed to be due to ischaemia of lower leg due to spasm of branches of posterior tibial and peroneal arteries. These vessels are abnormally sensitive to hot and cold weather similar to Raynaud's disease. In some cases, tubercle bacilli have been isolated, with ulcers responding to antituberculous treatment.
- These ulcers are managed conservatively.
- Sympathectomy may be beneficial in those patients who are hypersensitive to weather changes.
- Refer to page 181 also.

MADURA FOOT

- It is seen in tropical countries.
- History of trauma is usually present. It might have been forgotten also.
- Multiple nodules which later burst resulting in discharging pus, bony, spicules and red granules are characteristic. In fact, they are all sinuses.
- The limb is deformed and distorted, grossly thickened and swollen but painless unless secondarily infected (Fig. 3.32).

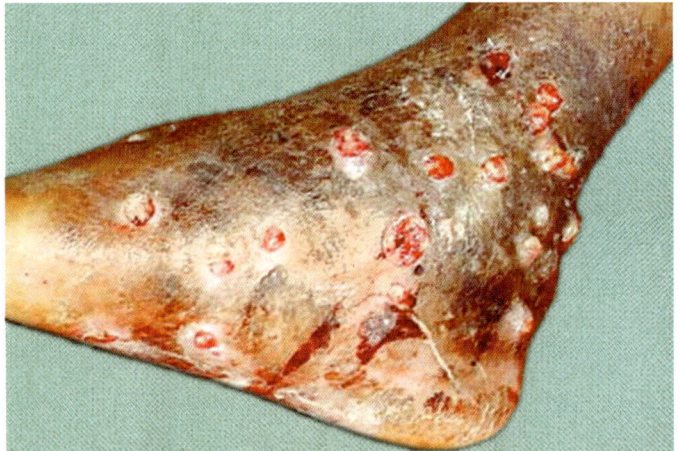

Fig. 3.32: Multiple sinuses with flattened plantar arch—typical of madura foot

PYODERMA GANGRENOSUM

- It is a primarily sterile inflammatory neutrophilic dermatosis. It starts with sterile pustules that rapidly progress and turn into painful ulcers of variable depth. The legs are most commonly affected. Inflammatory bowel disease, rheumatic or haematological disease and malignancy are risk factors.
- Areas rich in subcutaneous fat tissue bear a somewhat higher risk than others. One example is after breast surgery.

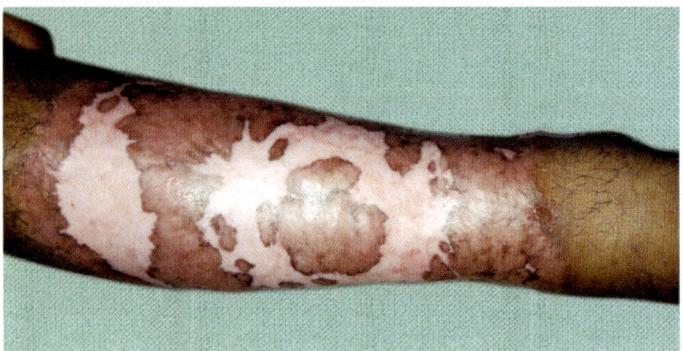

Fig. 3.33: Large ulcer in a patient with ulcerative colitis. He responded well to steroids

- These ulcers are treated by corticosteroids and cyclosporins (Fig. 3.33).

ULCER HEAD AND NECK INCLUDING FACE

History

- How and when did it start? History of trauma— any insect bites or any fall. Ask whether there was any trauma? Trivial trauma may be the precipitating factor for development of ulcers/ gangrene in the upper limb or in patients with occlusive arterial disorders such as TAO. Ulcers can occur spontaneously as in basal cell carcinoma (common site being the face). Sometimes, the patient may tell you that it started as a small nodule which ruptured and then resulted in an ulcer. This can happen in basal cell carcinoma (BCC) and in cutaneous tuberculosis also.
- Before the onset of ulcerations, presence of pain indicates inflammatory pathology such as cellulitis, boil and carbuncle. This history of a painful swelling which ruptures is typical of an abscess rupturing and forming sinus (Clinical Box 3.4).
- How is the progress? Is it becoming big, remaining the same or is it healing? An ulcer which is becoming big or progressive is malignant ulcer. Ulcers which are becoming small are healing ulcers. A non-healing and spreading ulcer can also be tubercular even though it is uncommon. When it occurs on the face, it is called lupus vulgaris. Sometimes, the patient may tell you that he has had the lesion for some time. It heals and ulcerates. This history is classical of basal cell carcinoma. Many of the BCC are extremely slow growing.
- Ask for nature of the discharge. Purulent discharge suggests infection. Serous discharge indicates healing ulcers.

Clinical Examination

- This should follow the same methods mentioned earlier such as inspection and palpation.
- Relevant examination should include oral cavity and lymph node examination.

DIFFERENTIAL DIAGNOSIS

1. Malignant ulcers

- **Basal cell carcinoma (BCC):** The most common malignant ulcer on the exposed white skin is BCC. History can be of a few months to years. Typically, the edge is raised and rolled with pearly white colour. Central ulceration is common. Lymph nodes are not enlarged. When it is pigmented BCC, it is difficult to differentiate from malignant melanoma.

- **Squamous cell carcinoma:** Lip is one of the common sites. Typically, short duration and rapidly growing, edges are everted, induration is present in the base and edge, fixity and lymph node enlargement are other features.

- **Malignant melanoma** with ulceration can present in the face. Pigmentation is classical, induration is minimal and big lymph nodes are palpable. They are mostly firm in consistency. Lentigo maligna melanoma is a slow growing indolent black patch in elderly patients typically in the exposed skin. Ulcerations and nodularity can occur slowly.

• Pigmentation is classical   • Induration is minimal   • Lymph nodes are palpable   • Diagnosis is clinical   • Treatment is surgical   • Early cases potentially curable   • Late cases miserable

Malignant melanoma

2. Tubercular ulcers

- Commonly occur after rupture of the cold abscess (more often presents as sinuses), edges are undermined. Underlying lymph nodes clinch the diagnosis
- Three types of cutaneous tuberculosis have been identified. They are *lupus vulgaris*, TB *verrucosa cutis*, and *scrofuloderma*. TB verrucosa cutis is an indolent warty plaque that occurs after direct inoculation—common in hands (anatomist's warts). Scrofuloderma results from breakdown of skin overlying a tuberculous focus, usually at a lymph node but also at the skin over infected bones or joints. Lupus vulgaris (Fig. 3.34) is a chronic and progressive form of cutaneous TB that occurs in tuberculin-sensitive patients. In most series, it is the most common form of cutaneous TB

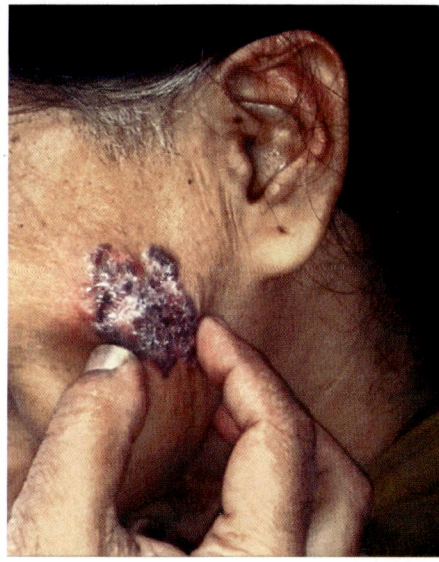

Fig. 3.34: Lupus vulgaris—cutaneous tuberculosis

and has the most variable presentation. Lesions appear in normal skin as a result of direct extension of underlying tuberculous foci, of lymphatic or hematogenous spread. Lesions usually are solitary, and more than 90% involve the head and neck. Small, sharply marginated, red-brown papules of gelatinous consistency (apple-jelly nodules) slowly evolve by peripheral extension and central atrophy into large plaques. Cartilage (nose, ears) within the affected area is progressively destroyed (lupus vorax). **Bone is never involved. (In BCC, SCC and in syphilis, bone is also involved.)**

Caseation necrosis is minimal, and acid-fast bacilli are rare.

3. Infective ulcers

- These will result after suppuration of the lesion which bursts open spontaneously or after surgical drainage (example of carbuncle) resulting in ulcer. They are very tender, edges are oedematous, purulent discharge is present. Movement of the part is greatly restricted and regional lymph nodes are enlarged and tender.
- Syphilitic chancre, gumma, and leishmaniasis are the other rare causes.

4. Benign tumours

Keratoacanthoma: It is a fleshy tumour that occurs on the lips (sun-exposed areas). It starts as a nodule, grows rapidly, ulcerates and mimics malignancy. Central keratin plug which is seen extruding out is characteristic.

ULCER IN THE BACK

Ulcers in the back are different group of problems encountered by surgeons because their aetio-pathogenesis and even management is different. No doubt they are not common but those cases can be short cases. Hence, they are discussed here. Most of them are of infective aetiology. History of pain, fever or toxicity and surgical procedure in the form of drainage or debridement is usually present. Clinical examination should be done like any other ulcer. Leucocytosis, and pus culture sensitivity are the relevant investigations.

Causes

- Carbuncle
- Following necrotising fasciitis
- Following pyomyositis
- Diabetes
- Traumatic

ANALYSIS OF A CASE OF ULCER IN THE BACK AND CLINICAL DISCUSSION (Fig. 3.35)

1. A 37-year-old male shopkeeper with no comorbid illness was admitted with severe backache, inability to move the back and fever of 3 days duration. He was diagnosed to have disc problems and MRI was done. It could not reveal any spine or disc pathology. He was put on traction. After 2 days, skin overlying the back started showing signs of inflammation such as redness. Examination revealed severe tenderness

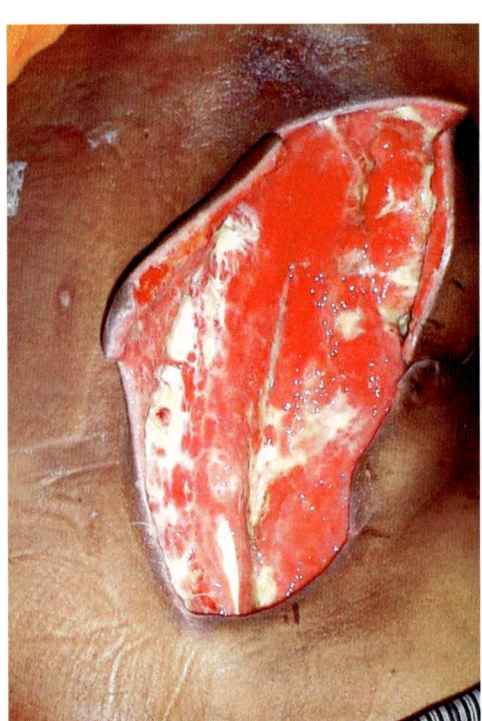

Fig. 3.35: Pyomyositis of the back muscles. The patient presented with high grade fever and renal failure. Photograph taken after debridement and drainage of pus

along the entire erector spinae muscles. Spine was normal. He underwent emergency exploration, 50 ml of pus and necrotic muscles were removed. Histopathology was acute pyomyositis. With regular debridement and dressings, wound started healing and later skin grafting was done.

Clinical Discussion

- Pain and fever indicate inflammatory pathology.
- Admitting orthopaedician did not give importance to fever and treated him for disc prolapse.
- Another good clinician diagnosed the case because of good clinical examination. Tenderness and redness were indicators of pus. Hence, it has been mentioned so often that local rise of temperature and tenderness should be checked first under palpation.
- Common swellings wherein local rise of temperature is present are abscesses including boil and carbuncle, cellulitis, pyomyositis, sarcoma (malignant tumour arising from soft tissues—it is vascular) and aneurysms.
- Once drainage was done, rapid recovery from toxicity took place.
- Why are back muscles involved? Skeletal muscles are rich in iron content which helps organisms to grow.

2. A case of carbuncle of the neck

Case History (Figs 3.36A and B):

- Typically a middle-aged man around fifties, a known diabetic since many years complaining of swelling in the nape of the neck 3–4 days duration and purulent discharge since 1 day duration.
- He also complains of fever since 3–4 days.
- On examination:

Inspection: Multiple openings, and discharging pus are seen in the nape of the neck.

- Swelling can also be visible.
- Other possibility is after treatment of carbuncle, ulcer results.
- On palpation, local rise of temperature and tenderness is present.
- Swelling is indurated and oedematous.
- Skin cannot be pinched out.
- Being an inflammatory swelling, it is not mobile.

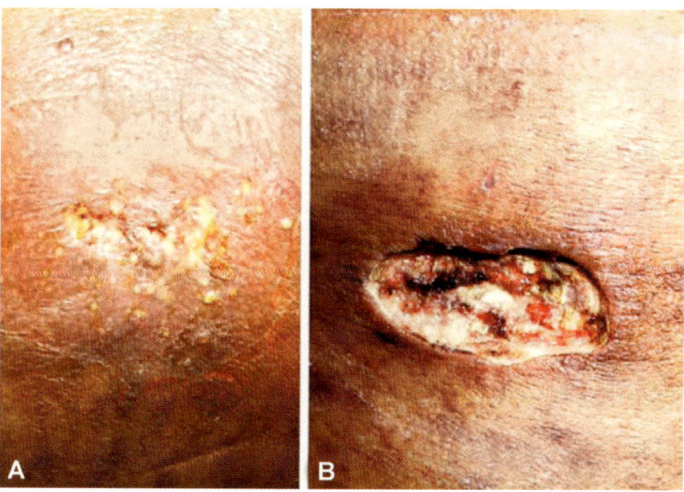

Figs 3.36A and B: Carbuncle of the back and second picture showing an ulcer after excision of the carbuncle

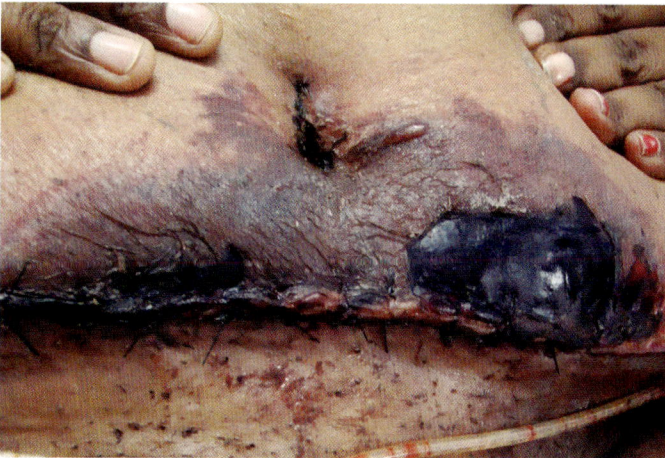

Fig. 3.37: Extensive abdominal wall gangrene—a case of incisional hernia repair—small bowel was injured. Faecal fistula developed which was repaired. Gangrene occurred after two weeks

- Regional lymph nodes such as axillary nodes may be enlarged.

Diagnosis: Carbuncle of nape of the neck—diabetic patient.

Features to say carbuncle
- Diabetic patient
- Nape of the neck
- Tender, red swelling
- Cribriform—multiple sieve-like appearance
- Slough or purulent discharge present.

Treatment
- Control of diabetes
- Excision of the carbuncle

ULCERS IN THE ABDOMINAL WALL

These are also special group of ulcers having a different aetiology. History and clinical examination should be done in the usual manner. Causes being:

1. *Diabetic ulcers:* These may follow after draining abscesses such as boil or carbuncle.

2. *Meleney's ulcer/necrotising fasciitis:* These follow abdominal surgery. It is also called synergistic gangrene (Fig. 3.37). Extensive gangrene of the abdominal wall followed by extensive ulceration can occur. Ulcers are tender, edges are undermined (because of a lot of destruction in the depth) and oedematous with copious discharge.

3. *Malignant ulcer:* Epithelioma (squamous cell carcinoma) can arise in the abdominal wall. Chronic irritation by *Saree* or *Dhothi* and by *Kangri* (earthen pot with hot charcoal applied to abdominal wall) can result in epithelioma. Malignant melanoma—superficial spreading variety commonly occurs in the abdominal wall.

Clinical Wisdom

1. Site-specific history and clinical examination is more relevant. Example: Exposure to venereal diseases is a more relevant question when there is a chancre in the genitalia but not when the ulcer is in the leg or back. Spine examination is more important when there is neuropathic ulcer and not in a venous ulcer.

2. Always after the clinical examination, a re-look into the history and some extra examination may have to be done in some selected patients. Example: Patient had a trophic ulcer foot. Only after the complete examination, re-look into the history revealed that the patient had a myelomeningocoele and it was operated when she was 3 years old.

3. Some examiners do not like to say squamous cell carcinoma because it is a histological diagnosis. Hence, better to say epithelioma.

4. Be thorough about the common leg ulcers such as diabetic ulcers, ischaemic ulcers and venous ulcers.

5. Please do observe how dressings are applied in the wards and find out what treatment and what surgery has been done in your patient. These are commonly asked questions.

6. H_2O_2 and eusol are not used nowadays. They are replaced by many agents.

VIVA FAVOURITE QUESTIONS AND ANSWERS

1. Why is it a healing ulcer?
- Sloping edge—granulation covered with epithelium and so slight bluish in colour
- Red granulation tissue
- Minimal or no discharge
- No oedema in the surrounding skin
- Minimal or no tenderness

2. Why is it a spreading ulcer?
- Edges are not sloping
- Slough in the floor
- Edge is tender
- Oedema present
- Purulent discharge

3. Why is it a callous ulcer?
- Minimal granulation tissue in the floor
- Pale granulation tissue
- Discharge absent or minimal
- Base is indurated
- Edge may be thickened or indurated

4. Why is it an arterial ulcer?
- Typically seen in distal parts of the body: Toes, fingers, etc.
- Tender and deep ulcers
- Floor—pale granulation tissue
- Edge not sloping, tender to touch
- Surrounding area may be cold, tender

5. Why is it a venous ulcer?
- Typically seen in gaiter areas—medial side of leg, lateral side of leg
- Superficial non-tender ulcers
- Sloping edge is seen when it is healing specially with rest to the part
- Floor granulation tissue/slough
- Surrounding area: Thickened, indurated—lipodermatosclerosis

6. Why is it a trophic ulcer?
- Located over the pressure points
- Punched out edges
- Pale granulation tissue present
- Edge and base may be indurated
- No sensations—touch /temperature/tenderness

⌐ Interesting Clinical Case Capsule

A 45 year old male was admitted in view of a trophic ulcer over the sole of his left foot. He had an intervertebral disc prolapse causing cauda equina syndrome in 2011, for which a decompressive laminectomy was done. Following this, he gradually regained power in his lower limbs, but developed a swelling in his lower back, at the operated site. The swelling is mostly asymptomatic but the patient develops a throbbing pain in the head on pressing the swelling.

On examination, a 6 × 4 cm swelling was noted in the midline back over the lower lumbar vertebrae, and the scar of the previous laminectomy was seen over the swelling. The swelling was soft and cystic with fluctuation present. Transillumination was also present. Based on the history and the examination findings, a diagnosis of postoperative pseudomeningocoele was made. This is a documented complication of posterior fossa and intradural spinal surgery and is most often asymptomatic.

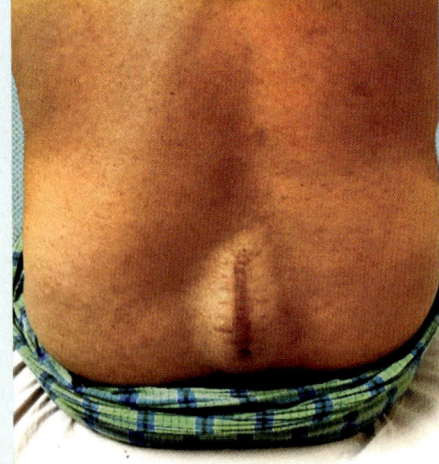

Fig. 3.38: Swelling in the lumbosacral region. You can see the laminectomy scar

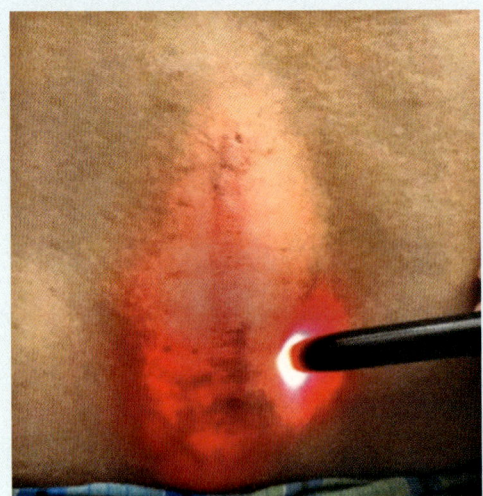

Fig. 3.39: Transillumination is positive

(*Courtesy:* Dr Devesh S Ballal, Dr Aneesh Suwarna, Dr Dinesh BV, Dr P Sampath Kumar, KMC, Manipal)

4

Examination of Swelling

INTRODUCTION

Swellings are common and interesting cases in the clinical examination. Swellings and lumps are commonly used terminology. Let us have some clear idea about these terms. A swelling refers to enlargement or protuberance of an organ or tissue. Example: Thyroid swelling means enlargement of thyroid gland, parotid swelling means enlargement of parotid gland. Lumps refer to a vague mass of body tissue or an irregular small palpable mass. Swelling in the neck, mass in the abdomen and lump in the breast sounds better (it is like telling that the boy is handsome and girl is pretty!) Broadly they are classified into solid swellings, cystic swellings and pulsatile swellings. This will help to sort out the swellings immediately. Cystic swellings are very interesting short cases which can be diagnosed often by history, some by inspection alone and some by palpation and others by auscultation.

Common solid swellings are fat tumours (lipoma), nerve tumours such as neurofibromas, malignant skin tumours, etc.

Have a broad idea about the origin of these swellings. Kindly go through classifications given below before examining these patients.

What is the cause of this swelling?

1. *Is it congenital?* Haemangioma, lymphangioma, dermoid cyst, branchial cyst, myelomeningocoele.

2. *Is it traumatic?* Haematoma, AV fistula

3. *Is it inflammatory?* Boil, carbuncle, chronic abscess

4. *Is it neoplastic?* Soft tissue tumours—lipoma, neurofibroma, malignant tumours such as metastasis in lymph nodes, soft tissue sarcoma.

5. *Is it tuberculous?* Cold abscess

6. *Is it parasitic?* Cysticercosis

If it is a cystic swelling, what is the cause of the cyst?

I. Congenital cyst

- Sequestration dermoid cyst
- Branchial cyst
- Thyroglossal cyst
- Lymphangioma
- Cysts of embryonic remnants: Cyst of urachus, vitellointestinal duct cyst

II. Acquired cyst

- Retention cyst—sebaceous cyst, galactocoele, spermatocoele, Bartholin's gland cyst
- Distension cyst—thyroid cyst, ovarian cyst
- Exudation cyst—hydrocoele
- Degenerative cysts—tumour necrosis
- Traumatic cyst—haematoma, implantation dermoid cyst
- Cystic tumours—cystadenoma of pancreas, cystadenoma of the ovary

III. Parasitic cyst

Cysticercosis, hydatid cyst

PATIENT DATA

They are recorded such as name, age, place, occupation, admitting complaints, etc.

History

1. *Site:* Where is the swelling? In many cases, when the patient points to the site of the swelling, diagnosis can be made out. Here are a few examples:
   - Dorsum of the hand: Ganglion (Fig. 4.1)
   - Outer canthus of the eye: External angular dermoid cyst (Fig. 4.2)
   - Nape of the neck: Carbuncle (Fig. 4.3)
   - In front of the tragus of the ear: Parotid swelling (Fig. 4.4)
   - Flanks: Lipoma (commonest site) (Fig. 4.5).

2. *What is the duration of the swelling?*

   When a patient says, 'I have a swelling', it is but natural to ask the duration—'When did you notice

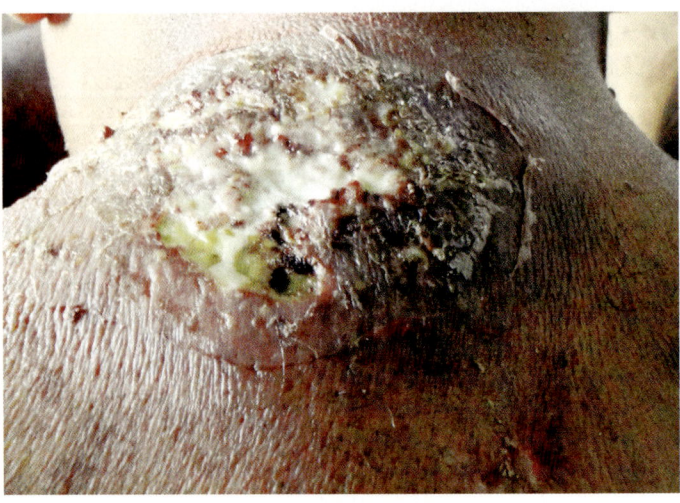

Fig. 4.3: Carbuncle

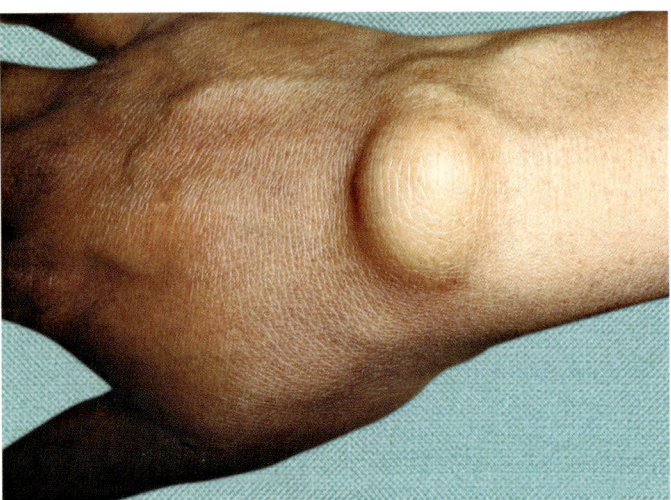

Fig. 4.1: Ganglion on the dorsum of the hand—common site

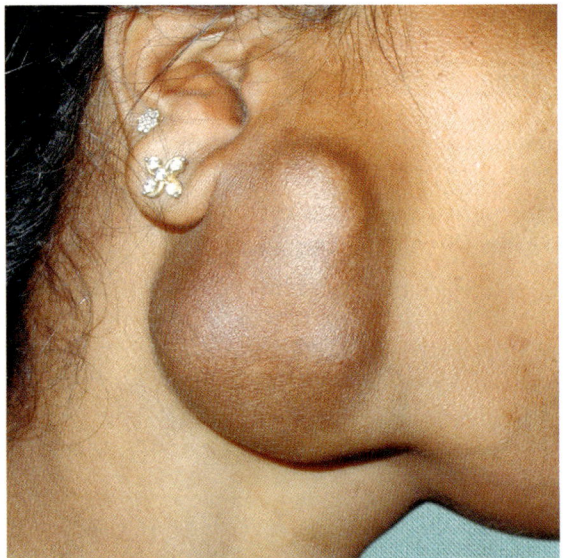

Fig. 4.4: Mixed tumour of parotid

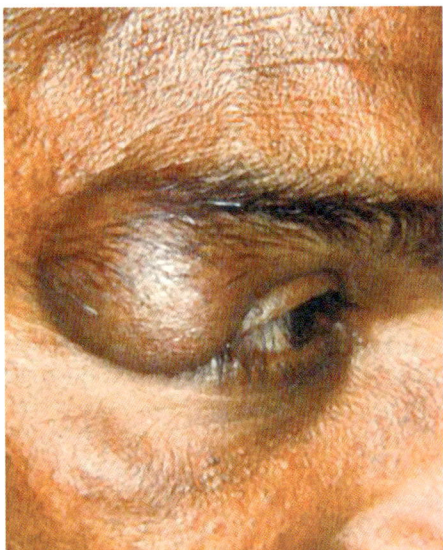

Fig. 4.2: External angular dermoid cyst—look for bony depression—it is pathognomonic of this swelling

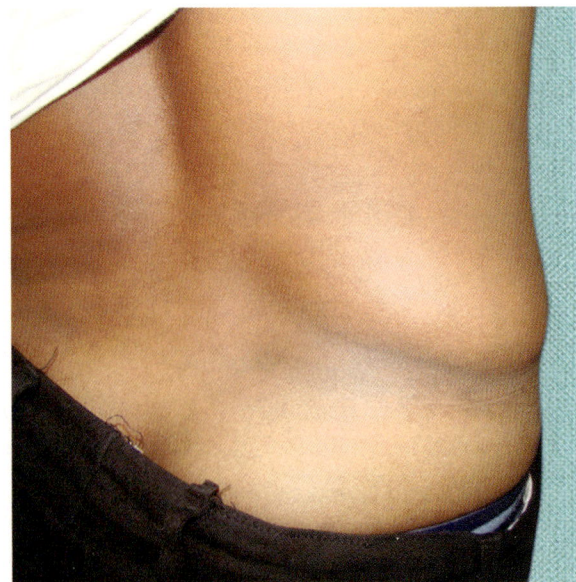

Fig. 4.5: Lipoma in the flank—commonest site of lipoma

this swelling first'? Some swellings are present since birth, some may have long duration and some may have short duration. Examples are given below.

I. Since birth

- Meningocoele (Fig. 4.6)
- Lymphangioma—cystic hygroma (Fig. 4.7)
- Dermoid cysts and branchial cysts. Very often they present in late teens.
- Haemangioma
- Hamartomatous lesions

II. Present since a few years

- Congenital: Branchial cyst
- Benign tumours: Lipoma, neurofibroma, dermoid cysts, sebaceous cysts

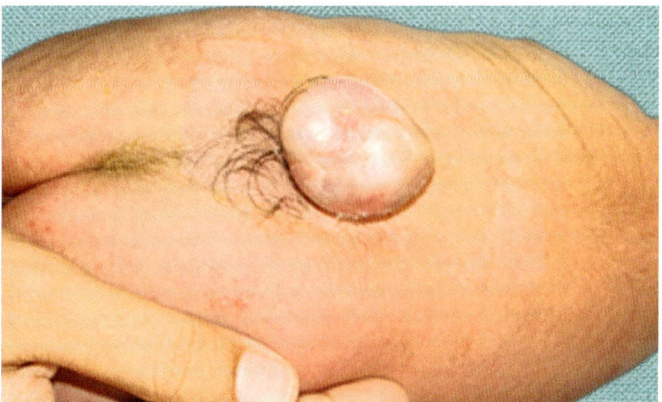

Fig. 4.6: Meningocoele

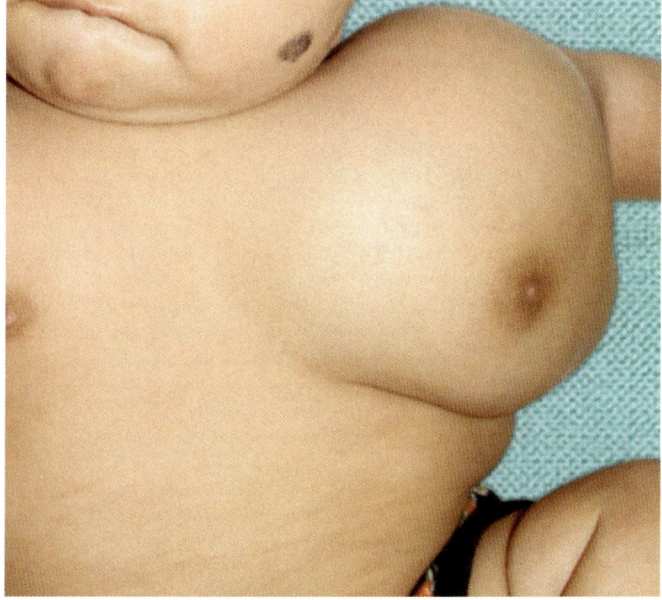

Fig. 4.7: Lymphangioma involving chest wall—brilliantly transilluminant swelling

III. Present since a few months

- With pain, short duration—inflammatory—carbuncle
- Without pain, short duration—malignant—soft tissue sarcoma

3. **Mode of onset:** How did the swelling start?

Insidious onset: When patient says he cannot recollect any special time or occasion, it is insidious in onset. Often thyroid swellings, benign tumours, and malignant tumours present as insidious in onset. During routine course of bathing, the patient might have noticed the swelling such as lipoma or neurofibroma. Very often others point out at thyroid swellings.

After trauma: Did you have any trauma? Fractures, dislocations and haematoma appear after trauma. Implantation dermoid cyst develops in the palms, fingers, sole and toes after sharp injury. Traumatic AV fistula develops after trauma. Keloids and hypertrophic scars develop over vaccination sites.

After any sting/bites: Snake bites, scorpion bites or sting bites are common in India. Resultant swelling is cellulitis which progresses later to an abscess.

With fever: Any swelling which appears along with fever is an inflammatory swelling such as pyogenic abscess (common in diabetics), boil or carbuncle.

4. **Do you have fever?** Fever and swelling together (Clinical Box 4.1) suggest inflammatory pathology. Fever since many days and recent swelling may suggest tuberculosis of lymph nodes. Lymph node swellings in the neck with fever can also be found in Hodgkin's lymphoma.

5. **Do you have pain?** Pain and swelling of short duration suggest inflammatory swellings. Causes have been mentioned below.

Nature of the pain

- Dull aching pain: Stretching of the capsule
- Throbbing pain: Abscess

Clinical Box 4.1

Swelling and fever together
- Boil—abscess
- Carbuncle
- Cellulitis, lymphangitis

Abdominal swelling (mass) and fever together
- Hepatoma
- Renal cell carcinoma
- Lymphoma

- Referred pain: Patients with parotid swellings may complain of itching or discomfort in the ear.
- *Swelling first and pain later* indicates following situations:
    a. *Infection in a sebaceous cyst*—secondary infection
    b. *Infection in a branchial cyst*—secondary infection
    c. Benign tumour transforming into malignant tumour—lipoma into liposarcoma
    d. Malignancy infiltrating nerves or bones.

Patients with osteosarcoma can have pain for a few days followed later by swelling of the bone.

6. *How is the progress of the swelling?* Is it rapidly growing, slow growing or stationary?

- *Rapid growth* in 1–2 months is suggestive of malignancies such as soft tissue sarcoma (Fig. 4.8).
- *Rapid growth within 5–10 days* is not from malignancy but from inflammatory swellings. It is interesting to note that phyllodes tumour of the breast grows more rapidly within 5–10 days to attain a size which will be much more than malignancy of the breast
- *Slow growing for many years:* 5–10 years are typically seen in lipoma, thyroid swellings and parotid swellings.

- *Slow growth and remain static:* Some lipomas, neural tumours may exhibit this property.
- **Slow growth for many years and recent rapid growth indicates malignant transformation of a benign lesion. A few examples are given below.**
    a. *Lipoma*—liposarcoma
    b. *Neurofibroma*—neurofibrosarcoma
    c. *Multinodular goitre (thyroid swelling)*—carcinoma thyroid

7. *Has the swelling regressed in size?*

- Inflammatory swellings will regress in size with treatment as happens in breast abscess or mastitis.
- Deeply situated abscess in the thigh may mimic sarcoma but diminishing size is a strong indication of inflammatory pathology.

8. *Any other symptoms associated with swelling?*

- Discomfort or tingling on pressure: Neurofibroma
- Recurrent bleeding after minor trauma: Haemangioma
- Whitish discharge—non-foul odour: Cold abscess (Fig. 4.9)
- Whitish discharge with foul odour: Sebaceous cyst (Fig. 4.10)

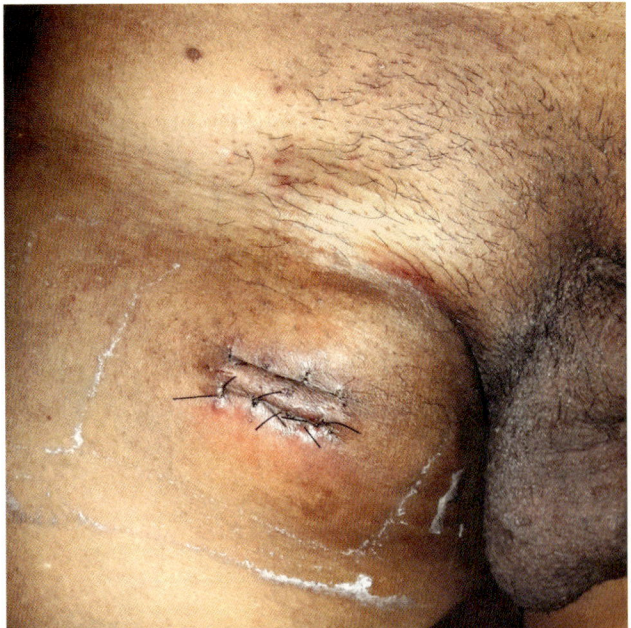

Fig. 4.8: High grade malignant fibrous histiocytoma arising from thigh muscles. You can see the incision biopsy mark

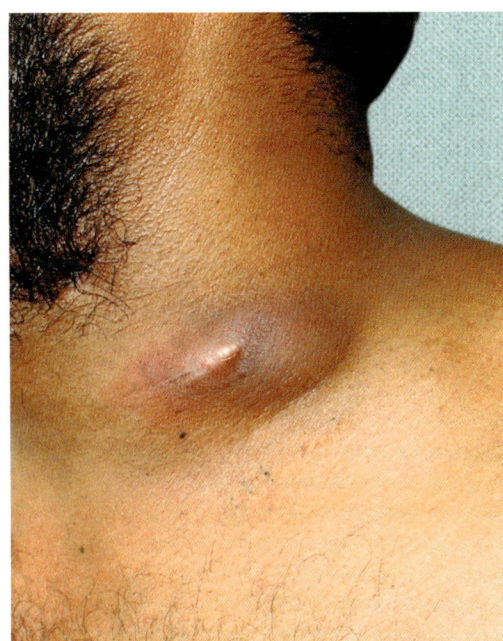

Fig. 4.9: Tuberculous cold abscess with sinus in the posterior triangle of the neck

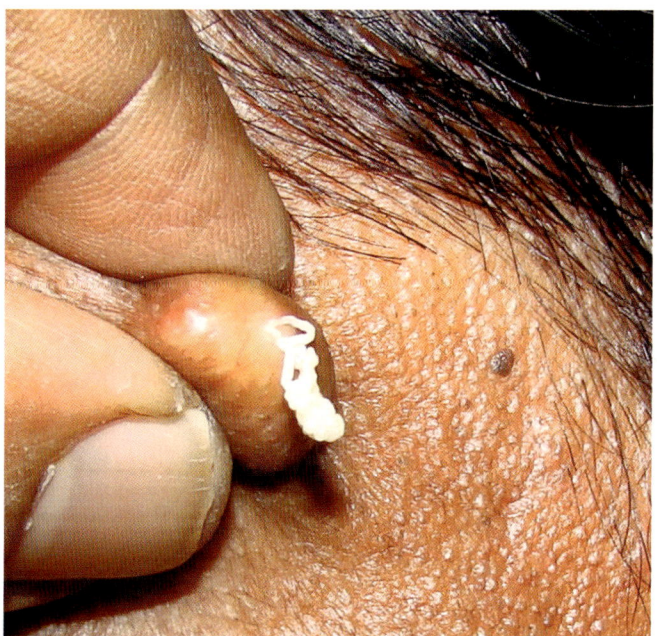

Fig. 4.10: Discharge from cyst-paste like

9. *Any other similar swellings elsewhere in the body?*

  • If present, they indicate multiple lipomatosis (Fig. 4.11) or multiple neurofibromatosis (Fig. 4.12).

  • Multiple lymph node swellings in multiple sites are typical of lymphoma.

  • Sudden appearance of multiple cutaneous nodules may indicate metastasis or non-Hodgkin's lymphoma (NHL, T cell/B cell) (Fig. 4.13).

10. *Any changes in the swelling?*

  Skin ulceration, and fungation are typical of malignancy infiltrating the skin.

11. *Has the swelling recurred after surgery?*

  • Benign tumours will not recur, if they are completely excised; but if they are not removed properly or completely, they may recur. Example being sebaceous cyst. If a part of the sebaceous cyst wall is left behind, it will recur not

Clinical Box 4.2

Benign swellings which recur
1. Desmoid tumour
2. Adamantinoma (Jaw tumour)
3. Keloid
4. Fibromatosis
5. Pleomorphic adenoma (after enucleation)

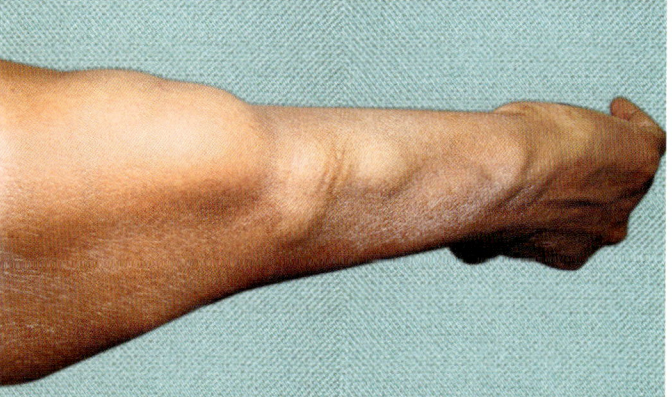

Fig. 4.11: Multiple lipomas—being subcutaneous in location, they become **prominent on contraction of muscles**

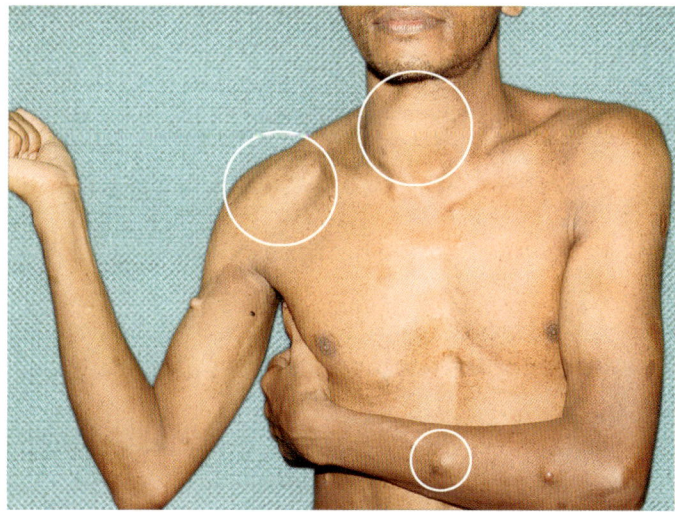

Fig. 4.12: Case of von Recklinghausen's disease with multiple nodules, pigmentation and schwannoma of vagus nerve (*Courtesy:* Dr Siddarth Bhandary, ex Professor, Department of Surgery, KMC, Manipal)

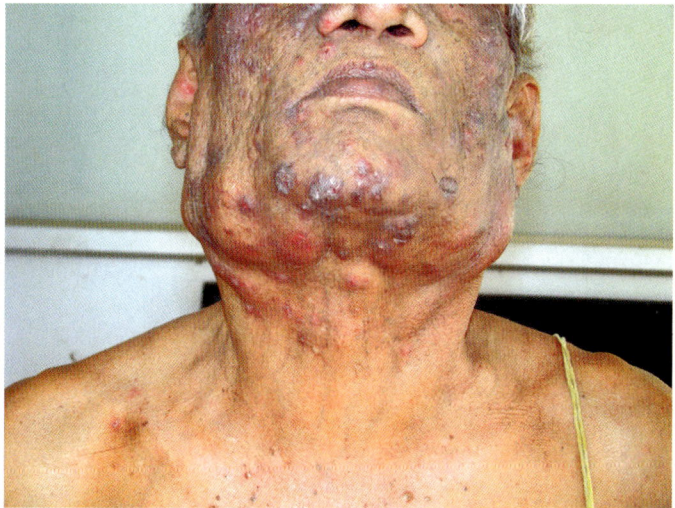

Fig. 4.13: NHL mycosis fungoides—'B' cell type

immediately—many months or years later. A few benign tumours have the property to recur. They are desmoid tumours, keloid and pleomorphic adenoma, if it is enucleated.

- Recurrence is the nature of malignant tumours even when they are removed with wide excision. Classical example being soft tissue sarcomas.

  Past history, personal history and relevant family history should be asked for.

LOCAL REGIONAL EXAMINATION

Inspection

Students should resist the temptation of palpating the swelling as soon as they see the swelling. Careful observation will help you arrive at the diagnosis in many cases.

Surgery short cases are so site-specific that you can often diagnose by first look at the swelling.

Location

- Thyroglossal cyst—midline, young, subhyoid (Fig. 4.14).
- Dermoid cysts occur in the line of fusion such as in the outer canthus of the eye, midline, etc. (Fig. 4.15).
- Most common site of ganglion is dorsum of the hand over scapholunate articulation (Fig. 4.16).
- Plexiform neurofibroma classically occurs over the distribution of ophthalmic division of trigeminal nerve.

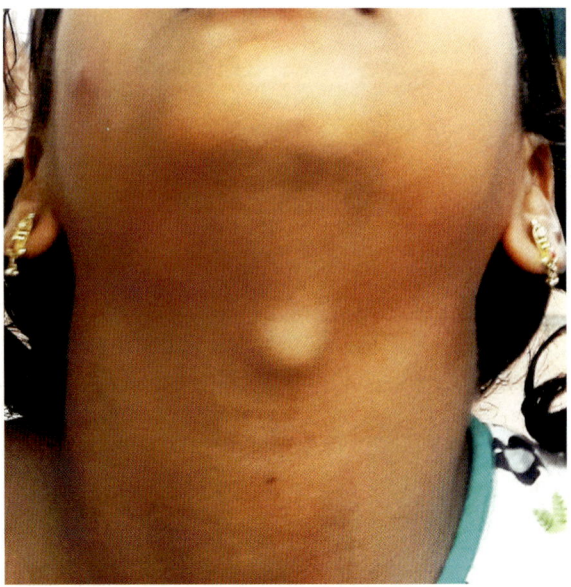

Fig. 4.14: Thyroglossal cyst

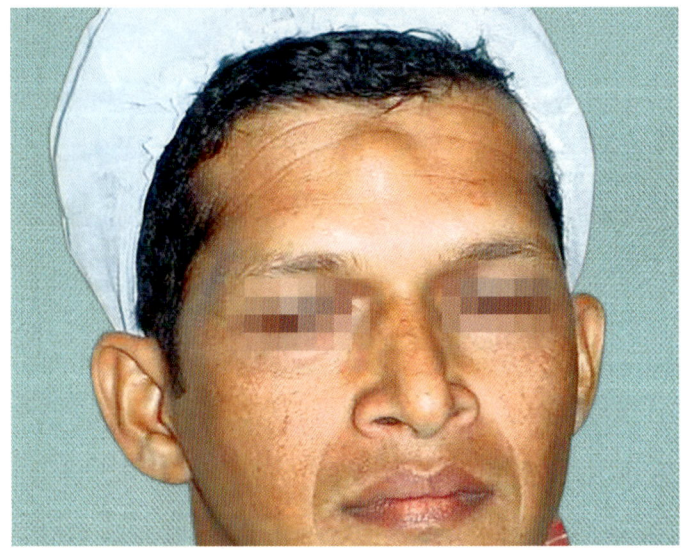

Fig. 4.15: Midline frontal dermoid cyst

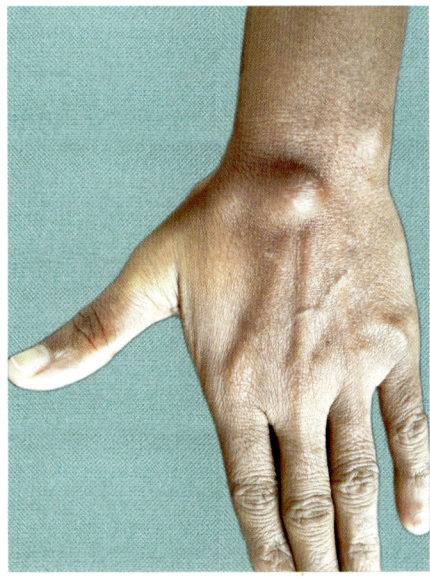

Fig. 4.16: Ganglion

- Classical location of branchial cyst—half in front and half behind the sternocleidomastoid is unremarkable.
- Typical site of the carbuncle is nape of the neck.

Number

- *A few swellings can be multiple such as*
  1. Sebaceous cysts in the scrotum, scalp or back (Fig. 4.17)
  2. Multiple lipomatosis
  3. Multiple neurofibromatosis
  4. Lymph node swellings as in lymphoma, tuberculosis, and infectious mononucleosis

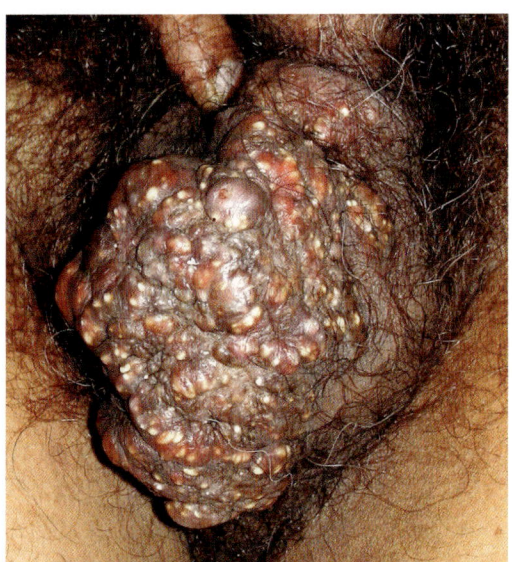

Fig. 4.17: Multiple sebaceous cysts on the scrotum—one of the common sites

5. Multiple abscesses in diabetic patients—they are very tender.
6. Metastatic deposits in the skin.

Extent, Size and Shape

- Describe the extent of the swelling (extending from where to where) in both transverse and vertical directions. Whenever possible describe in relationship to bony landmark.
- When you describe size, use the word approximately measuring about 3 cm or 4 cm, etc.
- A few swellings have some characteristic shapes.

  Examples

  1. *Sebaceous cyst:* Hemispherical
  2. *Thyroglossal cyst:* Vertically placed oval swelling
  3. *Subhyoid bursitis:* Horizontally placed oval swelling
  4. *Dermoid cysts*: Spherical or oval
  5. Epithelioma or squamous cell carcinoma (*cauliflower like*)

Surface

- *Smooth:* Branchial cyst, dermoid cyst—majority of cystic swellings have smooth surface and round borders.
- *Irregular:* In cases of malignant tumours
- *Nodular:* Multinodular goitre has classically nodular surface
- *Bossellated*: Large nodules (Clinical Box 4.3).

Edge: Edge or the margin is the outer limit of the swelling. It can be distinct and round as in thyroglossal cyst or irregular as in malignancies or indistinct (not well defined) as in inflammatory swellings.

Edge or margin cannot be felt clearly when the swelling arises from deeper structures.

Skin Over the Swelling

- *Erythematous:* Inflammatory swellings such as boil, carbuncle, and abscess.
- *Red shiny:* Soft tissue sarcoma.
- *Pigmentation:* May be present over the skin of neurofibroma. It is brownish in colour (Fig. 4.18).
- Blackish pigmentation is suggestive of mole or naevus.
- *Dilated veins:* Suggest increased vascularity as in soft tissue sarcoma (Fig. 4.19).
- Bluish colour, and port-wine colour may indicate haemangioma.
- *Blackish spot*: **Punctum is pathognomonic of epidermoid cyst** (sebaceous cyst) (Fig. 4.20).

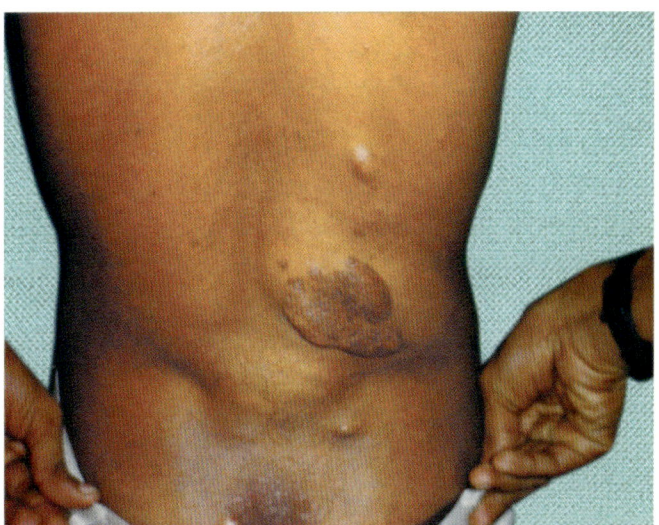

Fig. 4.18: The *café au lait* spots. More than five such spots will appear by early life (*Courtesy:* Dr Prashanth Shetty, Ex-Professor, KMC, Manipal)

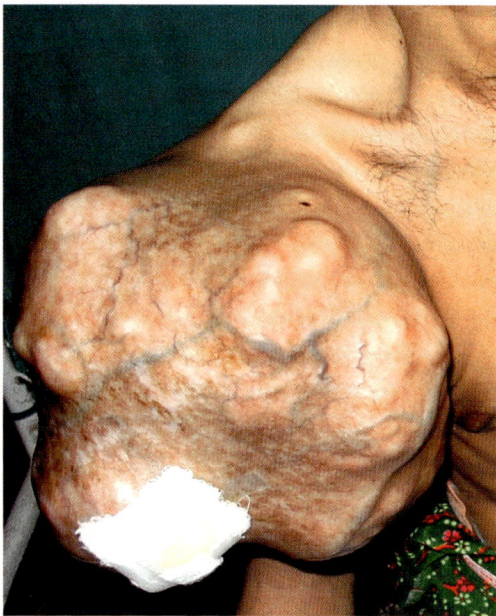

Fig. 4.19: Dilated veins—chondrosarcoma

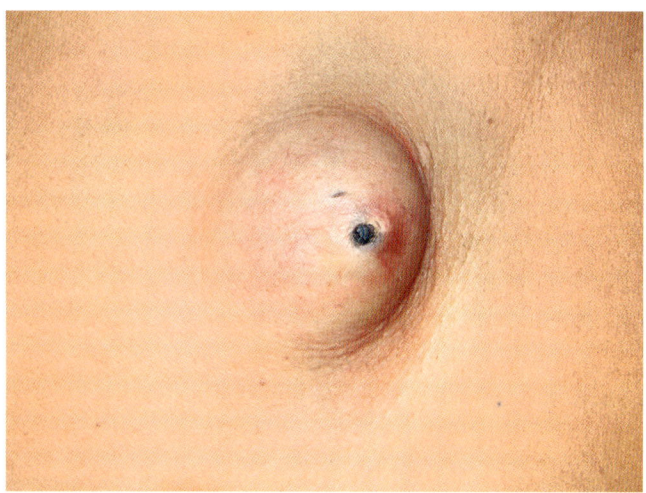

Fig. 4.20: Sebaceous punctum is diagnostic of sebaceous cyst

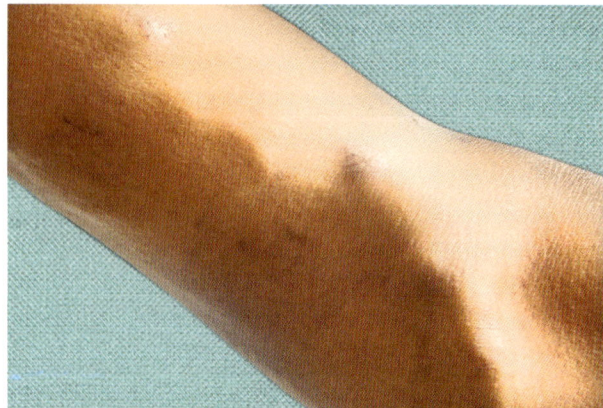

Fig. 4.21: Most common type of AV fistula you see today is in the nephrology ward—created to facilitate haemodialysis

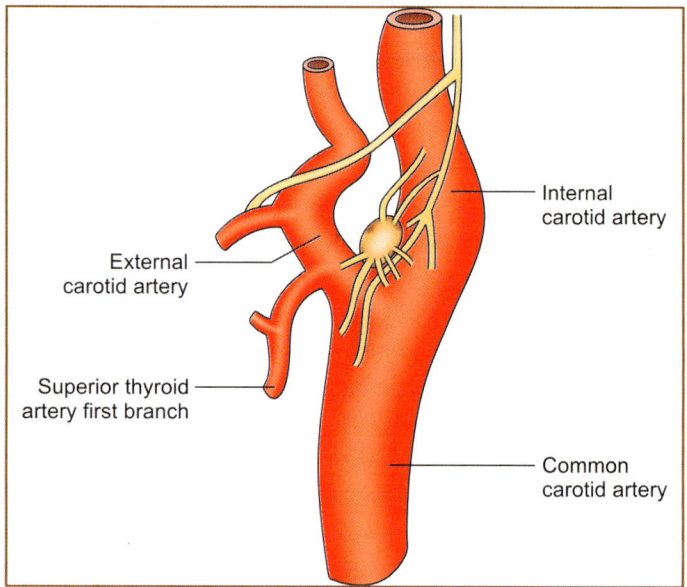

Fig. 4.22: Location of carotid body

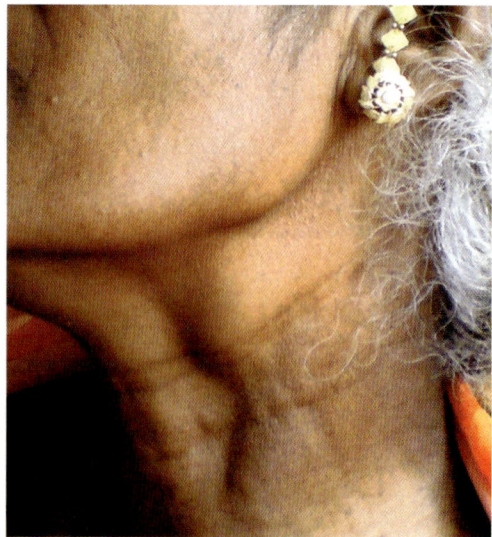

Fig. 4.23: 65-year-old lady with carotid body tumour. (*Courtesy*: Dr. Srivatsa, Dr. Bagali Baba Saheb, Prof. Bharathi, Dr Srikar Pai, MS Ramaiah Medical College, Bengaluru)

Pulsations

- *Aneurysm:* Will exhibit expansile pulsations—popliteal aneurysm in popliteal fossa, carotid aneurysm in the carotid triangle, and innominate aneurysm in suprasternal space of Burns. Please remember these 3 sites are also the sites of an abscess. Hence, carefully examine these areas and rule out pulsations and reconfirm before incising swellings in these locations.

- *AV fistula:* Most often you will see this in nephrology ward (fistula done for renal failure for dialysis (Fig. 4.21).

- *Pulsating tumour* in the neck is carotid body tumour (Figs 4.22 and 4.23).

Movement with Deglutition

This should be checked only when swelling is in the midline or anterior triangle of the neck. Swellings which are attached to or fixed to trachea or larynx move with deglutition. (More details are given in thyroid chapter.) Following are swellings which move with deglutition:

- Thyroid swellings (Fig. 4.24).
- Thyroglossal cyst
- Subhyoid bursitis
- Pretracheal and prelaryngeal lymph nodes.

Movement on Protrusion of the Tongue

This test also should be checked only when swelling is in the midline of the neck. Thyroglossal cyst classically moves on protrusion of the tongue (refer to page 255 for more details).

Pressure Effects

Pressure effects are common due to a swelling or due to lymph nodes which get enlarged in cases of malignant tumour. A few examples are given below.

- *Lymph node mass* in the neck can give rise to paralysis of nerves—hypoglossal nerve paralysis, cervical sympathetic chain involvement (Horner's syndrome, page 14, Fig. 1.23).
- *Soft tissue sarcoma* in the arm can give rise to radial nerve paralysis.
- *Swelling* can also compress a vein resulting in distal oedema and secondary varicosity (Fig. 4.25).

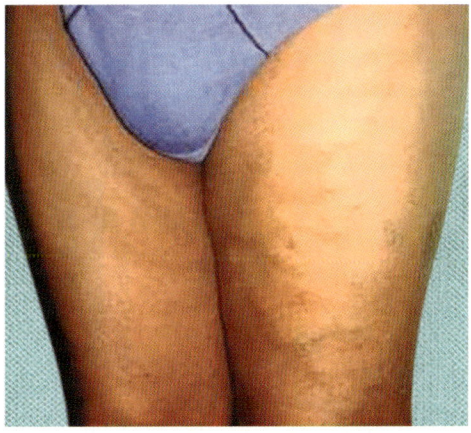

Fig. 4.25: Secondary varicosity thigh due to a pelvic tumour (*Courtesy*: Dr Prashanth Tubachi, Associate Professor, S.D.M. Medical College, Dharwar, Karnataka)

- *Femoral artery aneurysm* can compress the femoral vein and can give rise to tortuous veins in the thigh.
- *Popliteal aneurysm* can give rise to foot drop.

Surrounding Area

Mention if any abnormality is found such as pigmentation in neurofibroma or oedema in inflammatory swellings, etc.

Palpation

1. *Local rise of temperature* and tenderness should be checked first under palpation. Inflammatory swellings such as abscess will exhibit these signs—not found in cold abscess.

   Local rise of temperature is appreciated better with dorsum of the hand. It is more sensitive than palmar surface because of many cutaneous nerve endings and the skin is thinner (Fig. 4.26).

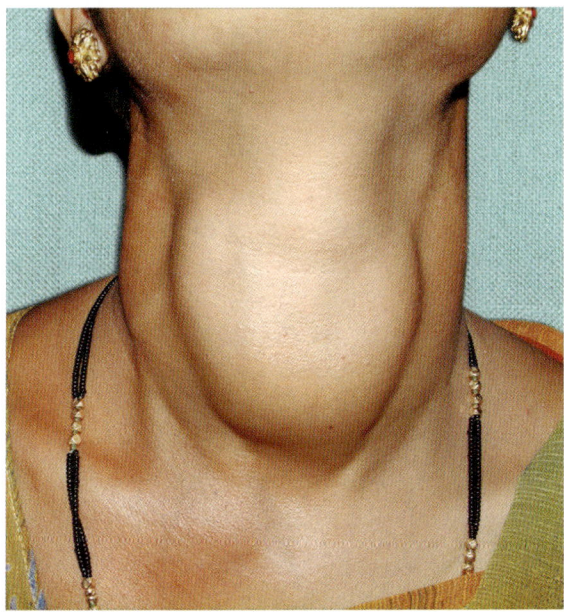

Fig. 4.24: Typical thyroid swelling

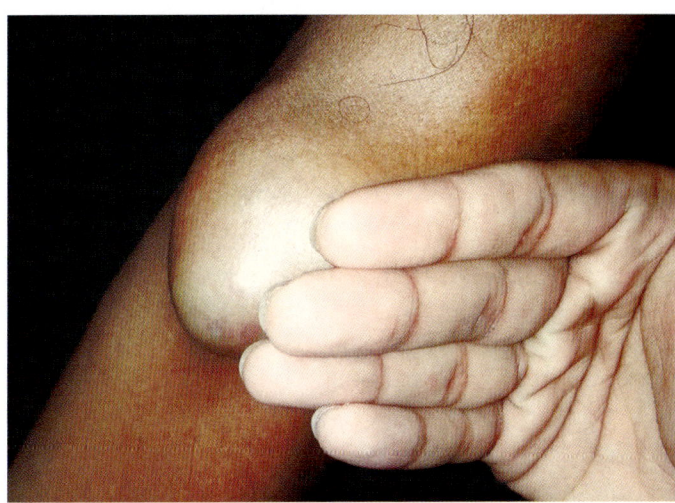

Fig. 4.26: Testing local rise of temperature

2. *Size and shape* have to be mentioned.

3. Again confirm **surface** and borders during palpation—smooth, irregular or nodular.

4. *Borders/edge*

- Round and distinct in benign swellings such as branchial cyst, thyroglossal cyst, neurofibroma.

- Edge slips under palpating fingers in a case of lipoma. This is pathognomonic sign of lipoma and is called slip sign (Fig. 4.27).

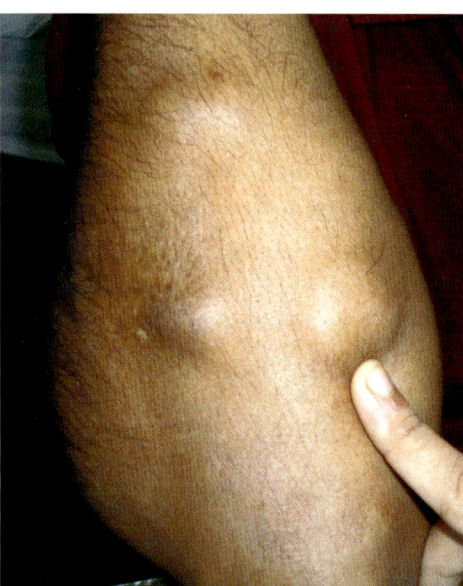

Fig. 4.27: Lipoma—slip sign is present. Also note multiple lipomas

5. *Consistency*

- *Soft:* Lipoma, cystic swellings are soft.

- *Firm* in cases of lymph node swellings, neurofibroma.

- *Hard* in metastatic nodes, bony swellings such as cervical rib and malignant swellings. A malignant swelling is not only hard but also indurated. Induration means hardness due to desmoplastic reaction caused by the tumour.

- A hard thyroid nodule can be malignant.

- *Putty consistency:* This is specially described for sebaceous cysts. These have sebum as content. Hence, these have consistency of toothpaste. Thus, change in the shape (sign of moulding) and sign of indentation are positive (Figs 4.28 and 4.29).

- *Variable:* Sometimes, swelling may have variable consistency such as a few areas are hard and few areas may be soft or firm. You should be able to explain why there is variable consistency.

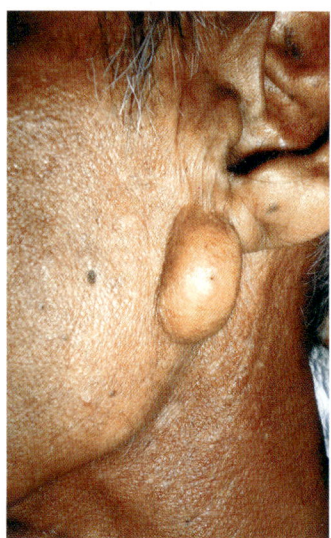

Fig. 4.28: Sebaceous cyst—sign of moulding—hemispherical cyst moulded into oval shape

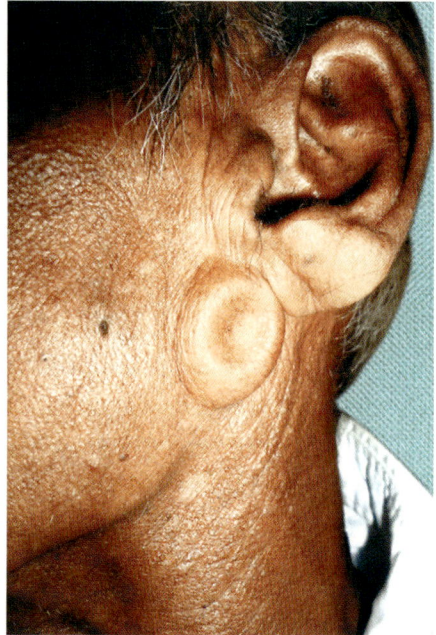

Fig. 4.29: Sebaceous cyst—sign of indentation

Example is given below: A large multinodular goitre may have areas which are hard—could be due to malignant changes or due to calcification and a few areas which are soft due to degeneration of the nodule. Variable consistency is also a feature of sarcomas when these grow rapidly because of tumour degeneration or tumour necrosis.

- *Rubbery consistency:* It has been mentioned for lymph nodes in Hodgkin's lymphoma.

6. *Fluctuation:* It should be done only when swelling is soft—to find out whether swelling contains fluid or not. Following are a few rules of fluctuation test:

- It should be done when the swelling is soft.

- Mobile swelling has to be fixed—first fix the swelling.

- Index and thumb from both hands are used. Press the swelling with the index finger (active finger) and the thumb will be raised (passive finger).

- Fluctuation should be elicited in both directions because muscles of the thigh can be fluctuant in the horizontal direction but not vertically (in the line of fibres) (Fig. 4.30).

- When the swelling is small—less than 2 cm, **Paget's test** is done. Use the index finger and press in the centre of the swelling. If it is soft, it is a cyst. Cystic swellings will feel soft in the centre and firm at the periphery, and solid swelling *vice versa* (Fig. 4.31).

Clinical Wisdom

- Tensely cystic swellings in the neck, breast and deeper planes (thigh) may feel firm but careful examination may reveal they yield and fluctuation may be positive.
- Do not try to elicit fluctuation for intra-abdominal cystic swellings.
- Lipoma does give rise to fluctuation even though it is a solid tumour because fat at body temperature behaves like fluid. Hence surgeons describe it as pseudofluctuant.
- Do not say sebaceous cyst is fluctuant even though it is a cyst, it yields and moulds but will not show fluctuation.
- If the swelling is hard, do not mention fluctuation and transillumination test.
- If you are wrong in eliciting and interpreting fluctuation test, entire sequence of the remaining tests and diagnosis will be wrong. Hence, do this test carefully.

7. *Transillumination test*: Swellings having clear fluid will transilluminate but those with blood (haemorrhage or haematoma) or pus (abscess) or thick contents such as cold abscess (tuberculous) will not (Fig. 4.32).

- This test should be done in a dark room.

- Pen torch is used to illuminate the swelling in one corner and look at the other side with illuminoscope (an X-ray sheet is rolled in) and observe whether the light is seen or not.

- Avoid surface transillumination.

- If the transillumination is positive, it is a cyst with clear fluid inside. Following are differential diagnosis:

  A. *Cystic hygroma:* Sites are neck, axilla and groin because lots of lymphatic tissues are present in these areas.

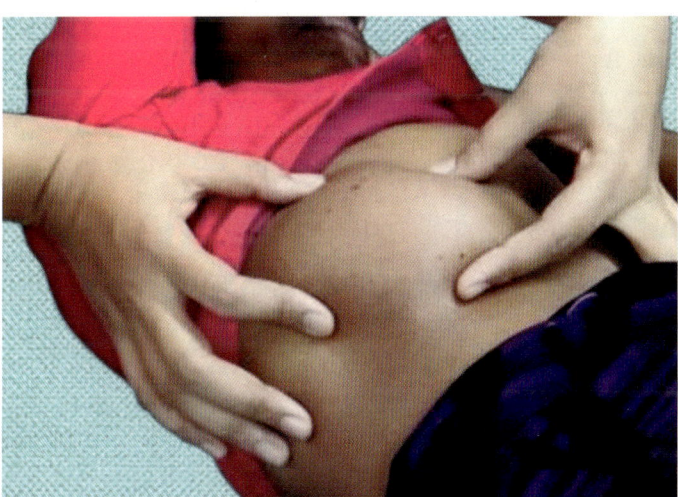

Fig. 4.30: Lipoma right side of chest

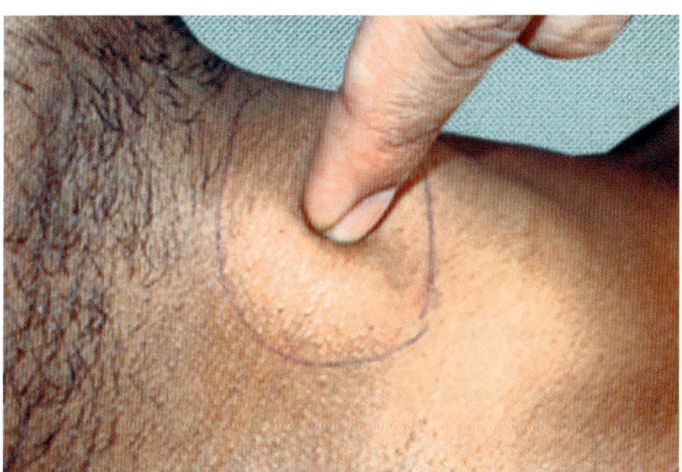

Fig. 4.31: Paget's test

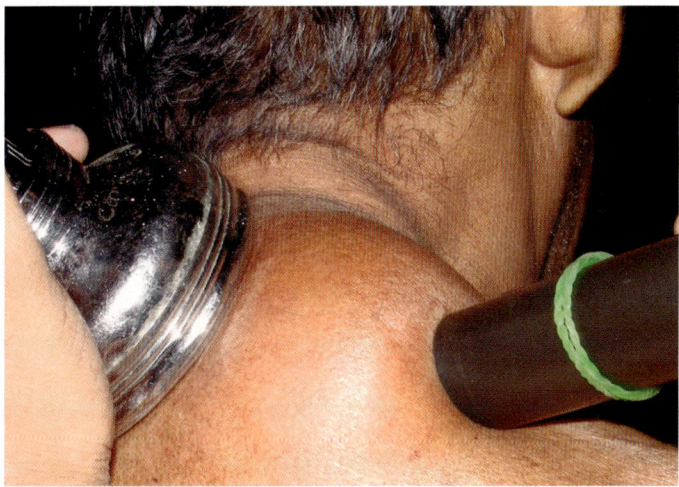

Fig. 4.32: Transillumination test

B. *Vaginal hydrocoele:* Scrotal swelling.

C. *Epididymal cyst:* Scrotal swelling behind the testis.

D. *Ranula:* Swelling in the floor of the mouth.

E. *Meningocoele:* Lumbosacral region.

Very rarely lipoma and thyroglossal cyst may exhibit transillumination (just know this, do not mention).

8. *Intrinsic mobility*

- Hold the swelling and gently move in horizontal and vertical directions. Majority of the subcutaneous swellings—dermoid cysts, neurofibromas, lipoma, etc. have free mobility (Fig. 4.33).

- **Restricted mobility is one of the early features of malignant tumours such as soft tissue sarcoma.**

- Also deep seated (deep to deep fascia or deep to muscles) benign tumours also may exhibit restricted mobility, especially when muscles are contracted.

- Bony swellings are unmistakably immobile. Example: Chondroma, cervical rib and metastasis in bones.

- Lipoma slips under palpating finger (slip sign)

Almost all the cystic swellings in the skin, subcutaneous tissue or in the deeper plane are benign and as a rule, these should have free mobility.

However, this is not true due to various anatomical factors.

- *Branchial cyst:* Restricted mobility is due to its **adherence to the sternomastoid muscle.**

- *Thyroglossal cyst:* Transverse mobility is absent because the cyst is **tethered by remnant of the thyroglossal duct.**

- *Sebaceous cyst:* Limited mobility due to the **adherence to the skin at the summit.**

9. *Sign of compressibility:* The swellings which have communication with tissue spaces or cavity give the positive sign of compressibility. Thus, a steady pressure is applied over the swelling. The swelling may disappear completely or may partially disappear. However, when pressure is released the swelling fills up slowly. Hence, it is also called the 'sign of refilling' (Fig. 4.34).

Examples are cavernous haemangioma, lymphangiomas, meningocoele, and empyema necessitans.

10. *Sign of reducibility:* We say hernias are reducible—it reduces into peritoneal cavity means these have been displaced into a different area. It requires coughing or straining for it to reappear. Whereas, compressible swellings reappear when compression is released.

11. *Pulsations:* Pulsations over the swelling are found in vascular swellings. These are of two types.

- *Expansile:* Aneurysms are characterised by expansile pulsations. When two fingers are placed over the swelling on the sides, the fingers are not only elevated but are also separated. Popliteal aneurysms typically give this sign (Figs 4.35 and 4.36).

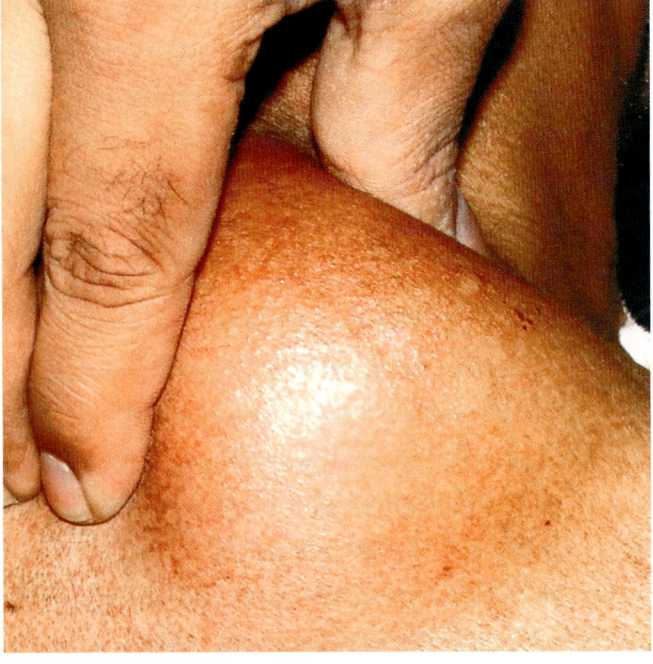

Fig. 4.33: Intrinsic mobility

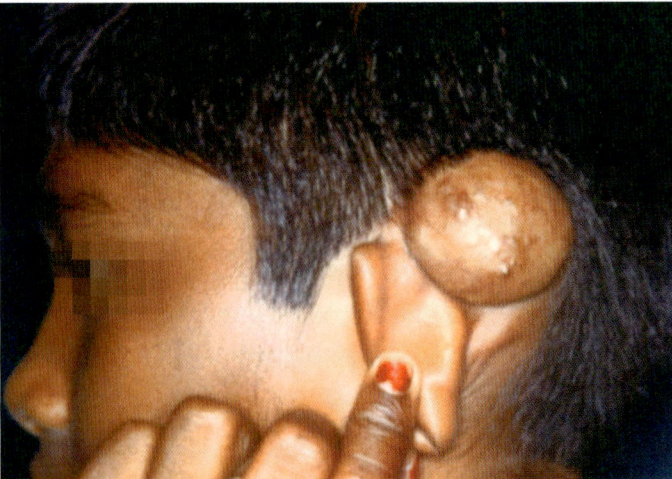

Fig. 4.34: Cavernous haemangioma. Sign of compressibility was present

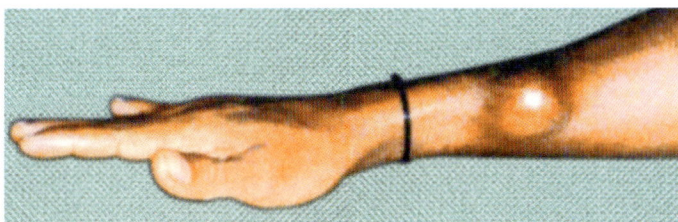

Fig. 4.35: Radial artery aneurysm

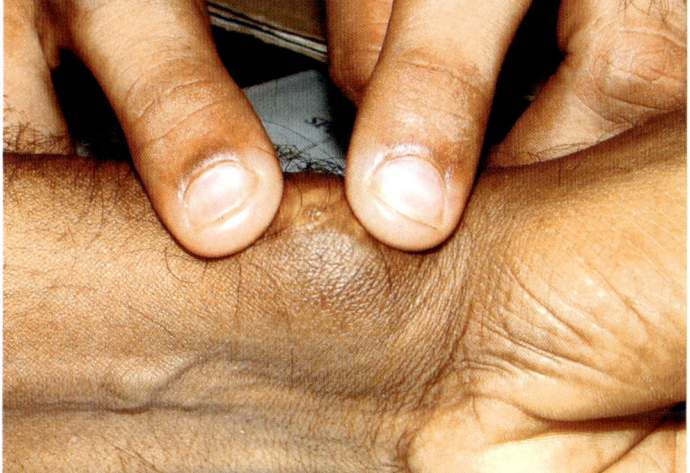

Fig. 4.36: Watch for elevation of finger

- *Transmitted:* When the swelling is situated over a vessel, the fingers are raised but not separated. Example: Jugulodigastric lymph node over carotid artery.

- When the swelling pushes the vessel anteriorly, transmitted pulsation can be obtained, e.g. cervical rib pushing the subclavian artery.

- *Pulsation* can also be present in vascular tumours such as osteogenic sarcoma or secondaries from carcinoma thyroid, etc.

- Pulsatile thyroid swelling is classical of primary thyrotoxicosis.

12. *Plane of the swelling*

   A. First lift the skin or pinch the skin. If it is not possible, lesion is arising from the skin or a swelling is deeper to it but fixed to it. Sebaceous cysts are attached to the skin at the site of punctum.

   B. Contract the muscles in the region of the swelling. If swelling becomes more prominent, it is superficial to the muscles (Fig. 4.37). Example: Subcutaneous lipomas in the forearm become more prominent when flexors are contracted.

C. Sometimes when the underlying muscle is contracted, swelling may remain same size but mobility may be restricted, This is either because swelling is arising from muscles or swelling is infiltrating muscles as in a soft tissue sarcoma. (Fig. 4.38). Refer to Figs 4.39 to 4.53 for more details.

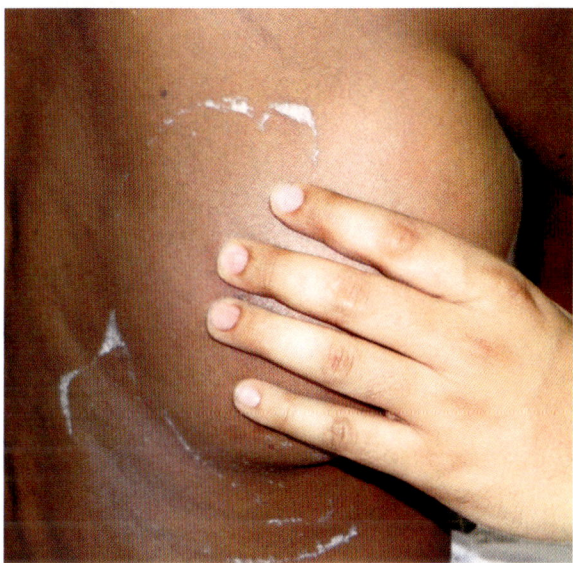

Fig. 4.37: Soft tissue sarcoma on the right side of the chest wall

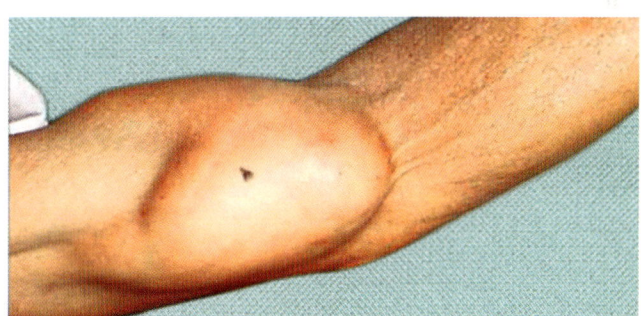

Fig. 4.38: Soft tissue sarcoma forearm

   D. Almost all significant cystic swellings in the neck are deep to deep fascia. Thus, contracting sternomastoid for laterally placed swellings and bending the chin against resistance for centrally placed swellings must be done to define the plane of swelling.

   E. Swelling due to semimembranous bursitis, almost disappears on flexion of knee and becomes more prominent on extension of the knee.

Clinical Wisdom

It is better to know the origin, insertion and action of a few important muscles in the chest, in the back and in the limbs. These are commonly asked in the university clinical exams, if you happen to get a swelling as a short case.

CONTRACTION OF THE MUSCLES AGAINST RESISTANCE

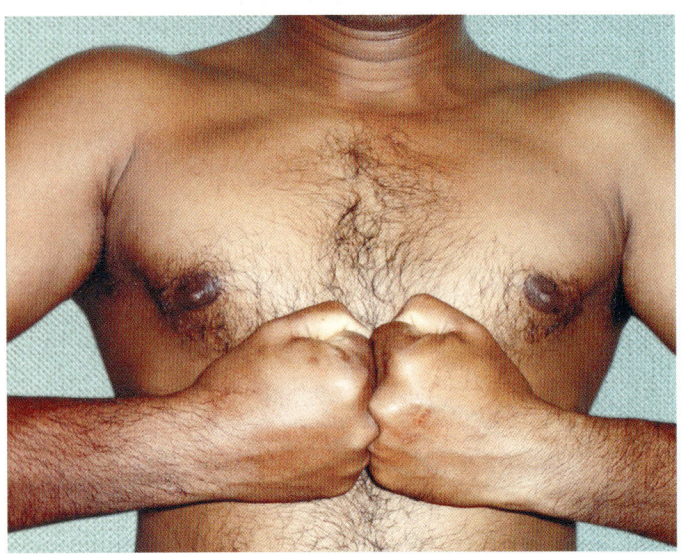

Fig. 4.39: Pectoralis major—two hands are pressed against each other

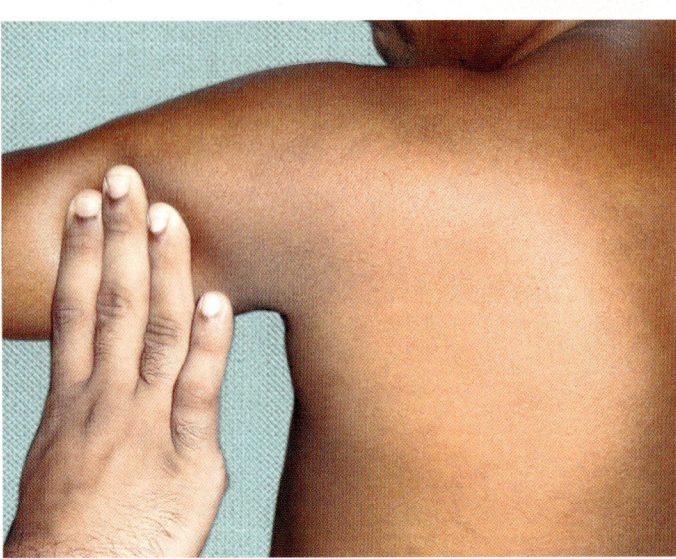

Fig. 4.42: Triceps: Extension of shoulder against resistance

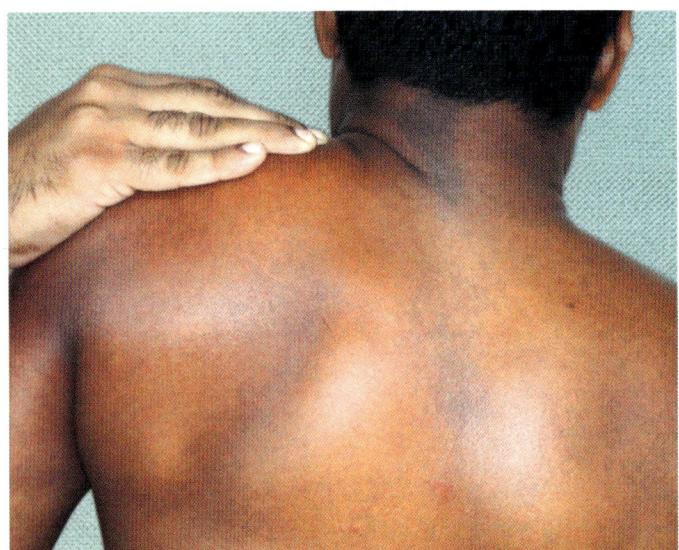

Fig. 4.40: Trapezius—raising the shoulder against resistance

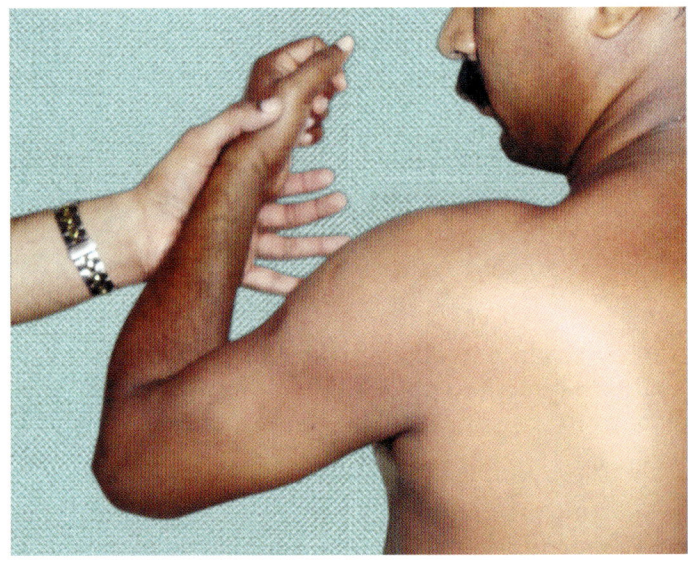

Fig. 4.43: Extension of elbow against resistance

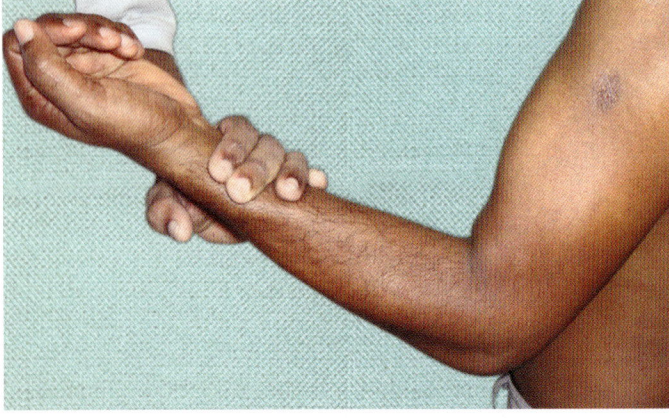

Fig. 4.41: Biceps brachii: Flexion of elbow against resistance

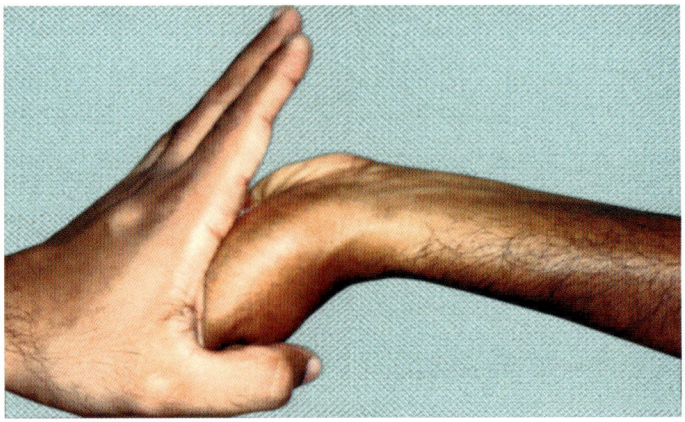

Fig. 4.44: Flexors of the wrist: Flexion against resistance

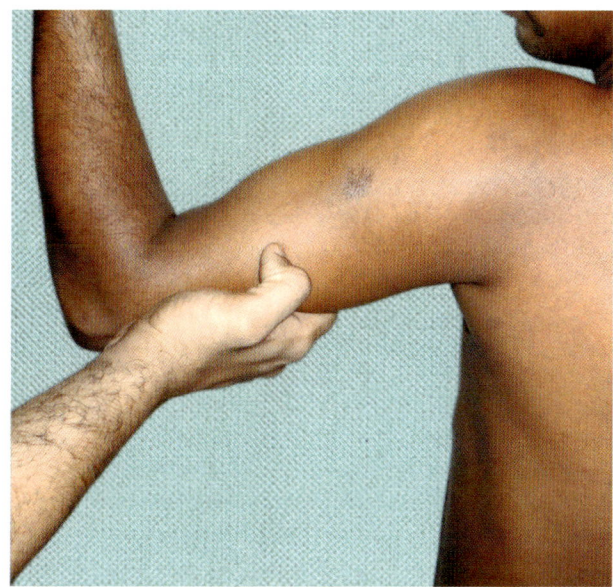

Fig. 4.45: Latissimus dorsi: Asking patient to push arm backwards and towards the trunk

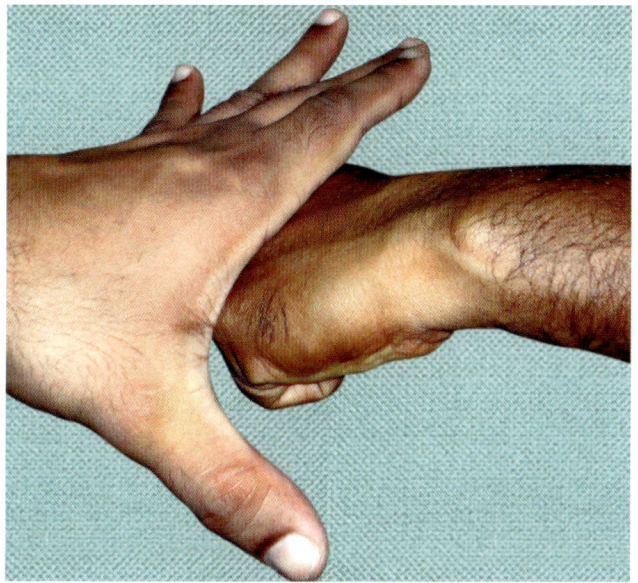

Fig. 4.46: Extension of the wrist—extend the wrist joint against resistance

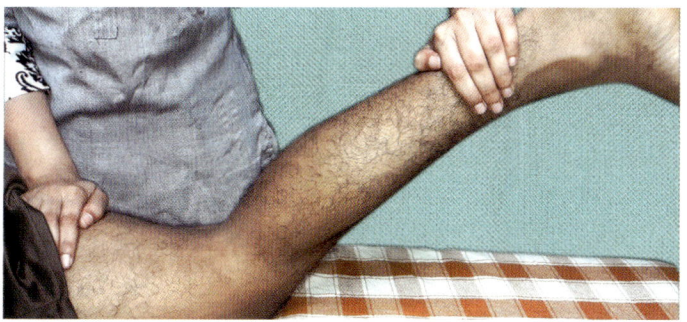

Fig. 4.47: Contracting gluteus maximus

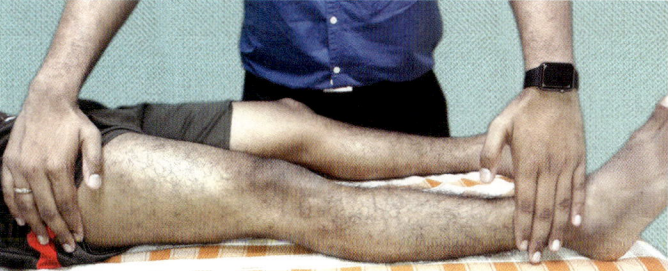

Fig. 4.48: Contracting gluteus medius by asking the patient to abduct the thigh against resistance

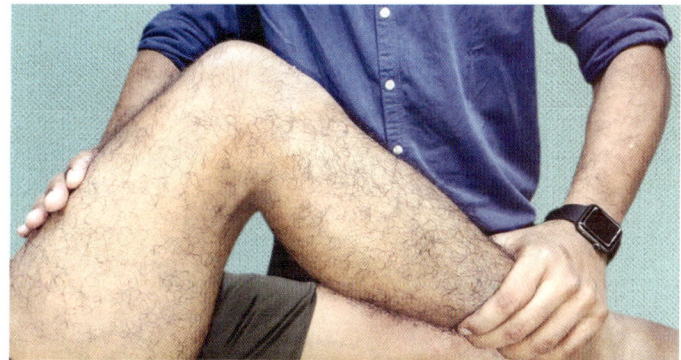

Fig. 4.49: Contracting quadriceps femoris

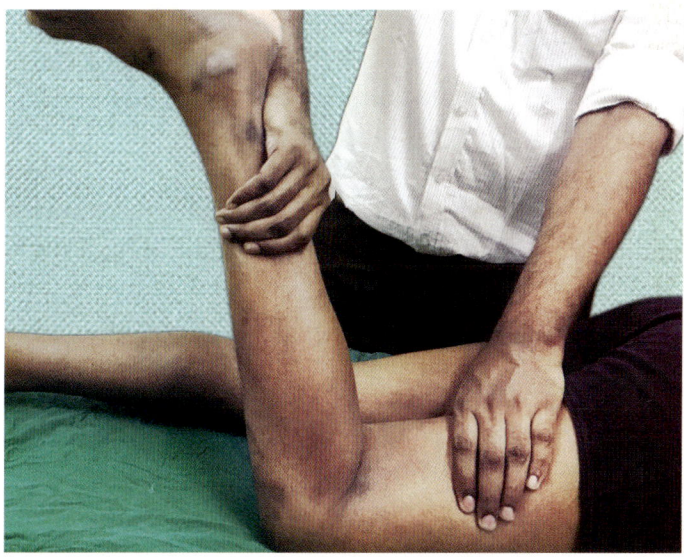

Fig. 4.50: Contracting hamstring muscles

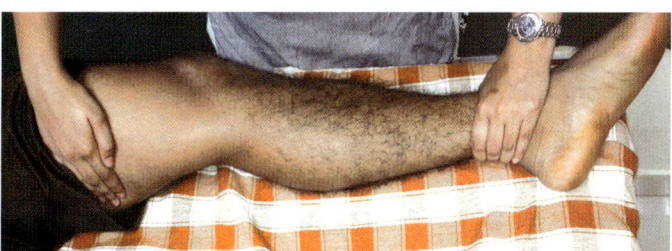

Fig. 4.51: Contracting adductors of the thigh against resistance

(*Courtesy:* Dr Navin Lella, Dr Kalyan Reddy and Dr Shruthi Pandith—Figs 4.39 to 4.51)

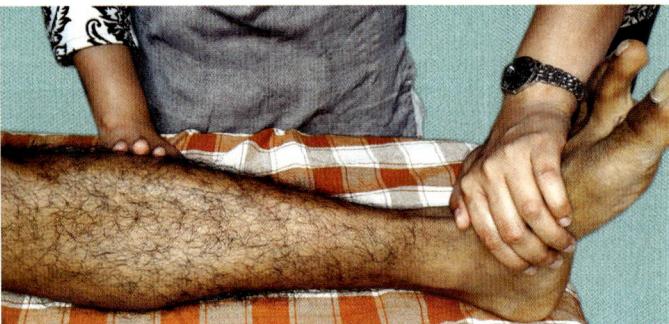

Fig. 4.52: Contracting extensors of the ankle against resistance

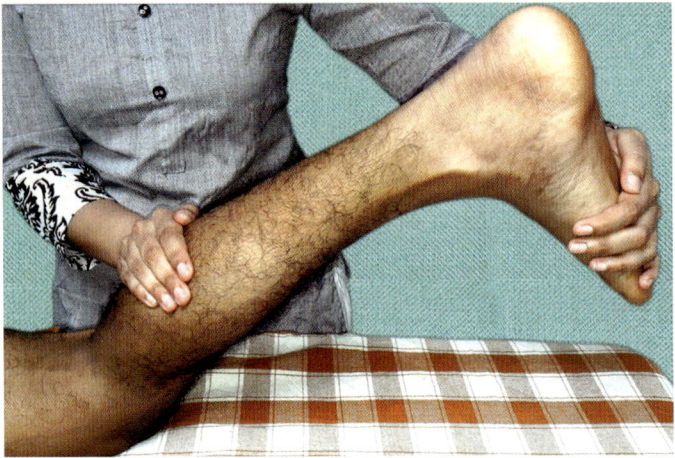

Fig. 4.53: Contracting flexors of the ankle joint against resistance

Before contraction of muscles, first move the swelling. Ask the patient to contract relevant muscles against resistance. Comment whether it is less prominent or more prominent and on its mobility.

13. *Any pressure effects*: Typically metastatic large fixed nodes in the groin/pelvis or tumours can give rise to distal neurovascular effects. Generally benign swellings do not give rise to oedema or wasting of the muscles but malignant swellings do. A few examples are given below.

- Sarcoma of the limbs may give rise to venous oedema distally.

- Sarcoma can also result in nerve palsy—which may give rise to wasting of muscles.

- Large lymph nodal mass in the axilla in Hodgkin's lymphoma or due to metastasis from carcinoma breast can give rise to swelling of the upper limb.

14. *Examination of regional lymph nodes*: Significant lymph nodes palpable are suggestive of malignancy. Nodes larger than 2 cm, firm or hard with

or without restricted mobility are suggestive of malignancy. Sometimes that may be the only vital clue for the diagnosis. Read the clinical notes below.

Clinical Case Capsule

MS exam case 1986. Government Wenlock Hospital, Mangalore. I was the candidate

A 50-year-old gentleman had a swelling in the elbow region for 2 months duration. He gave a history of trauma. On examination, it was firm and a few areas were soft. It was deep to deep fascia and had restricted mobility on contracting biceps. I gave a diagnosis of subfascial lipoma with haematoma and neurofibroma as differential diagnosis. Examiners agreed on my findings but asked me to examine axilla. There were 2 lymph nodes of 1–2 cm size and one of them was hard. I had done a mistake—blunder of not examining the axilla. I changed my diagnosis to synovial sarcoma. I passed MS examination because I had done other cases fairly well!

- In all cases of suspected tubercular cold abscess, look for any regional lymph nodes or look for any bony deformity or tenderness as in tuberculosis of spine.

15. *Examination of the joints for function*: Patients with soft tissue sarcomas or madura foot may have restricted movement of the limbs. At least affected joint function has to be mentioned.

- Patients with long-standing venous ulcers will have equinus deformity.

- Also examine the regional lymph nodes.

Clinical Wisdom

In case of soft tissue sarcomas of the lower limb, examine for distal pulsations, sensations, veins and function of the joints.

CLINICAL DIAGNOSIS

- Based on your findings, give 1 diagnosis as clinical diagnosis and 2–3 as differential diagnosis (DD).

- When you give a DD, think of common anatomical structures in the locality and common diseases affecting those structures. Importantly give a DD which matches most of the findings. Examples: For a sebaceous cyst, dermoid cyst can be the DD and for a cystic swelling, another cystic swelling can be the DD.

- In the following pages, you will come across site-specific differential diagnosis.

DIFFERENTIAL DIAGNOSIS

Swellings can be broadly classified into solid swellings, cystic swellings and pulsatile swellings.

PAPILLOMA

This is a benign tumour arising from skin or mucous membrane. It is characterised by finger-like projections with a central core of connective tissue, blood vessels, lymphatics and lining epithelium. It can be called hamartoma or a skin tag. It is an example of overgrowth of fibrous tissue.

Types

Skin papilloma (Fig. 4.54)

a. **Squamous papilloma** occurs in the skin, cheek, tongue, etc.
  - *Soft papillomas* are squamous papillomas. These are seen in elderly patients on the eyelid as small, soft, and brownish swellings.
  - *Squamous papilloma* can also be **congenital,** sometimes multiple in number and can be sessile or pedunculated.

b. **Basal cell papilloma** (seborrhoeic keratosis) is seen on the trunk of elderly patients as brownish elevated patch of skin and gives a semitransparent, oily appearance.

FIBROMA

Fibroma is a benign tumour, consisting of connective tissue fibres only. Clinically, it presents as a firm, subcutaneous swelling. However, **a true fibroma is rare.** These are combined with neural elements, muscle tissue or fatty tissue. **Do not give a clinical diagnosis of fibroma.**

Types

1. Soft fibromas—less fibrous tissue
2. Hard fibromas—more fibrous tissue
  - Neurofibroma—fibroma mixed with nerve fibres
  - Fibrolipoma—fibroma mixed with fat

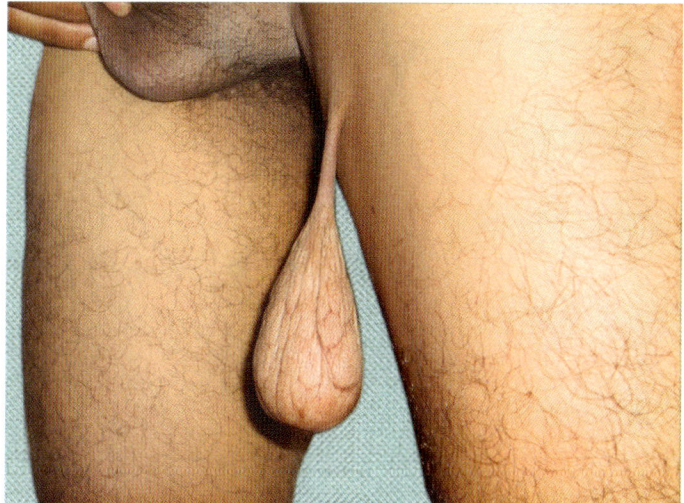

Fig. 4.54: Papilloma thigh with a narrow base—easy to remove it. Ulceration can be a problem here

- Myofibroma—Fibroma mixed with muscle fibres
- Angiofibroma—Fibroma mixed with blood vessels

LIPOMA (Universal Tumour)

Lipoma is a benign tumour arising from fat cells of adult type.

Types

1. Single Encapsulated Lipoma

- This is a single, soft, slow-growing, painless and semifluctuant swelling.
- Commonly present as a subcutaneous swelling, it *is **freely mobile.** The flank is the commonest site. Shoulder region, neck, back, and upper limbs are the other common sites (Figs 4.55 to 4.59).
- The swelling is soft, may feel cystic with fluctuation. This is also called pseudofluctuation because fat at body temperature behaves like fluid.
- Surface is **lobular** (Fig. 4.60). Lobulations are better appreciated with firm palpation of the swelling. Due to the pressure, lobules bulge out between the fibrous tissue strands.
- **The edge slips under the palpating finger which is a pathognomonic sign of lipoma.**
- **Dimpling sign**: Fibrous bands connect a lipoma to the skin. When the skin is **moved,** a dimple appears **on the skin.**

2. Multiple Lipomatosis

Such lipomas are multiple and very often tender because of *nerve elements* mixed with them. Hence, they are called *multiple neurolipomatosis.* **Dercum's disease** is one example of this variety *(adiposis dolorosa)* wherein tender, lipomatous swellings are present in the body, mainly the trunk.

3. Uncapsulated Lipoma (Diffuse)

- Diffuse variety is a rare type of lipoma. It is called pseudolipoma. It is an overgrowth of fat without a capsule.
- If lipoma is hard, it is liposarcoma.
- If lipoma is painful, it is neurolipoma and in cases of adiposis dolorosa.
- If lipoma is vascular, it is naevolipoma.
- Lipoma does not get infected because it is relatively avascular.
- Madelung disease refers to multiple lipomas developing in middle-aged alcoholic males in the neck and upper trunk region (Figs 4.58 to 4.60).
- **Lipoma arborescens** is a benign lipomatous mass which occurs most often in the knee joint.
- Abdominal emergency in a lipoma is intussusception.
- Dangerous complication of a lipoma is liposarcoma. A few retroperitoneal lipomas and lipoma in the thigh can turn into liposarcoma after many years of growth.

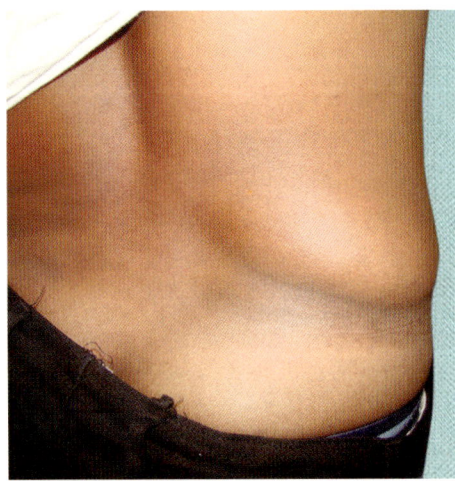

Fig. 4.55: Lipoma in the flank—**commonest site of lipoma**

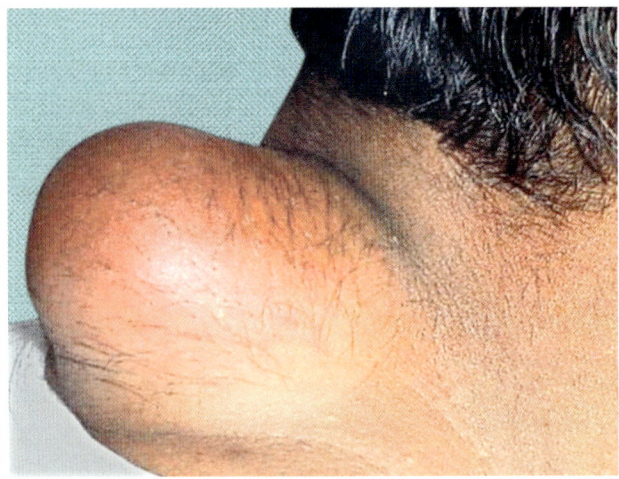

Fig. 4.58: Lipoma at nape of the neck

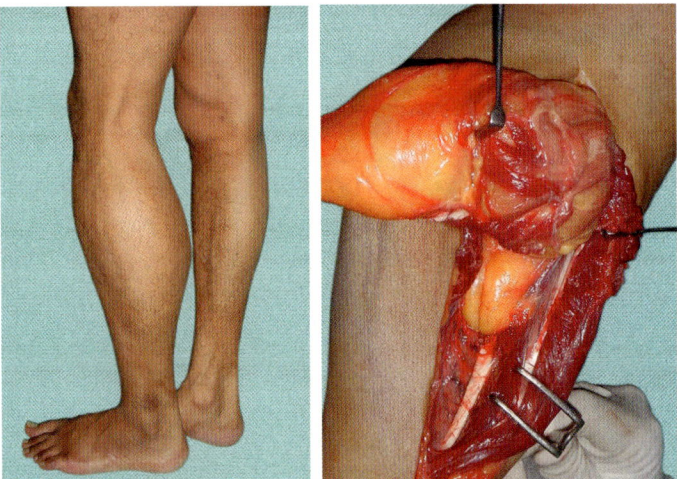

Fig. 4.56: Lipoma in the leg. Initially this patient was not evaluated but was started on anti-filarial drugs by general practitioner. One surgeon diagnosed this case as deep vein thrombosis and started on warfarin. Swelling was increasing in size. It was a case of intramuscular lipoma

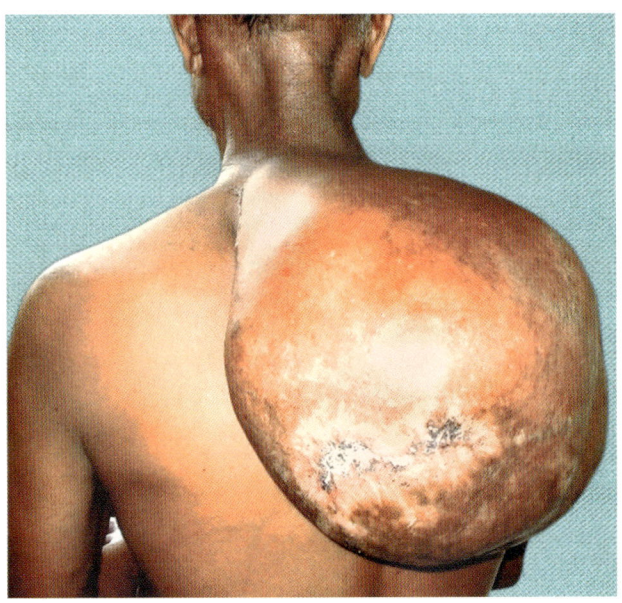

Fig. 4.59: Lipoma back region—posterior view

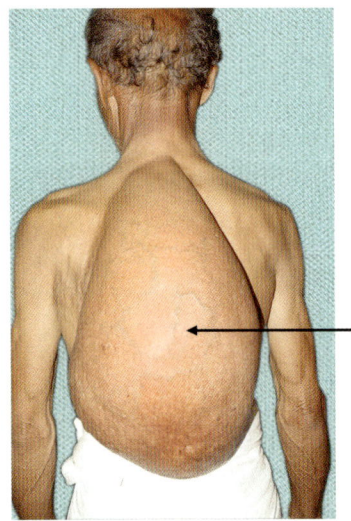

Since 3 months, it is rapidly growing, observe dilated veins and shiny skin. There is local rise of temperature. These features are suggestive of sarcoma

Fig. 4.57: Giant lipoma of the back of 15 years duration with features suggestive of sarcomatous change

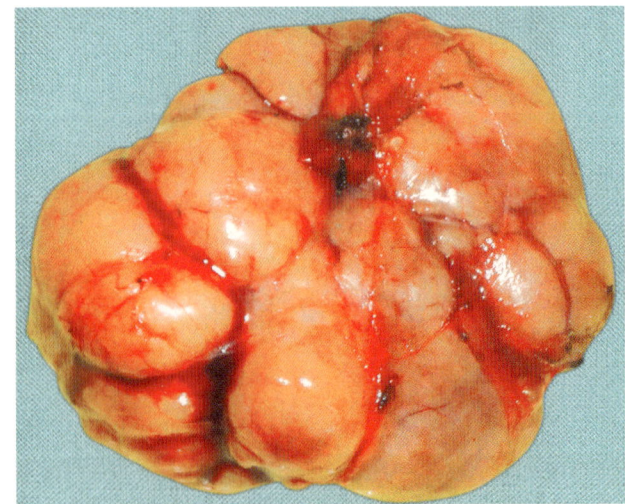

Fig. 4.60: Specimen of lipoma—lobular surface

Lipoma at the nape of the neck

- It is a common site, tends to grow to a large size.
- Lobularity and dimpling cannot be made out.
- Edge may not slip under palpating fingers.
- Can become giant lipoma—size of at least 10 cm in one dimension or weighing minimum of 1000 gm.

*Malignant transformation in a lipoma can be suspected when following features appear (Clinical Box 4.4)

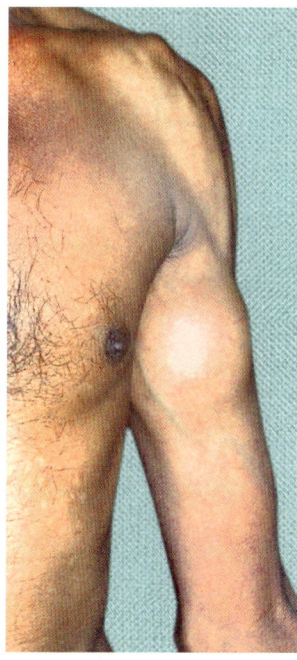

Fig. 4.61: Liposarcoma—rapidly growing, dilated veins on the surface

NEUROMA

These are uncommon benign tumours which arise from sympathetic nervous system or spinal cord. These can be classified into true neuromas (**ganglioneuroma, neuroblastoma, myelinic neuroma**) and false neuromas. False neuroma may be your short case.

False Neuroma

These tumours arise from the connective tissue of the sheath of nerve endings. These occur following nerve injuries, lacerations or after amputation. These are of two types:

1. *End neuroma:* It occurs after amputation due to proliferation of nerve fibres from the distal cut end of the nerve. This produces a bulbous swelling. If it is caught in the suture line or due to pressure of the prosthesis, it produces severe neuralgic pain. To avoid this, when an amputation is being done, the nerve is pulled downwards and cut as high as possible so that it retracts upwards.
2. *Lateral neuromas:* It occurs due to partial injury to the nerve on the lateral aspect.

NEUROFIBROMA

These are more common than true neuromas.

It is a benign tumour arising from the connective tissue of the nerve sheath. Typically, it produces a *fusiform swelling* in the direction of the nerve fibres. The tumour contains both neural (ectodermal) and fibrous (mesodermal) elements.

Clinical Types

1. **Single subcutaneous neurofibroma (local):** Commonly affects the peripheral nerves such as ulnar nerve, median nerve or cutaneous nerves. It occurs in adults.

   Clinical features
   - Presents as a painful, subcutaneous nodule.
   - Tingling and numbness, paraesthesia in the distribution of the nerve, specially when the nodule is compressed.
   - It is a round to oval swelling in the direction of nerve fibre.
   - It has a smooth surface with round border. The swelling moves at right angles to the direction of nerve fibres. Vertical mobility is absent.
   - The consistency is firm. Sometimes, it is hard.
   - Being a subcutaneous swelling, the skin can be lifted up.

2. **Generalised neurofibromatosis** [von Recklinghausen's (VR) disease (Type I)]:
   - This is an autosomal dominant disorder transmitted by both sexes. The whole body is studded with cutaneous nodules of varying sizes. They are soft and nontender.
   - Coffee brown pigmentation is characteristic of this condition (*café au lait* spots). *Café au lait* spots can be associated with involvement of cranial nerves—VIIIth nerve (auditory nerve) *acoustic neuroma*—**a cerebellopontine angle tumour. Popularly called vestibular schwannoma.**
   - Fibroepithelial skin tags are often present.
   - Type I is caused by **gene mutation on chromosome 17.**
   - The presence of skin pigmentation is an indication of the common neuroectodermal origin of nerve sheath cells and melanocytes.
   - Skeletal deformities such as kyphoscoliosis or osteoporosis are common.
   - It may be associated with phaeochromocytoma (high blood pressure).
   - Sarcomatous changes do occur.

3. *Plexiform neurofibromatosis (trigeminal)*

- In this condition, the branches of 5th cranial nerve are commonly affected. It can also involve the peripheries (Figs 4.62 to 4.65).
- The affected part is grossly thickened due to **fibro-myxomatous degeneration**.
- When it involves the branches of trigeminal nerve, following problems can occur:
  - **Tingling paraesthesia** in the distribution of Vth nerve, especially ophthalmic division.
- When it attains a huge size, it can **obstruct the vision**. As it grows bigger in size, it hangs in front of the neck, as a grossly thickened pendulous fold of skin.

4. *Elephantiasis neuromatosa*: This condition affects the limbs. It represents an advanced stage of plexiform variety. Gross thickening of subcutaneous tissue gives the appearance of elephant's leg. The skin is dry and coarse (Fig. 4.65).

5. *Pachydermatocele:* This refers to the plexiform lesions mainly found in the neck as a thickened, coiled single mass.

NEURILEMMOMA (SCHWANNOMA)

- This is a benign tumour arising from **Schwann cells.**
- Commonest site is the **acoustic nerve.** However, *vagus nerve is the most common peripheral site.*
- These can be single or multiple and present with a fusiform swelling in relationship with the nerves.

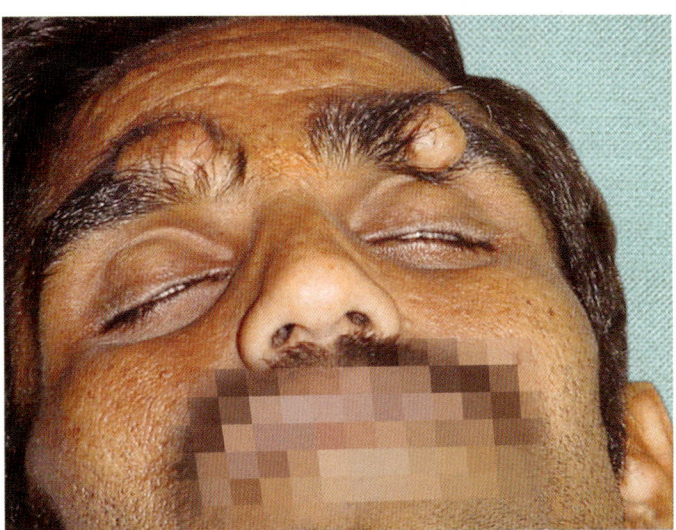

Fig. 4.62: von Recklinghausen's with plexiform neurofibromatosis (*Courtesy:* Dr Prashanth Shetty, Professor, Department of Surgery, KMC, Manipal)

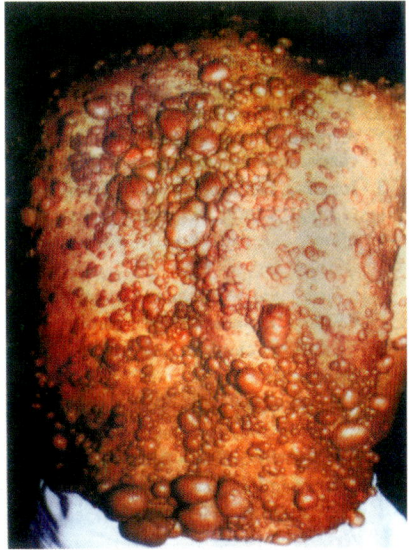

Fig. 4.63: von Recklinghausen's disease—tumours are multiple, congenital, and familial (*Courtesy:* Dr B Srinivas Pai, Professor, Department of surgery, SDM Medical College, Dharwad)

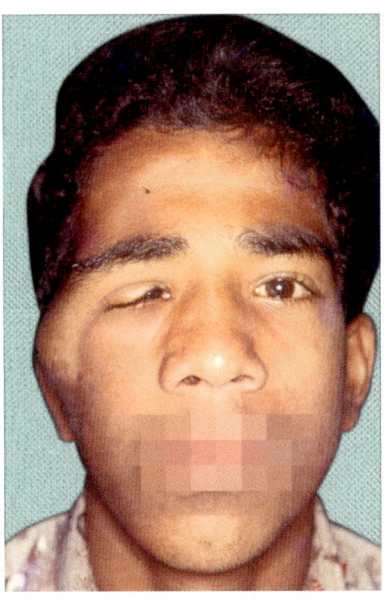

Fig. 4.64: Plexiform neurofibromatosis (*Courtesy:* Dr Rohit Jain, Assistant Professor, Dept of Surgery, KMC, Manipal)

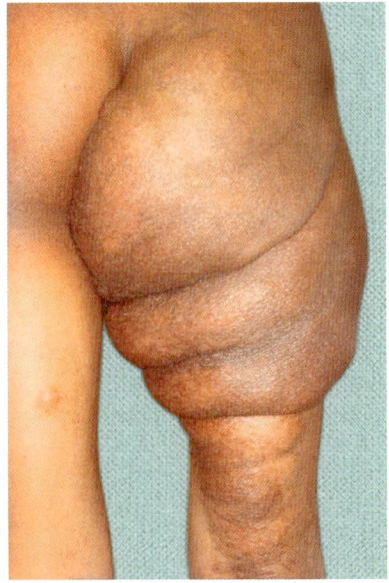

Fig. 4.65: Elephantiasis neuromatosa (*Courtesy:* Dr Balakrishna Shetty, Prof of Surgery, KS Hegde Medical Academy, Mangalore)

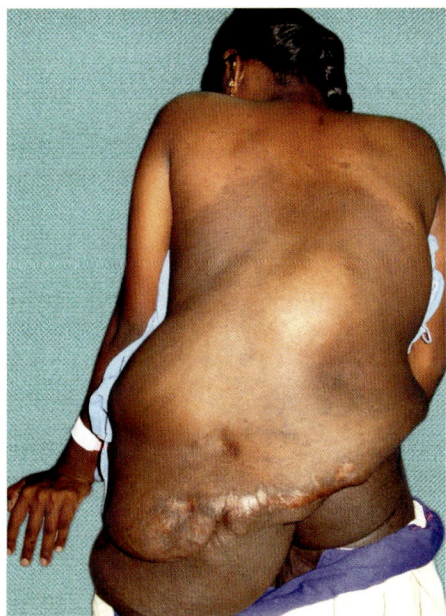

Fig. 4.66: Extensive neurofibromatosis, local gigantism kyphosis pigmentation are obvious. One attempt of decreasing the bulk and the disease has been done

- They can also arise from a peripheral nerve. **Sensory branches** are affected more frequently (Table 4.1).
- They can also be seen in mediastinum and retroperitoneum.
- They are **soft, lobulated, well encapsulated tumours.**
- They are **benign** and do **not turn into malignancy.**

CLINICAL DISCUSSION

How do you treat neurilemmoma?
- Excision of the tumour can be done without sacrificing the nerves because neurilemmoma is well encapsulated and displaces the nerve.

What about neurofibroma?
- In cases of neurofibroma, the nerve has to be sacrificed often.

HAMARTOMA

- It is a tumour-like developmental malformation of the tissues of a particular part of the body wherein it is arranged haphazardly.

- Hamartoma is a Greek word which means **fault or misfire.** It is not a clinical diagnosis.

A few examples of hamartoma: Haemangioma, neurofibroma, glomus tumour, benign naevus and lymphangioma.

Characteristic Features

- Being a developmental anomaly, these are seen at birth or in early childhood.
- In adults, there is a long history of swelling.
- Being a malformation (not a tumour), it does not have a capsule.
- These can be single or multiple.
- Some may regress as in strawberry angioma.
- These are benign lesions.
- Care should be taken when it contains vascular tissue such as haemangioma or neural tissue as in cases of neurofibroma.
- Facial nerve and its branches may be damaged while excising hamartomatous lesions over the face.

SOFT TISSUE SARCOMA—DIFFERENTIAL DIAGNOSIS

- How to suspect soft tissue sarcoma has been already discussed under lipoma. Any soft tissue swelling which is hard and irregular, of short duration, rapid growth should arouse suspicion of soft tissue sarcoma.
- Some important clinical features of sarcoma:
  1. Occurs in young patients
  2. Grows rapidly
  3. Swellings can have variable consistency—firm to hard and soft areas are due to tumour necrosis.
  4. Local rise in temperature and dilated veins indicate increased vascularity.
  5. Mobility is usually restricted
  6. Blood spread is a common feature

Sarcomas that metastasise to lymph nodes*
- **R**habdomyosarcoma
- **A**ngiosarcoma
- **C**lear cell carcinoma
- **E**pithelioid sarcoma
- **S**ynovial sarcoma

* You can remember as **RACES**

Table 4.1: Comparison between neurofibroma and schwannoma

Neurofibroma	Schwannoma
• More common	• Less common
• Ectodermal and mesodermal origin	• Ectodermal origin
• Subcutaneous (forearm) nerves are the commonest site	• Acoustic nerve is the commonest site
• Multiple lesions are common	• Very rare
• Feels firm or hard	• Soft
• Tender	• Nontender
• Can turn into sarcoma	• Does not turn into sarcoma
• Often nerve fibres are entangled with tumour. Hence, excision involves sacrificing nerve also	• Well encapsulated. Hence, enucleation is possible without sacrificing nerve

LIPOSARCOMA

- It is a malignant fatty tumour.
- **Common sites:** Proximal extremity, trunk or retroperitoneum.
- It is generally large at the time of diagnosis, e.g. retro-peritoneum. It results in gross swelling, which is firm to hard (more than 50% will be of >20 cm size).
- The compression on blood vessels may result in oedema of the limbs when it occurs in retroperitoneum.
- Well-differentiated myxoid liposarcomas are **notorious to recur** many times before spreading to lungs. **Hence, prognosis is good**.
- Pleomorphic and lipoblastic liposarcomas tend to be of higher grade and often present with metastasis.
- Wide excision/surgery is the primary treatment.
- They do respond to radiotherapy (Figs 4.67 and 4.68).

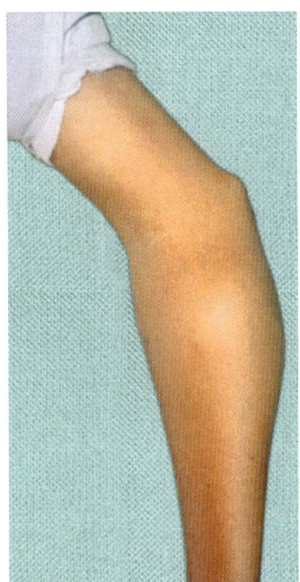

Fig. 4.67: Early stage of liposarcoma—this swelling had local rise of temperature and restricted mobility

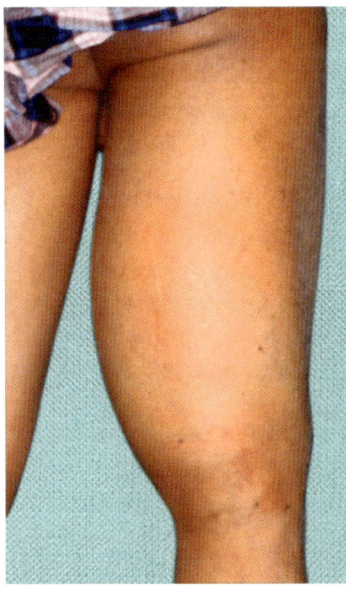

Fig. 4.68: Advanced case of liposarcoma—the swelling was hard and fixed. Dilated veins over the surface and location were characteristic

MALIGNANT FIBROUS HISTIOCYTOMA (MFH)

- Malignant tumour of mesenchymal tissue (fibrous tissue). This is the recent nomenclature of sarcoma. Fibrosarcoma or pleomorphic rhabdomyosarcomas are included under this. **Most of the so-called fibrosarcomas are presently included under MFH** (Figs 4.69 and 4.70).
- These are **high grade tumours** that lack differentiation.
- These can also arise from bone.
- **The MFH—superficial type rarely metastasises and carries good prognosis**.
- **Locations:** Retroperitoneum, trunks and limbs (intermuscular septa of adductors, scapulohumeral and pectoral muscles).

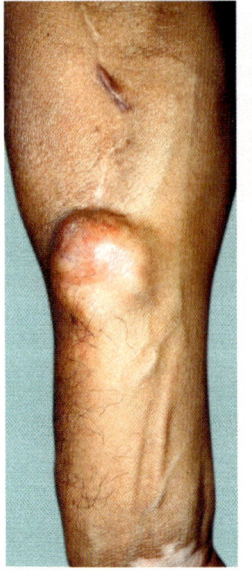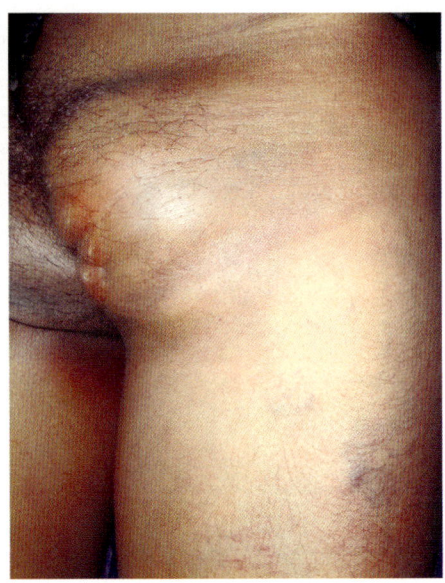

Fig. 4.69: Recurrent malignant fibrous histiocytoma. Look at the old scar and distal veins

Fig. 4.70: MFH in the groin region. Advanced with fixity to underlying structures (*Courtesy:* Dr Bharath Consultant Surgeon, Hassan)

Clinical Features

- Common in elderly patients (50 years) but can occur at any age.
- Slow-growing, firm to hard mass with restricted mobility.
- As the tumour is locally invasive, it infiltrates the muscles and adjacent structures. Thus, it can cause muscle weakness or pain, etc.
- **Spread:** Local spread is common. Distant metastasis by blood is late (lungs). Lymph node metastasis is rare.
- Like other sarcomas, dilated veins, local rise of temperature, restricted mobility and hardness will clinch the diagnosis.
- MRI is the investigation of choice to know the extent of the disease.
- Margin negative surgery should be the aim.

SYNOVIAL SARCOMA

- Any rapidly growing tumour in the region of joint/or near the tendons in young patients (20–40 years), synovial sarcoma is to be considered.
- Common site: Shoulder, wrist, knee, *etc.* (Fig. 4.71).
- Age: Young, between 20 and 40 years.
- Clinical features are similar to the other sarcomas—hard, painful mass.
- In addition to the local and blood spread, it also spreads by lymphatic route.
- Plain X-ray may show characteristic calcification
- It is aggressive, with high rates of recurrence.
- In the G-TNM staging system, these are grade 3.

EPITHELIOID SARCOMA

It is a soft tissue sarcoma. It is a high grade tumour spreads by all three routes—local, lymphatic and blood spread (Fig. 4.72).

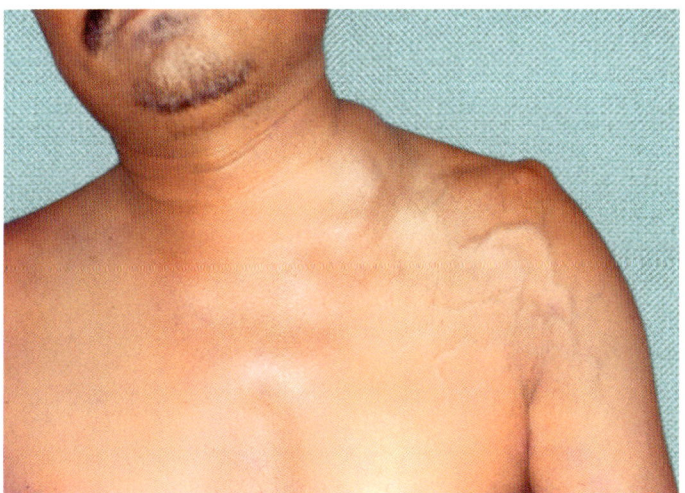

Fig. 4.71: Synovial sarcoma left shoulder region. *See the* secondary varicosity due to pressure effects. Non-extremity sarcomas have poor prognosis

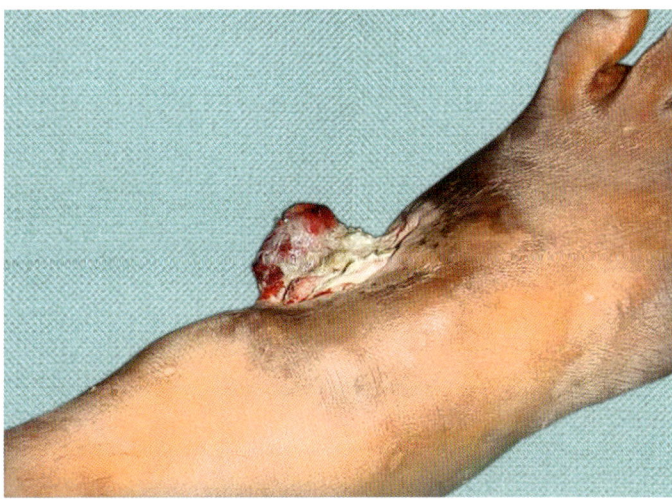

Fig. 4.73: Bleeding vascular lesion in the ankle region—angiosarcoma (*Courtesy:* Dr Mallikarjuna Desai, HOD, Surgery, SDMC, Dharwar, Karnataka)

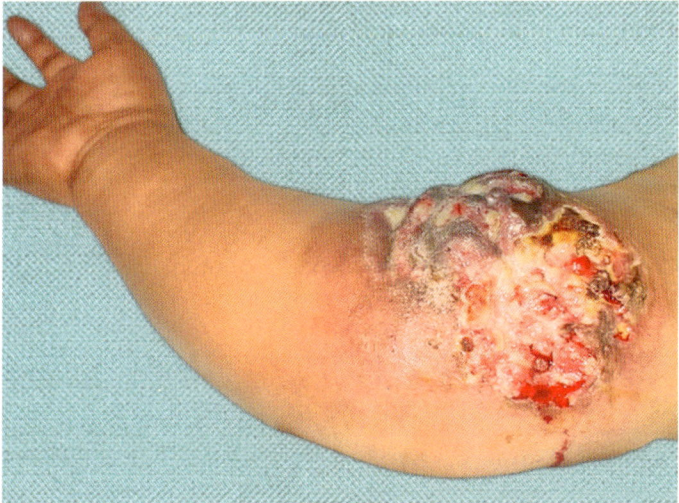

Fig. 4.72: Swelling in the elbow region for two years duration presented to the hospital with bleeding and fungation—advanced case of epithelioid sarcoma

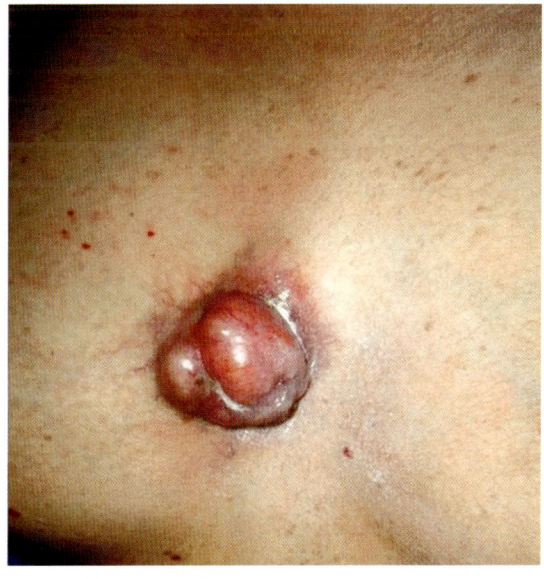

Fig. 4.74: Cutaneous angiosarcoma

ANGIOSARCOMA

- 1 to 2% of soft tissue sarcomas.
- Affects elderly patients (Fig. 4.73).
- These are high grade and aggressive tumours.
- These arise from skin and subcutaneous tissue rather than deeper tissues.
- Most of them occur in the head and neck, breast and liver.
- Surgery (excision) followed by radiotherapy/combination chemotherapy may have to be given (Figs 4.74 and 4.75).

RHABDOMYOSARCOMA

- It Is the **most common soft tissue sarcoma** seen in children, even though they are rare (under the age of 15).
- It arises from **striated muscle**—painless enlarging mass.

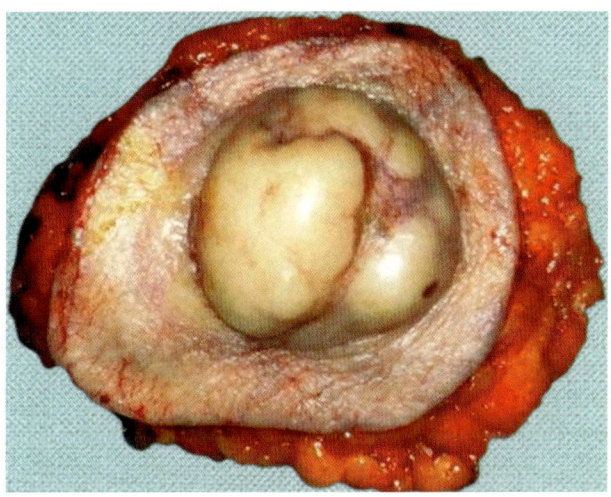

Fig. 4.75: Wide excision specimen

- Resection/chemotherapy/radiotherapy (combination) is tried depending on location.
- **Sites:** Head and neck (30%), genitourinary system (25%), and extremities (20%).
- All three varieties—embryonal, alveolar and pleomorphic are considered as Grade 3 in G-TNM staging. Hence, prognosis is not good.
- Complete tumour resection should be the aim. Chemotherapy and RT are also used.
- Rhabdomyosarcomas have a **high propensity for lymph node metastasis.**

KAPOSI'S SARCOMA

- Vulnerable section of people includes—Jews, immuno-compromised patients such as transplant recipients and AIDS.
- Typical sites: Legs other sites include chest, arm, and neck in epidemic form (Africa).
- It presents as **multiple pigmented sarcoma nodules** in the leg.
- It is interesting to note that **Kaposi's sarcoma is NOT SEEN in transfusion related 'AIDS'.**
- It manifests with purplish to red subcutaneous nodules in the leg followed by ulceration and bleeding.
- Combination chemotherapy with doxorubicin, etoposide and interferon have been used to control the disease.

DERMATOFIBROSARCOMA PROTUBERANS

- Clinically presents as nodular **exophytic 'mass' lesion—protuberans** (Figs 4.76 and 4.77).
- Locally aggressive tumour which does not metastasise.
- Wide excision should be the aim with negative margin to prevent local recurrence.

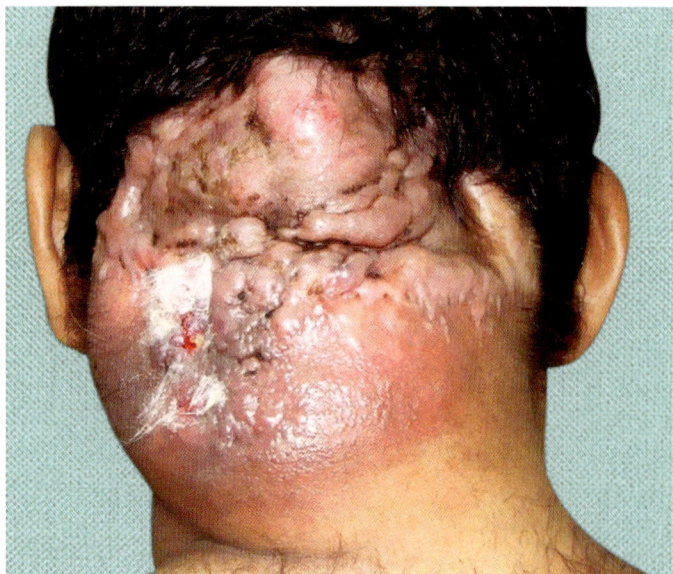

Fig. 4.76: Dermatofibrosarcoma in the nape of the neck

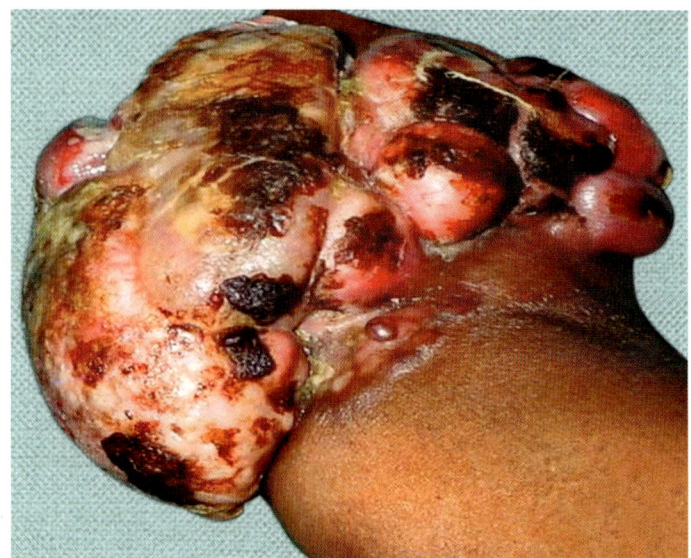

Fig. 4.77: Dermatofibrosarcoma protuberans in the elbow region

- Mohs' micrographic surgery, such as basal cell carcinoma, has been advocated to get negative margin and thus to get a low recurrence rates.
- It has a good prognosis, if treated early.

Investigations/Diagnostic Imaging

- Routine blood tests
- *Chest radiography:* Presence of cannon ball metastasis alters the staging, treatment policy and prognosis.

Clinical Wisdom

If STS is more than 5 cm (T2), computed tomography (CT) of the chest should be considered.

- **CT scan** is useful in evaluating retroperitoneal sarcomas. It can define structures, infiltration into neighbouring structures, hydronephrosis, etc. CT can guide a **core biopsy also.**
- **MRI** is the investigation of choice when STS occurs in **extremities to delineate muscle groups,** bones, vascular structures, etc.
- **Biopsy—FNA**
  - Acceptable first investigation to prove the diagnosis.
  - Useful to detect metastatic disease
  - To detect local recurrence
  - Ideal for superficial lesions
  - *Disadvantage:* Cannot assess tumour grading. Tissue is not sufficient for diagnostic tests.
- **Core needle biopsy**
  - Safe and accurate
  - Tissue is sufficient for grading, electron microscopes and flow cytometry
  - With CT guidance, core biopsy can be taken from deeper structures also.
- **Incisional biopsy**
  - When core biopsy tissue is not adequate, incisional biopsy is indicated (Clinical Box 4.5).

Guidelines while doing an incisional biopsy
- Incision should be oriented longitudinally in STS of extremities to facilitate removal of biopsy site, scar and tumour en bloc
- Flaps should not be raised
- Perfect haemostasis should be achieved
- Prevent dissemination
- Avoid drain

USEFUL TIPS IN A CASE OF SOFT TISSUE SARCOMA

In undergraduate clinical examination, students are advised to offer soft tissue sarcoma as the diagnosis. When asked the possible type, then only give a possible histological type based on various clinical features mentioned above. **Ask the following questions to yourself** to get ready for the clinical exams.

1. **Is it soft tissue sarcoma?** Tumour arising from soft tissue, dilated veins, reddish skin, increase in local temperature, firm to hard, rapidly growing swelling, with late involvement of skin (carcinoma starts in the skin).

2. **What is the age of the patient?**
   - In children   Rhabdomyosarcoma
     Undifferentiated sarcoma
   - In 20–40 years   Liposarcoma
     Synovial sarcoma
     Kaposi's sarcoma
   - In elderly   Angiosarcoma
     patients   Chondrosarcoma (bone)
     Malignant fibrous histiocytoma

3. **Which site has it occurred?**
   - Head and neck   Angiosarcoma
     Rhabdomyosarcoma
     Osteogenic sarcoma (jaw)
   - Distal extremity   Synovial sarcoma (limbs)
     Epithelioid sarcoma
     Clear cell sarcoma
   - Retroperitoneum   Liposarcoma
     and mesentery   MFH (malignant fibrous histiocytoma)/leiomyosarcoma

4. **Has it spread to lymph nodes?**
   - Rhabdomyosarcoma
   - Synovial sarcoma
   - Epithelioid sarcoma

5. **Has it spread to lungs or liver?**
   - Chest X-ray
   - Ultrasound

6. **What is the treatment? Can I preserve the limb? How?**
   - Wide excision with 2 cm margin or compartmental excision which includes all the muscles fascia in the compartment of the tumour. Also, amputation is done. Surgery is the main stay of the treatment for soft tissue sarcoma. Chemoradiation can be tried in selected cases preoperatively to save the limb.
   - Preoperative radiotherapy combined with surgery and postoperative radiotherapy is also given.

7. **What is the differential diagnosis of sarcoma? When it occurs in the thigh?**
   - Chronic abscess—may feel firm or hard, and tense.
   - Fever may be absent because of previous treatment with antibiotics.

CYSTIC SWELLINGS—DIFFERENTIAL DIAGNOSIS

A cyst is a swelling containing fluid. **True cysts** are lined by endothelium or epithelium. These contain clear serous fluid, mucoid material, pus, blood, lymph or toothpaste like material.

The **false cysts** do not have lining epithelium. These can be **degenerative cysts** as in the case of tumours which undergo tumour necrosis or tumour degeneration, or merely a **collection** of fluid which is walled off by coils of bowel as in tuberculous encysted ascites or an **exudation cyst** as in pseudopancreatic cyst.

DERMOID CYST

This is a cyst lined by squamous epithelium containing desquamated cells. The contents are thick, sometimes toothpaste-like which is a mixture of sweat, sebum and desquamated epithelial cells and occasionally, even hair. It is treated by excision.

Clinical Types of Dermoid Cyst

I. Congenital/Sequestration Dermoid

- These occur along the line of embryonic fusion, due to dermal cells being buried in deeper plane (Figs 4.78 to 4.82)
- The cells which are sequestrated in the subcutaneous plane proliferate and liquefy to form a cyst.
- As it grows, it indents the mesoderm (future bone) which explains the bony defects caused by dermoid cyst in the skull or facial bones.
- Even though these are congenital, these manifest as a swelling during childhood or later in life. Often these can be mistaken for lipoma and sebaceous cysts.
- These can occur anywhere in the midline of the body or the face.

  - Median nasal dermoid cyst: At the root of the nose at the fusion lines of frontal process.
  - External and internal angular dermoid cyst: At the fusion lines of frontonasal and maxillary processes.
  - In the suprasternal space of *Burns*
  - Sublingual dermoid cyst
  - Preauricular dermoid cyst—in front of the auricle
  - Postauricular dermoid cyst behind the auricle

Clinical features

- Though congenital, the cyst manifests in childhood or during adolescence. A few cases also manifest in 30–40 years of age group.
- Typically, the patient presents with a painless, slow-growing swelling.

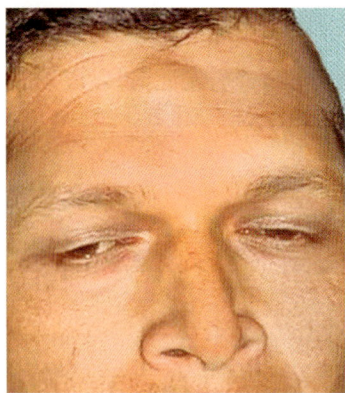

Fig. 4.78: Median frontal dermoid cyst—lipoma, and sebaceous cyst are other differential diagnosis

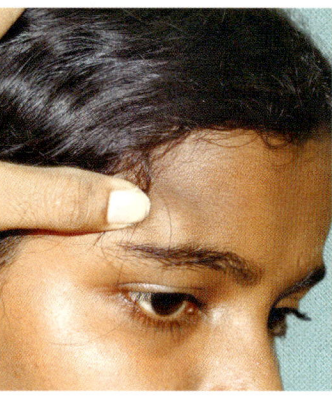

Fig. 4.79: Feeling for bony depression, if present it is a pathognomonic sign

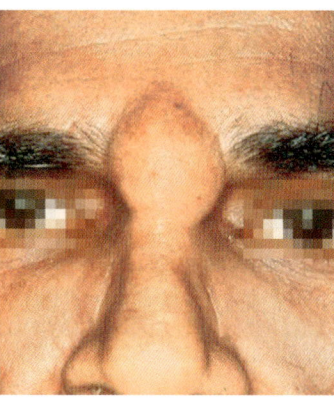

Fig. 4.80: Median frontal dermoid cyst at the root of the nose. Test for cough impulse

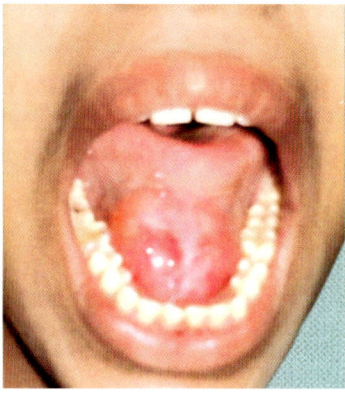

Fig. 4.81: Sublingual dermoid (*Courtesy:* Dr Sreejayan, Professor of Surgery, Calicut Medical College)

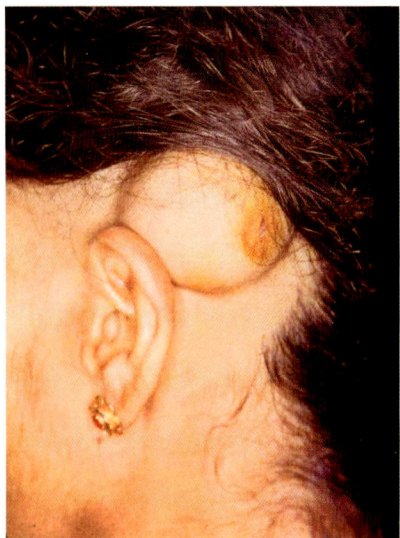

Fig. 4.82: Post-auricular dermoid cyst. Location and soft consistency are characteristic

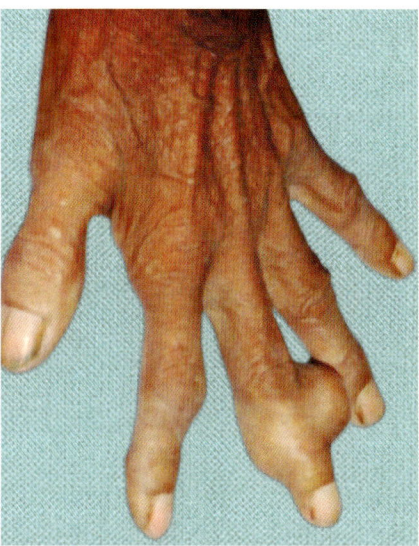

Fig. 4.83: Implantation dermoid cyst—classical sites are hand and foot which are prone for sharp injuries

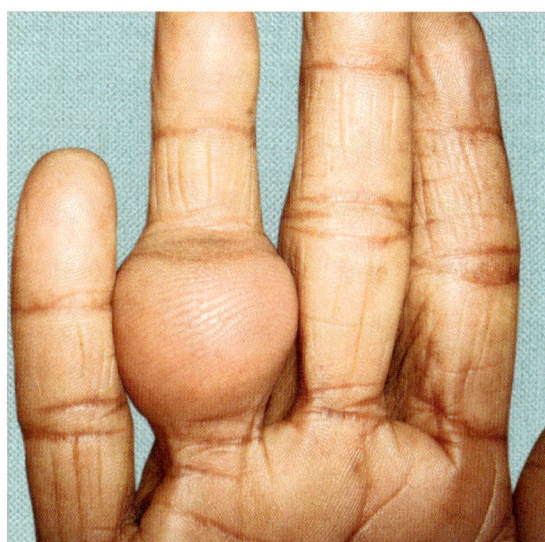

Fig. 4.84: Implantation dermoid cyst—TB synovitis and chronic abscess are the other differential diagnosis

- Soft, cystic and fluctuant, transillumination is negative.
- Rarely, it may be putty-like in consistency.
- **The underlying *bony* defect gives the clue to the diagnosis.**
- Classical location of the cyst (along the line of fusion) is a feature of sequestration dermoid cyst.

II. Implantation Dermoid Cyst (Figs 4.83 to 4.85)

- This is common in women, tailors, agriculturists who sustain repeated minor sharp injuries.
- Following a **sharp injury,** a few epidermal cells get implanted into the subcutaneous plane. There, they develop into an implantation dermoid cyst. Hence, it is typically found in the fingers, palm and sole of the foot. As the cyst develops in the areas where the skin is thick and keratinised, it feels firm to hard in consistency.

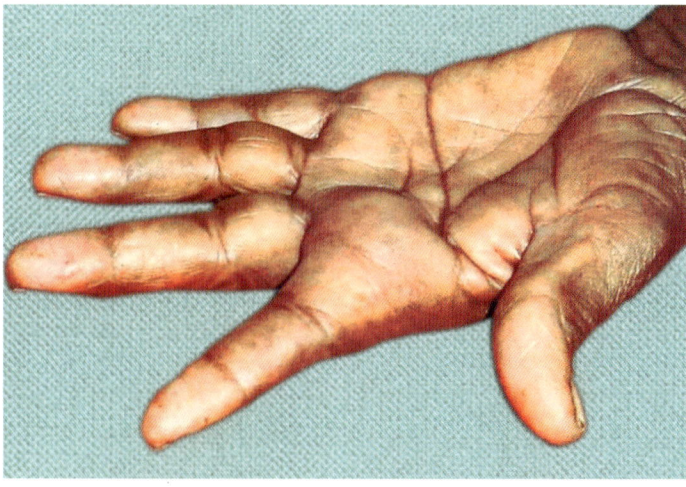

Fig. 4.85: Implatation dermoid cyst in the palm

III. Teratomatous Dermoid Cyst

- Teratoma is a tumour arising from **totipotential cells.** Thus, it contains ectodermal, endodermal and mesodermal elements—hair, teeth, cartilage, bone, etc.
- Common sites are ovary, testis, retroperitoneum and mediastinum.

    Rarely, due to errors in the neural tube closing dermoid cyst can also occur as spinal cord tumours.

Complications of Dermoid Cyst

1. Infection and suppuration—abscess
2. Ovarian dermoid can undergo torsion
3. External angular dermoid cyst can partially obstruct the vision—indication for surgery.

EPIDERMOID CYST/SEBACEOUS CYST/WEN

- This is popularly called **sebaceous cyst.** It is a misnomer. This occurs due to obstruction to one of the sebaceous ducts, resulting in accumulation of sebaceous material. Hence, this is an example of **retention cyst.**
- **Sites:** Scalp, face, back, scrotum, etc. **It does not occur in palm and sole,** where sebaceous glands are absent. In the back, scalp and scrotum, multiple cysts are often found.

Clinical Features

- They are slow-growing and appear in early adulthood or middle age.
- **Hemispherical** or spherical swelling located in the dermis. The central keratin filled **punctum** which is a **dark spot** is diagnostic feature of this cyst. The punctum indicates blockage of the duct (Fig. 4.86).
- In 20–30% of cases, instead of opening into the skin, sebaceous duct opens into the hair follicle. Hence, punctum is not seen (Fig. 4.87)
- Smooth surface, round borders, soft and putty in consistency, nontender.
- The cyst can be moulded into different shapes which is described as **sign of moulding.**

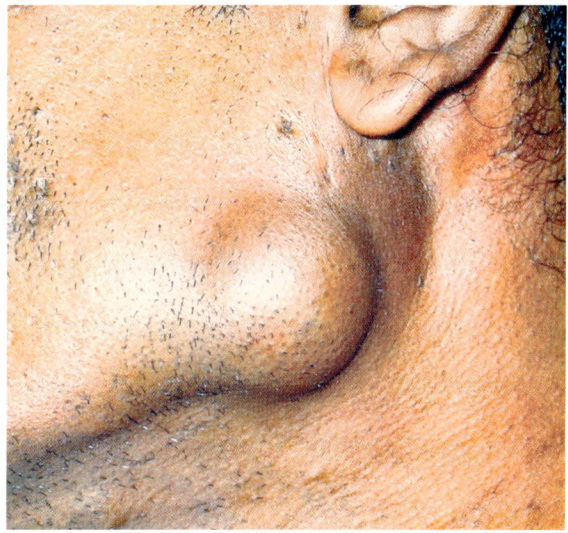

Fig. 4.87: Sebaceous cyst on the face—punctum is not seen

- **Sign of indentation** refers to pitting on pressure over the swelling.
- The swelling is mobile over the deep structures and the skin is free all around except an area of adherence at the site of punctum.
- When sebaceous cyst occur near the external canthus of the eye dermoid cyst is the differential diagnosis (Fig. 4.88). Differentiaing points between sebaceous cyst and dermoid cyst are given in Table 4.2.
- Very often cysts can be multiple (Figs 4.89 and 4.90).
- In the scalp, loss of hair (Fig. 4.90) is a feature over the swelling because of constant slow expansion of the cyst (Table 4.2).

Treatment

- Incision and **avulsion of cyst with the wall.** Very often, during dissection, the cyst wall ruptures. Care should be taken to excise the entire cyst wall. If not, recurrence can occur.
- * Infected sebaceous is treated like an abscess by incision and drainage (Figs 4.91 and 4.92)

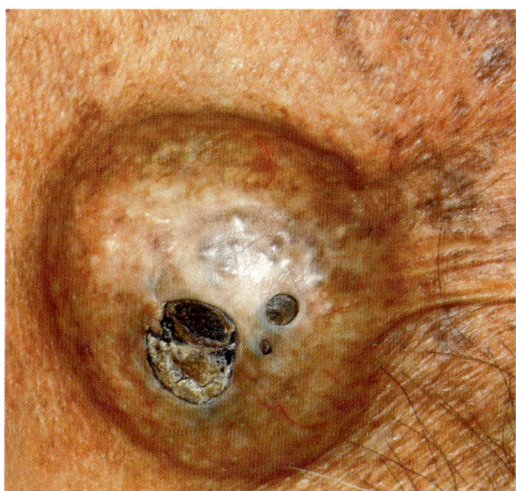

Fig. 4.86: Punctum is diagnostic

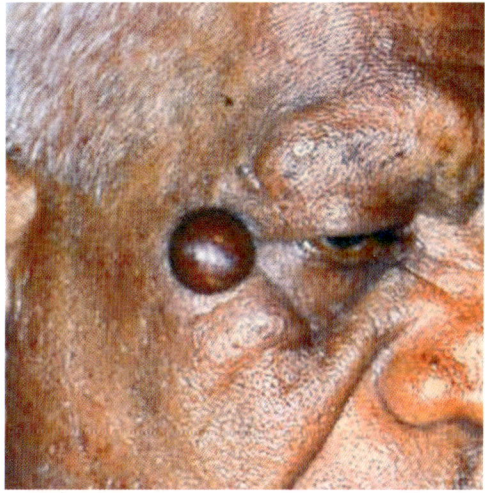

Figs 4.88: Sebaceous cyst near outer canthus of the eye

Table 4.2: Comparison of congenital dermoid cyst and sebaceous cyst

	Congenital dermoid cyst	Epidermal cyst
• Aetiology	Congenital—sequestration of dermal cells in the subcutaneous plane	Acquired—retention cyst due to accumulation of sebaceous contents
• Location	Midline of the body, along the line of fusion	Face, scalp, scrotum, back
• Sign of indentation, moulding	Uncommon	Very common
• Punctum	Absent	Present in 50% of cases—diagnostic
• Skin fixation	Absent	Skin is fixed at the site of punctum
• Bony defect	Present in majority of cases	Absent
• Intracranial communication	Rare, can be diagnosed by cough impulse test	Absent
• Treatment	Excision	Excision or avulsion

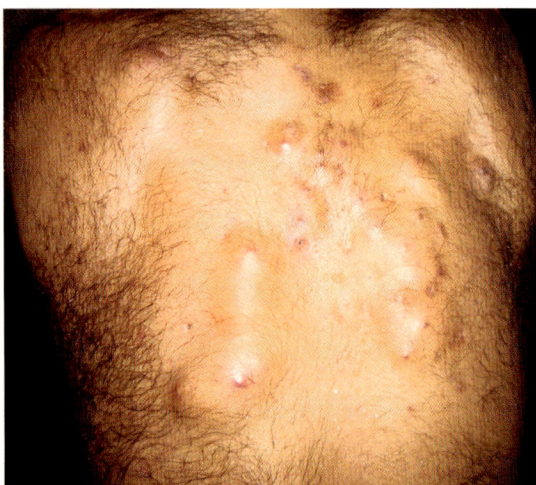

Fig. 4.89: Multiple sebaceous cysts on the back—troublesome situation

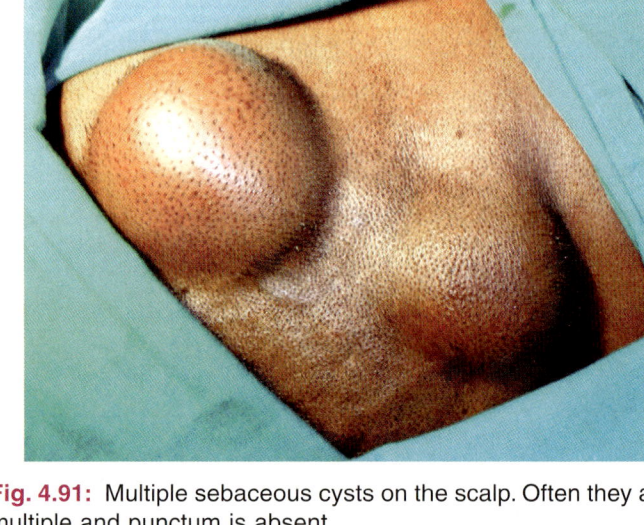

Fig. 4.91: Multiple sebaceous cysts on the scalp. Often they are multiple and punctum is absent

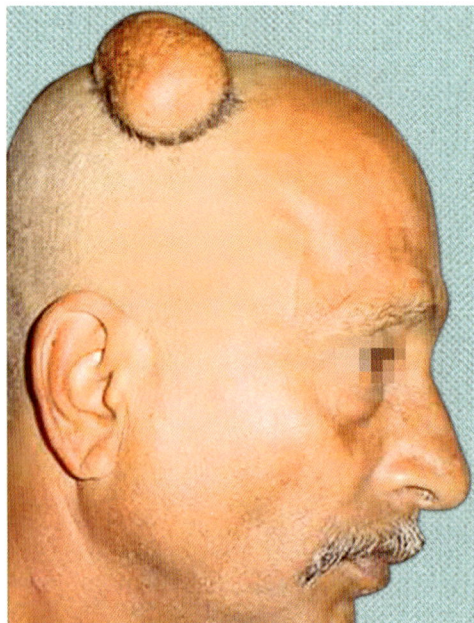

Fig. 4.90: Sebaceous cyst on the scalp—loss of hair is a feature. When punctum is absent, the differential diagnosis is lipoma

• When it is small it can be excised along with the skin (Fig. 4.92).

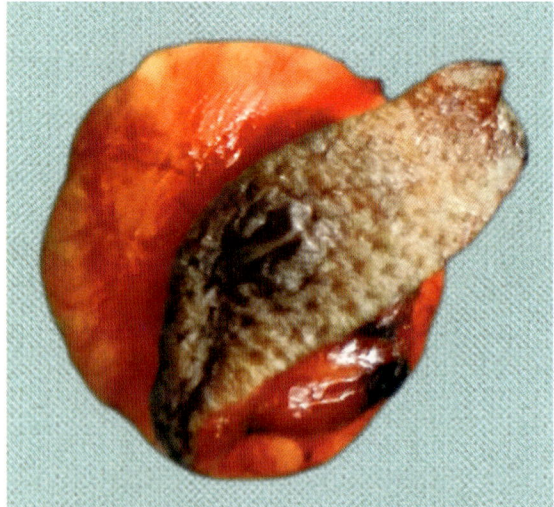

Fig. 4.92: Sebaceous cyst excised with skin

Complications

1. **Infection** can occur due to injury or scratch resulting in an abscess. The cyst will be tender, red and warm to touch. It should be treated like an abscess by incision and drainage. After one to two months, the cyst can be excised (Fig. 4.93).

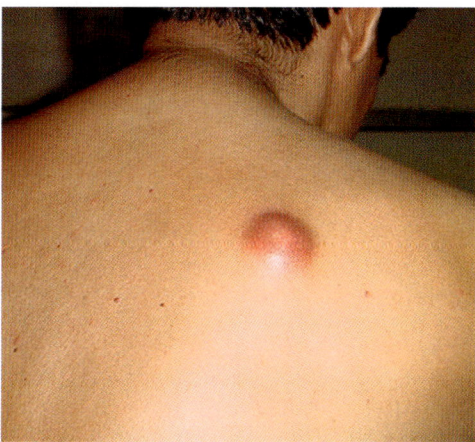

Fig. 4.93: Infected sebaceous cyst. You can see the local signs of inflammation

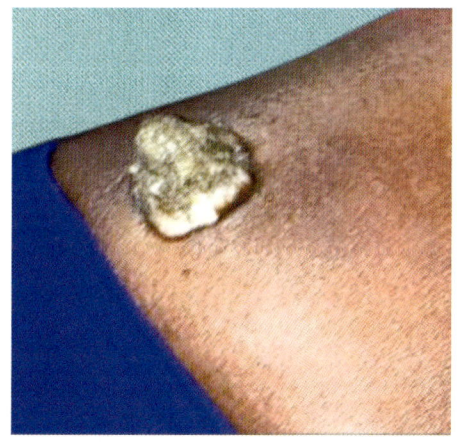

Fig. 4.94A: Sebaceous horn (*Courtesy:* Dr Haribabu MA, Associate Professor, SVMC, Tirupathi)

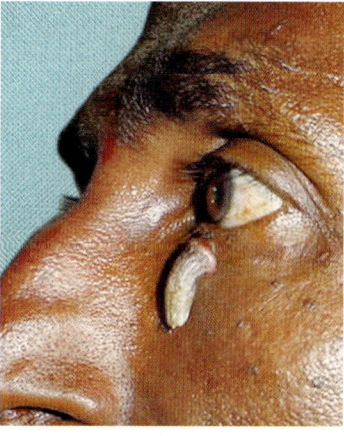

Fig. 4.94B. Sebaceous horn (*Courtesy:* Dr Prashanth Tubachi, SDM Medical College, Dharwar)

2. **Sebaceous horn** results due to slow drying of the contents which are squeezed out, specially if a patient does not wash the part. Thus, it is not common to find a large sebaceous horn nowadays because of better ways of living and sanitation (Figs 4.94A and B).
3. **Calcification**
4. **Cock's peculiar tumour** refers to infected, ulcerated cyst of scalp with pouting granulation tissue and everted edge resembling epithelioma (Clinical Box 4.6).

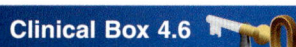

Clinical Box 4.6

Interesting—sebaceous cyst
- Syndrome: Gardner's syndrome
- Tumour: Cock's peculiar tumour
- Parasitic worm: Demodex folliculorum
- Strawberry scrotum: Multiple sebaceous cysts of scrotum

GANGLION

It is a tense, cystic swelling and occurs due to myxomatous degeneration of the synovial sheath lining the joint or tendon sheath. These are common around joints because of abundant fibrous tissue. These contain gelatinous fluid.

Common Sites

- The dorsum of the hand is the common site, at the **scapholunate** articulation (Figs 4.94 and 4.95).
- In the foot, dorsal or lateral aspect.
- Small ganglion in relation to flexor aspect of fingers.

Clinical Features

- Majority of patients are between 20 and 50 years.
- A round to oval swelling in the dorsum of the hand, with smooth surface and round borders. Skin over the swelling is normal.
- The swelling is tensely cystic and fluctuant. Transillumination is negative. It is mobile in the transverse direction.
- When the tendons are put into contraction, the mobility of the swelling gets restricted.

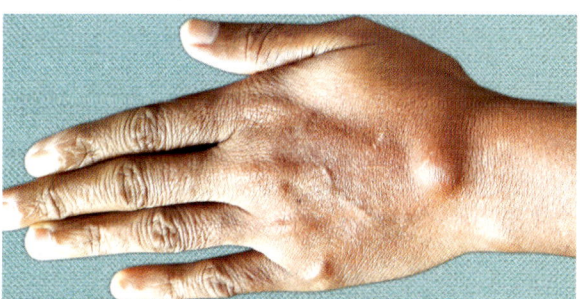

Fig. 4.95: Ganglion on the dorsum of the hand

- Ganglion is not connected with the joint space. Sometimes, it gives an impression of becoming small due to slipping away between bones.

Treatment

- Asymptomatic ganglion is **better left alone.**
- **Aspiration** of the ganglion and injection of sclerosants may reduce the size of ganglion.
- Sometimes, rupture of the cyst due to trauma may result in permanent cure.
- **Surgical excision** can be done. However, recurrence rate is high.

Differential Diagnosis (DD)

1. Implantation dermoid cyst, when it occurs in the feet or hand.
2. Exostosis of the bone, has to be considered, if *swelling is very hard.*
3. Bursa (*vide infra*)

COMPOUND PALMAR GANGLION

Aetiology

- **Tuberculous tenosynovitis** of the tendon sheaths affecting the flexor tendons. This is a common cause in India.
- **Rheumatoid arthritis** with involvement of multiple joints causing thickening of synovial membrane—common cause in Western countries.

Pathology

As a result of tuberculous tenosynovitis, typical caseous material collects within the flexor tendon sheaths. The tendons get matted, a swelling develops in the palm and another swelling develops in lower aspect of forearm. The thickening of synovial membrane, fibrin particles in the **fluid and melon seeds**, are characteristic of this condition.

Clinical Features

- Majority of patients are below 40 years of age.
- Concavity of the palm is obliterated.
- Soft, cystic, fluctuant, transillumination—negative swelling situated above and below the flexor retinaculum.
- **Cross-fluctuation test** (Clinical Box 4.7) between these two swellings is positive, which is diagnostic of compound palmar ganglion.

Clinical Box 4.7

Cross-fluctuation test positive in
- Plunging ranula
- Compound palmar ganglion
- Hydrocoele en bisac
- Iliopsoas abscess

- Restricted mobility of the fingers due to matting of the tendons.
- **Wasting of the small muscles** of the hand.
- **Paraesthesia** due to compression on median nerve.

Investigations

- ESR may be increased, if it is due to tuberculosis.
- Aspiration of the swelling and fluid can be sent for acid-fast bacilli.
- Synovial biopsy

Treatment

- **Antituberculous treatment** (ATT) in case of tubercular pathology. If the response rate is not satisfactory—exploration, decompression, synovectomy and release of matted tendons are the treatment.
- **Control of rheumatoid arthritis**, with complete excision of the synovial sheath, in cases due to rheumatoid arthritis.

Compound Palmar Ganglion
- Tuberculosis and rheumatoid arthritis—common causes.
- Synovial thickening will clinch the diagnosis.
- Cross-fluctuation test is an important clinical finding.
- Antituberculous treatment, if it is due to tuberculosis.
- Decompression or synovectomy may be required in both conditions mentioned above.

GLOMUS TUMOUR

This is also called glomangioma or angioneuromyoma. Glomus is a specialised organ.

Structure of Glomus (Glomus Body)

Abundant arteriovenous anastomosis surrounded by large clear cells (glomus cells) and medullated and non-medullated nerve fibres in between the cells are characteristics of glomus.

Clinical Features of Glomus Tumour

- Typical site: Under the nail beds of hands and feet.
- It is purple red in colour, usually single, the size does not exceed 1 cm in diameter.
- Glomus tumour is usually seen in the 5th decade.
- Excruciating pain either at rest or on movement of the finger or on pressure is pathognomonic feature of this tumour. Pain is due to compression of the nerve fibres by dilated glomus vessels.
- The tumour is compressible.

Treatment

Surgical excision results in *permanent cure.*

Differential Diagnosis

- Subungual melanoma: Painless and pigmented.
- Granuloma pyogenicum: Mild pain, bleeds on touch and evidence of infection is present.
- Chronic infection with granuloma.

BURSA

- Bursa means a sac or a sac-like cavity containing fluid lined by endothelium. It is meant to reduce the friction between the tendons of the muscle and the bone.
- Bursitis refers to inflammation of a bursa resulting in accumulation of excessive fluid inside the bursa. This results in a swelling in the anatomical sites of normal bursa.
- The causes of chronic bursitis include constant pressure, constant irritation or minor injuries.

Clinical Features

- A cystic swelling in a known anatomical site of a bursa is a chronic bursitis unless proved otherwise.
- Bursitis produces a soft, cystic, circumscribed or oval swelling with fluctuation.
- As majority of bursitis contains inflammatory fluid, they do not show transillumination.
- In a few cases, signs of inflammation may be present.

Complications

- Secondary infection may result in an abscess
- Frequent friction may result in ulceration

Treatment

- Excision is indicated only in the presence of symptoms such as pain or complications mentioned above.
- Chances of recurrence are high.

SEMIMEMBRANOSUS BURSITIS (Fig. 4.96)

This is the commonest swelling in the popliteal space. It presents as a tensely cystic swelling when the knee is extended and it becomes flaccid on flexion of the knee. It is not compressible as it does not communicate with the joint.

The differential diagnosis for semimembranosus bursitis is Morrant Baker's cyst, which is a herniation of the synovial membrane. The differences between these two swellings are given in Table 4.4.

Adventitious Bursae (Table 4.3)

This refers to a cyst which develops in an anatomical area where no bursa is present. These also occur due to constant pressure or friction. These are summarised in Table 4.4.

Subcutaneous Cysticercosis

- Cysticercosis is the most common parasitic infection of soft tissue.
- Pork consumption is the cause.
- These can occur in the subcutaneous plane—abdominal wall, chest wall, neck, etc.
- These can also present as calf muscle swelling. These can be deep beneath the subfascial layer.
- Clinically, these are diagnosed as lipoma and neurofibroma.
- In endemic areas, cysticercosis should be included in the differential diagnosis of nodular lesions.

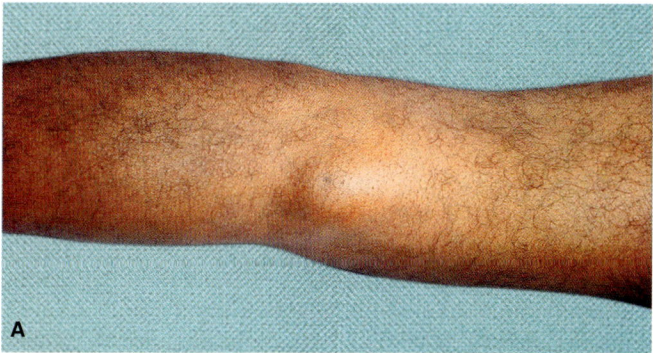

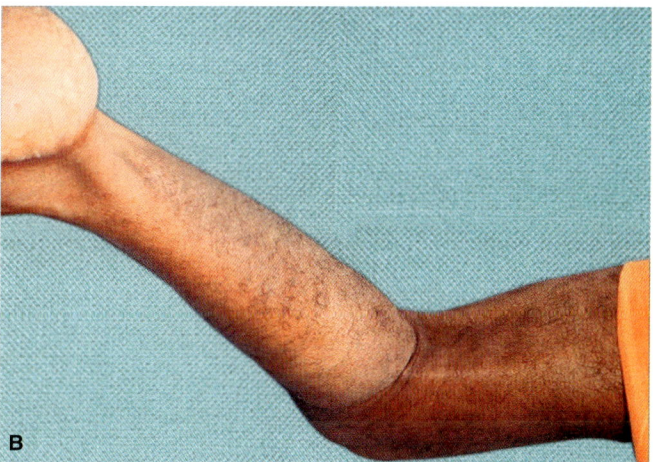

Figs 4.96A and B: (A) Semimembranosus cyst and (B) cyst disappears on flexing

Table 4.3: Adventitious bursae

Anatomical site	Popular nomenclature
1. Prepatellar bursa	Housemaid's knee
2. In front of patella tendon (infrapatellar)	Clergyman's knee
3. Olecranon bursa	Student's elbow
4. Under the insertion of tendons of sartorius, gracilis and semitendinosus muscle	Bursa anserina (extension of the bursa along with the sides of tendon—resembles goose's foot)
5. Between the tendon of the semimembranosus and the medial condyle of tibia	Semimembranosus bursitis

Table 4.4: Comparison of semimembranosus bursa and Baker's cyst (Fig. 4.97)

	Semimembranosus bursa	Baker's cyst
1. Aetiology	Friction or pressure	Rheumatoid or osteoarthrosis of knee joint
2. Age	Young patients	Middle aged
3. Location in the popliteal fossa	Higher up and more medial	Below and midline
4. On flexion of the knee	Disappears	Increases (Fig. 4.97)
5. On extension of the knee	Appears and is tense (Figs 4.96A and B)	Diminishes
6. Patellar tap	Absent	Present
7. Compressibility	Absent	Present partlally
8. Knee movements	Normal	Restricted

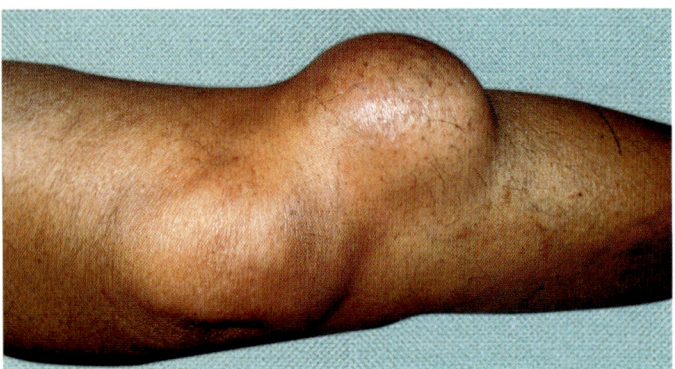

Fig. 4.97: Baker's cyst

CLINICAL ANALYSIS OF FOUR COMMON CASES

CASE 1: A 50-year-old man with painless swelling in the face near the inner aspect of the eye of 3 years duration.

Discussion: The swelling is of 3 years duration suggesting it is benign. The look of the swelling suggests possibility of sebaceous cyst but the punctum is absent. Although part of it is near midline, he says it did not start in the midline and he is 50 years old. On palpation, it had putty-paste like consistency. Hence, lipoma is ruled out. Thus, even in the absence of punctum, since the sign of indentation and moulding were positive, diagnosis of sebaceous cyst was made (Fig. 4.98).

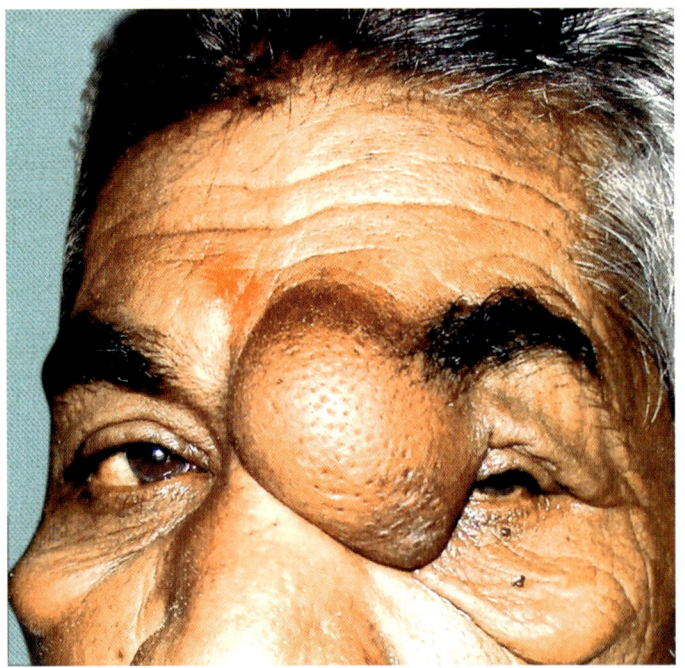

Fig. 4.98: Sebaceous cyst confused for mucocoele of frontal sinus

What else can occur in this location?

Mucocoele of the frontal sinus can present in this location with fluctuant swelling. With intracranial extension, cough impulse will be positive. Features of recurrent sinusitis, headache may clinch the diagnosis.

CASE 2: A 10-year-old boy with swelling behind the left ear of 5 years duration.

Discussion: Duration of 5 years suggests it is benign. Since he is only 10 years old, the swelling is possibly congenital in origin. Lymphangioma is unlikely because it is not the site. Diagnosis is by inspection—congenital dermoid cyst.

It was soft and so, dermoid cyst and haemangioma are likely. Slip sign is negative. Also remember that lipoma is very rare in children. Transillumination was negative. It was compressible. This one physical sign clinches the diagnosis of haemangioma. Dermoid cyst is ruled out (Fig. 4.99).

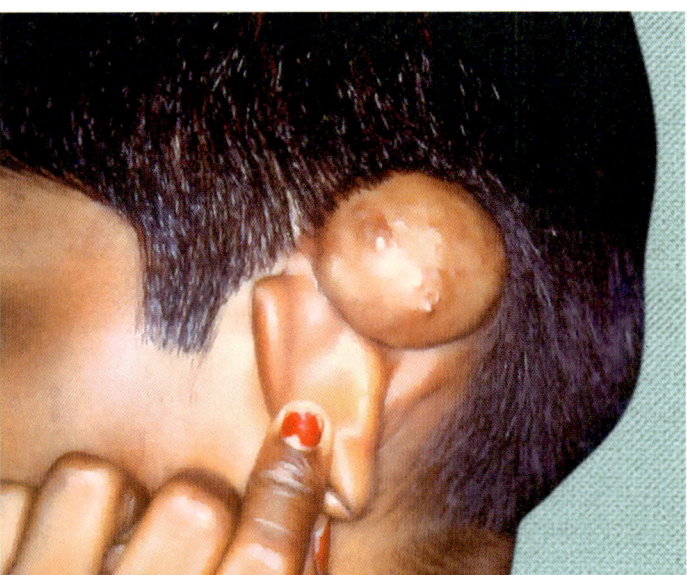

Fig. 4.99: Cavernous haemangioma

What else can occur in this location?

Lipoma and sebaceous cysts can be the differential diagnosis in adults.

CASE 3: A 35-year-old woman with swelling in the lower left arm of 1 year duration.

Discussion: She had a swelling in the inner aspect of lower arm of 1 year duration. It was painless to start with. Since the last two months, it is rapidly growing and is now painful. Since the last 15 days, it has

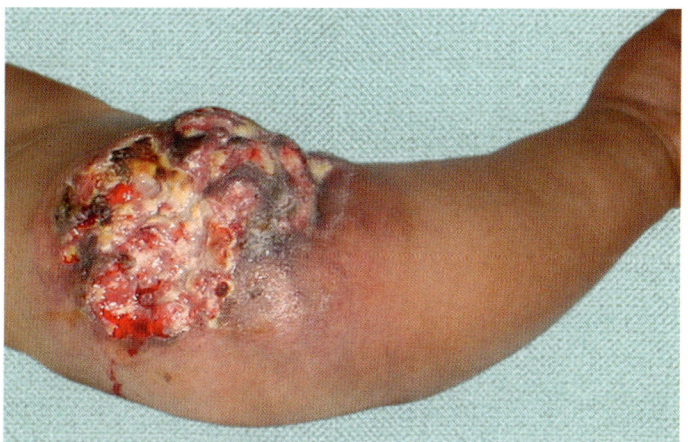

Fig. 4.100: Soft tissue sarcoma arm with distal oedema

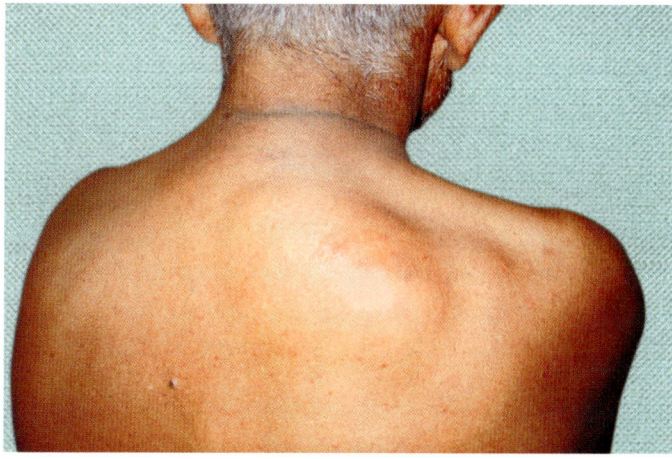

Fig. 4.101: MFH from scapular muscles

ulcerated and has started bleeding. This suggests malignant transformation in a benign lesion. Soft tissue sarcoma is likely. Pain suggests infiltration into skin underlying nerves or bones. Since the lesion is near the joint, synovial sarcoma is one possibility. However, malignant fibrous histiocytoma was the final diagnosis. Lesion was very extensive. Amputation of the arm was suggested but patient refused treatment. Since swelling started first in the deeper plane and skin was normal, malignant skin tumours are unlikely possibilities (Fig. 4.100).

CASE 4: A 55-year-old man with swelling in the upper part of the back on the right side—2 months duration.

Discussion: Look at the size—within 2 months means rapidly growing swelling suggests malignant swelling. On palpation, it was firm and a few areas were hard. Neurofibroma, and fibrolipoma were considered. Please note deep-seated lipoma may give feeling of hardness.

On contracting trapezius muscle, mobility of the swelling was restricted. It suggested that it is in a deeper plane and may be arising from muscles or infiltrating muscles. This sign is a strong indicator of malignancy along with rapid growth and hardness. Tru cut biopsy report was *malignant fibrous histiocytoma* (MFH). He underwent wide excision followed by chemoradiotherapy.

In some cases, tumours in this location may feel firm or soft, due to degeneration of the tumour. If it is near the mid-line, cold abscess is one of the differential diagnoses. Cough impulse and examination of the spine is mandatory (Fig. 4.101).

SITE-SPECIFIC DIFFERENTIAL DIAGNOSIS

Students should recollect various anatomical structures present in the given area for examination and try recollecting various pathological process affecting them. I have given you the list of swellings and DD when they occur in different sites. This will help you in your clinics for a quick reference.

Remember

- Agra is famous for Taj Mahal: Outer canthus of eye site for dermoid cyst
- Delhi is famous for India Gate: Floor of the mouth is site for ranula
- Nadankanan Zoo for white tigers: Carotid triangle is site for carotid body tumour
- Madurai is for Meenakshi temple: Flank is the common site for lipoma
- Kanyakumari for Vivekanand statue: Anterior triangle for cold abscess
- Udupi is famous for Krishna temple. Palm and sole for implantation dermoid cyst

- Then start asking questions rather than blindly asking all irrelevant questions. To give an example: A swelling in the axilla in an 18-year-old girl—*does it become big during menstruation* is a relevant and an important question. If this history is present, it is typical of axillary tail hypertrophy.

- Did you have a history of trauma—is a very relevant question specially in the legs because leg is vulnerable for trauma. Look at the list of swellings in the leg. You will find history of trauma in most of them.

COMMON SWELLINGS IN THE LEGS/FOOT

1. *Implantation dermoid cyst*: Foot, especially sole is more commonly affected. History of trauma to the foot is usually present. Negative history does not rule out implantation dermoid cyst because trivial trauma is forgotten. Slow-growing swelling of 1–2 years duration, feels little soft and sometimes firm because of the location (sole is cornified especially in agriculturists), deeper to skin and subcutaneous tissue with no other manifestations clinches the diagnosis (Fig. 4.102).

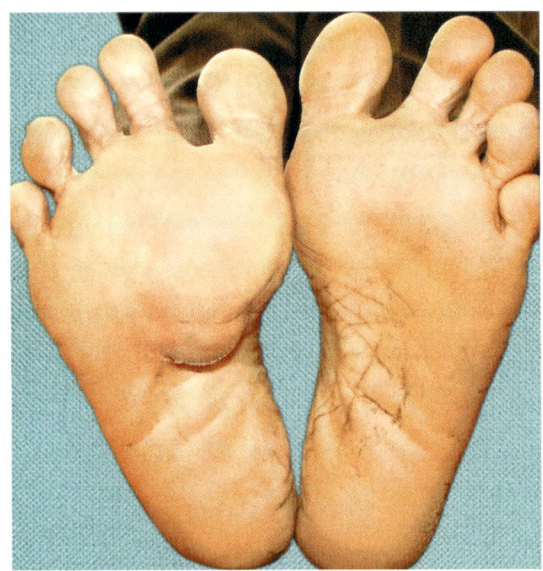

Fig. 4.102: Implantation dermoid cyst following sharp injury—value of comparison

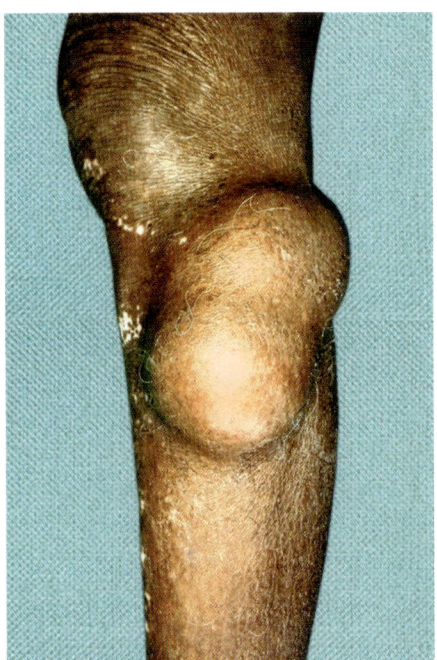

Fig. 4.103: Large cyst—lateral aspect of knee

2. *Bursa, bursitis*: It occurs in relation to joints/tendons, etc. It is soft and fluctuant. Hence, cystic swelling in relation to any joint should be considered as bursitis unless proved otherwise. Transillumination is negative because it contains inflammatory fluid. Some adventitious bursae have been given below.

   * *Tailor's ankle:* Above the lateral malleolus
   * *Porter's shoulder:* Between clavicle and skin
   * *Weaver's bottom:* Between gluteus maximus and ischial tuberosity
   * *Bunion:* Between prominent head of the first metatarsal and skin due to hallux valgus.

3. *Cystic swelling around knee joint*

   Anteriorly
   * Housemaid's knee (carpet-layer knee): Pre-patellar bursitis
   * Clergyman's knee: Intrapatellar bursitis

   Medially
   * Cyst of medial meniscus
   * Bursa anserina: It is a bursa between tendons of sartorius, gracilis and semitendinosus.

   Laterally
   * Cyst of lateral meniscus (4 times more common)
   * Synovial cysts (proximal tibiofibular joint)

   Posteriorly
   * Baker's cyst (popliteal cyst)
   * Semimembranosus bursitis.

4. *Haematoma*: This develops after trauma. Short duration of the swelling, sudden development of a swelling, pain and tenderness, and fluctuation will help in the diagnosis. Spontaneous knee haematomas are characteristic of haemophilia cases.

5. *Lipoma, neurofibroma*: Subcutaneous plane or in the deeper plane. Please note these two are common subcutaneous swellings. The characteristic features of both are present when these are in the subcutaneous plane. However, when these are deep, signs need not be classical. Example: Slip sign is difficult to elicit when lipoma is subfascial or intermuscular.

6. *Congenital AV fistula*
   * Present since birth
   * Soft, fluctuant, transillumination—negative, **pulsatile swelling**. A continuous bruit/murmur is characteristic.

- **Nicoladoni sign or Branham sign:** On compressing the feeding artery, the venous return to the heart diminishes, resulting in fall in pulse rate and pulse pressure.

- Proximal compression test: On compressing feeding artery, pulsation or **continuous murmur** may also disappear and swelling will diminish in size.

- The affected part is swollen (because of high pressure)—**local gigantism**. Thus, overgrowth of the limb or toe can occur.

- Distal to the AV fistula, there are **ischaemic ulcers**, due to comparative reduction in the blood supply.

- Angiography with **DSA** (digital subtraction angiography) pictures is essential before treating these patients.

- Therapeutic embolisation is the treatment of choice for arteriovenous fistula in congenital cases.

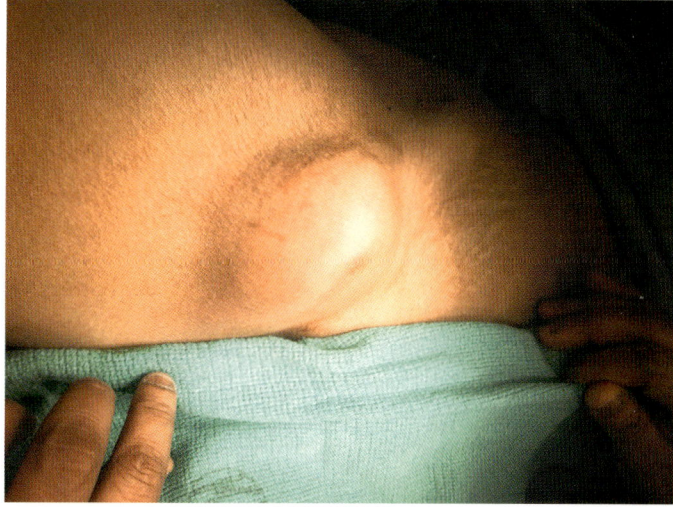

Fig. 4.104: Pseudoaneurysm femoral artery following angiogram

CLINICAL DISCUSSION

What is the danger of AV fistula?

- If the AV fistula is big, a high output cardiac failure can occur.

What are the other causes of local gigantism?

- Diffuse lipomatosis, diffuse neurofibromatosis and filariasis are the other causes of local gigantism.

What are the other pulsatile swellings?

- AV fistula, haemangiomas, aneurysms and vascular sarcomas.

7. *Traumatic AV fistula*: Leg is a common site for pseudoaneurysm because it is vulnerable for trauma. Trauma such as fracture of the tibia or fibula is followed a few years later by a swelling in the leg. Site of fistula may be little away from the fracture site. Careful examination reveals a sign of compressibility and continuous murmur. Acquired lesion may be observed or treated by quadruple ligation (Figs 4.104 to 4.106).

Thus, the old teaching/dictum, before you incise a swelling, look for

- **T**emperature
- **T**enderness
- **A**spiration
- **A**uscultation

You can remember as TATA

8. *Soft tissue sarcoma*: History of trauma is often present. Liposarcoma, MFH, and synovial sarcoma can occur in the leg. Short duration, rapid growth,

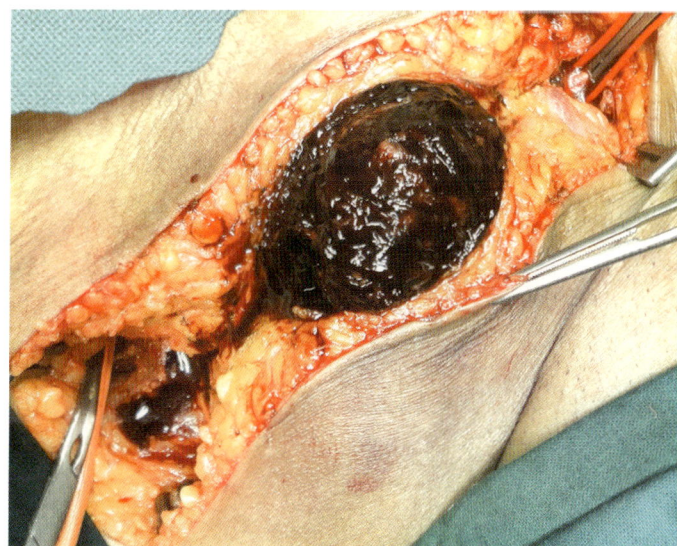

Fig. 4.105: Large clot at exploration

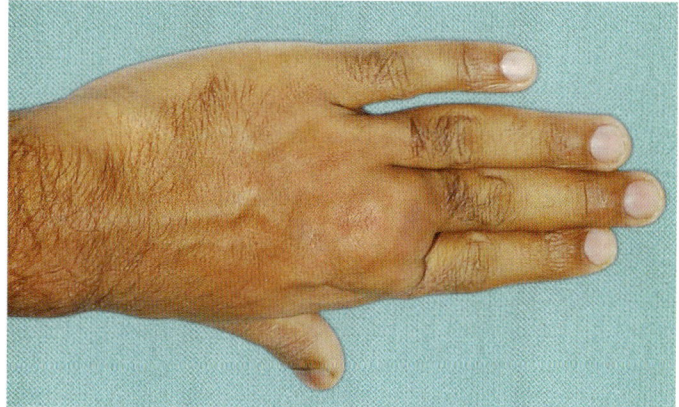

Fig. 4.106: Acquired AV fistula left hand

absent fever and pain are the symptoms. On examination, local rise of temperature, firm to hard swelling with restricted mobility and fixity are the features. Remember to examine regional lymph nodes.

COMMON SWELLINGS IN THE AXILLA

1. *Lymph node swelling*: Common causes of lymph node enlargement can be: (a) Metastasis, (b) lymphoma, and (c) tuberculosis.

   • Any round or nodular swelling in the known anatomical site of the lymph nodes should be considered as lymph node swelling unless proved otherwise.

   • Remember to examine all group of lymph nodes in such cases

   • Examine the drainage areas

   • Examine liver and spleen

   • Examine for any bony tenderness

   a. *Metastasis*: Classically nodes are hard, larger and with or without fixity. Try to recollect the drainage areas of the axilla. In a female, carcinoma breast should be considered first. Lump may not be palpable clinically. Bronchogenic carcinoma can metastasise to axillary nodes. It should be the diagnosis in male, elderly smokers. Cough, haemoptysis and age may give the clue. Search also for any cutaneous malignant lesions such as malignant melanoma of the chest or back and upper limb.

   • Left axillary lymph node enlargement in carcinoma of the stomach is called **Irish node.**

   b. *Lymphoma*: Both Hodgkin's and non-Hodgkin's lymphomas can have big lymph nodes in the axilla. These are firm or rubbery, not matted. Other lymph nodes in the neck with or without spleen and liver give the clue to the diagnosis (Fig. 4.107).

   c. *Tuberculosis*: Axilla is one of the sites. Spread is from pulmonary tuberculosis. Lymph nodes are firm, matted with or without cold abscess. Sinus formation is the hallmark of tuberculosis. Neck nodes are usually present.

2. **Lipoma**: Classically it is soft, lobular, and fluctuant swelling. You may get an impression of compressibility but in fact it is displacement. Being a universal tumour, any soft swelling in the axilla, lipoma should be one of the DD (Fig. 4.108).

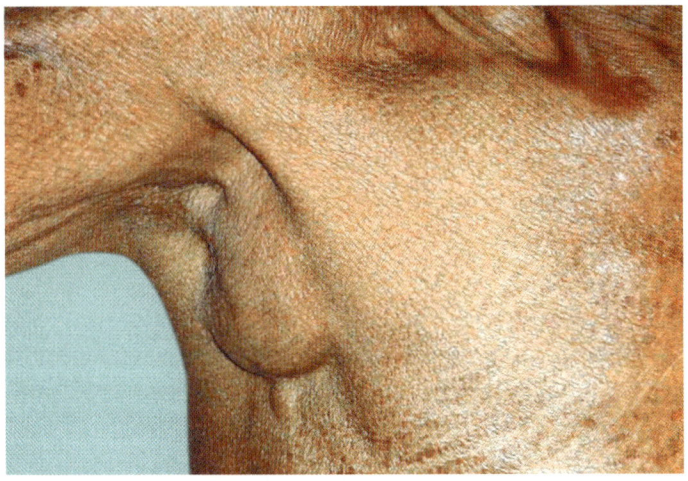

Fig. 4.107: Axillary nodes in lymphoma

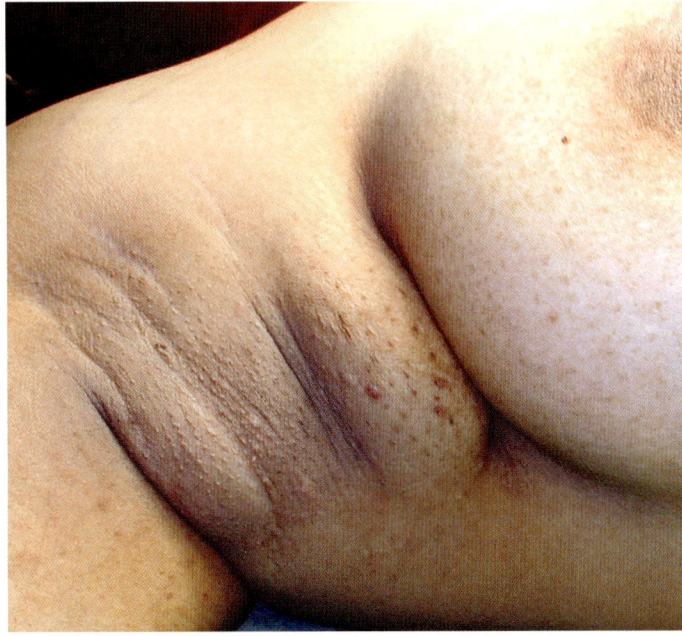

Fig. 4.108: Lipoma—axillary region

3. *Hidradenitis suppurativa*

   • It is an *infection of the apocrine sweat glands*. (Boil is an infection of hair follicles.)

   • Axilla is the commonest site. Groin is another site (in Caucasians).

   • Recurrent painful swelling with purulent discharge is characteristic (Fig. 4.109).

   • Chronic cases will have significant induration due to fibrosis.

   • Treatment is difficult—requires wide excision of the lesion with the overlying skin thus removing the focus of infection.

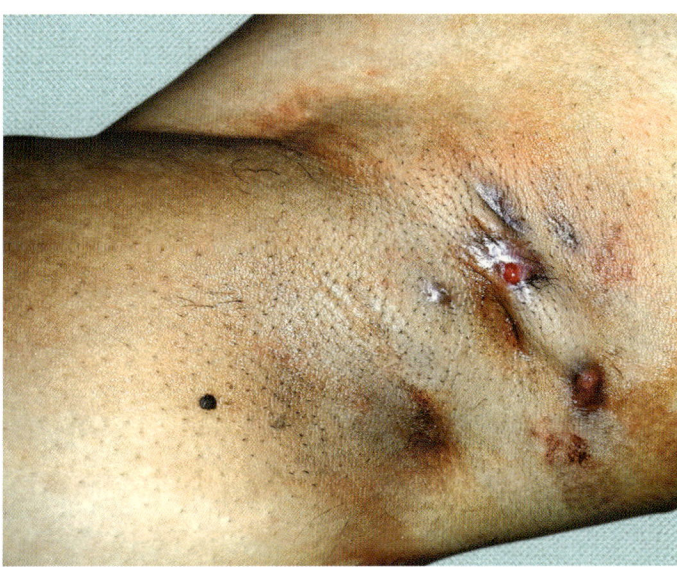

Fig. 4.109: Hidradenitis suppurativa

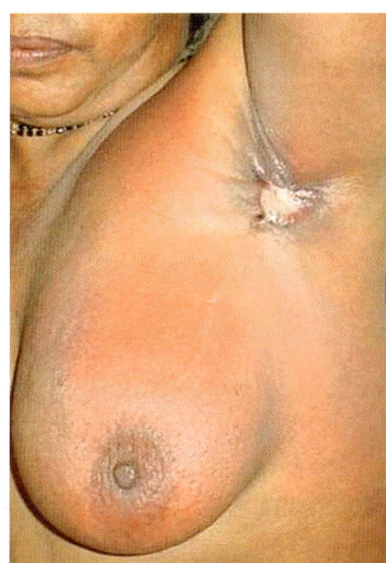

Fig. 4.111: Carcinoma axillary tail with fungation and lymphangitis of the breast

4. *Axillary tail hypertrophy*

- It is usually bilateral.
- Typically presents with pain in the axilla and increasing swelling during menstruation.
- Patients are usually young.
- Reassurance and symptomatic treatment should be given.

5. *Accessory breasts*: They are also called polymastia or supernumerary breasts. Axilla is one of the sites. It can be affected by all the diseases that can affect normal breast. Nipple/areola may or may not be present (Fig. 4.110).

6. *Carcinoma arising from tail of the breast*

- Typically presents as increasing swelling in the axilla which is painless (Fig. 4.111).

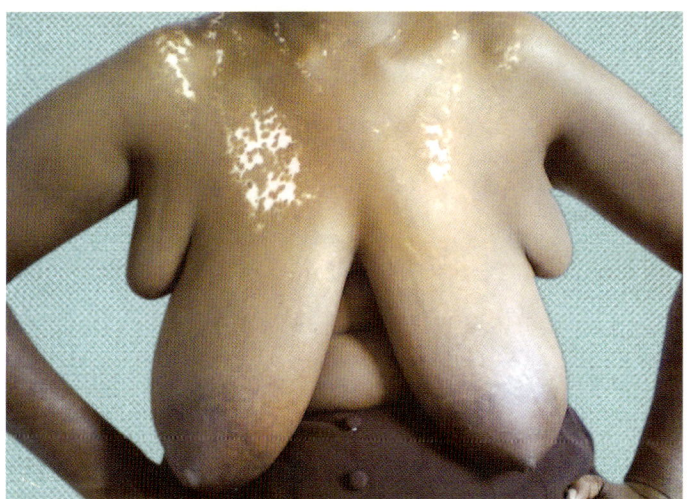

Fig. 4.110: Accessory breasts

- It is hard and irregular.
- Oedema of the breast in the infraclavicular region and palpable lymph nodes in the axilla clinch the diagnosis.

7. *Lymphangioma/lymph cyst*

- Failure of one of the lymphatics to join the major lymph sac of the body results in a lymphangioma. Hence, it occurs in places where lymphatics are abundant.

  The common sites: Posterior triangle of the neck, axilla, mediastinum, groin, etc. In the neck, it is called cystic hygroma of the neck. As the sac has no communication with lymphatics by the time swelling appears, the lymph is absorbed and is replaced by thin watery fluid (mucus) secreted by endothelium. Hence, it is also called hydrocoele of the neck.

- When it is largely confined to subcutaneous plane, it is called **cystic hygroma**.

CLINICAL DISCUSSION

What are the types of lymphangioma?

1. Lymphangioma circumscriptum: If it is less than 5 cm across.
2. Lymphangioma diffusum: If they are more widespread.
3. Lymphoedema ab igne: If they form a reticulate pattern of ridges.

Why do lymphangiomas have sign of compressibility?

- Lymphangioma is a multilocular swelling consisting of aggregation of multiple cysts. These cysts may intercommunicate and sometimes may insinuate between muscle planes. Hence, it gives the sign of compressibility! However, **complete reducibility is not a feature.**

What is the nearest DD for carcinoma tail of the breast?

- Lymph nodal mass because both are deep to deep fascia. (Breast is subcutaneous structure except axillary tail of Spence.)

- Soft, cystic, fluctuant, partially compressible swelling.
- The swelling is **brilliantly transilluminant** because it contains clear fluid (watery lymph).

8. *Neurilemmoma/neurofibroma*
- Uncommon sites of neural tumours.
- Neurilemmomas are soft and neurofibromas are hard.
- During palpation, the patient may complain of tingling and numbness along the distribution of the nerve—It suggests neural tumour (Fig. 4.112).
- Hard, smooth, oval swelling in relation to nerves is neurofibroma.
- These may be a part of von Recklinghausen's disease.

9. *Aneurysm of axillary artery*: It is one of the sites of an aneurysm but not a common site. The swelling is pulsatile, compressible with thrill and bruit. The patients are above 60 years of age and the cause is atherosclerosis.

COMMON SWELLINGS IN THE BACK

1. *Sebaceous cyst*
- Back is one of the common sites.
- Multiple cysts are common.
- Sign of moulding, indentation and punctum clinches the diagnosis.

2. *Carbuncle*
- Nape of the neck is the commonest site.
- Multiple abscesses which communicate and open to the exterior with multiple openings (cribriform or sieve-like) are characteristic.
- Typically, the patient is diabetic.
- Local rises in temperature, tenderness and redness are the other features.

3. *Cold abscess*
- Back—paravertebral space is one of the common sites (Fig. 4.113).
- Typically patient presents with cough, backache and swelling.
- It is on one side of the spine.
- Swelling is soft, and fluctuant. Transillumination is negative, not mobile.
- Spine deformity or tenderness clinches the diagnosis.

4. *Soft tissue sarcoma*
- Back has lots of skeletal muscles and so, it is but natural to suspect soft tissue sarcoma. Usually, it is malignant fibrous histiocytoma.

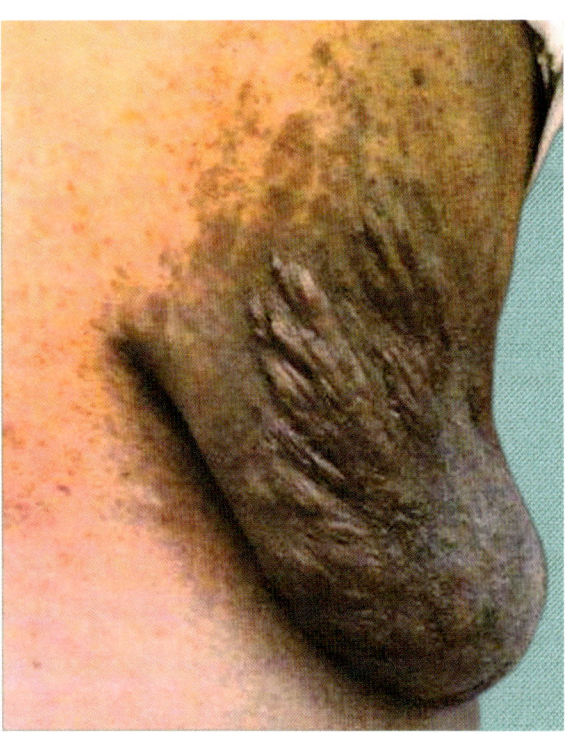

Fig. 4.112: Schwannoma in the axillary region

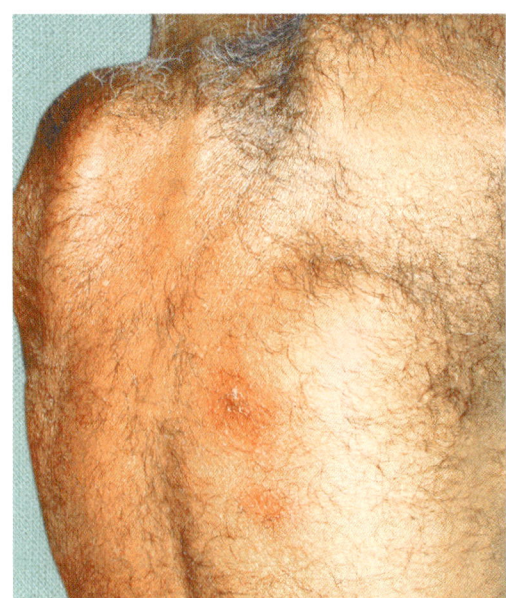

Fig. 4.113: Cold abscess back

- Typically rapidly growing, hard, irregular swelling with or without fixity.
- Chronic abscess, and cold abscess are DD.

5. *Lipoma*

- Soft to firm swelling with lobular surface and round borders, is a lipoma. If slip is present, it is a diagnostic sign.

6. *Meningocoele/meningomyelocoele (in newborns)*

A. *Meningocoele*

- **This is a type of spina bifida cystica.**
- In this condition, the neural arch is defective posteriorly. There is no visible swelling.
- It can be suspected when there is a tuft of hair, lipoma, naevus, pigmented patch of skin overlying the lumbosacral region.
- Child is normal at birth. Neurological symptoms, such as weakness, sciatica-like pain, may start appearing at puberty (neurogenic talipes equinus—club foot).
- During this time, because of growth, there may be traction on the spinal cord by a ligament called *membrana reuniens* (Fig. 4.114).
- X-ray can demonstrate the bifid spine.
- Surgical excision of the membrane gives permanent cure to the patient, if there are symptoms.

CLINICAL DISCUSSION

What are the complications of meningocoele?
- Skin covering the swelling is very thin and so, is prone for ulceration. Due to ulceration, secondary infection and meningoencephalitis can occur.
- Haemorrhage.

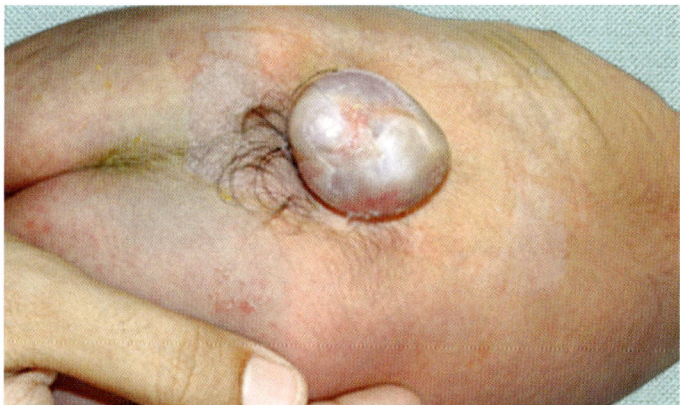

Fig. 4.114: Meningocoele. Lumbosacral region classical site

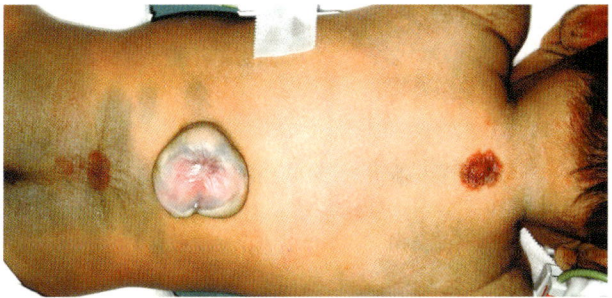

Fig. 4.115: Meningocoele, dermal sinus and pigmentation

B. *Meningomyelocoele:* Protrusion of meninges, with *nerve root of* **spinal cord or disordered spinal cord** results in meningomyelocoele. Neurological deficit such as **foot drop, talipes and trophic ulcer** of the foot (S1 root) may be present.

- Surgical excision may be followed by residual neurological deficit.

C. *Syringomeningomyelocoele*

- In this condition, in addition to the meninges, the central canal of spinal cord is also herniated out.
- Most of the children are stillborn.
- Very difficult to treat, if the child survives (Figs 4.115 and 4.116).

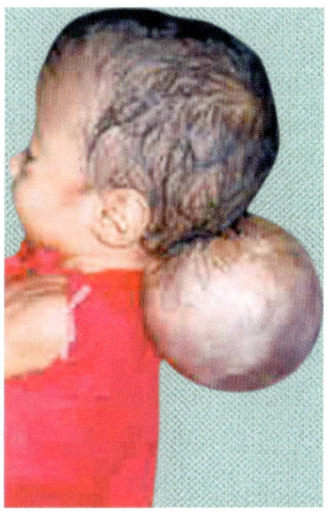

Fig. 4.116: Encephalocoele

COMMON SWELLINGS IN THE FACE

1. *Sebaceous cyst (lipoma is very rare in the face)*

- Face is one of the common sites of sebaceous cyst.
- All features mentioned earlier about sebaceous cyst will be present.

2. *Dermoid cyst:* Face is developed from 5 processes— two maxillary, two mandibular and one

frontonasal. Dermoid cysts tend to develop in the line of fusion of these processes.

- Typically, the swelling has a long duration (years).
- Slow-growing swelling in the midline or near the outer canthus of the eye.
- Swelling is soft and fluctuant, transillumination is negative and the swelling is mobile.
- On careful palpation, underlying bony depression can be felt. This is pathognomonic sign of congenital dermoid cyst.

3. *Plexiform neurofibroma*

- In this condition, branches of 5th cranial nerve are commonly affected.
- It can also involve the peripheries.
- The affected part is grossly thickened due to **fibromyxomatous degeneration**.
- Describe it as a swelling, with its extent and borders.
- Consistency will be soft to firm, and it is non-tender.

4. *Haemangioma*: It is an example for hamartoma. Capillary and cavernous—both varieties can occur here. Typical features of haemangioma are as follows:

- Most of them present since birth.
- Face, and lips are common sites.
- Either it is a patch or a swelling.
- Characteristic colour—bluish or purple.
- Soft, nontender, compressible swellings.
- Transillumination is negative.

Types of haemangioma

A. *Capillary haemangioma*: It consists of dilated capillaries and proliferation of endothelial cells. Hence, it commonly occurs in the skin. It can be of the following types (Fig. 4.117):

1. *Salmon patch* is a bluish patch over the forehead, in the midline, present at birth and disappears by 1 year of age. Hence, no treatment is required.
2. *Port-wine stain* is an extensive intradermal haemangioma. This is bluish purple in colour, commonly affects the face or other parts of the skin, is present at birth and usually progresses and does not regress (Fig. 4.118).
- It is a non-involuting capillary haemangioma.

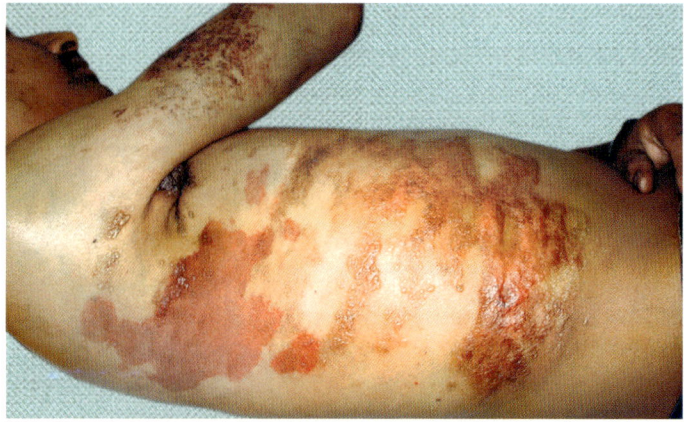

Fig. 4.117: Capillary haemangioma

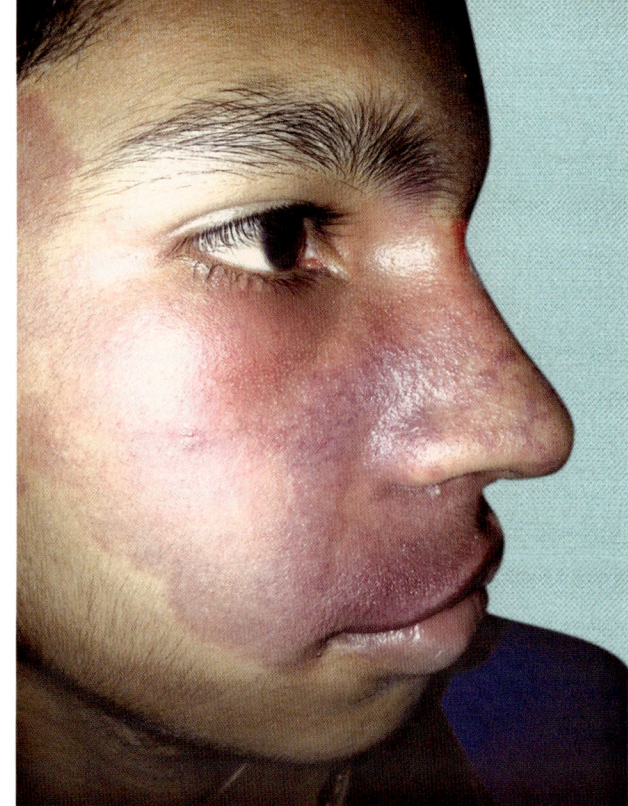

Fig. 4.118: Port-wine stain

- Area supplied by sensory branches of the fifth cranial nerve is involved.
- Start with light red colour and progress to deep colour.
- It may be associated with **Sturge-Weber syndrome.**

Clinical Wisdom

Flat, patchy lesion on the **face** in the area of **fifth** cranial nerve that **does not fade** is port-wine stain.

3. *Strawberry angiomas* produce swelling which protrude from the skin surface. The child is normal at birth. After a month, a **bright red swelling** appears over the head and neck region, which exhibits **sign of compressibility**. The lesion consists of immature vascular tissue. Even though the lesion grows initially, by 5–7 years of age, **swelling regresses and colour fades.** Hence, no specific treatment is necessary. The treatment is indicated only when the swelling persists. 70% resolve by 7 years of age.

B. *Venous (cavernous) haemangioma*

- This occurs in places where venous space is abundant, e.g. lip, cheek, tongue, and posterior triangle of the neck.

- History of a swelling in the neck of long duration. History of bleeding is present when it occurs in the oral cavity.

- The swelling is warm and **bluish in colour** but not pulsatile.

- Soft, fluctuant, transillumination is negative.

- **Compressibility** is present. This sign is also called 'sign of emptying' or 'sign of refilling'. When the swelling is compressed between the fingers, blood diffuses under the vascular spaces and when pressure is released, it slowly fills up. Compressibility is a diagnostic sign of haemangioma (Figs 4.119 and 4.120).

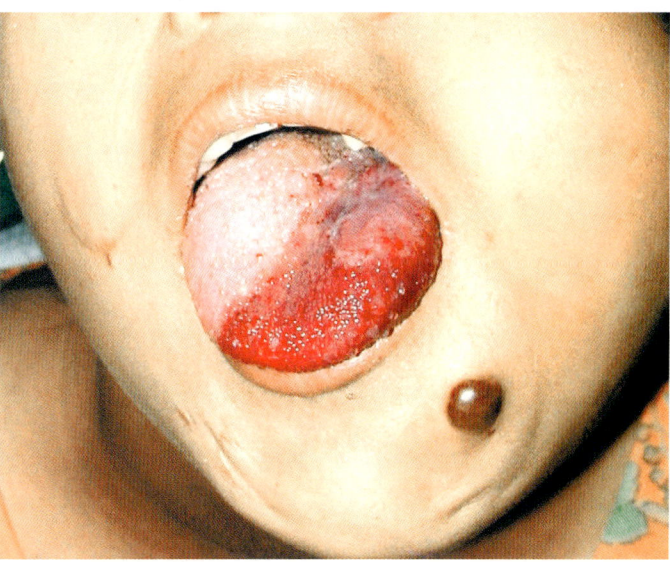

Fig. 4.120: You can also see the involvement of tongue

C. *Cirsoid aneurysm*

- Not an aneurysm.

- It is an AV fistula occurring in older people affecting the temporal region.

- The arteries and the veins are dilated and tortuous and are compared to pulsating bag of worms.

5. *Swellings in the parotid region*: Strictly speaking, parotid swellings are also swellings on the face—laterally. Since these are separate group of diseases, these are discussed in more detail along with salivary glands. For the sake of completion of the list, swellings in the parotid region are:

- Parotid tumours

- *Cysts in the parotid gland*: Haemangioma, lymphangioma

- *Preparotid lymph nodes*: Tuberculous, metastatic and lymphoma.

COMMON SWELLINGS IN THE CHEST WALL

1. *Common skin and subcutaneous swellings* can also occur here such as: Sebaceous cyst, lipoma, neurofibroma, and neurilemmoma.

2. *Cold abscess*: Lymph node swelling: Internal mammary nodes (also called sternal nodes) are present in the 4–5 intercostal spaces. The swelling is typically not in the midline but to one of the sides confined within first 3–4 intercostal spaces. It is soft, fluctuant, cystic and transillumination is negative. It is nontender (Figs 4.121 to 4.125).

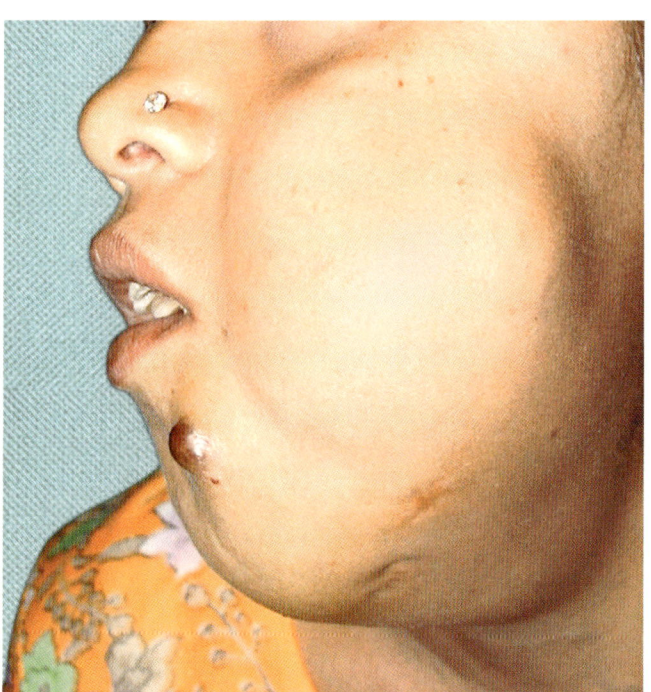

Fig. 4.119: Large haemangioma affecting cheek region

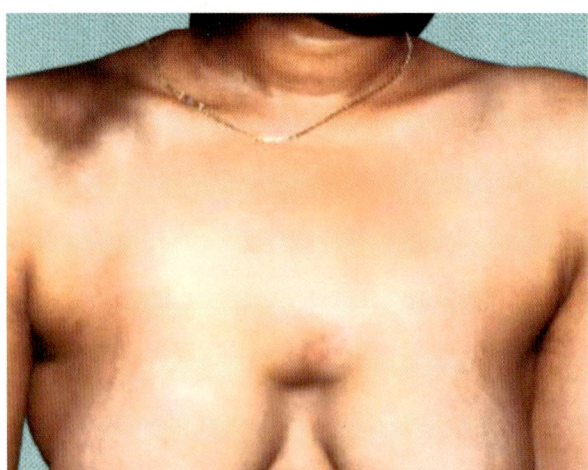

Fig. 4.121: Cold abscess—source is from internal mammary lymph nodes

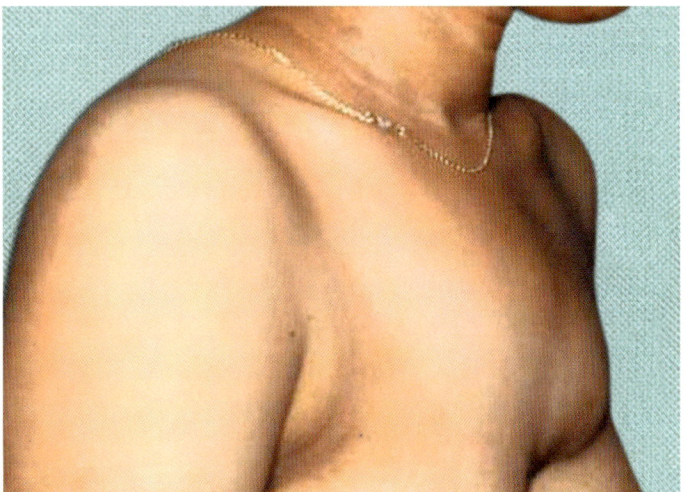

Fig. 4.122: Cold abscess chest wall lateral view (*Courtesy:* Dr Kshama Hegde, Assistant Professor, KMC, Manipal)

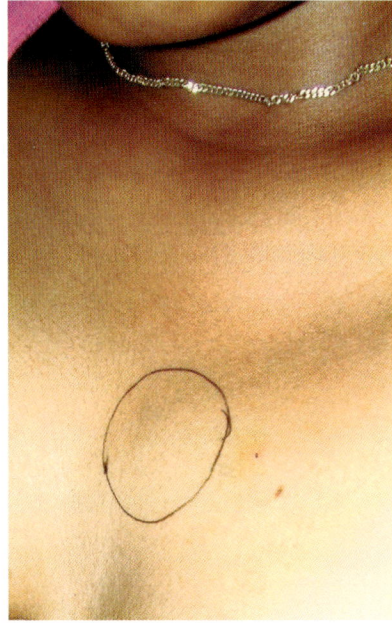

Fig. 4.123: Cold abscess from internal mammary lymph nodes

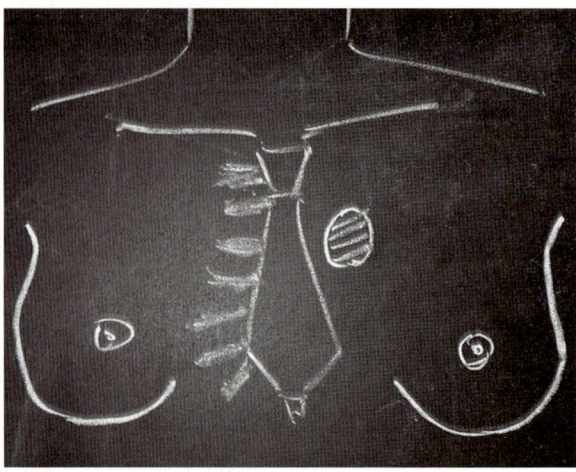

Fig. 4.124: Blackboard sketch to depict the exact site of internal mammary node as in Fig. 4.123

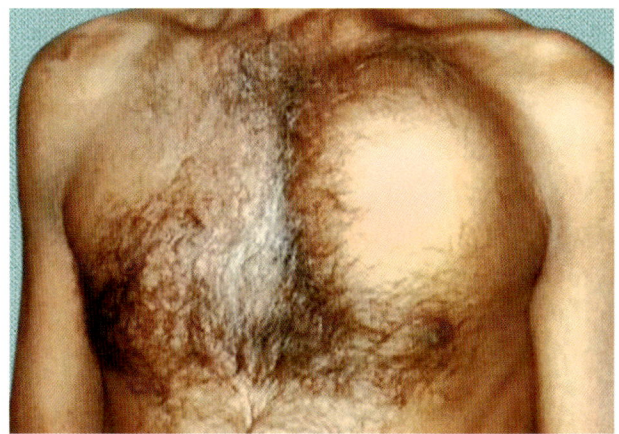

Fig. 4.125: Cold abscess—left chest wall (*Courtesy:* Dr Vidyadhar Kinhal, VIMS, Ballari): Check for impulse on coughing

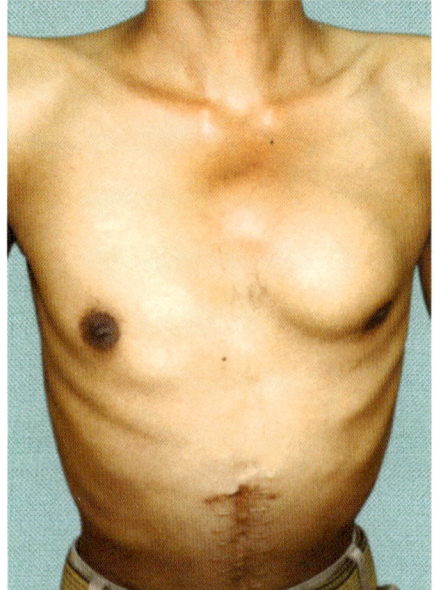

Any fluctuant swelling in the chest wall can be tuberculous cold abscess unless proved otherwise

Fig. 4.126: Cold abscess, the origin is from sternum. Look at the sternal bulge

- **Anatomy of the internal mammary nodes:** A node is one of the three groups of thoracic parietal lymph nodes. These are situated at the anterior ends of the intercostal spaces, adjacent to the internal thoracic artery. The afferent vessels of the sternal nodes drain the lymph from the breast, the diaphragmatic surface of the liver, and the deep ventral thoracic wall.

- **Cold abscess in the anterior chest wall:** It may be from any of the two sites:

  a. *Tuberculous rib or costal cartilage:* The involved rib will be tender and **rib is expanded.**

  b. *Tuberculous internal mammary nodes:* The internal mammary chain of lymph nodes does not extend below 6th intercostal space.

Clinical Wisdom

Suspect tubercular aetiology when an abscess is present in the neck, chest wall, paravertebral region, iliopsoas region and in mesentery.

Cold abscess in the posterior chest wall: It may be from any of the three sites:

a. Tuberculous rib or costal cartilage

b. Tuberculous dorsal vertebrae

c. Tuberculous perinephric abscess

3. *Soft tissue sarcoma:* Chondrosarcoma ribs are one of the common sites of chondrosarcoma. It presents as a slow-growing, painful enlargement and clinical examination reveals firm to hard, irregular swelling arising from bone (fixed to bone).

4. *Metastasis in the bones:* Pulsatile, tender bony swelling in the flat bones including ribs and sternum is usually from follicular carcinoma thyroid. Other causes are renal cell carcinoma, carcinoma branches, carcinoma breast, etc. (Fig. 4.127).

Clinical Wisdom

1. *Epidermoid cyst*: Sebaceous cyst: Punctum
2. *Dermoid cyst*: Location and bony depression
3. *Lipoma*: Slip sign
4. *Neurofibroma*: Swelling with coffee brown pigmentation (café au lait spots)
5. *Cystic hygroma*: Brilliantly transilluminant
6. *Haemangioma*: Sign of compressibility
7. *Metastasis in the bone*: Hard, irregular, pulsatile

SWELLINGS IN THE SCALP

Remember all the layers of the scalp and you can see that many swellings are related to these layers.

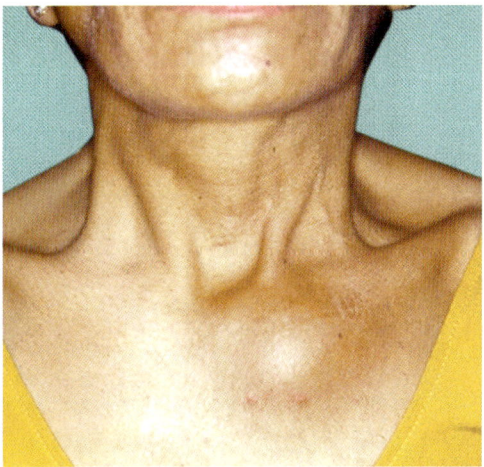

Fig. 4.127: Follicular carcinoma thyroid with metastasis in the ribs

Skin: Epidermoid cysts are very common. Epithelioma can also occur (Fig. 4.128).

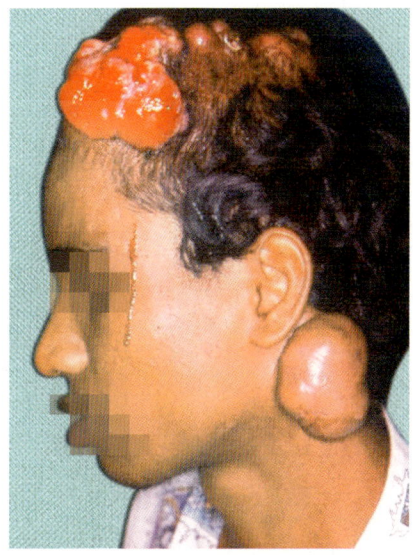

Fig. 4.128: Epithelioma of scalp with neck secondaries. Such large tumours are called as turbon tumours

Connective tissue: It is also a site of lipoma even though it is not common. Dermoid cysts (Fig. 4.129) can also occur along the line of fusion. These are common in young children but can also be found in adults. Multiple swellings in the scalp can also be part of multiple neurofibromatosis (Fig. 4.130).

Aponeurosis: It is called galea aponeurotica, the swelling deeper to it may not elicit any fluctuation.

Loose areolar tissue: Lipoma.

Periosteum: It is one of the sites of metastasis or secondary in the skull bone. They are vascular and pulsatile with bony erosion (Figs 4.131 and 4.132).

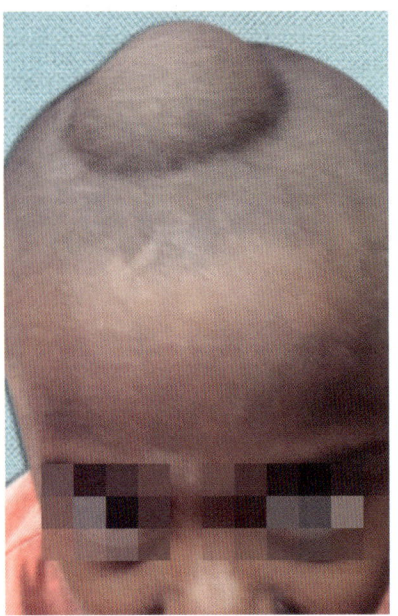

Any midline swelling over the scalp in young children impulse on coughing should be tested

Fig. 4.129: Dermoid cyst or lipoma? (*Courtesy:* Dr Srihari and Dr Ramaniah NV, Professors of Surgery, SVMC, Tirupathi)

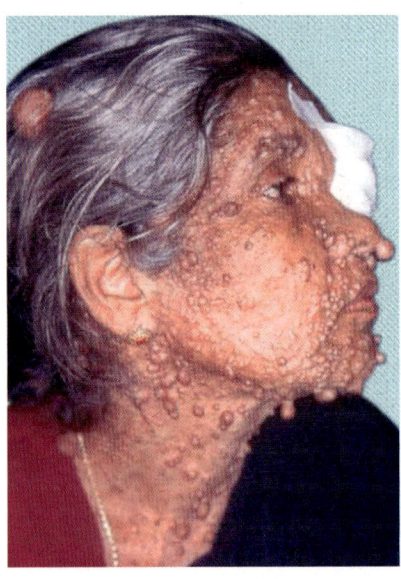

In cases of multiple neurofibromatosis examine the whole body. Presence of café au lait spots help in the diagnosis of von Recklinghausen's disease.

Fig. 4.130: von Recklinghausen's disease

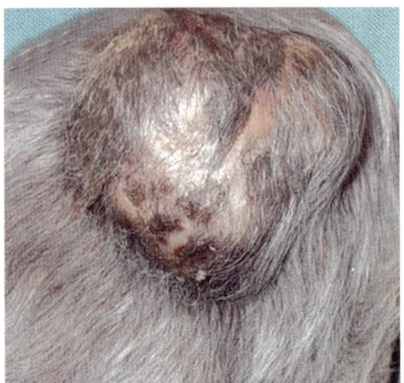

Skeletal metastasis in the scalp can be solitary or multiple. They are warm and tender and pulsatile with underlying bony erosion

Fig. 4.131: Metastasis from renal cell carcinoma—pulsatile, rapidly growing swelling in a 70-year-old man

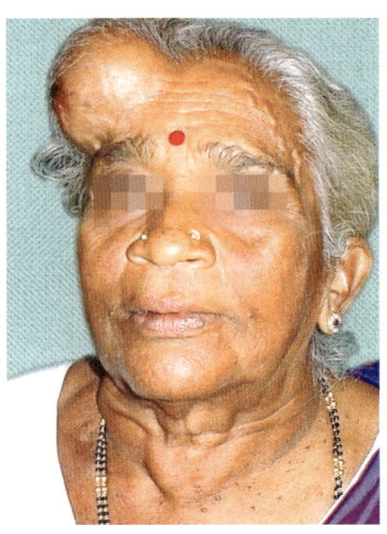

Fig. 4.132: Secondary deposit from follicular carcinoma thyroid—it was pulsatile

Turban Tumour

- This is referred to any large swellings/tumours over the scalp. Few features have been summarized in the Clinical Box 4.8 and Fig. 4.133.

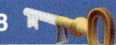

Clinical Box 4.8

Turban tumour of scalp
- Very rare
- They can be single or multiple
- Small or massive
- They arise from skin appendages
- Histologically they have thick hyalinised band of collagen
- They are benign
- Rarely may change to basal cell or squamous cell carcinoma

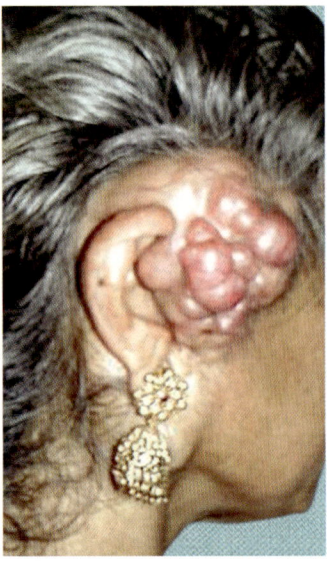

Fig. 4.133: Turban tumour of the temporal region (*Courtesy:* Dr Srijayan, Prof of Surgery, Calicut Medical College, Calicut)

Quick Analysis of Swellings Based on Consistency		
Soft	**Firm**	**Hard**
1. Sebaceous cyst • Putty • Sign of indentation • Sign of moulding	1. Neurofibroma • Firm • Mobile • Tender	1. Secondaries in the lymph nodes • Hard • Nodular • Restricted mobility
2. Underlying bony depression—dermoid cyst	2. Lymph nodes • Tuberculosis • Lymphoma	2. Fibromatosis • Hard • Irregular • Fixed
3. Fluctuant, slip sign is present—lipoma	3. Fibrolipoma	3. Bony lesion • Cervical rib • Metastasis in bones • Bony tumours
4. Fluctuant swelling anterior triangle of neck • Branchial cyst • Cold abscess	4. Carotid body tumour—pulsatile	
5. Transilluminant swelling A. Lymphangioma B. Ranula	5. Soft tissues sarcoma • Variable consistency—soft, firm, hard • Vascular • Local rise of temperature	
6. Transillumination negative compressible—haemangioma		
7. Continuous murmur/thrill—AV fistula		

5

Examination of a Sinus and Fistula

INTRODUCTION

Sinus or fistula can be short case in the examination. Often students get worried thinking what is there to examine? I am seeing only one opening. I do not know how to describe it. Yes, you are right. It is not like a swelling which can be described in its usual manner like size, shape, surface, etc. That is why it is important that you have a good idea about a sinus/fistula.

SINUS (Fig. 5.1)

Very often it is a spot diagnosis. Once you get the diagnosis, rest will be easy.

It is a blind track leading from the surface down into the tissues. It is lined with granulation tissue. Following are a few examples:

1. *Congenital sinus*: Preauricular sinus/postauricular sinus (Fig. 5.2).

2. *Acquired sinus*: Examples:

   • *Median mental sinus*: Occurs as a result of tooth abscess (Fig. 5.3).

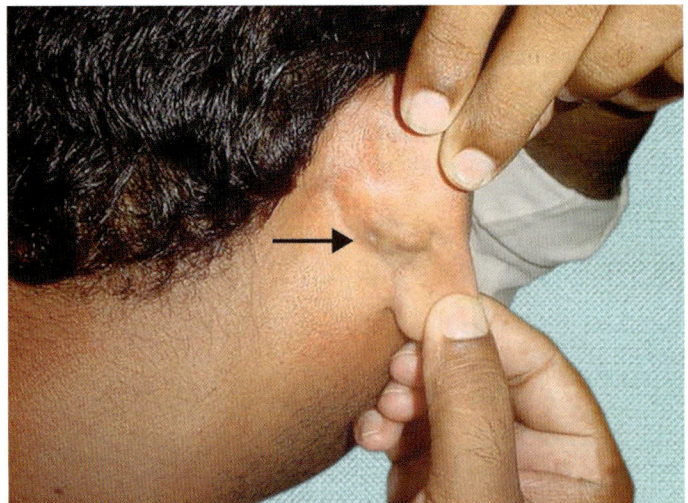

Fig. 5.2: Postauricular sinus

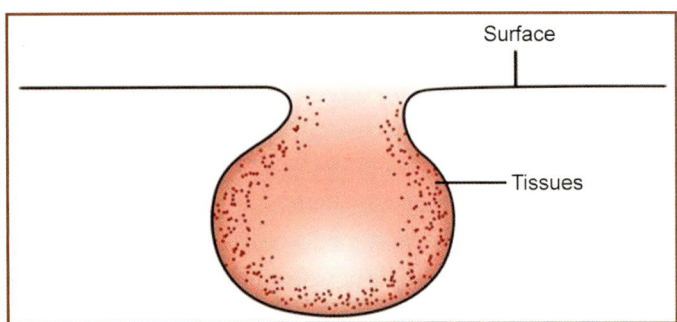

Fig. 5.1: Sinus

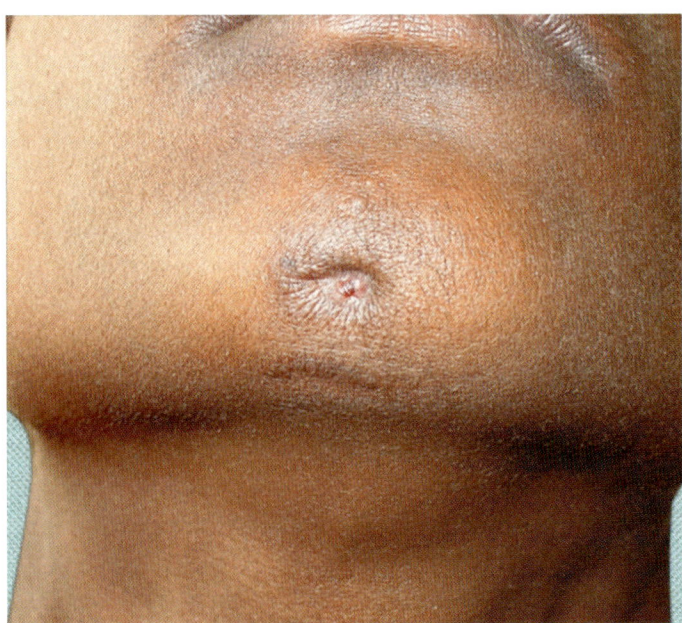

Fig. 5.3: Median mental sinus

- *Pilonidal sinus*: Occurs in the midline in the anal region (Fig. 5.4).
- *Osteomyelitis*: Gives rise to sinus discharging pus with or without bony spicules (Fig. 5.5).
- **Port site sinus:** It has become common now because of retained stones following laparoscopic cholecystectomy or due to persistent infected suture material.
- Commonest sinus in the neck is due to tubercular lymphadenitis. It discharges cheesy material. Skin surrounding the sinus shows bluish discolouration (Fig. 5.6).

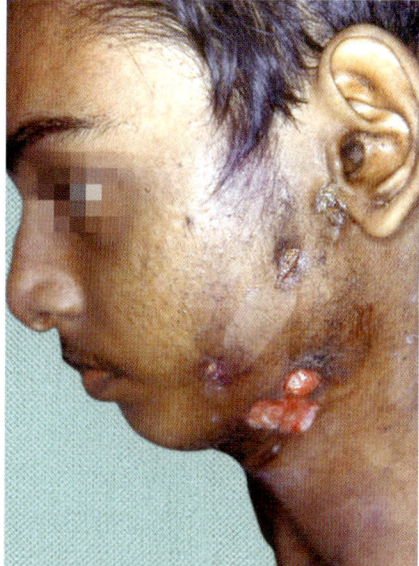

Fig. 5.6: Multiple tubercular sinuses

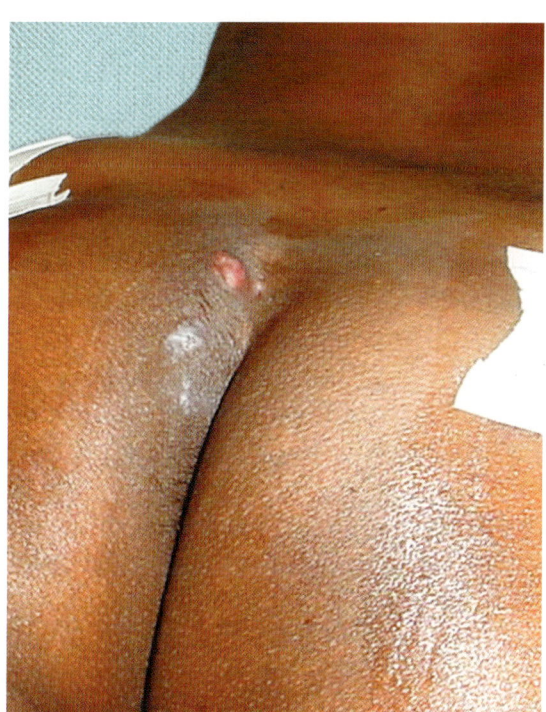

Fig. 5.4: Pilonidal sinus—multiple openings on one side of natal cleft

FISTULA

It is an abnormal communication between the lumen of one viscus and the lumen of another (internal) or communication of one hollow viscus with the exterior, i.e. body surface (external fistula) (Fig. 5.7).

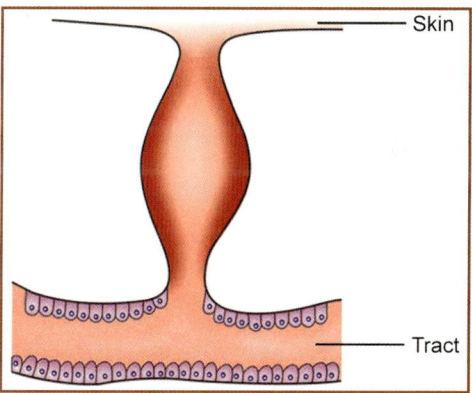

Fig. 5.7: Fistula

Examples of Internal Fistula

- Tracheo-oesophageal fistula
- Colovesical fistula

Examples of External Fistula

- Orocutaneous fistula due to carcinoma of the oral cavity infiltrating the skin
- Branchial fistula
- Thyroglossal fistula

*Causes of persistence of a sinus or fistula are given in Clinical Box 5.1.

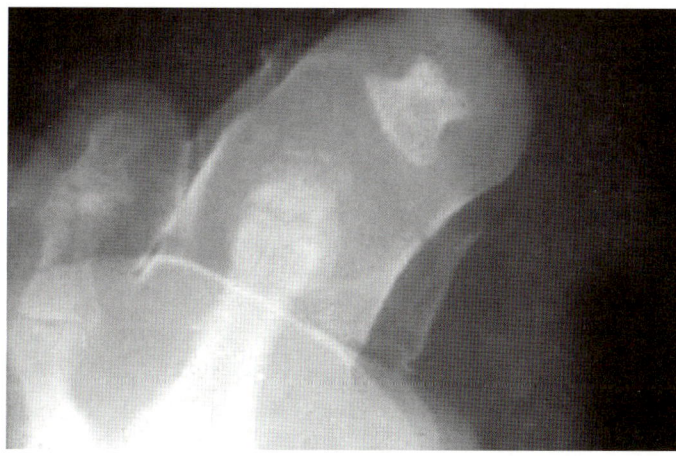

Fig. 5.5: Osteomyelitis of terminal phalanx in a diabetic patient

HISTORY

- When did you first notice the fluid (discharge) coming out? Is it since birth or did it develop later? Congenital causes are present since birth. Acquired lesions appear later.

- Did you have any trauma? Did you undergo any surgical procedure? Trauma and retained foreign body such as bullets, pellets, thorn and suture materials can give rise to sinus. In fact in the surgical wards, so-called the stitch granuloma is an example of a sinus—due to infected foreign body such as sutures. Repeated trauma (minor) is responsible for madura foot (Fig. 5.8).

- Did you have pain first and later swelling appeared and got ruptured? Typically seen in children and in osteomyelitis. Pain, fever, recurrent swelling and rupture are also seen in pilonidal sinus and umbilical sinus. Pilonidal sinus, cold abscess and vast majority present as a swelling first and rupture later (Fig. 5.9).

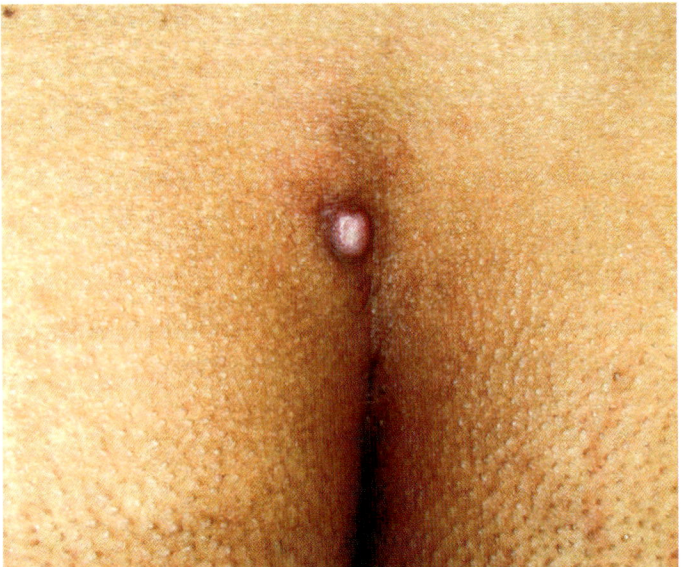

Fig. 5.9: Pilonidal sinus. This is how it starts—as an abscess, early case

- What is the colour and nature of discharge? Serous fluid is seen when there is no infection as in branchial cyst. White, thick, cheesy discharge is typical of tubercular sinus.

- Does it smell? Foul smell is typically due to mixed infections. In abdominal sinus, foul odour is not due to *Escherichia coli* but caused by the proteolytic activity caused by anaerobic organisms.

- Did you notice any bony spicules? If present, it indicates osteomyelitis. In surgical wards, often diabetic ulcer over the calcaneal region or over the great toe may present with osteomyelitis. (Dead bone is called sequestrum.) In madura foot, multiple sinuses discharging yellow granules are typical.

- Cough with expectoration, multiple sinuses in the region of lymph nodes, evening rise in temperature suggests tubercular aetiology.

- Discharge of faecal matter in faecal fistula and urine in urinary fisula are unmistakable (Fig. 5.10).

PAST HISTORY

- Specific chronic diseases in the past such as tuberculosis, actinomycosis.

- Ulcerative colitis, Crohn's disease.

- Any previous surgery: Post-appendicectomy fistula, laparotomy scar sinuses (foreign body—infected stitch, sinus following mesh repair is due to infected mesh) (Fig. 5.11).

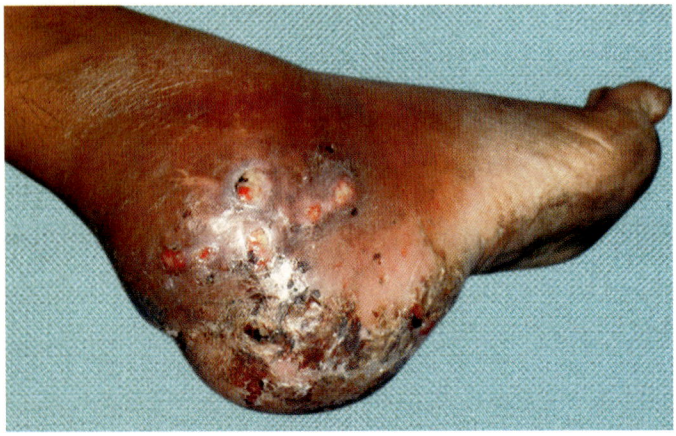

Fig. 5.8: Madura foot—multiple sinuses

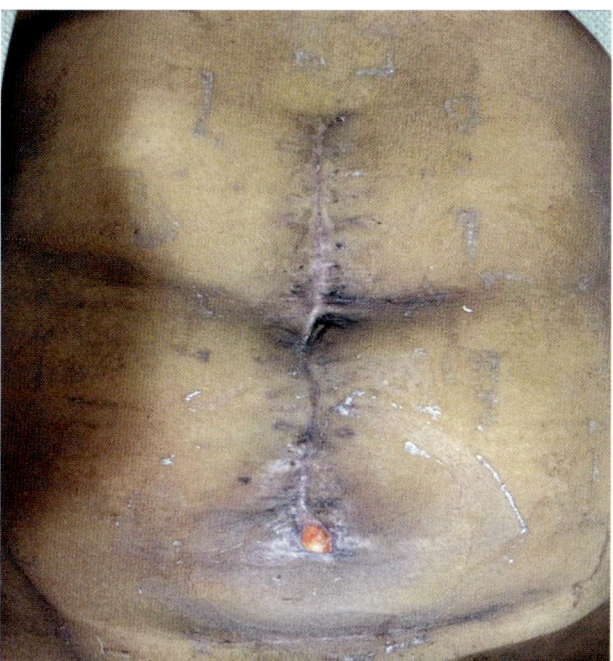

Fig. 5.10: Faecal fistula following resection anastomosis of ileal perforation. On 7th day, seropurulent fluid comes out and later, bile-stained fluid comes out. It is a fistula

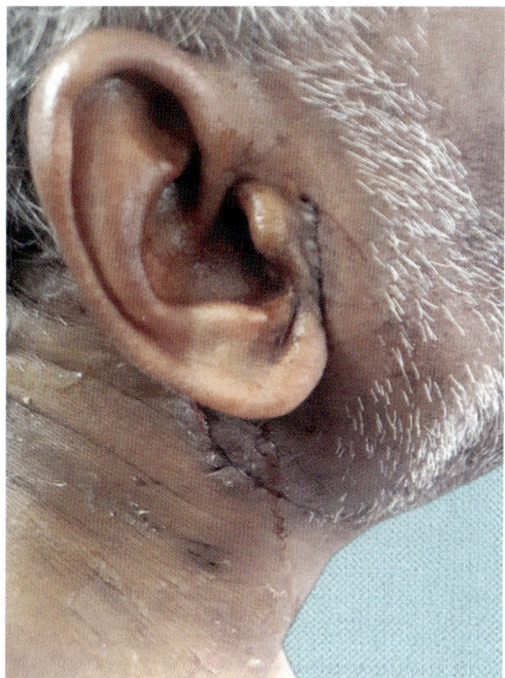

Fig. 5.12: Salivary fistula

Fistulas

- *Branchial fistula:* Anterior border of lower third of sternomastoid (Fig. 5.13).
- *Parotid fistula:* In the parotid region.
- *Thyroglossal fistula:* Midline of neck below hyoid bone.
- *Appendicular fistula:* Right iliac fossa.

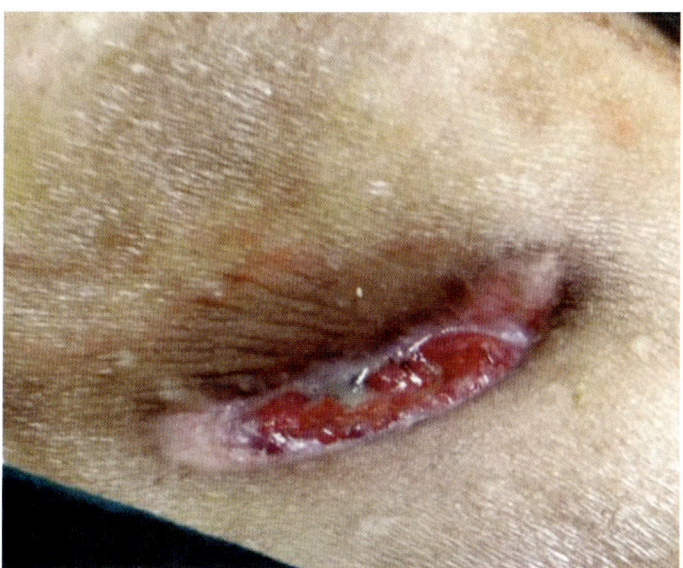

Fig. 5.11: Appendicular fistula

- Any laparoscopic surgeries.
- Salivary fistula may follow after superficial parotidectomy (Fig. 5.12).

LOCAL EXAMINATION

Inspection

1. *First mention the exact location/position of the sinus or fistula:* **Location** gives the diagnosis in majority of the cases of sinus or fistula.

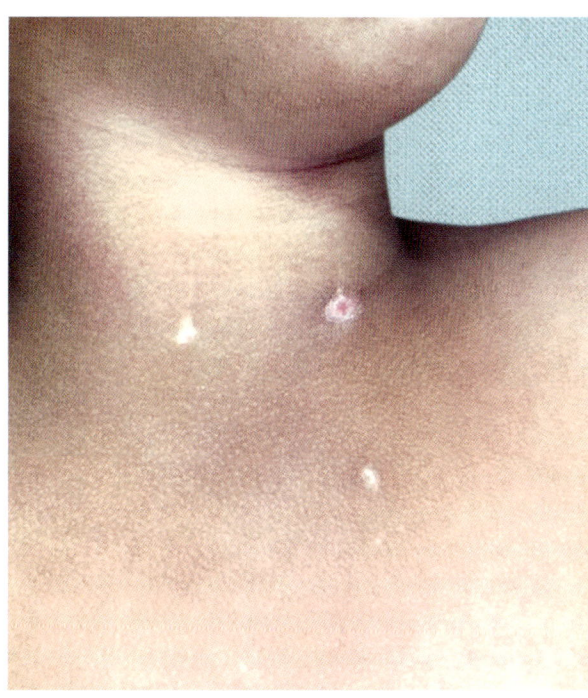

Fig. 5.13: Branchial fistula

- Sinus in the chest wall—could be a tubercular aetiology from *ribs*, cold abscess (Fig. 5.14).
- Multiple sinuses in the axilla are due to hidradenitis suppurativa (Fig. 5.15).

Sinuses

- *Preauricular sinus:* Front of root of helix of ear due to failure of fusion of ear tubercles. Direction of the sinus is upwards and backwards.
- *Median mental sinus:* Symphysis menti.
- *Tubercular sinus:* Neck, chest wall, groin, paravertebral (areas of cold abscess).
- *Lymphogranuloma:* Groin.

2. *Number:* It can be single or multiple.
   - Branchial sinus, median mental sinus, and preauricular sinus are single in number. On the other hand, actinomycotic and tubercular sinuses are multiple (Fig. 5.16).
   - One cannot mistake multiple sinuses in the scrotum due to stricture urethra, resulting in watering-can perineum.

3. *Opening*
   - Sprouting granulation tissue is also called proud flesh. It suggests underlying foreign body or infected bone (Fig. 5.17).
   - Flush with skin—tuberculosis (Fig. 5.18).

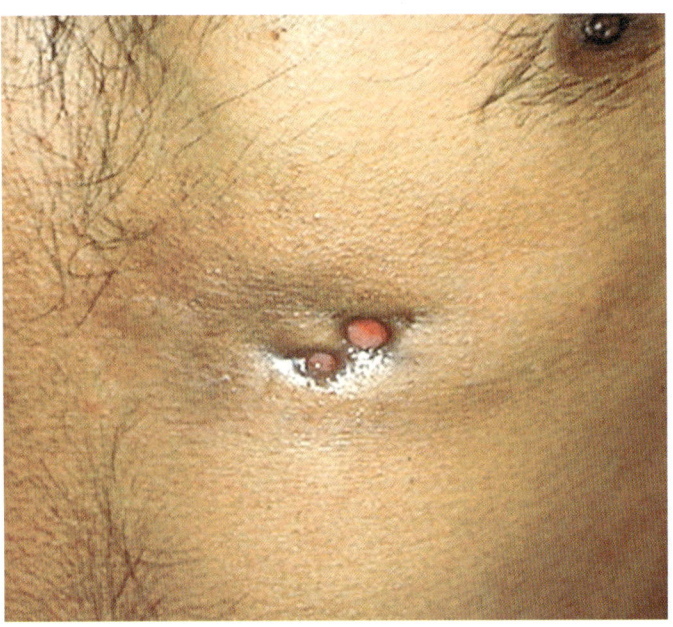

Fig. 5.14: Tuberculous sinus fixed to 6th rib. Bony erosion found on X-ray

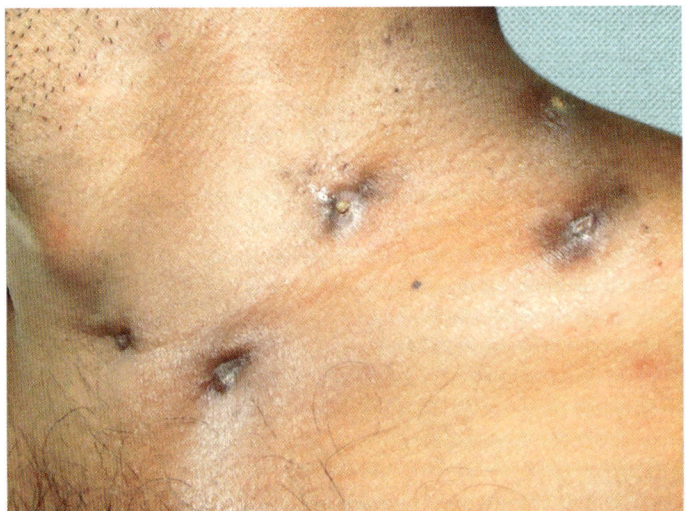

Fig. 5.16: Recurrent sinuses in drug-resistant tuberculosis

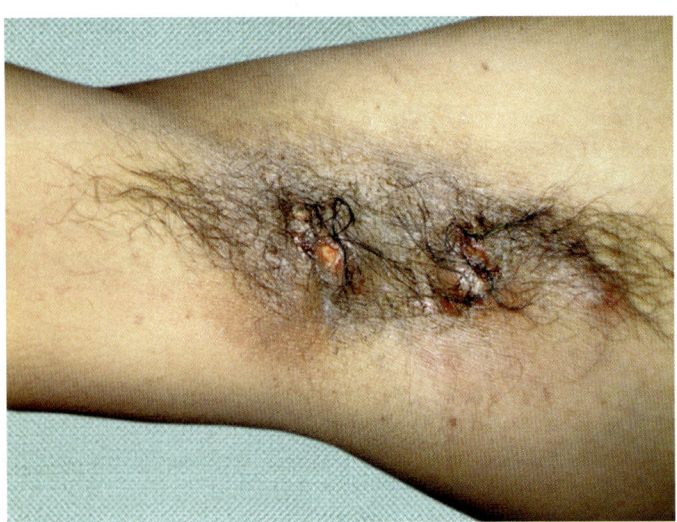

Fig. 5.15: Hidradenitis suppurativa

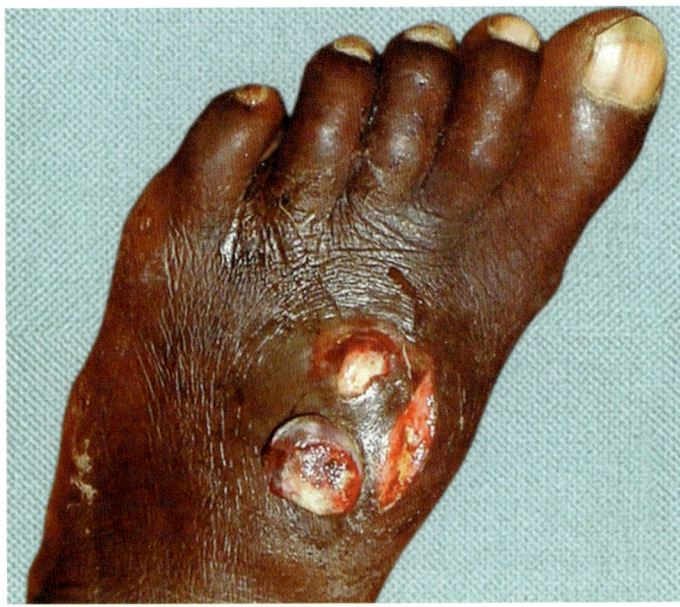

Fig. 5.17: Nonhealing multiple sinuses due to foreign body

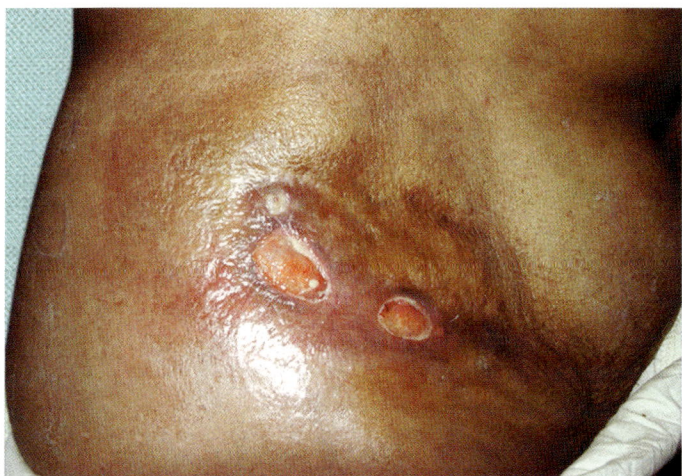

Fig. 5.18: Wide mouth sinus due to tuberculosis. The edge is in flush with the skin

4. *Discharge*

- White thin caseous—tuberculosis
- Yellow purulent—staphylococci
- Yellow granules—actinomycosis
- Thin mucus discharge—branchial fistula
- Urine—urinary fistula
- Faecal—faecal fistula

5. *Surrounding skin*

- Red, angry looking—inflammatory (Fig. 5.19)
- Bluish discolouration—tuberculosis
- Pigmentation—chronic sinus (Fig. 5.20)
- Skin excoriation—faecal fistula (Fig. 5.21)

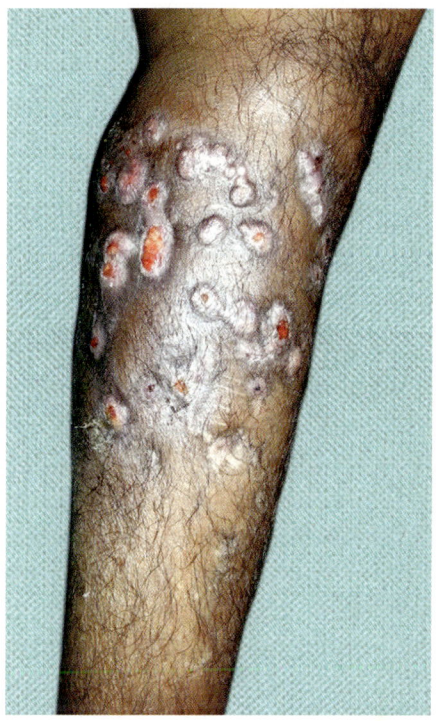

Fig. 5.20: Actinomycosis leg—multiple sinuses (*Courtesy:* Dr Reetesh Shetty, Dr Kshama Hegde, Dr Vijendra, Department of Surgery, KMC, Manipal)

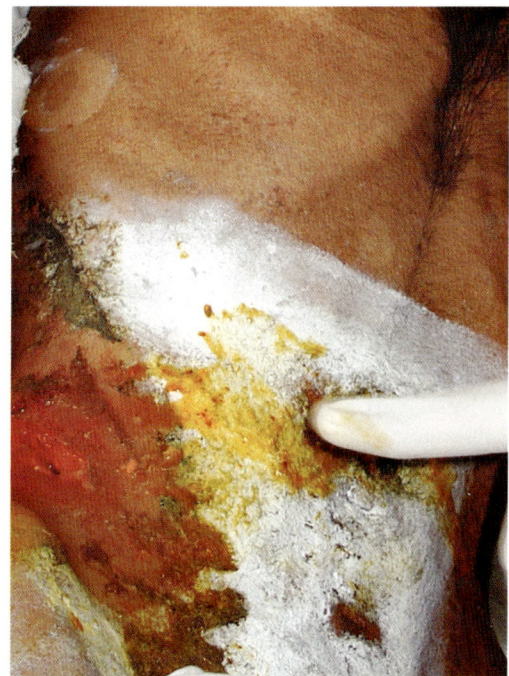

Fig. 5.21: Faecal fistula with extensive skin excoriation

6. *Any operative or traumatic scars*

- Mention the nature of the scar—length, location, healing, etc.
- Mention which part of the scar has sinus/sinuses.

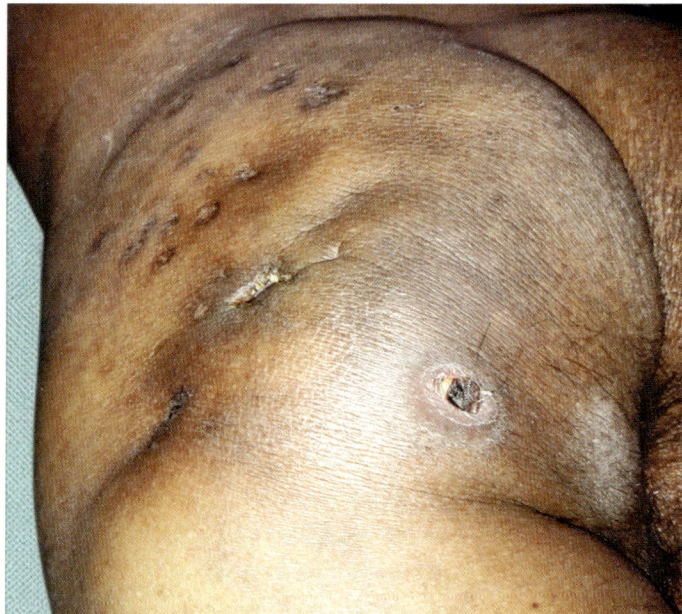

Fig. 5.19: Multiple sinuses in the gluteal region in a patient who was an addict to injection fortwin (pentazocine)

Palpation

1. Temperature and tenderness is increased, if there is inflammation of the sinus, e.g. pilonidal sinus.

2. Discharge after application of pressure. It suggests nature of fluid. White cheesy material can be due to TB sinus.

3. *Wall thickness*: Induration is present in chronic fistula, osteomyelitis, etc.

   • In tubercular sinus, induration is absent.

   • Marked induration is characteristic of actinomycosis.

4. *Fixity*: Try to pick the sinus opening and try moving. Osteomyelitis sinus is fixed to the bone and median mental sinus may be fixed to the jaw bone. The underlying bone in such cases is irregular and thickened.

5. *Palpation at a deeper plane*

   • Enlarged nodes in tuberculosis or lymphogranuloma venereum.

   • Thickening of mandible or bone

   • Submandibular stone may be palpable as in submandibular fistula.

   • Tenderness and lump at depth suggests an underlying abscess—secondary infection

6. *Examination with probe*: The only advantage of this test is one can assess the depth of the sinus and can also find out is it skin deep, muscle deep or bone deep. Probe test can cause discomfort, pain and minor bleeding also. *Since disadvantages are more* than *advantages, better not to probe* any *sinus or fistula.* (The final assessment of the track and depth can be assessed by *sinogram* or *fistulogram* with or without CT scan, Fig. 5.22).

7. *Regional lymph nodes*: Lymph nodes are generally palpable because of secondary infection. Matted nodes are diagnostic of tubercular aetiology.

   Typical site of sinus/fistula is given in Clinical Box 5.2.

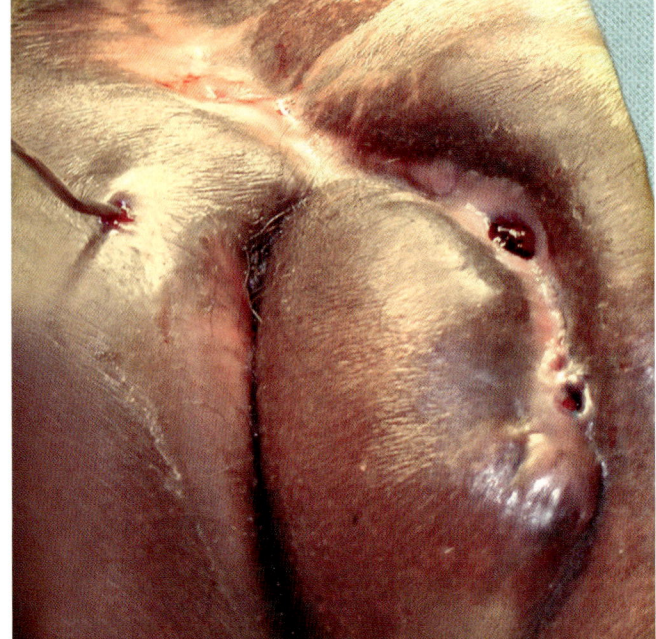

Fig. 5.22: Probe is passed into the opening of pilonidal sinus in the operation theatre

RELEVANT CLINICAL EXAMINATION

• Submandibular gland enlargement can be made out by bidigital examination.

• Alveolar abscess can be found as in median mental sinus—examine the mandible for thickness. Caries teeth may be present.

• Examine the long bones for thickness—osteomyelitis.

• Sinus in the loin: Examine ribs and spine to rule out tuberculosis. If there is urine smell in the discharge, examine the kidney. (Often it is not palpable but *it may harbor staghorn calculi.*)

• Chest examination in cases of sinus in the chest wall—empyema thoracis or tuberculous.

• Abdominal examination in abdominal sinus/fistula.

• Urethra, penis in cases of urinary fistula in the perineum.

• Per rectal examination and proctoscopy may reveal internal opening of the fistula (fistula in ano).

Clinical Box 5.2

Loin fistula/sinus: Staghorn

Intercostal space/chest: Tubercular

Anterior triangle neck: Branchial

Leg/foot: Osteomyelitis

Sinus chin: Median mental sinus

Clinical Wisdom

It is better to examine bones and joints (regional) in a case of sinus near the joint because tuberculosis is the most common cause of sinus in the body.

CLINICAL DISCUSSION

Why tuberculous sinuses take long time for healing?

- Because of the chronicity of the disease and often the track is lined by granulation tissue. Not only antituberculous treatment has to be given but also excision of the entire tract may have to be done.
- In actinomycosis, subcutaneous tissue is more involved than skin. Gross thickening of subcutaneous tissue with marked induration is characteristic.
- Wide mouth, blue colour, thin undermined edge and cheesy white discharge are characteristics of tuberculous sinus—often it looks like an ulcer.

What is watering-can perineum?

- Repeated dilatations of the urethral strictures can produce false passage and multiple openings in the skin. When these patients void urine, it flows out of these multiple openings in the perineal skin like a watering can. This is called watering-can perineum.

INVESTIGATIONS

1. Complete blood picture (**CBP**—haemoglobin %, total and differential count, erythrocyte sedimentation rate—**ESR**): **ESR** may be increased in cases of tuberculosis. Increased total count suggests infection.

2. Fasting blood sugar (**FBS**) and postprandial blood sugar (**PPBS**) to rule out diabetes.

3. **X-ray** of the part: Osteomyelitis of mandible; toe, also to look for foreign body (Fig. 5.5).

4. X-ray kidney, ureter, bladder region (**KUB**)—staghorn calculi as in lumbar urinary fistula.

5. Fistulography or sinography is done to know the exact extent or origin of the sinus or fistula.

6. Biopsy from the edge of sinus is done, if specific aetiology is suspected, e.g. tuberculosis, malignancy, etc.

DIFFERENTIAL DIAGNOSIS

1. *Tubercular sinus*: Common sites are neck, axilla, and groin. Source: Caseating lymph nodes, rupture and form collar stud and cold abscess. Sinuses in the vicinity of ribs, and costochondral junction originate from ribs. Sinus near the vertebral column originates from spine tuberculosis. Typically patients are young with constitutional disturbances such as fever with night sweats, loss of weight with or without cough and complain of discharging sinuses. Sinuses are single or multiple when they are originating from lymph nodes. Margin is undermined, edge is bluish in colour and opening is more like an ulcer with wide mouth. No induration. Underlying palpable lymph nodes, if present, clinch the diagnosis (Figs 5.23 to 5.25).

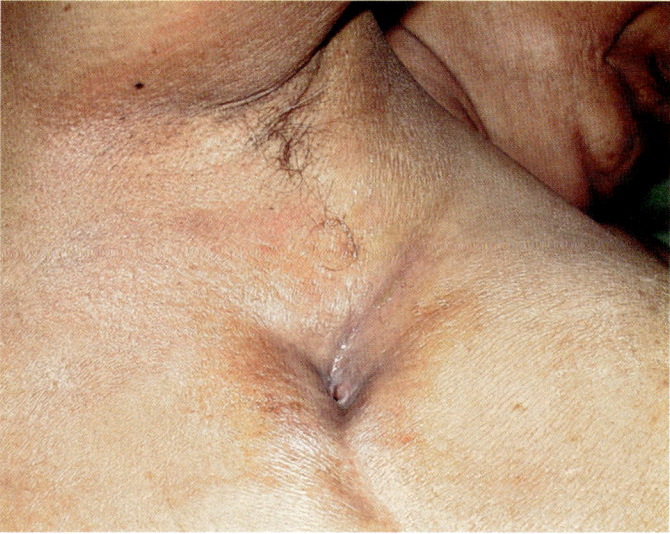

Fig. 5.23: Tubercular sinus in the axilla—source of infection is from axillary lymph nodes

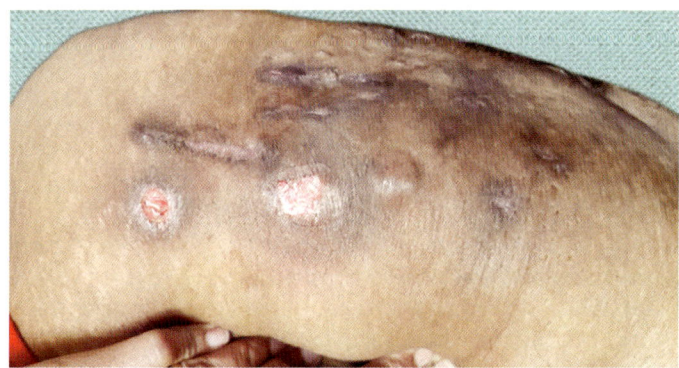

Fig. 5.24: Multiple sinuses in the abdominal wall due to infected mesh—case of incisional hernia repair. Mesh was removed and histopathology report was tuberculosis

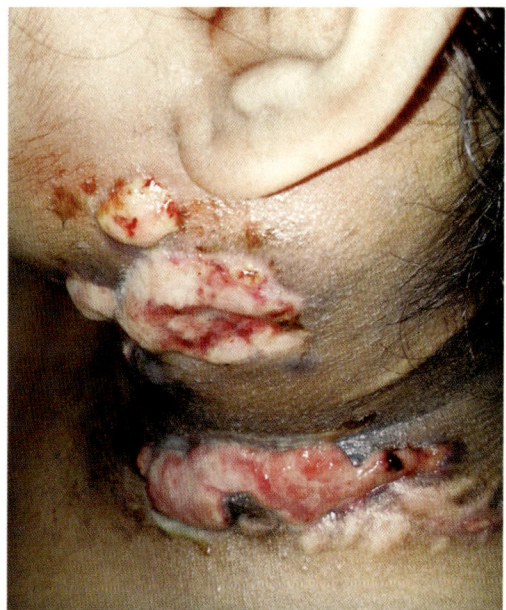

Fig. 5.25: Multiple sinuses due to tuberculosis of cervical lymph nodes

2. **Actinomycosis:** Rare cause of sinuses. **Extensive induration** (marked induration) of lower jaw (mandible) and gums, and **multiple subcutaneous nodules** over bluish-coloured skin of the jaw occur initially. The nodules rupture resulting in **multiple discharging sinuses.** The discharge contains **sulphur granules** which are gram-positive mycelia surrounded by gram-negative clubs. This requires wide excision and prolonged medications (Fig. 5.26).

When thorax and lungs are involved, multiple discharging sinuses occur over the chest wall. It is common in children caused by inhalation of ray fungus.

- *Lymph nodes are not involved in actinomycosis.*

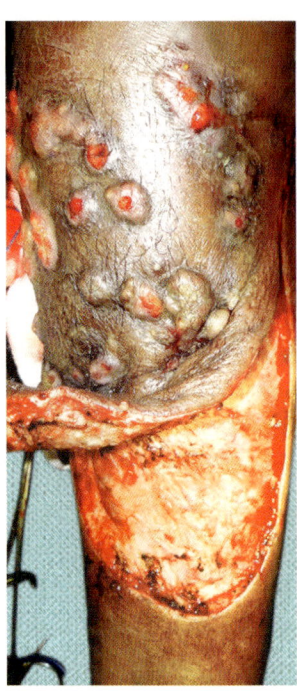

Fig. 5.26: Actinomycosis leg at surgery

3. **Chronic osteomyelitis:** Young children within 5–10 years of age are affected. Metaphyseal ends are often affected. It follows after acute osteomyelitis. History of fever for a few days and later swelling in the region of bone are suspicious of osteomyelitis. Once swelling ruptures, it results in sinus. Typically, it is a discharging sinus with pouting granulation tissue and discharging bony spicules. Bony spicules come from dead bone—sequestrum. Underlying bone is thickened and irregular (Fig. 5.27).

- *In older patients, it is secondary to some orthopaedic procedures resulting in persisting infection—any part of the bone may be affected.*

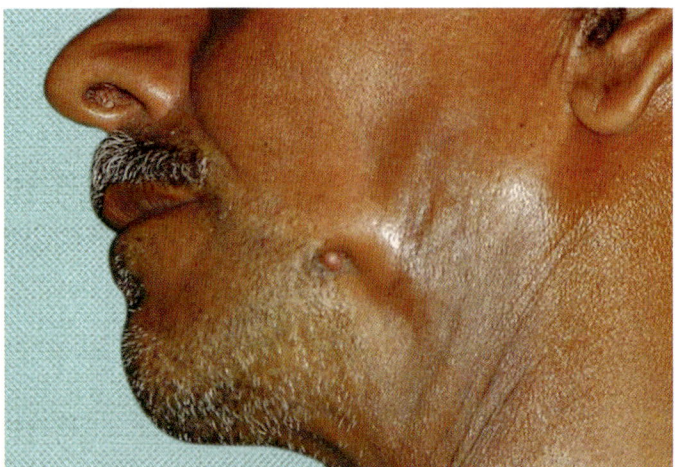

Fig. 5.27: Mandibular sinus due to osteomyelitis

4. **Median mental sinus:** This is a sinus in the midline just beneath the mentum produced by an apical abscess of lower incisors which penetrate buccal cortical plate below the origin of

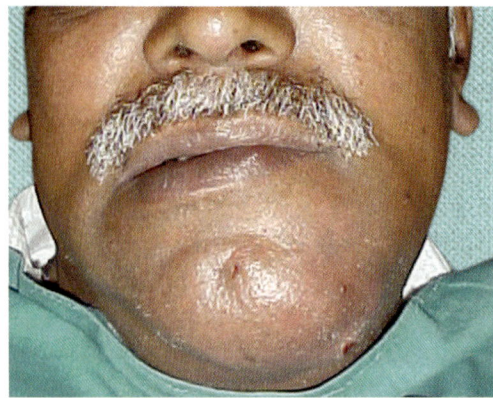

Fig. 5.28: Median mental sinus due to apical abscess of lower incisors

mentalis muscle. This muscle takes origin from labial surface of alveolar process just above the labial sulcus. Hence, pus discharges through a sinus in the centre of chin.

Patients present with recurrent swelling in the submental region which bursts open spontaneously discharging at times mucus and seropurulent fluid. Repeated history of swelling, discharge and healing are common presentations. Diagnosis is established by examination of the oral cavity which reveals evidence of caries tooth (Fig. 5.28).

- *Single opening exactly in the centre below the chin is median mental sinus.*

5. **Branchial sinus/fistula:** When internal opening of a branchial fistula is obliterated, it is a sinus. When internal opening is established (located in the anterior wall of posterior pillar of tonsils), it is a fistula. Typically, it is located in the junction of lower one-third and upper two-thirds of the sternocleidomastoid along the anterior border of the muscle. It can be bilateral also. It discharges serous fluid, may get secondarily infected. It is congenital and hence present since birth.

- Branchial sinus in relation to upper part of the sternocleidomastoid muscle is not congenital but acquired. It results due to infection following excision of branchial cyst.

6. **Preauricular sinus:** Preauricular sinuses and cysts result from developmental defects of the first and second *branchial arches. The first and second branchial arches each gives rise to 3 hillocks (tubercles); these structures are called the hillocks of His.* Preauricular sinuses are thought to occur as a result of incomplete fusion of these hillocks.

- Pinna is formed by 6 tubercles. Failure of fusion of one of the tubercles with the others will result in sinus or dermoid cyst. Usually sinus is located anterior to pinna. Hence it is called preauricular sinus. It can be found near the tragus of the ear or helix also. It will also be present since birth.

- Since it is a common congenital malformation characterized by a nodule, dent or dimple located anywhere adjacent to the external ear. They are inherited features and usually appear on one side, but may be bilateral in 25–50% of cases. Occasionally a preauricular sinus or a cyst can become infected.

- In almost all cases, the duct connects to the perichondrium of the auricular cartilage. They can extend into the parotid gland.

7. *Pilonidal sinus* (Fig. 5.29)

- Pilonidal sinus means **nest of hairs** in Greek. Also called **Jeep-bottom** because it was very common in jeep drivers.
- It is an acquired condition, commonly found in hairy males, more common in darker people.
- Appears between the age of 20–30 years.
- External opening of the sinus seen just above the anal verge in the midline over the coccyx.
- History of discharge of pus.
- History of recurrent abscesses which rupture, discharging pus.
- Can be asymptomatic.
- Osteomyelitis of the coccygeal bone.
- It is excised along with all tracks with involved portion of the skin

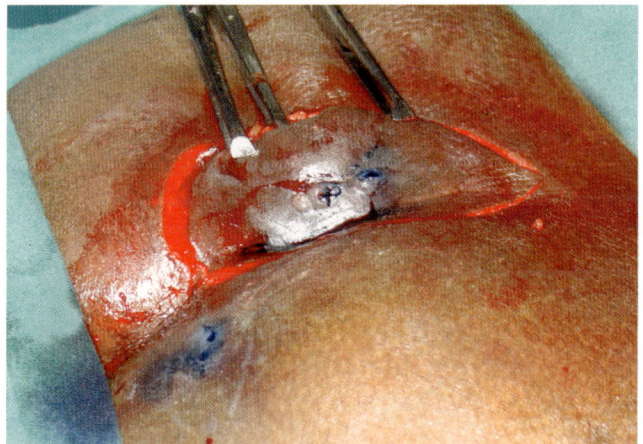

Fig. 5.29: Excision of the pilonidal sinus along with part of the skin and tracks

8. *Maduromycosis*: Mycetoma pedis

- Gross thickening of subcutaneous tisssue (*refer to page 181*)
- Chronic suppuration
- Multiple sinuses
- Discharging sulphur granules (Fig. 5.30).

CLINICAL DISCUSSION

- Long duration of a sinus (present since birth) indicates it is congenital.
- Pain and fever indicate inflammatory pathology as in actinomycosis or secondary infection as in pilonidal sinus.
- Tuberculous sinus is the most common acquired sinus in the body.
- Neck is the area of many branchial arches and clefts. No wonder it is the common site of congenital sinus.

Is pilonidal sinus congenital?

- No, the **hair follicle is never demonstrated in the wall of the pilonidal sinus** but hair is the content of pilonidal sinus. Hair accumulates due to vibration and friction causing shedding of the hair. Thus, it accumulates in the gluteal cleft and enters the opening of the sweat glands.

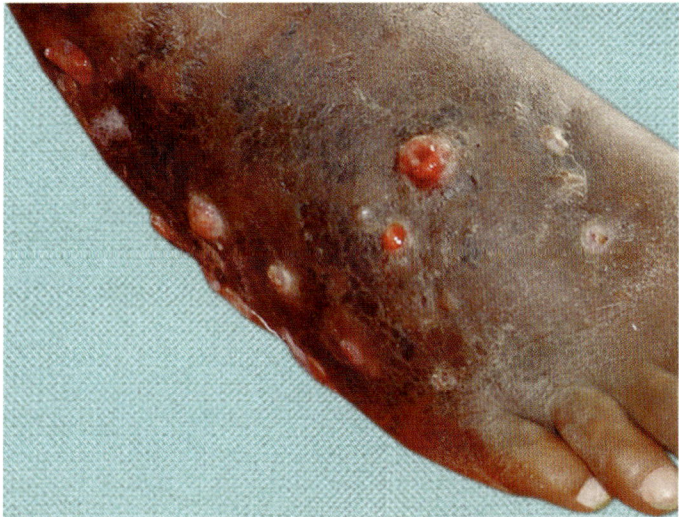

Fig. 5.30: Madura foot

1. CLINICAL ANALYSIS OF A CASE OF SINUS IN THE CHEST WALL (Fig. 5.31)

A 52-year-old man presented to the hospital with discharging opening in the chest wall of 30 days duration. There was no history of fever or cough with expectoration. He never complained of any pain or swelling before the onset of discharge.

On examination: Multiple openings—sinuses are seen in relationship to 6th intercostal spaces on the left side with wide mouth, and pale granulation tissue. On palpation, sinus was nontender and with gentle probing, it revealed undermined edge. Sinus was fixed to the costochondral junction. Underlying rib was thickened.

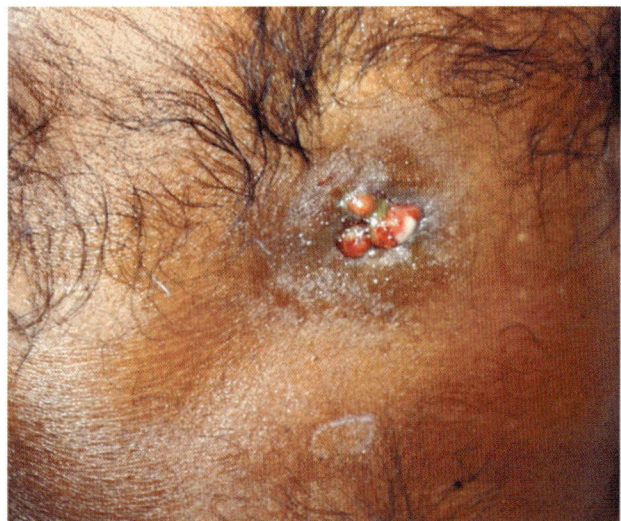

Fig. 5.31: TB (tuberculous) sinus in the chest wall (*Courtesy:* Dr Gopinath Pai, Dr Ganapathi Puranik, Professor of Surgery, KVG Medical College, Sullia, Karnataka)

Diagnosis: Tuberculous sinus

- Origin of the sinus may be from rib, intercostal or internal mammary lymph nodes, margin of the sternum.

- When you suspect tuberculosis in one site, always look for other common areas where tuberculosis can occur:

   1. Sinuses in the neck, axilla

   2. Cold abscess in the neck, axilla, paravertebral region

   3. Sinus in the scrotum—beaded vas and craggy epididymis

   4. Examine the spine

   5. Examine the chest

2. CASE OF MULTIPLE SINUSES IN THE LEG
(Fig. 5.32)

- A 60-year-old man presented to the hospital with multiple nodules in the leg with a few of them discharging some brownish pus-like material. This patient was operated for a swelling in the nasal cavity, 5 years back.

- On examination, multiple nodules were found, nontender, arising from skin. Biopsy of the nodules revealed it a case of disseminated rhinosporidiosis.

- The patient was prescribed Tablet Dapsone 100 mg/day for six months followed by wide excision and split skin grafting. Dapsone was continued for another six months.

- After six months, the patient returned with multiple cutaneous nodules over the skin of the grafted leg. He refused further treatment and was lost to follow up.

- Incidentally patient is a fisherman. He might have contacted this agent *Rhinosporidium seeberi*, an aquatic protozoa.

- The most common site of involvement is nasopharynx in about 70% of cases (Fig. 5.33).

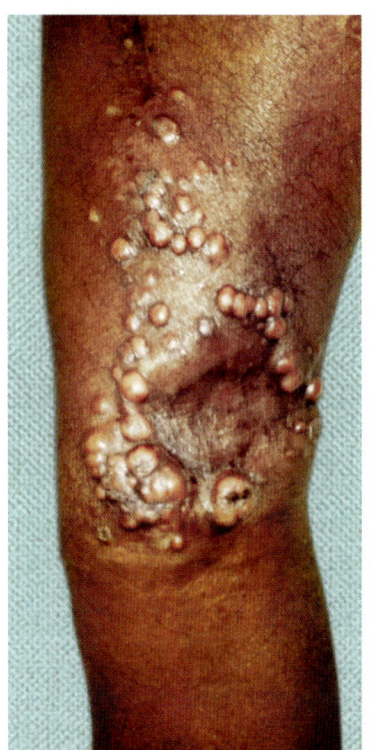

Fig. 5.32: Disseminated rhinosporidiosis

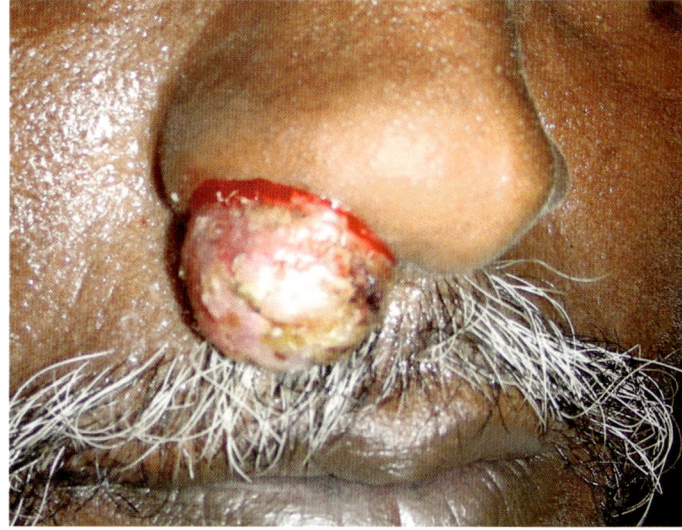

Fig. 5.33: Rhinosporidiosis (*Courtesy:* Dr Maruthu Pandyan, Prof and Head, Dept of Surgery, Madurai Medical College, Madurai, Tamil Nadu)

6

Examination of Keloid, Hypertrophic Scar and Contractures

INTRODUCTION

Keloid, hypertrophic scar and contractures represent exaggerated responses of wound healing. As the name suggests, there is hypertrophy of mature fibroblasts in hypertrophic scar. Blood vessels are minimal in this condition. However, in a keloid, proliferation of immature fibroblasts with immature blood vessels is found. These can be short cases specially when other swellings or ulcers are not available for clinical cases. Often students get worried thinking what is there to examine and how do I present this case. It is neither like a swelling nor like an ulcer. Hence, it is important that you have a good idea about these cases.

HISTORY TAKING

- Age, sex and race: Keloid is common in young children and adults. It is **very common in blacks** and least common in Caucasians.

- How did it happen? Often a history of injury over the sternum or a minor surgery (may be for sebaceous cyst) or injections in the deltoid region is present in cases of keloid. Enquire about the growth—typically it is very slow growing.

- History of itching is usually present.

- Enquire if there is pain: Typically, it is painless unless there is secondary infection.

- Often patient tells you that surgery has been done once or twice to remove the lesion. This is common history. In such cases, enquire about when it started growing again—recurrence. Keloid has a marked tendency for **local recurrence** after excision.

- Do any family members have this problem? Keloids can have inheritance.

- Is it growing even now? Keloid continues to grow after 6 months contrary to hypertrophic scar which does not grow after 6 months.

- History of operative scar (common) or accidental injury scar is present in cases of hypertrophic scars. In such cases, enquire details about the nature of surgery—emergency or elective, was there any wound infection—discharge of serous fluid, pus or any bowel contents (in cases of laparotomy scar)? How much time has the wound taken for healing? Wounds that take a long time to heal have more chances of hypertrophy.

INSPECTION

- Describe the lesion as an elevated lesion in the skin. Typically, keloid takes the shape of a butterfly over the sternum. It is the commonest site for a keloid.

- Describe its location, size and shape.

- Generally, it is an elevated lesion for about half centimetre with pigmented surface and the edge is vascular (reddish).

- Describe claw-like extensions. (Kelos means claw-like process.)

- If any ulcer is present over the keloid, describe it like an ulcer. Ulceration occurs due to surgery followed by break down of the wound or due to scratching.

- Look at other sites of keloid such as jaw, deltoid region, ear lobes and sites of piercing.

PALPATION

- First describe local rise of temperature and tenderness. Both these signs are present in keloid—not in hypertrophic scar.

- Describe the lesion as an elevated thickened lesion in the skin measuring about 3 × 5 cm.

- Feel the edge—it is thickened and may be tender.

- If any ulcer is present, describe the ulcer.

- Keloid moves with the skin and thus it is a lesion arising from the skin.

Examination of regional lymph nodes: Sternal keloid drains into axillary nodes. Keloids over vaccination sites from the arm drain into axillary nodes. Tender nodes are due to infection.

Diagnosis: Keloid.

Sternum, vaccination sites (arm), lower jaw, nape of the neck, scars are various sites of keloid (Figs 6.1 to 6.6)

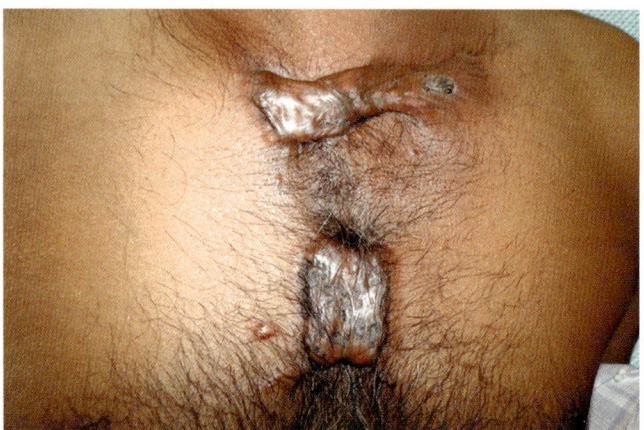

Fig. 6.1: Large keloid

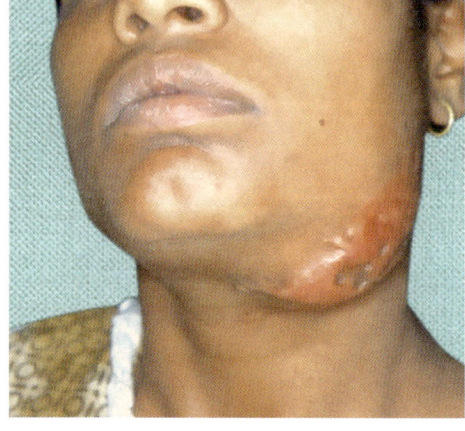

Fig. 6.2: Bad keloid over the jaw

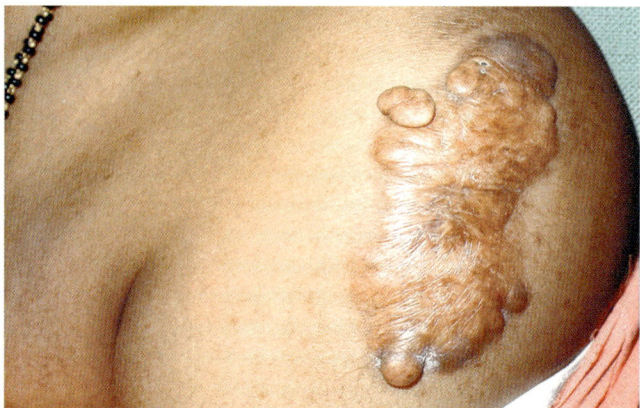

Fig. 6.3: Keloid—left deltoid region

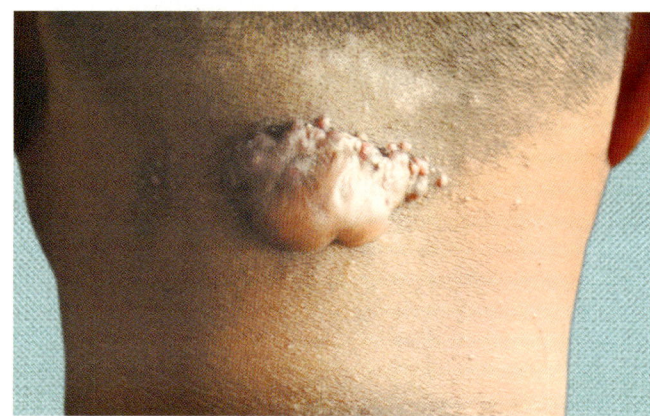

Fig. 6.4: Keloid—nape of the neck

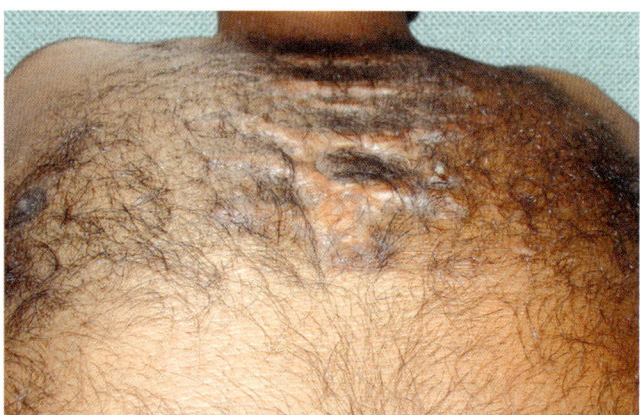

Fig. 6.5: Keloid over the sternum

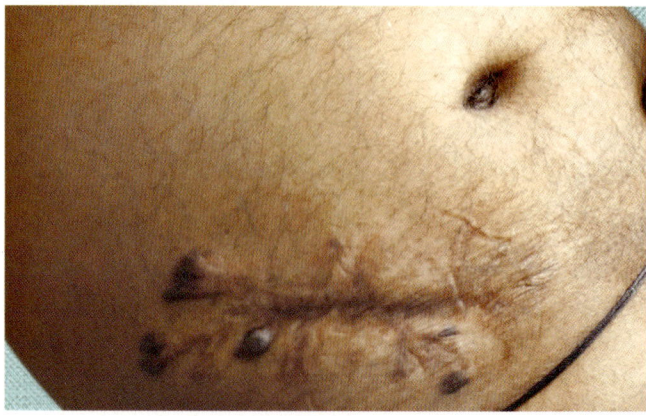

Fig. 6.6: Bad scar

Why do you say it is a keloid?
- Typical location, shape, skin lesion, edge is vascular. History of 1–2 surgeries and recurrence also helps in the diagnosis.

Why not hypertrophic scar?
- It arises from scar and generally does not grow after 6 months.

How do you treat keloid?
- Firstly no role for surgery. Injection triamcinolone acetate is given intrakeloidally.

A CASE OF POST-BURN CONTRACTURE (Fig. 6.7)

Specific History to be Taken

- Nature of primary injury: Thermal, electrical, chemical, traumatic
- History of treatment undergone (conservative, surgical reconstruction: grafting, flap cover)
- Specific symptoms, e.g. pain, itching, loss of function, cosmetic disfigurement
- Specific functional deficits, e.g. difficulty in upward gaze, mouth opening, incomplete
- History of physical therapy and interventions, e.g. splinting, compression garments, intralesional steroids.

General Examination

- Describe area of burn scars all over the body other than the principal scar being examined for the presentation in terms of:
  - **Size, shape, tenderness, erythema,** hyper- or **hypopigmented, hypertrophic** or **keloid** changes, **indurated** or supple, **blanching** or not blanching on touch, healed burn scar or healed graft scar.

- Describe the attitude of the patient:
  - Patient is supine/sitting
  - Joints in neutral position and/or
  - Joints in flexion/extension deformity.
- **Always examine donor sites!**

Local Examination

- **Describe the scar**
  - **Size, shape, tenderness, erythema,** hyper- or **hypopigmented, hypertrophic** or **keloid** changes, **indurated** or supple, **blanching** or not blanching on touch, healed burn scar or healed graft scar.
- Describe distortion or loss at the anatomical site (e.g. ear pinna, nostrils, eyebrows)
- Describe distortion of local landmarks (oral commissures, nasal alae, eyelids)
- Other pathological lesions at that site (e.g. ulcerations, calcifications)
- Specific tests to assess distortion or loss of function (e.g. hearing, vision, occlusion, airway compromise)
- Range of movements of joints in all the possible planes (different for each type of joint)
- Specific deformities (e.g. ectropion, microstomia)

Management

- Post-burn contracture of the parts of the body with specific deformities with pathological lesions and major anatomical distortions.
- Treatment plan: Correction of deformity/contracture release/skin grafting, etc.

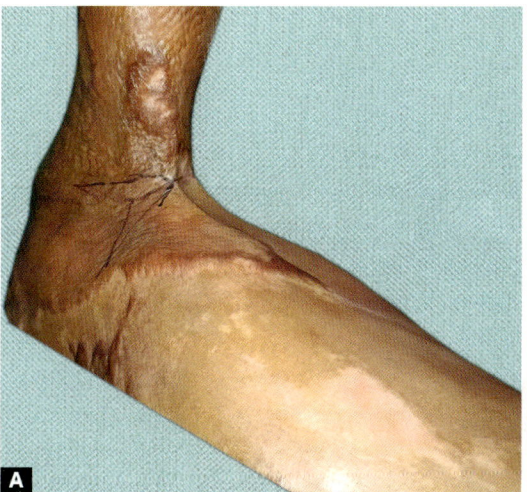
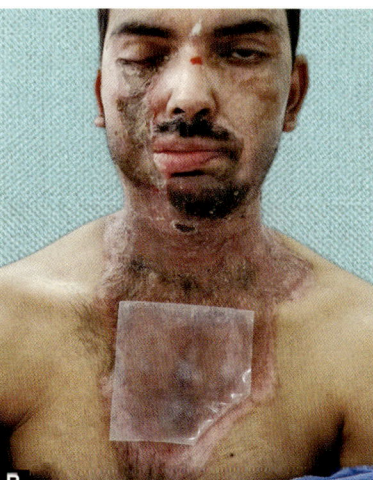
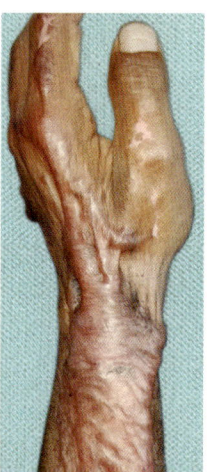
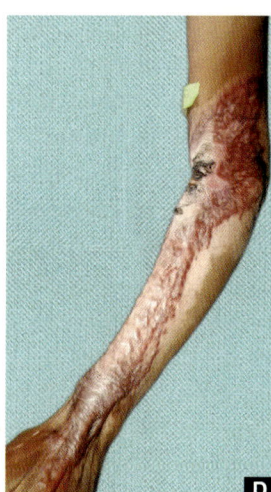

Figs 6.7A to D: Post-burn contractures (contributed by Dr. Joseph Thomas, Assistant Professor, Department of Plastic Surgery, Kasturba Medical College and Hospital, Manipal)

7

Examination of Lower Limb Ischaemia, Peripheral Arterial Occlusive Disease and Aneurysm

INTRODUCTION

- Though popularly called peripheral vascular disease, in fact these are occlusive arterial diseases. Thromboangiitis obliterans (TAO) also called Buerger's disease and atherosclerotic arterial disease are the two most common causes of occlusive arterial disease causing lower limb ischaemia. Diabetic patients are also vulnerable for developing various ischaemic problems to the leg in the form of ulcer, gangrene of the toes, gangrene of the leg, etc.

- Aetiopathogenesis, history, signs and symptoms and clinical tests differ significantly in the lower limb and upper limb and hence these have been discussed separately.

Clinical Box 7.1

Causes of lower limb ischaemia
- **A**therosclerosis
- **B**uerger's disease (TAO)
- **C**ollagen vascular disorders
- **D**iabetes mellitus
- **E**mbolic causes
  ABCDE of lower limb ischaemia

Figures 7.1 to 7.4

PATIENT DATA

- These are recorded such as name, age, place, occupation, admitting complaints, etc. A common question is, 'how old are you?' If the age group is between 20 and 40 years of age, mostly the leg ischaemia is caused by TAO. If patient is 50 years or above, mostly it is due to atherosclerotic vascular disease with or without diabetes. Young patients may have Raynaud's disease—a vasospastic disease caused by exposure to cold typically involving upper limb.

- If patient is 43-year-old, what can it be? Just find out when the symptoms started. Most of the TAO patients would have started smoking very early in teens and symptoms also would have been there in thirties or early forties. Signs of atherosclerosis are absent in such cases.

HISTORY OF PRESENT ILLNESS

1. *Pain* in the limb is the chief symptom of lower limb ischaemia. Get all the details about the pain—nature—what type—is it crampy, dull-aching or unbearable pain disturbing the asleep. When does it start? What is the relationship of the pain to walking? Is it present at rest? Where it is felt? Do you get sleep at night?

   - Popularly pain arising from circulatory insufficiency is called intermittent claudication. It is a severe cramp-like pain, due to ischaemia of the muscles brought on mainly by exertion. It is reproducible and stops completely on taking rest. It is called **intermittent claudication. (Claudius means, 'I limp'.** Name of the king who used to limp, probably due to poliomyelitis).

   - Boyd's classification of intermittent claudication:

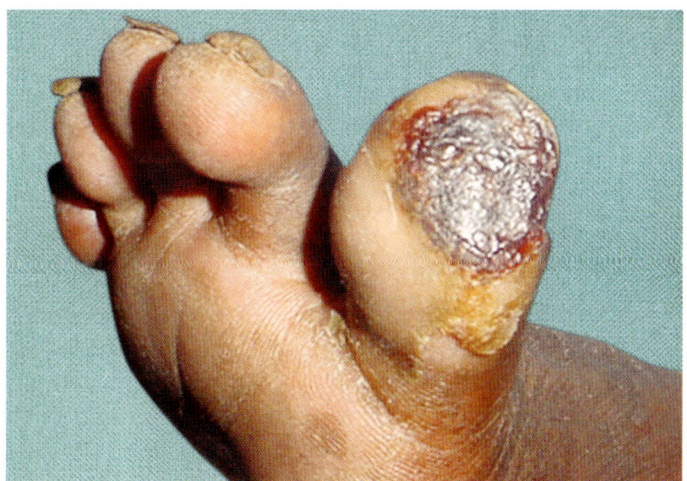

Fig. 7.1: Thromboangiitis obliterans with dry gangrene

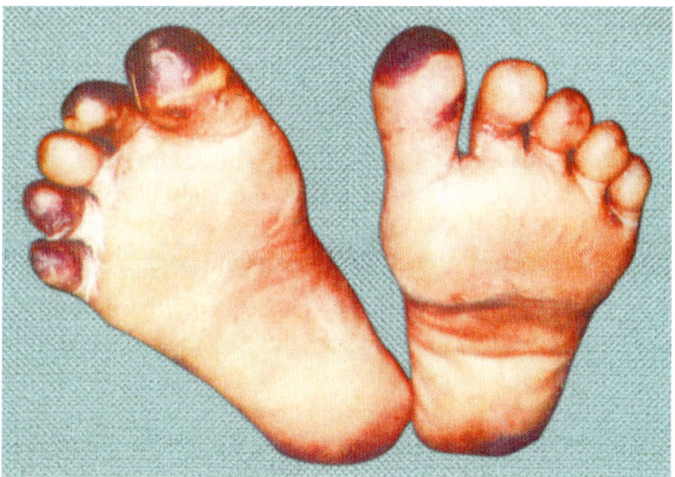

Fig. 7.3: Vasculitis with collagen vascular disorder. It had affected all the ten toes

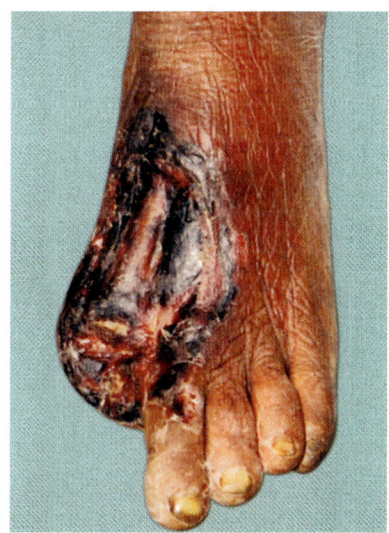

Fig. 7.2: Dry gangrene due to atherosclerotic arterial disease—part is dry, mummified and toe has been amputated

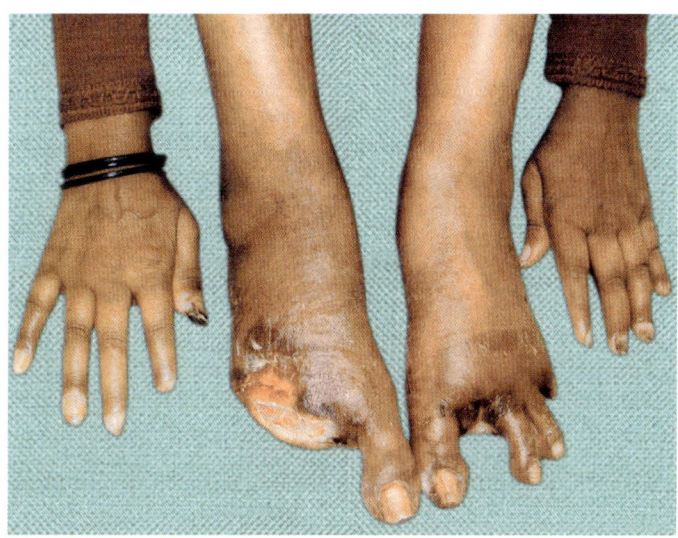

Fig. 7.4: SLE (systemic lupus erythematosus) involving all 4 limbs—female patient

---

Grades of intermittent claudication

Grade I: The patient walks for a distance, gets the pain, continues to walk and the pain disappears. As a result of ischaemia, anaerobic metabolism takes place, which produces ***substance P, lactic acid***, etc. These produce vasodilatation and the pain disappears.

Grade II: The patient walks for a distance, gets the pain and continues to walk with the pain. He has a limp.

Grade III: The patient walks and gets the pain. He has to take rest. This grade indicates severe muscle ischaemia.

Rest pain: **In late stages:** Pain at rest is due to ischaemia of nerves* in addition to ischaemia of the muscles.

*Cry of the dying nerves, due to involvement of vasa nervorum

- Often patients with rest pain are unable to sleep. They hang the foot below the level of the heart, downwards sitting on the bed. This results in venous stasis followed by reflex vasodilatation thus facilitating some blood flow to the ischaemic part.

- The location or site of the pain may suggest level of obstruction (Clinical Box 7.2).

Clinical Box 7.2 	
Level of occlusion	**Claudication site**
Aortoiliac obstruction	Claudication of both gluteal regions, thighs and calves
Iliofemoral obstruction	Claudication of thigh muscles
Femoropopliteal obstruction	Claudication of calf muscles
Popliteal obstruction	Claudication of the foot, muscles, Instep claudication

- *Rest pain:* It is an intractable type of pain usually felt in the foot (instep), toes, etc. It is an indication of severe ischaemia of the foot with impending gangrene. Typically, a patient with rest pain sits on the bed, holds his foot with both hands or may hang the foot out of bed. This gives him some kind of relief. Rest pain is worse at night time. It may lead to suicidal tendency.

- **Claudication distance** refers to the distance a patient is able to walk before the onset of pain. A patient with severe claudication may not be able to walk even a few yards.

- Any numbness or altered sensations like feeling pins and needles—this occurs when the muscle cramp starts. It is due to shunting of the blood from skin to muscle.

2. *How did it happen, suddenly or slowly?*

- Sudden appearance of colour changes, severe pain, etc. (Clinical Box 7.3) points at embolic gangrene. If this history is given, ask leading questions related to cardiac diseases such as previous myocardial infarction, hypertension, valvular heart disease, etc. (Figs 7.5 to 7.7 and Clinical Box 7.4).

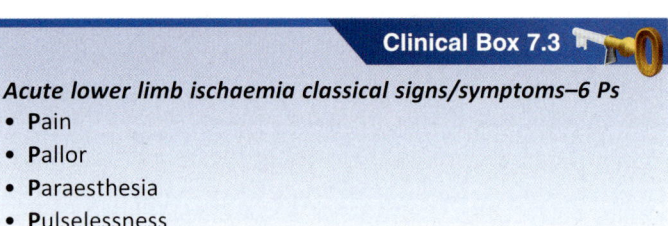

Clinical Box 7.3

Acute lower limb ischaemia classical signs/symptoms—6 Ps
- **P**ain
- **P**allor
- **P**araesthesia
- **P**ulselessness
- **P**aralysis
- **P**oikilothermia—loss of temperature

- Few causes of embolic gangrene are as follows:

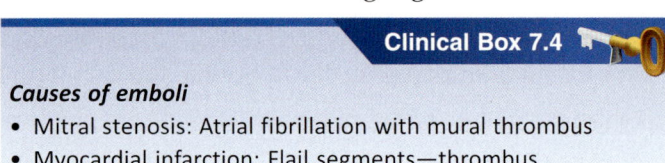

Clinical Box 7.4

Causes of emboli
- Mitral stenosis: Atrial fibrillation with mural thrombus
- Myocardial infarction: Flail segments—thrombus
- Myxoma of heart
- Atheromatous plaques

- **Common sites of emboli getting lodged are**

  a. Aortic bifurcation (saddle embolus)

  b. Common femoral bifurcation

  c. Popliteal trifurcation

- Slow development of pain, and colour changes suggest chronic occlusion as in TAO or atherosclerotic disease.

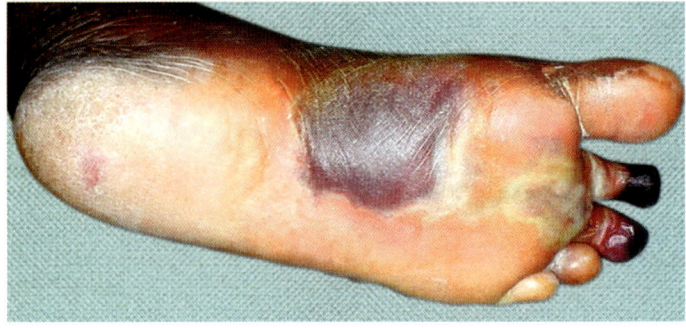

Fig. 7.5: Wet gangrene in a diabetic patient

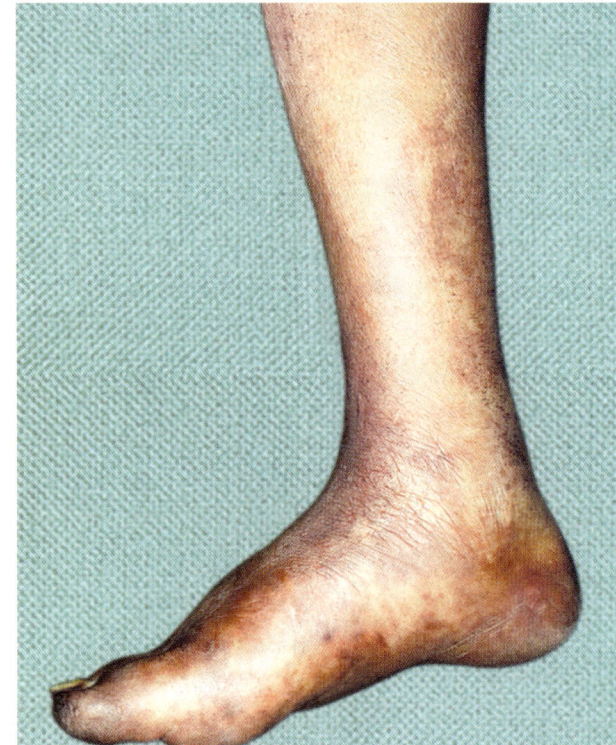

Fig. 7.6: Acute ischaemic limb

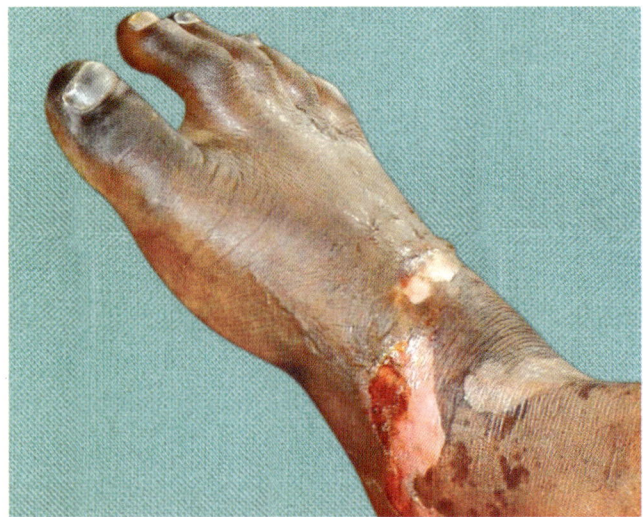

Fig. 7.7: Acute ischaemic gangrene

3. *If any ulcer is present, find out the duration and what caused it?*

   It is usually precipitated by a minor trauma and it occurs in the most distal part of the body such as the tip of toes. Ischaemic ulcers are deep and very painful. Often patient undergoes disarticulation of the toe for gangrene followed by wound which is left open to heal by granulation tissue. Such patients also will have ulcers.

4. If any black patches are found (gangrene), find out the duration. Some patients present with **gangrenous patches** of skin or subcutaneous tissue. Gangrene affects distal parts such as toes. However, gangrene is minimal because of collaterals.

   What are collaterals?
   - These are the branches of arteries which are very insignificant in normal conditions.
   - However, due to chronic ischaemia, these collaterals become big, dilated and thus some blood flow to the limb is maintained.
   - Chronic occlusions give adequate time for collaterals to develop.
   - Thus, gangrene which develops will be minor or small (in acute embolism, there is no time for collaterals to develop and hence the gangrene will be extensive).

5. Any symptoms related to heat/cold should be enquired into. *Example*:
   - Raynaud's disease attack can be precipitated by extreme 'cold' including insertion of hand into the refrigerator.
   - Symptoms may be increased after application of warmth.

6. History of **bilateral gluteal claudication** with impotence can occur in a young patient due to a saddle thrombus at the bifurcation of aorta. It is called **Leriche's syndrome.** Impotence is due to failure to achieve an erection due to paralysis of L1 nerve.

   Gluteal claudication is confused for sciatica and many patients are referred to orthopaedic department. Sciatica causes **neurogenic claudication** which is present even **at rest** and is aggravated on movements of the spine.

   Causes of neurogenic claudication are slipped disc, fracture vertebrae, tuberculosis of spine, etc.

7. History of coldness, numbness, paraesthesia and colour changes—indicates chronic ischaemia.

8. Sudden history of pain in the limb, redness and swelling indicates thrombophlebitis.

9. History suggestive of other organs involvement such as:
   - Chest pain—myocardial ischaemia
   - Fainting, transient black out—cerebral ischaemia
   - Blurred vision—retinal artery occlusion **(amaurosis fugax)**
   - Abdominal pain (post-prandial)—mesenteric ischaemia.

Clinical Wisdom

Other organ involvement is more common in atherosclerotic vascular disease.

10. Do you smoke? How many *beedi* or cigarettes per day? Majority of patients with peripheral vascular disease are smokers. TAO occurs exclusively in male smokers.

Smoking and TAO
- The severity of disease is related to number of cigarettes smoked. Here smoking index and pack years index is calculated.
- Smoking index (SI) = number of years of smoking × number of cigarettes smoked/day

  SI >300 is a risk factor
- **Pack year index (PYI)**
- Number of years of smoking × Number of packets of cigarettes/ day

  PYI >40 → Risk factor
- Shianoya's criteria—Buerger's disease:
  - Male tobacco user
  - Disease starts before 45
  - Distal extremities involved
  - No atherosclerosis, no diabetes, no hyperlipidaemia
  - With or without thrombophlebitis.

Past History
- History of cardiac diseases such as rheumatic heart disease, and previous myocardial infarction should be enquired.
- History of hemiparesis, or chest pain in the past which suggests atherosclerotic disease.

Family History

- Clotting disorders, such as protein S and protein C deficiencies, and sickle cell anaemia, can result in arterial thrombosis (more venous thrombosis).
- *Xanthelasma*: These are yellow plaques which occur most commonly near the inner canthus of both eyelids. (Upper eyelid is more common than lower eyelid.)

General Physical Examination

> **Clinical Clue**

- Pallor → poor tissue healing (anaemia)
- Xanthelasma → Atherosclerosis
- Nicotine stains → TAO
- Locomotor brachialis → Atherosclerosis
- Hypertension → Atherosclerosis
          → Polyarteritis nodosa
- Obesity → Atherosclerosis

LOCAL/REGIONAL EXAMINATION

Inspection

The *findings are appreciated* better, if a comparison is made with the opposite limb.

Attitude of the limb: Very often, patients hold the calf muscles or dorsum of foot with both hands (Fig. 7.8).

Commonly asked question—why does the patient hold his legs and hang them down the bed?

1. Venous stasis and reflex vasodilatation.
2. He compresses the muscles with his hands which may also help in venous return.
3. Warmth of hands is transferred to the limb.

These are explanations given by many experienced senior examiners and teachers. I request students to verify these explanations.

1. *Evidence of chronic ischaemia of the leg* (Fig. 7.9): It occurs due to shunting of blood from fascio-cutaneous compartment to muscle.
   - Flattening of the terminal pulp spaces of toes
   - Fissures, cracks in between the toes
   - Ulceration of toes, interdigital ulcers
   - Brittle, flat and ridged nails, shiny skin
   - Loss of hair and subcutaneous fat
   - The limb may appear more dark in dark-skinned patients or markedly pale in fair-skinned patients with vasospastic disease such as TAO.
   - The limb above may be congested, may be blue or pale in colour. Oedema may also be present. Skin lesions are also characteristic of ischaemia.
   - Limb above may show atrophy of muscles.
   - Colour change can be noticed.

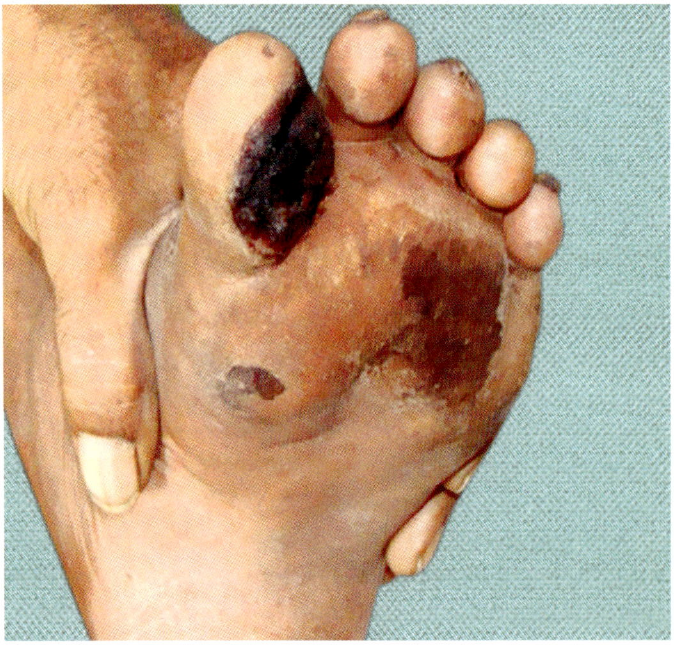

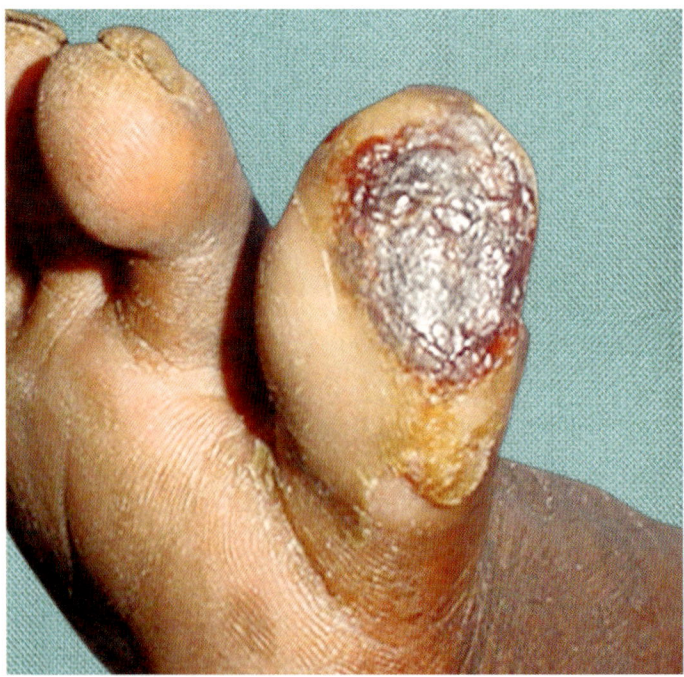

Fig. 7.8: Attitude of TAO patient—foot is tightly held by hand. Observe gangrene, ulcer, skin changes and ridged nails

Fig. 7.9: Evidence of chronic ischaemia of foot

2. *Mention, if there is gangrene*: Describe its location (usually tip of the toes), size and extent. Gangrene is usually dry with a clear line of demarcation in chronic ischaemia. It indicates the junction of dead and living tissue. Since the blood supply to the muscle is better, usually the **line of demarcation involves skin and subcutaneous tissue**. Line of demarcation is very well appreciated in senile gangrene **where it can be skin, muscle or bone-deep** (Figs 7.10 to 7.12 and Table 7.1).

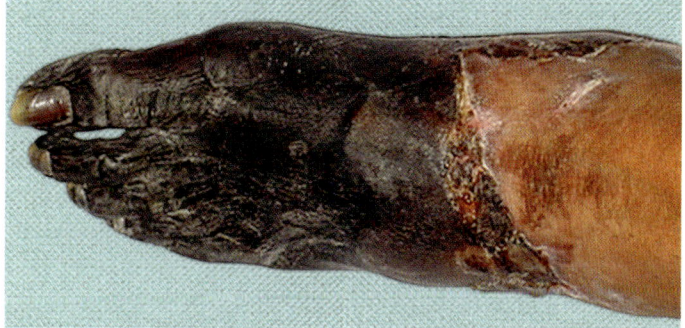

Fig. 7.10: Dry gangrene foot

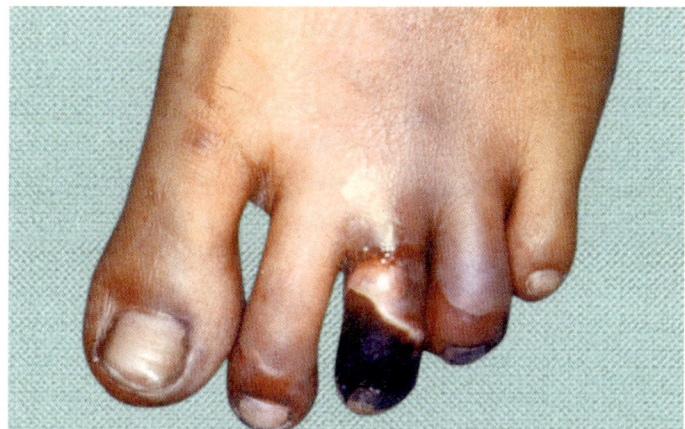

Fig. 7.11: Line of demarcation

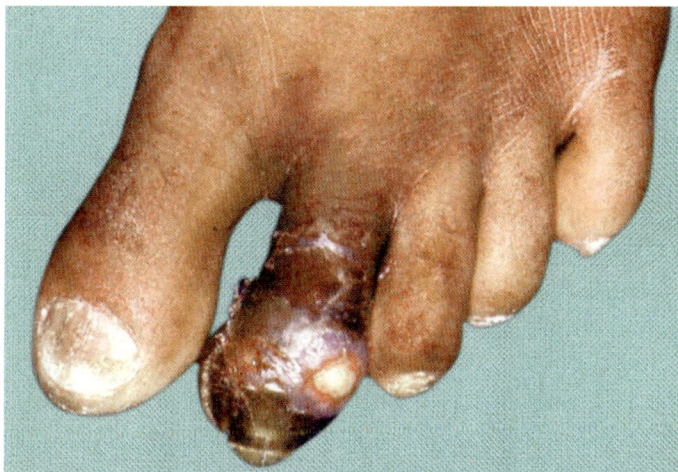

Fig. 7.12: Toe gangrene

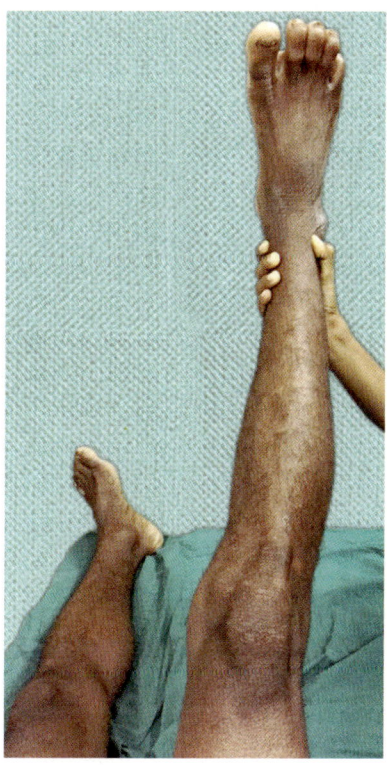

Fig. 7.13: Buerger's angle of circulatory insufficiency

3. *Other tests of minor importance*

   A. **Buerger's postural test** is relevant in fair-skinned patients. The patient (supine) is asked to raise his legs vertically upwards keeping the knees straight. In cases of chronic ischaemia, marked pallor develops within 2–3 minutes. The angle at which pallor develops is Buerger's angle of circulatory insufficiency (Fig. 7.13). In ischaemic limb, pallor develops even on elevation of leg up to 15–30°. A vascular angle of less than 30° indicates severe ischaemia.

   B. **Capillary refill test**: Apply pressure over the tip of the terminal pulp space for a few seconds and release the pressure. Rapid return of circulation is observed in normal persons (<2s).

   - The test can also be done in the ischaemic foot by asking the patient to sit up and hang his legs down and observe for colour changes. The time taken for the ischaemic foot to become pink is described capillary refill time. This is prolonged in an ischaemic foot (Fig. 7.14).

   C. **Venous filling**

   - Elevate the limb for a while and then lay it flat on the bed. Normal venous filling takes place within 5 seconds. In ischaemic limb, it is delayed.

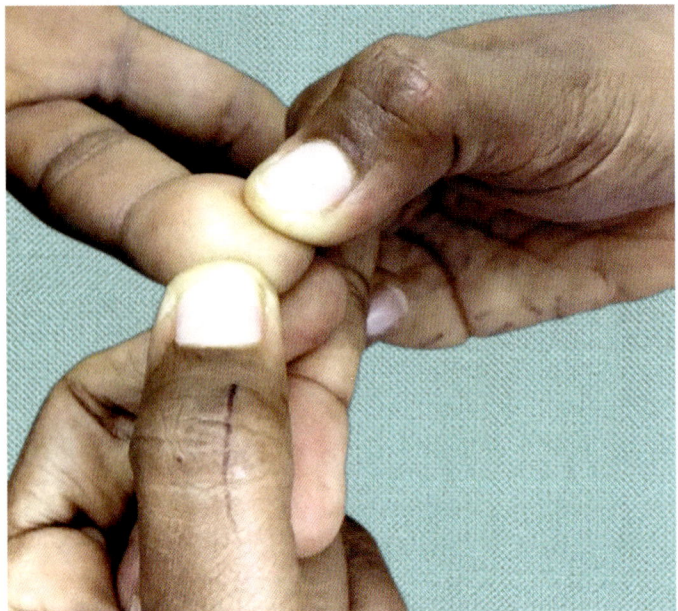

Fig. 7.14A: Capillary refilling test

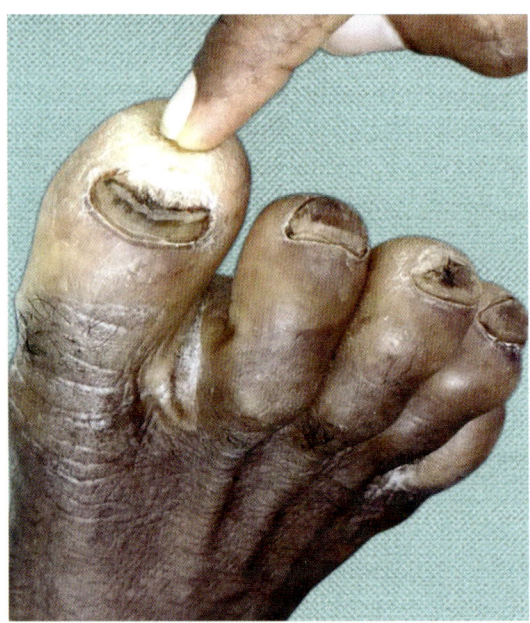

Fig. 7.14B: Capillary refilling test in great toe

- Elevate the limb above 90°—guttering of veins or normal collapse of veins is seen within a few seconds in normal persons. However, in an ischaemic limb, veins are collapsed in horizontal position or as soon as it is lifted to a small degree.

Palpation

1. *Ischaemic limb is cold*: Careful palpation from above downwards will reveal the change in temperature from warm to cold area. Temperature chan-ges are appreciated better with the dorsum of the hand which is more sensitive as it has thin skin with cutaneous nerve endings (Fig. 7.15).

2. *Tenderness*: It is tender due to the presence of inflammation—as in acute ischaemia.

3. *Ulcer*: Examination should be done as described in the chapter on ulcer. Ischaemic ulcers are very tender.

4. *Gangrene* is described according to its size, shape and extent. In dry gangrene, the part is dry and mummified or shrunken. Features of dry gangrene are summarised in Table 7.1 and Clinical Box 7.5.

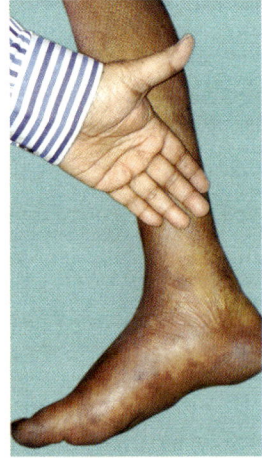

Fig. 7.15: Checking the temperature

Table 7.1: Comparison of dry gangrene and wet gangrene

	Dry gangrene	Wet gangrene
Cause	Slow occlusion of the arteries	Sudden occlusion of the arteries
Involvement of part	Small area is gangrenous due to presence of collaterals	Large area is affected due to absence of collaterals
Local findings	Dry, shrivelled and mummified	Wet, turgid, swollen, oedematous
Line of demarcation	Usually present	Absent
Crepitus	Absent	May be present
Odour	Absent	Foul odour due to sulphurated hydrogen produced by putrefactive bacteria
Infection	Not present	Usually present
Diseases	TAO, atherosclerosis	Emboli, ligatures, crush injuries
Treatment	Conservative amputation (minor)	Major amputation is necessary

---

Clinical Box 7.5

Signs of gangrene
- Loss of pulsation
- Loss of temperature
- Loss of function
- Loss of colour
- Loss of sensation

- Presence of crepitus indicates gas gangrene. However, crepitus is also found when there is anaerobic infections of leg.

5. *Sensation*: Due to the irritation of nerve endings, ischaemic limb is hypersensitive. When there is gangrene there will not be any sensation.

6. *Pitting oedema* can be due to thrombophlebitis or due to nonfunctioning of limb.

7. *Palpation of pulses* (Table 7.2 and Figs 7.16 to 7.26): After examining the pulses, results are interpreted in **a pulse chart.** Examine vessels in all four limbs and head and neck (Cinical Box 7.6). For example, pulse chart in a classical case of TAO left lower limb is given below

---

Clinical Box 7.6

Pulse chart

Lower limb pulses	Right	Left
Dorsalis pedis	++++	–
Posterior tibial	++++	–
Popliteal	++++	++
Femoral	++++	++++

++++ : Normal; ++ : Weak; – : Absent.

Table 7.2: Examination of peripheral vessels

Artery	Site where it is felt	Remarks
1. Dorsalis pedis is the continuation of anterior tibial artery	At the level of ankle joint, lateral to the tendon of extensor hallucis longus. It should not be felt distally where it dips into the plantar space	In 10% of cases, it can be absent. It is felt against head of talus, middle cuneiform or navicular tuberosity
2. Anterior tibial artery	Dorsiflex the foot. Artery is felt lateral to tendon of tibialis anterior or extensor hallucis longus. Felt above the ankle joint. It is felt on the surface of lower end of tibia	
3. Posterior tibial artery is a branch of popliteal artery	In between the medial malleolus and medial border of the tendo-Achilles	For circulation of the foot, any one of these arteries is sufficient
4. Popliteal artery, a continuation of femoral artery, extends from the hiatus in adductor magnus to the fibrous arch in soleus. It is about 20 cm long	It is felt in the prone or supine position with knee flexed. It is felt against tibial condyles (difficult to feel at the upper part)	The knee is flexed to relax popliteal fascia. Dorsalis pedis, posterior tibial and popliteal arteries are usually not palpable in patients with TAO
5. Femoral artery is the continuation of external iliac artery	It is felt midway between anterior superior iliac spine and pubic tubercle, just below the inguinal ligament against the head of femur	Abduction and external rotation of the hip joint may facilitate palpation in obese patients

Examination of head and neck vessels

1. Subclavian artery arises from the arch of aorta on the left side and brachio-cephalic artery on the right side	It is felt in the supraclavicular region in the posterior triangle against the first rib (just above middle of clavicle)	Difficult to feel in obese patients
2. Common carotid artery arises from arch of aorta on the left side and from brachiocephalic artery on the right side	It is felt against the carotid tubercle of sixth cervical vertebra (C6) in the carotid triangle (at the upper border of the thyroid cartilage)	Carotid artery bifurcates at the upper border of the lamina of thyroid cartilage (C3 vertebra)
3. Superficial temporal artery is the terminal branch of the external carotid artery	It is felt in front of tragus of the ear against the zygoma	This is involved in temporal arteritis, a type of giant cell arteritis

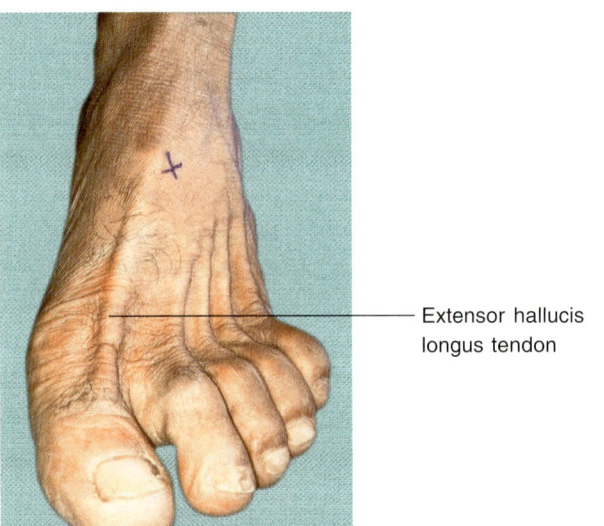

Extensor hallucis longus tendon

Fig. 7.16: Site of dorsalis pedis artery marked

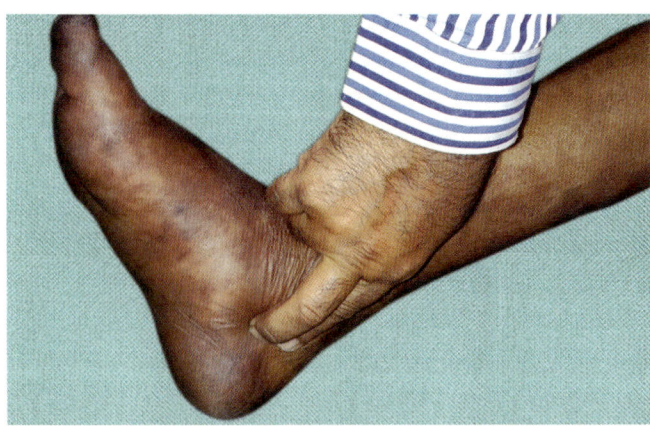

Fig. 7.19: Checking posterior tibial artery pulsations. It was absent here. Look at the foot

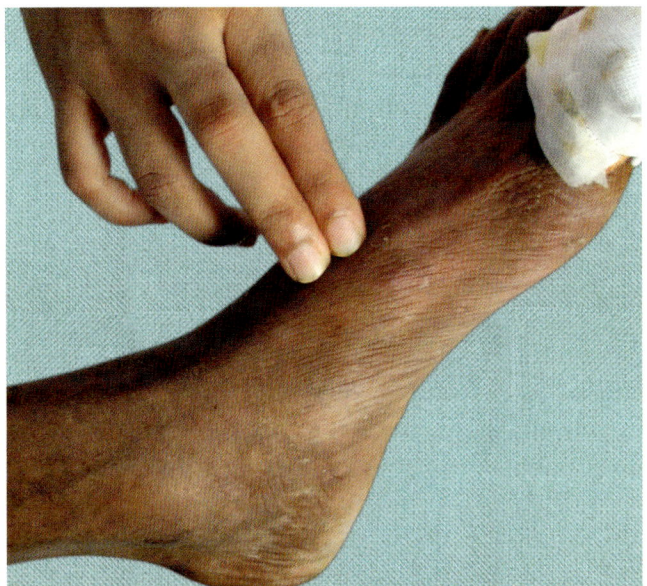

Fig. 7.17: Dorsalis pedis artery was not palpable in this patient with ulcer toe

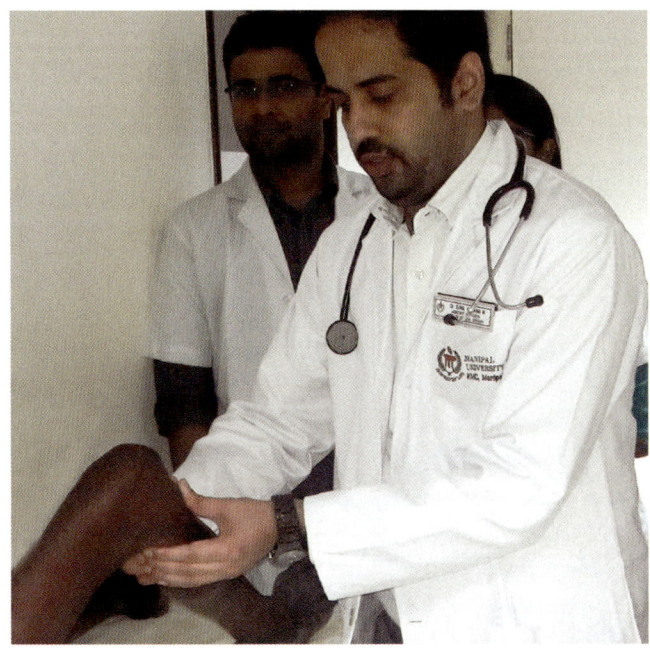

Fig. 7.20: Popliteal artery is palpable. Patient supine, knee fixed, both hands are used. Two thumbs anteriorly and fingers over tibial condyles

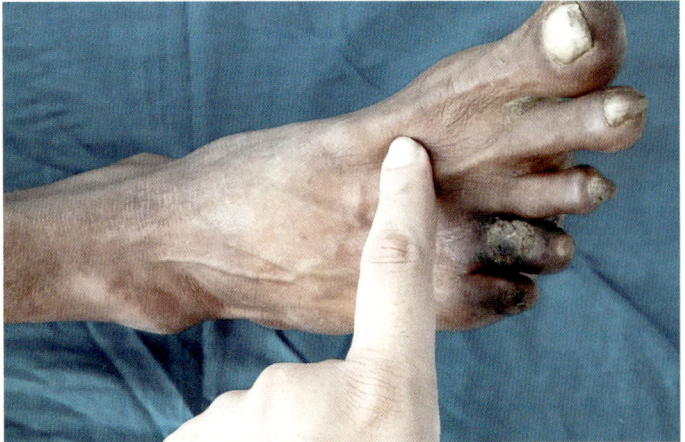

Fig. 7.18: Wrong method of palpation of dorsalis pedis artery. This artery dips into plantar space as it travels distally

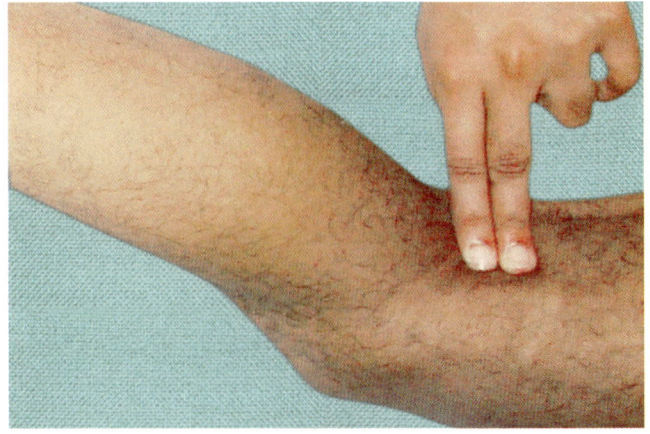

Fig. 7.21: Popliteal artery palpation in prone position

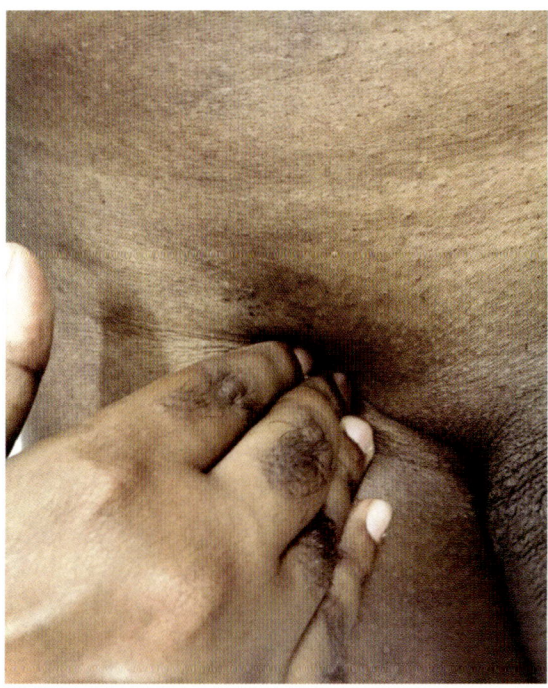

Fig. 7.22: Palpation of femoral artery

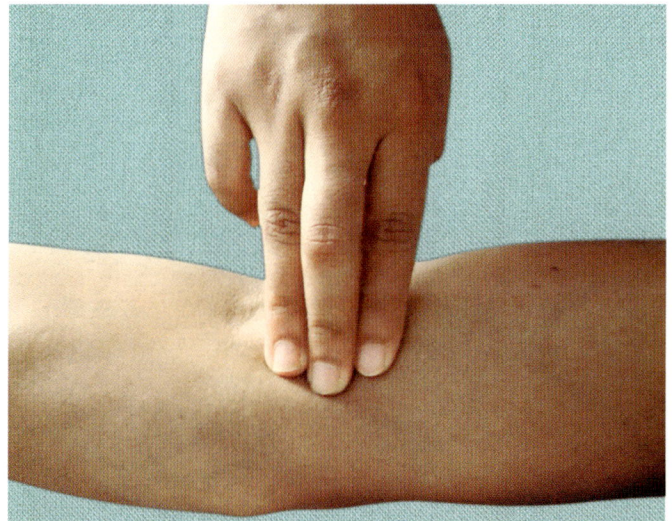

Fig. 7.23: Brachial artery is palpated on the medial side of arm

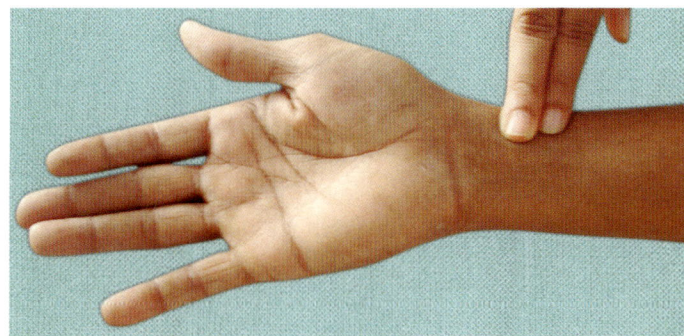

Fig. 7.24: Radial artery is palpated on the lateral side of the lower forearm

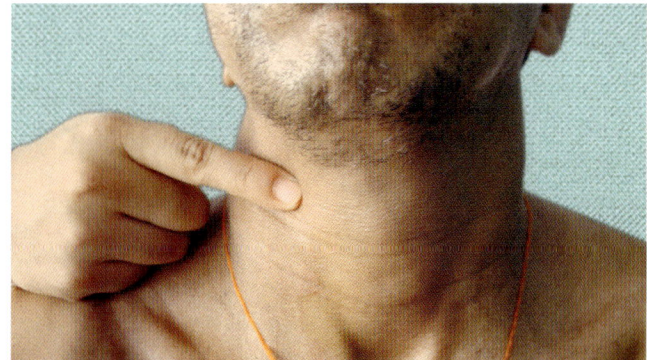

Fig. 7.25: Common carotid artery—upper border of lamina of thyroid cartilage (*refer* to Clinical Wisdom given below)

Clinical Wisdom

Carotid tubercle: It is called Chassaignac tubercle. It is the anterior tubercle of the transverse process of the sixth cervical vertebra. This tubercle is used to identify landmarks during deep cervical plexus block and stellate ganglion block.

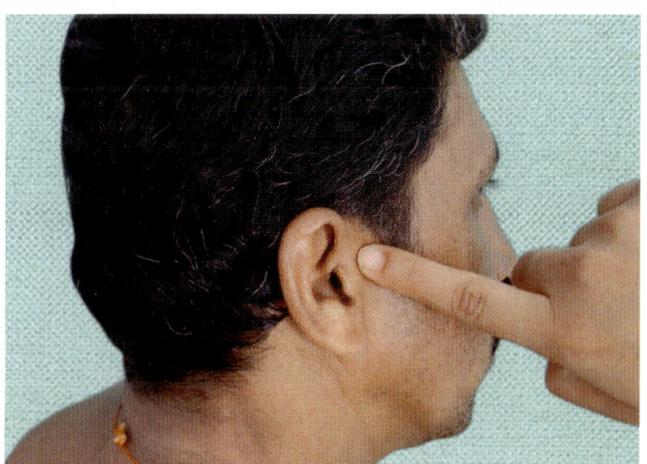

Fig. 7.26: Superficial temporal artery—in front of tragus of ear

8. ***Venous refilling*****:** Principle of this test is that blood flows towards the heart and in ischaemic limbs because of diminished arterial blood, there will be sluggish venous return.

   Method: Empty a section of the vein using index finger of each hand. Maintain compression on the vein with the finger closer to the heart and release the other to check for refill.

   Interpretation: In cases of ischaemia of the limbs, venous refilling is poor. It is increased in arteriovenous fistula. **This is called Harvey's sign.**

9. ***Fuchsig's test: Crossed leg test***

   Method: Patient sits with legs crossed so that popliteal fossa of one leg is partly compressed on the knee joint of other leg.

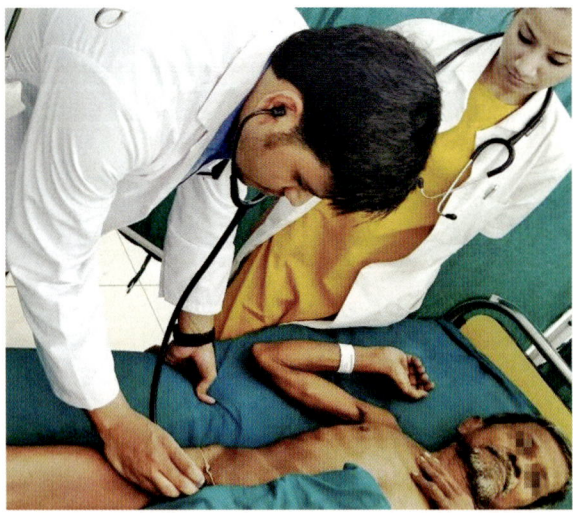

Fig. 7.27A: Auscultation over the femoral artery to look for bruit

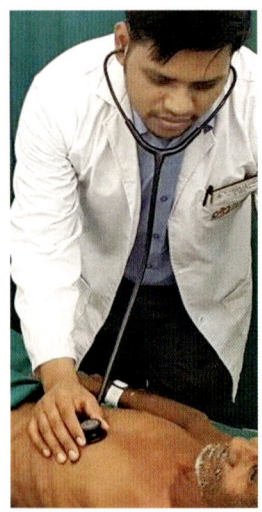

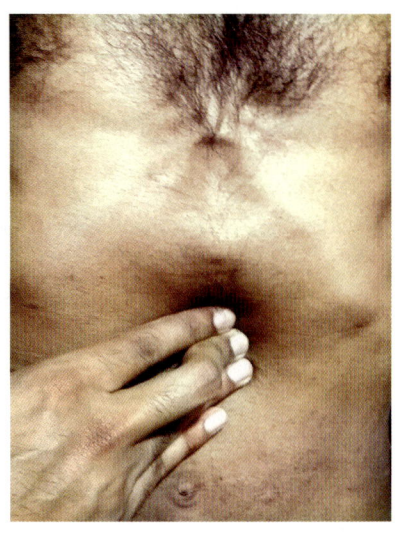

Fig. 7.27B: Auscultation of the heart to rule out valvular heart diseases

Fig. 7.28: Palpation of the aorta in the epigastrium

Start talking to the patient to draw his attention away.

Results: Oscillatory movements of foot can occur synchronising with popliteal artery pulsations.

Interpretations: No foot oscillations are found, if popliteal artery is blocked.

10. Systolic bruit over the femoral artery can be heard in atherosclerotic occlusion of iliofemoral segment, due to turbulence created by the blood flow (Fig. 7.27).

• Palpate the aorta above the umbilicus and to the left side (Fig. 7.28).

SYSTEMIC EXAMINATION

• *CVS:* Auscultate the heart to rule out valvular heart diseases such as mitral stenosis. Features of mitral

stenosis include mid-diastolic murmur, loud first heart sound, etc.

• *CNS:* If any specific complaint about CNS given by patient, examine spine.

• *Respiratory system:* Chronic smokers can have chronic bronchitis—manifesting clinically as cough, rhonchi and crepitations.

Clinical Checklist

In all cases of pain/ulcers in the leg, kindly examine:
• Pulsations of the limb
• Sensations of the limb
• Varicose veins of the limb
• Lymphatics of the limb
• Joints of the limb
• Function of the limb

DIFFERENTIAL DIAGNOSIS OF LOWER LIMB ISCHAEMIA/GANGRENE

Even though there are many causes of lower limb ischaemia, thromboangiitis obliterans (TAO) and atherosclerotic vascular disease are the commonest causes. Hence, they have to be considered first before giving other diagnosis specially in an undergraduate examination (Table 7.3).

1. **Buerger's disease:** It is also called TAO. Typically, a young male smoker aged between 20 and 40 years, coming from low socioeconomic group who has claudication of the calf and foot muscles and who has sleepless nights is usually suffering from TAO. On examination, small- and medium-sized vessels, such as dorsalis pedis artery, and popliteal artery, are not palpable. Arterial wall is not thickened, femoral thrill or a bruit is absent. Being a panarteritis, it affects veins and results in superficial migrating thrombophlebitis. Typically, it is a progressive inflammatory, segmental, occlusive, nonatherosclerotic disease with Raynaud's phenomenon. It also affects upper limb (Fig 7.29).

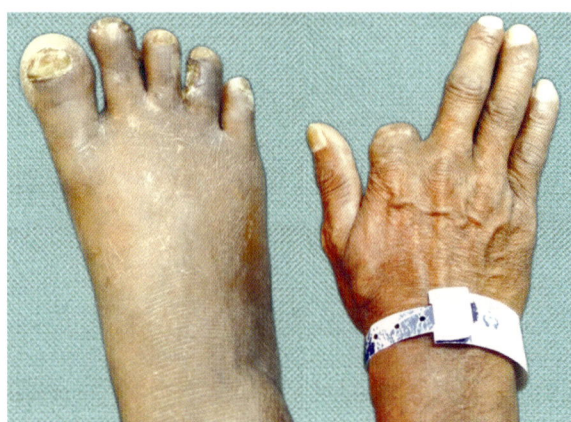

Fig. 7.29: Foot and hand involvement—case of TAO

Table 7.3: Differential diagnosis

	TAO (Buerger's disease)	Atherosclerosis
1. Age	20–40 years	Around 50 years and above
2. Sex	Exclusively males	Females are also affected
3. Aetiology	1. It is a smoker's disease. Excessive tobacco (nicotine) produces severe vasospasm of the vessels. 2. Excessive smoking produces increased levels of carboxy-haemoglobin which damages these vessels. 3. Low socioeconomic group, recurrent trauma to the foot, poor hygiene are additional factors. 4. Hypercoagulable state 5. Autonomic hyperactivity 6. Autoimmune factors	1. Atherosclerosis is a rich man's disease, who is usually a smoker, diabetic and hypertensive. 2. Strong family history is also present in a few cases. 3. Consumption of high fat diet leading to obesity, lack of regular exercises and hypercholesterolaemia are other factors.
4. Pathology	Diffuse inflammatory reaction involving all three coats of vessel (**panarteritis**) causing a thrombus, resulting in occlusion of lumen (**obliterans**). Polymorphs, giant cells and **micro-abscesses** are found within the thrombus. In severe cases, vein and nerve are bound by fibrous tissue.	Deposition of lipid-rich atheromatous plaque in the intima is the hallmark of atherosclerosis. Plaques tend to be more in **lower abdominal aorta**, coronary arteries, etc. Plaques may undergo **calcification**, ulceration and thrombosis, **dislodge** cholesterol emboli or may weaken the media and produce **aneurysm**.
5. Vessels involved	**Small- and medium-sized vessels,** such as dorsalis pedis, posterior tibial, popliteal, are commonly involved.	Medium-sized and large vessels such as aorta, common iliac, femoral, common carotid, etc. are involved.
6. Upper limb involvement	Not uncommon	Rare
7. Nature of vessel wall	Not thickened	Thickened
8. Blood pressure	Normal in the normal limb and low in diseased limb.	Hypertension is commonly present.
9. Superficial migrating thrombophlebitis	Seen in about 30% of cases of TAO. Veins of lower limb are involved and are tender and thickened.	Not seen
10. Raynaud's phenomenon	Can be present	Not seen
11. Auscultation—femoral artery	Bruit is not heard.	Bruit can be present as in aortoiliac disease.
12. Angiography	**Cork-screw pattern** of vessels	Shows site of block
13. Treatment	Lumbar sympathectomy Disarticulation of toe Treatment of ulcer	Bypass graft, repair of aneurysm or angio-plasty

Pre-senile Atherosclerosis

- I have seen this explanation given by many teachers when patient's age is around 45 years and femoral or iliac artery is blocked or narrowed. Many of these patients have been smoking since many years and the diagnosis of TAO is accepted. How to explain large artery involvement in TAO?

- The answer is: The small branches of femoral/iliac are affected in TAO and extension of the disease involves the origin of these arteries and thus the major arteries are involved.
- If patient has thickened vessel wall by 40–45 years of age, cardiac/neurological diseases, thrill/bruit/diabetes and femoral/iliac artery are involved → yes, it is pre-senile atherosclerosis.

2. **Atherosclerotic gangrene** is the commonest cause of lower limb ischaemia. Typically patients are above 50 years of age, with or without obesity and hypertension, who have pain and ulcer and gangrene of lower limb. Arterial wall is thickened, and medium- and large-sized arteries, such as femoral artery or even common iliac artery, are affected. It can manifest as simple ulcer to massive gangrene. Presence of chest pain, transient ischaemic attacks, post-prandial angina, etc. indirectly helps you in arriving at the diagnosis of atherosclerotic gangrene.

3. **Embolic gangrene**: It is a surgical emergency wherein the emboli have to be removed within 6–12 hours of arterial obstruction otherwise gangrene can occur. Gangrene can be massive in proximal obstructions such as femoral bifurcation or popliteal artery, etc. But in a few other cases, gangrene can be limited to small areas. Initial presentation is that of wet gangrene—part becomes oedematous, sudden change of colour to black, foul odour, with features of sepsis. If one examines these patients 2–3 weeks later, some demarcation would have developed and acute features will not be present such as foul odour and oedema. Sources of emboli have been discussed earlier but common sources being heart and atheromatous plaques.

4. **Diabetic gangrene** (Figs 7.30 and 7.31): Often the patient is elderly with many years of diabetes and develops gangrene after trivial trauma. Foot infections are common in diabetic patients because of following factors.

   A. Neuropathy: It commonly manifests after about 10 years of diabetes. Neuropathy can be distal and diffuse with a stocking type of distribution. Loss of vibration sense and deep tendon reflexes occur early. Later, joint position, touch, pain and temperature sensations are lost. As a result of this, trophic ulcer develops. It progresses and can penetrate deeper and deeper. Very often the patient is unaware of this. **Autonomic neuropathy** leads to absence of sweating and gives rise to anhydrotic skin.

   B. Resistance to infection is lowered in diabetes mellitus due to altered immune system. Uncontrolled diabetic patients are more susceptible for infection.

   C. Atherosclerosis: Diabetic angiopathy involving major vessels results in ischaemia of the foot **(macroangiopathy)**. These have accelerated atherosclerosis. In addition, it also produces small vessel disease in the form of nonspecific thickening of the basement membrane. It is described as **microangiopathy**. Thus, neuropathy or microangiopathy singly or in combination with secondary infection favours the development of diabetic ulcer. Ulcer starts due to minor trauma such as thorn prick, trimming of the nail or due to shoe bite. It may also start as a callosity in the sole of the neuropathic foot. Hence, utmost care should be taken to protect foot.

   • Typically, it is a wet gangrene involving great toe or many toes or dorsum of the foot, etc. Part is oedematous, and swollen with purulent discharge. There is no line of demarcation. (In dry gangrene, there is a line of demarcation.) Poor control of diabetes, and features of sepsis are other features.

5. **Traumatic gangrene**: Patients are young with history of road traffic accidents and with fracture dislocations of lower limb. Popliteal artery gets injured specially in a posterior dislocations of knee joint resulting in acute ischaemia of the leg.

6. **Vasculitis syndromes**: Often patients are young who have neither TAO nor atherosclerotic disease. Distal arteries/arterioles are involved, thus peripheral pulses may be normal. Women **are affected more than men. A few examples are given below.**

   A. *Systemic sclerosis—scleroderma* (Fig. 7.32):
   • Earlier called collagen vascular disorder because of obstruction of the small vessels by collagen deposition.

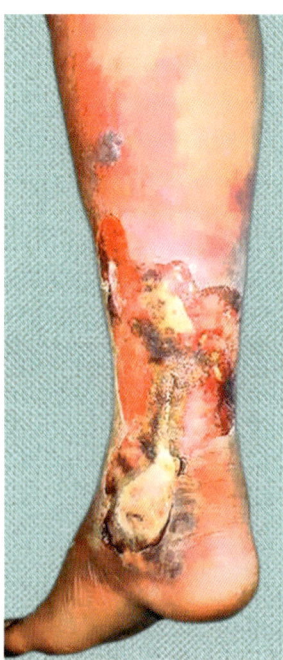

Fig. 7.30: Necrotising fasciitis and gangrene of the leg in a 50-year-old diabetic patient

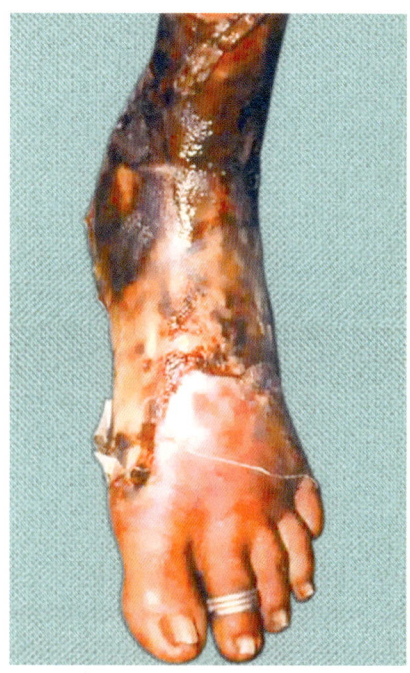

Fig. 7.31: Diabetic gangrene

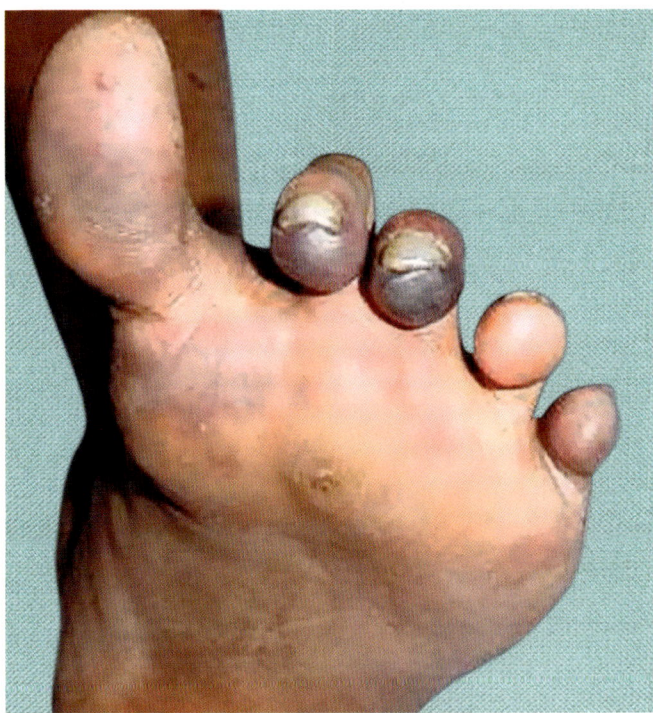

Fig. 7.32: Systemic sclerosis

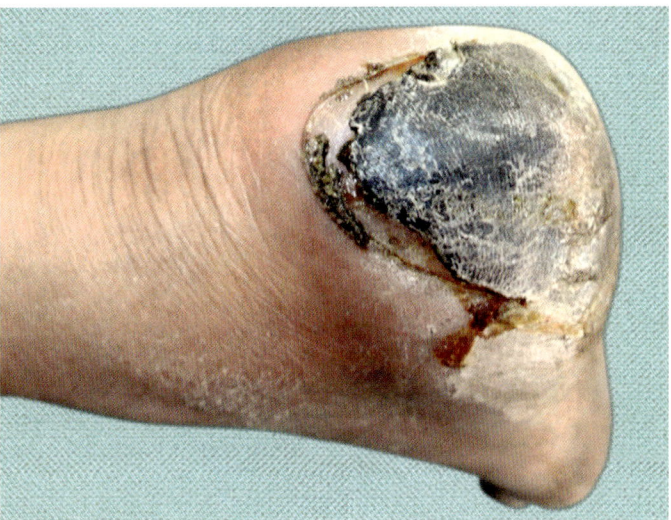

Fig. 7.33: Gangrene heel due to constant pressure in an unconscious patient

- Now it is included under vasculitis syndromes because of their association with inflammatory reaction.
- Ischaemic changes occur in the fingers and toes— necrosis and ulceration are common.
- Oesophageal involvement results in dysphagia.

B. *Polyarteritis syndrome:*

- This includes microscopic polyarteritis (commonly) and polyarteritis nodosa (less often).
- This syndrome also has an inflammatory reaction.
- Ischaemia of the lower limbs and upper limbs can occur due to involvement of small vessels.

7. **Frost bite**: It occurs due to too much of exposure to cold weather.

- High altitudes with excessive cold precipitates vasospasm and damage to the blood vessel wall. It causes sludging of blood and thrombosis.
- Malnutrition, and ageing process are the other precipitating factors. Severe burning pain, discolouration of foot, and development of blisters suggest that gangrene is imminent.

8. **Pressure sore/pressure gangrene** (Fig. 7.33)

- This occurs due to constant pressure.
- Immobilisation, unconscious patients, and comatose patients are vulnerable unless a good nursing care is given in changing the position of the patient.
- Bedsore is a classic example (decubitus ulcer).
- It occurs due to constant pressure resulting in focal necrosis of skin and subcutaneous tissues due to ischaemia.

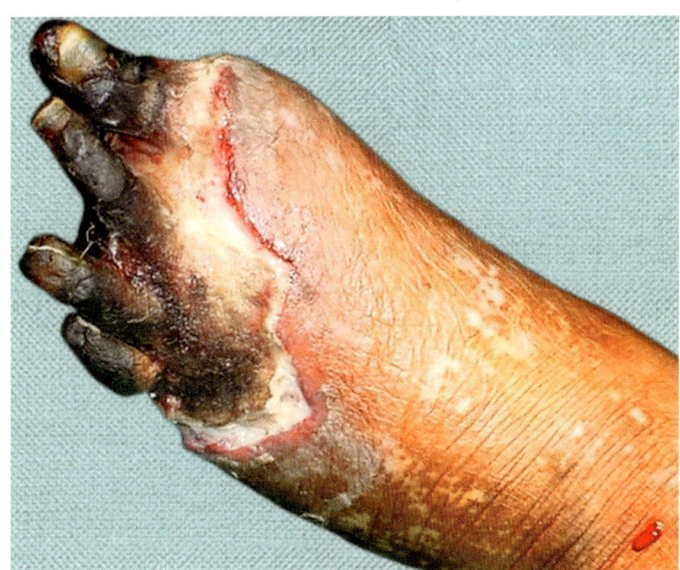

Fig. 7.34: Polycythaemia—gangrene foot

9. **Polycythaemia causing peripheral gangrene**

- It can be seen in neonates or even in elderly patients.
- It can be the first manifestation.
- Due to increased viscosity of blood, gangrene occurs.
- Toes and fingers are affected.
- It is important to rule out occlusive arterial diseases such as atherosclerosis and TAO.
- Peripheral pulses are normal.
- Repeated blood donation—venesection and treatment with Busulfan is the treatment of choice (Fig. 7.34)

10. **Ainhum**: It affects those who do not use footwear or walk barefooted. It starts as a fissure at the level of inter-phalangeal joint of a toe, usually fifth. Repeated trauma of minor degree may be present. The tissue becomes a fibrous band resulting in tight constriction and necrosis. If it continues, it may culminate in autoamputation (Fig. 7.35).

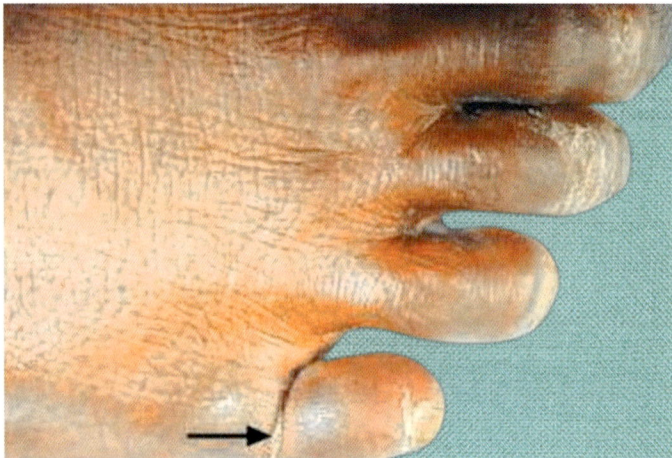

Fig. 7.35: Ainhum

CLINICAL DISCUSSION

What is disappearing pulse?

- When collateral circulation is very good, peripheral pulses may be normal. However, when the patient is asked to exercise, the pulse may disappear. Exercise produces vasodilatation below the obstruction and arterial inflow cannot keep pace with increasing vascular space, pressure falls and the pulse disappears.

What is Leriche's syndrome?

- **Bilateral gluteal claudication** with impotence can occur in patients due to a saddle thrombus at the bifurcation of aorta. It is called **Leriche's syndrome.** Impotence is due to failure to achieve an erection due to paralysis of L1 nerve. Gluteal claudication is due to diminished blood supply of the sciatic nerve.

Where do you feel popliteal artery?

- It is better felt in lower part of the popliteal fossa because in the upper part, two femoral condyles project outwards.

Does atherosclerosis affect upper limb?

- Usually it does not but TAO can. However, emboli can result in gangrene. When you have a patient who is 45-year-old but smoking since early teens, it can still be TAO. You have a patient who is 48-year-old whose radial artery pulsations are also not palpable, it is TAO not atherosclerosis. You have a patient who is 45-year-old smoker since many years but femoral artery pulsations are absent, it can be TAO.
- TAO affects the small and medium sized arteries. Disease (TAO) can spread contiguous to major artery and thus femoral artery can get affected.

What special tests do you have to do in a diabetic gangrene patients?

- In addition to examining ulcer and gangrene, one has to examine pulses to rule out atherosclerosis. Also, check the sensations of the foot including vibration sense and joint movement (Charcot's joints).

How do you suspect vasculitis syndromes?

- Middle age patients with no history of smoking, no features of diabetes or hypertension who have recurrent superficial ulcerations and gangrene of the toes and fingers may be having vasculitis syndrome. More common in women.

What is the significance of haematuria in a vasculitis patient?

- It indicates renal artery involvement (this is also responsible for hypertension)—polyarteritis nodosa.

What is venous claudication?

- It is rare. It can occur, if there is pelvic veins—iliac vein thrombosis.
- **How do you classify limb ischaemia?**
  Rutherford classification

Grade	Clinical feature
0	Asymptomatic
1	Mild claudication
2	Moderate claudication
3	Severe claudication
4	Ischaemic rest pain
5	Minor tissue loss
6	Major tissue loss

- **Any other classification?**
  Fontaine classification

Stage 1: No clinical symptom
Stage 2: Intermittent claudication
     2a: Well compensated: Can walk >200 metres
     2b: Poorly compensated: Walk <200 metres
Stage 3: Rest pain
Stage 4: Gangrene, ischaemic ulcer.

Clinical Wisdom

- When upper limb vessels are involved significantly, please rule out the causes of thoracic outlet obstruction also (these tests have been given in Chapter 8).
- If you see dancing brachialis—locomotor brachialis, it is likely to be a case of atherosclerotic arterial disease.

INVESTIGATIONS

1. *Complete blood picture:* Anaemia (low haemoglobin levels) decreases tissue oxygenation and delays wound healing. High total count indicates secondary infection and requirement of antibiotics. Elevated **platelet count** suggests that there is a risk of thrombosis.

2. *Fasting blood glucose* levels to detect diabetes. *Glycosylated haemoglobin* reflects how well it is controlled in the recent past (3 months). Increased serum creatinine indicates renal disease.

3. *Lipids:* (Total cholesterol, high density lipoprotein, low density lipoprotein and triglyceride concentration—hyperlipidaemia should be controlled to prevent progression of peripheral arterial disease, myocardial infarction, stroke and death.

4. *Hypercoagulable status:* Protein C deficiency is identified as a risk factor for arterial thrombosis especially in patients who will be treated with heparin. **Antiphospholipid antibody (APLA) syndrome is also called Hughes syndrome**. It is an

autoimmune hypercoagulable state resulting in thrombosis of veins (deep vein thrombosis), thrombosis of artery (stroke) and pregnancy related complications. It is treated by aspirin and heparin.

5. *Homocysteine levels more than 15 μmol/l:* It is a risk factor for arterial thrombosis.

6. *Doppler ultrasound blood flow detector:* Doppler probe can be used to detect the pulse even when the pulse is clinically not palpable. It is a bedside test and it is considered as extension of clinical examination in occlusive arterial disorder.

7. *Ankle Brachial Pressure Index* = (ABPI)

$$\frac{\text{Ankle blood pressure}}{\text{Brachial blood pressure}} = \text{It is always more than 1}$$

- By using sphygmomanometer, systolic blood pressure (SBP) of the limb can be measured by positioning the cuff at a suitable level and pressure index can be calculated. This is called ankle brachial index (ABI).

- Normal values are above 1. However, in patients with peripheral vascular disease of the lower limb, the values are below 1 which indicate vascular obstruction.

- When ankle pressure is less than 30 mmHg, gangrene may be imminent.

8. *Duplex scan:* This is the investigation of choice today. Duplex scan is a combination of Doppler with B mode ultrasound. With the availability of colour duplex, the direction of blood flow can be assessed. Red colour means direction of flow towards transducer and blue means away (standard settings).

9. *CT angiography:* It is good for vessels above the knee compared to those below knee (Figs 7.36 and 7.37).

10. *Magnetic resonance angiography (MRA):* It is more popular than arteriography because there is no need for arterial puncture and no contrast induced nephropathy.

TREATMENT

- **Buerger's disease:** First step is to stop smoking. Analgesics to control pain. Treatment of ulcer with dressings. Chemical sympathectomy is done by injection of sclerosants into the lumbar sympathetic ganglion. Phenol in almond oil is preferred. Effect is temporary. **When all measures fail, lumbar sympathectomy is done.**

- **Atherosclerotic vascular disease:** Bypass procedures are done specially for above knee blockages, examples being aortoiliac or aortofemoral or

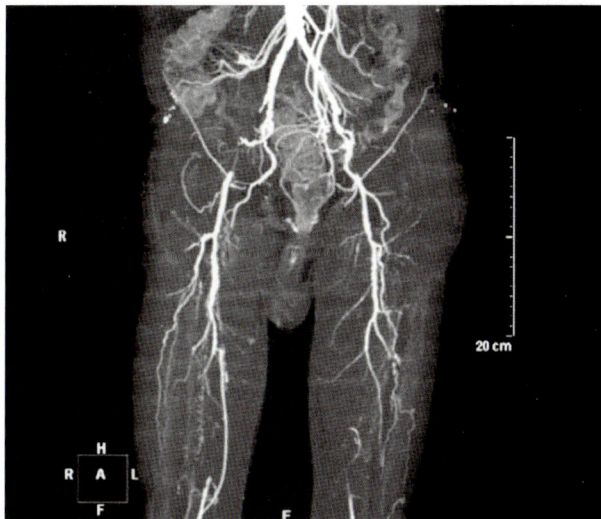

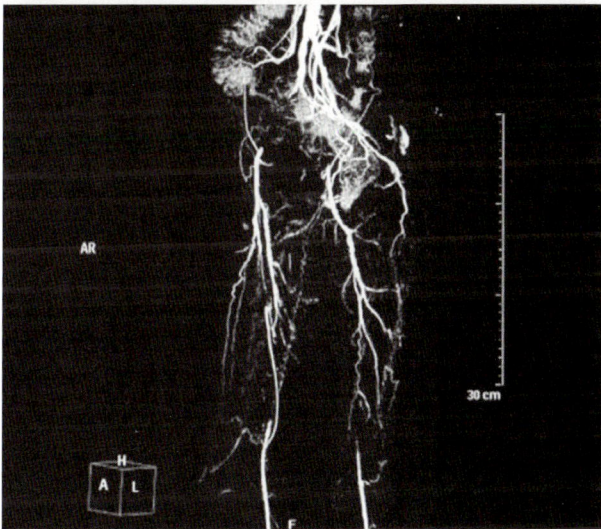

Figs 7.36 and 7.37: CT angiogram showing obstruction of common iliac artery on the right side and showing collaterals

iliofemoral, etc. Reversed saphenous vein or PTFE graft is used.

CLINICAL DISCUSSION ON MANAGEMENT

1. **How does lumbar sympathectomy help?**
- It helps by decreasing sympathetic tone of the lower limb vessels thereby promoting cutaneous circulation and healing of ulcers.

2. **What is the name of the balloon used for embolectomy?**
- Fogarty.

3. **What drug is used for intra-arterial thrombolysis?**
- Tissue plasminogen activator.

4. **Describe the graft used for revascularization.**
- It is called Y-graft or trouser graft. It has commonly 16 mm trunk and two 8 mm diameter limbs. Dacron or PTFE grafts are more commonly used.

5. **What is the 10-year patency rate?**
- 70–80%

6. **What are the differences between TAO and atherosclerosis?**
- *See* Table 7.3

ANEURYSM

Definition: Dilatation of a localized segment of an artery is called aneurysm.

- *Atherosclerosis* is the most common cause of aneurysm. This weakens the vessel walls uniformly and produces fusiform dilatation of the blood vessel. *Hypertension* is another factor which adds to the aneurysm.

- *Abdominal aorta* is the commonest of aneurysms followed by *popliteal artery. Femoral artery, carotid artery, splenic artery and renal artery can also be affected by aneurysm.*

Types

1. *True aneurysm:* It contains all the three layers of the arterial wall.

   A. Fusiform: Atherosclerosis, hypertension.

   B. Saccular: Due to injury.

   C. Dissecting: Due to rupture of intima by atheromatous plaques, blood dissects between layers of an artery—classically happens in aorta.

2. *False aneurysm:* In this condition, there is a sac lined by cellular tissue which communicates with the artery through an opening in its wall.

Causes (Clinical Box 7.7)

Clinical Box 7.7 🔑

Aneurysm: Causes

- **Congenital:** Berry aneurysm in the circle of Willis
- **Traumatic**
- **Degenerative:** Atherosclerosis
- **Rare causes**

  Syphilis: Endarteritis obliterans
  Mycotic: Infective emboli
  Subacute bacterial endocarditis
  Marfan's syndrome
  Polyarteritis

CLINICAL EXAMINATION

Patient Data

They are recorded such as name, age, place, occupation, admitting complaints, etc. A common question is: How old are you?

History

- Consider this as a swelling and ask common questions such as how it started, how is it progressing, was there any history of trauma? etc.

- Elderly man with no history of trauma who complains of dull aching pain in a swelling is common. Sudden severe bursting pain indicates rupture. Rupture will result in haematoma.

- Any referred pain indicates compression on the nerve. Popliteal aneurysm is known to cause foot drop due to compression on the common peroneal nerve. Patients with abdominal aneurysm can present with sciatica.

LOCAL EXAMINATION

Inspection

- If you see a swelling, describe all the details such as location, size, shape, surface, borders, etc. Classically aneurysmal swelling is a few cm in size, with smooth surface and round borders.

- *Look for pulsations:* Pulsations give you the first clue that swelling can be an aneurysm. Aneurysm, AV fistula, a few secondaries such as from follicular carcinoma thyroid, and a few sarcomas may exhibit pulsations.

- Mention surrounding area for any changes in the skin. Distal limb may have features of arterial insufficiency or venous changes.

Palpation

- **Once again confirm the size, shape, surface, and borders.**

- Aneurysms can be soft to firm, **compressible** swellings like arteriovenous malformations.

- **Expansile pulsations** are characteristic features of aneurysms. Place two fingers over the swelling, fingers are not only elevated but also separated. In transmitted pulsations, fingers are only elevated but not separated.

- **Proximal compression test:** When pressure is applied over the proximal artery, swelling diminishes in size—classically test is relevant in cases of popliteal aneurysms and femoral artery is compressed.

- **Thrill:** It is usually present unless thrombosis of the aneurysm has occurred.

Auscultation

- **Bruit** is also present.

Rest of the Limb

- Examination of the **veins**: Compression on the veins may cause oedema of the limb.
- Examination of the **nerves**: Tingling and numbness are the early features. Paralysis occurs later. Compression on the common peroneal nerve causing foot drop, due to paralysis of the peronei and the extensors of the foot.
- Examination of **bones**: Erosion can occur—may not be significant in popliteal aneurysm. One of the important features to differentiate tuberculous spine with cold abscess from aortic aneurysm is: *Erosion of vertebral bodies—is a feature of aortic aneurysm, not tuberculous spine.*
- Examination of **distal arteries**: Pulsations are weak or absent over the distal arteries.
- Evidence of any **gangrenous patches** in the skin or ulcers: Describe them. They are due to emboli from aneurysm.

Clinical Wisdom

Classical signs described above may be absent, if thrombus is present within aneurysm.

DIFFERENTIAL DIAGNOSIS OF SWELLING IN THE POPLITEAL FOSSA

1. **Popliteal Aneurysms**: They are the commonest peripheral aneurysms **because of the following reasons**:
   - Turbulence beyond stenosis at the adductor magnus hiatus
   - Repeated flexion at the knee.

   Clinical features
   - They affect elderly patients and atherosclerosis is the cause. Age at presentation is around 65 years.
   - **One-third** of the cases are associated with aortic aneurysm.
   - Striking preponderance in **males**. Male:female ratio is 20–30:1.
   - Presents as a swelling behind the knee.
   - Dull aching pain is common. Severe **bursting pain** indicates **rapid expansion** and impending rupture.
   - Pulsatile, tense, cystic, fluctuant swelling behind the knee, in the popliteal fossa and in the line of popliteal artery.
   - Its **size diminishes on extending the knee** as the aneurysm is deep to popliteal fascia.
   - **Proximal compression test**: On occluding the femoral artery proximally, the swelling may diminish in size.

- In all cases of popliteal aneurysm, abdominal examination should be done to rule out aortic aneurysm.

Clinical Wisdom

- In all cases of popliteal abscess, first insert a needle, aspirate and confirm that it is an abscess and not aneurysm.
- In all cases of popliteal aneurysm, please search for femoral and aortic aneurysm. (Refer to Clinical Case Capsule which is given below.)

Clinical Case Capsule

A postgraduate was asked to drain an abscess in the popliteal fossa. Total count was 8000 cells/cm^3. Local rise in temperature was present. Throbbing pain was absent. Incision was given only to get sudden bleeding. The popliteal artery was ligated. The patient developed gangrene of the leg and required amputation.

- Before incising any swelling better to auscultate and aspirate.
- Popliteal aneurysm may feel firm.
- In this case, careful clinical examination was not done.

2. **Semimembranosus bursitis/semimembranosus bursa**: This is the commonest swelling in the popliteal space. It presents as a tensely cystic swelling when the knee is extended and it becomes flaccid on flexion of the knee. **It is not compressible** as it does not communicate with the joint.

3. **Morrant Baker's cyst**: Usually **bilateral**. Patients are above the age of 40 years. It is soft, fluctuant, compressible but without transillumination. Transillumination is negative because of thick muscles covering the cyst. Basically, it is a protrusion of synovial membrane lining the knee joint (similar to pulsion diverticulum), hence compressible. Swelling disappears on flexion.

4. **Common subcutaneous swellings**: Lipoma, and neurofibroma can occur here. Lipoma is soft, lobular with slip sign positive. Neurofibromas are firm, transversely mobile swellings with or without pigmentation. Short saphenous varicosity can present as a dilated segment of vein—it disappears on elevation of the leg. Lymph nodal swelling may be due to some focus of infection in the lower leg or foot. Keep in mind malignant melanoma which can present as innocent lesion which the patient may not complain about. Presence of groin nodes, and skin nodules may clinch the diagnosis. Being subcutaneous swellings, many may exhibit transmitted pulsations. Lymph node swelling and neurofibroma can easily be lifted but not aneurysm of the popliteal artery.

5. **Popliteal abscess**: It is due to infection of the foot/sole, etc. During acute phase, severe pain on movement of the knee—extension, brawny swelling in the popliteal region. High grade fever with chills and rigors can occur. On palpation, tenderness is characteristic. Acute osteomyelitis of the lower end of the femur or upper tibia can present with infection of the popliteal node causing popliteal abscess. With antibiotics, abscess may well be organized and may feel more firm than soft.

   - In all cases of popliteal abscess, ruptured popliteal aneurysm should be ruled out (Clinical Case Capsule).

EXAMINATION OF A CASE OF ARTERIOVENOUS FISTULA

- An abnormal communication between artery and vein results in AV fistula.
- AV fistula can be congenital or acquired.
- Acquired are due to trauma or created in cases of chronic renal failure for dialysis purposes.
- Such AV fistula has got structural and functional effects.

Structural Effect

Since blood at higher pressure from an artery flows into the vein, the veins get dilated, tortuous and elongated. This arterialisation of the vein results in **secondary varicose veins**.

Physiological Effect

Increased pulse rate, increased cardiac output, and increased pulse pressure result due to increased venous pressure and arteriovenous shunt.

History

- How and when did it start? Often congenital lesions need not be present since birth. Parents may notice these lesions 1–2 years since birth (Fig. 7.38).
- Did you have trauma or injury? A few months later, patients come and show you a pulsatile lesion in the hand/foot/leg. Example: Treatment of fracture long bones in the leg.

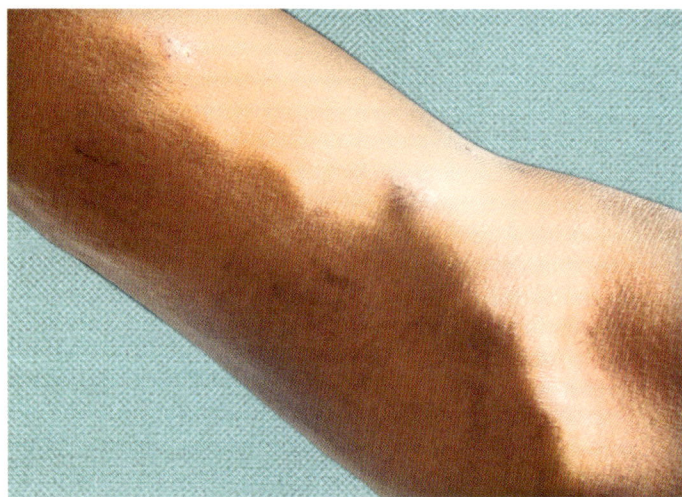

Fig. 7.39: Most common type of AV fistula you see today is in the nephrology ward—created to facilitate haemodialysis

- Has it been created for dialysis? Today more often AV fistulas you see in the hospital are done by urologists for dialysis (Fig. 7.39).
- Is there any bleeding?
- Patient may show you dilated veins for which he might have come to hospital.

LOCAL EXAMINATION

Inspection

- If you see a swelling, describe all the details such as location, size, shape, surface, borders, etc. Classically, swelling is a few cm in size, with smooth surface and round borders (Fig. 7.40).
- Look for **pulsations:** Pulsations give you the first clue that swelling is vascular in origin. Such swelling is usually superficial.

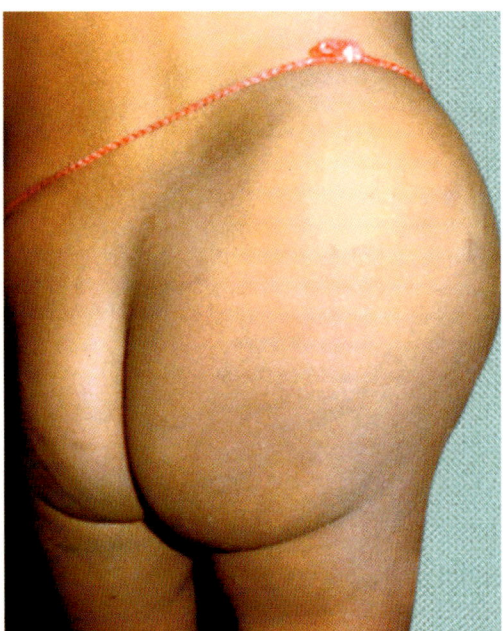

Fig. 7.38: Arteriovenous malformation in the gluteal region causing local gigantism

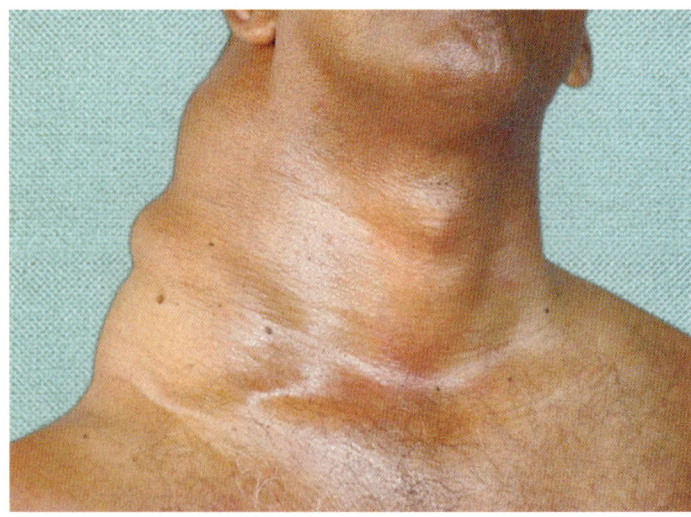

Fig. 7.40: Congenital AV fistula of 25 years duration

- Mention skin over the lesion—port-wine stain is seen in congenital AV fistula.

- The distal limb may have features of arterial insufficiency in the form of ulcers.

- Dilated veins are characteristic. (In aneurysm you will not see dilated veins.)

- The affected part is swollen (because of high pressure)—**local gigantism**. Thus, overgrowth of the limb or toe can occur specially in congenital AV fistula. However, below the fistula, limb muscles may show wasting.

Palpation

- **Once again confirm the size, shape, surface, and borders.**

- AV fistulas are **compressible** swellings like haemangiomas.

- **Pulsations are present.**

- **Proximal compression test:** When pressure is applied over the proximal artery, fistula diminishes in size and pulsations may disappear.

- **Nicoladoni sign or Branham sign:** On compressing the feeding artery, the venous return to the heart diminishes, resulting in fall in pulse rate and pulse pressure (rise in diastolic pressure). This sign is positive in long-standing, congenital large fistulas.

- **Thrill:** Continuous

- **Limb below is cold compared to above.**

- **If any ulcer is present describe the ulcer.**

Auscultation

Continuous bruit or murmur is characteristic and pathognomonic of AV fistulas.

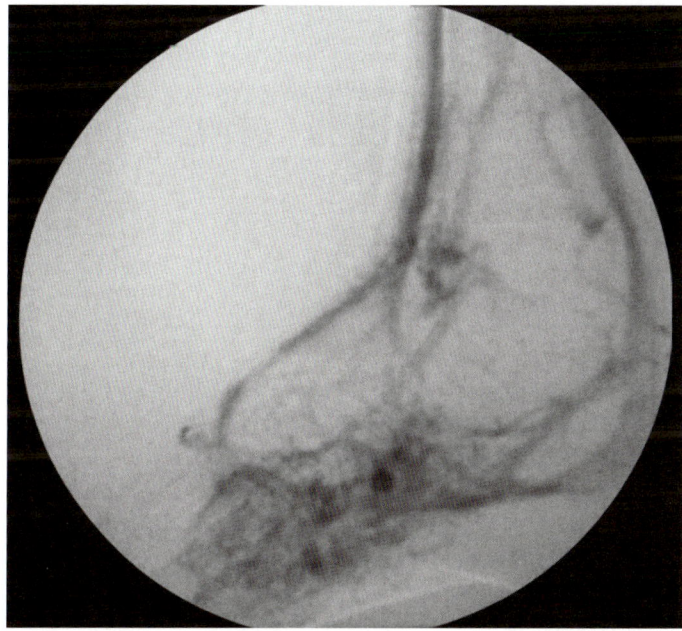

Fig. 7.41: DSA showing arteriovenous fistula

8

Examination of Upper Limb Ischaemia

INTRODUCTION

Upper limb ischaemia (ULI) is not an uncommon problem. Interestingly, there are many causes of ULI which are different from lower limb ischaemia. Generally, they are short cases in the university examinations. There are many special tests to be done in cases of upper limb ischaemia. Important causes have been given in Clinical Box 8.1. If you know the causes, then it is easy for you to ask leading questions. For example: Ergot drugs can give rise to gangrene. So, the question: Have you taken any drugs to treat your headache?

Pain in the upper limb can confuse many clinicians. If a 40-year-old man consults an orthopaedic surgeon, cervical spondylitis will be diagnosed. If he consults a physician, he will suspect Raynaud's disease. If he consults a surgeon, he will suspect TAO, and if he goes to a neurologist, he may suspect a spinal cord tumour.

Clinical Box 8.1

Causes of upper limb ischaemia
1. Raynaud's disease and Raynaud's syndrome: Usually bilateral
2. Embolic causes: Usually unilateral
3. Thoracic outlet syndrome: Unilateral
4. Trauma: Unilateral
5. Buerger's disease: May be bilateral
6. Axillary vein thrombosis: Unilateral
7. Vasculitis syndromes: Bilateral

PATIENT DATA

- Patient details such as name, age, place, occupation, admitting complaints, etc. are recorded. A common question is, 'how old are you?' If the age group is between 30 and 40 years, upper limb ischaemia is mostly caused by TAO (thromboangiitis obliterans) in men and vasculitis syndromes or Raynaud's disease in women.
- If patient is 50 years or above, ischaemia can be secondary to embolic process or trauma (atherosclerosis rarely affects upper limb arteries).
- 20–30 years old is the age group for cervical rib cases.

HISTORY

1. **Pain** in the limb is the chief symptom of lower limb ischaemia. When compared to lower limb, claudication in the upper limb is not common because of good collaterals and less vigorous muscular activity. Hence, pain may not be the first complaint. Often, it is mentioned as tiredness (sense of fatigue). If patient complains of pain, elicit all the details about the pain—nature, what type—is it crampy, burning, dull aching or unbearable pain disturbing sleep? When does it start? What is the relationship of the pain to usage of upper limb? Is it present at rest? Where is it felt? Does he sleep well at night?

   - Often a patient with rest pain holds his diseased hand with the other hand. This gives him some kind of relief. Rest pain is worse at night-time.

2. **How did it begin, suddenly or slowly?**

   - Sudden appearance of colour changes (pallor) and severe pain point at embolic gangrene (Fig. 8.1). If this history is given, ask leading questions related to cardiac diseases such as previous myocardial infarction, hypertension and valvular heart diseases.

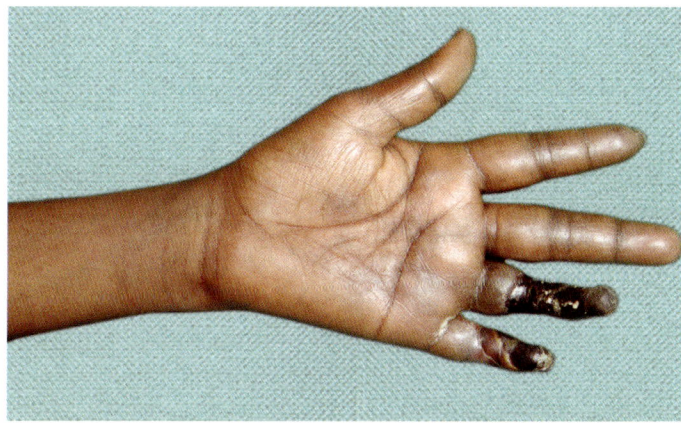

Fig. 8.1: Acute embolic gangrene—a case of cervical rib

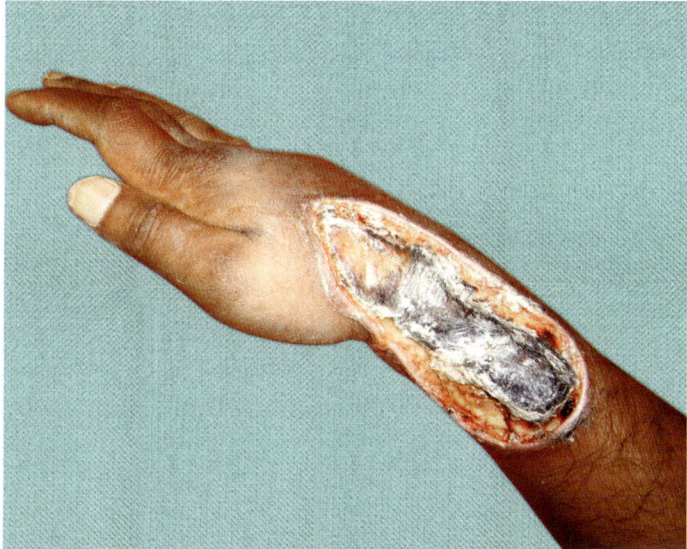

Fig. 8.2: Acute infective gangrene of the upper limb in a diabetic patient

- Slow development of pain, colour changes suggest chronic occlusion as in TAO.

3. **If any ulcer is present, find out the cause and duration.** It is usually precipitated by minor trauma and it occurs in the most distal part of the body such as the tip of the fingers. Ischaemic ulcers are deep and very painful. Enquire history of diabetes (Fig. 8.2).

4. If any black patches are found, enquire about the duration. Some patients present with **gangrenous patches** of skin or subcutaneous tissue. Gangrene affects distal parts such as fingers and nail beds.

5. History of coldness, numbness, paraesthesia and colour changes indicates chronic ischaemia. Excessive sweating is a vasomotor symptom.

6. History of any swelling in the lower neck or any dull pain suggests cervical rib.

7. Tingling and numbness, or paraesthesia in the distribution of C8, T1 **suggest features of ulnar nerve paralysis** or weakness. Lower nerve roots involvement, mainly first thoracic nerve can cause paralysis of interosseus muscles and wasting of hypothenar muscles. It includes sensory disturbances, motor disturbances (performing fine action—writing, buttoning), etc. (Clinical Box 8.2).

Clinical Box 8.2

Common causes of weakness of small muscles
1. **C**ervical rib
2. **C**arpal tunnel syndrome
3. **C**ervical disc (central protrusion)
4. **C**ervical spondylitis
5. **C**hronic disease—leprosy

Observe 5 Cs

---

8. Have you taken any medications for headache? Ergot alkaloids can cause peripheral gangrene.

9. Did you have any trauma to the upper limb or fingers? Trauma might have resulted in thrombosis or cut in a few arteries. Examples:
   - Supracondylar fracture of humerus: Brachial artery
   - Supracondylar fracture of femur: Popliteal artery
   - Dislocation of shoulder: Axillary artery
   - Dislocation of knee: Popliteal artery

10. History suggestive of other organ involvement is seen in atherosclerosis.
    - Chest pain—myocardial ischaemia
    - Fainting, transient black out—cerebral ischaemia
    - Blurred vision—retinal artery occlusion (*amaurosis fugax*)
    - Abdominal pain (post-prandial)—mesenteric ischaemia

11. Does he smoke? If yes, how many beedi or cigarettes per day? Majority of patients with peripheral vascular disease are smokers. TAO occurs exclusively in male smokers (Figs 8.3A and B).

Clinical Wisdom

Intermittent claudication of the masseter muscles can be caused by obstruction of ipsilateral common carotid or external carotid artery. It is more characteristic of Takayasu's arteritis.

Past History

- History of cardiac diseases, such as rheumatic heart disease and previous myocardial infarction, should be enquired.
- History of hemiparesis or chest pain in the past suggests atherosclerotic disease (embolic gangrene, Fig. 8.4).

Family History

Clotting disorders, such as protein S and protein C deficiencies, and sickle cell anaemia, can result in arterial thrombosis. They can also give rise to venous thrombosis.

Personal History

Important point is to enquire history of smoking and usage of nicotine.

CLINICAL EXAMINATION OF A CASE OF UPPER LIMB ISCHAEMIA

Inspection

- *Hand, fingers and entire upper limb*: Look for evidence of ulcer or gangrene. If present, describe them. Look for evidence of muscle wasting. Like lower limb look for evidence of chronic ischaemia of upper limb like ridging of nails, loss of pulp space, muscle wasting, etc. (trophic changes).

  Look for any prominent veins and oedema which may be caused by axillary vein thrombosis. In acute embolic gangrene, veins are empty.
- Mention muscle wasting/limb girth.
- Look for any swelling in the neck (supraclavicular region) which may be pulsatile. It may be post-stenotic dilatation of subclavian artery caused by cervical rib.

Palpation

- Palpate for any loss of sensation, tenderness and muscle wasting.
- Describe the ulcer such as location, size, shape, floor, edges, etc. Ulcers are typically located in the distal fingers and nail beds. They are usually small in size and irregular in shape. The floor of the ulcer may contain unhealthy (fresh case) and healthy granulation tissue in delayed cases. Edges can be sloping in healing ulcers or oedematous in spreading ulcers.

- Palpate brachial artery and radial artery: Mention beats per minute, volume, irregularities. Arterial wall is thickened in atherosclerosis.
- *Neck:* Bony mass or prominence caused by *cervical rib. It will be bony hard and fixed.*

  A. If a pulsatile swelling is found, mention whether the pulsations are transmitted or expansile.

  B. Other mass—lymph nodal mass.

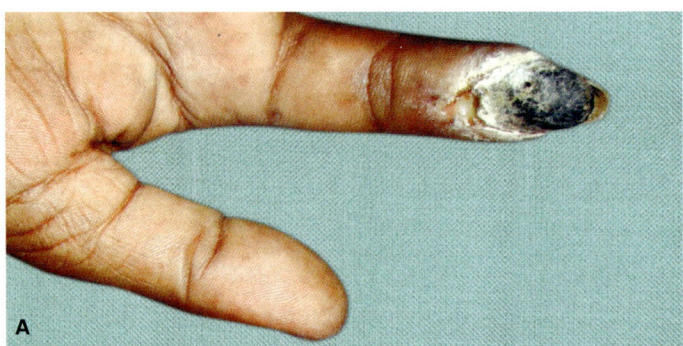

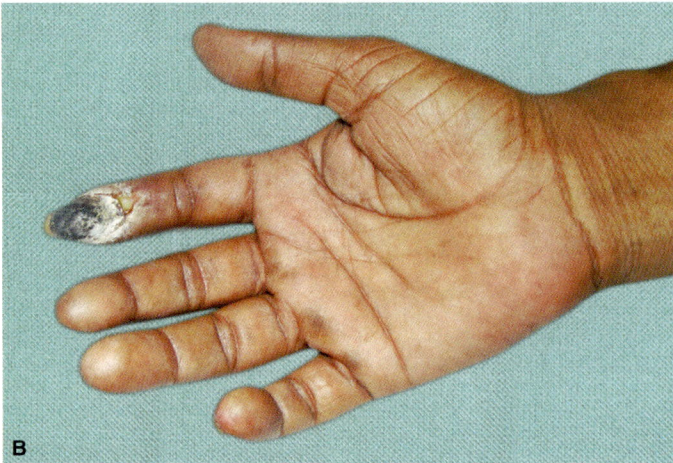

Figs 8.3A and B: Gangrene and secondary infection—TAO patient

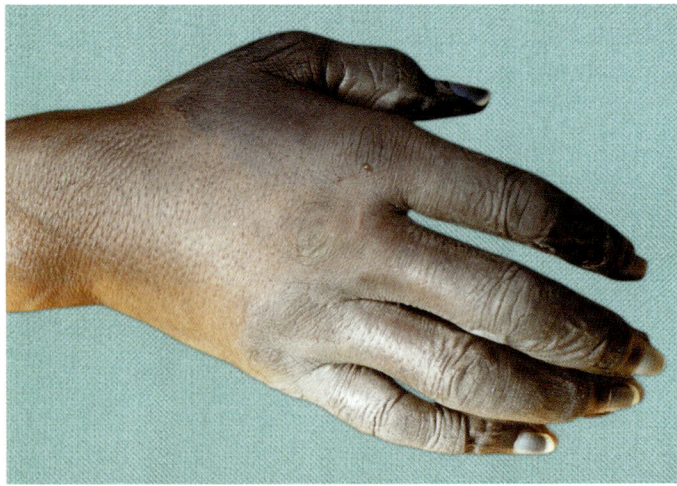

Fig. 8.4: Embolic gangrene—patient presented late to the hospital

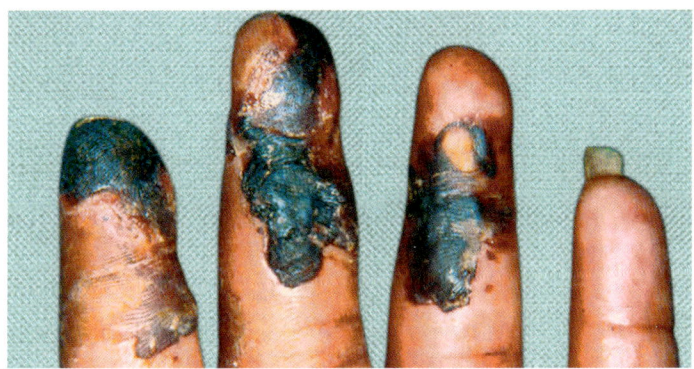

Fig. 8.5: Embolic gangrene of the fingers in a patient with mitral stenosis

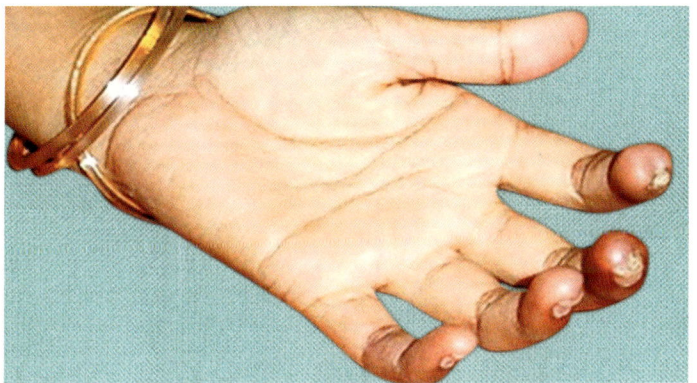

Fig. 8.6: Ischaemic ulcers and deformity of fingers—a case of systemic lupus erythematosus

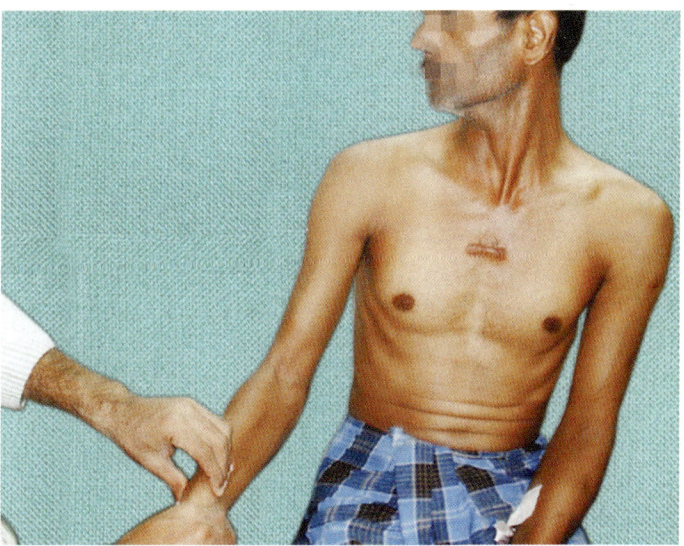

Fig. 8.7: Adson's test

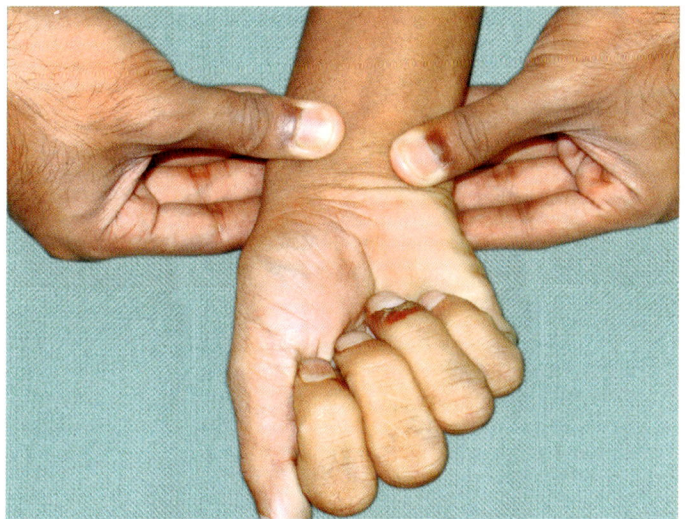

Fig. 8.8: Allen's test

- If gangrene is present (Fig. 8.5) or deformity (Fig. 8.6) is seen, describe them.
- **Special tests for thoracic outlet syndrome** (page 130)
  1. **Adson's test:** Feel radial pulse, ask the patient to take deep inspiration and turn the neck to the same side. The pulse may disappear or it may become feeble. This test indicates compression of subclavian artery (Fig. 8.7).

  2. **Allen's test:** The patient is asked to clench his fist tightly. Compress the radial and ulnar arteries at the wrist with your fingers. Wait for 10 seconds and then ask him to open his hand. The palm will appear pale. Now, release pressure on the radial artery and watch the blood flow into the hand. If there is radial artery occlusion, the colour changes to pink very slowly. You can repeat the test, releasing the pressure on ulnar artery this time, to check its patency (Fig. 8.8).

  3. **Military attitude test** (Fig. 8.9): When shoulders are set in backward and downward position, the radial pulse becomes weak. This is due to the compression of subclavian artery between the clavicle and first rib. **This is seen in costo-clavicular syndrome.**

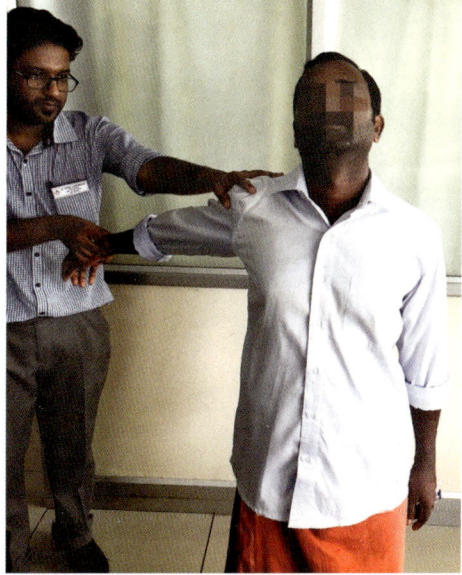

Fig. 8.9: Military attitude test

4. **Hyperabduction test (Halsted test):** This test is done to rule out hyperabduction syndrome caused by pectoralis minor. The radial pulse becomes weak on hyperabduction due to angulation of axillary vessels and brachial plexus, which gets compressed between pectoralis minor and its attachment to the coracoid process (Fig. 8.10).

5. **Elevated arm stress test (EAST) (Roos):** The patient is asked to abduct the shoulders to 90° and to flex the elbow. Then he is asked to pronate/supinate forearms continuously. Appearance of symptoms suggests thoracic outlet syndrome (Fig. 8.11).

Evidence of Nerve Paralysis

A. **Card test:** Patient is asked to hold a thin paper or a card in between the fingers. In cases of ulnar nerve paralysis, due to weakness of interossei muscles, patient is unable to hold the card tightly (Fig. 8.12).

B. **Froment's sign:** Patient is asked to hold a book between the hand and the thumb. In cases of ulnar nerve paralysis, since the adductor pollicis is paralysed, there is flexion at the distal interphalangeal joint of the thumb. This is because **flexor pollicis longus** which is **supplied by median nerve contracts** (Fig. 8.13).

Clinical Wisdom

Ulnar nerve involvement with ischaemia of fingers may suggest cervical rib as a cause of gangrene

---

Clinical Box 8.3

- Inspect hand for colour changes, ulcers, gangrene and muscle wasting
- Palpate upper limb arteries for pulsations
- Palpate supraclavicular region for bony mass
- Auscultate supraclavicular region for thrill
- Examination of peripheral nerve
- Examine the heart for murmur

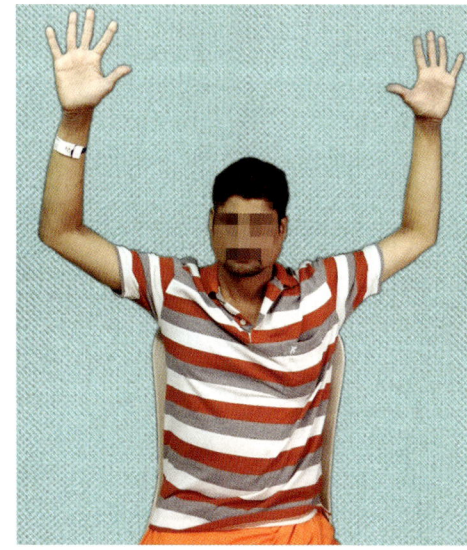

Fig. 8.11: Elevated arm stress test (EAST)

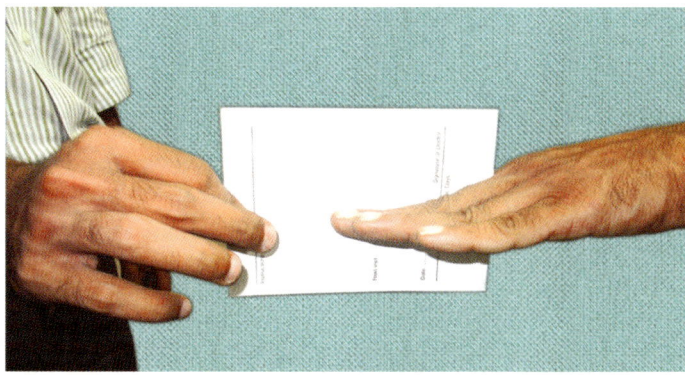

Fig. 8.12: Card test

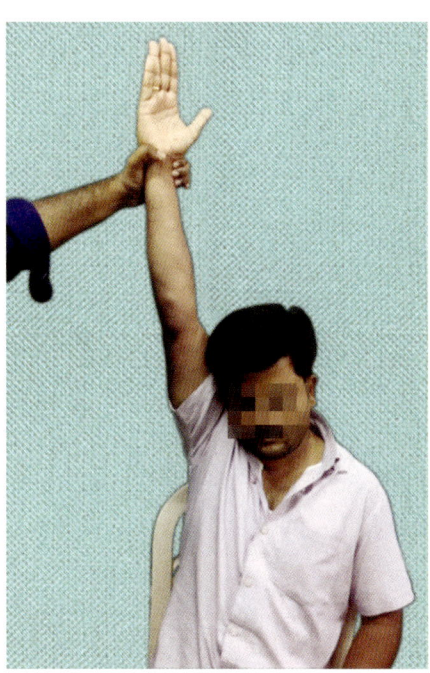

Fig. 8.10: Hyperabduction test (Halsted test)

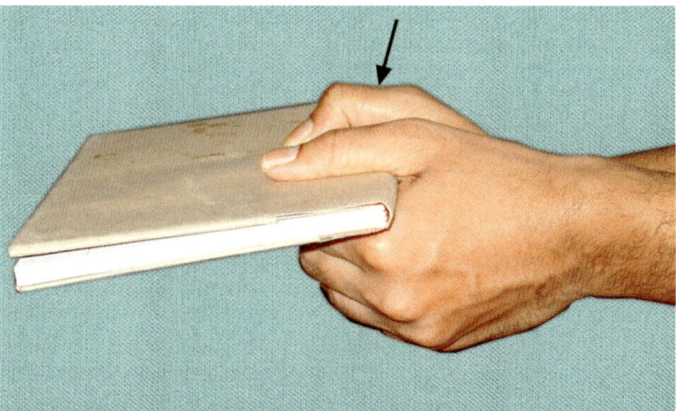

Fig. 8.13: Froment's sign

Examination of Regional Lymph Nodes

Enlargement of axillary lymph nodes can be due to infection associated with the gangrene.

Examination of Peripheral Vessels in all other Limbs

Upper limb involvement in addition to lower limb involvement is common in patients with TAO (Buerger's disease).

Examination of Cardiovascular System

Murmur and loud first heart sound are suggestive of mitral stenosis.

DIFFERENTIAL DIAGNOSIS

1. **TAO**: TAO can also affect upper limbs. It is a segmental occlusive inflammatory panarteritis. Usually involves the lower limb arteries first and later progresses to upper limb arteries. Typical features include: Chronic smoker, age between 25 and 40 years, involvement of small- and medium-sized arteries such as radial and brachial arteries in the upper limbs. If lower limb arteries also involved, it will add to the diagnosis. More details are given in Chapter 7.

2. *Raynaud's disease*
   - Affects young women.
   - Typically, it is described as **bilateral episodic digital ischaemia on exposure to cold.** Three stages have been described.
     a. *Stage of syncope:* Arterioles undergo constriction as an abnormal response to cold. As a result of this, the part becomes blanched and severe pallor develops.
     b. *Stage of asphyxia:* After a brief period of vasoconstriction, capillaries dilate, filling with deoxygenated blood resulting in bluish discolouration of the part (cyanosis).
     c. *Stage of recovery or stage of rubor:* As the attack passes off, relaxation of the arterioles occur, circulation improves and redness occurs. Because of dilatation of capillaries, red engorgement of the part occurs, which causes tingling, burning or bursting pain in the fingers.
   - **Thumb is usually spared.**
   - **Peripheral pulses are normal.**
   - Pallor, cyanosis and rubor are the colour changes occurring during the attack along with pain.
   - In a few patients, because of **recurrent attacks,** gangrenous patches occur on the tip of the fingers (superficial necrosis).

3. *Acute embolic gangrene*
   - **Brachial artery is the most common site of thrombo-embolism.**
   - It is a surgical emergency wherein the emboli have to be removed within 6–12 hours of obstruction. Otherwise gangrene can occur. Gangrene can be massive in proximal obstructions such as brachial artery. In a few other

cases, gangrene can be limited to small areas. Initial presentation is that of wet gangrene—part becomes oedematous, sudden change of colour to black, foul odour, with features of sepsis. If one examines these patients 2–3 weeks later, some demarcation would have developed and acute features will not be present such as foul odour and oedema. Sources of emboli are heart and atheromatous plaques.

   - In upper limb, source can also be from cervical rib with aneurysmal dilatation of subclavian artery harbouring thrombus.

4. *Vasculitis syndromes*:
   A. *Giant cell arteritis*: Elderly women presenting with **severe headache** is the common presentation. Involvement of various arteries will result in various symptoms. Palpable, **pulsatile, tender temporal arteries** will clinch the diagnosis. Relapses and remissions are common.
   B. *Polyarteritis syndrome*: Ischaemia of the lower limbs and upper limbs can occur due to involvement of small vessels. Abdominal pain is due to involvement of visceral vessels.
     - Involvement of renal arteries causes loin pain, haematuria and hypertension (Clinical Box 8.4).
   C. *Systemic sclerosis—scleroderma*
     - Ischaemic changes occur in the fingers and toes— necrosis and ulceration are common.
     - Oesophageal involvement results in dysphagia.
     - Raynaud's symptoms can be controlled using calcium channel blockers and nitrates.

Vasculitis syndrome **Clinical Box 8.4**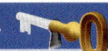

- Ischaemia and headache—giant cell arteritis
- Ischaemia with haematuria—polyarteritis syndrome with bruit in the loin
- Ischaemia with dysphagia—scleroderma with changes such as Raynaud's phenomenon in fingers
- *Upper limb claudication*, hypertension, visual disturbances in a woman with absent pulses—Takayasu's arteritis

---

Clinical Case Capsule

- A 40-year-old lady who had been getting recurrent episodes of pain and pallor of the digits of both upper limb and lower limb was admitted to the hospital this time for gangrene of the digits. On examination, all the four limbs were involved. All peripheral pulses were normal. It rules out atherosclerotic disease. A typical Indian woman and a nonsmoker, practically TAO is ruled out.
- Raynaud's disease was considered but lower limb involvement is extremely uncommon.
- Special tests for collagen vascular diseases were done, they were positive. In fact, she showed some improvement with steroids.

5. Cervical rib

- It is **more frequently** encountered on the **right side**. It is common in **young females**. Even though congenital, symptoms appear only at or after puberty. This is because of the development of shoulder girdle muscles and sagging of the shoulder which narrows the root of the neck. Nerve roots C8,T1 are stretched by completion of growth around 25 years.

- Tingling and numbness in the distribution of ulnar nerve can occur.

- Dull-aching pain in the neck is caused by expanded bony end of cervical rib.

- Claudication pain is apparent when the arm with muscle wasting is used. Low temperature, pallor, excessive sweating (vasomotor disturbances), **splinter haemorrhages**, ischaemic ulcers in fingers and gangrene of the skin of the fingers are the other features. Peripheral pulses may be absent/feeble. Oedema and venous distension are very rare. These are called vascular symptoms of cervical rib.

- Sensory disturbances and motor disturbances (performing, etc.) can also occur.

Types of Cervical Rib (Fig. 8.14)

Type I   The free end of the cervical rib is **expanded** into a hard, **bony mass** which can be felt in the neck (Fig. 8.15).

Type II   **Complete** cervical rib extends from C7 vertebra posteriorly to the manubrium anteriorly.

Type III Incomplete cervical rib, which is partly bony, partly fibrous.

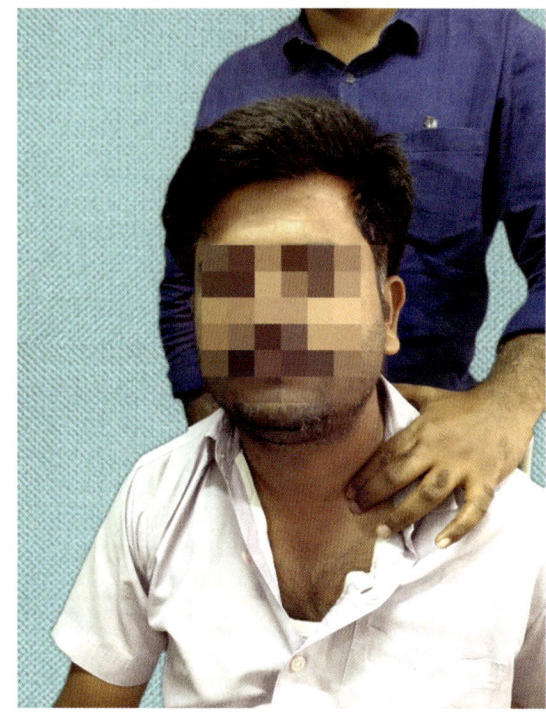

Fig. 8.15: Palpating for cervical rib

Type IV   A complete fibrous band which gives rise to symptoms but cannot be diagnosed by X-ray.

Investigations

1. X-ray neck: May show cervical rib (Fig. 8.16).
2. Duplex scan to detect post-stenotic dilatation and thrombus.

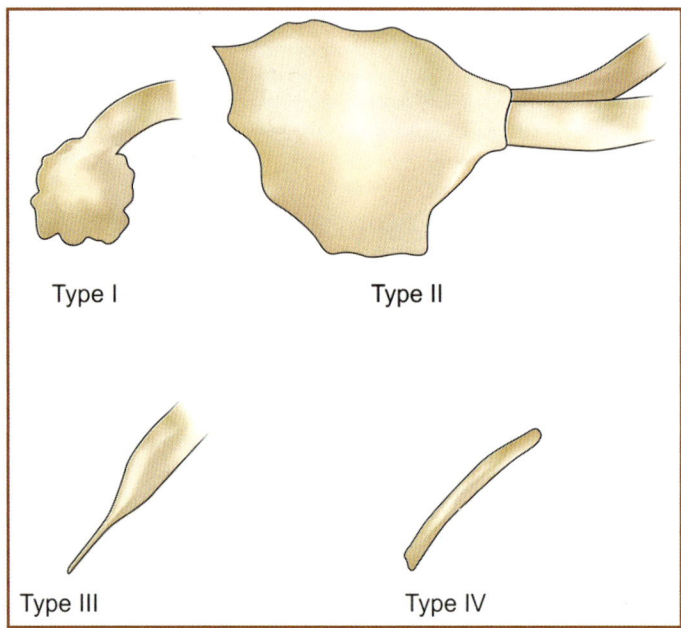

Fig. 8.14: Four types of cervical rib (*see* text)

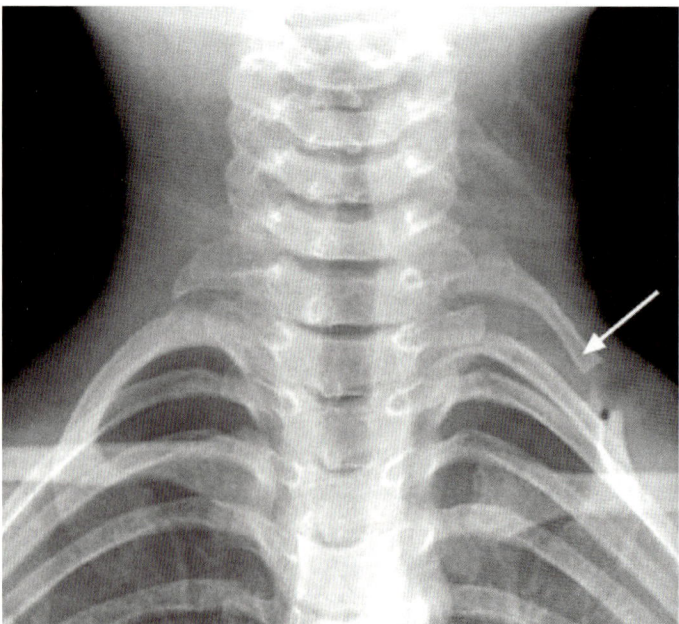

Fig. 8.16: Cervical rib

CLINICAL DISCUSSION

1. What is the definite indication for cervical rib excision?
- Presence of vascular symptoms such as ischaemic pain, pallor and gangrenous patches.

2. What is the treatment for cervical rib with symptoms?
- Extraperiosteal excision because if periosteum is left behind, recurrence can occur.

3. If hyperabduction test is positive, how do you treat?
- It is due to compression by pectoralis minor. In such cases, pectoralis minor has to be divided.

4. Which artery gets involved in Raynaud's disease?
- Usually all named arteries are normal because it affects arterioles. Hence, radial and ulnar artery will still be palpable but digital arteries are affected resulting in ischaemic changes.

5. How do you test for costoclavicular syndrome?
- It is by **military attitude test**.

6. If patient has severe headache, what is the diagnosis?
- Giant cell arteritis

7. Which nerve is affected in cases of cervical rib?
- Ulnar nerve

8. Why does post-stenotic dilatation occur?
- Due to jet-like effect or venturi effect

9. What is the treatment for post-stenotic dilatation?
- Repair

10. Why add cervical sympathectomy?
- To decrease the vasospasm.

GANGRENE

Definition

It is defined as macroscopic death of tissue with superadded putrefaction. It can affect the limbs intestines, appendix, etc. In this chapter, differential diagnosis of causes of gangrene of the limbs is considered.

Pregangrene

Rest pain, colour changes at rest and at exercise, oedema, hyperaesthesia, and skin ulcerations are due to inadequate blood supply to the limb. These changes are described as pregangrenous changes in the limb.

Classification of Gangrene

1. Cardiovascular causes

- TAO
- Atherosclerotic gangrene
- Acute embolic gangrene
- Syphilitic gangrene
- Raynaud's disease
- Cervical rib
- Vasculitis syndrome
- Polycythaemia

2. Neurological causes: Hemiplegia, paraplegia, bedsore

3. Traumatic gangrene: Direct—thrombosis; indirect—crushing injuries.

4. Physical causes: Sun rays, radiation, corrosive acids

5. Drugs: Ergotamine

6. Diabetic gangrene

7. Acute infective gangrene: Boil, carbuncle, cancrum oris, gas gangrene.

Clinical Types (Table 8.1)

Basically there are of two types:

- *Dry gangrene*: Non-infective
- *Wet gangrene*: Infective

Clinical Features of Gangrene
(Clinical Box 8.5)

- A part which is gangrenous is a dead portion of the body. It has **no arterial pulsations**, **venous return or capillary filling.**

- It has no sensation.

- The colour initially will be pale and later it changes to dusky grey and finally black. The **black colour** is due to disintegration of haemoglobin and formation of iron sulphide.

- The gangrenous part has to be treated by surgical excision or debridement, which may amount to either disarticulation of the toe or even an amputation.

- The gram-positive, gram-negative and anaerobic organisms multiply in this segment and can produce septicaemia. Thus, this may precipitate multiorgan failure such as renal failure, adult respiratory distress syndrome (ARDS), etc.

Special Types of Gangrene

Cancrum Oris

- It is an extensive ulcerative disease of cheek mucosa occurring in malnourished children.

Clinical Box 8.5

- No pulsations
- No sensations
- No venous return
- No capillary filling
- No function

Table 8.1: Comparison of dry gangrene and wet gangrene

	Dry gangrene	Wet gangrene
Cause	Slow occlusion of the arteries	Sudden occlusion of the arteries
Involvement of part	Small area is gangrenous due to presence of collaterals	Large area is affected due to absence of collaterals
Local findings	Dry, shrivelled and mummified	Wet, turgid, swollen, oedematous
Line of demarcation	Usually present	Absent
Crepitus	Absent	May be present
Odour	Absent	Foul odour due to sulphurated hydrogen produced by putrefactive bacteria
Infection	Not present	Usually present
Diseases	TAO, atherosclerosis	Emboli, ligatures, crush injuries
Treatment	Conservative amputation	Major amputation is necessary

- **Precipitating factors** are
  - Malnourishment
  - Major such as diphtheria, whooping cough, typhoid, measles, kala-azar, etc.
- As a result of these factors, opportunistic organisms such as Vincent's organisms—*Borrelia vincentii* and *fusiformis* multiply and cause multiple ulcers, erosions, later fibrosis.
- As the disease progresses sometimes the whole thickness of the cheek may be lost.

Treatment of cancrum oris
1. Ryle's tube feeding
2. Improve the nutrition
3. Appropriate antibiotics: Metronidazole 400 mg three times a day for 7–10 days.
4. Reconstructive surgery may be necessary later.

Complications of cancrum oris
1. Fibrosis causing restriction of the movement of jaw
2. Septicaemia, toxaemia and death

Acrocyanosis
- It is also called hereditary cold extremities.
- Persistent cyanotic discolouration of hands when exposed to cold is a feature.
- This is brought about by intermittent spasm of small peripheral vessels—commonly affects hands, rarely feet also.
- Generally, it is mild and nonprogressive.

Drug Abuse and Gangrene
- Abuse of the drugs is an important cause of gangrene in the modern days.

- Inadvertent injection of drugs into artery, results in thrombosis of the artery and acute ischaemia—commonly in the femoral artery.
- Emergency treatment in symptomatic cases includes heparinisation, and infusion of dextran 40.
- In severe cases, emergency angiography and intra-arterial thrombolysis is considered.

Iatrogenic Drug-induced Gangrene
- Inadvertent **intra-arterial injection of thiopentone** into one of the high divisions of brachial artery, (*congenital anomaly*) usually the ulnar, will result in severe burning and blanching of the hand (Fig. 8.17).
- After the injection, initial signs and symptoms occur very fast (within 15–20 seconds). It consists of intense forearm pain and mottling of the skin on his hand.
- Minutes later, discolouration and nail bed pallor become evident. Approximately 3 to 4 hours later, the symptoms progress to paraesthesias and pronounced hand weakness.

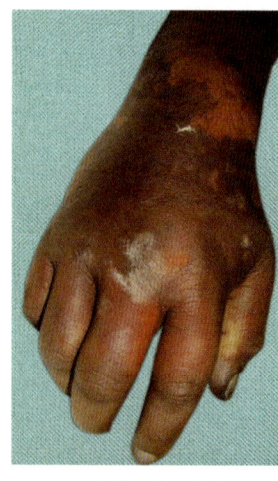

Fig. 8.17: Gangrene following intra-arterial injection

- Rapid development of signs indicative of necrosis (by the eighth day) may require the patient to undergo fasciotomies, multiple debridements and skin grafts for cosmesis.
- If this complication is noticed, following steps (measures) have to be taken immediately.

  Step 1: If iatrogenic, maintain the intra-arterial catheter in place—do not remove it.

  Step 2: Identify the progress of the disease—colour changes, necrosis, and gangrene.

  Step 3: Initiate anticoagulation—with unfractionated heparin intravenously.

  Step 4: Institute symptomatic relief and plan for rehabilitation—analgesics, physiotherapy.

  Step 5: Elevation of extremity, antibiotics.

  Step 6: Perform specific interventions—angiogram, intra-arterial thrombolysis, vasodilators, prostacyclins, sympathectomy, and corticosteroids.

  Step 7: Aim is to save the limb—last will be amputation.

Ergot and Gangrene

- Ergot preparations are used by patients with migraine over a long period.
- Ergotamine gangrene occurs in those who eat bread infected with *Claviceps purpurea*. *Example:* Dwellers on the shores of the Mediterranean sea and the **Russian Steppes.**

Axillary Vein Thrombosis

Patients present with swelling of arm after intense activity from the dominant hand.

- **Hypertrophy of subclavius muscle** also can cause compression of subclavian—axillary vein (sportsman).
- Peripheral pulses will be normal.
- Venography to diagnose thrombus.
- Thrombolysis or if necessary venotomy, removal of the thrombus and 1st rib (if it is the cause of obstruction) are the treatment modalities.
- Axillary vein thrombosis is also a complication of axillary block dissection especially where extensive nodal dissection has been done.

Bilateral Peripheral Symmetrical Gangrene

The most common cause of this is prolonged shock status. Septic shock in surgery can result due to peritonitis, bowel gangrene, mesenteric ischaemia,

etc. Septic shock results in a state of low perfusion to peripheries. It is a systemic derangement affecting all organ systems including coagulation and micro-circulation, resulting in hypoperfusion to peripheries. Long duration of low perfusion pressures might lead to peripheral ischaemia. Symmetrical peripheral gangrene is described as multiple extremity ischaemia at two or more sites in the absence of large vessel obstruction (Figs 8.18 and 8.19). Possible aetiological factors include obstructive sepsis, small vessel obstruction, use of vasopressors, etc. Aggravating factors are diabetes mellitus, cold injury to extremities, renal failure, and use of vasopressors. **It presents typically in intensive care unit and hence called as ICU gangrene. While treating the patient with vasopressors and other drugs in ICU, it is important look for pallor, cyanosis or colour changes in the extremities. If colour changes are seen, discontinue vasopressors as soon as possible. Debridement, amputations, skin grafting may be required depending upon severity.**

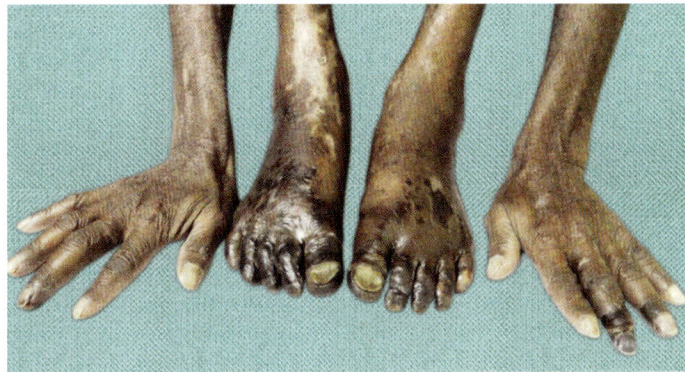

Fig. 8.18: All the four limbs developed gangrene following severe hypotension and shock due to gangrene of the bowel—resection and anastomosis

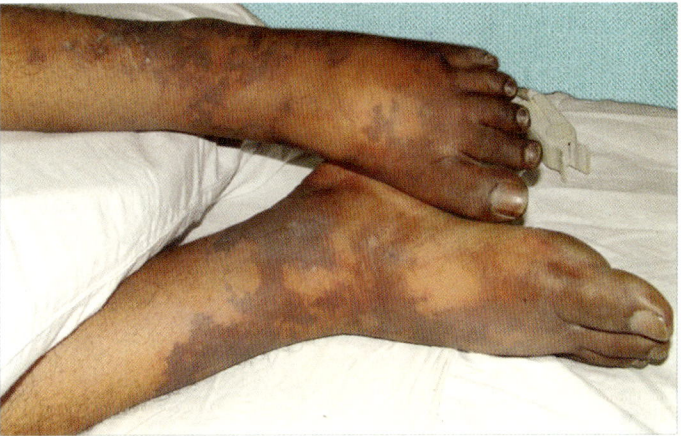

Fig. 8.19: Gangrene of the lower limbs in a patient who had myocardial infarction

9

Examination of Varicose Veins

INTRODUCTION

"Varicosity is the penalty for verticality against gravity". This is the common statement made in lecture classes. The blood has to flow from the lower limbs into the heart against gravity because of the upright posture of human beings. In many cases, varicose veins are asymptomatic. The raised intra-abdominal pressure also precipitates varicose veins, more commonly in females due to repeated pregnancy. The complications of varicose veins are responsible for hospitalisation of the patient. It is a common problem, more often encountered in males who stand for a long time—agriculturists, hotel workers, security guards, and traffic police.

- Students should have a clear idea about anatomy and physiology of venous drainage of lower limb before reading this chapter. In this chapter, examination of lower limb varicosity is being discussed.

Definition

Dilated (more than 3 mm), tortuous and elongated superficial veins of the limb are called varicose veins.

Examples of Varicosity

- Long saphenous varicosity (Fig. 9.1)
- Short saphenous varicosity (Fig. 9.2)
- Oesophageal varices and fundal varices
- Haemorrhoids
- Varicocoele
- Vulval varix and ovarian varix

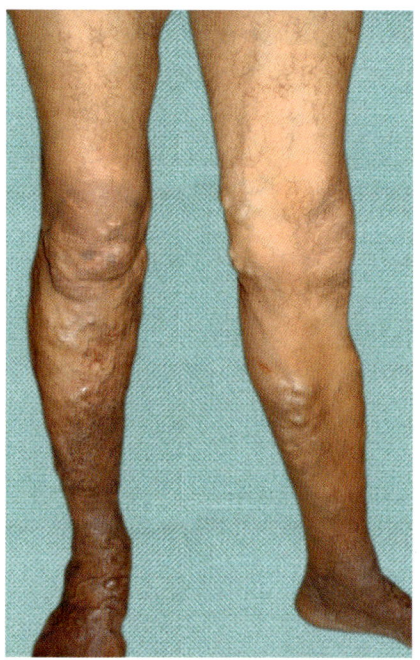

Fig. 9.1: Long saphenous varicosity

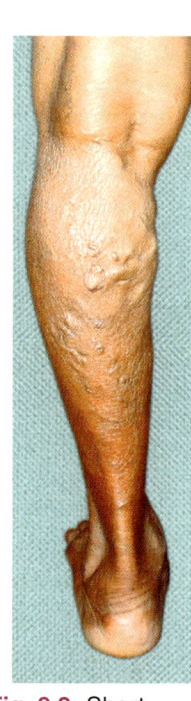

Fig. 9.2: Short saphenous varicosity

Types

I. *Primary:* Here varicosity develops due to incompetence of the valves at saphenofemoral junction or at saphenopopliteal junction or due to valves at the site of perforators, popularly called perforator incompetence.

II. *Secondary:* Here varicosity develops due to proximal obstruction of the venous system such as common iliac obstruction or inferior vena caval obstruction as happens in pregnancy, pelvic tumours, etc.

III. *Congenital AV fistula:* Appearance of varicose veins in young patients and in unusual locations in the leg may suggest congenital arteriovenous fistula.

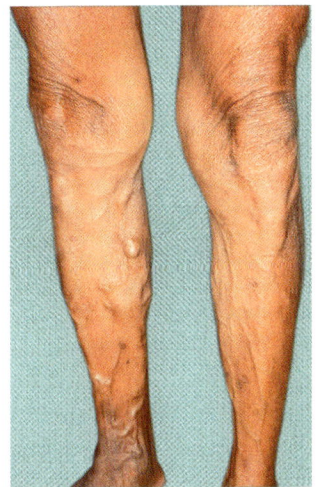

Fig. 9.3: Bilateral varicose veins

CLINICAL EXAMINATION OF A CASE OF VARICOSITY OF THE LEG

Patient Data

1. *Name and age:* Varicose veins are common in middle age group patients.
2. *Sex:* Women (10 times more common) are affected more than men.
3. *Occupation:* Hotel workers, traffic police, agriculturists who stand for a long time are vulnerable.
4. *Body build:* Tall individuals are more susceptible. Obesity is also one of the causes for varicosity of leg veins.

Symptoms

- Many patients are referred to the hospital because of the dilated veins (Fig. 9.3). When you ask them whether they have pain, they may acknowledge heaviness/dragging pain more so at night.
- Ask common questions such as where did the swelling or varicosity appear first? What is the progress? Do you have any pain? Do you have itching, skin changes, bleeding? etc.

Clinical Wisdom

Please do not describe the veins as swelling even though the patient may describe it as a swelling. You present as dilated veins. Rest of the history must be described in the patient's own words as given in various books.

- Majority of the patients present with dilated veins in the leg. They are minimal to start with and at the end of the day they are sufficiently large because of the venous engorgement.

Clinical Box 9.1

Common causes of cramps in the leg
1. Occlusive arterial diseases
2. Varicose veins
3. Dehydration
4. Hypocalcaemia, hypokalaemia, hypomagnesaemia
5. Medications such as:
   a. Diuretics, can cause loss of fluid and minerals
   b. Statins, which lower cholesterol and can cause muscle injury
6. Muscle fatigue or strain from overuse, too much exercise
7. Holding a muscle in the same position for a long time

- **Dragging pain** in the leg or dull ache is due to heaviness.
- **Night cramps** occur due to change in the diameter of veins. Aching pain is relieved at night on taking rest or elevation of limbs (Clinical Box 9.1).
- Often pain in the leg is disproportionate to the varicose veins and pain may be assumed to be 'psychological'. **In such cases, rule out occlusive arterial disease.**
- Sudden pain in the calf region with fever and oedema of the ankle region suggests deep vein thrombosis (DVT). Often pain in DVT has been described as bursting type of pain. Some patients with DVT may be asymptomatic. The pain is sometimes worse when varicose veins are developing than when they are fully stretched. Chronic DVT can present as dilated veins.
- Patients can present with ulceration, eczema, dermatitis and bleeding.
- Enquire about pruritus/itching and skin thickening.

Clinical Wisdom

Interestingly, pain due to varicose veins occurs on standing for a long time and is relieved on exercise in contrast to pain due to arterial diseases, which get worse on exercise. Pain in the legs can be due to arthritis, ischaemia or due to sciatica (neurogenic claudication). It is important to keep in mind these possibilities.

GENERAL PHYSICAL EXAMINATION AND ITS RELEVANCE IN VARICOSE VEINS

- Tall thin individuals
- Obese patients
- Port-wine stains, malformations can be associated with Klippel-Trenaunay syndrome (Clinical Box 9.2)

Past History

- Any surgical procedures in the past for varicosity—not uncommon.

Klippel-Trénaunay syndrome
- Port-wine stains capillary malformation
- Venous/lymphatic malformations
- Soft tissue hypertrophy of the limb
- Called valveless syndrome
- Typically the veins are large, lateral, superficial, valveless, unilateral or bilateral

- Any trauma to the leg such as road traffic accidents can lead to development of DVT. In such cases, varicose veins can be secondary to DVT.

Personal History

- Enquire about history of smoking in men. Smokers have an increased incidence of varicose veins. It may be due to the damage caused to veins by toxins present in tobacco.

- In women, elicit obstetric history including number of pregnancies, usage of contraceptive pills, when were the varicose veins noticed, was it during pregnancy or after the birth of the first child, should be enquired.

Clinical Wisdom

Varicosity is more common in women than in men, probably due to progesterone.

Family History

Family history can be present in a few patients. They have an early onset of varicose veins. Congenital absence of valves or weakness of the wall of the vein is responsible in such cases.

LOCAL EXAMINATION/REGIONAL EXAMINATION

Inspection (Clinical Box 9.3)

Saphenous vein
- Greeks knew the caudal part of the vein and called the vein saphenous. This word is derived from Greek word SAFAINA which means *evident*—easily seen (Fig. 9.4).
- On the other hand, proximal saphenous vein is called el safin or concealed by *Arabic physicians*.

1. *Veins*
   - **Dilated and tortuous veins** are present in the medial aspect of leg and the knee. Sometimes they are visible in the thigh also. These are due

Inspection
- Should be examined in the standing position
- Inspect both legs, groin and abdomen
- Inspect front, lateral and posterior parts of the leg
- Veins on the medial side are due to long saphenous varicosity and veins on the lateral and posterior side are due to short saphenous varicosity.
- Look for any inflammatory signs
- Look for any sign of deep vein thrombosis.

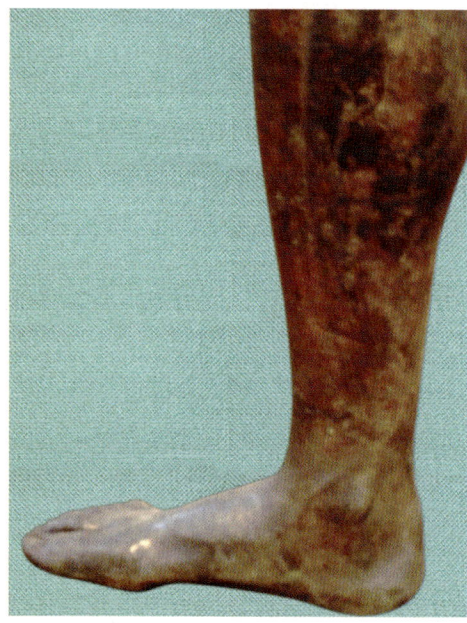

Fig. 9.4: Photograph of a bronze statue in National Archaeological Museum, Athens (Greece) showing long saphenous vein crossing anterior to medial malleolus

to long saphenous varcisosity. Classically veins can be seen running in front of medial malleolus. (Fig. 9.5)

- Single dilated varix at SF junction is called saphena varix. It is due to **saccular dilatation** of the upper end of long saphenous vein at the saphenous opening.

- A localised, dilated segment of the vein, if present, is an indication of a **blow out**. It signifies underlying perforator incompetence (Fig. 9.6).

- **Ankle flare** is a group of veins near the medial malleolus (Fig. 9.7).

- In the lower part of the leg and ankle, itch marks, ulcer or scarring may be present. Describe the ulcer, if it is present (Fig. 9.8).

- Healed scar indicates previous ulceration (Fig. 9.9).

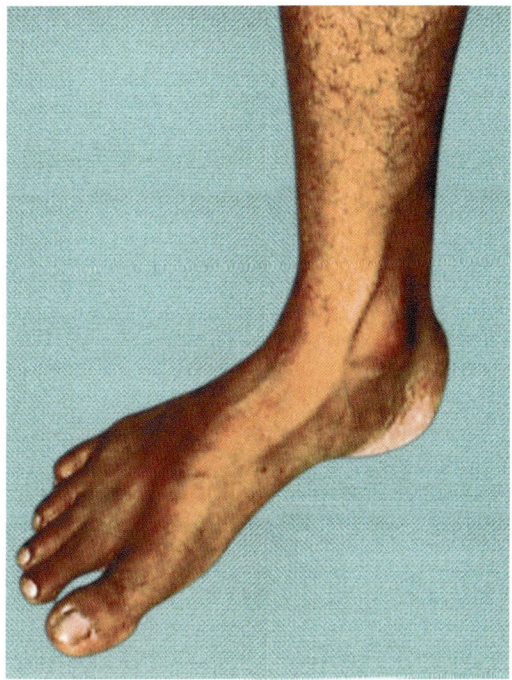

Fig. 9.5: Veins on the medial side of leg

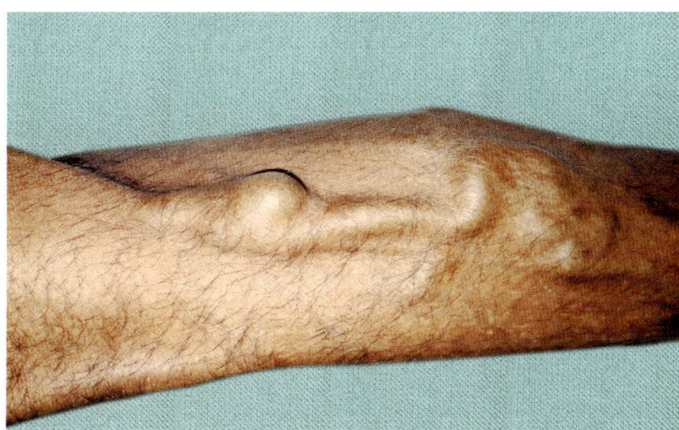

Fig. 9.6: Classical blow out

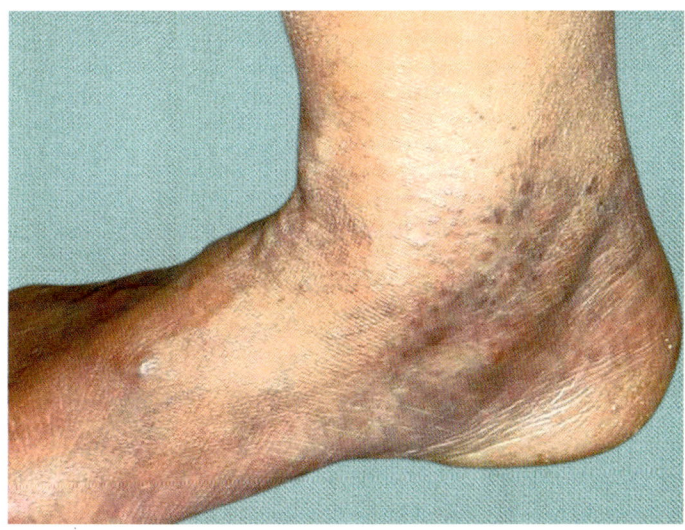

Fig. 9.7: Malleolar flare

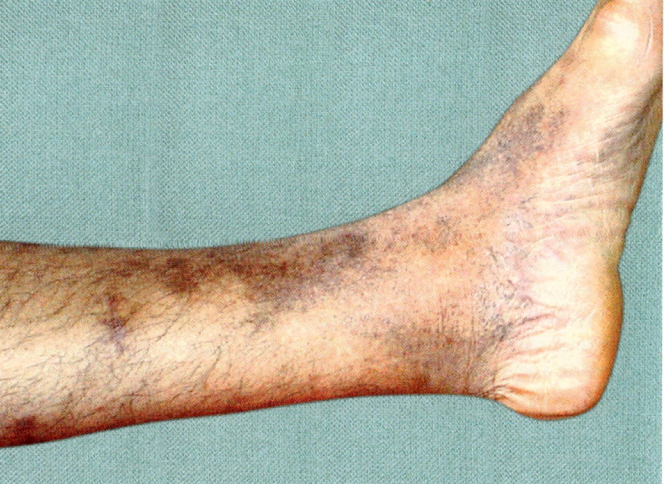

Fig. 9.8: Early skin changes—pigmentation and shiny skin

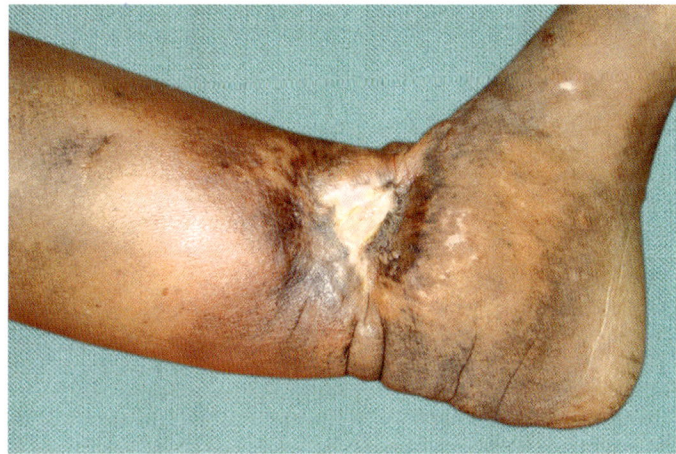

Fig. 9.9: Scarring ulcers, swollen lower leg

2. *Skin of the limb*
   - It can be normal in early cases.
   - Skin can be dry in long-standing cases.
   - Brownish pigmentation is due to loss of red blood cells into the tissues.

   - *White leg*: It is called phlegmasia alba dolens (PAD). It is due to lower limb deep vein thrombosis causing critical limb ischaemia.
   - *Blue leg*: It is called phlegmasia cerulea dolens. It is a more severe form of venous obstruction resulting in blue-cyanosed leg and swelling.

   - Local redness can be due to superficial thrombophlebitis. (Migratory thrombophlebitis is also seen in Buerger's disease and in visceral malignancies such as carcinoma pancreas.)

3. *Ulcers:* If ulcers are present, describe them in the usual manner—location (gaiter's area), size and

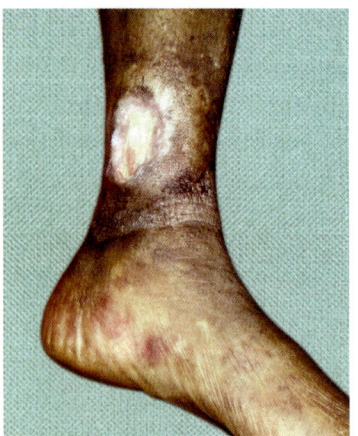

Fig. 9.10: Classical site of venous ulcer with pigmentation

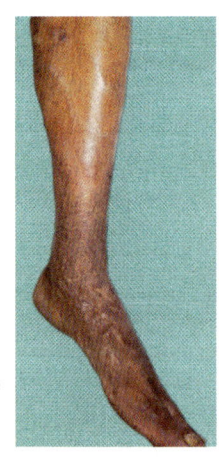

Fig. 9.11: Gaiter area pigmentation

shape, floor, edge, etc. Typically venous ulcers are located in the lower third of leg—on the medial side in long saphenous varicosity and on the lateral side in short saphenous varicosity. Sloping edge, pale/pink granulation tissue and pigmentation surrounding the ulcers are classical (Figs 9.10 and 9.11).

4. *Cough impulse test (Morrissey's test):* This test should be done in the standing position. Look for any impulse on coughing at the saphenous opening.

5. In a few cases of treated varicose veins, the ulcer would have healed with thin scar and you may see some residual veins.

*Some important findings have been mentioned in Clinical Box 9.4

Palpation

Before demonstrating the various tests for varicose veins, palpate the entire leg and look for:

- Tenderness along the vein—thrombophlebitis.
- Firm/hard nodule like feeling—calcification.
- Thickening of lower leg and tenderness, red shiny skin—chronic venous hypertension.
- Grossly thickened leg is due to lipodermatosclerosis.
- Tests for varicose veins can be classified as given below.

1. *Cough impulse test (Morrissey's test):* This test should be done in the standing position. First locate the SF junction (2.5 cm below and lateral to pubic tubercle). The examiner keeps the finger at SF junction and asks the patient to cough. Fluid thrill, an impulse felt by the fingers, is indicative of *'sapheno-femoral incompetence'* (Fig. 9.12).

2. *Brodie-Trendelenburg test:* This test is done in two parts:

- *Trendelenburg I:* The patient is asked to lie on the couch in the supine position. The leg is elevated above the level of heart and the vein is emptied. SF junction is occluded with the help of the thumb (or a tourniquet) and the patient is asked to stand. In Trendelenburg I, release the thumb or tourniquet immediately. *Rapid gush of blood from above downwards indicates saphenofemoral incompetence* (Figs 9.13 and 9.14).

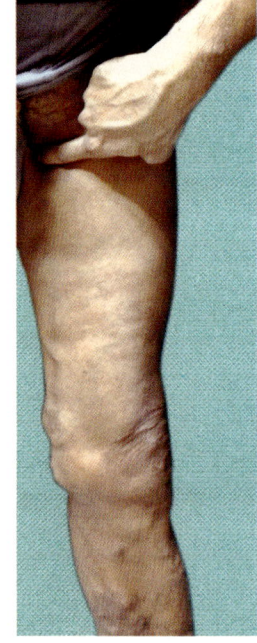

Fig. 9.12: Morrissey's cough impulse test

Test		
For SFJ	**For perforators**	**For DVT**
1. Morrissey's test	1. MTT	1. Perthes' test
2. Brodie-Trendelenburg test	2. Schwartz test	2. Modified Perthes' test
	3. Pratt's test	3. Homans' sign
	4. Fegan's method	4. Moses' test

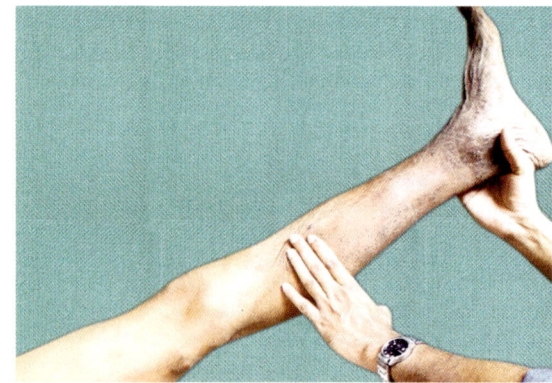

Fig. 9.13: Elevation of leg to empty the vein

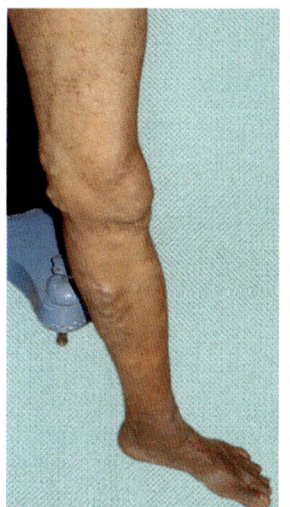
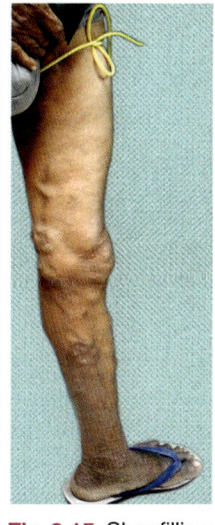
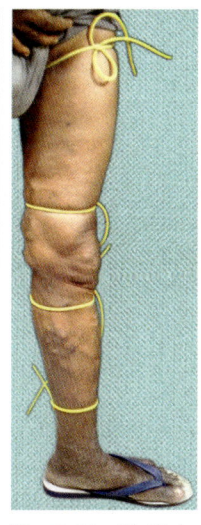

Fig. 9.14: Rapid filling in Trendelenburg I

Fig. 9.15: Slow filling in Trendelenburg II

Fig. 9.16: Multiple tourniquets test

- *Trendelenburg II*: The pressure at the SF junction is maintained without releasing the thumb or tourniquet. The patient is then asked to stand. ***Slow filling of the long saphenous vein from below upwards is seen. It is due to perforator incompetence*** (retrograde flow of blood) (Fig. 9.15).

3. **Multiple tourniquet test (Oschner—Mahorne test)** is done to find out exact site of perforators (Fig. 9.16).

   - *Method*: The patient is asked to lie supine on the couch. The vein is emptied by elevation. As the name suggests, 3–5 tourniquets (multiple) can be applied. However, if more tourniquets are applied, the exact localisation of the perforators can be made out. It is not practical. There are mainly ankle, knee and thigh perforators. Hence, four tourniquets can be applied at various levels as mentioned below:

     - *1st tourniquet*: At the level of saphenofemoral junction (SF junction).

     - *2nd tourniquet*: At the level of middle of the thigh, to occlude perforator in the Hunter's canal.

     - *3rd tourniquet*: Just below the knee.

     - *4th tourniquet*: Palm breadth (lower third of the leg) above medial malleolus/ankle.

   Ask the patient to stand and observe for appearance of veins.

   Inference: Appearance of veins between first and second tourniquets indicates incompetence of thigh perforators, between second and third indicates incompetence of knee perforators and below the fourth tourniquet indicates incompe-

tence of ankle perforators. Usually, below knee and ankle perforators will be incompetent.

On releasing the tourniquets one by one from below upwards, sudden retrograde filling of the veins occurs.

4. **Schwartz test**: It is done with the patient in the standing position and can be done by 2 methods

   - *Tap below*: Place the fingers of the left hand over a dilated segment of the vein and with the right index finger tap the vein below. A palpable impulse suggests *continuous column* of *blood in the vein* and it also *suggests incompetence of the valves* in that segment of the vein (Fig. 9.17).

   - *Tap above*: Tapping above the most prominent part of the vein, one can get the impulse or wave below. It suggests absent or incompetent valves between tapping fingers and the palpating finger.

5. **Modified Perthes' test** is done to rule out deep vein thrombosis. The patient is asked to stand, the tourniquet is applied at SF junction and he is asked to take a brisk walk (Fig. 9.18).

Inference: If the patient complains of severe pain in the calf region or if superficial veins become more prominent, it is an indication of **deep vein thrombosis** and is a contraindication for surgery.

Clinical Wisdom

Please note: Vein is not emptied in this test

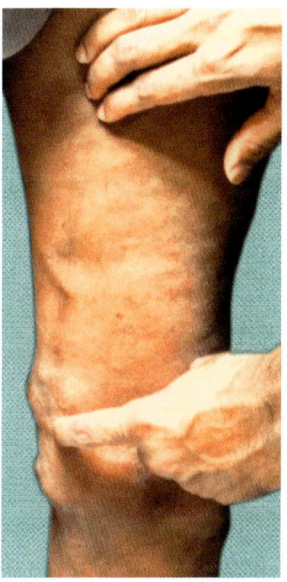
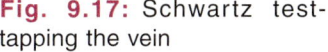
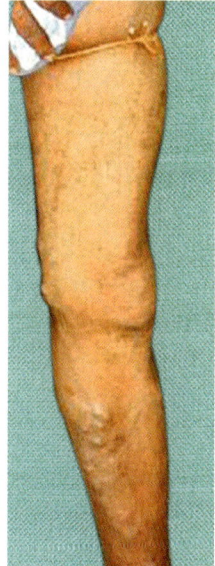

Fig. 9.17: Schwartz test- tapping the vein

Fig. 9.18: Vein is not emptied in Perthes' test

6. *Pratt's test*: This test helps to reconfirm what has been inferred by multiple tourniquet test such as the site of perforators.

Procedure: An Esmarch elastic bandage is applied from toes to groin. A tourniquet is applied superior to the Esmarch's bandage in the groin. Thus, veins are emptied. Now Esmarch's bandage is removed. Now the same bandage is applied from above downwards.

Results: Prominence of the veins is seen, especially the blow outs where there are incompetent perforators. They can be marked before the surgery with the help of Duplex scan.

Historical

Esmarch bandage (also known as **Esmarch's bandage for surgical haemostasis** or **Esmarch's tourniquet**) in its modern form is a narrow hard rubber tourniquet with a chain fastener that is used to control bleeding by applying it around the limb in such a way that blood is expelled from it. This prevents the flow of blood to or from the distal area, making it easier to operate. The limb is often elevated as the elastic pressure is applied. The original version was designed by Friedrich von Esmarch, Professor of Surgery at the University of Kiel, Germany, and is generally used in battlefield medicine. Esmarch himself had been Surgeon General to the German army during the Franco-German War.

7. *Fegan's method (test)*: It is done to detect the site of perforators. The patient is asked to stand. The varicosity is marked with methylene blue and he is asked to lie down. The leg is elevated to empty the vein and the vein is palpated throughout its course. The defects in the deep fascia have a circular, button hole consistency (Fig. 9.19).

   Please note: *All these tests have lost importance because of very subjective interpretations and inconvenience caused to the patients. Duplex scan is more reliable, credible and convenient to the patients. However, for the sake of passing examinations, one should know them.*

8. Inspection of posterior surface of leg to rule out short saphenous varicosity (Fig. 9.20).

9. *Examination of varicose ulcer* by inspection and palpation should be done. Typically, it is an ulcer with sloping edge and nontender.

10. *Examination of groin nodes*: These are enlarged in venous ulcers.

11. *Evidence of deep vein thrombosis*: Homans' test and Moses' test (*vide infra*) must be done in chronic DVT.

12. *Examination of the abdomen*: To rule out pelvic tumours. Look for inferior vena caval obstruction

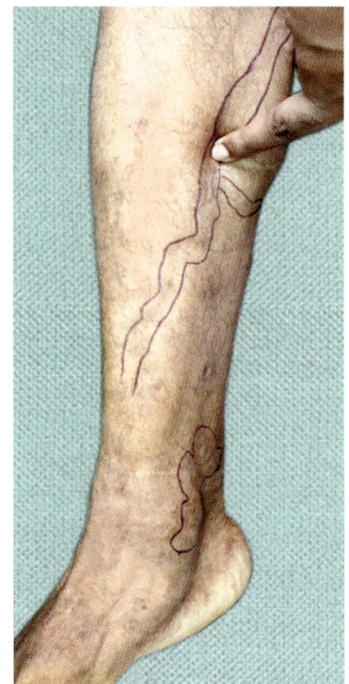

Fig. 9.19: Fegan's method

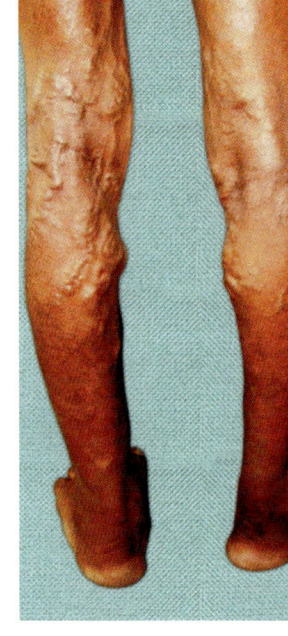

Fig. 9.20: Posterior part of leg showing dilated veins due to long saphenous varicosity

in the form of dilated veins in the lateral abdominal wall.

- *Harvey's test*: When veins are visible in the abdominal wall, this test helps in determining the direction of the blood flow. Place two fingers over the vein and slide one finger along vein to empty it. Then release the finger and watch which way blood flows. Now do the reverse and you can then conclude which way the blood flows (Figs 9.21 and 9.22).

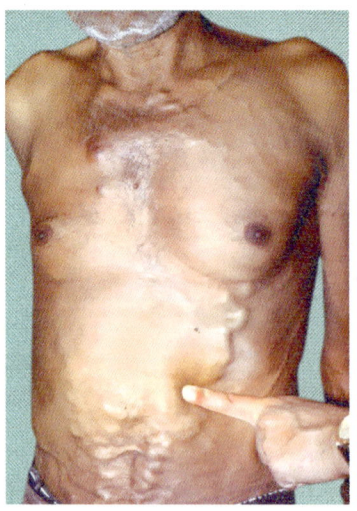

Fig. 9.21: Checking for direction of blood flow

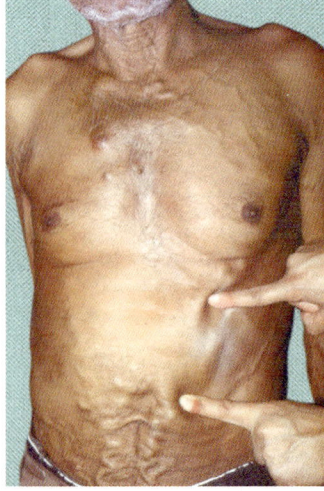

Fig. 9.22: Veins of anterior abdominal wall—testing for refilling

A few examples of this test are given below

1. **In caput medusae** (veins around umbilicus in portal hypertension), blood flow is towards the heart from veins above umbilicus but blood flow is towards groin from veins below the umbilicus.
2. **In cases of inferior vena caval obstruction,** prominent veins will develop in the flanks. They are called inguinoaxillary veins. Blood flow is from below upwards.
3. **In superior vena caval obstruction :** Prominent veins will develop over the chest and neck. Blood flow is towards the heart.

Examination of peripheral arteries: Palpate for the presence of at least a few lower limb arterial pulsations such as dorsalis pedis and posterior tibial artery (refer to Clinical Case Capsule).

■ Clinical Case Capsule

A 35-year-old chronic smoker who had cramps in the leg presented to the surgeon with dilated veins in the leg. Trendelenburg's operation was done as he had saphenofemoral and perforator incompetence. A tight elastic crepe bandage was applied to the foot. The surgeon had to leave his hospital for some personal work for another 2 days. The patient had excruciating pain in the first 2 days postoperatively which was attributed to surgery and analgesics were given. When the surgeon saw him after 2 days, he had gangrene of the limb for which he underwent below knee amputation. The surgeon had to pay huge sum following the verdict of the court as a compensation. The entire problem could have been avoided, if he were to examine his peripheral pulses which were weak. It was a case of Buerger's disease and veins were asymptomatic.

Auscultation: This is relevant only in cases of tortuous veins due to arteriovenous fistulas with high pressure flow.

Diagnosis: Mention the side, the vein which is involved status of SF junction, perforators and complications if any

- Refer to Tables 9.1 and 9.2 for classification and grades of varicose veins. When you are giving the diagnosis you can mention the grade and the CEAP classification also.

TESTS FOR SHORT SAPHENOUS VARICOSITY

Inspection

- Typical location is on the lateral side of the foot and the vein ascends behind lateral malleolus. A few

Table 9.1: Classification of chronic lower extremity venous disease

Classification	Definition
C	Clinical signs (grade 0–6): A for asymptomatic or S for symptomatic
E	Etiologic classification (congenital, primary or secondary)
A	Anatomic distribution (superficial, deep or perforator, alone or in combination)
P	Pathophysiologic dysfunction (reflux or obstruction, alone or in combination)

This classification is from International Consensus Committee on Chronic Venous Diseases.

Table 9.2: Clinical classification of chronic lower extremity venous disease

Grade	Characteristics
0	No visible or palpable signs of venous disease
1	Telangiectases, reticular veins, or malleolar flare
2	Varicose veins
3	Oedema without skin changes
4	Skin changes ascribed to venous disease (e.g. pigmentation, venous eczema, or lipodermato-sclerosis)
5	Skin changes as defined above with healed ulceration
6	Skin changes as defined above with active ulceration

communicating veins may be found joining and ending in the popliteal vein (posterior aspect of knee).

- Impulse on cough at SP (saphenopopliteal) junction can be tested but may be difficult to appreciate since it is a small vein and the SP junction is not constant in position.
- Pigmentation, skin changes including ulcer, if present, should be described.

Palpation

- Impulse on cough at SP junction can be tested by keeping the fingers over SP junction and asking the patient to cough.
- Trendelenburg's test can be done by applying tourniquet over the SP junction and looking for veins in the leg.
- Schwartz test is also done in a similar way as done for long saphenous varicosity.
- Comparison between long saphenous varicosity and short saphenous varicosity is given in Table 9.3 (next page).

Table 9.3: Comparison between long saphenous and short saphenous veins

Features	Long saphenous vein	Short saphenous vein
1. Origin	Medial part of dorsal venous arch	Lateral part of dorsal venous arch
2. Location	Front of medial malleolus	Behind lateral malleolus
3. Relation with nerve	Saphenous nerve	Sural nerve
4. Number of valves	15–20 valves	10–15 valves
5. Termination	Saphenofemoral junction	Saphenopopliteal junction

CLINICAL DISCUSSION

At the end of clinical examination, you should be able to answer the following questions:

1. **Which system is involved?**
   - Medial veins—LSV
   - Lateral veins—SSV

2. **Is SF junction incompetent?**

   Yes—Trendelenburg I is positive.

   No—Trendelenburg I is negative.

3. **Is there perforator incompetence?**

   Yes—Trendelenburg II is positive.

   No—Trendelenburg II is negative.

4. **Which group of perforators are incompetent?**

   According to the results of multiple tourniquet test (mostly ankle and below knee).

5. **Is there deep vein thrombosis?**

   Yes—Perthes' test is positive.

   No—Perthes' test is negative.

6. **Is there any abdominal mass?**

   Pelvic tumours can compress iliac veins and can result in secondary varicosity and distal oedema.

7. **Are there any visible veins in the abdominal wall?**

   If so, is there inferior vena caval obstruction?

8. **Are there any complications?**

   Eczema, dermatitis, ulcer, etc.

9. **Is it unilateral or bilateral?**

10. **What about short saphenous varicosity?**

    Veins on lateral and posterior part of leg.

11. **What is the first investigation apart from routine investigations?**

    Hand-held Doppler, when kept over the saphenofemoral junction (SF) and calf is squeezed, will show the direction of flow and reversal in saphenofemoral incompetence. In the similar way, saphenopopliteal (SP) reflux can also be demonstrated.

12. **What is role of Valsalva manoeuvre?**

    Valsalva manoeuvre is asking the patient to exhale or blow air with nose and mouth closed (airway closed). Venous reflux can be demonstrated at SF junction.

13. **What next?**

    Colour Doppler or duplex Doppler imaging: This is an excellent investigation to get the anatomical details about the veins including abnormalities such as accessory long saphenous vein, to know the luminal narrowing, to define the reflux (Valsalva manoeuvre), to localise the perforators and mark them (before surgery). Colour coding will help to identify the veins (blue) and artery (red). Importantly, it is the investigation of choice for deep vein thrombosis.

14. **What is the treatment for SFI?**

    Trendelenburg's flush ligation followed by stripping of long saphenous vein up to below knee.

15. **What are the tributaries to be ligated?**

    Superficial circumflex iliac, superficial epigastric and superficial external pudendal veins.

16. **What if only perforators are involved?**

    Subfascial ligation of perforators (Cockett and Dodd).

17. **Any other tests?**

    Routinely not done but in cases of unusual veins, unnatural veins, unexpected veins, e.g. sudden appearance of veins in the thigh, proximal obstruction is suspected and an abdominal ultrasound is obtained to rule out pelvic tumours.

18. **Should we do any tests to rule out hypercoagulable state?**

    These are not routinely done but patients having recurrent deep vein thrombosis, recurrent embolism, as in limb ischaemia, stroke, myocardial infarction. Various tests that are done are: Activated protein C, homocysteine levels, anti-phospholipid antibodies (APLA), factor V Leiden.

19. **What nutrient deficiency can give rise to hyperhomocystinaemia?**

    Vitamin B_6, vitamin B_{12} and folate.

20. **What is postphlebitic limb?**
    - Due to increased pressure in the venous system and due to long-standing disease, limb undergoes several changes which are grouped together as postphlebitic limb (Fig. 9.23).

21. **How do you suspect deep vein thrombosis (DVT)?**
    - Sudden pain in the calf region with oedema of the ankle region.

22. **What is May-Thurner syndrome?**
    - Iliofemoral thrombosis is common on the left side because left common iliac vein is compressed by common iliac artery.

23. **Why is varicose vein more common in medial side?**
    - Because of plenty of perforating veins.

24. **What is the complication of long-standing varicose ulcer?**
    - Marjolin's ulcer.

25. **What are the tests to detect deep vein thrombosis?**
    - Doppler ultrasound can detect 95% of cases of DVT which are proximal to calf muscles but sensitivity comes down for calf veins DVT. Measurement of D-dimer crosslinked fibrin degradation products as a noninvasive test has 90–

92% sensitivity. Ascending venography is still the standard but is invasive.

26. What are the causes of secondary varicose veins?

- Obstruction, destruction or high pressure flow.

    Obstruction—mass

    Destruction—DVT

    High pressure—arteriovenous fistula.

27. What is Trendelenburg's operation?

- It involves ligation of tributaries at saphenofemoral junction followed by juxtafemoral flush ligation of long saphenous vein.

28. What are tributaries to be ligated at SF junction?

- Superficial external pudendal, superficial epigastric and superficial external iliac

29. What will happen if they are not ligated?

- Blood can flow back from these named tributaries into the unnamed tributaries and can result in development of varicosities. These are called secondary varicosities.

30. What will happen if SF junction is not ligated juxta-femoral?

- It will result in saphena varix

DEEP VEIN THROMBOSIS (DVT)

It is also called phlebothrombosis. It is an acute thrombosis of deep veins. Deep vein thrombosis is very common in the Western countries, the exact cause of which is not known. Postoperative immobilisation, pressure on the calf muscles, sluggish blood flow and prolonged bedrest are the various factors which precipitate deep vein thrombosis. Commonly, it affects venous sinuses in the soleal muscles. It is a common starting place. It can also involve pelvic veins. Important causes have been summarised in Clinical Boxes 9.5 and 9.6.

Clinical Box 9.5 🔑

- Postoperative immobilisation
- Pressure on calf muscles
- Poor (sluggish) blood flow
- Prolonged bedrest

Clinical Box 9.6 🔑

Major hypercoagulable syndromes
- Factor V Leiden mutation—activated protein C resistance
- Antithrombin III deficiency
- Protein C deficiency
- Protein S deficiency
- Dysfibrinogenaemia
- Antiphospholipid syndrome

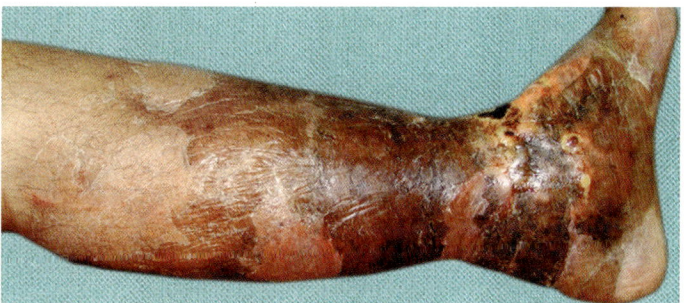

Fig. 9.23: Postphlebitic limb

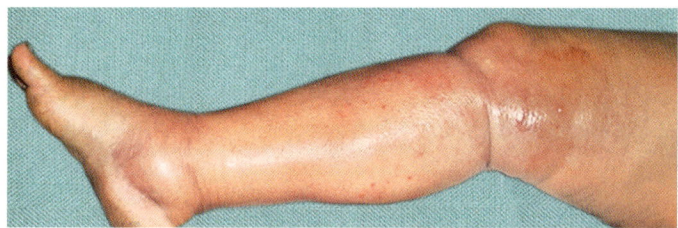

Fig. 9.24: Acute DVT

▌ Clinical Case Capsule

A case of deep vein thrombosis

A 56 year old gentleman came to surgery outpatient department with unilateral swelling of the limb of 2 months duration. He was a smoker which prompted a consultant to ask for arterial Doppler which showed atherosclerotic changes. However, he never had any claudication of the foot or thigh muscles.

Careful examination revealed chronic deep vein thrombosis with minor secondary veins. History, examination and usual investigations could not reveal the cause of thrombosis. A special thrombosis work up was done including protein C, protein S and homocysteine. Serum homocysteine level was elevated 10 times the normal. He was put on capsule Homocyst. He improved.

Clinical Features of Acute DVT

- The maximum incidence occurs on the 2nd day and 5th–6th days in the postoperative period.

- First complaint is usually oedema, erythema, and dilated veins of the leg (Fig. 9.24).

- Dull aching or nagging pain in the calf muscles is present.

- Superficial blebs in the skin.

- Low grade fever with increased pulse rate is characteristic.

- *Phlegmasia alba dolens refers to white leg. It occurs when the thrombus extends from calf region to iliofemoral vein.*

- Phlegmasia cerulea dolens refers to blue leg with loss of superficial tissues of the toes.

Table 9.4: Pharmacological management of DVT

Drug	Dosage	Timing
DVT prophylaxis		
LMWH		
• Enoxaparin	40 mg SC OD	Start 12 hours preoperatively
• Dalteparin	2500–5000 IU SC OD	12–24 hours postoperatively
• Danaparoid	750 U SC BD	12–24 hours postoperatively
• Nadroparin	38 U/kg SC OD	12–24 hours postoperatively
• Tinzaparin	50–75 U/kg SC OD	12–24 hours postoperatively
Factor Xa inhibitor		
Fondaparinux (Arixtra)	2.5 mg SC OD	6–8 hours postoperatively
DVT treatment		
Enoxaparin (Clexane)	1 mg/kg BD or 0.6 ml SC BD	
Fondaparinux (Arixtra)	<50 kg: 5 mg SC OD	
	>50 kg: 7.5 mg SC OD	
Nadroparin (Fraxiparine)	50 kg: 0.5 ml SC BD	
	60 kg: 0.6 ml SC BD	
	70 kg: 0.7 ml SC BD	

SC: Subcutaneous
OD: Once a day
BD: Twice a day

Signs (Acute DVT)

1. **Homans' test:** Forcible dorsiflexion of foot results in severe pain in the calf region.
2. **Moses' test** (ideally should not be done for fear of embolism): Tenderness over calf muscle on squeezing the muscle from side-to-side.

   *Prophylaxis of DVT and drug treatment are given in Table 9.4.

Clinical Features of Chronic DVT

A DVT which is present longer than 4 weeks of duration is defined as 'Chronic DVT'. The signs and symptoms include pain, oedema, telangiectasia, hyperpigmentation, lipodermatosclerosis, ulceration and venous claudication. The clinical manifestations are secondary to Post Thrombotic Sequelae (PTS) that occurs after an episode of DVT as thrombosis leads to venous hypertension from venous obstruction and reflux.

The diagnosis of a chronic DVT is usually made by ultrasound duplex scan which shows a hyperechoic, non-compressible material in a narrow irregular lumen with collateral vein formation.

Treatment

- Graded compression stockings along with anticoagulation therapy. Compression stockings (30-40 mmHg) should be worn daily for 2 years from onset of DVT.
- Parenteral anticoagulation initially and oral anticoagulation is added which is titrated with measuring the INR. Vitamin K antagonist Tab Warfarin 5–10 mg per day is given with monitoring of the INR (International Normalised Ratio) with a therapeutic target INR between 2.0 to 3.0.
- In patients with proximal DVT (ilio-femoral), recurrent episodes or secondary to malignancy should be treated for a period of 6 months – 1 year. Indefinite therapy is recommended for patients with recurrent episodes of venous thrombosis regardless of the cause.

Surgical Management

- Open surgery: Femoro-femoral bypass (Palma bypass when saphenous vein is used)
- Femoroiliac infrahepatic inferior vena cava bypass.

10

Examination of the Lymphatic System

INTRODUCTION

The lymphatic system consists of aggregation of lymphoid tissue—lymph glands (nodes), tonsils and lymphatic channels which help in circulation as well as production of lymphocytes in the thymus, liver, spleen and bone marrow. 500 to 700 lymph nodes are present in the body out of which about 300 are present in the neck. Common causes of enlargement of lymph nodes are tuberculosis, tumours and infections. Normal shape of lymph nodes is *bean*-shaped. When enlarged, lymph nodes become round/oval in shape. Significant lymph nodes are present deep to deep fascia of the neck. It is important that in every case of lymph node enlargement, clinical examination should cover following examinations as given in Clinical Box 10.1.

Clinical Box 10.1

Checklist for lymphatic system examination
- All group of lymph nodes: Cervical, axillary, para-aortic, iliac, inguinal
- Special location nodes: Popliteal and epitrochlear
- Waldeyer's ring: Palatine tonsil and lingual tonsil, pharyngeal tonsil (adenoids) and tubal tonsils (where eustachian tube opens)
- Liver and spleen
- Skeletal system—bones
- Drainage areas

TERMINOLOGY

- *Generalised lymphadenopathy*: It is defined as enlargement of more than two noncontiguous lymph node groups.

- *Normal enlargement*: In children, anterior cervical (1 cm), axillary (1 cm), inguinal (up to 1.5 cm) nodes are defined as normal.

- *Significant lymphadenopathy*
  - Any palpable node in the drainage area of malignancy is significant.
  - Supraclavicular lymph nodes of any size and any consistency should be considered as significant. Often enlargement is due to malignancy or lymphoma. It can also be due to tuberculosis (TB).
  - Any lymph node which is hard with or without mobility should be considered as significant.

PATIENT DATA AND HISTORY OF PRESENT ILLNESS

1. *Age of the patient*
   - In young children, common cause of lymph node enlargement is due to **viral aetiology.** Tuberculosis can also occur. Acute leukaemia can present with lymph node swelling and fever.
   - *Adults:* TB lymphadenitis is common in this age group. Typically, *jugulodigastric* cervical nodes are enlarged.
   - *Middle age:* Hodgkin's lymphoma
   - *Old age:* Metastasis from known and unknown primary.

2. *Duration of the swelling*: Common questions asked include when was the swelling noted and what is the duration.
   - *Short:* In cases of pyogenic infections, e.g. in acute tonsillitis, you may get enlargement of tonsillar node, jugulodigastric node in a few days.

- *Long:* In tuberculosis and metastasis (secondaries), the duration is long—may be one or two months.

3. *Other such similar swellings*
   - Often lymph node swellings can be in multiple sites. In such cases, find out which one started first, e.g. in Hodgkin's lymphoma. The patient may say that the swelling started in the neck first and was followed by axillary swelling (lymph nodes).
   - The patient may show multiple sites wherein swellings have appeared simultaneously, e.g. submental, submandibular, preauricular, etc. which suggests it could be a case of non-Hodgkin's lymphoma.

4. *Speed of growth*
   - Short duration and rapid growth usually suggests metastasis in lymph nodes.
   - Slow growth suggests tuberculosis or even lymphomas.

5. *Fever*
   - High grade fever suggests acute suppurative lymphadenitis.
   - Mild fever with *evening rise,* sometimes with chills suggests *tuberculosis.*
   - *Remittent bouts* of intermittent fever suggest *lymphoma.*
   - Metastasis in the lymph nodes usually does not give rise to fever.
   - Often leukaemia and lymphomas can present as fever with or without lymph nodes.
   - Fever with *multiple nodes* and *pain* may be a feature of *infectious mononucleosis. Sore throat* gives a clue to the diagnosis.
   - *Recurrent chills and rigors, and groin swelling:* Such attacks are common in our country and the most probable cause is *filarial lymphangitis and lymphadenitis of lymph nodes in the groin.* They are very tender.

6. *Weight loss*
   - Fever with weight loss suggests chronic diseases such as tuberculosis or metastasis.
   - Significant weight loss refers to loss of 10% or more of body weight in the last 6 months.

7. *Pain*
   - Pain indicates inflammation as in pyogenic lymphadenitis. Pain can be very severe as in

axillary lymphadenitis due to hand infections or sometimes so severe to mimic acute appendicitis as in external iliac lymphadenitis due to foot trauma, more so in children.
   - Painless enlargement of cervical nodes in an elderly person may suggest metastasis (secondaries—more common) or lymphoma. Tubercular lymphadenitis is also not painful.

8. *Find out the primary focus*
   - History of dysphagia in patients with cervical lymph nodes suggests it can be metastasis and primary may be in posterior third of the tongue—pyriform fossa, upper oesophagus, etc.
   - History of change in voice or breathing difficulty can be due to carcinoma larynx.

9. *History suggestive of chronic disease in the past or present should be asked*
   - TB: Evening rise in temperature, weight loss, cough with or without haemoptysis (TB).
   - Exposure to sexually transmitted diseases such as HIV or syphilis (rare nowadays). *HIV is more significant today.* It decreases the immunity and predisposes to tuberculosis as well as lymphoma.
   - Enlargement of groin lymph nodes with or without suppuration may be due to sexually transmitted infections such as granuloma inguinale or lymphogranuloma venereum infections.

GENERAL PHYSICAL EXAMINATION

It should be done from head to toe. Only relevant points or examination findings in cases of lymph node swellings are given below.

a. *Pallor:* It suggests chronic disease such as tuberculosis or malignancy.

b. *Jaundice:* It can be seen in late cases of lymphoma with involvement of liver.

c. *Skin rashes:* Coppery red skin rashes with lymphadenopathy may be an indication of secondary syphilis (rare nowadays).
   - Rashes and patches are seen in cutaneous T cell lymphoma (mycosis fungoides).

d. *Dilated veins* over the chest and congestion of the face suggest superior vena caval obstruction—may be caused by mediastinal lymph nodes. Suspect lymphoma.

e. **Bony pains** with lymph nodes in the neck may be due to leukaemia or lymphoma, or due to disseminated malignancy.

f. **Unilateral pedal oedema** can be caused by enlarged iliac nodes—may be malignant or lymphoma.

LOCAL/REGIONAL EXAMINATION

Inspection

• *Swelling:* First describe the exact location, e.g. anterior triangle or posterior triangle. In anterior triangle, upper part—upper deep cervical (jugulo-digastric) or lower part (juguloomohyoid) (Fig. 10.1). If it is posterior triangle, is it in the upper part—posterior upper deep cervical nodes or is it in the lower part— supraclavicular group. Is it inguinal—vertical chain of lymph nodes or horizontal. Multiple site involvement is common in lymphoma (Figs 10.2 to 10.7).

• Swellings which occur in the anatomical location of the lymph nodes have to be considered as lymph node origin unless proved otherwise.

• Describe their number. When more than 1 node is present just say multiple nodes are seen.

• Lymphoma can present as massive enlargement of lymph nodes, what has been described as bullneck appearance (Fig. 10.3).

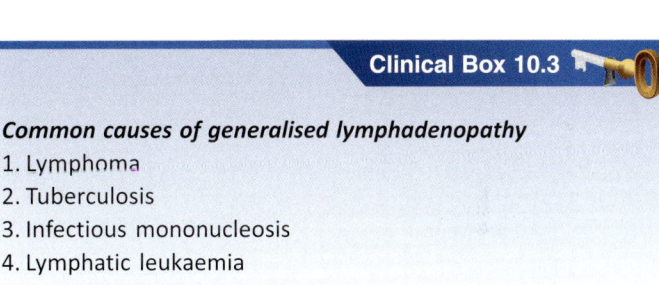

Clinical Box 10.2

Disease and common sites
1. Tuberculosis: Upper deep cervical (Fig 10.1)
2. Hodgkin's Lymphoma: Supraclavicular/posterior triangle/ axillary lymph nodes (Fig. 10.2)
3. Bronchogenic carcinoma: Supraclavicular lymph nodes
4. Filariasis: Inguinal lymph nodes
5. Secondary syphilis: Epitrochlear or occipital (Fig. 10.9)
6. Non-Hodgkin's lymphoma: Waldeyer's ring. However, atypical presentations should be kept in mind

Clinical Box 10.3

Common causes of generalised lymphadenopathy
1. Lymphoma
2. Tuberculosis
3. Infectious mononucleosis
4. Lymphatic leukaemia
5. Sarcoidosis
6. Brucellosis

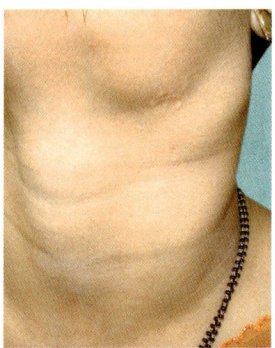

Fig. 10.1: Tuberculous lymphadenitis (*Courtesy*: Dr Sunil Krishna, Associate Professor, KMC, Manipal)

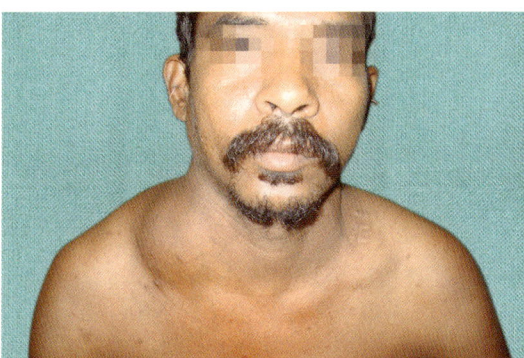

Fig. 10.2: Hodgkin's lymphoma: Involving right supraclavicular region

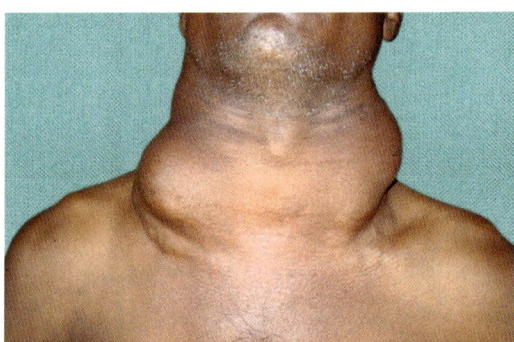

Fig. 10.3: Hodgkin's lymphoma (bullneck appearance) (*Courtesy*: Dr Vijay Kamath, Prof of Surgery, KIMS, Hubballi,Karnataka)

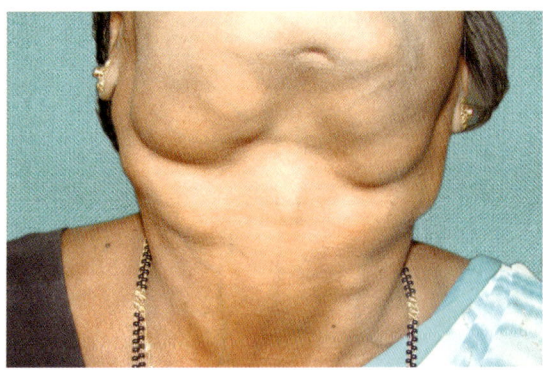

Fig. 10.4: Submental, submandibular, anterior and posterior cervical nodes—Hodgkin's lymphoma

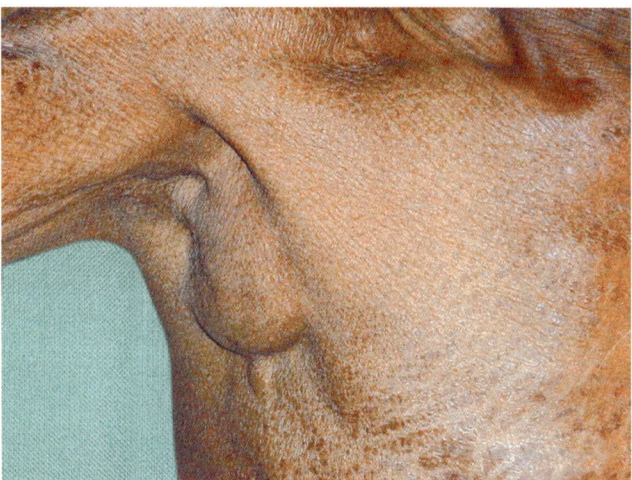

Fig. 10.5: Axillary lymph nodes—non-Hodgkin's lymphoma

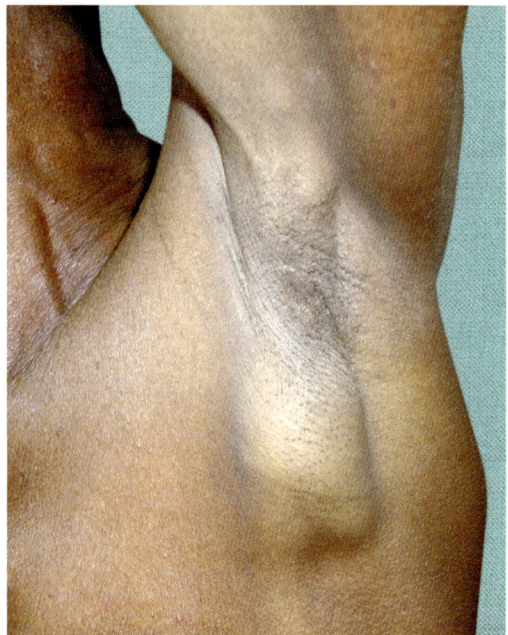

Fig. 10.6: Large axillary nodes

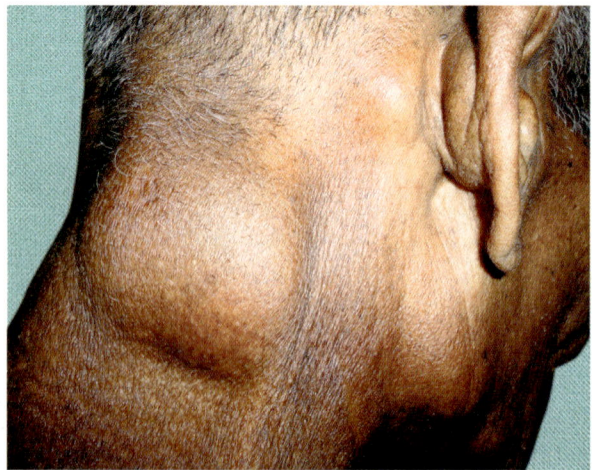

Fig. 10.7: Large occipital lymph node: A case of non-Hodgkin's lymphoma

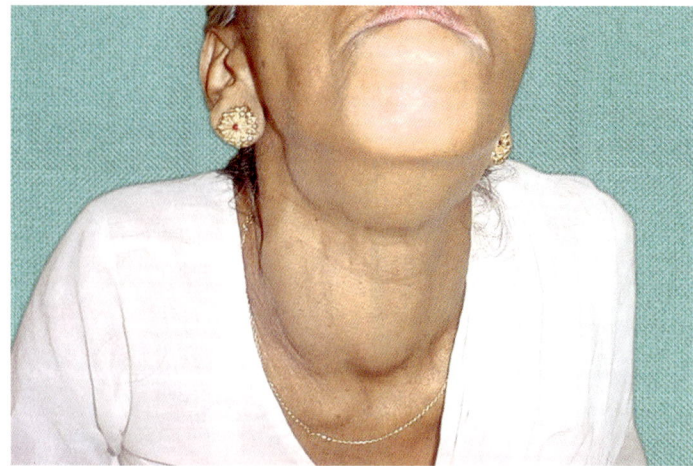

Fig. 10.8: Level I and II nodes: Metastatic lymph nodes

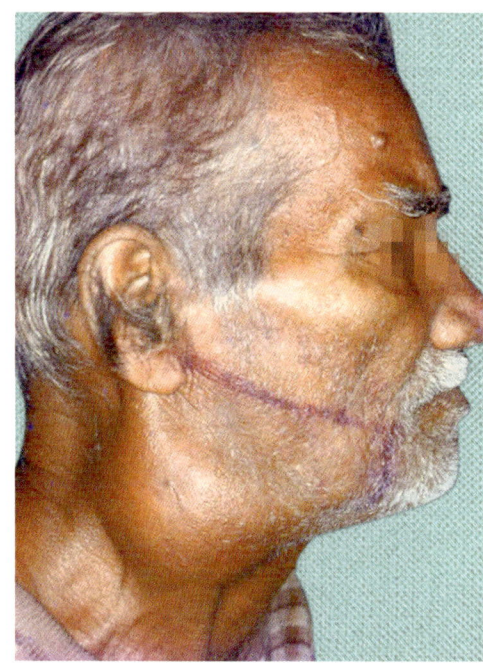

Fig. 10.9: Level I, II and III nodes: Metastatic lymph nodes. You can see the radiation mark in this patient.

- *Size:* When the size is variable, describe the largest and the smallest one and mention that they vary from, say 1 to 3 cm.
- *Surface:* Like any other swelling describe them as—smooth—isolated enlargement of lymph node or cold abscess (tubercular), nodular in lymphoma or secondaries or may be uneven as in secondaries (Figs 10.8 and 10.9).
- *Skin over the swelling*
  a. **Red:** Inflammatory in acute lymphadenitis.
  b. **Yellowish:** Inflammatory with formation of pus. Please note both these signs are absent in cold

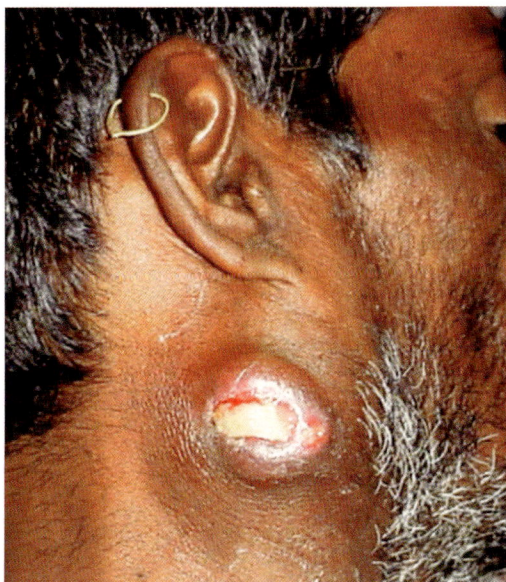

Fig. 10.10: Cold abscess with secondary infection in a patient with HIV (*Courtesy:* Dr Vijendra, SR Dept of Surgery, KMC, Manipal)

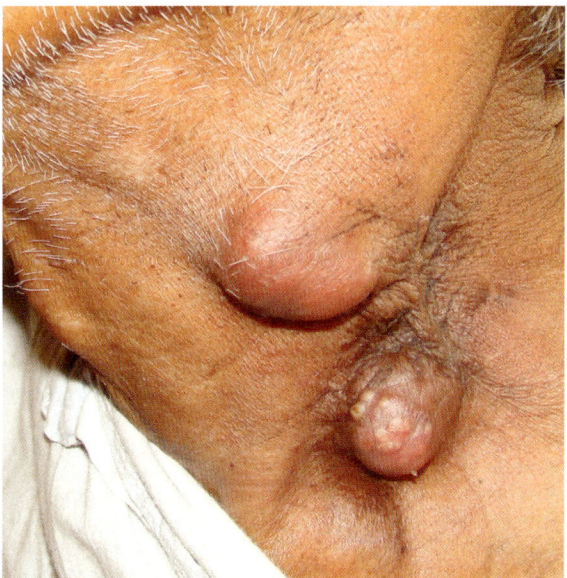

Fig. 10.12: Predominantly level II, III and V nodes: From naso-pharyngeal carcinoma

abscess due to tuberculosis, hence the name cold abscess.

c. **Sinus:** This is due to tuberculosis (Figs 10.10 and 10.11). Describe discharge also in such cases. Sinus in the groin can be also due to lympho-granuloma inguinale.

d. **Tethering of skin or dimpling** or peau d'orange means skin is infiltrated by the underlying disease and it is *most likely secondaries or metastasis* (Fig. 10.12).

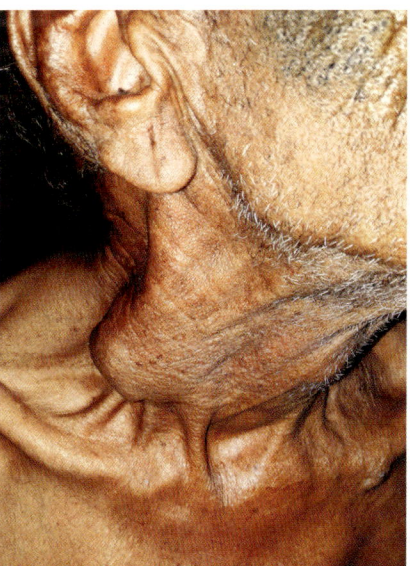

Fig. 10.13: Platysma sign

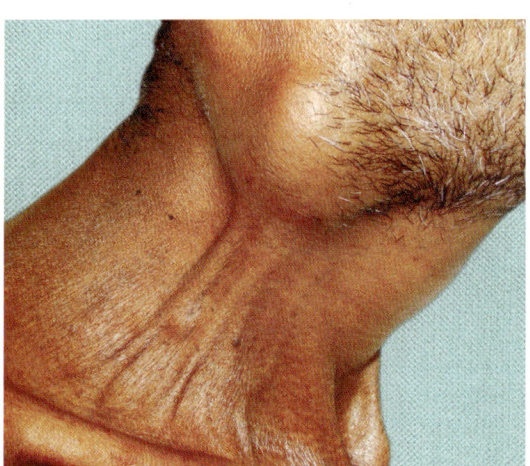

Fig. 10.11: Tethering of skin

e. Sometimes a fold of prominent skin is seen in the neck in advanced cases of secondaries in the neck. It is due to *infiltration of skin including platysma by the underlying secondaries. It is called platysma sign* (Fig. 10.13).

f. Fungating ulcer over a lymph node mass is typical of *late cases of secondaries.*

g. Dilated veins over the skin reflects increased vascularity, usually seen in secondaries.

- *Pressure effects*

a. Lymphoedema of the leg and arm is common as a result of pressure by groin nodes and axillary lymph nodes, respectively.

b. Large lymph node masses, especially media-stinal nodes from Hodgkin's lymphoma can compress the trachea and bronchus resulting in difficulty in breathing.

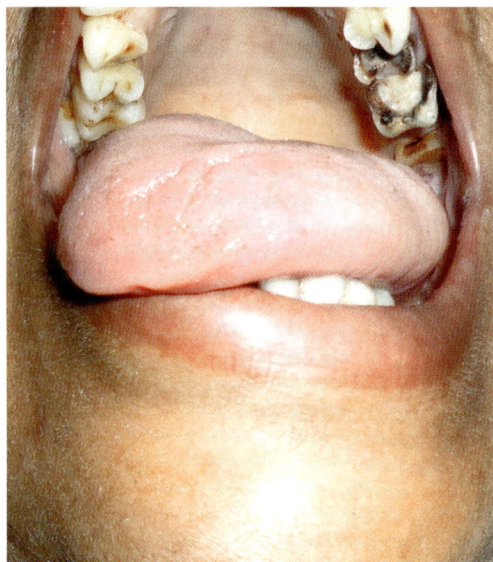

Fig. 10.14: Hypoglossal nerve palsy

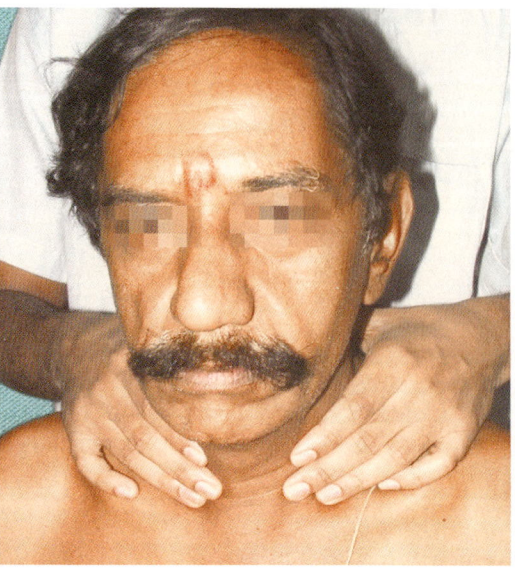

Fig. 10.15: Neck nodes should be examined from behind

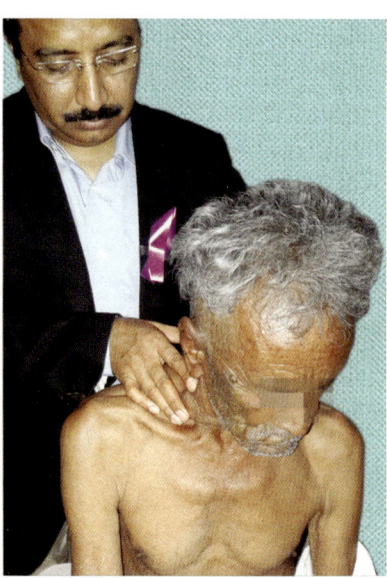

Fig. 10.16: Neck is flexed and bent towards the same side

c. Metastatic nodes in the upper jugular chain may infiltrate or compress hypoglossal nerve causing hypoglossal nerve paralysis, resulting in deviation of tongue to the same side (Fig. 10.14).

Palpation

- Palpation of the neck lymph nodes should be done from standing behind the patient, with *slight bending of the neck to relax strap muscles and deep cervical fascia* (Figs 10.15 and 10.16).

- *First describe like any other swelling:* Local rise in temperature and tenderness. If these signs are present, it may be infective aetiology—acute lymphadenitis.

- Since lymph nodes form a swelling, description should be like examination of swelling (page 52) in the form of site, size, shape, surface, borders, consistency, mobility, etc. A few typical examples are given below. Consistency is an important sign.

1. *Location:* Describe the exact location. A few examples are given below.

   a. 2 cm above the clavicle on the left side in the posterior triangle.

   b. 1 cm below the thyroid cartilage in the midline.

2. *Local rise in temperature and tenderness*

   a. If present they indicate inflammatory pathology such as acute suppurative lymphadenitis.

   b. Increased vascularity in a nodal swelling is seen in acute lymphadenitis.

   c. Secondaries in the neck are nontender unless they are advanced.

   d. Tuberculous lymphadenitis is nontender unless it has secondary infection.

3. *Consistency*

   a. Nodes are soft and usually tender in acute lymphadenitis. They may be soft also when the tubercular nodes undergo caseation necrosis which is called **cold abscess (no signs of inflammation).** Even malignant lymph nodes undergo degeneration and may feel soft. It is due to lack of blood supply specially in the centre. This is an ideal situation to do Paget's test (page 57). You will find hard lymph nodes underneath or indurated area underneath a soft area in cases of malignancy.

   b. Firm nodes are seen in chronic infection classically tuberculous or even filarial nodes in the groin (Fig. 10.17).

   c. Rubbery is a word to be used only in lymphomas (Hodgkin's lymphoma).

   d. *Hard nodes are characteristic of malignancies.* It is also mentioned that chronic tuberculous lymph nodes sometimes may feel hard due to calcification but that situation is very rare.

4. *Matting* (Fig. 10.18)

   a. This refers to adherence of one lymph node to the other so that they cannot move independent of each other. Classically described for tuberculous nodes in stage II wherein there is periadenitis which is responsible for matting.

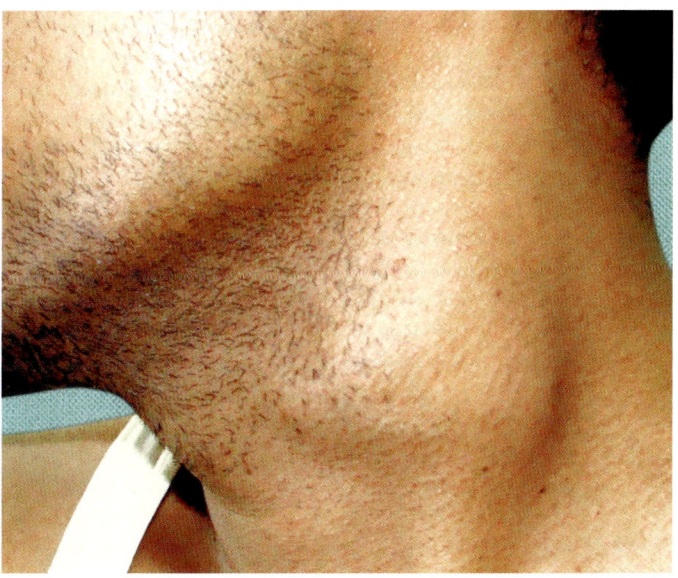

Fig. 10.17: Matted lymph nodes in tuberculosis

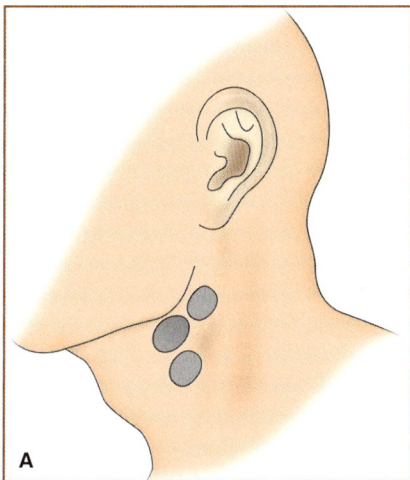

A

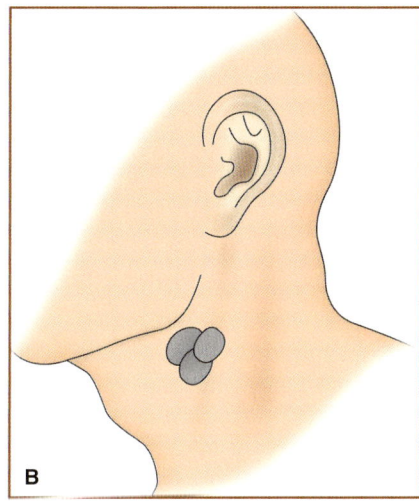

B

Fig. 10.18: (A) TB lymphadenitis—discrete nodes; (B) TB lymphadenitis—matted nodes

b. In malignancies, lymph nodes get adhered together due to infiltration (it is better not to use the word matting in malignancies). Matting is sometimes seen in acute infections other than tuberculosis.

5. *Mobility and fixity:* Mobile nodes are seen in chronic infections, e.g. tuberculous and filarial nodes in the groin. In early stages of secondaries in the lymph nodes, nodes may be mobile. However, once infiltration starts, mobility gets restricted and later they become immobile. In this situation, it is called fixed. *It should be remembered that in cases of acute enlargement of nodes, mobility may be restricted due to inflammatory reaction. Such nodes are often tender. Refer to* Clinical Case Capsule *which is given below.*

Clinical Box 10.4

Para-aortic node enlargement—common causes
- Lymphoma
- Testicular tumours
- Malignant melanoma
- Gastrointestinal malignancy

■ Clinical Case Capsule

A 55-year-old lady presented with hard, but tender nodes in the posterior triangle of 8 days duration. She had flu-like syndrome of 5 days duration. The lymph nodes had restricted mobility.

The treating physician explained to the relatives about possibility of malignancy and he even told about poor prognosis. However, FNAC revealed it to be a case of **Kikuchi disease**. Within 2 months, the patient was back to normal.

---

6. *If the nodes are fixed, mention to what structures they are fixed, for example*

a. *Lift the skin* (lifting is a better word than pinching). If it is not possible to lift the skin, it is fixed to skin. It happens typically in secondaries in the neck. The skin may not be liftable also in cold abscess or pyogenic abscess (pyogenic lymphadenitis) if they involve skin.

b. *Contract the muscle* in relation to the nodes and see for movement. Restricted mobility indicates infiltration into the muscles as in secondaries. In cases of cervical nodes (jugulodigastric and jugulo-omohyoid nodes, contract the sterno-mastoid muscle and mention the plane of the swelling (Fig. 10.19).

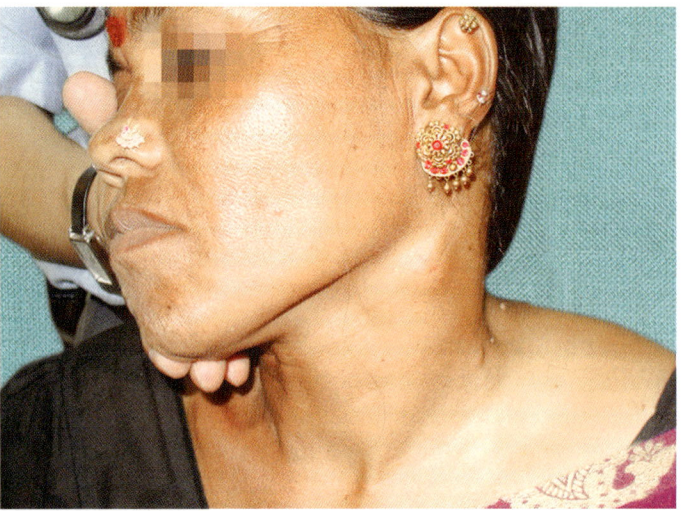

Fig. 10.19: Sternomastoid contraction test

7. *Infiltration into the nerves*: Large neck node mass due to *secondaries can infiltrate the hypoglossal nerve* and cause paralysis of the intrinsic muscles of the tongue. In such cases, *the tongue deviates to the same side* of the lesion.

- A few examples of primary malignant tumour and lymph nodes involving the various nerves are given in Clinical Box 10.5.
- Surrounding area: Palpate for oedema or induration.

8. *Palpate for all other group of lymph nodes*
- Cervical
- Axillary (usually forgotten)
- Para-aortic/mesenteric/iliac (abdominal)
- Inguinal
- Special (supraclavicular, epitrochlear/popliteal, scalene node)

9. *Examine for any oedema distally and dilated veins due to venous obstruction caused by lymph node mass.*

Clinical Box 10.5

Malignancies and nerve paralysis
- *Carcinoma parotid*: Facial nerve paralysis
- *Carcinoma thyroid*: Recurrent laryngeal nerve paralysis
- *Metastatic nodes in neck*: Hypoglossal nerve paralysis
- *Sarcoma of the arm*: Radial nerve paralysis
- *Maxillary antral carcinoma*: Infraorbital nerve paralysis
- *Osteosarcoma fibula*: Lateral popliteal nerve paralysis

Relevant Tests for Nerve Paralysis

1. *Hypoglossal nerve*: Ask the patient to protrude the tongue and see for any deviation. Tongue will point out the side of the lesion because of the contraction of the opposite side muscle.

2. *Recurrent laryngeal nerve paralysis*: Decreased pitch, dyspnoea on exertion and dysphagia.

3. *Facial nerve paralysis* (refer to page 210): Ask the patient to clench the teeth and see for any deviation of the angle of the mouth.

4. *Infraorbital nerve paralysis*: Anaesthesia over the prominence of the cheek.

5. *Lateral popliteal nerve paralysis*: Foot drop.

SPECIAL LYMPH NODES

SUPRACLAVICULAR LYMPH NODE—VIRCHOW'S NODE

Involvement of supraclavicular lymph node in visceral malignancies such as carcinoma stomach represents spread through lymphatics (thoracic duct) and it suggests inoperability of the disease. It has been described as *Troisier's sign*. Hence, it is very important to carefully look for enlargement of supraclavicular nodes—the reason why a few special methods have been followed. They are given in Clinical Box 10.6.

Clinical Box 10.6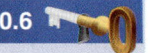

Different methods to detect/feel supraclavicular node
1. **Inspection:** Look for any fullness in the posterior triangle just above clavicle.
2. **Palpation from behind:** This is more commonly followed. Stand behind the patient and carefully palpate for nodes above the clavicle in the posterior triangle.
3. **Patient elevating and hunching shoulders:** This will help to insinuate finger just behind clavicle to detect a node which may be just enlarged and partly behind clavicle.
4. **Palpation from front:** With slight bending of neck towards the same side, standing in front of the patient, 3 middle fingers can be used to palpate the lymph node.

Virchow's Node

- It is also called left supraclavicular lymph node, or signal node.

- Originally described by Rudolf Virchow, a German pathologist, who correlated this lymph node to gastric cancer.

- However, it is also involved in other malignancies such as colon, pancreas, testicular tumour, etc. Hence, the palpable Virchow's node in visceral malignancies is called **Troisier's sign**.

- Enlargement of Virchow's node occurs due to following reasons:

  1. Blockage of the thoracic duct near the entry into left subclavian vein resulting in regurgitation of the cells into surrounding nodes (Virchow's node).

  2. Another possibility is that one of the transverse lymph nodes is the blind end of the thoracic duct itself.

EPITROCHLEAR NODE ENLARGEMENT (Fig. 10.20)

Osler noted that epitrochlear nodes were a prominent clinical feature of secondary syphilis. Today specially in African countries, HIV infection has to be considered as first diagnosis instead of syphilis. It is classically located on the *anterior surface of the medial intermuscular septum, 1 cm above the base of the medial epicondyle (Clinical Box 10.7).*

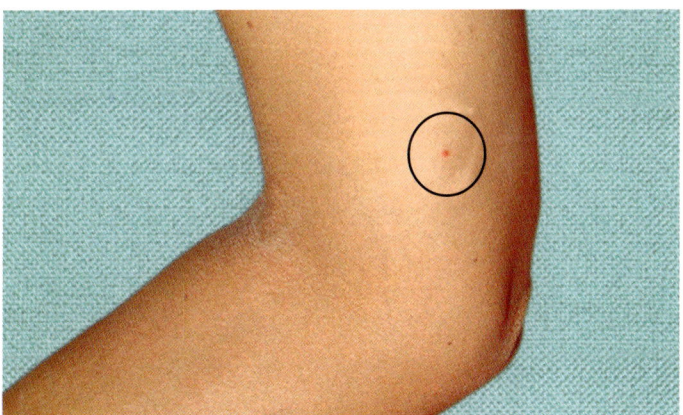

Fig. 10.20: Epitrochlear node

Clinical Box 10.7

Causes of epitrochlear node enlargement
- Cat scratch disease: Irritation
- Non-Hodgkin's lymphoma
- Glandular fever: Infectious mononucleosis
- Secondary syphilis
- Hand infections
- Rheumatoid arthritis—when active joint disease is present in the joints: Inflammation

In most instances, any lymph node up to 1 cm can still be considered normal. The two exceptions to this rule include the epitrochlear node in which up to 0.5 cm is normal and the inguinal nodes in which up to 1.5 cm is normal.

SCALENE NODE

It is located in between two heads of sternocleido-mastoid. It is typically enlarged in bronchogenic carcinoma (*refer* to page 27).

It is also the member of the medial nodes of the transverse cervical nodes (supraclavicular nodes).

LOOK FOR EVIDENCE OF THE PRIMARY

- This specially refers to when metastasis or secondaries should be suspected. You must ask yourself why is this lymph node enlarged?

- Hence, when neck nodes are enlarged, a thorough examination of the oral cavity should be done. Examine buccal mucosa, anterior and posterior third of the tongue, retromolar trigone, etc. Look at the tonsils also.

- Think about which area is drained by this lymph node and what pathology may be present. A few examples are given below:

  1. A young female, 30 years old with firm mobile multiple nodes in the upper part of the neck— oral cavity examination revealed enlargement of the tonsils—it was a case of non-Hodgkin's lymphoma (Fig. 10.21).

  2. A 50-year-old male smoker and pan chewer, presented with hard lymph nodes in the lower

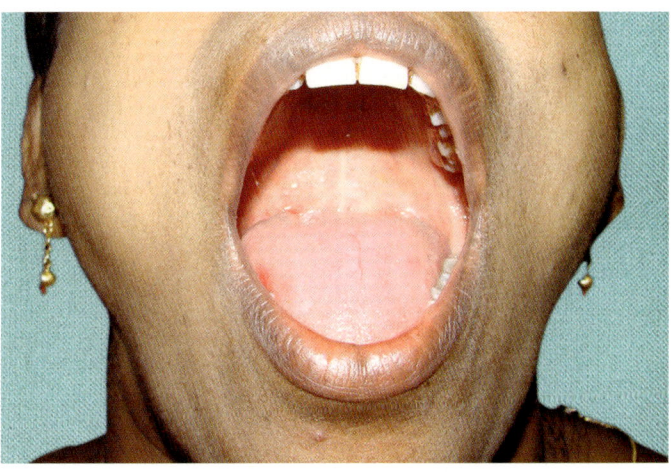

Fig. 10.21: Examine the oral cavity

deep cervical region (juguloomohyoid). The diagnosis is metastasis. Where is the primary? Inspection and palpation of the anterior third of the tongue revealed a hard indurated lesion in the tongue. Diagnosis is carcinoma of the tongue (Fig. 10.22).

3. Young lady of 30 years presented with palpable jugulo-omohyoid nodes and nodes in the posterior triangle. One should carefully examine the thyroid gland. She had a nodule in one of the lobes. The diagnosis is **papillary carcinoma thyroid** (Fig. 10.23).

4. Elderly lady presents with axillary lymph node enlargement—consider not only lymphoma but also carcinoma breast (Fig. 10.24).

5. Young female presented to the hospital with groin nodes which were firm and a few were hard. Examination of the lower limb was normal. On careful questioning, she said she had some itching, burning and discharge per anal canal. Separation of the buttocks and proctoscopy revealed an **ulcerated malignant melanoma**.

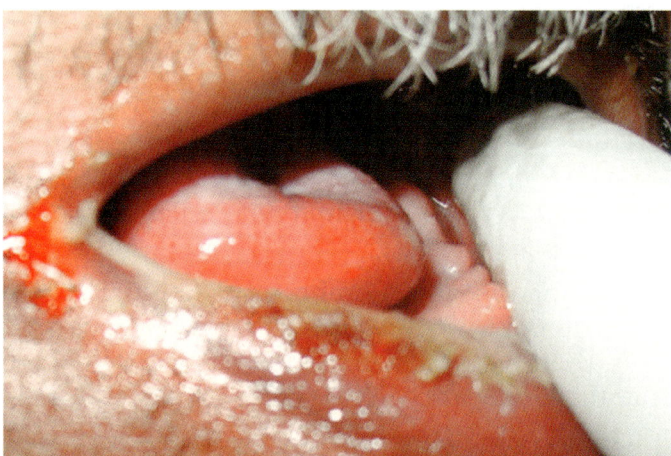

Fig. 10.22: When you suspect metastasis in the cervical lymph nodes, examination of the oral cavity should be done—as you see here, there is a cancerous growth in the tongue. Carcinoma in posterior one-third is easily missed

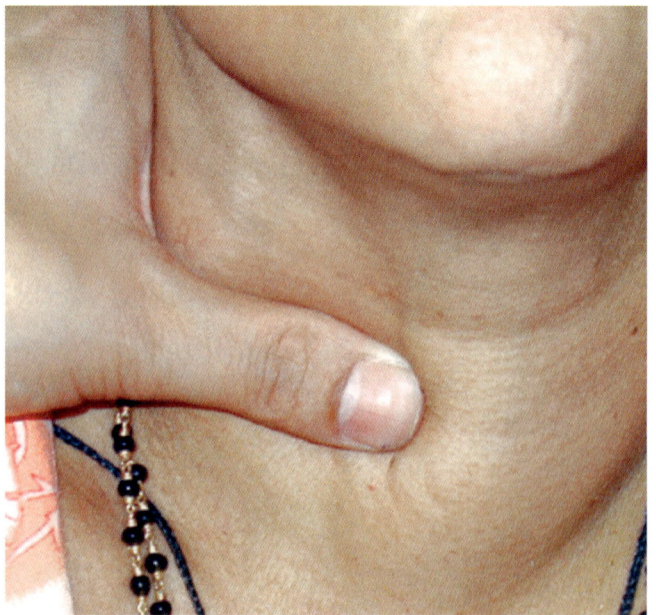

Fig. 10.23: When you get a young patient with firm lower deep cervical nodes (sometimes they can be soft and cystic), carefully look for thyroid nodule—presence of which suggests papillary carcinoma thyroid

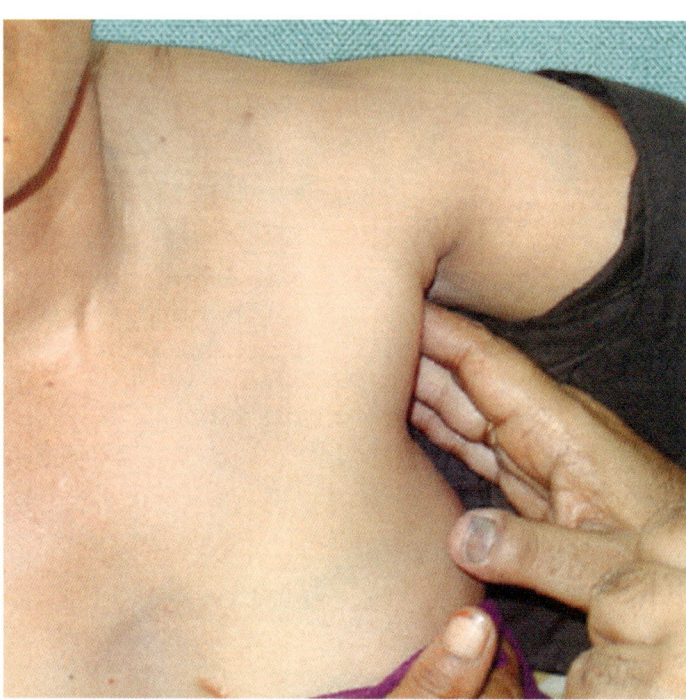

Fig. 10.24: Examination of the lymph nodes in the axilla—when these are involved, examination of the breast should be done

EXAMINATION OF ABDOMEN

- In cases of cervical lymphadenopathy, abdomen should be examined for enlargement of spleen, liver, para-aortic nodes and external iliac nodes.

- Various interpretations of the abdominal signs with lymph node enlargement findings are:

  1. Cervical group of lymph nodes on the left side with palpable spleen: Most likely it is Hodgkin's lymphoma.

  2. Cervical nodes with para-aortic and iliac nodes: Hodgkin's lymphoma.

  3. Hepatosplenomegaly with lymph nodes: Lymphoma, chronic lymphocytic leukaemia and autoimmune disorders.

Clinical Features of Enlarged Liver

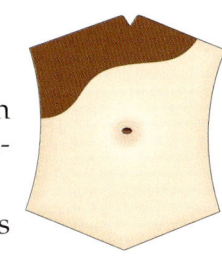

- When liver is enlarged, it is felt in the right hypochondrium, epigastrium and left hypochondrium.
- It is dull to percuss and dullness continues over the mass below.
- Finger insinuation between the liver mass and costal margin is not possible.
- It has no intrinsic mobility because it is covered by ribs.

Clinical Features of Enlarged Spleen

- It is located in the left hypochondrium and *enlarges towards right iliac fossa.*
- It moves with respiration.
- It is dull on percussion.
- Fingers cannot be insinuated between splenic mass and costal margin.
- Splenic notch, if felt, is characteristic of spleen—it is felt in the anterior border.

Clinical Features of Para-aortic Lymph Node Mass

- Located in the epigastrium and umbilical region.
- Typically nodular, firm to hard mass.
- Does not move with respiration.
- Aortic pulsations may be felt over the swelling—transmitted pulsations.
- It does not fall forwards in the knee elbow position because they are retroperitoneal.

DIFFERENTIAL DIAGNOSIS OF LYMPHADENOPATHY

- **Tuberculous lymphadenitis:** It commonly affects upper deep cervical nodes or nodes in the anterior triangle. When infection is haematogenous, medulla of the lymph node is affected. When lymphatic spread is the cause, cortex is involved and periadenitis occurs fast. Basic pathology is fibrous, proliferative or caseous. Nodes are firm and matted. Within 1–2 months, cold abscess occurs which ruptures resulting in sinus formation. It is typically seen in children and young adults. Evening rise of temperature, weakness, anorexia, loss of weight provide the clue to the diagnosis. Liver and spleen are not involved unless it is miliary tuberculosis. Rarely lymph nodes are hard due to calcification. To summarise lymphadenitis, matting, cold abscess, collar stud abscess and sinus formation are the various ways of presentation. Retroviral infections should be ruled out in these cases. Tuberculous lymphadenitis of the **neck is called scrofula—king's evil. It refers to tuberculous and non-tuberculous (atypical) mycobacteria** (Figs 10.25 to 10.31).
- **Lymphoma**—Hodgkin's lymphoma affects lymph nodes in the posterior triangle, axillary nodes, groin nodes and para-aortic nodes. Nodes are classically rubbery or firm, not matted and nontender. Nodes are large in size. Multiple sites of involvement with or without liver and spleen involvement clinch the diagnosis. Recurrent bouts of remittent fever is characteristic of this condition.
- **Lymphoma**—non-Hodgkin's lymphoma (NHL) primarily affects circular chain of lymph nodes in the neck, namely submental, submandibular, preauricular, postauricular, and suboccipital. It also affects Waldeyer's ring, namely palatine and lingual tonsils. Epitrochlear node enlargement also helps in diagnosing non-Hodgkin's lymphoma (Figs 10.32 to 10.39).
- **Metastasis or secondaries in lymph nodes:** This should be always borne in mind whenever an elderly patient presents with hard swelling in the neck of recent onset. Typically one group of lymph nodes are enlarged. (In lymphoma, multiple sites involvement is common.) The nodes are hard and indurated. Late cases will have restricted mobility, ulceration, fungation and fixity giving rise to many other signs. *Example*: Hypoglossal nerve paralysis from large metastatic deposits in the upper deep cervical nodes and submandibular nodes from carcinoma tongue.

  Please note: Papillary carcinoma usually presents in a young girl or woman with level 3 or 4 group of nodes and often **without enlargement of thyroid gland**. Lymph nodes are firm and not matted. When thyroid gland is clinically not palpable, this situation is described as **occult primary**.
- When in doubt, ultrasound examination of neck can pick up early nodal enlargement. It also helps in guiding a FNAC (Clinical Box 10.8).
- **Chronic pyogenic lymphadenitis:** This is not uncommon in the neck and in the groin. Often the lymph nodes are 1–2 cm in size and tender on palpation. No other constitutional features are present. However, dandruff, scalp infections or middle ear infections, and chronic sinusitis are the causes (even oral cavity infections).

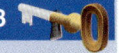

Clinical Box 10.8

Characteristic of neoplastic lymph node in ultrasound examination

- Loss of normal shape—oval to round
- Loss of fatty hilum
- Loss of regular margin
- Necrosis
- Blood flow on Doppler ultrasound
- Punctate calcification in papillary thyroid cancer
- Reticulated appearance in lymphoma

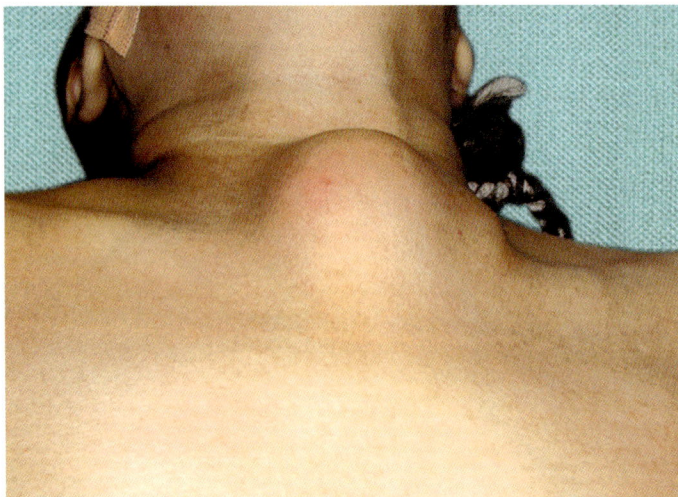

Fig. 10.25: Cold abscess in the suprasternal space of Burns with rupture into the subcutaneous plane. It was confused for lipoma

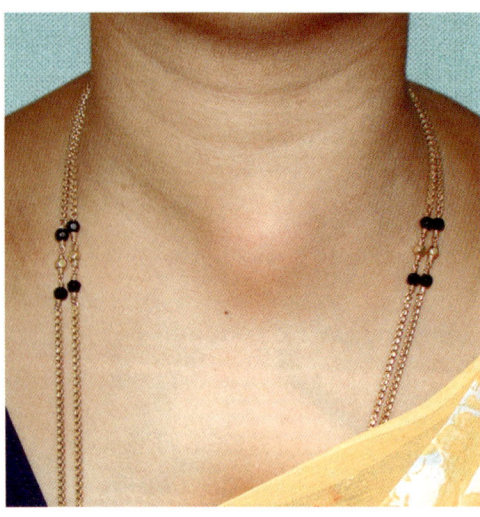

Fig. 10.26: Cold abscess in the suprasternal space of Burns. Patient had evening rise of temperature

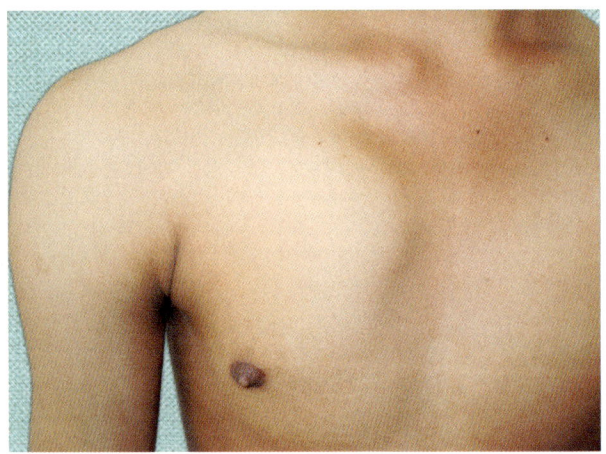

Fig. 10.27: Cold abscess in right chest wall. Source is from internal mammary lymph nodes. Swelling is confined to upper intercostal spaces

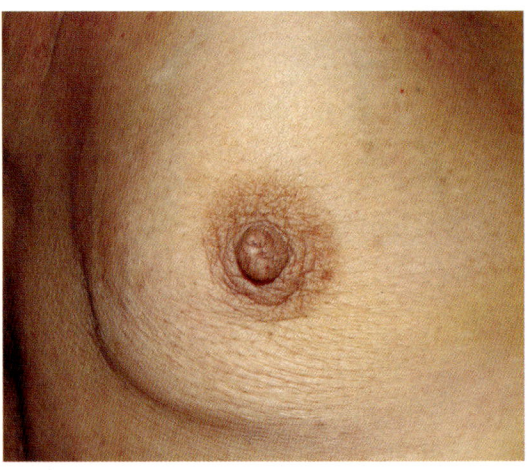

Fig. 10.29: Tuberculous cold abscess confused for carcinomatous lump in a 45 year old lady. You can also see dilated veins. It was a fluctuant swelling

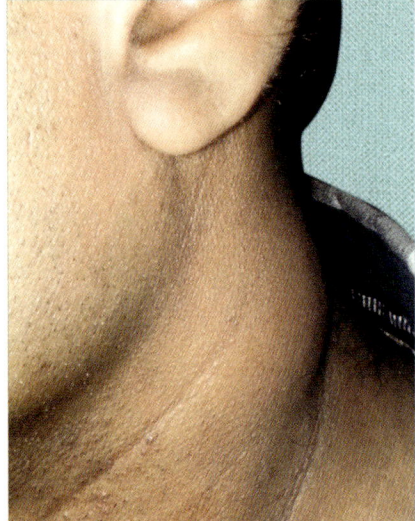

Fig. 10.28: Cold abscess in the posterior triangle. Source is usually from adenoids

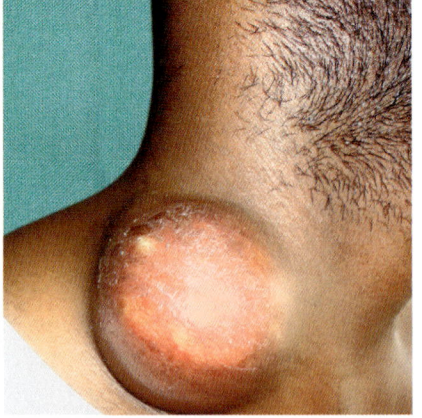

Fig. 10.30A: Cold abscess with secondary infection in a patient with HIV, that is why it is red

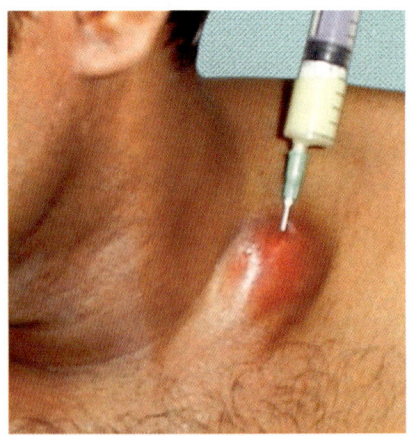

Fig. 10.30B: Nondependent aspiration of the cold abscess by using wide bore needle

(*Courtesy:* Dr Bharat, Dr Vijay, Dr Vamshi, Department of Surgery, KMC, Manipal)

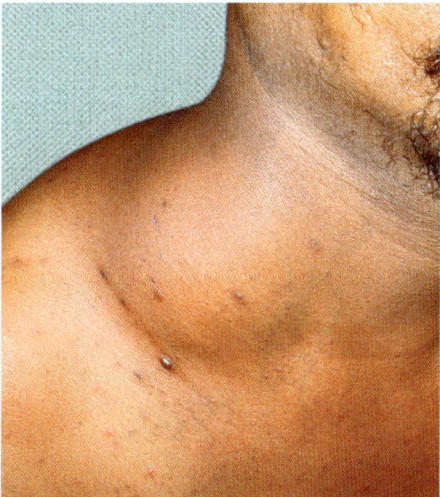

Fig. 10.31: Hodgkin's lymphoma affecting lymph nodes in the posterior triangle. A common site

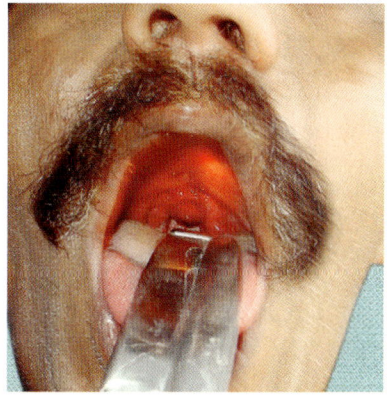

Fig. 10.32: Examination of the oral cavity is not only to look for evidence of primary but also to look for enlargement of the tonsils which suggests it may be a case of non-Hodgkin's lymphoma

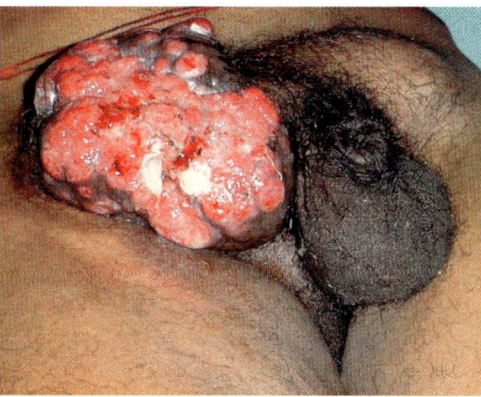

Fig. 10.33: Examine the groin nodes—rubbery nodes suggest Hodgkin's lymphoma, firm nodes suggest chronic infections and hard nodes suggest metastasis. In this picture you can see fungating lymph nodes. It is due to metastasis from carcinoma penis.

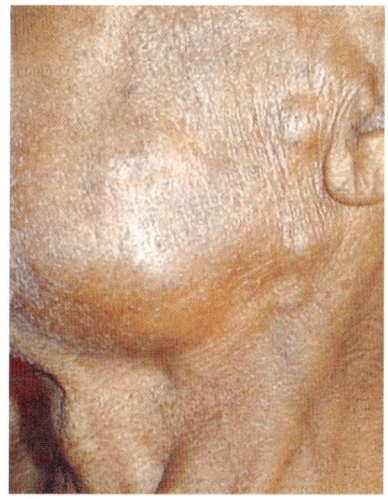

Fig. 10.34: Examine the horizontal chain of lymph nodes which get enlarged in cases of non-Hodgkin's lymphoma

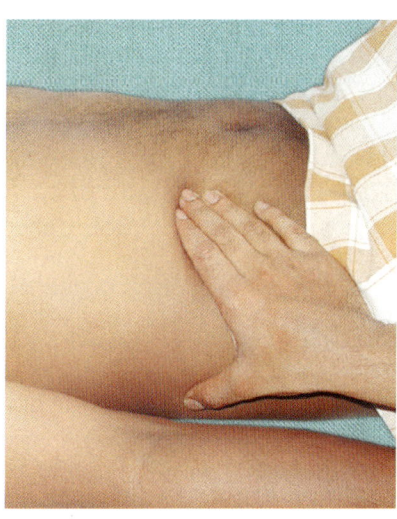

Fig. 10.35: Palpation of the liver—Liver will be smooth and firm without any nodularity in cases of lymphoma

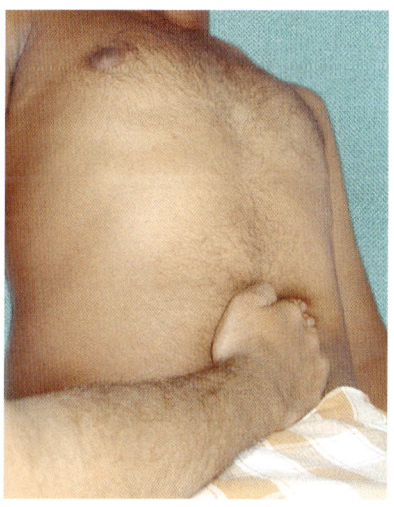

Fig. 10.36: Examination of the spleen in the left hypochondrium—Enlarged spleen will be smooth and firm in cases of lymphoma

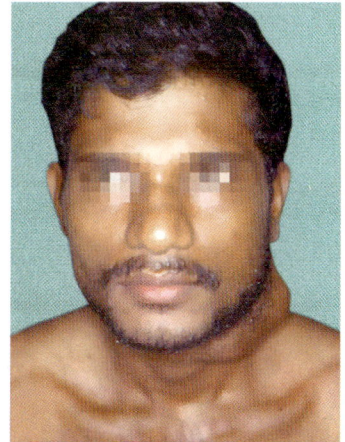

Fig. 10.37: Hodgkin's lymphoma affecting submandibular, jugulodigastric group of lymph nodes

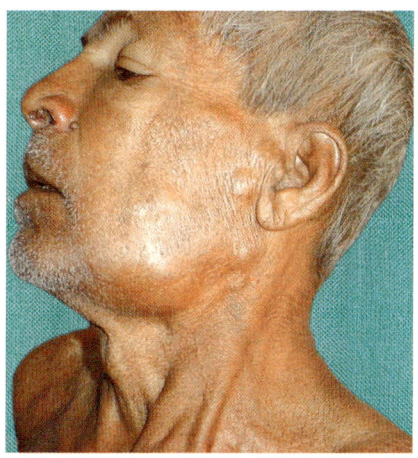

Fig. 10.38: NHL affecting preauricular, jugulodigastric, submandibular lymph nodes

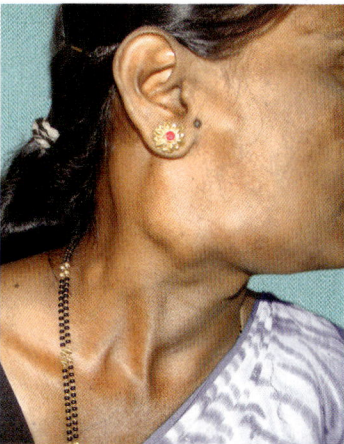

Fig. 10.39: Submandibular, upper jugular pre-parotid, facial and posterior triangle nodes

- **Chronic lymphocytic leukaemia:** The affected individuals are usually more than 50 years of age. This blood disorder presents as multiple lymph node swellings, fever, weight loss and anorexia. On examination, nodes are not matted, firm, mobile and nontender. Hepatosplenomegaly and bony tenderness, if present, confirms the diagnosis. **It typically progresses more slowly than other types of leukaemia.**

- **Infectious mononucleosis (glandular fever):** Firm, nontender (slightly tender) lymph node enlargement in the neck is common presentation. Sore throat, rashes and splenic enlargement clinch the diagnosis. Involvement of axillary, inguinal and mediastinal lymph nodes is not uncommon.

- **Kikuchi disease,** also called histiocytic necrotizing lymphadenitis or Kikuchi-Fujimoto disease, is an uncommon, idiopathic, generally **self-limited cause of lymphadenitis.** Infectious and autoimmune aetiologies have been proposed. Cervical nodes are affected in 80% of patients; of these, 65–70% involve posterior triangle cervical nodes. Lymphadenitis results from apoptotic cell death induced by cytotoxic T lymphocytes. Lymphadenopathy most often resolves over several weeks to 6 months. A flu-like prodrome with fever is present in 50% of cases. Condition will resolve by a few weeks to months. It is the cause of anxiety that nodes can be firm to hard thus mimicking tuberculosis, lymphoma or metastatic deposits (head and neck). Only a biopsy will help in confirming the diagnosis and more importantly to rule out other diseases.

A FEW SPECIFIC SITES: DIFFERENTIAL DIAGNOSIS

LYMPHADENOPATHY IN THE GROIN

Surgical Anatomy

Inguinal lymph nodes are classified into superficial lymph nodes which are superficial to deep fascia and deep groups which are deep to deep fascia—fascia lata. Classification is given below.

Superficial: These nodes are behind and parallel to the inguinal ligament. They are further classified into:
1. *Horizontal*
   - A. *Medial:* Drain penile skin and skin of vulva
   - B. *Lateral:* Lower limb and abdominal wall on the lateral side.
2. *Vertical chain:* Along the upper end of the long saphenous vein.

Deep: Deep nodes are along femoral vein. They are 2 or 3 in number. One of them is **lymph node of Cloquet** in the femoral canal. They receive lymph vessels running along with the femoral vein, lymph from glans penis or clitoris and from superficial lymph nodes. From deep inguinal nodes, drainage is to the external iliac nodes.

Clinical method of palpation is given below

- The patient is lying down on the couch. Hip is flexed to relax muscles and fascia of the thigh. Exposure should be adequate from umbilicus to upper thigh. First palpate with flat of the hand and later use fingertips to feel the enlarged nodes.

- Often, enlargement of groin nodes is due to different aetiology (*refer to* Clinical Box 10.9). A few specific diseases have to

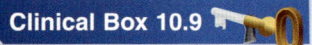

Clinical Box 10.9

When inguinal lymph nodes are enlarged, check the following
- *Infections:* Acute—lymphangitis, ulcers, cellulitis in the leg
- *Neoplastic:* Lymphoma, metastatic
- *Glans penis:* Ulcers, growth
- *Urethra:* Terminal urethritis
- *Infection:* Chronic filariasis
- *Navel:* Examination of umbilicus
- *Anal canal:* Ulcers, moles
- *Lower limb:* Epitheliomas, malignant melanoma

be kept in mind. They are filariasis, malignant melanoma, sexually transmitted diseases, etc. Hence, it has been discussed separately.

Differential Diagnosis

1. **Filarial lymphadenitis:** The disease is caused by *Wuchereria bancrofti*. Males in endemic areas are commonly affected. Filariasis is caused by mosquito bites. Recurrent attacks of lymphangitis and groin swelling are characteristic. Ultimate result is chronically enlarged nodes with or without tenderness. Lymph nodes are large-sized and firm. Pain in the leg, fever and groin swelling have periodicity. Swelling and tenderness of the spermatic cord and scrotum gives the clue to the diagnosis.

2. **Metastatic nodes:** Inguinal nodes are the common site of lymph node metastasis from squamous cell carcinoma and malignant melanoma of the lower limb. Often, a mole is silent but lymph nodes are bulky and firm to hard. Hence, search for the mole or ulcer in the entire limb. Only when it is negative, search for an ulcerated mole in the anal canal. Refer chapter on examination of skin malignancies.

3. **Lymphoma:** Inguinal nodes along with cervical and paraaortic nodes help in the diagnosis of lymphoma. Nodes are rubbery or firm without matting. Palpable liver and spleen if present, clinches the diagnosis.

4. **Lymphogranuloma venereum (LGV):** It is a sexually transmitted disease caused by psittacosis type of organisms. Primary lesion is small but lymph nodes are big. Iliac nodes also get enlarged. Slowly suppuration develops resulting in a swelling both above and below the inguinal ligament—cross fluctuation can be elicited.
   - *Groove sign:* Swelling above and swelling below the inguinal ligament separated by inguinal ligament has been described as groove sign.
   - In late stages, it will burst resulting in multiple discharging sinuses. Pus is thick yellow. (In tuberculosis, pus is white and cheesy.)

   Please note that in granuloma inguinale, lymph nodes are not involved.

5. **Chancroid or soft sore:** It is a sexually transmitted disease caused by *Haemophilus ducreyi* (Ducreyi's bacillus). Short incubation period and rapid development of painful ulcer in the penis and inguinal nodes are characteristic. **Inguinal nodes suppurate often resulting in an abscess. Usually one side is affected. Suppurated soft swelling in the groin is called bubo.**

LYMPHADENOPATHY IN THE AXILLA

- Axilla or armpit is one of the common sites of abundance of lymphatics and lymph nodes. Hence, any swelling in the axilla should be diagnosed as lymph node swelling unless proved otherwise.
- Also remember, in any young female, swelling in the axilla which is mimicking a node or lipoma should be considered as *hypertrophy of the axillary tail of the breasts* unless proved otherwise. It is usually bilateral and painful specially during menstruation.
- Remember the other structures which are present in the axilla. They are sweat glands, fatty tissue, nerves and blood vessels. Swellings arising from these structures will become differential diagnosis. Tender swelling in the axilla is usually *hidradenitis suppurativa*.

Differential Diagnosis

1. **Chronic lymphadenitis:** Upper limb is common site of trauma in the form of cuts, injuries, abrasions, etc. Specially in manual labourers, agriculturists, recurrent infection may result in enlargement of axillary nodes. Middle finger infections spread straight into central nodes. Such nodes are firm without matting and usually are 1 cm in size.
2. **Tuberculous lymphadenitis:** Route of infection is from mediastinal lymph nodes. Typically nodes are matted with or without cold abscess. At the stage of cold abscess, differential diagnosis should include fluctuant swellings such as lymphangioma and lipoma.
3. **Hodgkin's lymphoma:** Enlargement of cervical and axillary nodes is common in Hodgkin's lymphoma. Nodes are big—more than 2 cm and firm or rubbery without matting.

    The disease starts in the left posterior triangle as a group of lymph nodes with a 'bunch of grapes' appearance (Fig. 10.31). This is seen in about 80% of cases. By means of contiguous and centripetal spread, other lymph nodes in the neck, axillary, mediastinal, para-aortic and inguinal lymph nodes get enlarged. Abdominal pain can occur due to hepatosplenomegaly, which are smooth and firm with round borders. Typically para-aortic nodes are enlarged.

    Multiple bony pains can occur due to secondary deposits, especially in the lumbar vertebrae. The secondary deposits are usually osteoblastic giving rise to **ivory vertebrae.** **Superior vena caval obstruction** indicates enlarged mediastinal nodes. This is tested by asking the patient to raise the hand above the head. Engorgement of the veins indicates obstruction and the test is said to be positive **(Pemberton's test).**
4. **Metastatic nodes (secondaries):** It is not a common site of metastasis. However, in a female, if hard nodes are present in the axilla, primary should be considered to be from breasts unless proved otherwise.

*Refer to Clinical Wisdom and Clinical Box 10.10 also

LYMPHOEDEMA OF LEG

Accumulation of the lymph in the subcutaneous tissues results in enlargement of the limb. Fluid collects in the **extracellular, and extravascular compartments.**

Clinical Box 10.10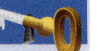

Common lymph node sites involved in various diseases
1. Posterior auricular node—rubella
2. Anterior auricular—lesion is conjunctiva, eyelid
3. Epitrochlear—non-Hodgkin's lymphoma
4. Scalene node—bronchogenic carcinoma
5. Bilateral upper cervical—tuberculosis
6. Bilateral lower cervical—lymphoma
7. Axillary nodes—carcinoma breast female
8. Left axillary node in carcinoma stomach—Irish node
9. Popliteal node—malignant melanoma

Common Sites of Lymphoedema

1. Lower limbs are the most common sites.
2. Upper limbs
3. Scrotum: Elephantiasis of the scrotum is caused by filarial organism *(Wuchereria bancrofti)*.
4. Elephantiasis of penis caused by filarial organisms produces **Ram's horn penis**.

Causes of Lower Limb Elephantiasis

I. Primary

1. **Lymphatic aplasia:** Number of lymphatic channels and nodes are grossly reduced.
2. **Lymphatic hypoplasia:** In this variety, the lymphatic channels are of small calibre.
3. **Milroy's disease** is a type of lymphoedema congenita which runs in families.
4. Depending upon the time at which the lymphoedema appears, it can be classified as follows:

    Birth: Lymphoedema congenita.

    Puberty: Lymphoedema precox.

    Later life: Lymphoedema tarda (Fig. 10.40).

II. Acquired (Secondary Lymphoedema)

1. **Filarial elephantiasis** (Fig. 10.41) is caused by **Wuchereria bancrofti**, transmitted by the mosquito *(Culex fatigans)*. The disease is caused by adult worms which have the affinity towards lymphatic vessels and lymph nodes. **Microfilariae do not produce any lesion.**

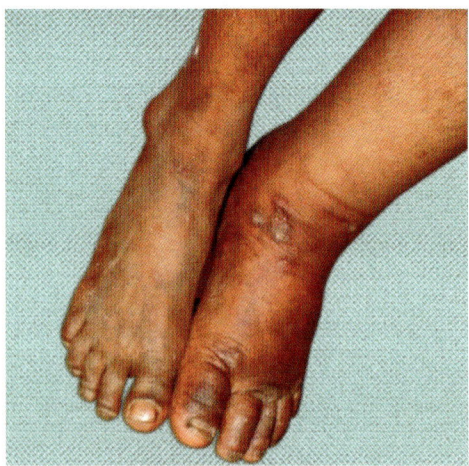

Fig. 10.40: Lymphoedema tarda

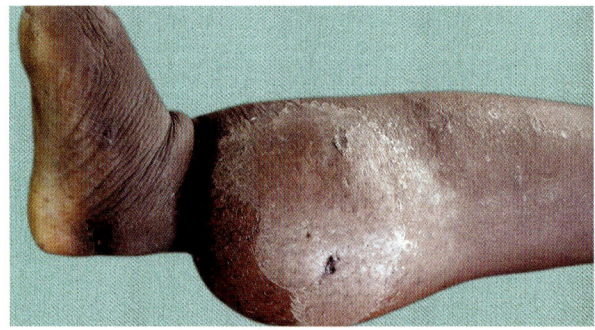

Fig. 10.41: Filariasis—elephant leg

Flowchart 10.1: Elephant leg

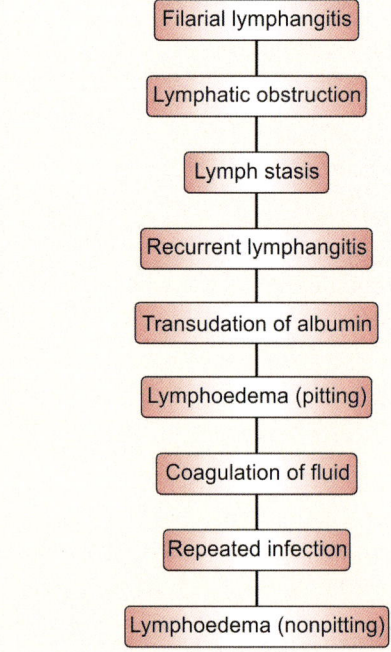

- Initially, it causes lymphangitis which clinically presents with high grade fever with chills and rigors, red streaks in the limb, with tenderness and swelling of the spermatic cord and scrotum.

- The lymph nodes are swollen and tender. Retro-peritoneal lymphangitis produces acute abdominal pain. Flowchart 10.1 shows various lymphatic manifestations)

- Due to such repeated infections, fibrosis occurs resulting in lymphatic obstruction. This later gives rise to lymphatic dilatation. Lower limb lymphatics are dilated and tortuous (lymphangiectasis).

- To start with, lymphoedema is pitting in nature and after some time becomes non-pitting in nature. Lymph (protein) provides good nourishment for fibroblasts.

- After repeated infections, the skin over the limb becomes *dry, thickened,* thrown into folds and even *nodules* which *break open* and result in ulcers, hence called "elephant leg". Lack of nutrition and infection precipitate lymphoedema. Oedema is also due to reflux of lymph from para-aortic vessels into the smaller lymphatics draining the lower limb. Subcutaneous tissue is grossly thickened. The presence of deep fascia prevents involvement of the deep muscles of the lower limb.

2. After inguinal block dissection for secondaries in lymph nodes (upper limb lymphoedema following axillary block dissection).

3. Following radiotherapy to lymph nodes

4. Advanced malignancies

5. Repeated infections due to barefoot walking.

Differential Diagnosis of Unilateral Elephantiasis of the Leg

1. **Filariasis** is the most common cause of elephantiasis of the leg in endemic areas such as Coastal Karnataka, Coastal Andhra Pradesh, Tamil Nadu, etc.

2. **Congenital AV fistula** can present with unilateral gigantism of the leg. Dilated veins, continuous murmur, gigantism, and non-healing ulcer in the leg in a young boy give the clue to the diagnosis.

3. **Elephantiasis neuromatosa** of the leg can cause diffuse enlargement of the leg. The leg is tender on palpation with soft to firm diffuse swelling.

4. **Extensive lipomatosis** of the leg.

EXAMINATION OF LYMPHATIC VESSELS

- Examine the leg and upper limb for any red streaks or lines which is one of the features of filarial lymphangitis.

- Examine the limbs distally:

  1. For example: When there is enlargement of axillary group of lymph nodes, the upper limb may be swollen—it is due to *lymphatic obstruction called lymphoedema.*

  2. For example: When there are multiple inguinal lymph node enlargement, there may be lymphoedema of the leg.

  3. For example: In cases of malignant melanoma, multiple cutaneous nodules may be found

between the primary lesion and secondaries (groin nodes). These are called *in transit deposits.* This occurs due to the spread of malignant cells through lymphatics.

A CASE OF LYMPHOEDEMA OF THE LEG

A 60-year-old housewife, coming from Kundapur presented to the hospital with following complaints:

1. Swelling of the right lower limb—10 years duration (Fig. 10.42).
2. Ulceration in the leg since 30 days
3. Fever with rigors since 3 days

History of Present Illness

- The patient complains of swelling of the right lower limb since 10 years. To begin with, she used to get recurrent attacks of fever with chills and rigors. Initially she had not taken specific treatment. By the time she went to hospital, her leg had swollen to a reasonable size. She also used to get recurrent swelling in the groin. In the last 10 years, she has been hospitalized several times for fever and swelling for which she has been treated with some tablets and injections (anti-filarial) treatment.

- The patient complains of ulcer over the lower part of the leg since 30 days. To begin with she noticed some redness over the leg. Following a few days, skin ulcerated resulting in ulcer. Last few days, it is discharging purulent fluid.

- Fever with chills and rigors since last 3 days. It is high grade with severe pain and redness over the leg.

- Patient had no history of trauma but she scratched the skin over the leg which resulted in ulcer.

CLINICAL DISCUSSION

- Swelling of 10 years duration and the patient is 60 years old which means this problem is not congenital but acquired. Recurrent attacks of fever suggest filarial infection. Swelling in the groin means inguinal lymph node enlargement. Skin changes in the leg such as gross thickening, rugosity, cracks precipitate itching which might have resulted in secondary infection. Thus, cellulitis, abscess, and ulceration have occurred.

What are the causes of gross oedema in this patient?

- Initial lymphangitis and later recurrent attacks result in fibrosis of the lymph nodes and obstruction to the lymphatics.

Inspection

- The right leg is swollen. The swelling is confined to the leg and lower thigh. Affected part is grossly

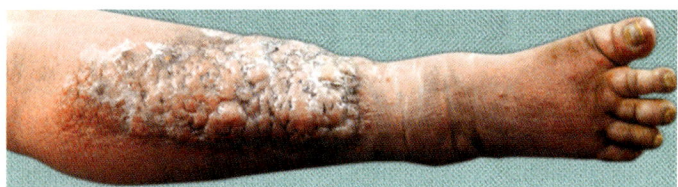

Fig. 10.42: Skin changes and lymphangitis

Clinical Wisdom

- In all cases of lymph node swelling, remember to examine drainage area.
- Lymphoedema of the lower limb affects toes more than any other part. This is not a feature in oedema due to cardiac, renal or venous causes.

thickened with rugosity resembling elephant leg. Skin is thickened, pigmented, nodular with cracks and ulceration.

- A few red streaks are visible.

- Ulceration is seen on the medial side with floor of the ulcer having slough and the edge is not sloping—almost punched out like.

- Seropurulent discharge is present.

Palpation

- There is local rise in temperature and tenderness is limited to a few cm surrounding the ulcer.

- Part is grossly thickened, oedematous and is non-pitting in nature.

- Base of the ulcer is fixed to subcutaneous tissue.

- Bones cannot be appreciated.

Other Relevant Examination

Movements of the ankle joint: Restricted because of swelling and inflammation.

Examination of groin nodes: Vertical group of inguinal nodes are enlarged and about 2 cm in size and they are firm and tender on palpation.

Examination of peripheral pulses: Dorsalis pedis and posterior tibial arteries are normal.

Management

1. Rest and elevation
2. *During acute stage :* Diethyl carbamazine 100 mg 3 times /day for 21 days and Injectable cephalosporins are given.
3. Treatment of chronic cases depend upon the severity—Swiss-roll operation, excision and grafting and amputation are some of the surgeries.

11

Examination of Peripheral Nerves

INTRODUCTION

Majority of the patients present with some form of weakness involving the concerned muscles supplied by a nerve when it is involved by disease, or divided by trauma. One example is a patient says I am having difficulty in buttoning my shirt or doing the typing work. It means small muscles of the hand are weak. Thus, a careful examination revealed weakness of the muscles supplied by ulnar nerve. Patient had a swelling in the region of ulnar nerve. Final diagnosis was ulnar nerve abscess affecting ulnar nerve with ulnar nerve paralysis caused by leprosy. Apart from the various diseases affecting nerve, an important cause of nerve weakness is nerve injury caused by fractures involving limb bones or sharp penetrating injuries. Nerves may be inadvertently damaged during surgery or sometimes sacrificed after a radical procedure for carcinoma.

Extensive discussion and details are not discussed here. Please refer orthopaedic books.

HISTORY OF PRESENT ILLNESS

- First question is like any other case: What are your complaints? Why have you come here? What happened? When did you notice this?
- History of intramuscular injections given in the deltoid and gluteal regions should be taken in suspected radial nerve and sciatic nerve weakness.
- Any accidents and any fractures or dislocation? A few fractures and dislocations with nerve paralysis are given below: Supracondylar fracture of the humerus—all the 3 nerve injuries—ulnar, median and radial. Fracture shaft of humerus—radial nerve

palsy. Fracture neck humerus—axillary nerve. Posterior dislocation of the hip—sciatic nerve. Fracture neck fibula—lateral popliteal nerve.

- Is the weakness progressive? Is there any tingling and numbness? Is there any specific type of work which you cannot do?
- Have you undergone any operations or surgery? Surgeries done for a swelling or a tumour in the known anatomical site of the nerve can give rise to nerve paralysis or weakness. A few examples are given below.

  - Parotidectomy and facial nerve paralysis
  - Thyroidectomy and recurrent laryngeal nerve paralysis
  - Groin dissection and femoral nerve injury
  - Hypoglossal nerve after submandibular gland tumour
  - Wrist drop following excision of a swelling in the posterior triangle (Figs 11.1 and 11.2)

- Any tingling and numbness? (Fig. 11.3) or any other skin lesions, nodules? It may be a case of leprosy (Fig. 11.3)

INSPECTION

1. *Attitude of the limb*: Following are some characteristic attitudes of the limb that help in diagnosis:
   - *Wrist drop*: Paralysis of radial nerve.
   - *Foot drop*: Paralysis of lateral popliteal nerve.
   - *Claw hand*: It is also called main en griffe. This occurs due to paralysis of interossei which are supplied by ulnar nerve and lumbricals which are supplied by median nerve.

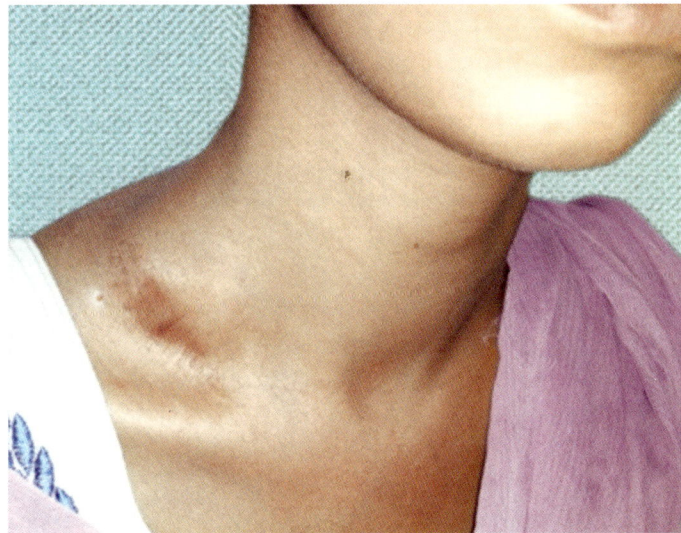

Fig. 11.1: Posterior triangle—neurilemmoma excised

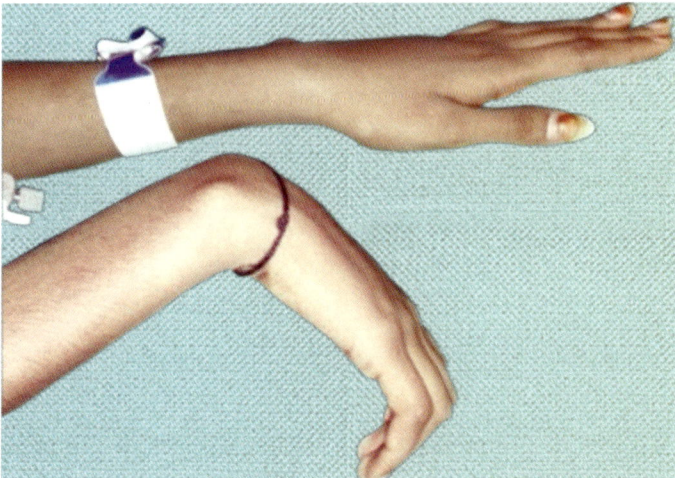

Fig. 11.2: Right radial nerve paralysis—wrist drop following excision of the tumour

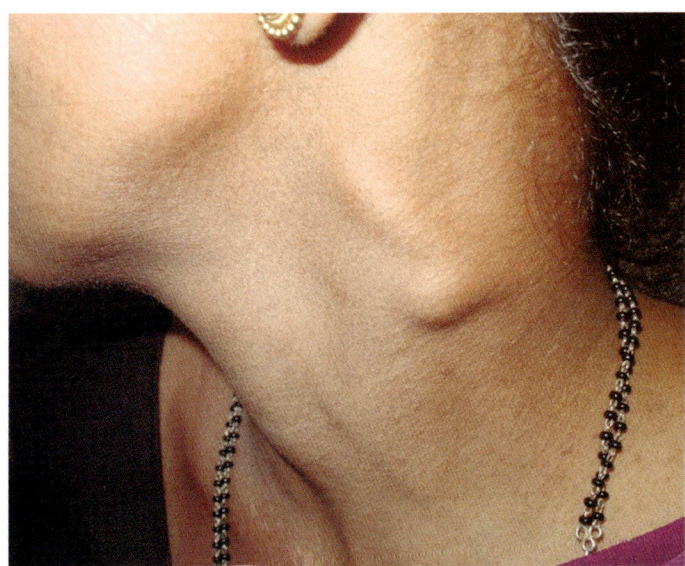

Fig. 11.3: Thickened posterior auricular nerve with nerve abscess

- *Ape thumb deformity*: It is due to paralysis of the opponens pollicis which is supplied by median nerve.

- *Pointing test*: It is due to paralysis of lateral half of the flexor digitorum profundus.

- *Winging of scapula*: Paralysis of long thoracic nerve results in prominent vertebral border of the scapula due to paralysis of serratus anterior.

- *Erb's paralysis*: It is due to lesion of the upper brachial plexus commencement of 5th and 6th cervical nerve roots, and suprascapular nerve, nerve to subclavius, abductors and lateral rotators of the shoulder, flexors and supinators of the elbow. Typical attitude of the limb has been described as policeman receiving a tip—the arm is adducted, internally rotated and hangs by the side of the body whereas the forearm is extended at the elbow and fully pronated.

2. **Wasting of the muscles**: This is best done by comparing with the other side. To give a few examples: Hypothenar eminence wasting in ulnar nerve paralysis and thenar eminence wasting in median nerve paralysis (Fig. 11.4).

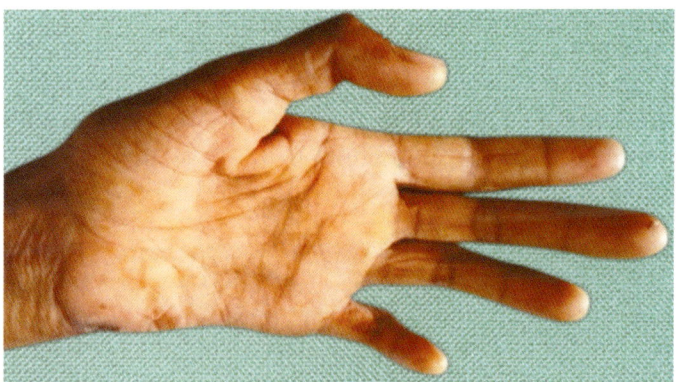

Fig. 11.4: Wasting of muscles

3. *Skin changes*: Skin will be dry because of absence of sweating due to sympathetic paralysis. The skin will be glossy and smooth. Trophic ulcers will develop over the pressure point as in leprosy, diabetic neuropathy, etc. Other changes are ridged nail, brittle nail and scaly skin. Vasomotor changes are pallor, cyanosis, excessive sweating.

4. *Any wound or scar*: This may point at the cause such as nerve injury.

PALPATION

1. *Temperature changes*: Paralysed part always feels cold when compared to the other side. Back of the hand is used to check the temperature changes.

2. *Muscles*: Feel the wasted muscles and normal muscles. Wasted muscles are flabby and soft. No muscular contractions. Grading of the motor activity is given below. It is called as Oxford/MRC (Medical Research Council) grading scale.

Grade	Muscle activity
0	No contraction
1	Flicker/trace contraction
2	Active movement with gravity eliminated
3	Active movement against gravity
4	Active movement against gravity and resistance
5	Normal power

3. *Skin*: Feel the skin and find out any loss of sensation. Hence, students should have the perfect knowledge of sensory distribution of various nerves. Details are given later. One example is given here. Deep peroneal nerve (anterior tibial nerve) supplies a small portion of the dorsum of the feet (space between the great toe and second toe.)

4. *Swelling*: Check for any swelling in the distribution of nerve or any swelling compressing the nerve. Thus neuromas, nerve abscess due to leprosy or a sarcoma should be looked for. Neuroma or neurofibromas are tender, firm to hard oval swellings. Sarcoma is very vascular with variable consistency

and nerve abscesses are tense firm swellings in relation to nerve. Look for other features of leprosy in such patients (Fig. 11.5).

EXAMINATION OF NERVES OF UPPER LIMB

1. *Axillary nerve*: Abduct the shoulder against resistance. Examiner can feel for the contracted deltoid to check whether patient is contracting the muscles or not? Axillary nerve (C5, 6) may be injured from fracture of surgical neck of humerus or scapula and sometimes by misplaced intramuscular injection. There is deltoid palsy and wasting with loss of sensation around its insertion (regimental patch) (Table 11.1).

2. *Radial nerve*: Radial nerve injury results in wrist drop. Radial nerve supplies triceps, brachioradialis and extensor carpi radialis longus (only extensor of the wrist joint supplied by radial nerve). It has a major branch—posterior interosseous nerve. Posterior interosseous nerve supplies supinator, extensor carpi radialis brevis, extensor digitorum, extensor digiti minimi, extensor carpi ulnaris, extensor pollicis longus, extensor indicis, abductor pollicis longus and brevis (Tables 11.2 to 11.4 and Fig. 11.6).

Tests for radial nerve injury or paralysis

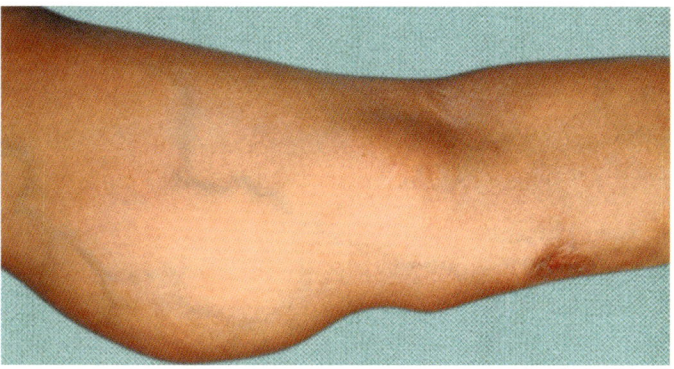

Fig. 11.5: Neurilemmoma of ulnar nerve

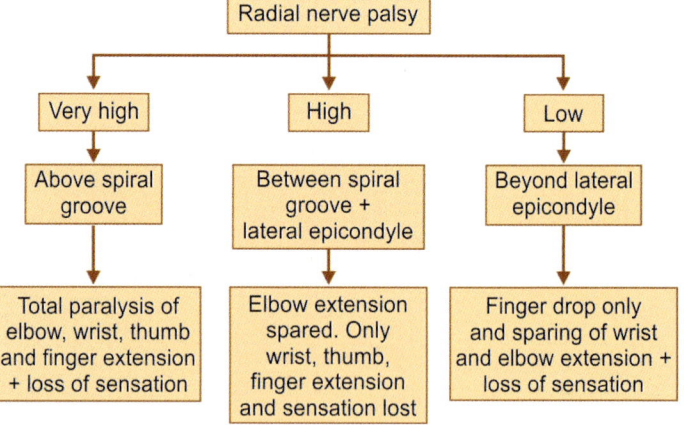

Table 11.1: Branches of axillary nerve

	Trunk	Anterior division	Posterior division
Muscular	—	Deltoid (most part)	Deltoid (posterior part) and teres minor. The nerve to teres minor is characterised by the presence of a pseudoganglion
Cutaneous	—	—	Upper lateral cutaneous nerve of arm
Articular and vascular	Shoulder joint	—	To posterior circumflex humeral artery

Table 11.2: Branches of radial nerve

	Axilla	*Radial sulcus*	*Lateral side of arm*
Muscular	Long head of triceps brachii	Lateral head of triceps brachii	Brachioradialis
	Medial head of triceps brachii	Anconeus	Extensor carpi radialis longus (ECRL)
			Lateral part of brachialis (proprioceptive)
Cutaneous	Posterior cutaneous nerve of arm	Posterior cutaneous nerve of forearm	—
		Lower lateral cutaneous nerve of arm	
Vascular	—	To profunda brachii artery	—
Terminal	—	—	Superficial and deep or posterior interosseous branches

Table 11.3: Branches of deep division of radial nerve

	Cubital fossa	*Back of forearm*	*Wrist*
Muscular	Extensor carpi radialis brevis and supinator	Abductor pollicis longus, extensor pollicis brevis (ECRB), extensor pollicis longus, extensor digitorum, extensor indicis, extensor digiti minimi and extensor carpi ulnaris (ECU)	—
Articular	—	—	To inferior radioulnar, wrist and intercarpal joints

Table 11.4: Branches of superficial division of radial nerve

	Forearm	*Anatomical snuff box and dorsum of hand*
Cutaneous and vascular	Lateral side of forearm and radial vessels	Skin over anatomical snuff box, lateral half of dorsum of hand and lateral 2½ digits till their distal interphalangeal joints
Articular	—	To wrist joint, 1st carpometacarpal joint, metacarpophalangeal and interphalangeal joints of the thumb, index and middle fingers

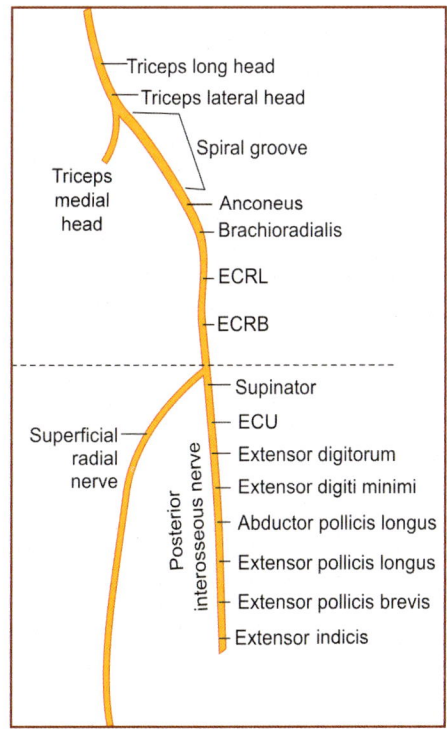

Fig. 11.6: Muscles supplied by radial nerve

- *Triceps*: Main action is extension of the elbow. Ask the patient to extend the elbow and surgeon resists the extension—extension against resistance.

- *Brachioradialis*: Action of this muscle is flexion of elbow in the mid-prone position of the elbow. Ask the patient to flex the elbow in the mid-prone position against resistance. Muscle can be seen and felt as a prominent band. In fact this is how valley of brachioradialis can be demonstrated to students. Radial nerve after supplying brachioradialis is divided into superficial and deep (posterior interosseous nerve). This means if brachioradialis is weak, the lesion is above the division and vice versa.

- **Extensors of the wrist**: Posterior interosseous nerve supplies all the muscles of the wrist joint **except extensor carpi radialis longus**. Wrist drop is the important and obvious complaint of these patients with radial nerve paralysis. Interphalangeal joint extension is possible because it is done by interossei through extensor expansions which are supplied by ulnar nerve.

- **Extensor digitorum:** Extension of metacarpophalangeal joint is possible mainly by extensor digitorum. Hence, this action is not possible when this muscle is paralysed.

3. **Median nerve:** Muscles supplied by median nerve are flexor pollicis longus, flexor digitorum superficialis and lateral half of flexor digitorum profundus. These muscles help in clasping the fingers, opposition of thumb, etc. (Table 11.5 and Fig. 11.7).

- **Flexor pollicis longus (FPL):** Clinician will hold the proximal phalanx steady and the patient is asked to bend the terminal phalanx against resistance. This muscle is paralysed when injury to median nerve occurs high in the forearm. It is supplied by anterior interosseous branch from median nerve.

- **Flexor digitorum superficialis (FDS) and lateral half of flexor digitorum profundus:** The patient is asked to clasp the hand. Index finger of the hand fails to flex and hence it will be straight. It is called the pointing index finger and is also called Oschner's clasping test.

- **Abductor pollicis brevis:** Contraction of this muscle produces abduction of the thumb. This means that the thumb will move straight upwards and outwards from the palm. This can be demonstrated by pen test. The hand is kept flat and supinated on the table. A pen is kept at a vertically slightly higher level than the tip of the thumb. The patient is then asked to touch the tip of the pen with his thumb.

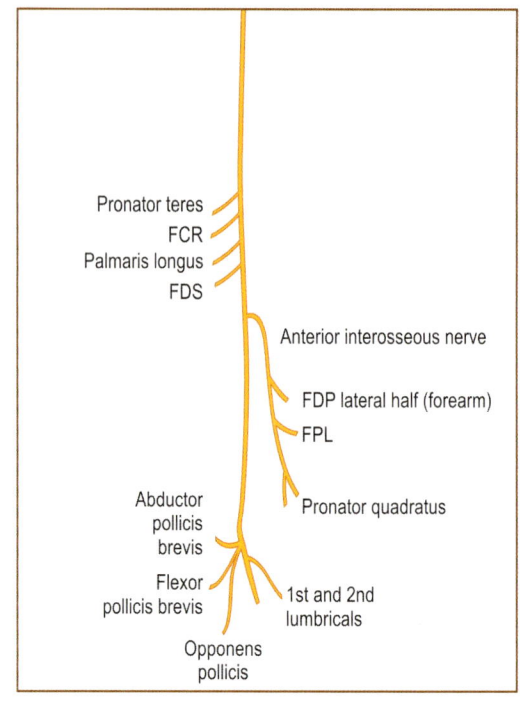

Fig. 11.7: Muscles supplied by median nerve

- **Opponens pollicis:** The patient is asked to touch the pulp space of all fingers by using the thumb. This is not possible, if this muscle is paralysed. One should watch carefully when this movement is done because adductor pollicis supplied by ulnar nerve can produce adduction which should not be confused for opponens.

4. **Ulnar nerve:** It arises from medial cord of brachial plexus comprising of C8 and T1. It is also called musician's nerve because it controls fine movements of the fingers through interossei muscles. Muscles supplied by ulnar nerve are flexor carpi ulnaris,

Table 11.5: Branches of median nerve

	Axilla and arm	Cubital fossa	Forearm	Palm
Muscular	Pronator teres in lower part of arm	Flexor carpi radialis, flexor digitorum superficialis, palmaris longus	Anterior interosseous which supplies—lateral half of flexor digitorum profundus, pronator quadratus, and flexor pollicis longus	Recurrent branch for abductor pollicis brevis, flexor pollicis brevis, opponens pollicis. 1st and 2nd lumbricals from the digital nerves
Cutaneous	—	—	Palmar cutaneous branch for lateral two-thirds of palm	• Two digital branches to lateral and medial sides of thumb • One to lateral side of index finger • Two to adjacent sides of index and middle fingers • Two to adjacent sides of middle and ring fingers. These branches also supply dorsal aspects of distal phalanges of lateral 3½ digits
Articular and vascular	Brachial artery	Elbow joint	—	Give vascular and articular branches to joints of hand

Table 11.6: Branches of ulnar nerve

	Forearm	Hand
Muscular	Medial half of flexor digitorum profundus, flexor carpi ulnaris	Superficial branch; palmaris brevis. Deep branch—muscles of hypothenar eminence, medial two lumbricals, 1–4 dorsal interossei and 1–4 palmar interossei and adductor pollicis
Cutaneous/digital	Dorsal cutaneous branch for medial half of dorsum of hand. Palmar cutaneous branch for medial one-third of palm. Digital branches to medial 1½ fingers, nail beds and dorsal aspects of distal phalanges	
Vascular/articular	Also supplies digital vessels and joints of medial side of hand	

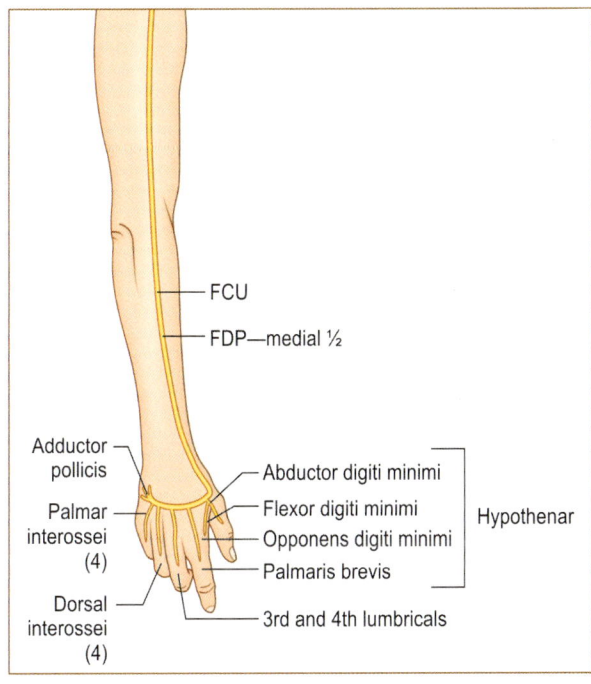

Fig. 11.8: Muscles supplied by ulnar nerve

interossei, adductor pollicis (Table 11.6 and Fig. 11.8).

- *Flexor carpi ulnaris*: This muscle flexes the hand and adducts the hand at the wrist joint. When patient is asked to flex the hand against resistance, hand deviates to the radial side when this muscle is paralysed.

- *First palmar interosseous and adductor pollicis*: Chief action of both these muscles is adduction of the thumb. The patient is asked to hold a card or book between extended thumb and the other fingers. If these muscles are paralysed, the patient will try to hold the book by using flexor pollicis longus which is supplied by median

nerve. In this situation, one can see the flexion of the terminal phalanx. It is called *Froment's sign*.

- *Interossei*: PAD and DAB are the favourite mnemonics to remember the action of interossei. Palmar interossei with adduction and dorsal interossei with abduction. More importantly, interossei along with lumbricals, flexes the metacarpophalangeal joint and extend both proximal and distal inter phalangeal joints.

  a. Ask the patient to abduct the fingers or ask him to separate the fingers against resistance. Other test is ask him to hold a card in between the fingers **(card test)**. When he fails in the first test, dorsal interossei are paralysed and in the second test, palmar interossei are involved.

  b. The patient is asked to extend the middle and terminal phalanx against resistance, and the clinician steadies the proximal phalanx. Weakness of the muscles indicates paralysis of the nerve.

CLINICAL DISCUSSION

1. What is Erb's palsy?
- It occurs due to traction injury to C5, 6 roots (upper trunk), due to forced lateral flexion of neck (to the opposite side) and depression of shoulder. The limb is typically adducted, internally rotated at shoulder, extended at elbow and flexed at wrist, assuming the so-called 'waiter's tip' (policeman's tip) position.

2. What is Klumpke's palsy?
- It is the lesion of C8, T1 roots (lower trunk), resulting from forced traction of abducted shoulder. This can occur during delivery or grabbing a support, while falling from a height. The intrinsic muscles of hand are mainly affected, with impaired sensations over the medial forearm and hand. If the T1 root is injured before giving the rami communicans to the sympathetic chain, Horner's syndrome may be seen, but not in distal lesions.

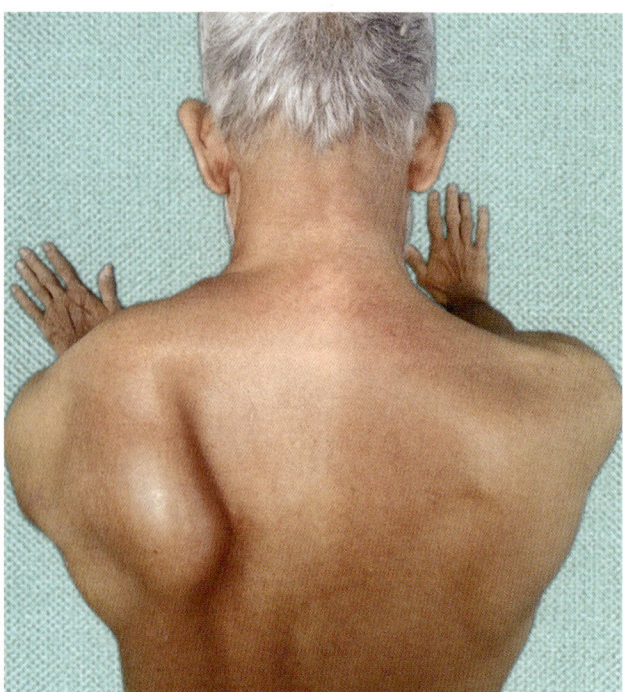

Fig. 11.9: Winging of scapula

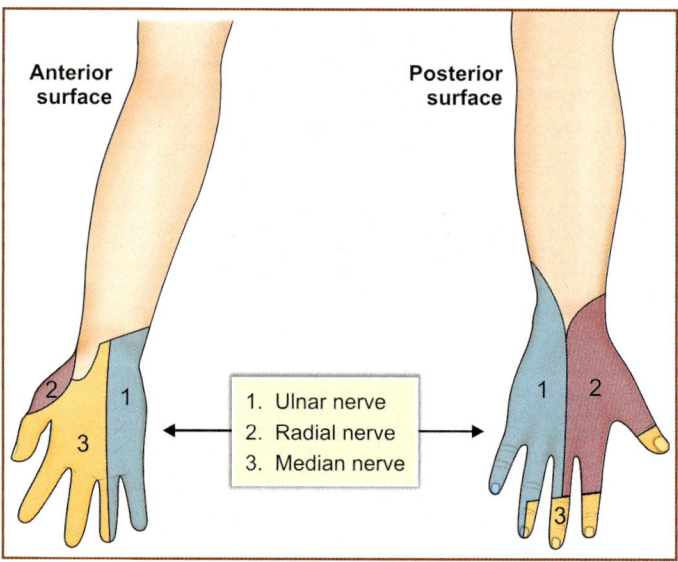

Fig. 11.10: Sensory loss in median, ulnar and radial nerve paralysis

3. What is winging of scapula?
* Long thoracic nerve of Bell (C5, 6, 7), supplying the serratus anterior, may be injured during heavy lifting or axillary surgery such as axillary dissection during modified radical mastectomy done for carcinoma breast. The muscle helps to push the scapula forwards. *Winging of scapula* is seen when it is paralyzed, while the patient pushes against a wall, with outstretched hands, but the shrugging of shoulder is retained, to differentiate from winging due to trapezius palsy (Fig. 11.9).

SENSATIONS OF THE UPPER LIMB

Sensations: All the three nerves of the upper limb have sensory supply to the hand (Fig. 11.10).

* *Median nerve*: Palmar aspect of the thumb, index and middle fingers.

    Dorsal aspect of the distal phalanx and half of the middle phalanx of same fingers mentioned above the variable amount of the radial side of the palm of the hand, including thenar eminence.

* *Ulnar nerve*: Skin on the anterior and posterior surfaces of the little finger and ulnar side of the ring finger.

    Skin over hypothenar eminence and similar strip of skin posteriorly.

* *Radial nerve*: Skin over the lateral aspect of the first metacarpal and back of the first web space.

NERVES OF THE LOWER LIMB

SCIATIC NERVE

It is formed by ventral and dorsal divisions of L4, 5 and S1, 2, 3. Total paralysis is not common. A few causes of injury are by intramuscular injections in the gluteal region and posterior dislocation of the hip. Sciatic nerve supplies all the muscles of the entire lower limb below the knee. It also supplies hamstring muscles. Common injuries which affect this nerve are subtrochanteric fracture of femur and posterior dislocation of the hip. These injuries are incomplete and they almost always affect common peroneal nerve.

Sciatica is a common condition that affects the sciatic nerve.

Sciatica: It is not a disease but a symptom complex consisting of radicular type of pain in the entire leg, caused by nerve root compression. A few important causes of nerve root compression are: Herniated disc, tumour, metastasis, abscess, granuloma or an osteophyte. Tuberculous spine is also an important cause in India.

Typically pain radiates from the lumbar spine or gluteal region to the foot, and is aggravated by coughing, sneezing or stooping forwards.

Straight leg raising (SLR): Pain of root compression or irritation may also be elicited by SLR. It is made worse by dorsiflexion of foot (Lasegue's sign); both manoeuvres exert traction on nerve roots, through the sciatic nerve.

Depending upon the level, tendon reflexes may be abolished (knee jerk—L4 and ankle jerk—S1) and weakness of extensor hallucis longus (EHL), innervated by deep peroneal nerve (L5, S1) may be present.

Sciatic nerve divides into smaller common peroneal nerve (lateral popliteal nerve) and larger tibial nerve.

Common Peroneal Nerve (L4, 5, S1, 2)

It is also called **lateral popliteal nerve**. The common peroneal nerve divides into superficial peroneal and deep peroneal nerves after it winds around neck of fibula.

- It is highly vulnerable to injury as it goes around the fibular neck, in fractures, lacerations or tight plaster casts. It is also involved very often in Hansen's disease and palpating a thickened nerve against the neck of fibula is a diagnostic point. Its superficial location makes it a convenient point for nerve block, for surgery on the foot.

- Common injury which affects this nerve is fracture neck of the fibula. This nerve supplies extensor and peroneal muscles of the leg. Patient is asked to dorsiflex the foot and evert. He will not be able to do so. Thus, foot goes for a deformity called **talipes equinovarus**.

- Like the wrist drop in upper limb, there is a foot drop with slapping gait.

- It is also sensory to anterior and lateral aspects of leg and dorsum of the foot through its musculo-cutaneous branch, except the skin between the great toe and the second toe. This space is supplied by deep peroneal nerve which is also called anterior tibial nerve.

Tibial Nerve (L4, 5, S1, 2, 3)

It is the larger of the two and is injured less often. It is also called **medial popliteal nerve**. This nerve supplies mainly plantar flexors of the ankle joint such as soleus, gastrocnemius, popliteus, tibialis posterior, flexor digitorum longus and flexor hallucis longus. The patient is asked to flex the ankle against resistance. He will not be able to do the flexion at ankle joint. In an attempt to do so, invertors of the foot will act resulting in **talipes calcaneovalgus deformity.**

The tibial nerve is sensory to lateral part of the leg and sole through plantar nerve. Plantar nerves also supply plantar muscles and hence clawing takes place.

In lesions at the ankle level, the small muscles of foot are involved and by the unopposed action of long flexor of toes and dorsiflexors of foot, it produces a high-arched or claw foot (pes cavus).

SENSATIONS

One of the important part of clinical examination of peripheral nerves is checking for sensations. Various sensations to be checked are tactile sensations, pain, temperature, position sense, ability to recognize object size, shape, etc.

Tactile sensations: Use cotton and touch the area of the skin and then use pulp of the finger and put some degree of pressure find out from patient whether he can appreciate touch sensation or not. Two-point discrimination is another test specially useful in loss of sensation in cases of nerve injuries. Here two points at 2 mm distance should be appreciated by a normal person.

Pain: Use pinhead and gently prick and find out from the patient whether he appreciates pricking type of pain. Similarly, press on the bone or muscles to check out deep pain sensation.

Temperature: Two tubes, one containing warm water and the other, cold water are used. The patient is asked to close his eyes and announce the type of temperature sensation he is feeling.

Size, shape, and form of the object: Give a common familiar object to the patient. Ask him to close his eyes and recognize the object. *Example:* Pen, pencil, ball, etc. Loss of this property is called **astereognosis**.

Position sense: Ask the patient to lie supine. Move his great toe up or down to check position sense. Ask him in which position is the great toe and in which direction is it moved. Ask the patient to stand up straight with closed eyes. If he sways, it is an indication that posterior column is involved and Romberg's sign is said to be positive.

Vibration sense: One of the early sensation which is lost in diabetic neuropathy is vibration sense. Tuning fork is made to vibrate and kept over the part to be tested and the patient is asked to tell whether he can feel vibrations or not.

12

Examination of the Hand and Foot

INTRODUCTION

Examination of hand involves swellings related to tendons, bones, nerves, soft tissues and vessels. Diseases of the hand can be broadly classified into acute and chronic cases from clinical point of view. Acute cases are the ones which are called hand infections. Short accounts of hand infections are included here because they are common and sometimes you may encounter these cases in the clinical examination. Nerve injuries are discussed under peripheral nerve examination (*refer* to Chapter 11). Various deformities, congenital or acquired, are orthopaedic disorders and beyond the limits of this chapter. Common short cases encountered in day to day practice are discussed in this chapter.

CLASSIFICATION

1. *Cystic swellings*: Implantation dermoid cyst, syno-vitis, bursitis, ganglion, compound palmar ganglion, chronic tubercular synovitis, pyogenic granuloma.

2. *Solid swellings*: Osteoma, bone tumours, gouty arthritis

3. *Pulsatile swellings*: Traumatic AV fistula

4. Ulcers/gangrene

5. Contractures

Table 12.1 shows common swellings in the hand and foot.

HISTORY OF PRESENT ILLNESS

- **Patient may complain of swelling. Ask about the duration, progress and pain.** How did it start? History of trauma is common. Is there a history of thorn prick? If present, it may be an implantation dermoid cyst. Also remember acquired AV fistulas can develop after penetrating injuries (sharp cut). Suppurative tenosynovitis develops after pricking type of injury. Pain is an important feature. Presence of a foreign body may be the cause of swelling.

- How is the growth of the swelling? Slow growth is typical of implantation dermoid cyst, ganglion and AV fistula, rheumatoid disease and tubercular tenosynovitis. Rapid growth may indicate soft tissue sarcoma. (It is not common in the hand).

- History of fever suggests tuberculosis or chronic abscess.

Table 12.1: Common swellings in the hand and foot

Solid swellings	Cystic swellings	Vascular
1. Neural tumours	1. Implantation dermoid cyst	1. Haemangioma
2. Lipoma	2. Pyogenic abscess Chronic abscess	2. Traumatic AV fistula/ pseudoaneurysm
3. Osteomas, exostosis	3. Tenosynovitis	3. Pyogenic granuloma
4. Soft tissue sarcomas	4. Ganglion	4. Glomus tumour
5. Malignant skin tumours	5. Compound palmar ganglion	(A very small tumour suspected but not felt)
6. Maduromycosis (foot only)		
7. Elephantiasis (common in foot)		

- Slow growing swelling which may give rise to bleeding is pyogenic granuloma.

- Ulcerations over the capillary and cavernous haemangioma can also give rise to bleeding.

- Chronic pain in the fingers and hand with ulcerations and gangrene suggests occlusive arterial diseases. *When you do not find any swelling or any specific cause of pain, think of the possibility of glomus in the tip of the fingers.*

■ Clinical Case Capsule

A 45-year-old smoker, obese patient with a short neck presented to an orthopaedic surgeon with pain in the forearm and fingers. Examination revealed tenderness in the muscles of the forearm and fingers. Pain was severe. The patient also said that he had pain in the neck on turning. He was diagnosed to have cervical spondylosis and was given a cervical collar. After 48 hours, he presented with colour changes and gangrenous patches of skin over the digits. The diagnosis was now obvious. It was an occlusive arterial disease. The orthopaedician had not palpated the pulses. Radial artery was not palpable. Brachial arterial pulsations were weak. It was a case of TAO.

CLINICAL EXAMINATION

I. *Swelling*: All the basic principles of inspection, palpation and auscultation should be done. Some swellings have specific findings that help clinch the diagnosis. They are:

- Compressibility in haemangioma and AV fistula

- Continuous murmur in AV fistula

- Tenderness and tense cystic nature of chronic abscess

- Cross-fluctuation of compound palmar ganglion

- Tense, cystic (may feel firm), nontender implantation dermoid.

- Other specific tumour in the hands is glomus tumour which is an extremely painful tumour. Details are given in page 179.

II. Examination of Hand: 'ABCDEF' of Hand

A. Anomalies or abnormalities of fingers (Figs 12.1 to 12.4): Sinuses may be due to osteomyelitis and when they are multiple, may be due to tubercular aetiology. Osteomyelitis of terminal phalanx can present with persistent sinus in the tip of the finger.

- Any muscle wasting should be carefully looked for. *Example*: Small muscles wasting—hypothenar muscles in ulnar nerve paralysis caused by cervical rib.

- Intermetacarpal hollowness indicates muscle wasting also.

B. Bony projections or bony contour must be mentioned, if present. Bony swelling is immobile and hard. *Example*: Osteoma.

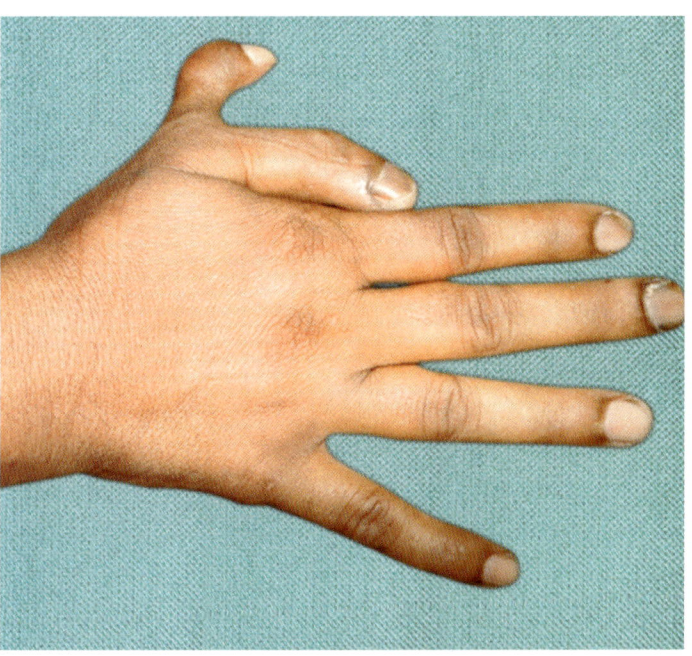

Fig. 12.1: Polydactyly—extra thumb

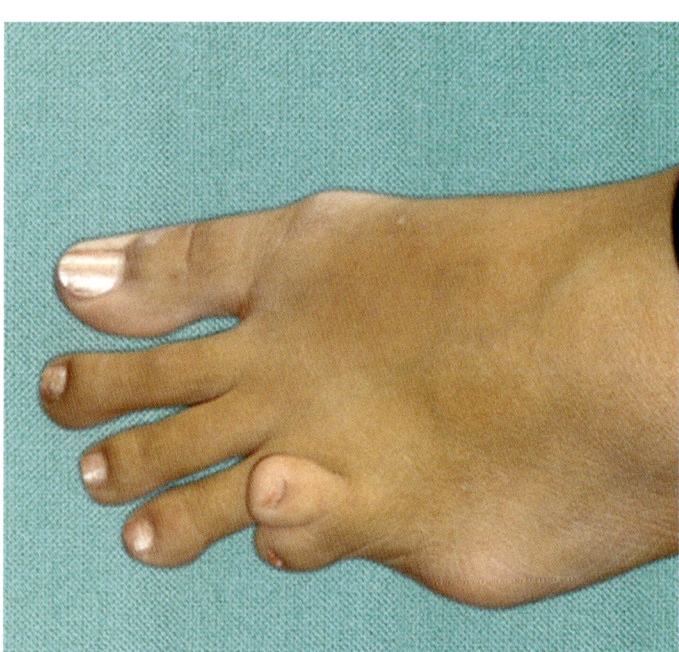

Fig. 12.2: Webbed toes

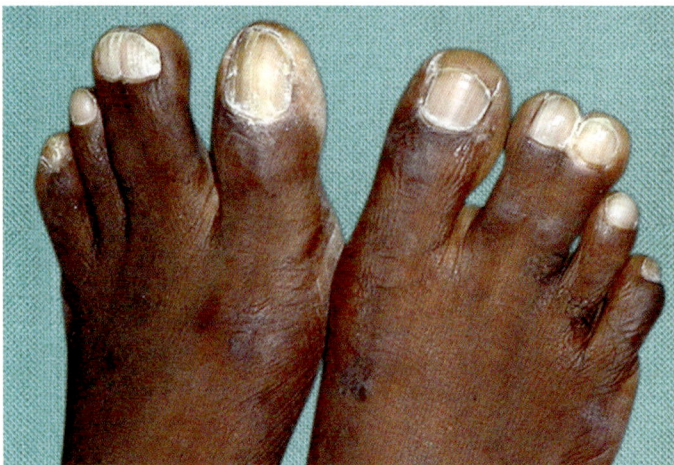

Fig. 12.3: Webbed toes

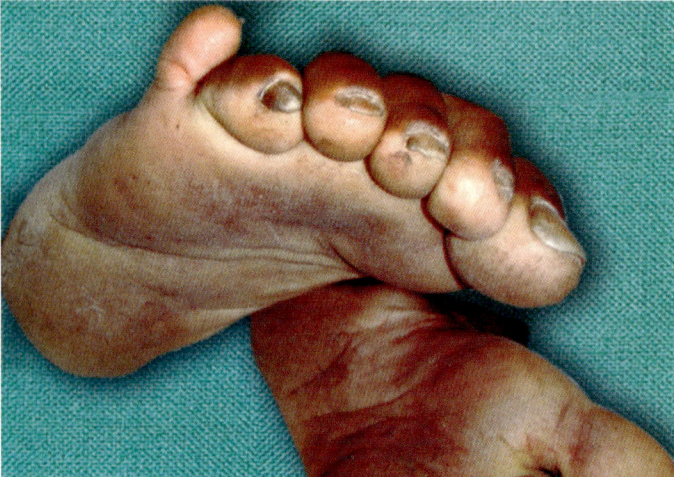

Fig. 12.4: Polydactyly feet

C. Circulation: Please refer to chapter on upper limb ischaemia. Pulsation of radial artery, and brachial artery must be checked.

- Slow ischaemia can be easily missed if proper clinical examination is not done. Hence, examination of peripheral pulses is mandatory when a patient complains of pain in the hand and upper limb.

D. Deformities: Details are given in Chapter 11.

E. Examination of nerves

- *Sensory nerves*: Details are given in Chapter 11 (*refer* to Fig. 11.10).

- *Motor nerves*
  - *Median nerve palsy* causes wasting of thenar eminence and loss of abduction of the thumb.
    - Flexion of the terminal interphalangeal joint of the little finger is absent.
    - Absent opposition of the thumb.

- *Ulnar nerve palsy* causes wasting of hypothenar eminence.
  - Absence of flexion of the little and ring fingers.
  - Hollows between the metacarpals.
  - Absence of adduction and abduction of the fingers.
- *Radial nerve palsy* causes absence of wrist extension, and absence of extension of the meta-carpophalangeal joints.
  - Absence of the extension of the thumb.

F. Function/movements

- *Thumb*: Flexion, extension, abduction, adduction and opposition at carpometacarpal joint.
- *Fingers*: Flexion, extension, abduction, adduction at metacarpophalangeal joint.
- *Fingers*: Flexion, extension at interphalangeal joints.

DIFFERENTIAL DIAGNOSIS

Differential Diagnosis for Hand Infections

1. *Acute paronychia*

- It occurs due to trimming of the nail or ingrowing nail (Figs 12.5 and 12.6).
- Infection starts in the lateral sulcus and *spreads all around.* (Paronychia means near the nail or run around.) This is because eponychium (skin overlying the nail base) is adherent to the nail base. Hence, the infection spreads beneath the nail base. The affected finger is painful. Throbbing pain suggests presence of pus. Low grade fever may be present.

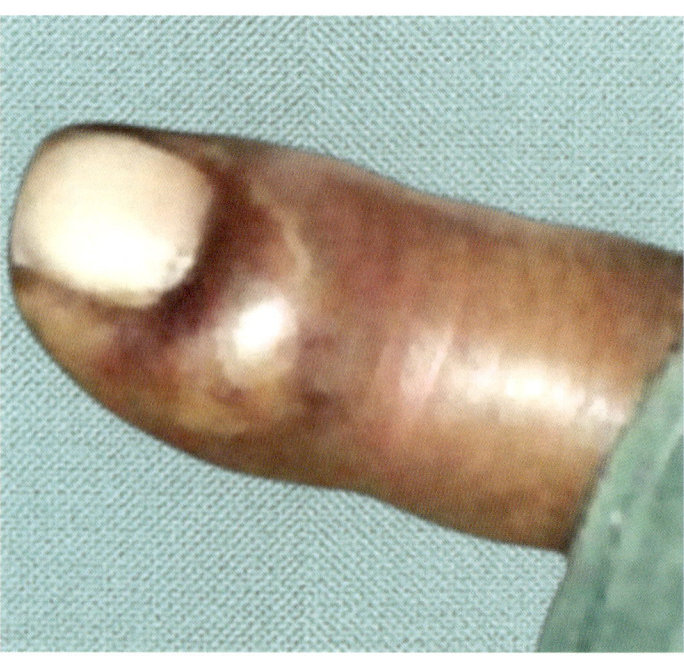

Fig. 12.5: Acute paronychia

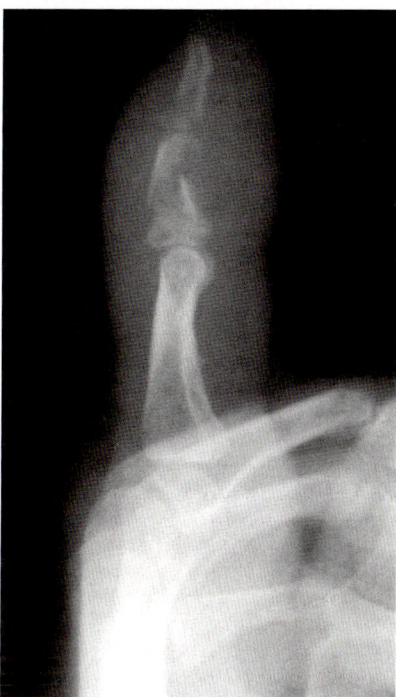

Fig. 12.6: Plain radiography of hand showing osteomyelitis of terminal phalanx

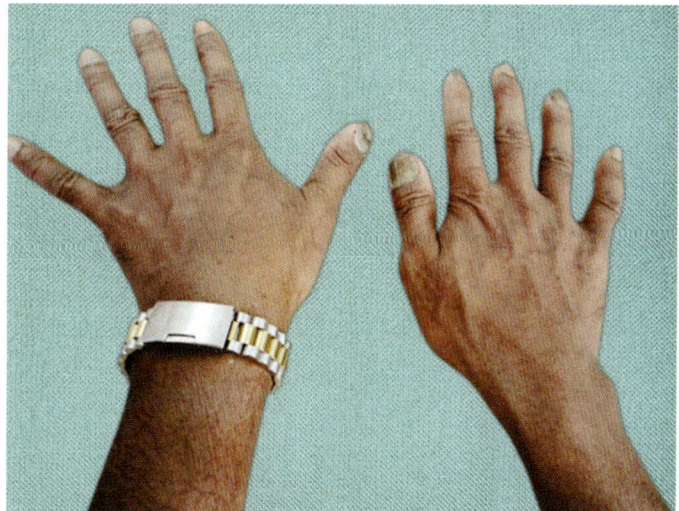

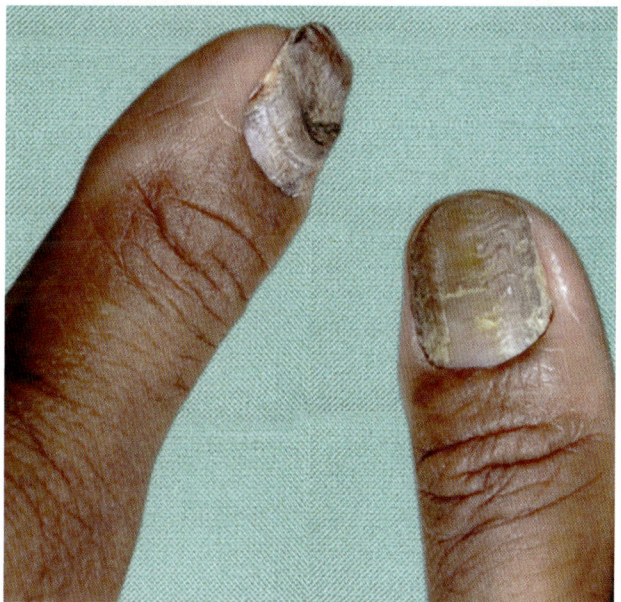

Figs 12.7 and 12.8: Chronic paronychia

Early cases (before formation of pus) can be managed by soaking, elevation and antibiotics. If it does not respond to treatment, it can be drained by incising the eponychium using a digital block (with 5 ml of 2% *plain lignocaine* injected into the root of the digit).

2. Chronic paronychia: It is due to fungal infection—moniliasis or due to *Candida* infections. It is common in women who wash the clothes, utensils, etc. and have constantly wet fingers. As a result of this, fungal infection takes place. The infection is insidious in onset, chronic and difficult to eradicate. It produces a dull nagging pain in the fingers. Antifungal agents are used (Figs 12.7 and 12.8).

3. Acute lymphangitis of hand: It is caused by a minor abrasion. The causative organism is *Streptococcus*. Severe pain in the hand with fever, chills and rigors and gross oedema of dorsum of hand are usual features. Red, hot streaks over the limb which indicates route of lymphatics, is characteristic of this condition. Regional lymph nodes are swollen and tender. It is treated by injection crystalline penicillin 10 lakh units IV or IM for 5–7 days.

- *Infection of little finger*—epitrochlear lymph nodes are enlarged.
- *Ring and middle finger*—nodes above the clavicle are affected.
- *Index and thumb*—axillary nodes are enlarged.

4. Infection of the terminal pulp space (felon): This space commonly gets infected due to prick injuries which are relatively deep. It is the second common infection of the hand seen in about 25% of the patients. Injury to the affected finger is usually present. Thumb and index are commonly involved. Throbbing pain is worse in the dependent position, with nocturnal exacerbations. The pulp is indurated, red and tense and is characteristic of this condition. Touch, movement, dependent position worsen

the pain. Incision and drainage is the treatment of choice. *Thrombosis of digital artery resulting in osteomyelitis and necrosis of the terminal phalanx is a complication* (Fig. 12.8).

5. Apical subungual infection: Infection is confined to the space between the distal quarter of the subungual epithelium and periosteum of the distal phalanx. Penetration by a sharp object is the cause for this condition. It manifests very often as a tender yellow spot beneath the distal portion of the nail. Pain, redness and minimal swelling are the features. Tenderness is maximum at the free edge of the nail. Pulp and distal parts of fingers are relatively painless. It is treated by "V" excision of a portion of nail and opening of the abscess cavity with antibiotic cover.

6. Web space infections: Web spaces are the triangular spaces in between the four divisions of the palmar aponeurosis. *They are 3 in number.* Thumb has no palmar aponeurosis. They are filled with subcutaneous fat and posteriorly by metacarpal bones. This space can be infected due to penetrating injuries, or due to lumbrical canal infection—suppurating tenosynovitis. It is an extremely tender and a hot swelling. Finger separation sign—

adjacent fingers are separated due to gross oedema of the hand. It is treated by incision and drainage. The skin edge is trimmed in such a way as to leave *diamond*-shaped opening to get better drainage.

7. *Deep palmar abscess*: Infection of mid-palmar space results in deep palmar abscess. Mid-palmar space is the space behind the palmar aponeurosis and in front of the metacarpal bones. Since palmar fascia is thick, strong and unyielding, pus collects deep to palmar fascia. Palmar fascia covers long flexors. Apex of the triangular palmar aponeurosis is continuous with flexor retinaculum and palmaris longus tendon. Distally, it forms four longitudinal digital bands and attaches to bases of proximal phalanges. Two fibrous septa extend from medial and lateral margins of palmar aponeurosis. They are medial and lateral fibrous septa. The septum is attached to 5th and 3rd metacarpals, respectively. Deeper to flexor tendons, digital arteries and nerves, lies the midpalmar space. The mid-palmar space is continuous with anterior compartment of the forearm *via* carpal tunnel. This space is called 'Space of Parona'. Clinically, it presents as obliteration of *normal concavity of the palm, gross oedema* of the dorsum of the hand, and extreme tenderness in mid-palmar space.

Fingers are held in *flexion* at the *metacarpophalangeal* (MP) joint because the palmar aponeurosis gets relaxed in this position (frog hand). *MP joint movements are painful.* Interphalangeal (IP) joint movements are not painful. It is treated by drainage of the pus by placing a transverse crease incision over the area of maximum tenderness and splitting the palmar aponeurosis *longitudinally* in the direction of the fibres (*to avoid damage to nerves and vessels*).

8. *Acute suppurating tenosynovitis*: Infection of the flexor tendon sheath occurs due to pricking type of injuries. The flexor tendon sheaths which enclose the tendons run along the whole length of the finger. In the palm, the medial tendons are enclosed by a common synovial pocket called "ulnar bursa" and on the lateral side by "radial bursa". These two are communicating in 80% of the cases. In 25% of cases, the flexor tendon sheath of the thumb is communicating with radial bursa and of the little finger with ulnar bursa. Thus, infection of the fingers (flexor tendon sheath) can involve the entire hand (Fig. 12.9).

- The patient gives history of symmetrical, fusiform painful enlargement of finger. Flexed, fixed finger (hook sign) is a characteristic feature. *IP joint movements are very painful.*
- Severe pain on passive finger extension is described as **signe du crochet**.
- *MP joint movements are not painful.* This sign differentiates suppurating tenosynovitis from deep palmar abscess.
- When there is infection of ulnar bursa, the maximum tender spot is in between the two palmar creases. This sign is described as 'Kanavel's sign'. Similarly, there is tenderness over lateral side, over the flexor pollicis longus sheath when radial bursa is involved.

Differential Diagnosis of Soft Tissue Swelling in the Hand

When a patient presents with swelling in the hand, compare it with the other hand. If both are symmetrically swollen, it could be a medical problem such as hypothyroidism (carpal tunnel,

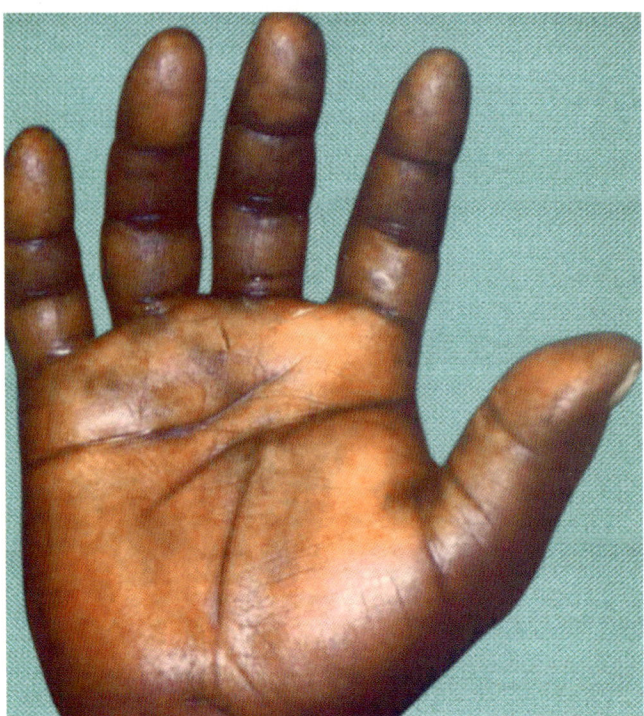

Fig. 12.9: Suppurating tenosynovitis

etc.), general anasarca from nephrotic syndrome, etc. The discussion that follows below is related to localized swelling in the hand and fingers of surgical interest.

- Lipoma (universal tumour), even though not common in the palm, can still present as a tense swelling without slip sign because it will be deeper to palmar aponeurosis (subfascial).

Some important swellings are discussed below.

1. *Implantation dermoid cyst*: This is common in women, tailors, agriculturists who sustain repeated minor sharp injuries. Following a sharp injury, a few epidermal cells get implanted into the subcutaneous plane. There, they develop into an implantation dermoid cyst. Hence, it is typically found in the fingers, palm and sole of the foot. As the cyst develops in the areas where the skin is thick and keratinised, it feels firm to hard in consistency. From the clinical point, the swelling feels firm but Paget's test may be positive. It is treated by excision (Figs 12.10 and 12.11).

Clinical Wisdom

Do not consider sebaceous cyst as a differential diagnosis for a swelling in the palm and hand because there are no sebaceous glands in these locations. *Refer* to page 71, for details on dermoid cyst.

2. *Ganglion*: It is a tense, cystic swelling and occurs due to myxomatous degeneration of the synovial sheath lining the joint or tendon sheath. They are common around joints because of abundant fibrous tissue. They contain gelatinous fluid. **The dorsum of the hand is the common site, at the scapholunate articulation.** It may also be seen in the flexor aspect of fingers and dorsal or lateral aspect of the foot. Majority of patients are between 20 and 40 years. A round to oval swelling in the dorsum of the hand, with smooth surface and round borders. Skin over

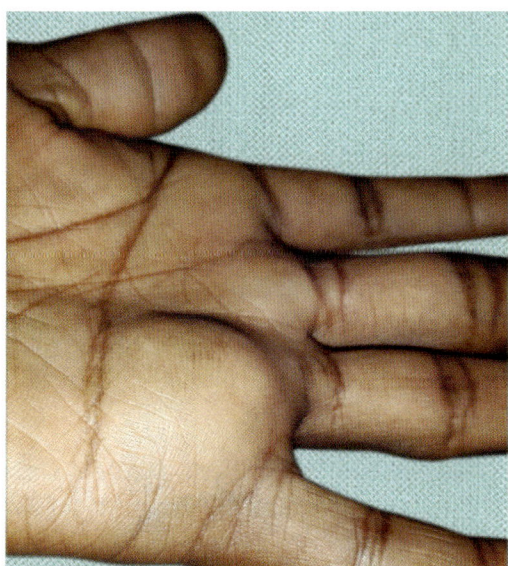

Fig. 12.10: Implantation dermoid cyst of 2 years duration following a rose thorn prick

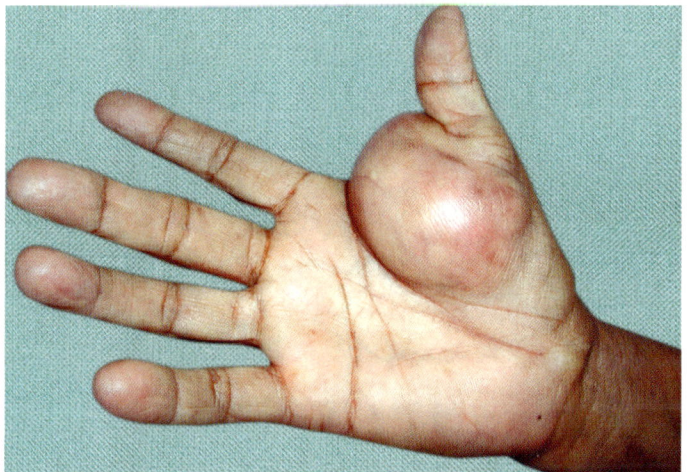

Fig. 12.11: Infected implantation dermoid cyst in the palmar aspect of thenar space since 4 months. It was slow-growing. Neural tumours, lipoma and chronic abscess are differential diagnosis.

the swelling is normal. The swelling is tensely cystic and fluctuant. Transillumination is negative. It is mobile in the transverse direction. When the tendons are put into contraction, the mobility of the swelling gets restricted. Ganglion is not connected with the joint space. Sometimes, it gives an impression of becoming small due to slipping away between bones. (Do not get confused this sign with sign of emptying.) Asymptomatic ganglion is *better left alone.* Aspiration of the ganglion and injection of sclerosants may reduce the size of ganglion. Sometimes, rupture of the cyst due to trauma may result in permanent cure. *Surgical excision* can be done. However, recurrence rate is high (Fig. 12.12).

Clinical Wisdom

Small tense ganglion may feel hard suggesting it may be a sesamoid bone. However, bony swelling is immobile.

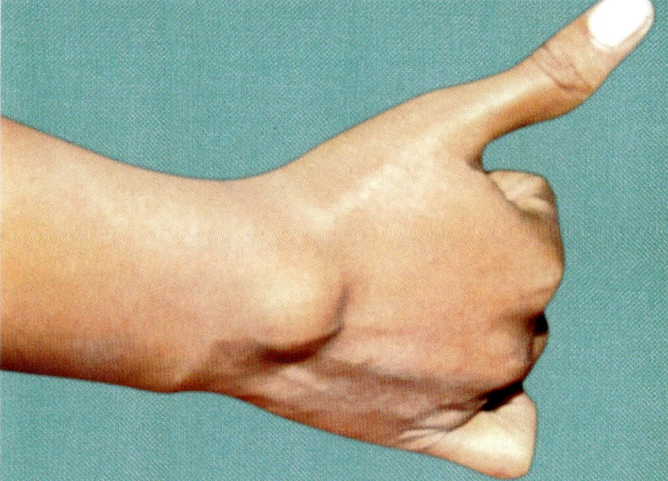

Fig. 12.12: Ganglion dorsum of the hand. Scapho-lunate articulation is the common site

3. *Chronic tuberculous tenosynovitis/compound palmar ganglion*: Tuberculous tenosynovitis is a common cause in India. As a result of tuberculous tenosynovitis, typical caseous material collects within the flexor tendon sheaths. The tendons get matted, a swelling develops in the palm and another swelling develops in lower aspect of forearm. The thickening of synovial membrane, fibrin particles in the fluid and melon seeds (sometimes they can be felt as moving small bodies) are characteristics of this condition. Patients can present with typical symptoms and signs of carpal tunnel syndrome. At operation, multiple large rice bodies can be seen along the flexor tendons with adherent synovitis involving the index finger. Widespread surgical debridement with excision of involved synovium is the treatment of choice. This is followed by anti-tuberculous treatment.

Rheumatoid arthritis with involvement of multiple joints causing thickening of synovial membrane is a common cause in Western countries.

Clinical features

- Majority of patients are below 40 years of age. Concavity of the palm is obliterated.
- It is a soft, cystic, fluctuant, transillumination—negative swelling situated above and below the flexor retinaculum, classically described as hourglass swelling. Cross-fluctuation test between these two swellings is positive, which is diagnostic of compound palmar ganglion. Restricted mobility of the fingers is due to matting of the tendons.
- Wasting of the small muscles of the hand.
- Paraesthesia due to compression on median nerve.

4. *Traumatic AV fistula*: It is more common in this location than a congenital AV fistula (Figs 12.13 to 12.18).

- It is a soft, pulsatile swelling and feels cystic. Sign of compressibility is present (Clinical Box 12.1).
- A continuous bruit/murmur is characteristic.
- *Nicoladoni's sign or Branham's sign*: On compressing the feeding artery, the venous return to the heart diminishes, resulting in fall in pulse rate and pulse pressure. On compressing feeding artery, pulsation or continuous murmur may also disappear and swelling will diminish in size.

Clinical Box 12.1

Signs of congenital AV fistula

Pulsatile swelling
Sign of compressibility
Arterialisation of veins
Thrill or bruit—machinery murmur
Ischaemic ulcers distally (in congenital AV fistula)
Overgrowth of limb
Nicoladoni sign

You can remember as
PULSATION

■ Clinical Case Capsule

A 24-year-old man had a fall with bruising on the left palm 4 months back. After about 2 months, he noticed mild discomfort and pain in the palm. He also noticed a swelling about the same time. It has attained the present size in 4 months' duration. Initially the clinician who saw the case diagnosed it as implantation dermoid cyst because it developed after a fall on the palm but there was no sharp injury. Clinical examination revealed sign of emptying/compressibility. The diagnosis changed to vascular swelling, a low output traumatic AV fistula following trauma.

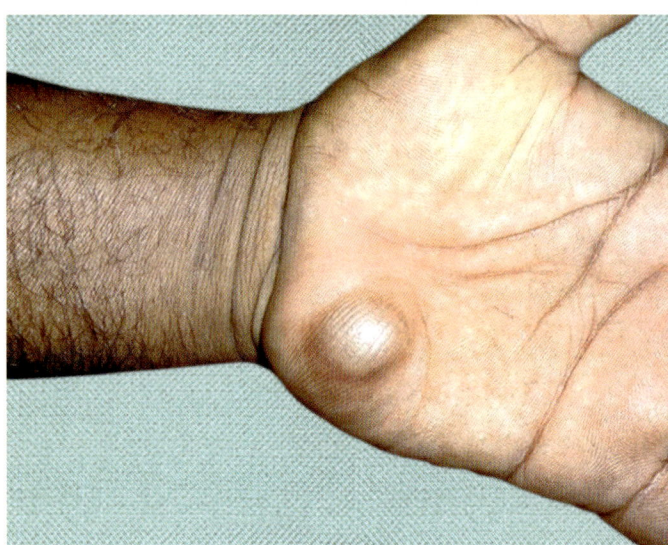

Fig. 12.13: Traumatic AV fistula

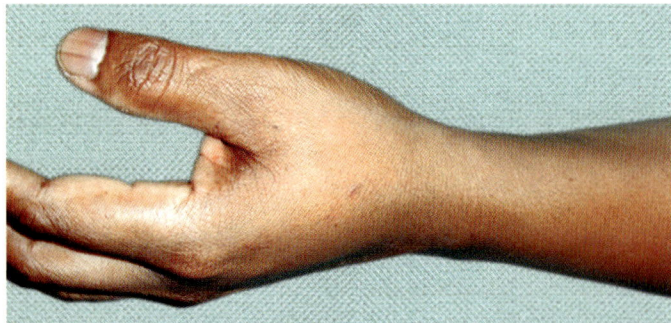

Fig. 12.14: Another case of a swelling in the dorsum of the hand following trauma

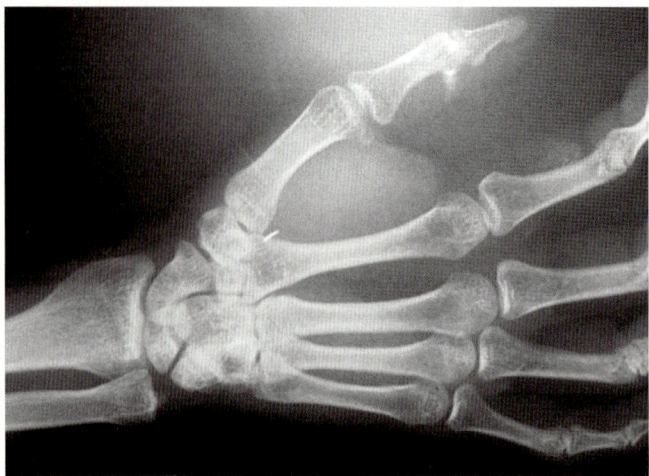

Fig. 12.15: X-ray hand showing soft tissue swelling

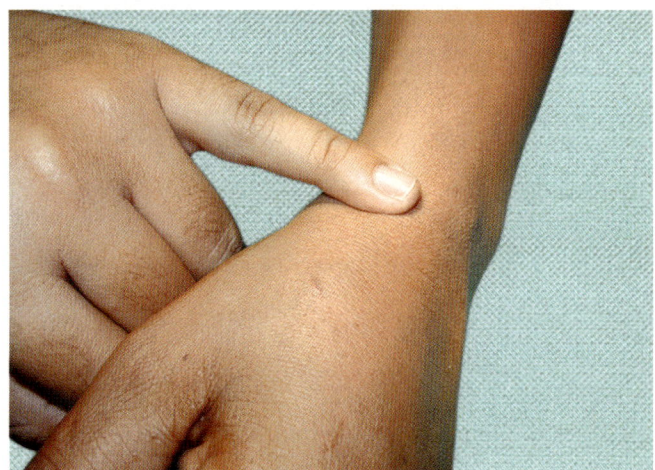

Fig. 12.16: Proximal compression test to check any reduction in the size of the swelling

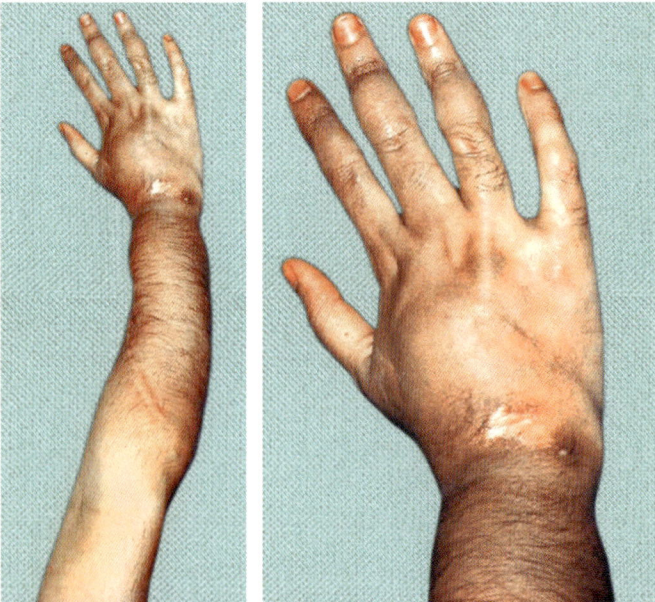

Figs 12.17 and 12.18: Local gigantism and prominent veins due to AV fistula

- Secondary varicose veins occur when blood at high pressure from an artery flows into the veins. Consequently, the veins get dilated, tortuous and elongated. This is called arterialisation of the vein.
- If the AV fistula is big, a high output cardiac failure can occur.
- The affected part is swollen—local gigantism. Thus, overgrowth of the limb or toe can occur.
- Can be remembered as PULSATION (Clinical Box 12.1).

5. Glomus tumour

- This is also called glomangioma or angioneuromyoma. Glomus is a specialised organ with abundant arteriovenous anastomosis surrounded by large clear cells (glomus cells) and medullated and non-medullated nerve fibres in between the cells (Clinical Box 12.2).

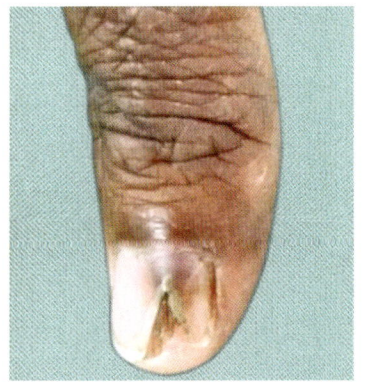 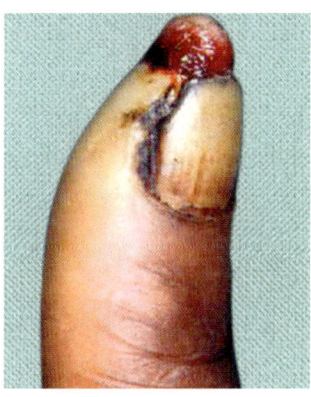

Fig.12.19: Glomus tumour (*Courtesy:* Dr Satish Pai, Head, Dept of Dermatology, KMC, Manipal)

Fig. 12.20: Pyogenic granuloma

Clinical Box 12.2 🗝️

Glomus tumour

- Rare and benign tumour
- The most painful tumour
- The smallest benign tumour, does not turn malignant
- Nail bed is the commonest site (Fig. 12.19)
- Histologically, it is an *angioneuromyoma*
- It is radioresistant
- Excision gives permanent cure
- Function of glomus is concerned with heat regulation

- *Typical site*: Under the nail beds of hands and feet.
- It is purple red in colour, usually single and *the size does not exceed 1 cm in diameter*.
- Glomus tumour is usually seen in the 5th decade.
- Excruciating pain either at rest or on movement of the finger on pressure is pathognomonic feature of this tumour. Pain is due to compression of the nerve fibres by dilated glomus vessels.
- The tumour is compressible.
- *BP cuff test*: When blood pressure cuff is applied and *inflated over systolic pressure*, pain will be decreased to great extent.

6. Pyogenic granuloma: Chronic recurrent infections of the hidden wound of the nail bed produces protuberant granulation tissue. It is also called proud flesh. It presents as red, fleshy, soft and fluctuant swelling. Patients can present with bleeding and swelling. Histologically, it is an example for haemangioma (Fig.12.20).

7. Bony swellings such as exostosis and sesamoid bone are other 2 diagnosis to be kept in mind: Both these swellings are bony hard. In the hand—two sesamoid bones are located in distal portions of the first metacarpal bone (within the tendons of adductor pollicis and flexor pollicis brevis). The pisiform bone of the wrist is a sesamoid bone as well (within the tendon of flexor carpi ulnaris). It is not uncommon to find exostosis of carpal bones and confusing it for ganglion.

Differential Diagnosis of Hand Deformity

1. Hand in leprosy: *Hands*: Involvement of ulnar nerve at the elbow and median nerve at wrist gives rise to 'claw hand' with extension at MP joint and flexion at IP joint. Wasting of hypothenar eminence is quite common when ulnar nerve is involved. Wasting of thenar muscles results in flattening of thenar eminence. In the foot, posterior tibial nerve is involved at the ankle leading to clawing of the toes. Foot drop occurs when lateral popliteal nerve below the knee joint is involved (Figs 12.21 to 12.24).

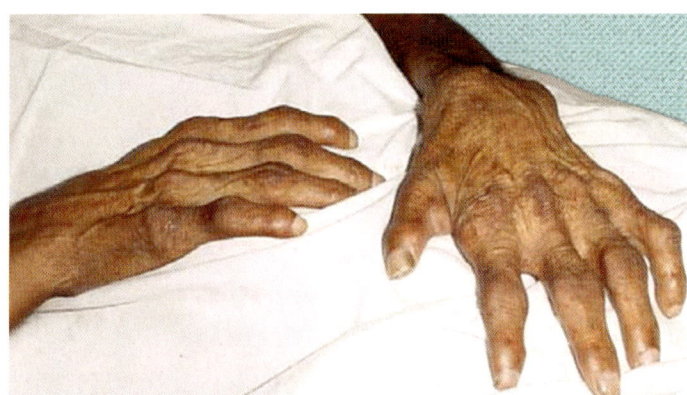

Fig. 12.21: Claw hand in leprosy—dorsal view

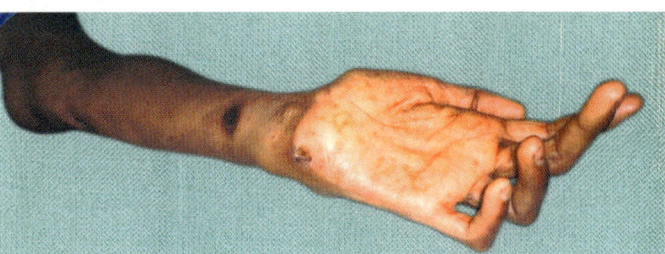

Fig. 12.22: Claw hand in leprosy

2. Hand in rheumatoid arthritis (Fig. 12.25): Initially pain and swelling are characteristic due to inflammation. Eventually, swan-neck deformity occurs. It is a deformed position of the *finger*, in which distal interphalangeal joint is permanently bent while proximal interphalangeal joint is extended. Other causes of swan-neck deformity are: *Congenital*, or *Ehlers-Danlos syndrome*.

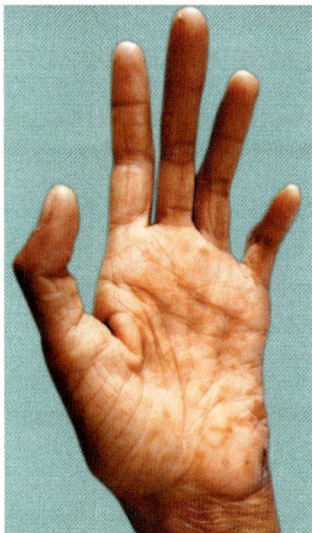

Fig. 12.23: Palmar view of hand in leprosy. Gross muscle wasting is obvious

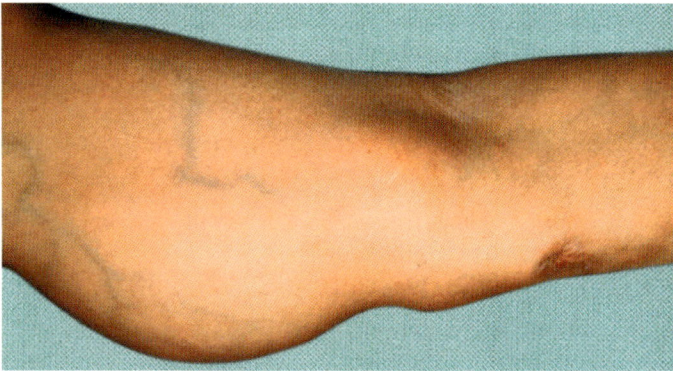

Fig. 12.24: Cold abscess of ulnar nerve at the elbow region. Swelling was soft to firm in consistency. Soft tissue sarcoma can also be considered as differential diagnosis

When it affects only thumb, the deformity has been described as duck-bill deformity.

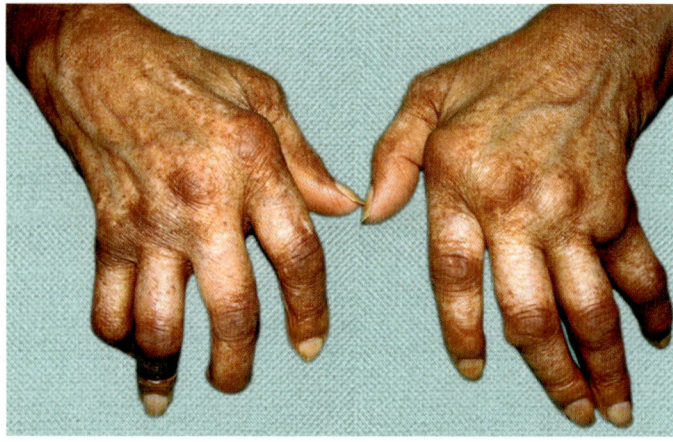

Fig. 12.25: Hand in rheumatoid arthritis

2. *Vascular malformations*: Haemangioma—low output can occur from birth in the limbs and hand also resulting in enlargement of the limb. The disease is often present since birth. Basically,

it is a hamartoma. Slow enlargement of the organ or the part is a feature. Patients present late because it does not produce any pain. Often patients come for cosmetic complaints. Rarely a trivial injury will result in bleeding. They are investigated by Doppler to assess the feeding vessels. MRI is another useful investigation. High output malformations are treated by embolisation followed by surgery. Low output malformations can be treated by surgery.

Malignant Skin Tumours in the Hand

1. *Epithelioma*: Epithelioma can occur in the hand. Though not a common site, if the part is irritated, example by coal tar, it can occur. Typically as seen in the picture, it is a cauliflower like growth with everted edges, indurated base and with restricted mobility. As it advances, it fixes to the tendons and then bones. Wide excision followed by skin grafting is ideal in early cases. When it involves deeper structures as in neglected cases, amputation may be necessary (Fig. 12.26).

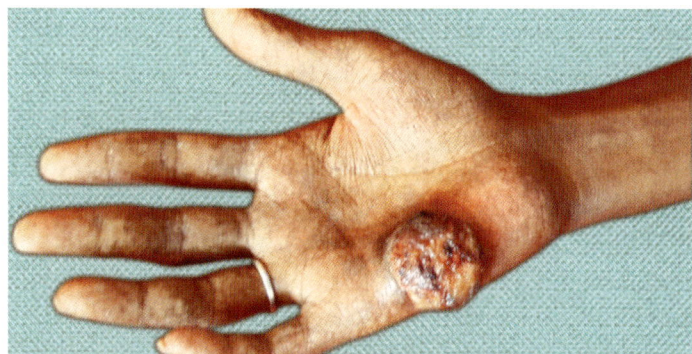

Fig. 12.26: Epithelioma. Watch the hand carefully. You can see skin freckles. It was a case of xeroderma pigmentosa (*refer* to page 187 also)

2. *Malignant melanoma of the nail unit or digit*: Acral lentigenous variety can occur in the nail unit under the nail and can involve the adjacent nail fold. This sign has been described as Hutchinson's sign. It is more common in sole than palm and fingers. More details are given in chapter on skin tumours (*refer* to page 193, Chapter 13).

Contractures in the Hand: Differential Diagnosis

1. *Burns*: A contracture scar is a permanent tightening of skin that may affect the underlying muscles and tendons limiting mobility. In most of the cases, there is a possible damage or degeneration of the nerves. Contractures develop when normal elastic connective tissues are replaced with inelastic fibrous tissue. This makes the tissues resistant to stretching and prevents normal movement of the affected area.

Physical therapy, pressure and exercise in many cases can aid in controlling contracture in burn scars. If these treatments do not control the effects of contracture scars, surgery may be required. A skin graft or a flap procedure may be performed. Additionally, a new technique such as Z-plasty or tissue expansion may be recommended.

2. *Volkmann's ischaemic contracture*: The contracture is mainly in the flexor group of muscles of the forearm consequent to ischaemia. The causes can be too tight a plaster following supracondylar fracture of the humerus (mainly in children), direct compression of the brachial artery by the displaced bone or due to severe vasospasm. Fingers are flexed. They can be partially extended when wrist is flexed. It is important to diagnose this condition in early cases by noting pallor, pulselessness, paralysis and puffiness (oedema).

3. *Dupuytren's contracture* (Clinical Box 12.3): The tissues under the skin on the palm of the hand thicken and shorten so that the tendons connected to the fingers cannot move freely. The palmar aponeurosis becomes hyperplastic and undergoes contracture. Incidence increases after the age of 40; at this age men affected more often than women. A few conditions associated with Dupuytren's contracture are given in Clinical Box 12.4.

Clinical Box 12.3

You can remember as PALMAR
- **P**almar aponeurosis is fibrotic and contracted
- **A**dherent to skin (palmar aponeurosis)
- **L**ittle finger gets affected later
- **M**en are affected 10 times more than women.
- **A**ssociated lesions or conditions—cirrhosis of liver, Riedel's thyroiditis, minor recurrent trauma to tendons
- **R**ing finger is commony affected.

Clinical Box 12.4

Some conditions or factors associated with Dupuytren's contracture are as follows. You can remember as **DREAM:**
- **D**iabetes
- **R**epeated trauma
- **E**pilepsy
- **A**lcoholism
- **M**embers in the family (family history).

---

4. *Congenital contracture of the little finger*: It is usually bilateral and develops during childhood. Soft tissues are involved in this condition, not palmar aponeurosis.

CLINICAL DISCUSSION

What are Heberden's nodes?
- They are seen in osteoarthritis. Tiny hard knob-like swelling in relation to terminal interphalangeal joints of 4 digits. Thumb is not involved. Interestingly thumb is not involved in Raynaud's disease, and Dupuytren's contracture also. Women at menopause are commonly affected.

What is pannus?
- Hypertrophy of the synovial membrane of the joints in cases of rheumatoid arthritis.

What are the changes in the hand in rheumatoid arthritis?
- Proximal interphalangeal joint space of index finger is most commonly affected with fusiform swelling. It is firm to hard, tender and is called rheumatoid nodule. Ulnar deviation of the fingers occurs due to pull by gravity and push of the extensor tendons by the synovium. The next stage is stage of deformities (swan-neck) due to atrophy of the small muscles of the hand.

What are Beau's lines?
- They are transverse furrows seen in nails in general debilitating illness.

EXAMINATION OF FOOT

Common lesions in the foot which general surgeon encounters can be classified into benign and malignant lesions. Common benign lesions are:

1. *Ingrowing toenail (onychocryptosis)*
- It is also described as embedded. Exact aetiology is not clear. However, a few patients have family history of this condition. Trimming the nail too much may result in ingrowing toenail.
- As the nail grows inside, some degree of infection sets in, resulting in development of granulation tissue which starts pouting. The condition is painful, disturbing and unsightly.

2. *Mycetoma pedis*
- It refers to chronic granulomatous lesions of the foot involving skin and subcutaneous tissues. The disease not only involves skin and subcutaneous tissue but also the deeper structures such as bones resulting in osteomyelitis (Figs 12.27 and 12.28).
- **Gross thickening of subcutaneous tissue results in convexity of the instep of the foot** that is characteristic of this condition. Chronic suppuration, **multiple sinuses,** and sulphur granules in the discharge are characteristics of mycetoma pedis.
- Barefoot walking, which results in repeated minor trauma, implants the organisms within subcutaneous tissue. It starts as a **pale, painless single nodule**. Later multiple nodules develop and rupture resulting in multiple sinuses.

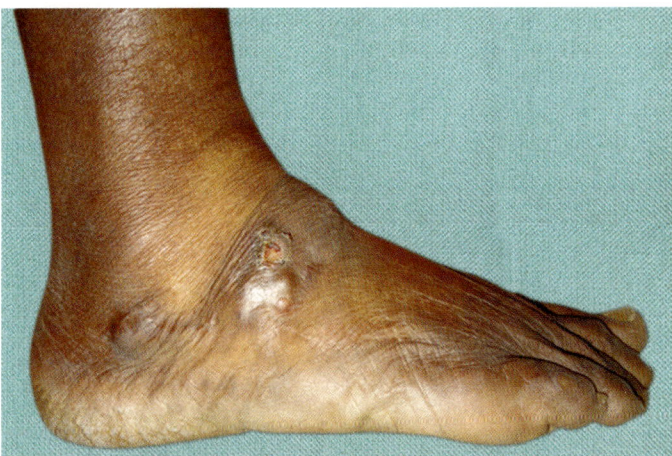

Fig. 12.27: Initial stage of mycetoma pedis presenting as multiple subcutaneous nodules

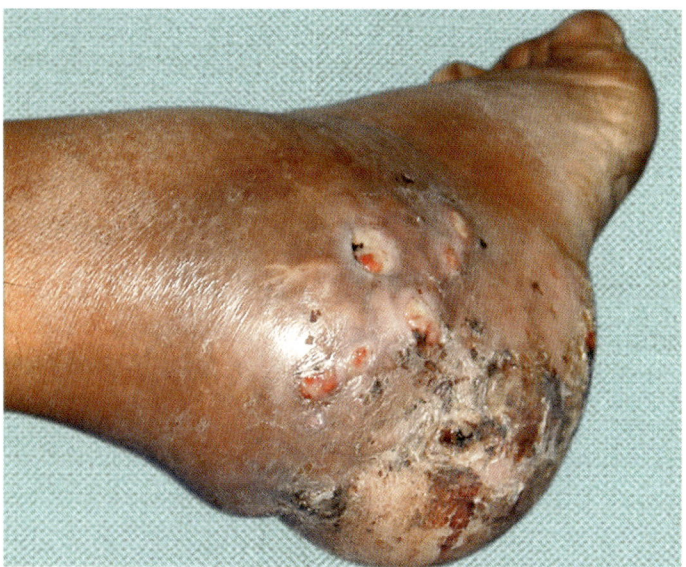

Fig. 12.28: Madura foot with multiple sinuses

Types

1. *Bacterial mycetoma*: It is due to *Nocardia madurae* or due to *Actinomyces*. These organisms are normally present in the soil.

2. *Fungal mycetoma*: It is caused by *Madurella mycetoma*, etc.

Diagnosis: Sulphur granules in the discharge, X-ray of the foot.

Treatment

- Broad-spectrum antibiotics to treat secondary infection along with **dapsone 100 mg, twice daily are the choice.** Treatment may have to be continued for 1–2 years.
- Fungal mycetoma may not respond to antibiotics.
- Amputation may be necessary, in refractory cases, to get rid of a deformed, diseased limb.

3. *Diabetic ulcer foot*: Detailed evaluation of ulcer leg/foot has been given in the chapter on leg ulcers. Diabetic foot ulcers are common. Uncontrolled diabetes, trivial injuries including nail paring, diminished blood supply due to atherosclerosis, loss of sensation (neuropathy), and infection are the major contributing factors. Loss of sensation typically contributes to the development of ulcers in the sole of the foot. Sensations and pulsations must be checked in all cases of ulcer leg (Figs 12.29 to 12.31).

4. *Feet in leprosy*: Leprosy is one of the causes of total anaesthetic feet. It is still common in India. Loss of sensation is the hallmark of the disease. Thickening

of the lateral popliteal nerve can be appreciated in the leg against fibula. Trophic ulcers are common. Auto-amputation occurs slowly (Fig. 12.32).

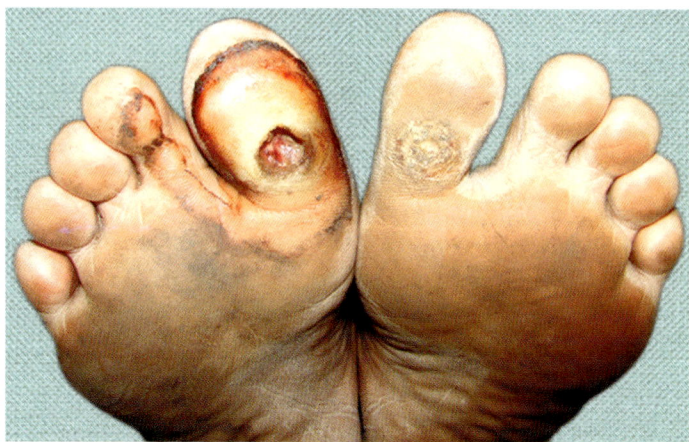

Fig. 12.29: Trophic ulcers of foot due to diabetes mellitus

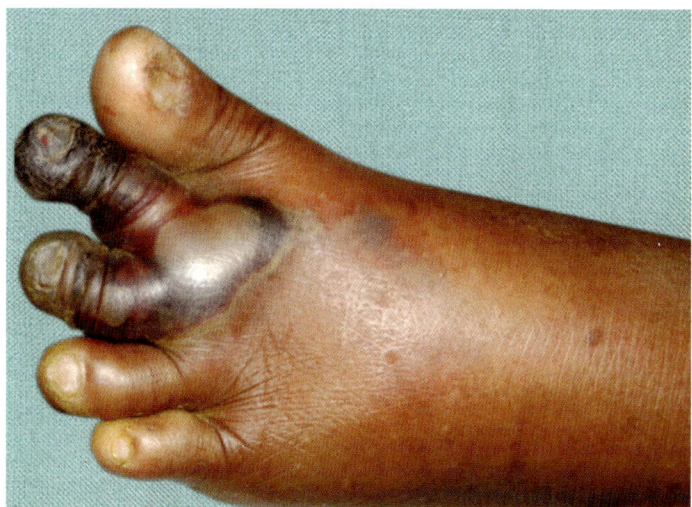

Fig. 12.30: Wet gangrene due to diabetes mellitus

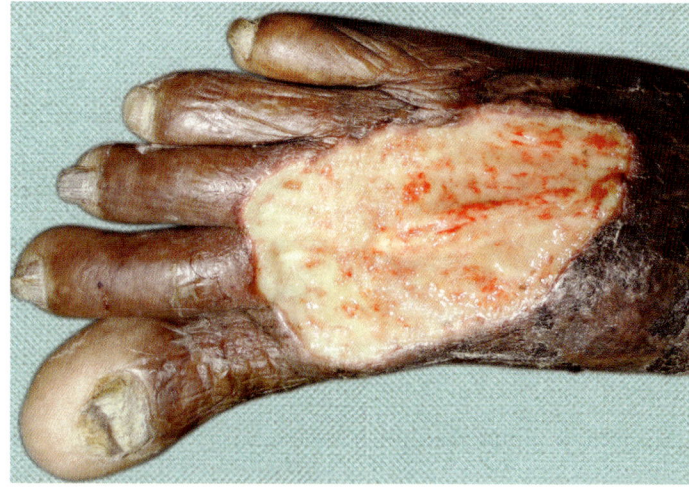

Fig. 12.31: Diabetic ulcer due to atherosclerosis and spreading infection. Started after trauma

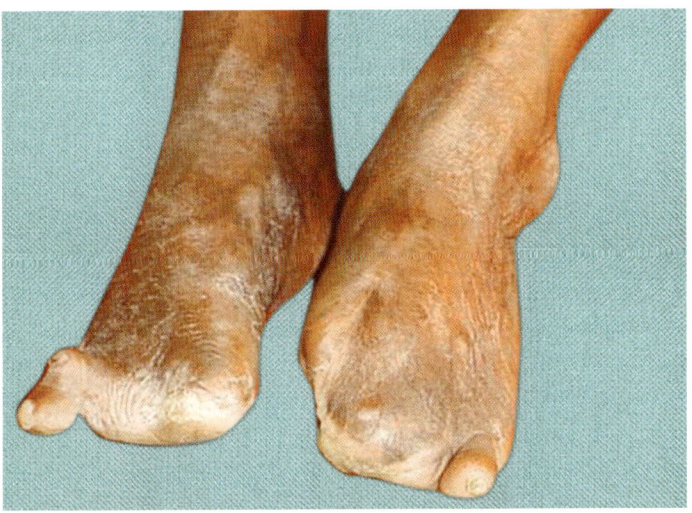

Fig. 12.32: Autoamputation of toes in leprosy

MALIGNANT TUMOURS IN THE FOOT

1. *Moles and malignant melanoma*: Sole of the foot is one of the common sites of malignant melanoma. Any mole which is enlarging or ulcerating should arouse suspicion of malignant melanoma (Figs 12.33 and 12.34). Details are given in the chapter on skin tumours. Typically, the lesion is ulcerated mole with irregular margin and edge. Induration is much less than epitheliomas. Satellite nodule is a nodule within 5 cm of the primary lesion. In-transit deposits occur due to spread along the lymphatics. When pigment is not found such melanomas are called as amelanotic melanoma (Fig. 12.35). Regional lymphadenopathy is common including popliteal and inguinal lymph nodes. Superficial spreading, nodular, acral lentiginous and amelanotic melanoma are the various types which can occur in the foot. When melanoma starts under nail, it slowly involves the nail fold. It has been described as **Hutchinson's sign** (Fig. 12.36).

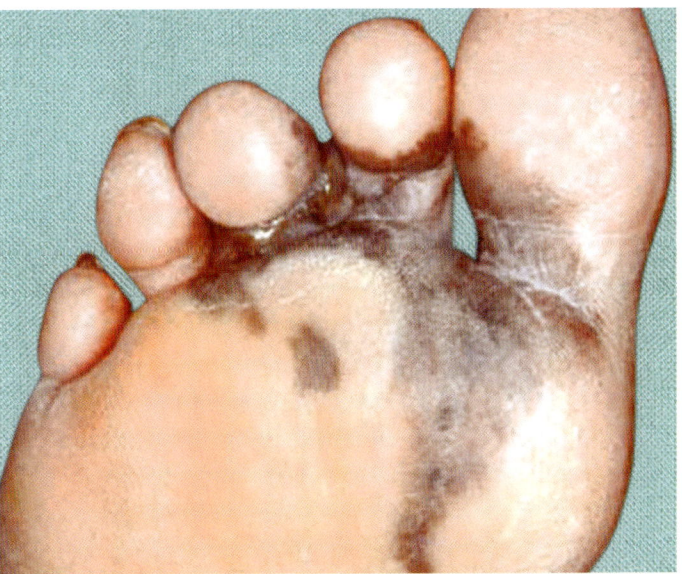

Fig. 12.34: Superficial spreading variety of malignant melanoma

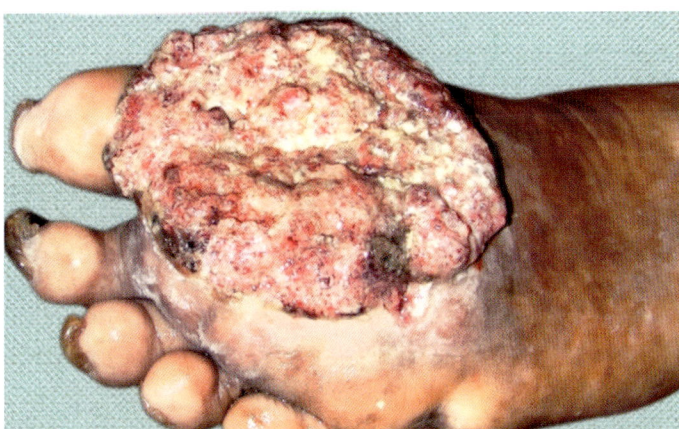

Fig. 12.35: Tumour resembles epithelioma. Biopsy proved to be amelanotic melanoma

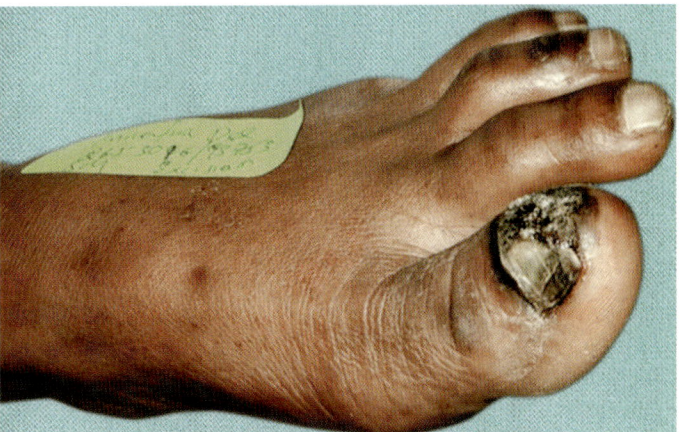

Fig. 12.36: Hutchinson's sign

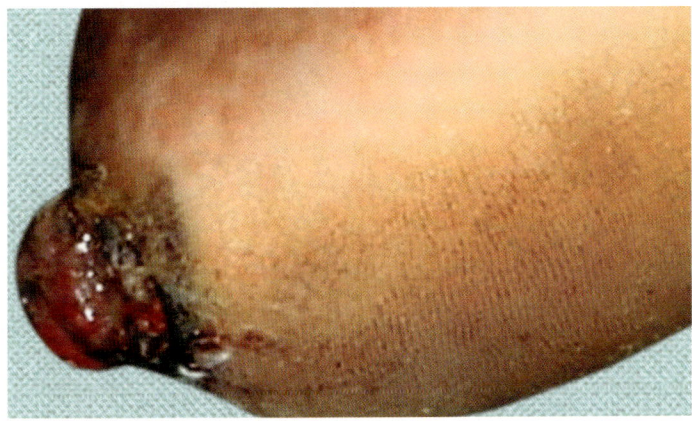

Fig. 12.33: Melanoma in the sole region—growing since 3 months

2. *Epithelioma*: Foot is one of the sites of epithelioma—squamous cell carcinoma. Repeated trauma to the barefoot has been blamed as one of the causative factors. Typically, it is a cauliflower-like growth factor with everted edges and induration. It is very friable. Neglected cases involve deeper structures such as tendons, muscles and bone. Wide excision in early cases and amputation in late cases is the treatment (Fig. 12.37).

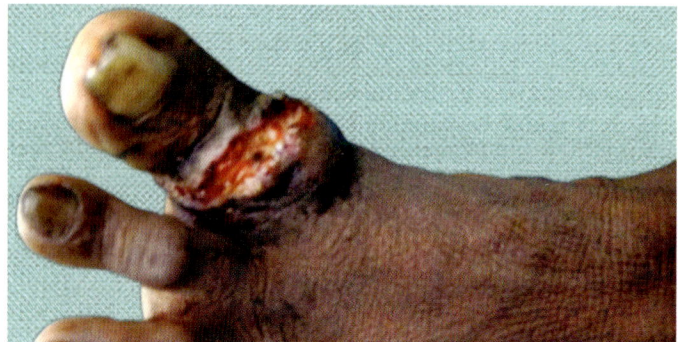

Fig. 12.37: A small nonhealing ulcer at the metatarsophalangeal joint space. The patient was a smoker and it was initially diagnosed as TAO. However, careful examination revealed everted edges. Biopsy confirmed squamous cell carcinoma

3. *Elephantiasis*: Filariasis is the cause for elephantiasis. Details are given in the chapter on lymphoedema. Initial swelling is due to oedema. It is pitting in nature. Repeated attacks of lymphangitis and lymphadenitis result in fibrosis. Slowly oedema becomes nonpitting in nature. As the disease advances, the skin becomes thick, wrinkled and develops folds resembling elephant leg (Fig. 12.38).

4. *Soft tissue sarcomas*: Details have been given in the chapter on examination of swelling. Just to remind, foot is not a common site of sarcomas but a few can still occur here. A basic rule is that any swelling growing in and around joint should be considered as synovial sarcoma unless proven otherwise. Thus, synovial sarcoma, angiosarcoma, etc. can occur in the foot. Increasing size of swelling, later involvement of skin ulcerations, nodularity, and bleeding are the characteristic features (Figs 13.39 to 13.41).

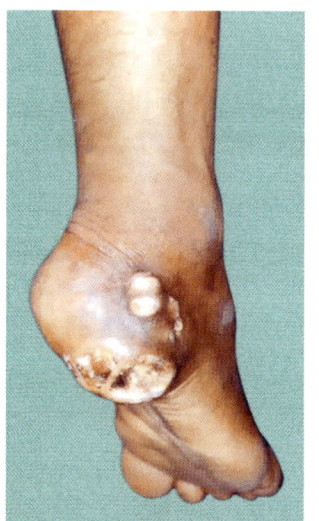 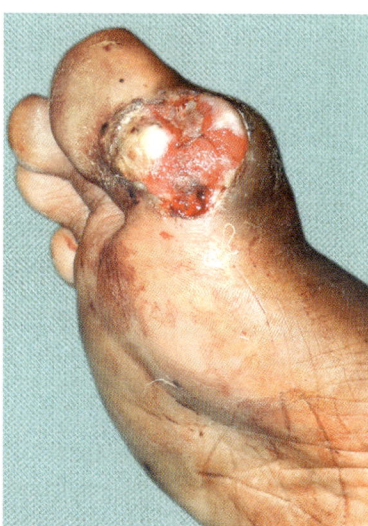

Fig. 12.39: Angiosarcoma—ankle region   **Fig. 12.40:** Synovial sarcoma—toe

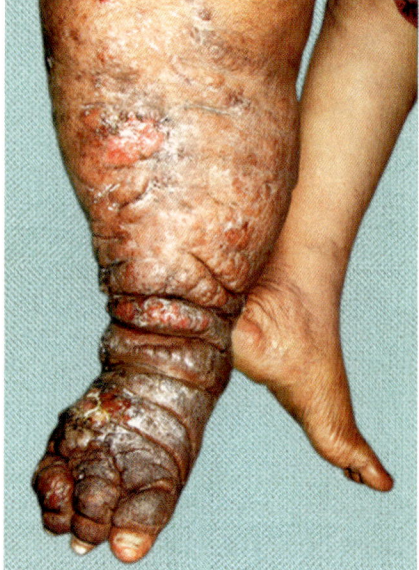

Fig. 12.38: Right lower limb elephantiasis

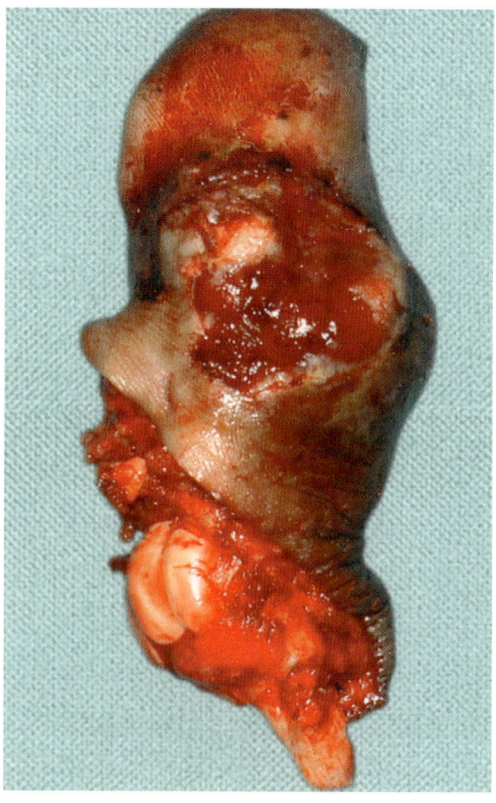

Fig. 12.41: Disarticulation of the toe

13

Examination of Skin and Skin Tumours

INTRODUCTION

Skin malignancies (basal cell carcinoma), epithelioma (squamous cell carcinoma) and malignant melanoma (malignant skin tumour arising from melanin pigment) are common cases in the university clinical examinations. No doubt, they are classified under malignant ulcers. However, a discussion of these malignancies in the chapter on ulcer dilutes the clinical examination of these malignant ulcers more so with reference to malignant melanoma. For students, it is important first to realize that given ulcer or a lesion is malignant, then only they should refer and follow this chapter for further clinical methods. Students are expected to be thorough with the chapter on ulcer by the time they read this chapter.

HISTORY OF PRESENT ILLNESS

- **Where are you from and what is your occupation?** Specially in whites, malignant melanoma is common in patients who are exposed excessively to sunburns (outdoor occupations). Those who are exposed to chemicals, such as tar or dye industries, are more susceptible for epithelioma because of chronic irritation of the skin.

- **How did it start?** Often malignant melanoma in the leg, more so on the sole starts as an ulcer or an itchy lesion in a pre-existing naevus. **Did you have any mole?** Patient may say that he started scratching or itching over the mole and ulcer developed. **Is there any trauma?** Trivial trauma might have brought the attention of the patient to the lesion (Figs 13.1 and 13.2).

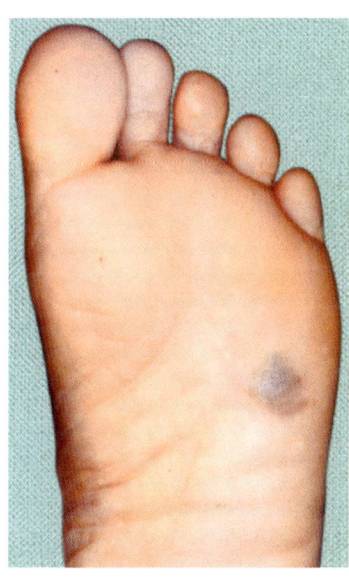

Fig. 13.1: Acral lentiginous variety with early changes—never incise or cauterise such melanomas

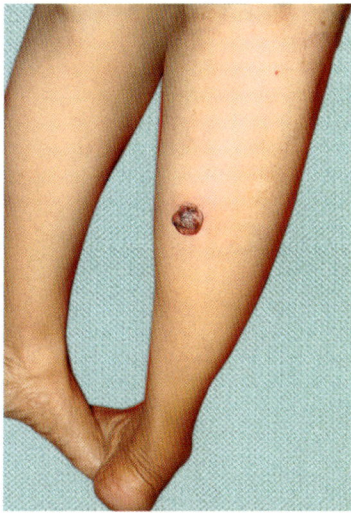

Fig. 13.2: Only complaint of this 28-year-old lady was increase in the size and oozing from the lesion

- **How is the progress?** Often patient may show you a lesion which has been growing so slowly that you may not believe it. Such lesions are **basal cell carcinomas (BCC) which are very slow growing** (Figs 13.3 and 13.4). Melanomas grow faster. **Is it becoming bigger, remaining the same or is it healing?** An ulcer which is becoming bigger is a spreading ulcer. A nonhealing and spreading ulcer can be malignant unless proved otherwise.

- **Do you have any pain?** Pain is not a feature of skin malignancies unless they are secondarily infected or have infiltrated sensitive structures such as bone. This is the reason why many patients come late to the hospital.

- **Did you see any blood coming out of the wound?** Malignant ulcers particularly squamous cell carcinomas are very friable and bleed easily, especially on touch.

- **Has the ulcer healed for some time?** Healing is the property of benign ulcers *but basal cell carcinoma is an exception to this rule.* Healing with scab formation and then re-ulcerating is typical of basal cell carcinoma. It reflects the slow indolent nature of the tumour (Fig. 13.5).

- **Do you have any other swelling?** Presence of swelling suggests enlargement of inguinal, iliac or cervical lymph nodes.

- **Do you have any other complaints?** Epithelioma is relatively slow growing and *distant metastasis is uncommon* but malignant melanoma can grow rapidly and spread to other organs. Thus, history taking must include symptoms suggestive of metastasis. Examples are given below.

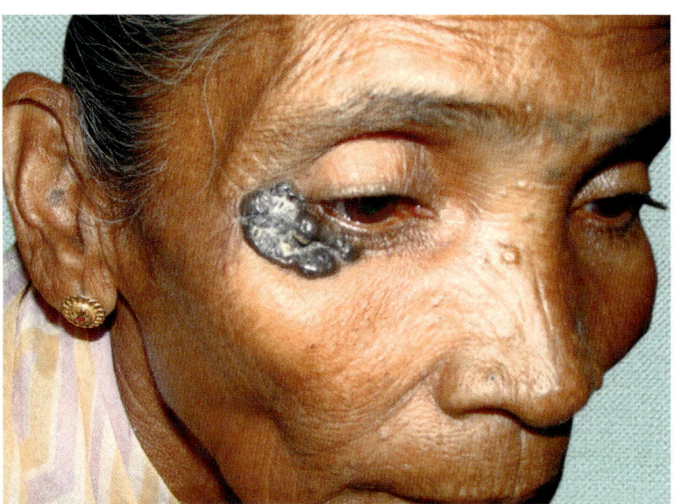

Fig. 13.3: Slow growing mole of 5 years duration

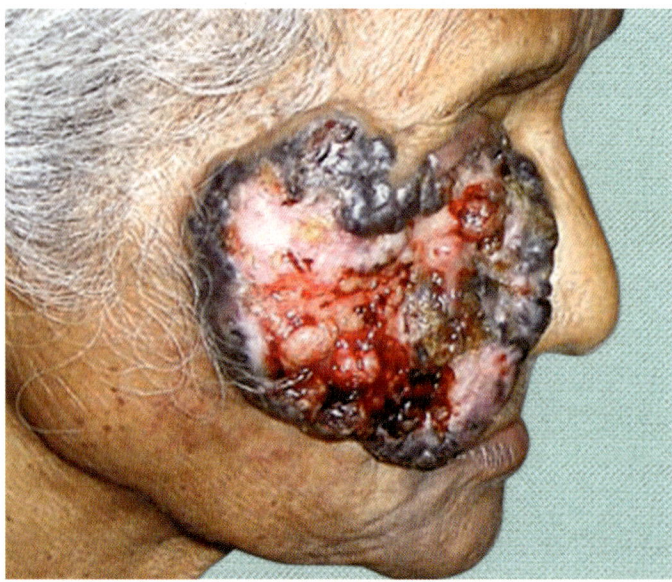

Fig. 13.4: BCC lateral view (*Courtesy*: Dr Vidyadhar Kinhal, Professor and Head, Dept of Surgery, VIMS, Bellary, Karnataka)

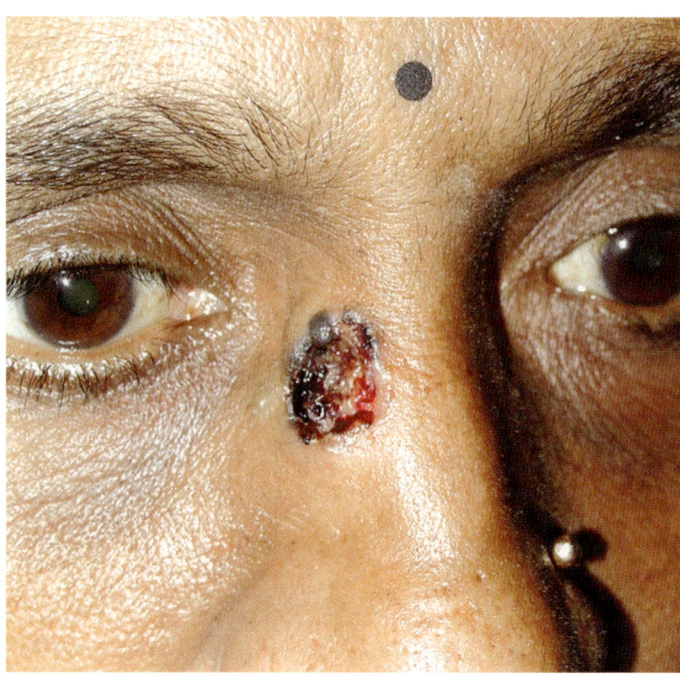

Fig. 13.5: BCC showing scabbing

Treatment History

- **Have you taken any treatment for this condition?** The patient may tell you about hospitalisation, biopsy or FNAC, etc. Try getting the reports from the patient.

- **Did you undergo surgery in the past?** (Fig. 13.6) The patient may show groin region for swelling or a few lesions in the leg but he says he has undergone surgery in the past for a pigmented lesion in the leg/sole. The diagnosis is quite obvious.

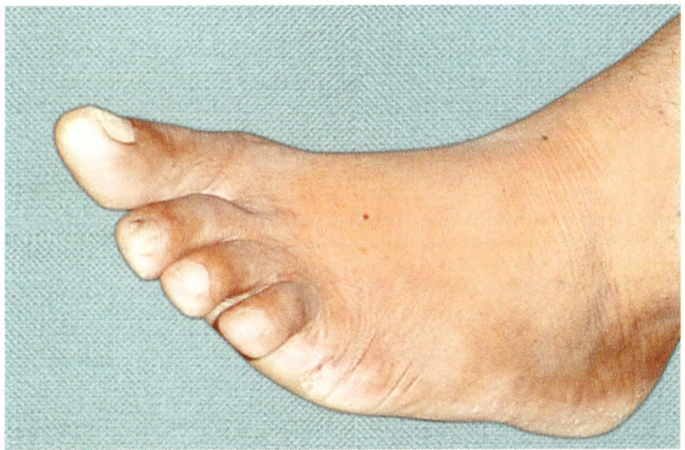

Fig. 13.6: Observe the foot. Little toe has been amputated five years back for malignant melanoma

Past History

Ask for any history suggestive of chronic ulcers or history of burns. Be aware that squamous cell carcinoma arises in a scar tissue **specially burns scar**. Such lesions are called **Marjolin's ulcer** (Fig. 13.7).

Family History

- Family history of xeroderma pigmentosum (Figs 13.8 and 13.9) and albinism (Fig. 13.10) may be present in cutaneous malignancies.

- Fitzpatrick scale types I and II: Skin of these types (almost always burn, rather than tan, in response to UV light) is considered at risk for malignant melanoma.

Ultraviolet 'B' waves produce sunburns.

Gorlin's syndrome: It is an inherited condition in which multiple basal cell carcinoma can occur. Other systems involved are nervous system, eye, bones and endocrine. Ovarian fibromas can occur.

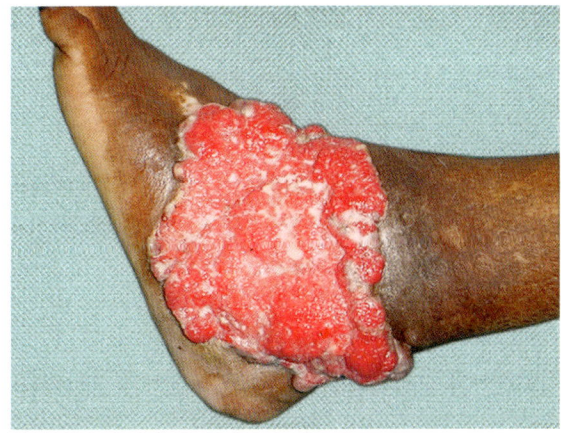

Fig. 13.7: Marjolin's ulcer—squamous cell carcinoma arising from burn scar

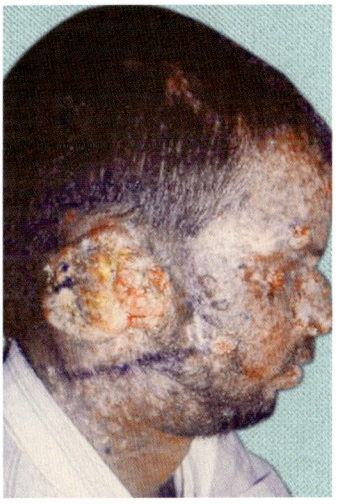 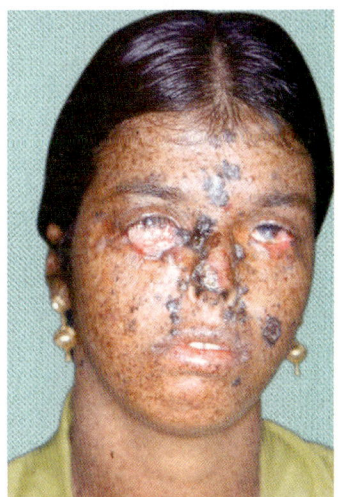

Fig. 13.8: Basal cell carcinoma involving the right ear

Fig. 13.9: Basal cell carcinoma involving skin of the nasolabial fold

A brother and sister with **xeroderma pigmentosum** developed 33 and 26 skin malignancies respectively which included basal cell carcinoma, squamous cell carcinoma and malignant melanoma, since the age of 5 till 22 years. Eventually the boy died at 22 years of age. This is the sad part of this distressing and frustrating disease. I have not seen this girl since 20 years now.

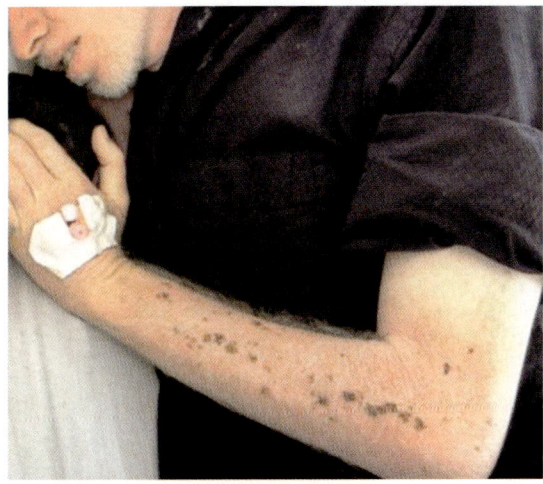

Fig. 13.10: Albinism with photophobia

PERSONAL HISTORY/OCCUPATION

- **Chimney sweep's cancer** refers to scrotal cancer found due to exposure to 'soot' in chimney sweepers. **Sir Perciviall Pott observed it first**.
- Those who work in coal tar industries also have high incidence of skin cancers.
- Chemicals responsible for cancerous changes of skin include arsenic and polycyclic aromatic hydrocarbons.
- Ionising radiation is also a known carcinogen. Gamma rays are the most penetrating carcinogenic and alpha rays are the least penetrating.

GENERAL PHYSICAL EXAMINATION

1. *Attitude*: The patient has photophobia and freckles over the body—xeroderma pigmentosum and albinism (Figs 13.10 and 13.11).
2. Glassy eye/enucleation of eye—could be enucleation done for malignant melanoma of the choroid.

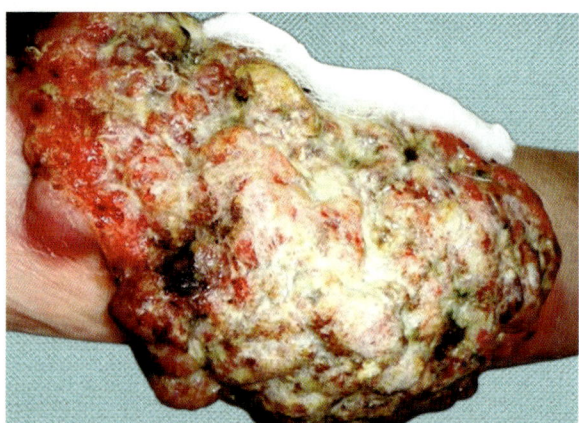

Fig. 13.11: A patient with albinism presented with large epithelioma

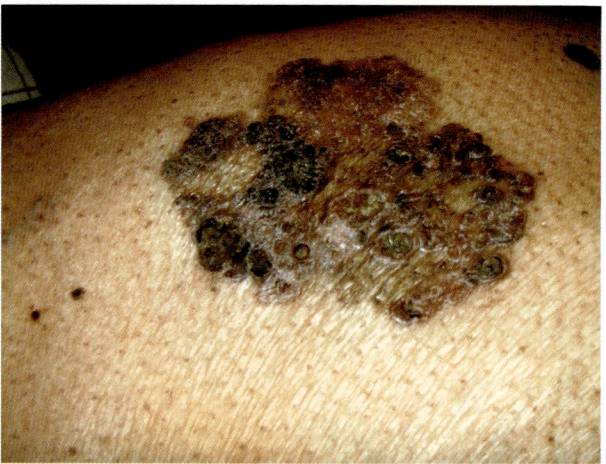

Fig. 13.12: Bowen's disease of the skin

3. Scaly erythematous multiple brownish raised patches—Bowen's disease (Fig. 13.12).
4. Missing toe/amputated foot/leg (the patient may have inguinal metastatic nodes).
5. Perianal ulcerated pigmentation.
6. Chronic anaemia: Poor wound healing

LOCAL EXAMINATION

Inspection

First decide whether the lesion is a swelling, an ulcer or an ulceroproliferative lesion (growth). Describe it in the usual manner such as location, size, shape, surface as for a swelling and floor as for an ulcer. Describe the discharge. Serous and serosanguinous discharge is common for any ulcer. Mention any pigmentation in the lesion or the surrounding area. Malignant ulcers are friable and bleeding is a feature. Then describe surrounding area for any swelling, pigmentation, scarring. Some typical examples/lesions are described below.

Clinical Wisdom

- First swelling, then ulcer:
  - Sebaceous carcinoma
  - Sweat gland carcinoma
  - Nodular malignant melanoma
- First ulcer, then swelling: Epithelioma melanoma

---

1. **Malignant melanoma in the sole of the foot** (Figs 13.13 to 13.18): A pigmented ulcer is present in the sole of the foot measuring about 5 cm in size which is irregular in shape, floor is covered with unhealthy tissue, edges are everted, and pigmented. Bloody discharge is seen in the floor of the ulcer. Surrounding area is pigmented and oedematous (if lymphatics are blocked or due to secondary infection). You may find nodules surrounding the lesion. They are called satellite nodules which are characteristics of malignant melanoma. They are due to lymphatic spread. Also many such nodules may be present in the leg which are called in-transit deposits.

- It can also present as a pigmented ulcerated nodule.

- Malignant melanoma can present as proliferative growth without pigment. They are called amelanotic melanoma.

[1]Sir Perciviall Pott observed the direct relationship of 'soot' to the scrotal cancer and he is responsible for bringing a change in the chimney sweep workers

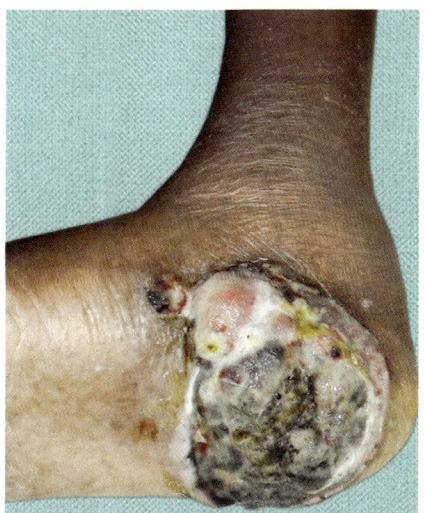

Fig. 13.13: Ulcerated melanoma (*Courtesy:* Dr MA Balakrishna, Dr Madhu BS, Dr Dinesh, Dr Ramaswamy, Govt Medical College, Mysore)

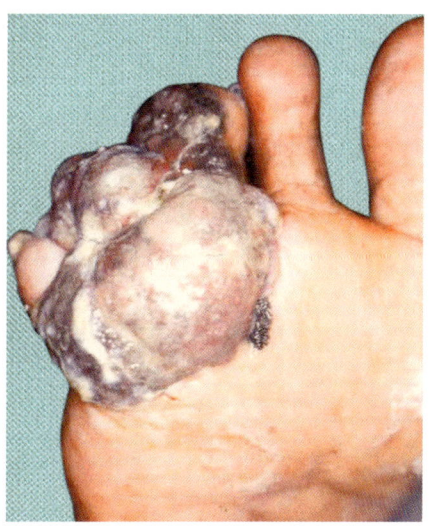

Fig. 13.14: Nodular melanoma (*Courtesy:* Dr BH Anand Rao, Professor of Surgery, KMC, Manipal)

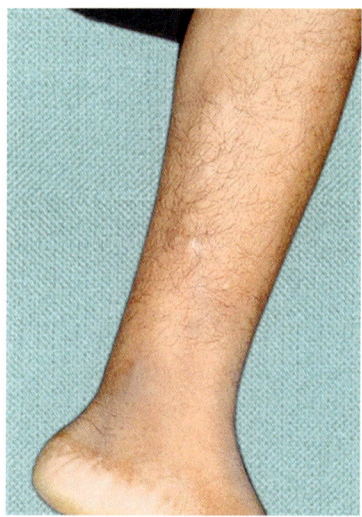

Fig. 13.15: In-transit deposits (*Courtesy:* Prof U Santhosh Pai, KMC, Manipal)

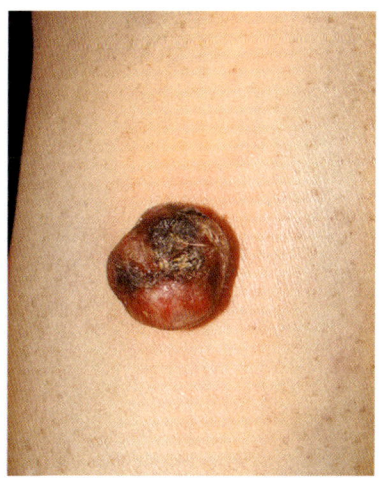

Fig. 13.16 Pigmented nodular lesion in the leg. Itching was present. Early changes of transformation of a mole. (Clinical Box 13.1)

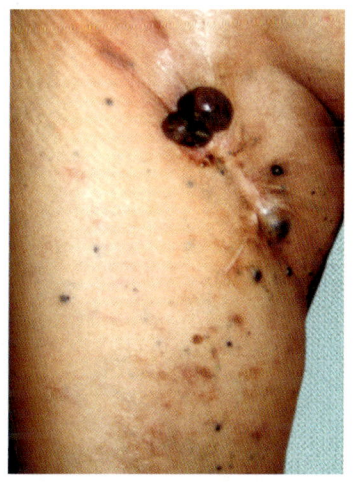

Fig. 13.17: Disseminated melanoma (*Courtesy:* Prof BS Madakatti, Head Department of Surgery, KIMS, Hubballi 2005)

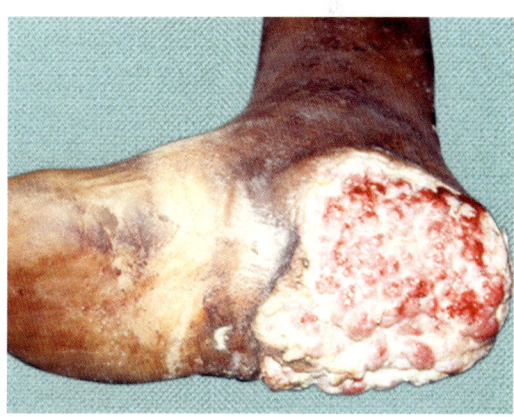

Fig. 13.18: The lesion resembles squamous cell carcinoma. Punch biopsy reported as amelanotic melanoma

---

Clinical Box 13.1 🔑

Special checklist for malignant melanoma in inspection
- Pigmentation
- Loss of normal skin marking (crease)
- Oozing
- Brown halo is due to pigment produced by the tumour which spreads into the normal skin
- Flat mole changes to nodule or plaque
- Normal impalpable mole becomes palpable.

Clinical Wisdom

Multiple circumoral moles are seen in Peutz-Jeghers syndrome. They are actually patches of lentigo and they do not turn malignant. However, hamartomatous polyps in intestines and stomach rarely can turn malignant.

2. **Typically ulceroproliferative lesions** are due to epitheliomas. They have characteristic nodular or proliferative tissue and everted edges. Blood also may be seen (Figs 13.19 to 13.23).

3. **Basal cell carcinoma** can start as ulcer nodule which can be pigmented and slow growing. Edges are typically elevated (Figs 13.24 and 13.25).

4. **Marjolin's ulcer:** Ulceroproliferative growth with everted edges, floor covered with necrotic tissue or tumour tissue, with serous or bloody discharge, and oedematous surrounding area. Scarring is present in Marjolin's ulcer. Marjolin's ulcers have good prognosis (Fig. 13.25 and Table 13.2).

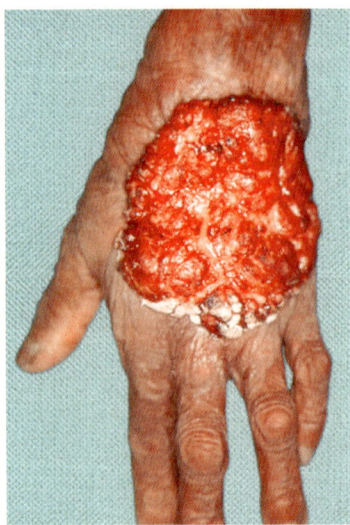

Fig. 13.19: Squamous cell carcinoma affecting dorsum of the hand—ulceroproliferative lesion

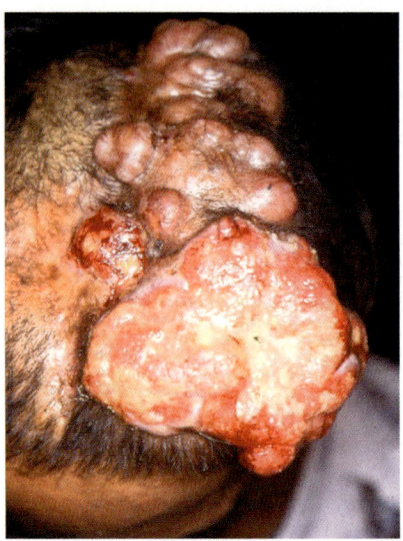

Fig. 13.22: Squamous cell carcinoma affecting scalp region—such large tumours are called as turban tumours

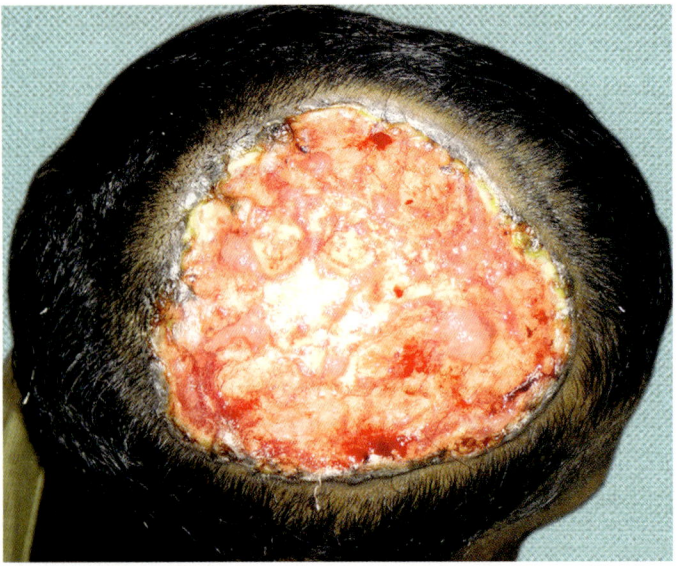

Fig. 13.20: Squamous cell carcinoma (epithelioma) of the scalp

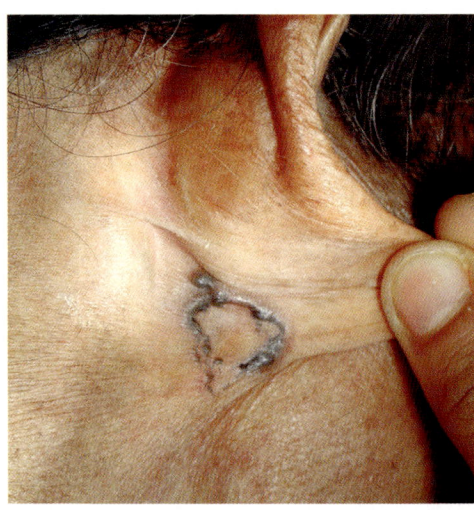

Fig. 13.23: Pigmented basal cell carcinoma—morphoeic variety

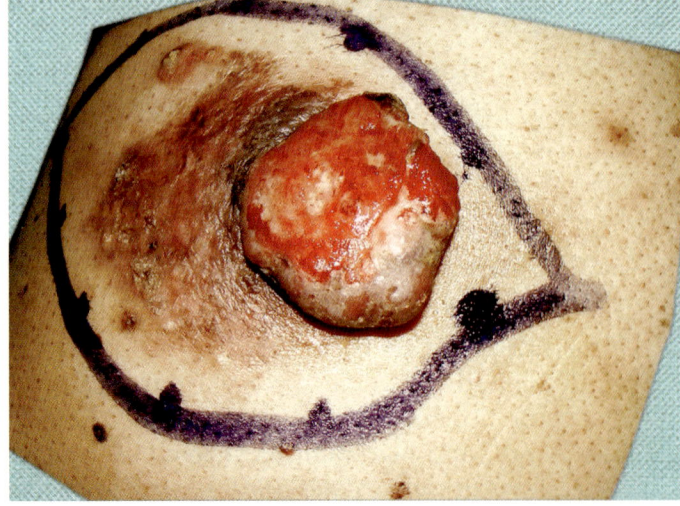

Fig. 13.21: Bowen's disease—precancerous condition of the skin giving rise to sebaceous carcinoma

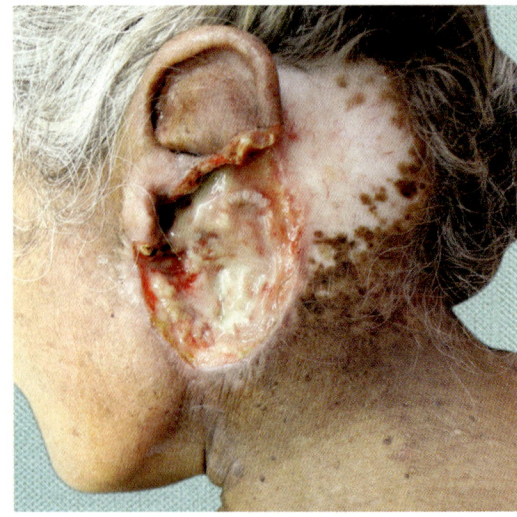

Fig. 13.24: Rodent ulcer with destruction of pinna. Poverty and the ulcer led to isolation of this 83-year-old lady

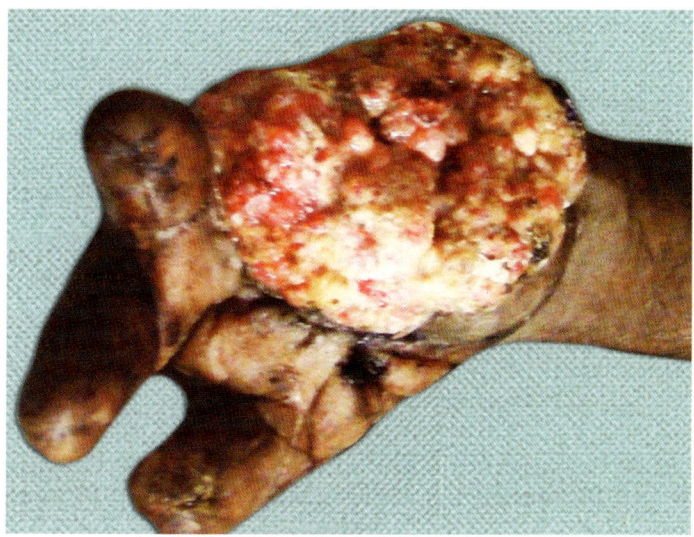

Fig. 13.25: Squamous cell carcinoma arising in leprosy patient who had extensive scarring and deformity

Palpation

- First look at the lesion. Is it an ulcer or growth?
- If it is a swelling/nodule—describe like a swelling—size, shape, surface, borders (edge), consistency, mobility plane of the swelling. Nodule in the skin—examples malignant melanoma, nodular variant of basal cell carcinoma, sebaceous carcinoma and cutaneous T cell lymphoma.
- If it is an ulcerative growth, local rise in temperature must be mentioned not over the growth, but in the surrounding skin.

1. *Tenderness and local rise in temperature*: Malignant ulcers are *nontender unless they are infected or have infiltrated bones*. Local rise of temperature is indicative of increased vascularity due to inflammation or in vascular tumours.

2. *Edge*: Induration (hardness) of the edge is characteristic of squamous cell carcinoma. Induration occurs due to extensive fibrosis. The fibrosis delays lymphatic spread and is believed to be a host defense mechanism.

3. *Base*: The base can be tendons, muscles or bone depending upon the site of ulcer. *Marked induration at the base is diagnostic of squamous cell carcinoma.*

It is interesting to note that induration is comparatively less in malignant melanoma as it induces less desmoplastic reaction. This also explains easy spread.

4. *Depth*: It is not an important sign. However, if possible, try to assess the depth of the ulcer. Penetrating or perforating malignant ulcers in the sole of the foot will be very deep up to the bone. Assessment can be done by probing but is not recommended for the fear of risk of spread.

5. *Nodule*: Describe it. Hard nodule can be suggestive of malignancy (Clinical Box 13.2).

Clinical Box 13.2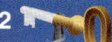

Differential diagnosis of a nodule in the skin

- Malignant melanoma—satellite nodule or in-transit deposits
- T cell lymphoma
- Metastasis in the skin
- Keratoacanthoma
- Sebaceous carcinoma
- Kaposi's sarcoma
- Nodular basal cell carcinoma

Clinical Wisdom

Malignant lesions and nodes are usually hard but when the tumour and nodes grow rapidly, necrosis occurs. They may feel firm or even soft in such situations. Hence it is better to use the term variable consistency.

---

6. *Mobility*: Gentle attempt is made to move the ulcer or growth to know its fixity to the underlying tissues. Malignant ulcers or growths arise from skin and hence they move with skin. Immobility is a feature of infiltration into the deeper structures such as deep fascia or bones.

7. *Bleeding*: Epithelioma is friable like a cauliflower. On gentle palpation, it bleeds.

8. *Surrounding area*
   - Thickening and induration are found in squamous cell carcinoma.
   - Tenderness and pitting on pressure indicate spreading inflammation surrounding the ulcer.

9. *Satellite nodule and in-transit deposits*: If present, describe them—they are nontender, firm swellings which are black in colour (Fig. 13.26).

10. *Function of the joint*: Movements of the involved joint are restricted either due to pain, involvement of the joint or due to infiltration into the joint by malignant ulcers.

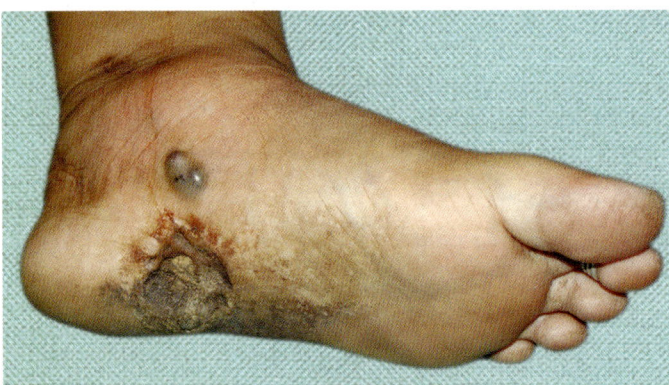

Fig. 13.26: Satellite nodules

11. *Regional lymph nodes*

- *Tender and enlarged*—acute secondary infection
- *Nontender and hard*—squamous cell carcinoma
- *Nontender, large, firm to hard, multiple*—malignant melanoma (Fig. 13.27).

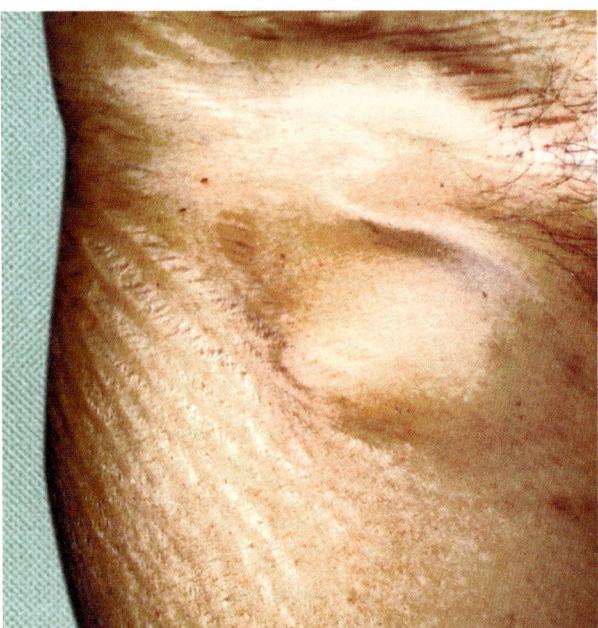

Fig. 13.27: Lymph nodes in the groin

12. *Systemic examination*: It is very important specially in cases of malignant melanoma. Metastasis in the liver can present as palpable liver—nodular, rapidly enlarging liver.

Malignant Melanoma of Toes

What is Hutchinson's sign?

- Subungual melanoma, a variant of acral lentiginous melanoma, arises from the nail matrix.

- Most commonly in the great toe or thumb.

- Subungual melanoma can present as a pigmentation under the nail fold. Often these are confused for ischaemic areas as in Buerger's disease or atherosclerotic vascular diseases. Sometimes it is confused for haematoma under the nail.

- Unless and until carefully examined and observed under good daylight, this type of melanoma can be easily missed.

- Slowly the nail fold pigmentation widens as the disease progresses (Figs 13.28 and 13.29).

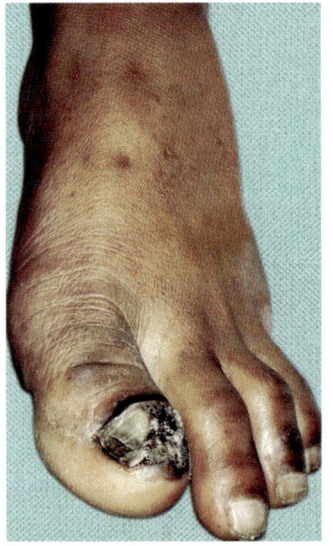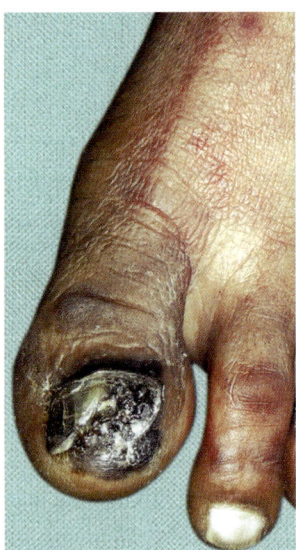

Figs 13.28 and 13.29: Hutchinson's sign—close up view

DIFFERENTIAL DIAGNOSIS

Malignant Melanoma (Figs 13.30 to 13.35)

It is a malignant tumour arising from neural crest and so ectodermal in origin. It is common in whites, however, also seen in other races. Exposure to sunlight has been blamed as one of the factors. It is rare before puberty. *About 30–40% of the malignant melanomas arise in pre-existing moles.* It starts as an

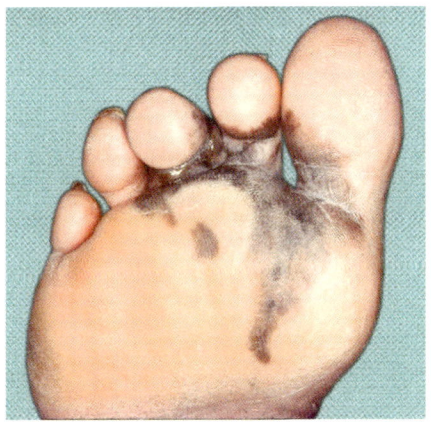

Fig. 13.30: Nonulcerated melanoma

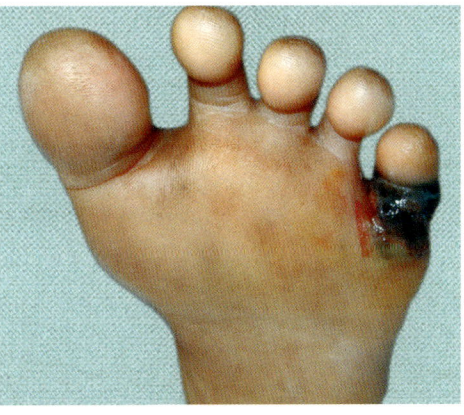

Fig. 13.31: Ulcerated, pigmented, very innocent-looking lesion

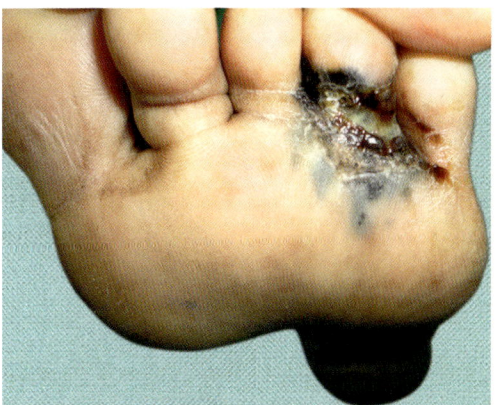

Fig. 13.32: Malignant melanoma of toes

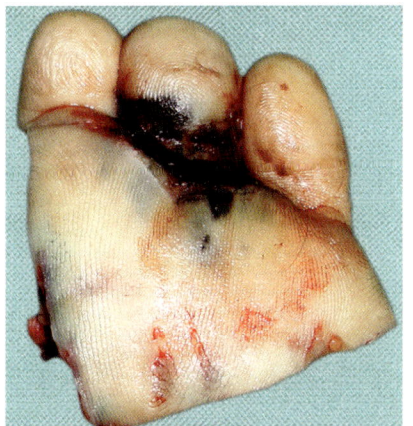

Fig. 13.33: Plantar surface of specimen

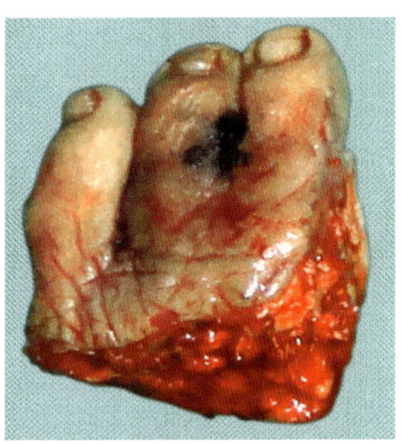

Fig. 13.34: Amputation of three toes

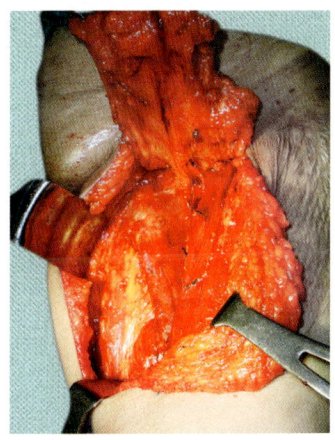

Fig. 13.35: Block dissection in progress

itchy lesion or with ulcerations and bleeding. Classically lesion is pigmented (amelanotic is without pigmentation) with or without satellite nodules and in-transit deposits. Groin nodes are enlarged and they are big size too. They give clue to the diagnosis.

Important clinical signs to look for in malignant melanoma:

1. Asymmetry/irregularity of borders in a mole.
2. Look for satellite nodule.
3. Look for in-transit deposits.
4. Palpate popliteal group of lymph nodes inguinal, iliac, para-aortic and nodes in the neck.
5. Look for Hutchinson's sign: Brown or black pigmentation spreads from subungual nail fold to adjacent cuticle and nail folds. This will not happen in cases of subungual haematoma.
6. Look for enlarged liver.

   Table 13.1 shows clinical/histological types of melanoma.

Diagnosis

It is by clinical examination and excision biopsy for small lesions. FNAC of the lymph nodes can be done. Metastatic work up includes abdominal ultrasound/CECT, chest X-ray, etc. It is treated by wide excision (1–2 cm) /amputation. Inguinal lymph nodes are treated by inguinal block dissection.

Table 13.1: Clinical/histological types of melanoma

1. Superficial spreading	Most common 70%	Trunk, proximal extremity	Ulceration	Least aggressive
2. Nodular	10–20%	More in leg (any part)	Raised nodule	More invasive
3. Acral lentigenous	4–8% most common in blacks	Palm, sole, digits, subungual	Ulceration	Late presentation aggressive
4. Lentigomaligna melanoma	3–5%	Sun exposed parts—temporal region. Elderly	Pigmented lesion	Slow growing
5. Desmoplastic or amelanotic	3–5%	Foot/trunk	Nonpigmented	

Melanoma—Initial features/evaluation

A: Asymmetry

B: Border irregularity

C: Colour variation

D: Diameter >6 mm

E: Evolution/change over time (ugly duckling)

Epithelioma/Squamous Cell Carcinoma and Marjolin's Ulcer

It is common in elderly patients. Chief precipitating factor is chronic irritation (Clinical Box 13.4). Thus, kangri cancer, kang cancer, chimney-sweep cancer, saree and dhothi cancers are names given to epithelioma occurring in different locations (Fig. 13.36). Typical lesion is an ulceroproliferative growth resembling cauliflower with everted edges. Floor bleeds on touch. Base is indurated. Slowly growth infiltrates the deeper structures and gets fixed. Satellite nodules and intransit deposits are not a feature of epithelioma. Regional lymph node enlargement is an important feature. Affected nodes are hard and indurated. Tender nodes suggest secondary infection which is more common in epithelioma than malignant melanoma. It should be noted that *Marjolin's ulcer does not spread to lymph nodes because lymphatics are obliterated* due to scarring. However, when the *lesion invades normal skin, lymph nodes do get enlarged*. Wide excision and regional block dissection of lymph nodes is the treatment of choice (Table 13.2).

In squamous cell carcinoma, look for

• Chronic exposure to ultraviolet rays

• Chronic immunosuppression

• Chronic scar

• Chronic irritation—tar, chemicals

• Chronic radiation damage

Basal Cell Carcinoma (Rodent Ulcer)

It is the most common malignant skin tumour arising from basal cell of the pilosebaceous adnexa. It is diagnosed by long duration of the history of a nonhealing ulcer and typical location. Majority of the lesions are found on the face above a line from lobule of the ear to the angle of mouth. In some cases, it can present as locally penetrating, ulcerative and destructive lesion. The ulcer has raised and beaded edge, induration may be present, and bleeds on touch. The base can be subcutaneous fat or deeper structures such as muscle or bone depending upon invasion. Scabbing also takes place suggesting a slow indolent nature of the disease. It can also present as a painless, firm, nodule, which is pigmented with fine blood vessels on its surface. Lymph nodes are not enlarged (Figs 13.37 to 13.39).

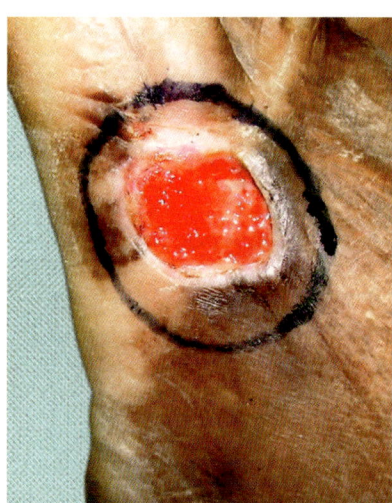

Fig. 13.36: Wide excision of squamous cell carcinoma

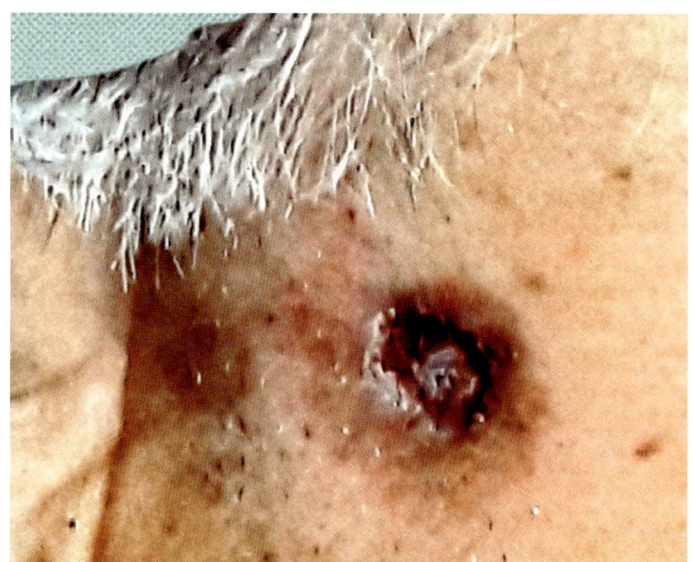

Fig. 13.37: Basal cell carcinoma treated as seborrhoeic keratosis

Table 13.2: Comparison of Marjolin's ulcer and squamous cell carcinoma

Marjolin's ulcer	*Squamous cell carcinoma/epithelioma*
1. Grows very slowly because of scar tissue	Grows slowly
2. It is painless as scar does not contain nerves	It can be painful, if it infiltrates the nerve fibres
3. Lymphatic metastasis does not occur because lymphatics are destroyed or occluded	Lymphatic metastasis is the chief method of spread
4. It is less malignant	Comparatively more malignant
5. Wide excision (Fig. 13.36) cures the disease, radiotherapy is not very useful	Both surgery and radiotherapy are used

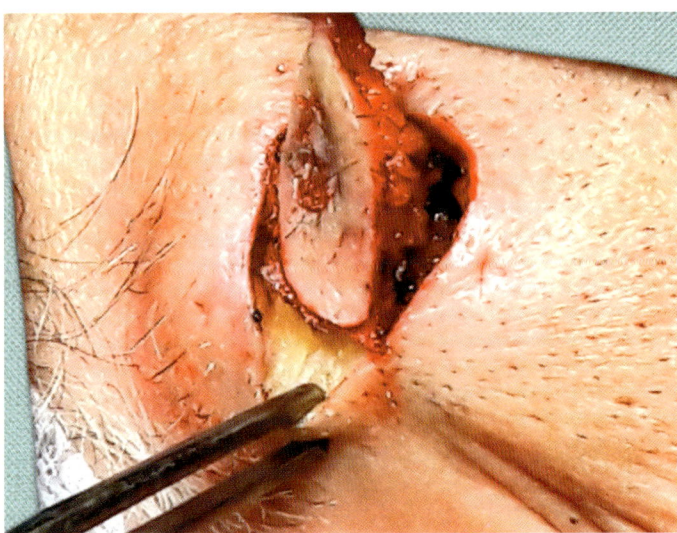

Fig. 13.38: Wide excision for basal cell carcinoma

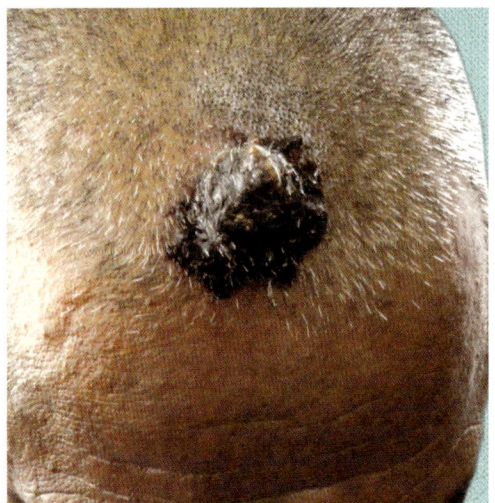

Fig. 13.40: Seborrhoeic keratosis

Dermatofibrosarcoma Protuberans

- This is a locally malignant tumour arising from the dermis.
- **Common sites:** Trunk, flexor region of limbs. It presents as nodular (bossellated) ulcerative lesion of many years duration (Fig. 13.41).
- Regional lymph node involvement is uncommon.
- It is less aggressive, hence curable.
- Treatment is by local wide excision followed by primary closure or skin grafting.

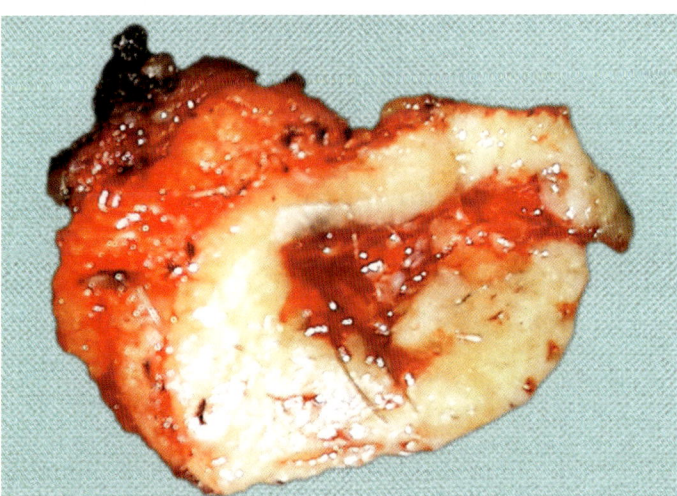

Fig. 13.39: Resected specimen

Clinical Wisdom

- In well differentiated squamous cell carcinoma, keratin pearls are found within the masses extending into the dermis.
- In seborrhoeic keratosis, keratin pearls are seen in epidermis.

Differential Diagnosis for Basal Cell Carcinoma

- **Keratoacanthoma:** It occurs only in the face. Edge can be raised with ulceration, thus resembling basal cell carcinoma.
- **Sclerosing angioma.**
- **Malignant melanoma:** Pigmented basal cell carcinoma may be mistaken for malignant melanoma.
- **Squamous cell carcinoma:** Face is not a common site of epithelioma. Everted edge, induration and significant nodes confirm the diagnosis.
- **Seborrheic Keratosis:** It is a benign condition of the skin presents as a round or oval elevated brown to black skin lesion. It mimics basal cell carcinoma. It arises from keratocytes. Excision is indicated if it is increasing in size or itching or if it gets infected (Fig. 13.40).

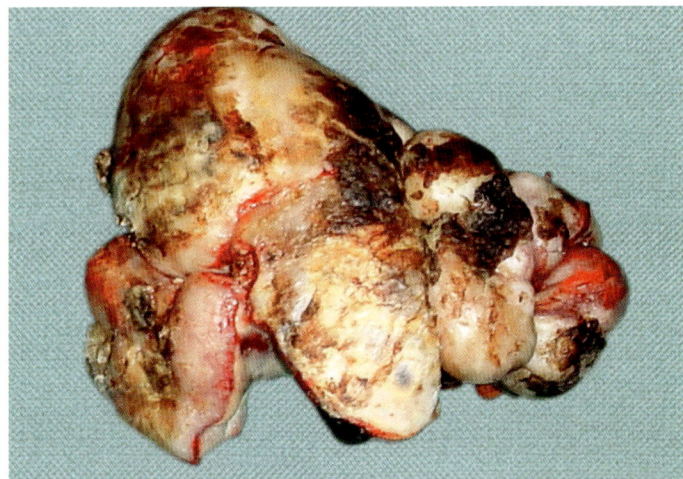

Fig. 13.41: Specimen of dermatofibrosarcoma protuberans

Kaposi's Angiosarcoma (Clinical Boxes 13.5 and 13.6)

- Common in **Black population**
- This neoplasm arises from **proliferating capillary vessels** and **perivascular connective tissue cells.**
- **Multiple, purplish nodules** that appear in the limb and ulcerate with bleeding is characteristic feature.
- Regional lymph node involvement can occur
- Increasing incidence due to AIDS.

Differential Diagnosis

1. Malignant melanoma
2. Soft tissue sarcoma
3. Multiple cutaneous metastases
4. T cell lymphoma

BENIGN LESIONS OF THE SKIN

1. *Keratoacanthoma* (molluscum sebaceum, molluscum pseudocarcinomatosum):
   - Self-limiting benign neoplasm of viral origin (probably).
   - Arises due to overgrowth of hair follicle and subsequent *spontaneous regression is characteristic.*
   - It is painless swelling in the skin with central dark brown core. After initial rapid growth of 2–4 weeks, spontaneous regression occurs in 24 hours. After separation of the central core, lump diminishes in size leaving a deep indrawn scar.
   - Usually single, face is the commonest site.
   - Like sebaceous cyst, it presents as hemispherical swelling.
   - Treated by excision.

2. *Turban tumour*: It is the **blanket term** used to describe a tumour occupying the whole of the scalp thus resembling a **turban**.
   - Most often used to describe *multiple cylindromata.*
   - They produce *pink nodular masses.*
   - Diagnosis is confirmed by biopsy.
   - Treatment includes excision and reconstruction by skin grafting or rotational flaps.

3. *Corn* (Fig. 13.45)
   - It is a **painful lesion in the plantar surface (sole) of the foot.**
   - It affects the plantar surface of toes and sole of the feet.
   - Corn develops due to intermittent pressure over a limited area.
   - Basically, it is a localised hyperkeratinisation of the skin with a hard central core.
   - It will be a cone-shaped lesion, broad on the surface and narrow at deeper plane.
   - They are **painful and very tender.**
   - Most of these are **hard corns.**
   - **Soft corn** can occur in between the toes.
   - Symptomatic corns have to be excised, one has to **excise a good cone**-shaped tissue for permanent cure. Otherwise **recurrence can occur.**

4. *Wart* (Fig. 13.46)
   - A wart is a rough excrescence on the skin.
   - Papillomaviruses are responsible for this.
   - They are pigmented, keratinised, irregular lesions and common in young adults.
   - *Common sites*: Fingers, feet, genitalia, beard area, etc.
   - They are multiple and sometimes are painful.
   - When it occurs in the feet there will be difficulty in walking.
   - *Venereal warts*: They are also called **papilloma acuminata**. They can occur in the anal region, perineum and in the coronal sulcus of the penis.
   - Some of the warts may regress spontaneously. **Fulguration** with diathermy is the treatment.

CLINICAL DISCUSSION

1. **What are the ectodermal sites of melanoma?**
   Anal canal, choroids, meninges.

2. **What are the areas of junctional naevus?**
   Palm, sole, face, neck, subungual digits and genitalia.

3. **What is amelanotic melanoma?**
   In 10% of patients, pigment is absent. It is called amelanotic melanoma.

4. **Which are the areas wherein basal cell carcinoma cannot occur?**
   It cannot occur in the mucosal surfaces which do not have pilosebaceous adnexa, e.g. cervix, lips, tongue.

5. What are the common sites of basal cell carcinoma?

Nasolabial fold, inner canthus of eye (Clinical Box 13.7)

6. What are satellite nodules?

Satellite nodules (within 2 cm of the primary) may be found surrounding the lesion which are due to *spread through intradermal lymphatics*.

7. What is temozolamide?

It is an oral analogue of dacarbazine. It is supposed to decrease incidence of cerebral metastasis.

8. What is Merkel cell carcinoma?

It is highly malignant tumour derived from *neuroendocrine cells* which function as *touch receptors*.

9. What is a dysplastic naevus?

It is 6–15 mm macular spot. Majority do not turn into malignancy.

10. What are giant congenital nevi?

Nevi larger than 20 cm. They have increased incidence of malignant melanoma and even sarcoma.

11. What is a Spitz naevus?

Rapidly growing pink or brown, benign skin lesion. It is also called epithelioid/spindle cell naevus.

12. What are the clinical features of epithelioma (squamous cell carcinoma)?

Growing ulcer or growth, edges are everted, base is indurated, mobility is restricted. Lymph nodes, if enlarged, also favours the diagnosis.

13. What features will be there in basal cell carcinoma (BCC)?

Typical site is in the face—nasolabial fold, inner canthus of eye, etc. Elevated edge, sometimes beaded or even pigmented, very slow growing lesion. Lymph nodes are not enlarged.

14. How do you investigate?

Edge biopsy is done because it is the fast growing area so that adequate tumour cells can be seen.

15. What are the findings in SCC and BCC?

Epithelial pearls are typical of SCC and pallisading of cells is typical of BCC.

16. In which type of SCC epithelial pearls are not seen?

In undifferentiated carcinoma, epithelial pearls are not seen.

Clinical Box 13.7

Typical sites
1. Inner canthus of the eye
2. Outer canthus of the eye
3. Eyelids
4. Bridge of the nose
5. Around nasolabial fold
These sites are the areas where the tears roll down. Hence, it is also called **tear cancer**.

17. What about ultrasound?

It can be used to detect lymph nodes. Loss of normal shape of lymph node (bean shape), increased vascularity may suggest malignant nature. It can also guide FNAC.

18. What other investigations can be done?

X-ray of the part (in limbs), CT scan can also be done.

19. How do you treat SCC?

- SCC is treated by wide excision of 1 cm margin all around and at depth. It has been called 3-dimensional wide excision. If defect is small direct closure is done, otherwise split skin grafting can be done. Large fungating tumours may require some form of amputation depending upon the location of tumour. Large tumour infiltrating calcaneous is treated by amputation. Large tumours in the hand are treated by amputations.
- Early cases can be treated by radiation of 4000 to 6000 cG units over a period of 4 to 6 weeks.

20. How do you treat BCC?

Wide excision with 1 cm margin is adequate. Most of them are in the face, slow growing and well differentiated. Direct closure is possible mostly. Otherwise flap reconstruction has to be done.

21. When do you give radiotherapy in the adjuvant setting?

In SCC, if perineural spread is detected or positive surgical margins or multiple nodes or extracapsular spread is present.

22. How do you manage malignant melanoma?

- Growing mole is excised with few mm margin and then subjected for biopsy.
- However chest X-ray /CT scan of lung or abdomen may be required to know the spread of the disease.

23. What are the recommended margins for malignant melanoma? (Figs 13.42 and 13.43)

Depending upon Breslow thickness. It is more reliable and usable—thin melanoma—less than or equal to 1 mm, intermediate between 1 to 2 mm and 2 to 4 mm and thick more than 4 mm.

Size of melanoma	Excision margin
Melanoma *in situ*	5 mm
<1.0 mm	1 cm
1.0–2.0 mm	1–2 cm
2.0–4.0 mm	1–2 cm
>4.0 mm	2 cm

24. What are the treatment options available?

- Surgery is the main form of treatment. Excision with adequate margin followed by regional lymph node block dissection is the treatment of choice.

25. What are Heberden's nodes?

They are seen in osteoarthritis. Tiny hard knob-like swelling in relation to terminal inter-phalangeal joints of 4 digits. Thumb is not involved. Interestingly thumb is not involved in Raynaud's disease, and Dupuytren's contracture also. Women at menopause are commonly affected.

MISCELLANEOUS—FEW PICTURES

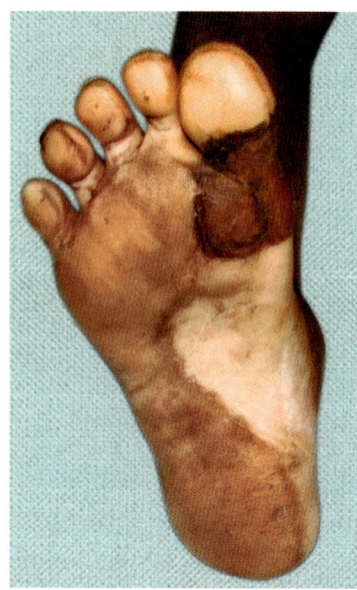

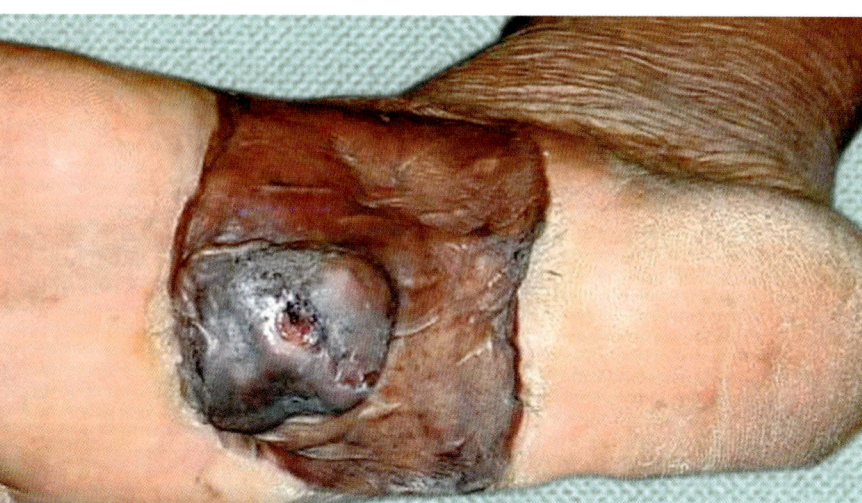

Fig. 13.42: Wide excision and skin grafting was done for a 1 cm lesion—malignant melanoma. **Fig. 13.43:** Recurrence of malignant melanoma. Hence careful follow up is a must and examine not only for metastasis but also for recurrence at the operated site

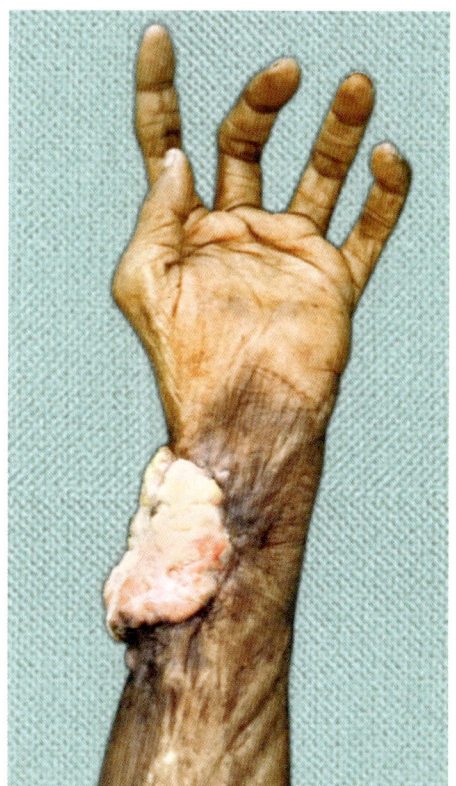

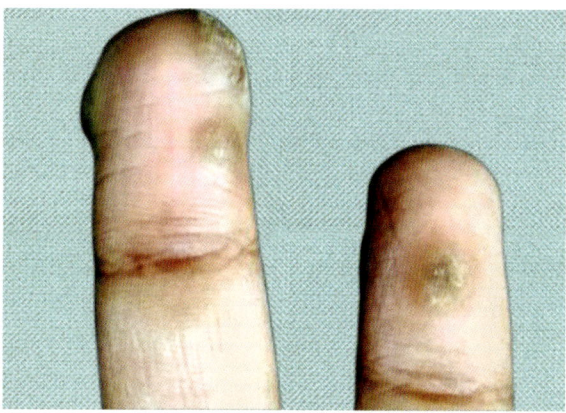

Fig. 13.45: Multiple corns. (*Courtesy:* Dr Satish Pai, Head, Dept of Dermatology, KMC, Manipal)

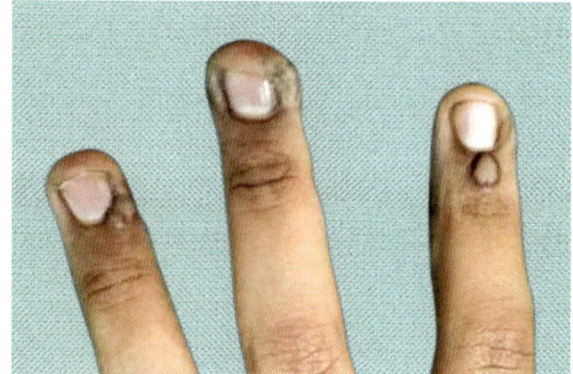

Fig. 13.44: Marjolin ulcer with contracture: The patient had burns 25 years back. He developed nonhealing ulcer with growth of six month duration. You can see contractures caused by burns

Fig. 13.46: Warts (*Courtesy:* Dr Satish Pai, Head, Dept of Dermatology, KMC, Manipal)

14

Examination of Face, Pinna and Scalp

INTRODUCTION

Face is developed from 1 frontonasal process, 2 maxillary processes and 2 mandibular processes. During the development, line of fusion may not develop properly or some cells may get trapped underneath, resulting in development of various anomalies. To give a few examples—dermoid cysts, cleft lip, cleft palate, etc. Face also reflects various diseases—classical being Cushingoid facies in Cushing's syndrome. Capillary haemangiomas are also common on the skin of the face. Face is the site of basal cell carcinoma. Most of these are short cases. Thus, a swelling or an ulcer description should follow in the usual manner.

Broadly for clinical purposes, swellings/ulcers over the face can be classified as follows:

1. *Congenital*
   - Dermoid cyst
   - Vascular—haemangiomas
   - Hamartoma
   - Neural tumours—von Recklinghausen's disease
2. *Acute inflammatory*
   - Boil/furuncle
   - Facial cellulitis
   - Erysipelas
3. *Chronic inflammatory*
   - Lupus vulgaris
   - Cold abscess facial/parotid lymph nodes
   - Actinomycosis of face and jaw—sinuses, nodules
   - Rhinosporidiosis
4. *Traumatic*
   - Abrasions, contusions, haematoma
   - Traumatic AV fistula

5. *Neoplastic*
   - *Benign*: Lipoma, salivary gland tumours
   - *Malignancy*: Basal cell carcinoma, sebaceous carcinoma, melanoma, etc.

DIFFERENTIAL DIAGNOSIS

Swelling Over the Face

1. **Capillary haemangioma**: They consist of dilated capillaries and proliferation of endothelial cells. Hence, it commonly occurs in the skin. **Salmon patch** is a bluish patch over the forehead, in the midline, present at birth and disappears by 1 year of age. Hence, no treatment is required. **Port wine stain** is an extensive intradermal haemangioma. This is bluish purple in colour, commonly affects the face or other parts of the skin, is present at birth and usually progresses and does not regress. Area supplied by sensory branches of the fifth cranial nerve is involved. It starts with light red colour and progresses to deep colour. It may be associated with Sturge-Weber syndrome.

> **Clinical Wisdom**
>
> Flat, patchy lesion on the face in the area of fifth cranial nerve that does not fade is port-wine stain.

Why do you say it is capillary haemangioma?
1. Location—face is one of the common sites
2. Arising from skin
3. Typical colour—bluish to red
4. Compressibility
5. Present since birth/childhood.

2. **Strawberry angiomas** produce swelling which protrude from the skin surface. Child is normal at birth. After a month, a bright red swelling appears over the head and neck region, which exhibits *sign of compressibility*. They are common in younger age group, typical locations including face, colour (mostly red) and are compressible (Fig. 14.1).

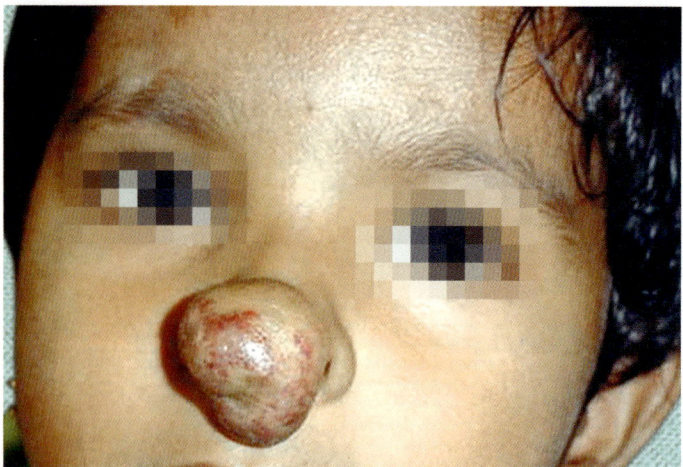

Fig. 14.1: Strawberry angioma—haemangioma nose

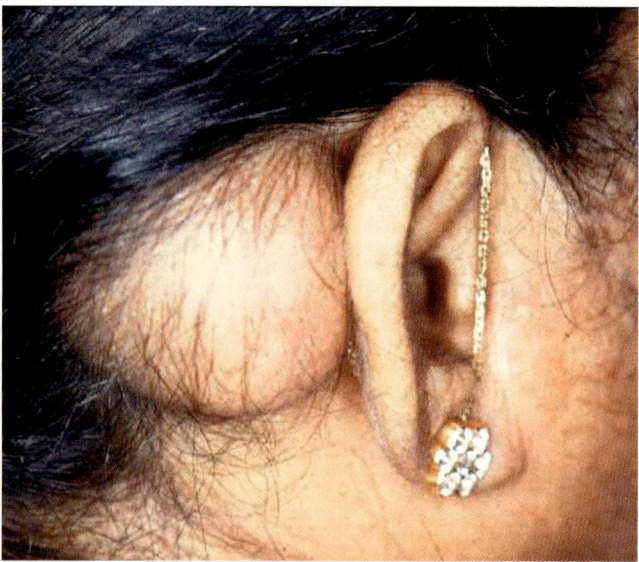

Fig. 14.2: Postauricular dermoid cyst

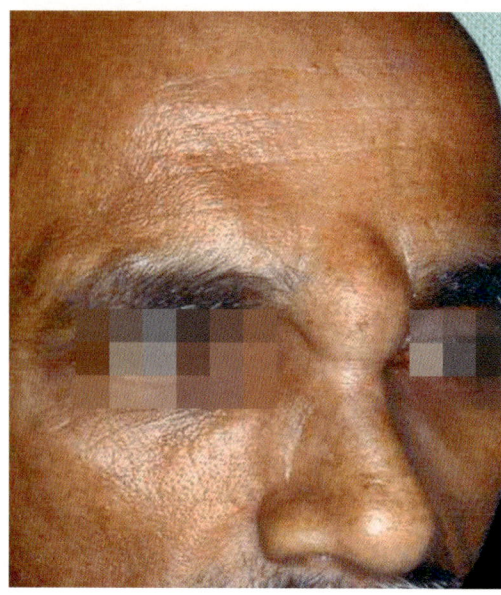

Fig. 14.3: Median frontal dermoid cyst at the root of nose

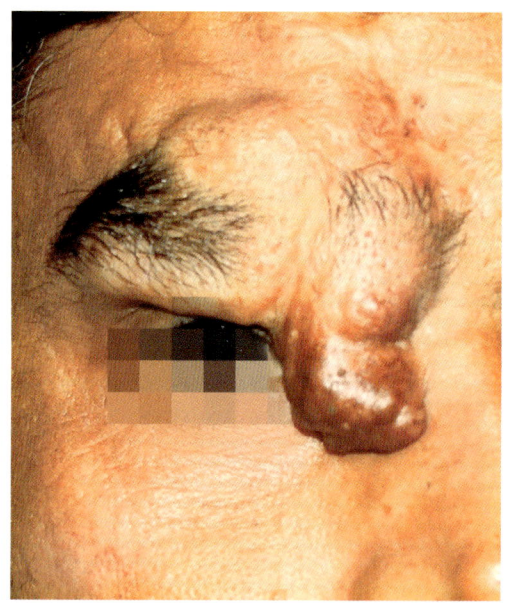

Fig. 14.4: Plexiform neurofibromatosis

3. **Dermoid cyst**: External angular dermoid cyst, preauricular dermoid cysts, and frontal dermoid cysts are common on the face. These have been dealt in detail in page 73 (Figs 14.2 and 14.3).

Why do you say it is dermoid cyst?
• Congenital—long duration
• Painless slow growing swelling
• Smooth surface, round borders
• Typical location—a line of fusion (sequestration dermoid)
• Bony depression is felt underneath.

4. **Plexiform neurofibroma** *(page 67)*: Any swelling which is pendulous hanging in the form of folds, infront of the eye is mostly plexiform neurofibromatosis. In this condition, branches of 5th cranial nerve (trigeminal nerve) are commonly affected. It can also involve the peripheral nerves. The affected part is grossly thickened due *to fibro-myxomatous degeneration* (Fig. 14.4).

When it hangs down in the form of folds it is called pachydermatocoele (Fig. 14.5).

Why do you say it is plexiform neurofibroma?
• Swellings are congenital and multiple—long duration of history.
• Typical location—branch of trigeminal nerve—ophthalmic division is involved.
• Pigmented spots—such as café au lait spots are seen.
• Swelling is soft to firm in consistency.

5. **Boil:** Infection of hair follicle is common over the face resulting in a boil. Carbuncle is not common over the face may be because it is richly vascular.

6. Other swellings such as parotid gland tumours can also occur on the face. Very often it can be confused for sebaceous cyst and lipoma (Fig. 14.6).

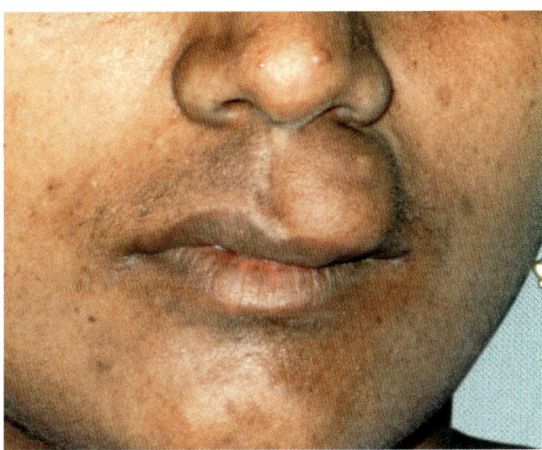

Fig. 14.5: Neural tumour of the lip (*Courtesy:* Dr Deepti Pai, PG student, KMC, Manipal)

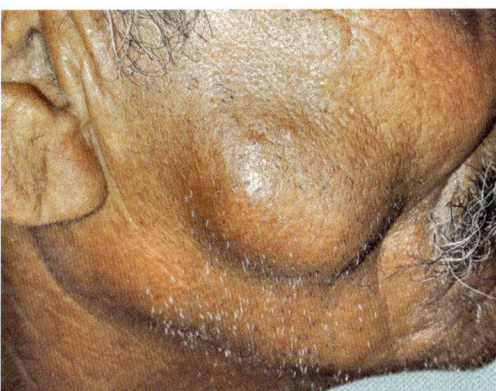

Fig. 14.6: Warthin's tumour in a 65 year old male which was confused for lipoma

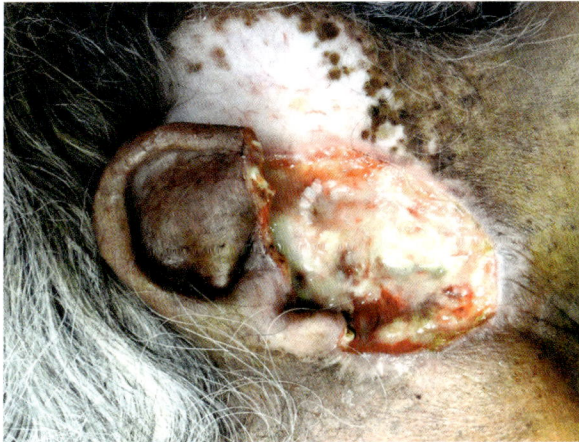

Fig. 14.7: Penetrating basosquamous cell carcinoma with destruction of the left ear

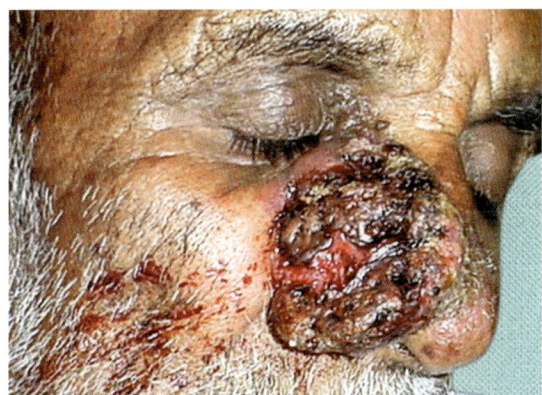

Fig. 14.8: Basal cell carcinoma—the classical site. Ulcer of 18 months duration

Ulcer Over the Face

1. ***Basal cell carcinoma:*** Typical location, nonhealing ulcer, very slow growth, typical elevated edge and no significant lymphadenopathy (Figs 14.7 and 14.8).

2. ***Sebaceous carcinoma:*** It is almost like squamous cell carcinoma as far as lesion is concerned—everted edges, cauliflower-like growth, induration, fixity and significant lymphadenopathy.

3. ***Keratoacanthoma***
   - Self-limiting benign neoplasm of viral origin (probably).
   - Arises due to overgrowth of hair follicle and subsequent spontaneous regression is characteristic.
   - It is painless swelling in the skin with central dark brown core. After initial rapid growth of 2–4 weeks, spontaneous regression occurs in 24 hours. After separation of the central core, lump diminishes in size leaving a deep indrawn scar.
   - Usually single, **face is the commonest site.**
   - Like sebaceous cyst, it presents as hemispherical swelling.
   - Treated by excision.
   - Keratoacanthoma, if associated with sebaceous carcinoma and visceral malignancy (colon cancer), constitutes **Muir-Torre syndrome.**

4. ***Lupus vulgaris:*** Tubercular ulcer over the face, rare to find now (Fig. 14.9 and Clinical Box 14.1):
   - Various lesions in the face affected by tuberculosis are called lupus vulgaris.
   - Common sites affected are around nose, cheeks, ears, and eyelids.

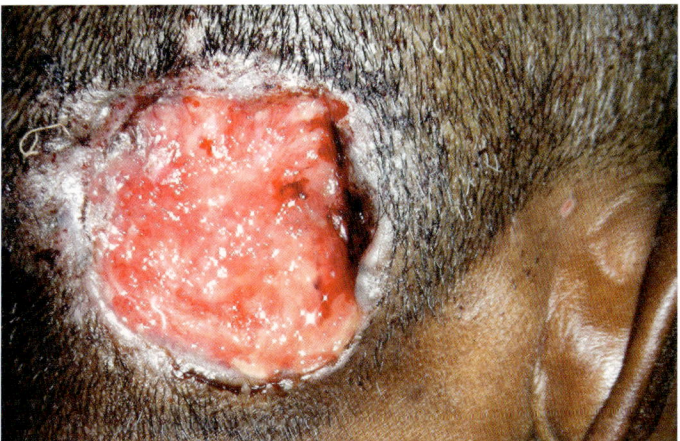

Fig. 14.9: TB ulcer in scalp (*Courtesy:* Dr Maruthu Pandyan, Head, Dept of Surgery, Madurai Medical College, Tamil Nadu)

Clinical Box 14.1 🗝

Tuberculous lesion in the skin
1. *Lupus vulgaris*: Face
2. *Verruca cutis*: Warty lesions hand, foot neck, joint
3. *Miliary tuberculosis*: Multiple skin lesions/ulcers
4. *Tuberculid*: Reddish nodules, good immunity, erythema induratum

- Lesions start as a nodule and progress to ulcers with significant disfigurement. Lupus means hungry like a wolf. Typically small, sharp, reddish brown nodules and ulcers, apple jelly nodules.

5. ***Traumatic ulcers***: They are not common, however, road traffic accidents and fall resulting in crushing injury to the face can result in ulcers.

Inflammatory Lesions in the Face

1. ***Facial cellulitis***: It can occur due to infections. Face will be swollen, and signs of inflammation will be present. Causative organisms are *Streptococcus* and *Staphylococcus*. Since infection affects deep layers of the skin, it is painful. Significant oedema results in gross swelling of face and peau d'orange appearance.

2. ***Boil or furuncle***: Inflammation of the hair follicle results in boil (an abscess). Diabetes is the chief precipitating factor. It is a very painful tender, hot swelling. Face is also one of the sites (Fig. 14.10).
   - *Danger area of the face*: It is the triangle between the two corners of the mouth and the bridge of the nose. Infections from this site can spread through facial veins to ophthalmic veins to the cavernous sinus. This will result in cavernous sinus thrombosis.

3. ***Erysipelas***: Infection of skin with cutaneous lymphangitis is called erysipelas. Red raised rash is almost diagnostic. When it affects the face area adjacent to pinna, erysipelas will not affect pinna because of lack of subcutaneous tissue in the ear. It is called as Milian's ear sign. It is caused by beta-haemolytic group 'A' Streptococcus.

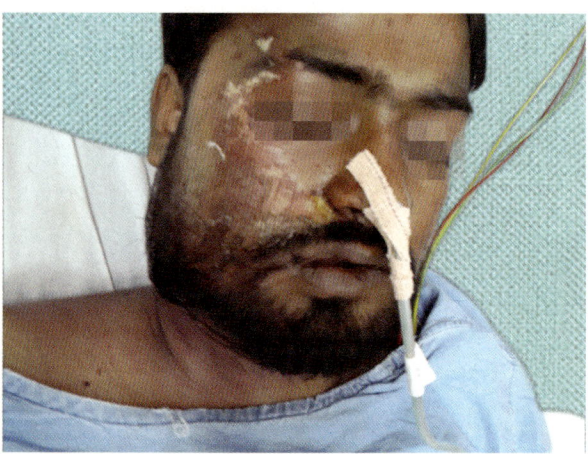

Fig. 14.10: Facial trauma resulting in cellulitis and pustules in the danger area of the face

SOME CHARACTERISTIC FACIES

1. ***Hippocratic facies*** (Fig. 14.11): This is seen in terminal cases of septic shock. Eyes are sunken, drawn in cheeks, tongue is dry and coated, forehead is cold and clammy.

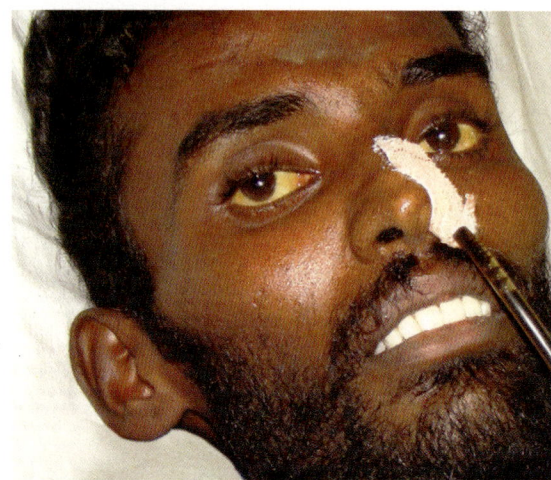

Fig. 14.11: Hippocratic facies (*Courtesy*: Dr Raghunath Prabhu, Associate Professor, Department of Surgery, KMC, Manipal)

2. ***Moon face*** (Fig. 14.12): This is seen in Cushing's syndrome. Most of the cases have adrenal adenoma, others have pituitary adenomas. Face is round like a moon and lips are pursed.

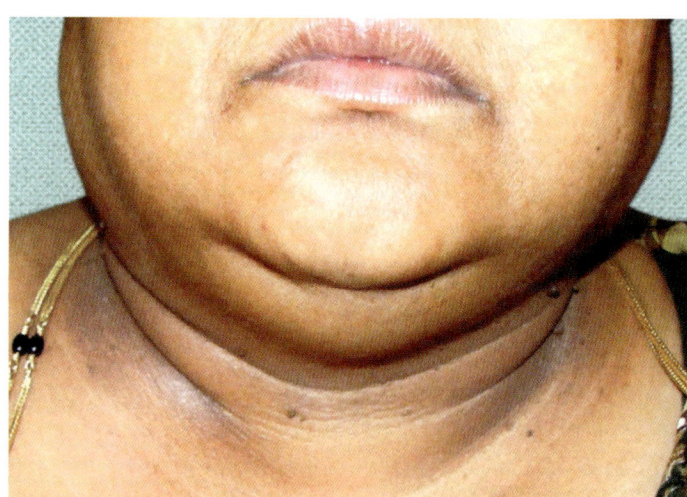

Fig. 14.12: Moon face of Cushing's syndrome

3. ***Facies of cretinism***: Pale, puffy face with protruding tongue is classical of cretinism.

4. ***Facies of myasthenia gravis***: Intermittent ptosis, drooping of jaw and sneezing smile are seen due to weakness or rapid exhaustion of muscles particularly of the face. After rest they usually recover.

CLEFT LIP AND PALATE (Figs 14.13 to 14.15)

- It is also called hare lip.
- Cleft lip results from abnormal development of the median nasal and maxillary processes.
- Cleft palate results from a failure of fusion of the two palatine processes.

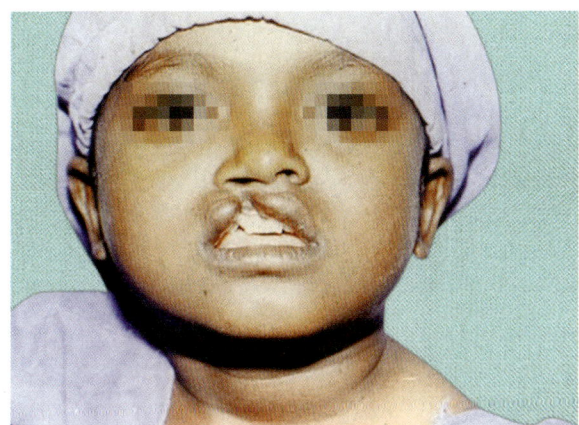

Fig. 14.13: Cleft lip (*Courtesy*: Dr CG Narasimhan, Consultant Surgeon, Mysore)

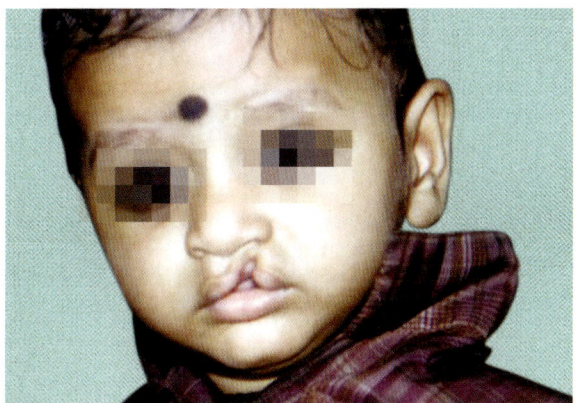

Fig. 14.14: Cleft lip (*Courtesy*: Dr CG Narasimhan, Consultant Surgeon, Mysore)

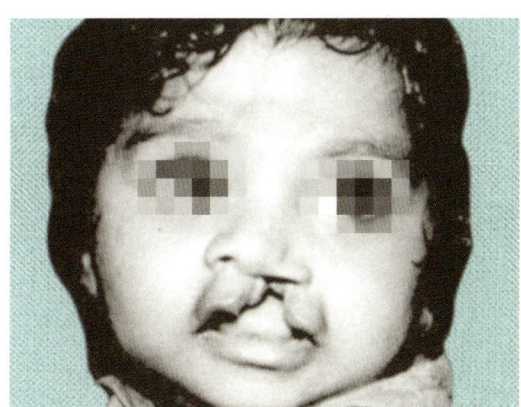

Fig. 14.15: Cleft lip (*Courtesy*: Dr CG Narasimhan, Consultant Surgeon, Mysore)

Types of Cleft Lip (Figs 14.16 and 14.17)

I. *Central*: It is very rare and occurs due to failure of fusion of two median nasal processes.

II. *Lateral*: It is the commonest variety wherein there is a cleft between the frenulum and the lateral part of the upper lip. This is due to imperfect fusion of maxillary process with median nasal process. The lateral variety can be unilateral or bilateral.

III. *Complete or incomplete*: In cases of complete variety, cleft lip extends to the floor of the nose. In cases of incomplete variety, the cleft does not extend up to the nostril.

IV. *Simple or compound*: Compound refers to cleft lip associated with a cleft in the alveolus.

- *Cleft lip is more commonly found lateral—not in the midline.* Cleft lip is formed in the tip of the lip as either a small gap or an indentation in the lip (partial or incomplete cleft) or it continues into the nose (complete cleft). Lip cleft can occur as one-sided (unilateral) or two-sided (bilateral). It is due to the failure of fusion of the *maxillary and medial nasal processes* (formation of the primary palate) (Figs 14.18 to 14.20).

- *Cleft palate* is a condition in which the two plates of the *skull* that form the *hard palate* (roof of the mouth) are not completely joined. The *soft palate* is in these

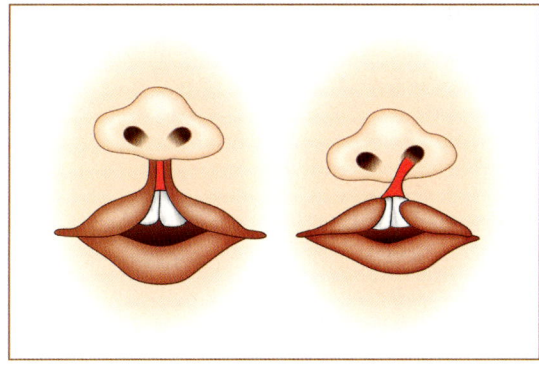

Figs 14.16 and 14.17: Types of cleft lip (I and II)

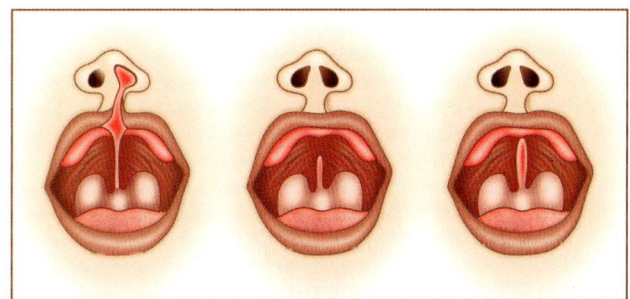

Figs 14.18 to 14.20: Types of cleft palate (I, IIa and IIb)

cases cleft as well. In most cases, cleft lip is also present. Cleft palate occurs in about one in 700 live-births worldwide. Palate cleft can occur as complete (soft and hard palate, possibly including a gap in the jaw) or incomplete (a 'hole' in the roof of the mouth, usually as a cleft soft palate). When cleft palate occurs, the *uvula* is usually split. It occurs due to the failure of fusion of the lateral palatine processes, the nasal septum, and/or the median palatine processes (formation of the *secondary palate*). The hole in the roof of the mouth caused by a cleft connects the mouth directly to the *nasal cavity.*

- In your institution, you may be given a case of cleft lip and cleft palate as short cases. What students need to know is they are neither swellings nor ulcers but describe them in the usual manner as cleft of the lip or palate, etc.

- *History*: Some important history should be taken such as maternal smoking, maternal *alcohol abuse* or *antihypertension* treatment. Other causes include—pesticide exposure.

- Following points to be noted when you examine a case of cleft lip and palate:
    1. Is it unilateral or bilateral?
    2. Is it complete or incomplete?
    3. Is there cleft palate or not?
    4. Is there any anomalies of the maxilla?
    5. What about the nasal septum?
    6. Enquire about functional problems—problems with feeding, ear infections, ear blockade, and speech.

Clinical Features

In 80% of the cases, cleft lip is unilateral and in about 60% of the cases it is associated with cleft palate. In many cases, nostril is widened. Maldevelopment or malalignment of the teeth in relation to the cleft is common.

Functional Effect

Presence of cleft lip does not interfere much with sucking. However, there may be some difficulty in bottle feeding. Some degree of difficulty in speech (disarticulation) is present.

CLEFT PALATE

Development of Palate

- Palate is developed around 6–8 weeks of intra-uterine life from **3 components**. The premaxilla

which is developed from the median nasal processes. 2 and 3. Maxillary process which contributes one palatine process on each side.

- The line of fusion of these processes is in the form of a letter Y.

- Imperfect fusion or developmental anomalies result in cleft palate.

Types

I. *Complete*: Failure of fusion of palatine processes and premaxilla results in complete cleft palate. In such situations, the nasal cavity and mouth are interconnected. When premaxilla is not fused with both palatine processes, it hangs down from the septum of nose. Thus, complete cleft can be of two types as shown in Figs 14.16 and Fig. 14.17.

II. *Incomplete*: When the fusion of three components of palate takes place, it starts from uvula and then backwards. Thus, various types of incomplete fusion result.

- Bifid uvula
- The whole length of soft palate is bifid
- The whole length of soft palate and the posterior part of hard palate are involved. On the other hand, anterior part of palate is normally developed. In about 25% of cases, cleft palate alone and in 50% of cases, both cleft palate and cleft lip are encountered.

Effects of Cleft Palate

1. Presence of cleft palate interferes with swallowing to some extent.

2. They are unable to make the consonant sounds like B, D, K, P, T.

3. **Teeth:** Upper lateral incisors may be small or even absent. The maxilla tends to be smaller. Teeth are crowded.

4. **Nose:** Oral organisms contaminate the upper respiratory mucous membrane through cleft palate.

5. **Hearing:** Even with repair, acute and chronic otitis media and hearing problems can occur.

Treatment of Cleft Lip

1. **What is rule of 10 for cleft lip and palate?**

   At the time of cleft lip repair, child should weigh 10 lbs (4.54 kg), age around 10 weeks, haemoglobin >10 gm% and total count less than 10,000 cells/mm^3—this is called **Millard's rule of 10.**

2. What is an ideal surgery for unilateral cleft lip repair?

Millard rotation advancement flap.

3. What are the 3 layers involved in cleft lip repair?

Mucosa, muscle layer and skin.

4. What about bilateral cleft lip repair?

Single or two stage repair?

5. What is the ideal time for cleft palate repair?

18 months.

6. What is the type of repair?

V-Y palatoplasty.

TRIGEMINAL NERVE AND SURGEON

- If *anterolateral wall of maxillary antrum* is involved in carcinoma, asymmetry of the face results in pain in the cheek. Anaesthesia over the skin of the cheek including upper lip occurs due to involvement of infraorbital nerve, a branch of maxillary division of the trigeminal nerve.
- Plexiform neurofibromatosis affects the branches of 5th cranial nerve—ophthalmic division.
- Flat, patchy lesion on the face in the area of fifth cranial nerve that does not fade is port-wine stain.

Examination of Fifth Cranial nerve

Motor: Pterygoid, temporal and masseter muscles are supplied by 5th cranial nerve. Hence, following tests for motor function:

1. Ask patient to clench the teeth. Look for contraction of temporal and masseter muscles.
2. Ask patient to open the mouth. Look for deviation of the jaw. If it deviates to one side, it indicates paralysis of pterygoids on the same side.

Sensory: Trigeminal neuralgia affects 2nd or 3rd division of fifth cranial nerve. Eating, talking, etc. will trigger the neuralgia. During the attack, hyperaesthetic area can be detected easily.

CLINICAL DISCUSSION

1. What are the trigger zones of Patrick?

These are the areas which on touch trigger trigeminal neuralgia.

2. What is diagnostic sign of dermoid cyst?

Bony depression (indentation) underneath the swelling.

3. What test is done when a dermoid cyst occurs in a young child specially in the midline over scalp bones?

Check for expansile impulse on cough to rule out intracranial communication.

4. How are large haemangiomas on the face managed? (Fig. 14.21)

- Because of vascularity, therapeutic embolization should be done first after doing CT angiogram.
- Once the vascularity diminishes, surgery can be attempted. Vascular surgeon's help is required. Adequate blood to be arranged. In all vascular tumours, high output haemangiomas (AV malformations) are dangerous.
- Patient in Fig. 14.21, was diagnosed as lipoma and explored. Suddenly, rapid gush of blood started pouring out and surgeon had to cancel the procedure. He packed the swelling and referred to higher centre.

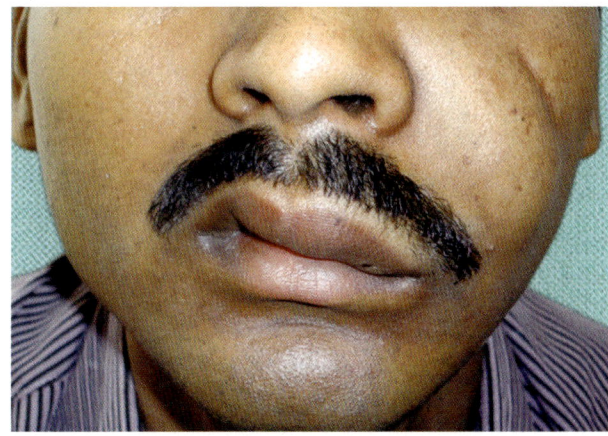

Fig. 14.21: Haemangioma face

15

Examination of the Salivary Glands

INTRODUCTION

It should be remembered that if one salivary gland is enlarged, examine all three salivary glands and on both sides because, some diseases can affect all glands on both sides. Salivary gland tumours are common swellings encountered in the clinical examination. If one follows the common plan which has been described for examination of swellings, it is easy to diagnose the case.

PATIENT DATA

Age: Salivary gland tumours commonly occur in the middle age group patients. Sialectasis is congenital, manifests early in the childhood and in adult life. Calculous disease is common on the submandibular salivary gland, can occur between age group of 20 and 50 years. Autoimmune disorders, such as Mickulicz's disease, occur in the age group between 20 and 40 years.

Sex: All salivary gland lesions are common in women.

HISTORY OF PRESENT ILLNESS

1. *Swelling*: When did you notice the swelling? Was there any pain or fever to start with? How is it progressing? These are the usual questions. Most often parotid or submandibular gland lesions present as swelling. In such a case you have to ask the *duration* of the swelling and *growth pattern*. Slow-growing neoplasm of the parotid gland is *pleomorphic adenoma*. Generally, patient says it has been there since 3–5 years and it is slow growing. If such a tumour *grows rapidly*, it is due to *malignant transformation* of the tumour. It means pleomorphic adenoma is turning into carcinoma. In such cases, it also causes pain.

- Slow growth is for pleomorphic adenoma (Fig. 15.1).
- Medium-moderate is for low grade mucoepidermoid carcinoma.
- Rapid growth is for adenoid cystic carcinoma (Figs 15.2 and 15.3).
- If patient complains of recurrent swelling, get all the details about the initial swelling, surgical procedure and treatment such as radiotherapy, etc. Pleomorphic adenoma is known for recurrences, if it is just enucleated. Such recurrent swellings are difficult to treat.

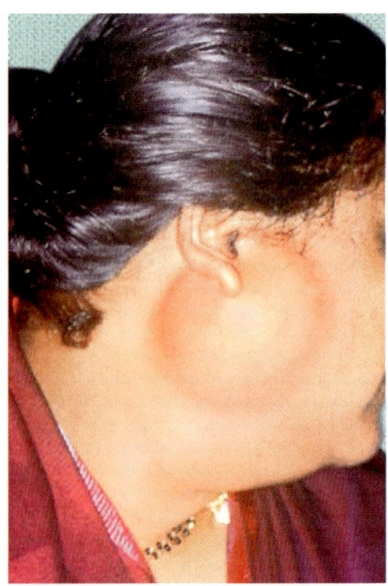

Fig. 15.1: Slow-growing swelling since 10 years—pleomorphic adenoma

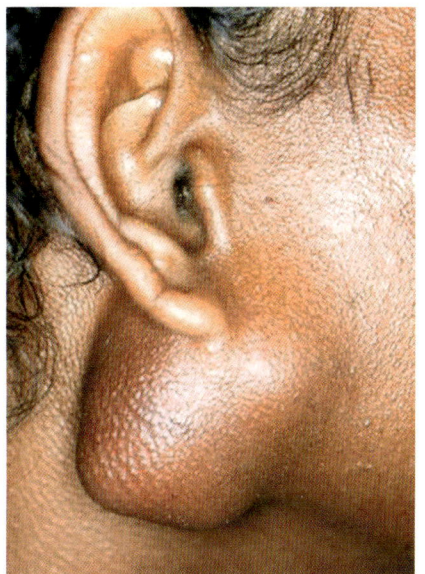

Fig. 15.2: Swelling since 18 months—low grade mucoepidermoid carcinoma

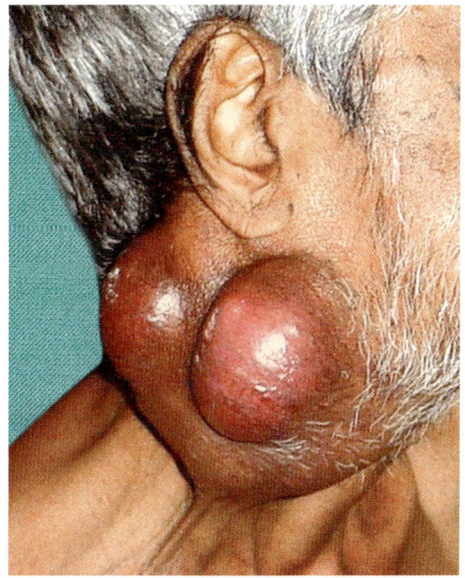

Fig. 15.3: Rapidly growing swelling since 4 months—adenoid cystic carcinoma

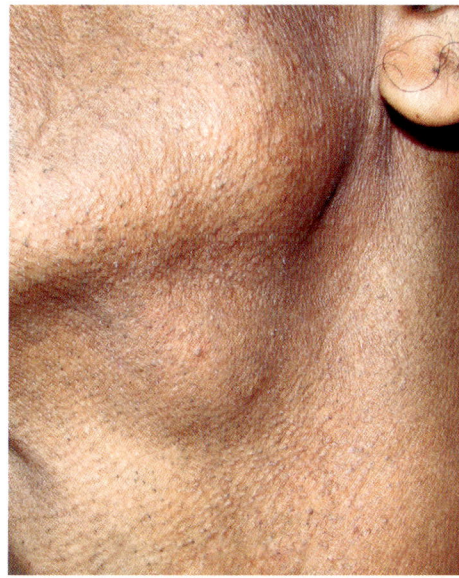

Fig. 15.4: Swelling becomes more prominent when he chews the food. Classical history of stone in the submandibular gland

- If the initial surgery is for malignancy, history of radiation can be elicited.

- In cases of submandibular swellings, swelling *may appear or may increase* in size *following a meal.* It is also associated with *pain* which is *characteristic of calculi in the duct* (Fig. 15.4).

2. *Pain:* Pain can be due to following conditions. In acute parotitis, gland is enlarged and patient has significant pain. Usually it is bilateral. Parotid abscess can give rise to throbbing pain. Mild pain can also be due to malignant transformation in a pleomorphic adenoma.

   - Recurrent parotitis in a child is suggestive of HIV infections.

3. *Discharge: Watery* flow from a sinus in the region of parotid gland is a *parotid fistula.* It occurs when parotid duct is damaged or injured. In such cases, elicit *history of surgery in the parotid region*—maybe for a *swelling* (lymph node) or following drainage of *parotid abscess or following surgery on the parotid gland* (refer to page 220).

4. *Any drooling of saliva:* This should be enquired only when you suspect malignancy such as in a rapidly growing parotid swelling. If present, it indicates facial nerve paralysis.

5. Frequent enlargement of submandibular gland suggests **autoimmune disorder.** In such patients, enquire about joint pain.

6. Are there any other swellings in the neck? It can be lymph node enlargement and it suggests malignancy.

Clinical Wisdom

Recurrent parotitis, recurrent pancreatitis, recurrent panosteitis (bone pains)–Suspect autoimmune aetiology.

Past History

- History of surgery for parotid tumours. Invariably it is pleomorphic adenoma. It has recurred because of enucleation (should not be done) or adequate parotidectomy had not been done. Rapid recurrence is due to malignant parotid tumour.

- Recurrent pain and swelling of parotid glands since childhood suggest congenital sialectasis—a difficult problem to treat.

Inspection

1. **Swelling:** If you see a swelling, describe it in the usual way like location, size, shape, surface and borders. Parotid swellings are usually situated *below, in front of and behind the lobule of the ear.* Often ear lobule is raised (Figs 15.5 to 15.7).

   - Ear lobule may not be raised in a few cases because the tumour may be arising from lower pole of the parotid.

   - Typically, *pleomorphic adenoma* will have *nodular surface. Adenolymphoma* will have *smooth surface* and *carcinoma* will have *irregular surface.* As upper attachment of the parotid fascia is to the zygomatic arch, upper extent of the swelling is limited (Fig. 15.6) to a maximum of up to the zygomatic process.

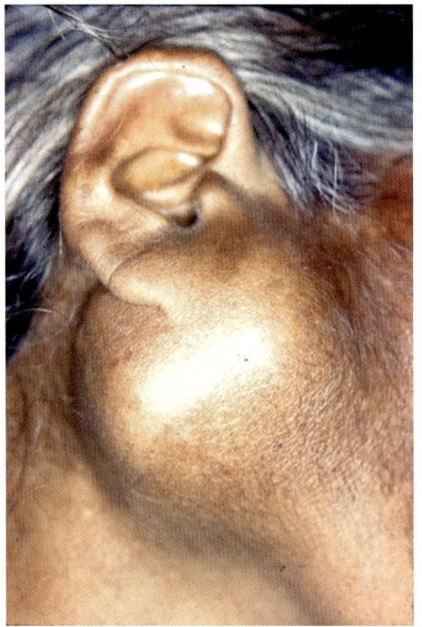

Fig. 15.5: Typically, swelling is located below, in front and behind the ear lobule and lifting the ear lobule

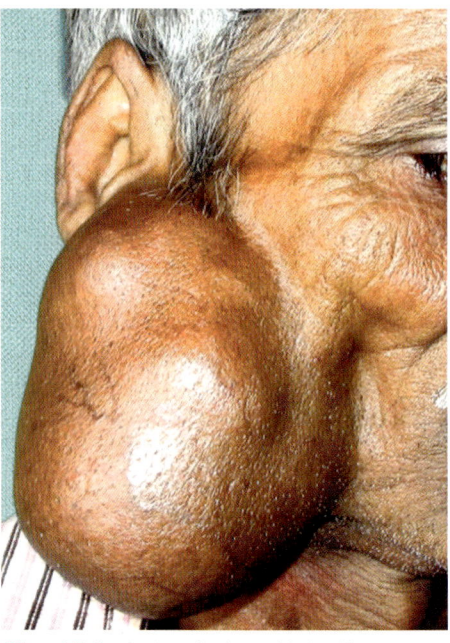

Fig. 15.6: Lateral view. Note the upper extent limited up to zygomatic process, described as **curtain sign positive**

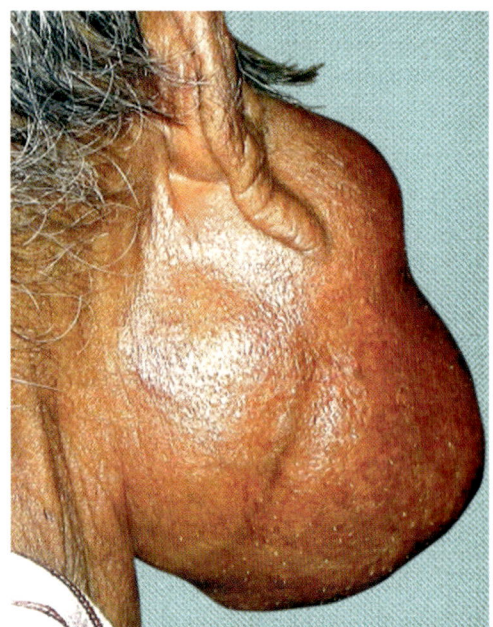

Fig. 15.7: Ear lobe is raised and obliteration of retromandibular groove (*Courtesy:* Dr Vijay Kamath, Professor of Surgery, KIMS, Hubballi)

2. Look for the **retromandibular groove** (between mandible and mastoid process) which is usually obliterated in parotid swellings (Fig. 15.7).

3. Check the extent carefully all around anteriorly also (Fig. 15.8).

4. Presence of **dilated veins** (Fig. 15.9), redness over the swelling, indicates malignancy of the parotid gland. However, if redness and skin oedema are present with short duration of swelling, it indicates parotitis or parotid abscess.

5. **Ask the patient to close the eyes.** Look for rolling of the eyeball above (Bell's palsy). If present, it indicates facial nerve paralysis—a sign of malignancy of the parotid gland.

6. Ask the patient to clench his teeth and make a note of any deviation of the angle. It suggests facial nerve paralysis (Fig. 15.10).

7. Mention, if any lymph node swelling, if it is visible in the neck.

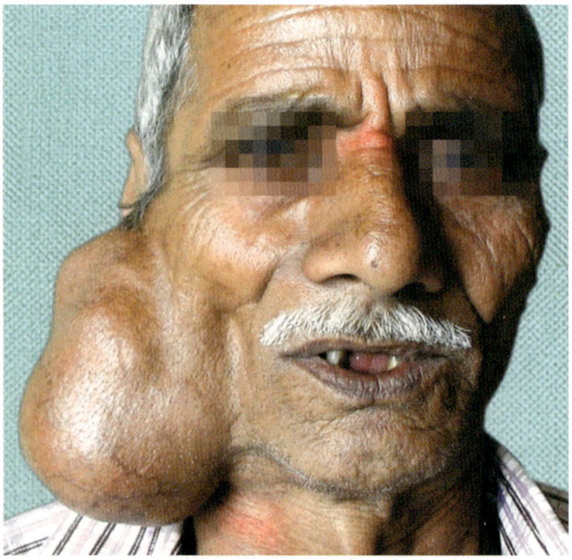

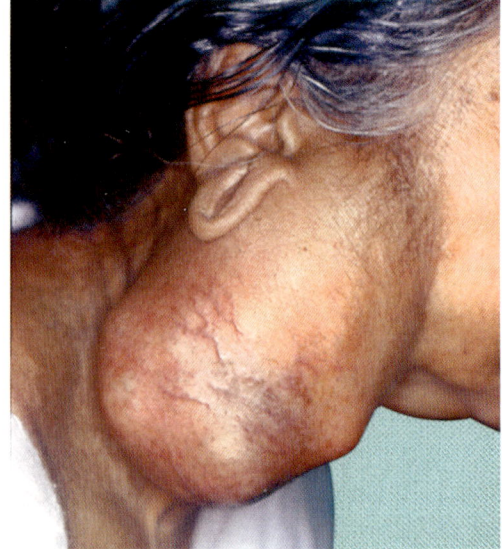

Fig. 15.8: Nodular surface—large pleomorphic adenoma (*Courtesy:* Dr Vijay Kamath, KIMS, Hubballi)

Fig. 15.9: Rapidly growing swelling with dilated veins

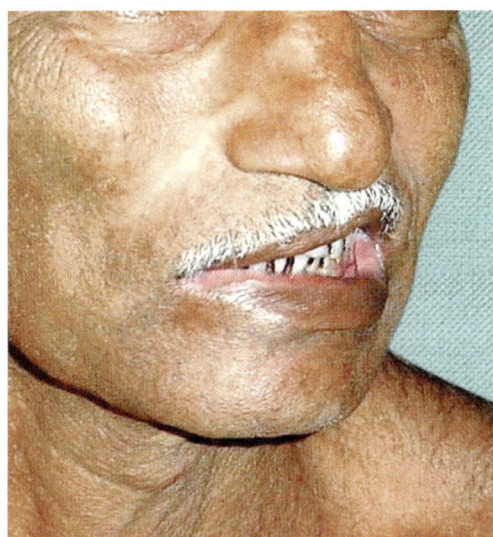

Fig. 15.10: Deviation of the angle of the mouth on clenching the teeth, suggestive of facial nerve paralysis

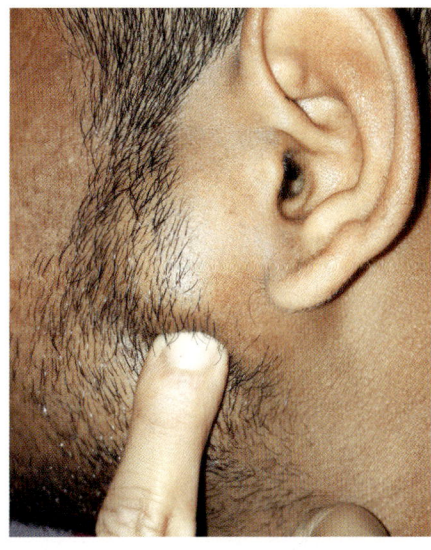

Fig. 15.12: Feeling the lower limit of the swelling (*Courtesy:* Dr Kalyan Reddy, PG student, KMC, Manipal)

8. Ask the patient to open the mouth. Parotid fascia gets stretched. The gland becomes less prominent. It means parotid swellings are deep to parotid fascia.

Palpation

- First look for local rise of temperature and tenderness. If present, they indicate inflammation such as parotitis or parotid abscess. When such features are present in submandibular gland, it suggests sialoadenitis mostly due to calculi. Other causes of enlargement with pain have autoimmune mechanism.

- *Extent*: Check the extension behind mandible and lower limit (Figs 15.11 and 15.12).

- Look for surface, borders and consistency. Consistency is soft in cases of haemangioma, lymphatic cysts or even cold abscess in the intraglandular lymph nodes (rare). Variable consistency is common in rapidly growing neoplasms because of degeneration or necrosis. Typically, carcinomas are stony hard.

- *Intrinsic mobility*: Move the gland in both directions. Generally benign swellings are mobile. It should be remembered that vertical mobility (Fig. 15.13) is up to zygomatic arch because the deep fascia after enclosing the parotid gland is attached to zygomatic arch. This sign is called *curtain sign* (Fig. 15.14).

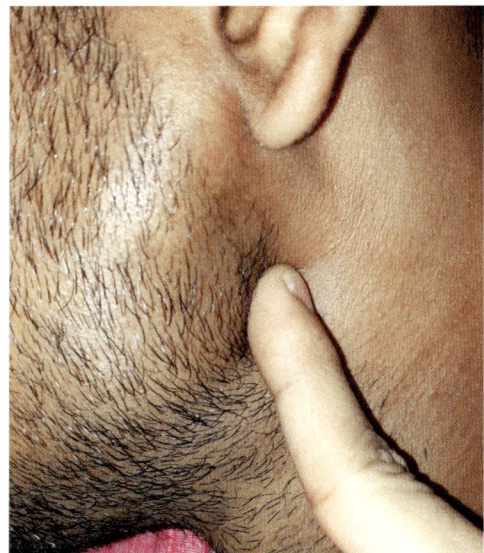

Fig. 15.11: Checking for extension into the retromandibular groove (*Courtesy:* Dr Bharath, Consultant Surgeon, Hassan)

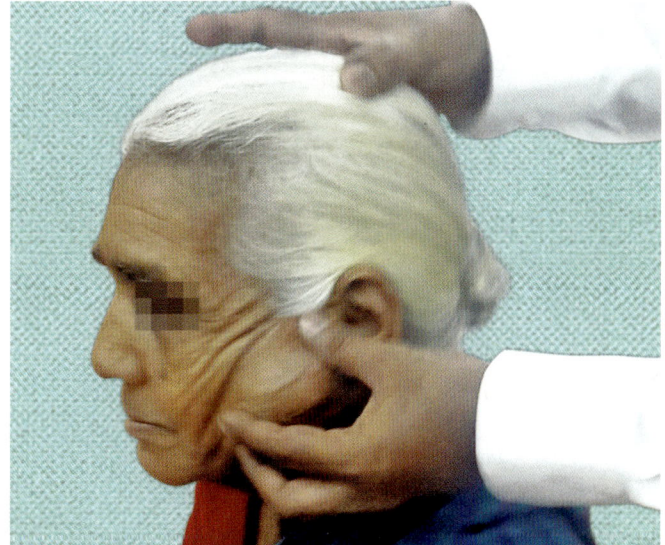

Fig. 15.13: Intrinsic mobility test (*Courtesy:* Dr Ramaniah NV, Principal, SV Medical College, Tirupathi)

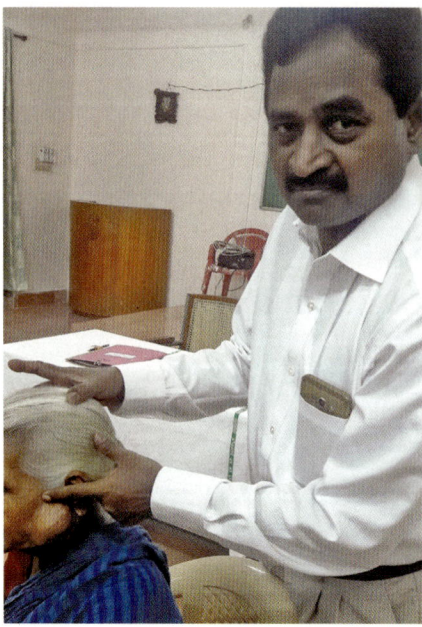

Fig. 15.14: Upper border can reach only up to zygomatic process—curtain sign positive. (*Courtesy*: Dr Ramaniah NV, Principal, SV Medical College, Tirupathi)

- *Masseter contraction test*: Ask the patient to clench the teeth and check the mobility of the gland. *Restricted mobility* suggests swelling infiltrating the muscle. It suggests a malignant lesion (Fig. 15.15). If swelling becomes more prominent, it is super-ficial to masseter (Figs 15.16 and 15.17).

- *Examine mastoid for tenderness*: If present, it suggests spread of malignant tumour. This happens mainly in adenoid cystic carcinoma wherein perineural spread can occur at a distant site resulting in bony resorption (Fig. 15.18).

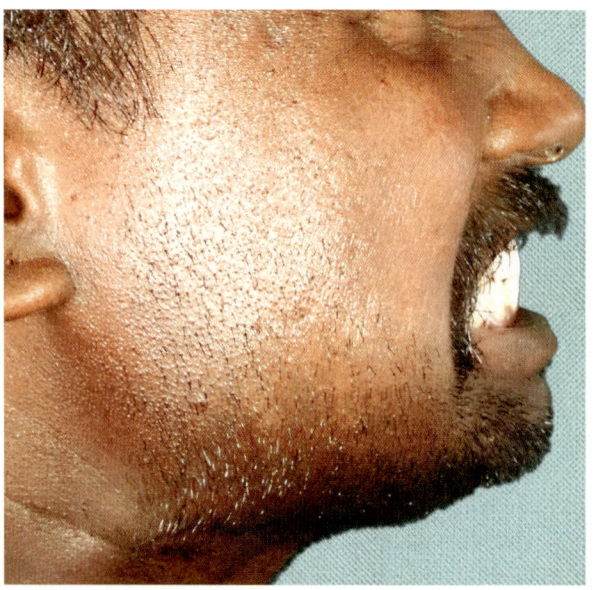

Fig. 15.15: Masseter contraction test

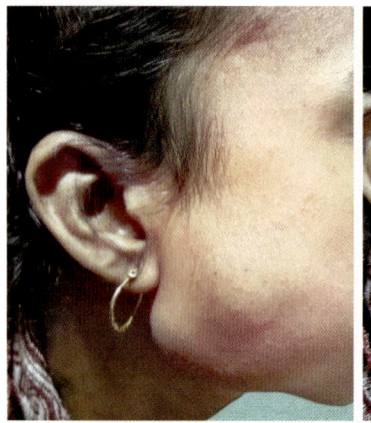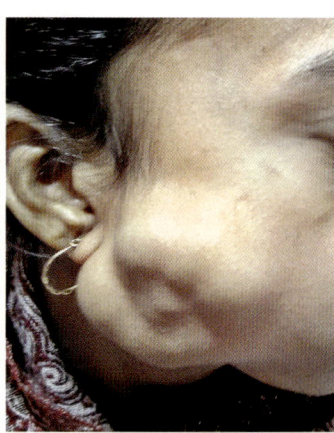

Fig. 15.16: Parotid lymphangioma, **Fig. 15.17:** Plane of the swelling. The patient is asked to contract masseter. Swelling becomes more prominent. (*Courtesy*: Dr Iniyan Samarasan, Dr Sukriya Nayak, Professors of Surgery, CMC, Vellore)

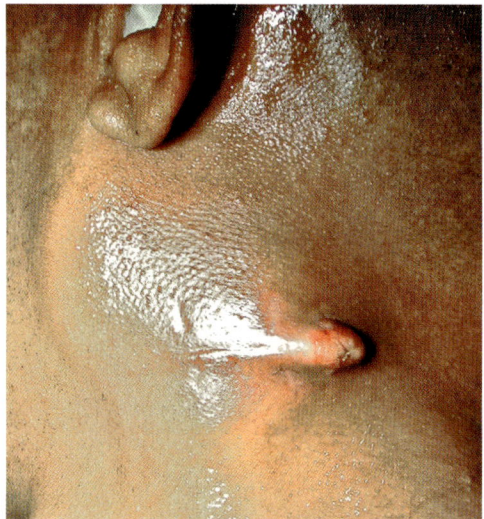

Fig. 15.18: Adenoid cystic carcinoma spreads along perineural sheath distally into bones. Look for mastoid tenderness

* Features of parotid swelling are given in Clinical Box 15.1.

Clinical Box 15.1 🗝️

Classical features of the parotid swelling
1. It presents as a swelling in front, below and behind ear
2. Raises ear lobule
3. Retromandibular groove is obliterated
4. Upper limit is confined to zygomatic arch
5. On opening the mouth, gland becomes less prominent

Examination of Regional Lymph Nodes

- Parotid glands drain into lymph nodes in the posterior triangle (upper) level-5. When the nodes are enlarged due to metastasis, they are hard and with restricted mobility.

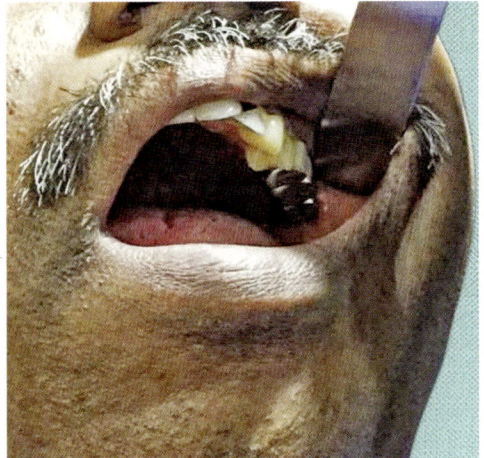

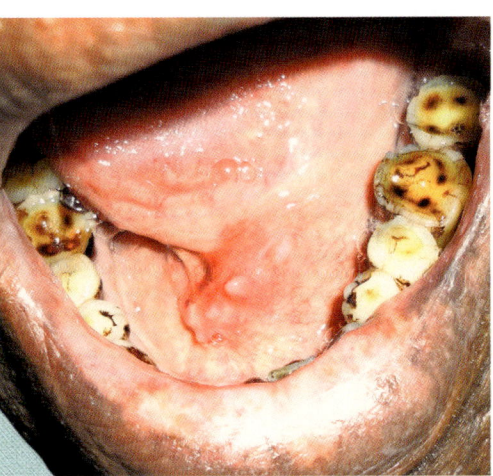

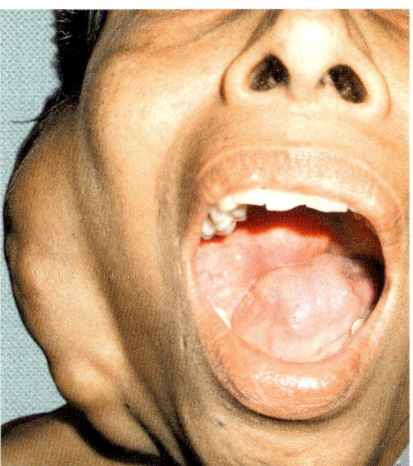

Fig. 15.19: Examination of opening of the parotid duct

Fig. 15.20: Inflamed opening of submandibular duct

Fig. 15.21: Deep lobe tumour

- When lymph nodes in the region of parotid are enlarged—preauricular, possibilities of tuberculosis or lymphoma also to be kept in mind.

Examination of other Salivary Glands

- Autoimmune disorders (Mikulicz disease), metabolic disorders (diabetes, acromegaly), granulomatous disorders (sarcoidosis, toxoplasmosis), and alcoholic cirrhosis affects glands on both sides.
- Tumour, such as Warthin's tumour, affects both parotid glands.

Intraoral Examination

With good illumination, following points to be noted:

- **Examination of the parotid duct (Stensen's duct) opening:** Opposite the upper 2nd molar tooth (Fig. 15.19). Redness surrounding the orifice suggests inflammation. If pus is seen coming out, it is a case of suppurative parotitis specially when you apply gentle pressure over the surface. **Surface marking of Stensen's duct:** One finger breadth below the lower border of zygomatic bone.
- **Examination of the orifice of the** submandibular duct **(Wharton's duct)** by asking the patient to move the tongue and to touch the palate and look at the undersurface of the tongue on either side of the frenulum of tongue (Fig. 15.20).
- **Examination of the tonsils and pharyngeal wall:** In deep lobe enlargement of the parotid gland, the tonsils and pharyngeal wall may be pushed medially. Tongue should be depressed with tongue depressor. This test should be done in good light (Fig. 15.21). If you get these intraoral finding, then palpate behind the mandible with another finger as shown in Fig.15.22. This is called as bidigital method of palpation of the parotid gland.

- **Bidigital examination for deep lobe of the submandibular gland** (Figs 15.23).
- **Examination of hard palate to look for accessory glands** (Fig. 15.24).

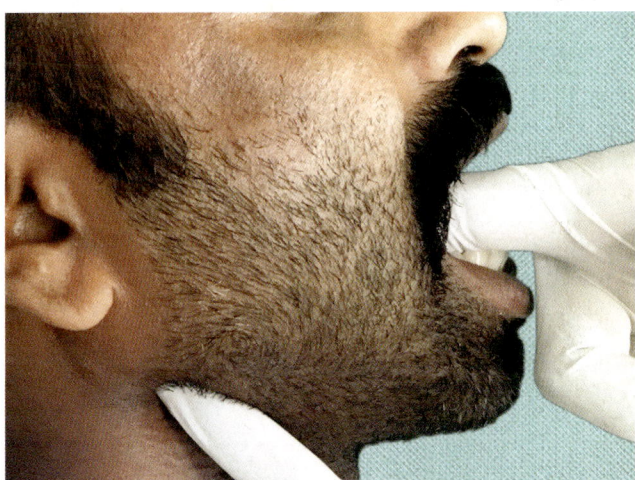

Fig. 15.22: Bidigital palpation for deep lobe tumours

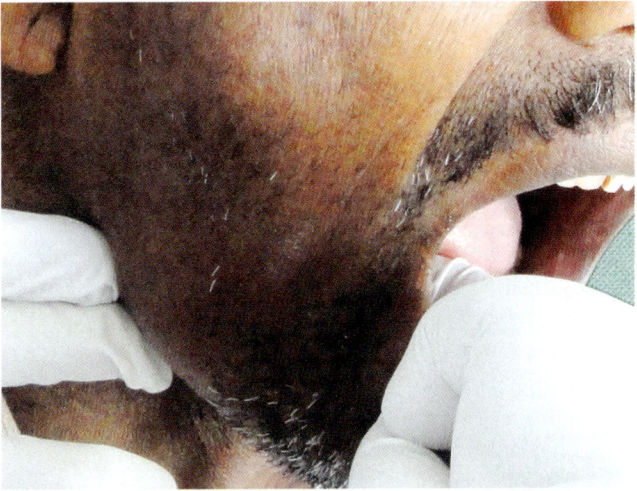

Fig. 15.23: Bidigital palpation of submandibular gland

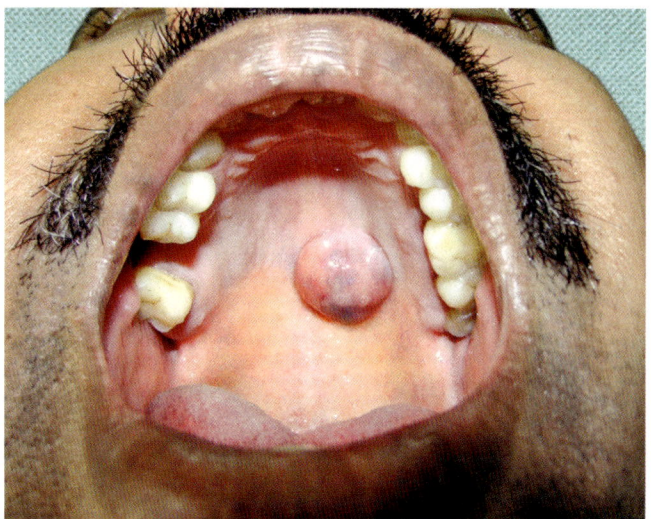

Fig. 15.24: Palate is the most common site of accessory salivary gland

Intraoral examination in salivary gland
1. *Parotid duct* opening—opposite the crown of 2nd upper molar tooth.
2. *Papilla* of the submandibular duct opening—side of frenulum of the tongue.
3. *Parapharyngeal shift*—due to deep lobe enlargement.
4. *Palate*—ectopic tissue—commonest site.
5. *Floor of mouth*—for enlargement of deep lobe of submandibular gland.

Clinical Wisdom

Submandibular gland has a large cervical and a small buccal part. The buccal part is above the mylohyoid muscle. By bidigital method, one should ascertain that both parts are contiguous swellings.

- **Bidigital palpation of the submandibular duct and gland:** It can be done by inserting the finger between the alveolus and tongue. The other finger is placed under the jaw. Slowly *both fingers are withdrawn*. If there is a calculus in the duct, it can be appreciated.

- The *finger inside the oral cavity* can also feel the *deep part* of the submandibular salivary gland, if it is enlarged but not when submandibular lymph node is enlarged because deep lobe is situated *above mylohyoid muscle* and lymph node below the muscle (Clinical Box 15.2).

- Differential diagnosis (Table 15.1)

CLINICAL CHECKLIST IN SALIVARY GLAND SWELLINGS

1. Examination of swelling in general—size, shape surface, borders, consistency, mobility, and plane of the swelling.
2. Look for facial nerve paralysis in case of parotid tumours.
3. Examination of the mastoid process.
4. Look for enlargement of lymph nodes in the neck.
5. Look for all other salivary glands in the neck on both sides.
6. Intraoral examination for deep lobe enlargement in parotid and submandibular tumours.
7. Look for openings of the salivary ducts.
8. Palpate spleen, if you suspect autoimmune aetiology.

Table 15.1: Differential diagnosis of a 2 cm swelling in front of tragus of the ear		
	Solid swelling	*Cystic swelling*
1. Parotid—benign	Pleomorphic adenoma	Warthin's tumour
2. Parotid—malignancy	Mucoepidermoid carcinoma	Adenoid cystic carcinoma
3. Lymph node—benign	Tuberculosis—matted nodes	Cold abscess
4. Lymph node—malignancy	Non-Hodgkin's lymphoma	Metastasis
5. Neural tumour	Neurofibroma	—
6. Fat	Lipoma	—
7. Congenital	—	Dermoid cyst, haemangioma Lymphangioma

*Parts drained by preauricular lymph node can be remembered as **SCALP**
- **S**calp
- **C**heek, conjunctiva
- **A**uditory meatus external
- **L**id—upper eyelid, eyebrow
- **P**art of face—forehead

- Parotid swelling is deep to capsule of the parotid gland hence has restricted mobility
- Parotid lymph node is superficial to capsule of the parotid gland and hence it has free mobility

TESTS FOR FACIAL NERVE PARALYSIS

1. **Ask the patient to close the eyelids.**

   He will not be able to close eyelids and eyeball is rolled upwards. This is called Bell's phenomenon. It indicates lower motor neuron palsy of facial nerve.

2. **Ask the patient to show his teeth.**

   Angle of mouth is drawn to normal side due to contraction of muscle on normal side.

3. **Ask the patient to blow out with closed lips.**

   Paralysed side blows out more than normal side.

4. **Ask the patient to move eyebrow upwards.**

   He will not be able to do.

CLINICAL DISCUSSION

1. **Where do you feel parotid duct?**
   One finger breadth below the inferior border of the zygomatic bone.
2. **When do you suspect malignant changes in pleomorphic adenoma?**
   Refer to Clinical Box 15.3.
3. **Facial nerve comes out of which foramen?**
   Stylomastoid foramen.
4. **How is the retromandibular vein formed?**
   Formed by union of superficial temporal vein and maxillary vein.
5. **What is pes anserinus?**
   5 terminal branches of facial nerve resembling foot of a goose is called pes anserinus.
6. **Chronic parotitis in children is pathognomonic of what condition?**
   HIV infection.
7. **Bilateral parotid enlargement is due to what tumour?**
   Warthin's tumour.
8. **What specific organ enlargement should be looked for in the abdomen?**
   If there is any suspicion of autoimmune disease, look for enlargement of spleen.
9. **How does an enlarged deep lobe reach parapharyngeal part?**
   It is through stylomandibular tunnel of Patey.
10. **What is the most common parotid gland tumour?**
    Pleomorphic adenoma.

Clinical Box 15.3

Malignant changes in pleomorphic adenoma
- It starts growing rapidly
- Skin infiltration occurs
- Facial nerve paralysis occurs
- Gets fixed to masseter muscle
- Red, dilated veins over the surface
- Presence of lymph nodes in the neck
- Tumour feels stony hard

DIFFERENTIAL DIAGNOSIS

PAROTID SWELLING

I. Painful Parotid Swellings

1. ***Mumps parotitis***: Mumps is an acute generalised viral disease with painful enlargement of salivary glands, chiefly the parotids. The virus belongs to Paramyxoviridae family and only one serotype is known. Incubation period is 10–24 days. Fever, headache and muscular pain are usually found. Both parotids are enlarged with pain and temperature. Swelling starts subsiding by 3–7 days of time.

2. ***Acute bacterial parotitis***: *Staphylococcus aureus* infection of parotid produces serious illness with marked engorgement of parotid. Typically, it produces parotid abscess. Diabetes, malignancy, and malnutrition increase the risk. Decreased salivary secretion is an important predisposing factor (Fig. 15.25).

3. ***Postoperative parotitis*** can be prevented by good mouth care and good oral hygiene. Due to poor oral hygiene, ascending infection occurs from the oral cavity resulting in parotitis. A patient who is recovering in the postoperative period may complain of pain and swelling in the parotid region. Presence of severe pain with a very sick, toxic look and high grade fever, chills and rigors indicates parotid abscess. **Diffuse brawny swelling is characteristic.** Fluctuation is a late feature. The opening of the parotid duct may be inflamed and on gentle compression of the parotid gland, pus can be seen coming out of the parotid duct.

4. ***Recurrent parotitis of childhood***
   - Children between ages of 3 and 6 years are commonly affected. Aetiology is unknown. It may be due to sialectasis (dilatation of branches of salivary duct). Recurrent pain and

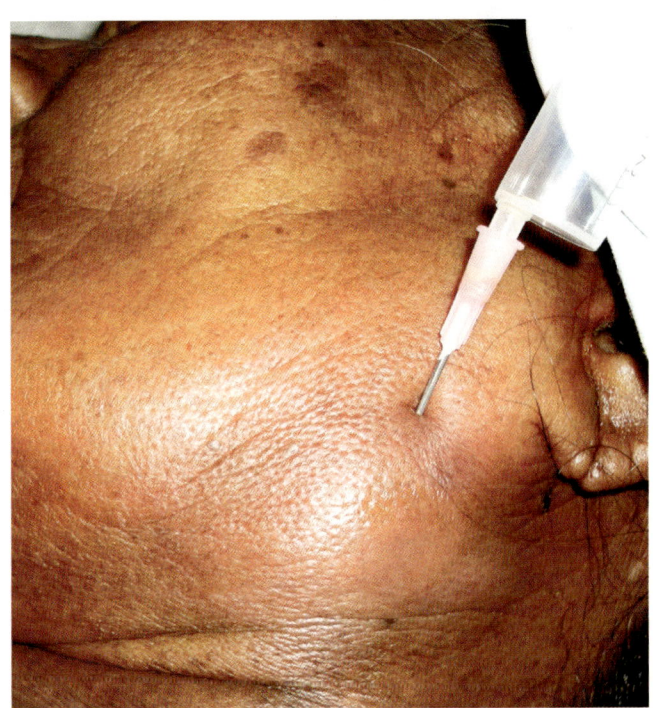

Fig. 15.25: Bacterial parotitis, needle is inserted to check for pus

swelling of one or both parotids are common. Each attack may last for 3 to 7 days. It is **self-limiting** (if the attack is minor).

- *Sialography* shows **punctate sialectasis**—called **snowstorm** appearance. A short-course of antibiotics has to be given to cover *Staphylococcus viridans*.

5. Sialoadenitis due to autoimmune disorders

a. *Sjögren's syndrome*: This disease is 10 times more common in females and presents with painful enlargement of the glands. It is the diffuse infiltration of salivary and lacrimal glands with lymphocytes resulting in enlargement of glands and slow destruction of acini. Thus, clinical features include dry eyes (keratoconjunctivitis sicca) and dry mouth (xerostomia). Lingual papillary atrophy is also an important feature. These along with a third component rheumatoid arthritis, form the triad of **Sjögren's syndrome**. 30% of patients with systemic lupus erythematosus and all patients with primary biliary cirrhosis develop Sjögren's syndrome. This is termed as **secondary Sjögren's syndrome**.

b. *Mikulicz disease*: Due to autoimmune mechanism, symmetrical enlargement of all salivary glands and lacrimal glands occur. Dry mouth and narrow palpebral fissures are diagnostic of this condition.

Clinical Wisdom

Autoimmune thyroiditis will predispose to lymphoma of the thyroid and autoimmune sialoadenitis will predispose to lymphoma of the parotid gland.

II. Painless Parotid Swellings

1. Pleomorphic adenoma of parotid gland (mixed tumour):
It is the most common benign salivary gland neoplasm which occurs in middle-aged women, around 40 years (Figs 15.26 to 15.29).

Clinical Wisdom

Female, fifth decade and fullness near ear lobule.

Pathology: Epithelial cells proliferate in strands, or may be arranged in the form of acini or cords. There are also myoepithelial cells which proliferate in sheets. They are called spindle-shaped cells. The tumour produces mucoid material which displaces and separates the cells resembling cartilage in histological section.

Clinical features: Typically, a history of a very slow-growing swelling (for a few years) is usually present. **The swelling is painless.** Any painless swelling near the ear is best assumed to be parotid gland neoplasm unless proved otherwise on examination.

Swelling has the following classical features:

- It presents as a **swelling in front**, below and behind ear.
- **Raises ear lobule.**
- **Retromandibular groove** is obliterated.

It is rubbery or firm. Soft areas indicate necrosis. In long-standing cases, it can be hard. Surface can be nodular or sometimes bosselated. Skin is stretched and shiny. However, being a benign tumour, it is neither adherent to the skin nor to the masseter.

After a few years, pleomorphic adenoma may show features of transformation into malignancy (carcinoma expleomorphic adenoma).

It should be suspected when

- It starts growing rapidly
- Skin infiltration occurs
- Facial nerve paralysis occurs
- Gets fixed to masseter muscle
- Red, dilated veins over the surface
- Presence of lymph nodes in the neck
- Tumour feels stony hard
- Once clinically suspected, ultrasound followed by FNAC is done to confirm the diagnosis and conservative superficial parotidectomy is the treatment of choice.
- In large tumours, deep lobe tumours and suspected malignancies, CT scan/MRI is done to assess for operability. Treatment in malignant cases is total parotidectomy.

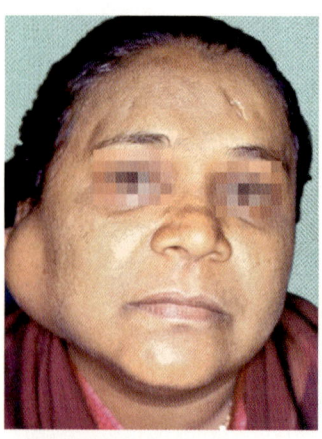

Fig. 15.26A: Anterior view of pleomorphic adenoma

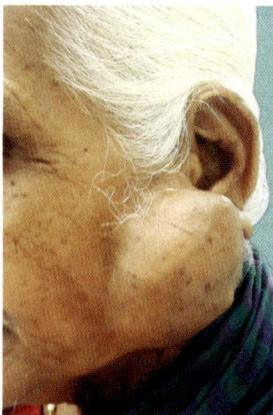

Fig. 15.26B: Classical site and classical features

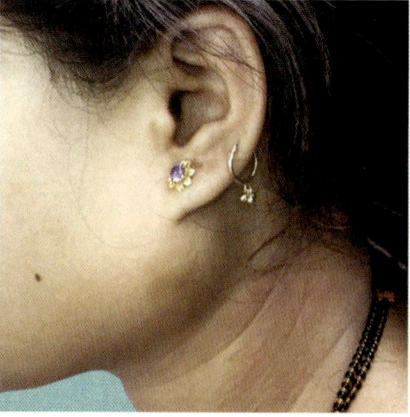

Fig. 15.27: Pleomorphic adenoma arising from lower pole of the parotid gland

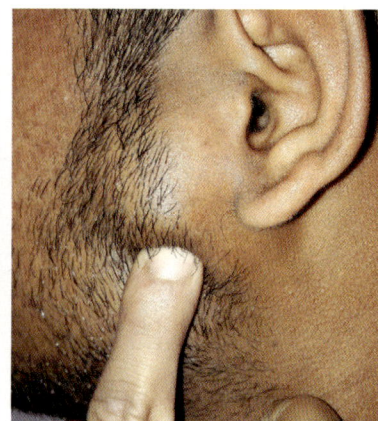

Fig. 15.28: In front of ear lobule—ear lobule is not raised

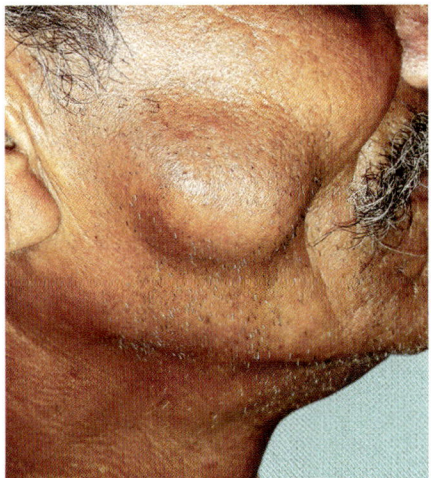 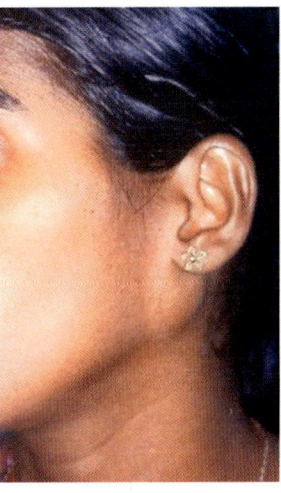 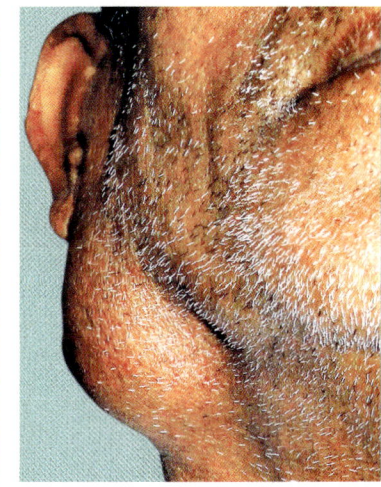

Fig. 15.29: Swelling is quite a distance from the ear lobule but FNAC—pleomorphic adenoma

Figs 15.30A and B: Typical site of Warthin's tumour. Ear lobule is also raised (*Courtesy*: Dr Vijendra, Assistant Professor, KMC, Manipal)

Fig. 15.31: Adenolymphoma—view from the front

Always conserve facial nerve if possible. Postoperative radiotherapy may be required.

2. *Adenolymphoma (Warthin's tumour, papillary cystadenoma lymphomatosum)*

- Adenolymphoma is not a lymphoma. It is a benign parotid tumour and next common to pleomorphic adenoma. **Origin of adenolymphoma:** During development, some parotid tissues get included within lymph nodes (preparotid) which are present within the parotid sheath.

- Interestingly, they do not occur in blacks.

- Middle-aged or elderly males are commonly affected—usually **they are smokers**.

- Can be **bilateral**, in some cases (10%).

- It has smooth surface, round border with soft, cystic consistency (Figs 15.30 and 15.31).

- Classically, it is situated at the lower pole of parotid elevating the ear lobule. Sometimes it may be **multicentric**.

- **This tumour affects only parotid gland** (very, very rarely other glands may be affected) (Table 15.2).

Treatment: It has got a well-defined capsule. Hence, enucleation used to be done earlier **but not now. Superficial parotidectomy is the treatment of choice** (Fig. 15.32).

3. *Adenoid cystic carcinoma*

- It is a highly malignant tumour consisting of cords of dark staining cells with cystic spaces containing mucin. It also consists of myoepithelial cells and duct epithelium.

- Even though **slow-growing**, it spreads along the **perineural tissue,** may invade periosteum or medullary bone at a distance. This bone resorption results in bony tenderness (Figs 15.33 and 15.34).

Table 15.2: Comparison between pleomorphic adenoma and adenolymphoma

Features	Pleomorphic adenoma	Adenolymphoma
1. Incidence	70–80%	10%
2. Sex	Common in females	Common in males
3. Number	Single	Sometimes multiple
4. Site	Unilateral	Bilateral
5. Clinical feature	Nodular, firm	Smooth, soft cystic
6. Histology	Pleomorphism	Double layer epithelium and lymphoid tissue
7. ^{99m}Tc-pertechnetate scan	Cold spot	Hot spot
8. Treatment	Superficial parotidectomy	Superficial parotidectomy
9. Can progress into	Carcinoma	No
10. Location	Parotid gland	Near the tail of parotid
11. Age	30–40 years	60–70 years
12. Strong association with smoking	+	–

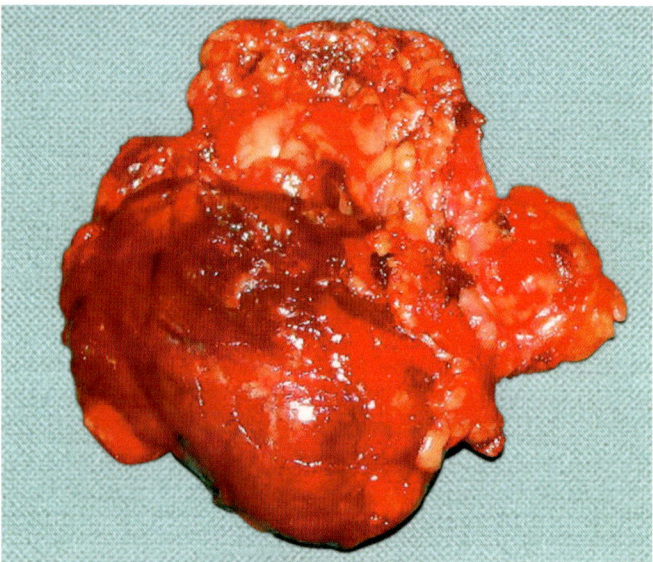

Fig. 15.32: Adenolymphoma

- These tumours have **high incidence of distant metastasis** but in general **they display indolent growth**. Local infiltration, lymphatic and blood spread and local recurrence are important features.

- It is **hard and fixed** and can produce **anaesthesia of the skin overlying the tumour**.

4. *Mucoepidermoid tumour*

- As name itself suggests, it consists of sheets of epidermoid cells and cystic spaces lined by mucus secreting cells. **In childhood, it is the commonest parotid tumour.** They are benign, slow growing but hard in consistency. (Adenolymphoma and mixed tumours are firm but mucoepidermoid tumour is hard.) Parotid is the commonest site. In cases of minor salivary glands, palate is the commonest site.

- Mucoepidermoid tumours can infiltrate local tissues, lymph nodes or skin. Hence, a few consider that **mucoepidermoid tumours are always carcinomatous** (Figs 15.35 to 15.37).

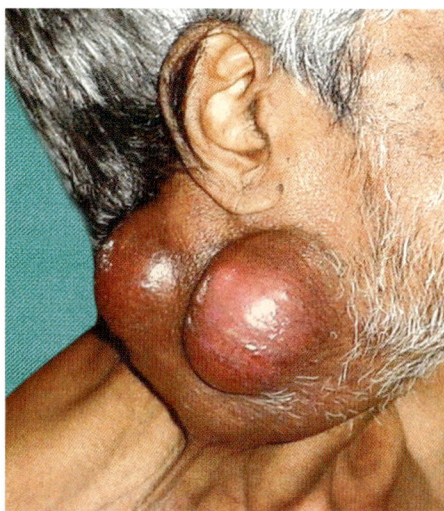

Fig. 15.33: Adenoid cystic carcinoma—rapidly growing. Skin and platysma involved

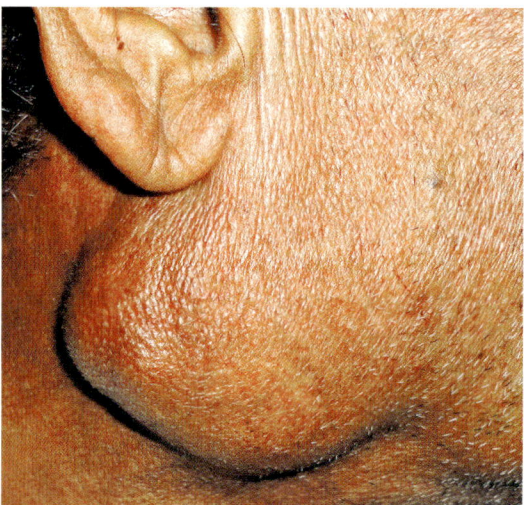

Fig. 15.35: Mucoepidermoid carcinoma—low grade 1 year duration

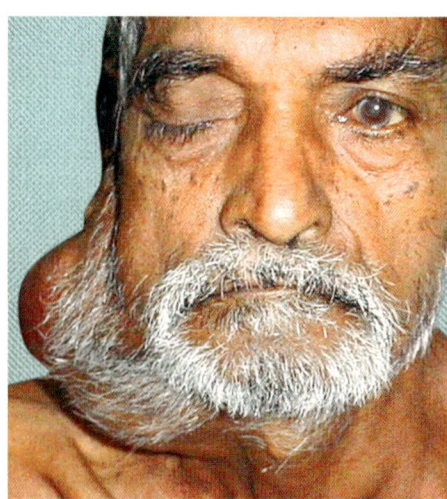

Fig. 15.34: Same patient in Fig. 15.21 with facial nerve paralysis

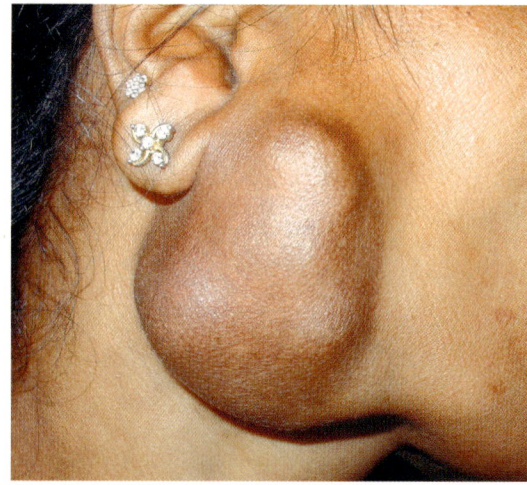

Fig. 15.36: Intermediate grade mucoepidermoid tumour. (*Courtesy*: Dr Dilip Amonkar, Head, Department of Surgery, Government Medical College, Goa)

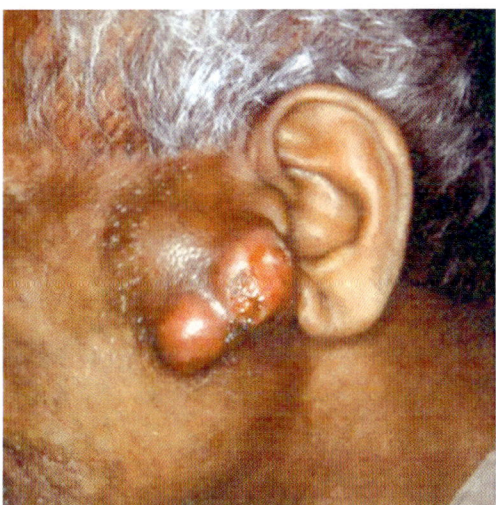

Fig. 15.37: High grade mucoepidermoid tumour with skin ulceration

<table>
<tr><td>

Clinical Wisdom

- Well-differentiated tumours behave like benign tumours, intermediate ones are aggressive and undifferentiated tumours, metastasise early.
- Mucoepidermoid carcinoma is the most common malignant epithelial neoplasm of salivary gland.

</td></tr>
</table>

5. *Miscellaneous swellings arising from parotid gland*

a. *First branchial cleft cysts:* These cysts can occur within the lymph nodes in the parotid gland and on the surface of the gland. They are painless, cystic lesions about a few cm in size. They usually affect superficial lobe. These cysts occur due to the inclusion of branchial apparatus remnants or due to the remaining cervical sinus. Other theory is that cysts are due to changes in the epithelium trapped in the cervical node.

b. *AIDS related—benign lymphoepithelial lesions:* These are due to obstruction of the intraglandular ducts due to

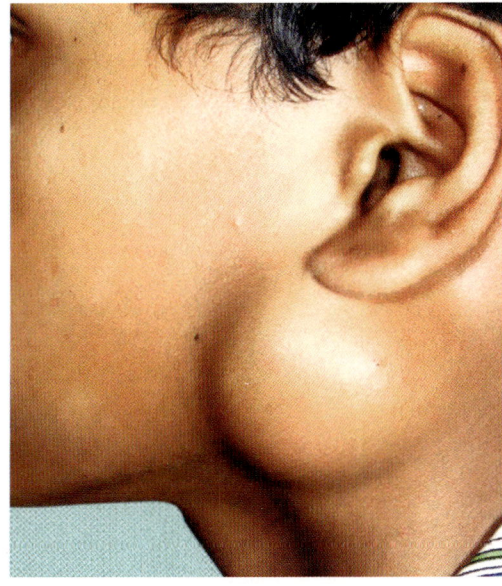

Fig. 15.38: Haemangioma of the parotid gland

lymphoid hyperplasia as it occurs in AIDS patients. They are mixed swellings with and solid cystic components.

c. *Haemangioma:* It is the most common benign tumour in children. Typically, a soft fluctuant swelling which is cystic but not transilluminant (Fig. 15.38).

d. *Lymphangioma:* Parotid lymphangiomas are very, very rare unlike haemangioma. Fluctuation and transillumination are the key clinical signs (*see* Fig. 15.16, page 210).

CLINICAL DISCUSSION

1. **What are dumbbell tumours?**

   Deep lobe tumours present as dysphagia. Such tumours may not show gross swelling on the outer aspect but as they grow, they pass through the stylomandibular tunnel of Patey and push the pharyngeal wall, tonsil and soft palate. These tumours are called **dumbbell tumours.**

2. **Why should superficial parotidectomy be done for pleomorphic adenoma?**

   - As the tumour grows, it compresses the normal parotid tissue and the branches of the tumour penetrate the thin capsule and enter the substance of the parotid.
   - These are called pseudopods. Simple enucleation will result in a recurrence. Hence, superficial parotidectomy has to be done.

3. **Why slow-growing parotid tumours should not be subjected to biopsy?**

   - Because of the fear of injury to the facial nerve and seeding of tumour cells in the subcutaneous plane which causes recurrence in about 40–50% of the cases.
   - Chances of salivary fistula are present.

4. **Why the name adenolymphoma?**

   Presence of lymphatic tissue in the stroma and lymph follicles is characteristic of adenolymphoma (hence the name).

5. **What are the drugs causing enlargement of salivary glands?**

   Carbimazole and thiouracil.

6. **What are the metabolic disorders causing enlargement of salivary glands?**

   Diabetes and acromegaly.

7. **What is the role of lingual nerve?**

   Lingual nerves, supply parasympathetic innervation by way of the chorda tympani nerve (from cranial nerve VII) and the submandibular ganglion.

8. **What is the role of myoepithelial cells?**

   When they contract they help saliva enter into the ducts.

9. **What are the causes of granulomatous sialoadenitis?**

   These are rare, painless swellings. Following are the causes:

   - Tuberculosis, sarcoidosis—commonly affects parotid gland wherein it is called pseudotumour.
   - Toxoplasmosis, cat-scratch disease.
   - Wegener's granulomatosis.

10. **What are the causes of sialoadenosis?**

    It refers to non-neoplastic non-inflammatory swelling in association with acinar hypertrophy and ductal atrophy. Five major groups are as follows:

    - Metabolic (e.g. obesity, cirrhosis, malabsorption)

- **E**ndocrine (e.g. diabetes mellitus, hypothyroidism)
- **D**rug induced (e.g. thiourea)
- **I**nflammatory
- **A**utoimmune (e.g. Sjögren disease)
- **N**utritional (e.g. vitamin deficiency, bulimia)

> You can remember as **MEDIAN**

11. What about recurrent parotid tumour?

Recurrent parotid tumour

- Very often, it is due to inadequate primary surgery (first surgery). Enucleation can give rise to up to 60% recurrence (Figs 15.39 and 15.40).

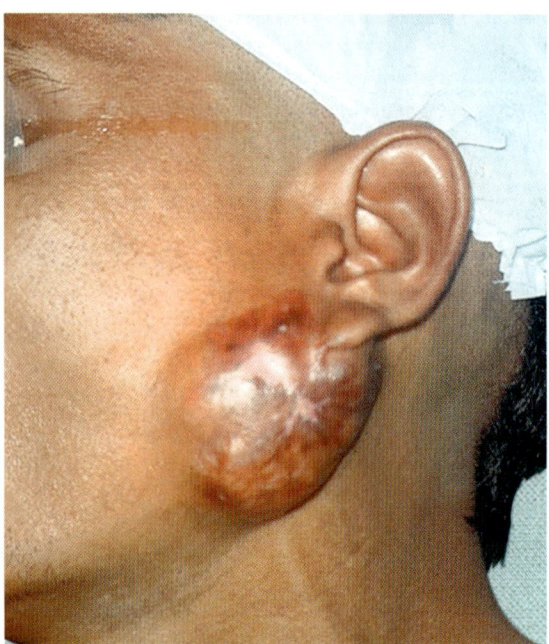

Fig. 15.39: Recurrent parotid tumour

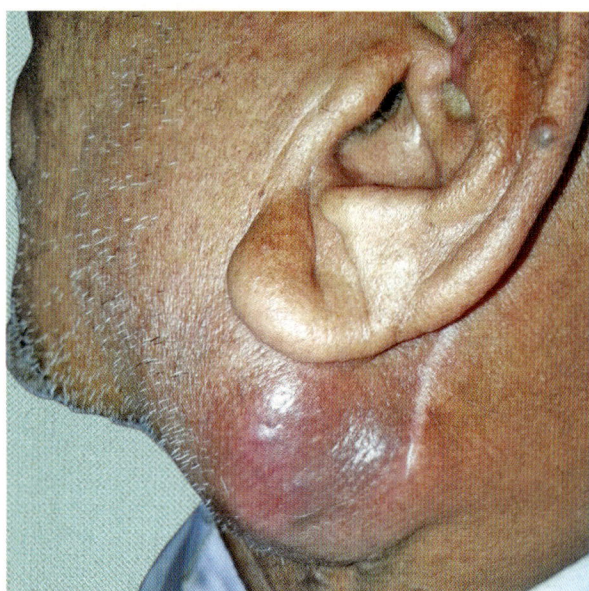

Fig. 15.40: Recurrent highly malignant parotid tumour—adenoid cystic carcinoma

- In 5 to 10% cases, it can occur after adequate parotidectomy (superficial parotidectomy).
- Recurrence is due to pseudopods of the tumour.
- Even though single, recurrent tumours are multicentric, hence multiple.
- Recurrences are often beyond the scar lines.
- During re-excision, plane may be difficult, chances of injury to facial nerve is high.

SUBMANDIBULAR SWELLING

1. *Chronic submandibular sialoadenitis*

- Obstruction is the most important cause of submandibular sialoadenitis. Obstruction can be due to stone—the most common cause, other causes being stricture of the duct, or fibrosis of the papilla. The causative organism is *Staphylococcus*.
- Calculi (80% of them occur in the submandibular salivary gland) commonly occur in the duct and also within the gland and produce recurrent sialoadenitis. Calculi are more common in the submandibular salivary gland than in the parotid gland because of **higher mucin content** in the submandibular salivary gland secretions, rich **calcium and phosphate** content in the secretions, **nondependent drainage** of the secretions and **kinking or hooking** of submandibular duct by lingual nerve (Fig. 15.41).

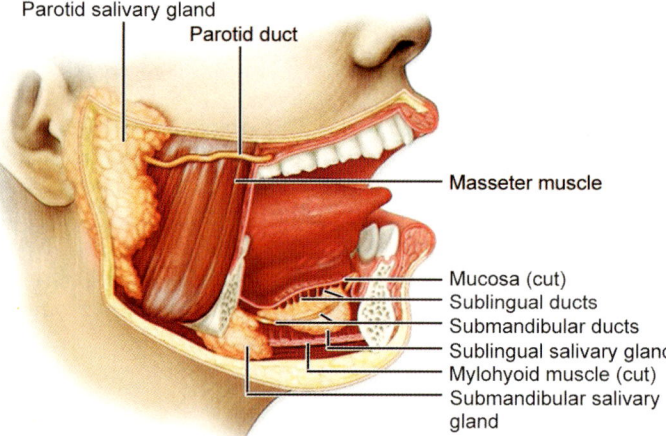

Fig. 15.41: Parotid duct is horizontal but submandibular duct has an upward course

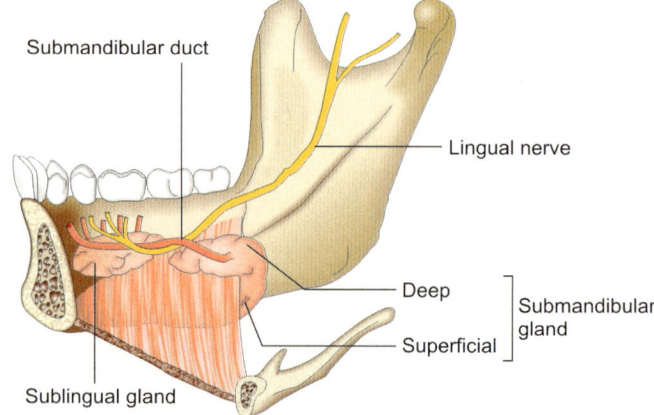

Fig. 15.42: Submandibular duct and lingual nerve

- *Salivary colic*: It is a severe pricking type of pain due to increased tension within the gland which is exaggerated at the time of meals. This results in **enlargement of salivary gland during meals** which **is the characteristic feature of salivary calculus.** Salivary secretions are induced by a meal or lemon (lemon juice test). **Lingual colic:** If a calculus is situated within the submandibular duct where it is hooked by lingual nerve, the pain can radiate to the tongue as a result of irritation to the lingual nerve (Fig. 15.42).

- Classically, submandibular salivary gland swelling is located in the submandibular region. It is firm in consistency with a lobular surface. It is tender and both lobes are enlarged. **It is bidigitally palpable (submandibular lymph node is palpable only in the neck)** both inside the oral cavity and in the neck. The swelling reduces in size once the stimuli are withdrawn (after meals) (Figs 15.43 to 15.47).

- The stone may be palpable within the gland (in the neck), within the duct (intraorally), or sometimes it may be seen at the orifice of the submandibular duct on the side of lingual frenulum.

- Chronic sialoadenitis can give rise to rubbery or hard gland. It can also give rise to stricture of the salivary duct.

2. *Submandibular salivary gland tumours* (Figs 15.43 to 15.47):

- Very often it will be a case of carcinoma. Incidence of carcinoma is more compared to parotid gland. Typically, patients are between 40 and 60 years of age, who complain of slow-growing submandibular surely which is hard and irregular, bidigitally palpable. Infiltration into the skin, lymph node enlargement is not common (Fig. 15.48).

- Differential diagnosis is metastatic submandibular nodes. They are bidigitally not palpable.

- Refer to Clinical Box 15.4 for features of submandibular salivary gland enlargement.

3. *Sublingual and ectopic salivary gland tumours*

- Even though they are called minor, numberwise they are major (many) about 450 in number.

- They are mucus-secreting.

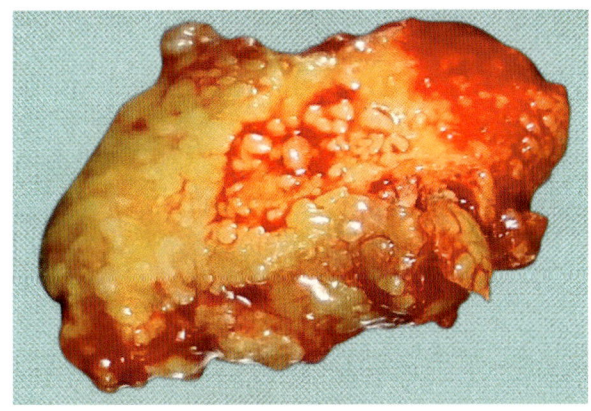

Fig. 15.46: Large stone embedded in the Wharton's duct

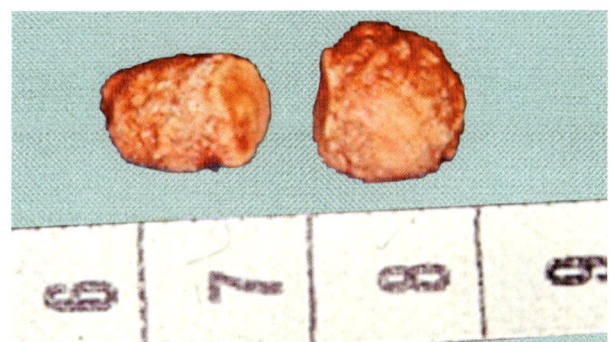

Fig. 15.47: Submandibular duct stones removed by intraoral approach by incising the papilla

---

Clinical Box 15.4

Submandibular salivary gland enlargement
- Location—submandibular region
- Lobular, firm swelling
- Bidigitally palpable
- Stone may be palpable within the duct, intraorally

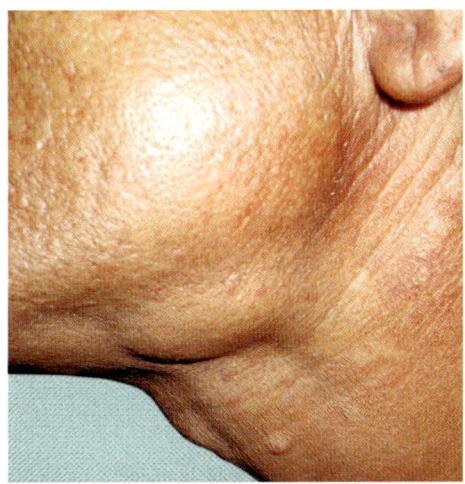

Fig. 15.43: Classical location of submandibular swelling

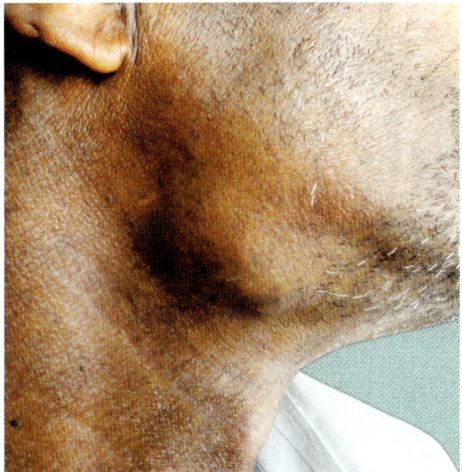

Fig. 15.44: Submandibular sialoadenitis due to a stone. You can see the round border

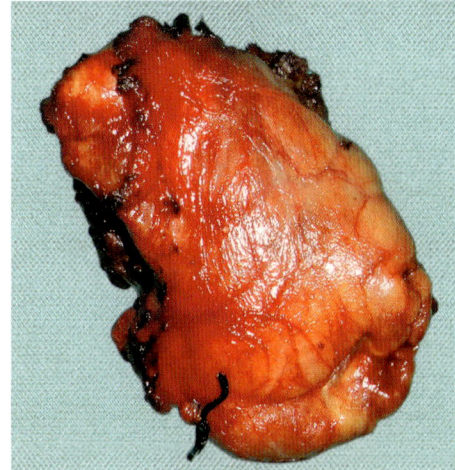

Fig. 15.45: Excised submandibular gland

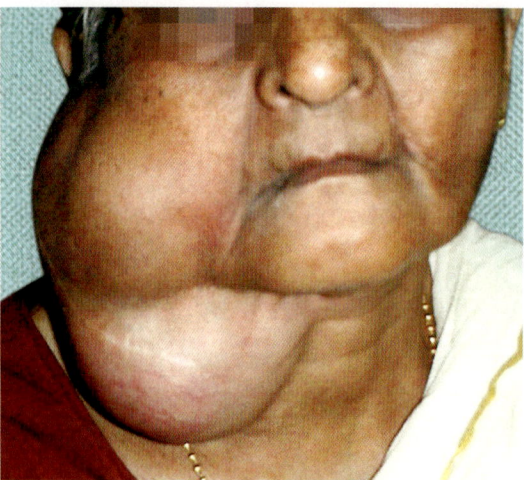

Fig. 15.48: Very large submandibular salivary gland tumour extending onto the face. FNAC suggested pleomorphic adenoma. Such tumours are uncommon in the submandibular salivary gland. (*Courtesy:* Dr Srijayan, Prof of Surgery, Calicut Medical College, Calicut)

• They can present as mucus retention cyst (common in lip) or as malignant tumour.

• 90% of minor salivary gland tumours are malignant.

• Since they are submucosal, they start as a submucous nodule (very important point in the history) to differentiate from carcinoma buccal mucosa/lip, etc.

• As they grow, they ulcerate. Ulceration is a feature of malignancy.

• Slowly lymph nodes get enlarged.

• Treatment of benign cyst/tumour is by simple excision and malignant tumour is by wide excision.

• Other sites of ectopic salivary tissues are buccal mucosa (commonest), nasopharynx, pharynx, lips tongue, etc.

Clinical Box 15.5 🔑

Parotid fistula

• Any surgery on the parotid gland—superficial parotidectomy, drainage of abscess, surgery for carcinoma cheek, and facio-maxillary trauma are the causes.

• Discharging watery fluid, exaggerated by keeping lime in the mouth.

• Fistulogram confirms the diagnosis.

• Exploration and excision of fistula and ligation of duct is required.

Interesting Two Cases—Clinical Case Capsule

I. A case of parotid fistula/sinuses (Clinical Box 15.5)

• **What is the duration of the fluid discharge in front of ear?**

If it is since childhood, often it is a pre-auricular sinus.

• **Have you undergone some surgery in this region.**

If yes, it is a salivary fistula due to ductal damage (Fig. 15.49).

• **Does it increase while eating/during meals?**

If yes, it is a fistula. If not, it is a sinus.

• **What is the differential diagnosis?**

Tubercular sinus.

• **What is it due to?**

It is due to tuberculous lymphadenitis of preparotid group of lymph nodes progressing to cold abscess and rupture.

• **How will you differentiate parotid fistula/sinus from tuberculous sinus?**

 – History of a swelling, rupture (cold abscess)

 – Nature of discharge—cheesy thick (cold abscess)

 – Edge of the sinus—undermined.

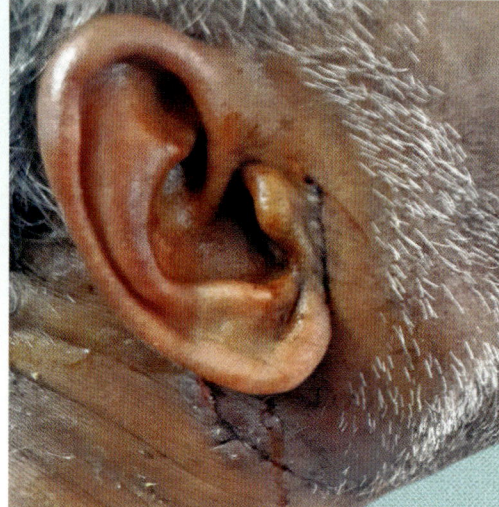

Fig. 15.49: Parotid fistula following superficial parotidectomy

II. A 42-year-old old patient complains of a swelling in front of tragus of the ear mimicking parotid gland enlargement.

• **How will you rule out swelling arising from the parotid gland?**
It is difficult. However, if the swelling is freely mobile, round to oval, it has not raised the ear lobule nor obliterated the retro-mandibular groove, it could be a lymph nodal swelling.

• **If it is a lymph node swelling, what are the causes?**

 – In tuberculosis, lymph nodes are matted with or without cold abscess and sinus formation.

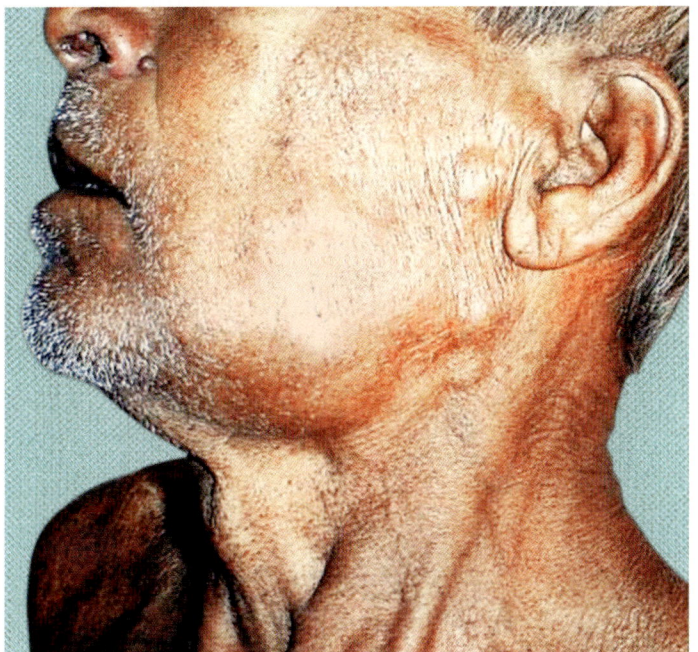

Fig. 15.50: Preauricular lymph node. Is it parotid gland? Look carefully. Submandibular lymph node and other lymph nodes in the neck are also palpable. It is a case of Non-Hodgkin's lymphoma

– Non-Hodgkin's lymphoma can affect preparotid lymph nodes. However, other lymph nodes, such as post-auricular, occipital neck nodes, clinch the diagnosis (Fig. 15.50).

• **If these are metastatic lymph nodes, what are the primary sites (drainage areas)?**
   – Eyebrow—trichilemmal tumours
   – Eyelid
   – Conjunctiva—part of eye
   – External auditory meatus

CLINICAL DISCUSSION

1. **What is the most common cause for submandibular sialoadenitis?**
   It is stone.
2. **Why are stones more common in submandibular gland?**
   • Calcium contents are more.
   • Secretions are more alkaline and mucus.
   • Drainage (opening of gland) is antigravity.
   • Duct has two bends—first at posterior border of mylohyoid muscle and second near the duct orifice.
   • The opening of the duct is narrow.
3. **What are the nerves related to submandibular salivary gland?**
   • Lingual nerve: It is related to the duct.
   • Hypoglossal nerve is in the bed of the gland (deeper). When the gland is mobilised and lifted upwards during excision, this nerve will come into view.
   • Cervical branch of facial nerve may be damaged while incising through the fascia of neck.
4. **What muscle separates superficial and deep parts of the submandibular salivary gland?**
   Mylohyoid muscle
5. **What is mylohyoid muscle also called as?**
   Oral diaphragm
6. **Where are lymph nodes located?**
   They are in the submandibular triangle deep to deep fascia but superficial to mylohyoid muscles. Hence, they are palpable only in the neck.
7. **What test is done to differentiate enlarged lymph nodes from enlarged submandibular salivary gland?**
   Bidigital method of palpation
8. **What is Manipal Rule of '2'**
   Refer to Table 15.3.

Table 15.3: Submandibular salivary gland excision—**Manipal Rule of 2**

• **2** common indications	→ Stone and as a part of radical neck dissection
• **2"** long incision	→ Curved incision over the swelling
• Protect **2** superficial nerves	→ Cervical and marginal mandibular branches of facial nerve
• Protect **2** deep nerves	→ Lingual and hypoglossal nerve
• Ligate facial artery **2** times	→ First at deeper plane and then at superficial plane
• Divide **2** muscles	→ Superficial—platysma; Deep—fibres of mylohyoid
• Remove **2** lobes	→ Superficial and deep
• Incision is **2** cm medial to mandible, **2** cm anterior to angle of the mandible	→ To protect 2 superficial nerves

16

Examination of the Oral Cavity

INTRODUCTION

Malignancies of the oral cavity are common short or long cases in the university examination. They include carcinoma buccal mucosa, carcinoma alveolus, carcinoma floor of the mouth, carcinoma lip and carcinoma tongue. All these lesions start as ulcer or a growth. Any lesion which begins as a swelling in the oral cavity and later ulcerates but has features of malignancy is most likely a malignant ectopic salivary gland tumour. Other lesions such as epulis, mucous cysts, submucous fibrosis, and leukoplakia, are also included under short cases. Specific tongue lesions which manifest as swellings have also been included.

Clinical examination should be done using an oral cavity kit (Fig. 16.1).

Oral Cavity Examination Kit

- *Pen torch*: Good light to visualise.
- *Tongue depressor*: To depress tongue.
- *Spatula*: To retract cheek.
- *Biopsy forceps*: To take biopsy from the ulcer.
- *Pair of gloves*: To conduct clinical examination. (specially intraoral) and posterior one-third of the tongue.

I have given 5 photographs (Figs 16.2 to 16.6) in the beginning of the chapter. These are the 5 types of oral cavity malignant lesions. Look at them carefully and decide if it is an ulcer or growth.

PATIENT DATA

Age: Carcinoma buccal mucosa or tongue occurs in the middle age group and elderly patients. Mucous cysts are retention cysts occur in young patients (Fig. 16.7).

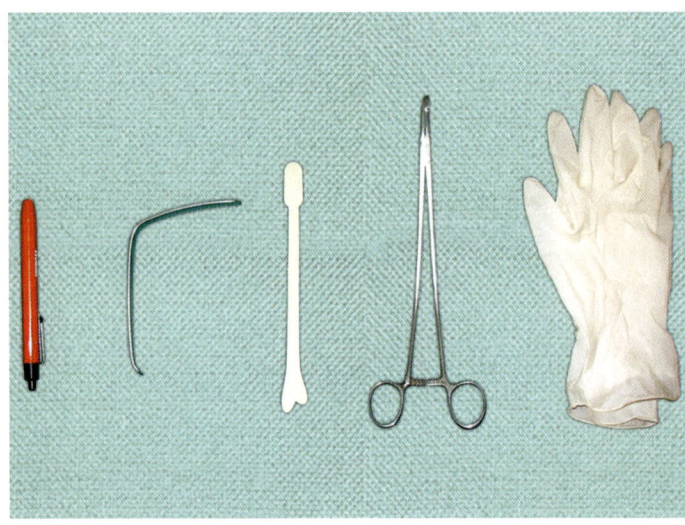

Fig. 16.1: Oral cavity examination kit

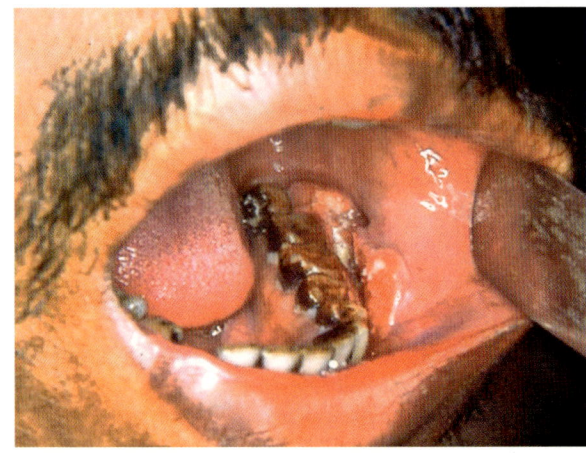

Fig. 16.2: Carcinoma buccal mucosa—ulcerative variety

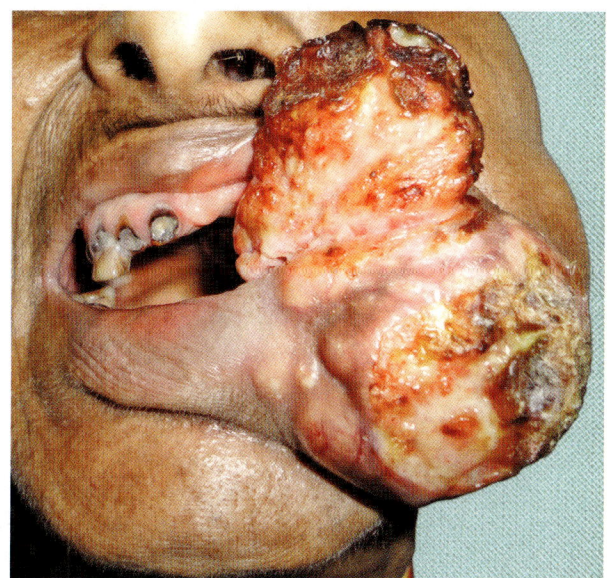

Fig. 16.3: Carcinoma buccal mucosa—**ulceroproliferative variety**

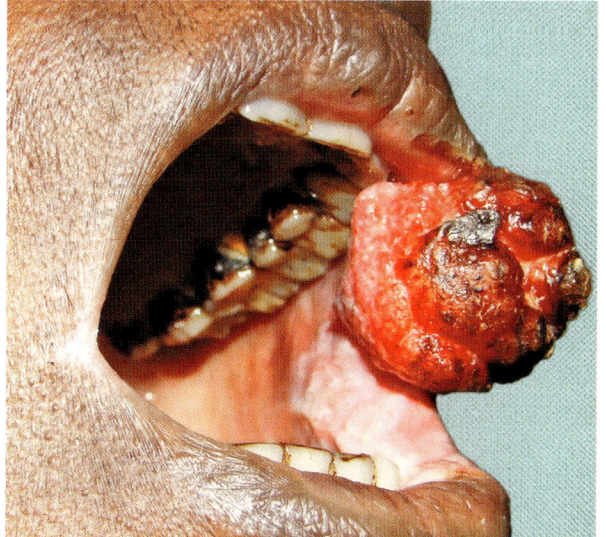

Fig. 16.4: Exophytic lesion arising from commissure. Also observe leukoplakia in the surrounding buccal mucosa

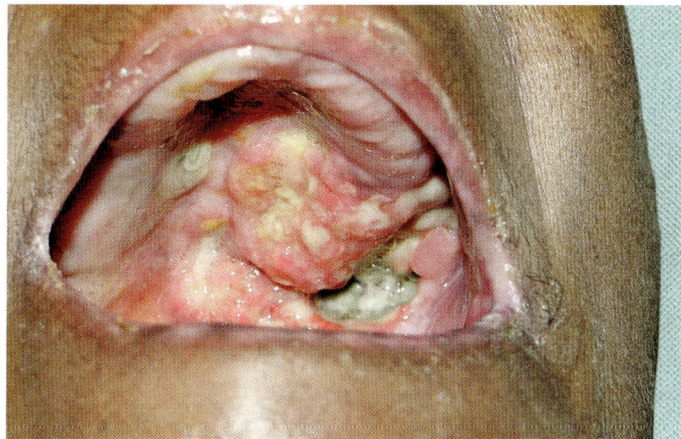

Fig. 16.5: Carcinoma alveolus—**excavating ulcer**. Such lesions are advanced at the time of presentation

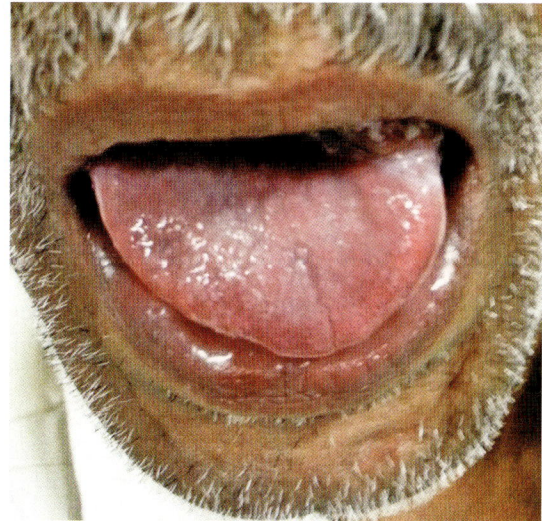

Fig. 16.6: Carcinoma tongue **indurated** variety. Cannot protrude the tongue outside—ankyloglossia

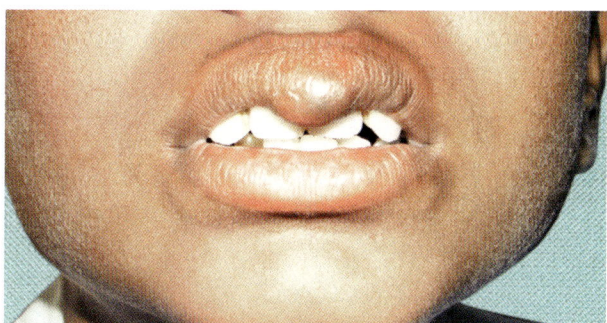

Fig. 16.7: Mucous cyst

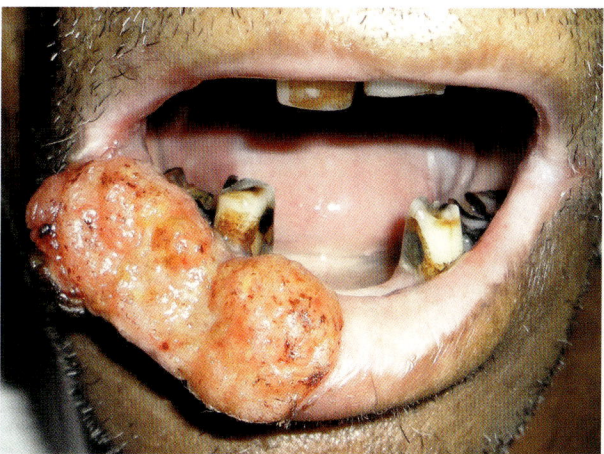

Fig. 16.8: Countryman's lip—70-year-old agriculturist with this lesion of 8 months duration

Sex: Oral cancers are more common in men.

Occupation: Carcinoma lip is more common in patients with outdoor occupation such as agriculturists—lower lip is more commonly affected than upper lip. Hence, it is called **countryman's lip** (Fig. 16.8).

HISTORY OF PRESENTING ILLNESS

1. **Ulcer:** First complaint is usually a painless ulcer. 'When was the ulcer first noticed, was it associated with any pain, how is it progressing', are the usual questions? If an ulcer has started with pain, it is aphthous ulcer. Malignant ulcers are painless to start with. Although initially painless, secondary infection is very common in the oral cavity and results in pain later. Rapidly growing ulcer is most likely malignant ulcer. Generally the patient says it has been there since 2–3 months and it is spreading and not healing. If the ulcer shows evidence of healing or becoming smaller, it means it is not malignant ulcer. For example, patient had an ulcer on the lateral border of the tongue. It started healing once the sharp tooth was removed (Fig. 16.9).

2. **Pain:** It is due to secondary infection. Referred pain is due to involvement of nerve. Often patients with carcinoma tongue complain of pain in the ear and temporal region which is the area of distribution of auriculotemporal nerve. This is because lingual nerve and auriculotemporal nerve are the branches of mandibular nerve. Severe pain over the jaw indicates periostitis.

   Pain is also a feature of stomatitis, dental ulcers and tubercular ulcers of tongue (rare).

3. **Bleeding:** Did you notice any bleeding? Malignant ulcers **bleed on touch**, when there is a minor trauma from the teeth or due to the food bolus. Drops of blood may be seen during mastication or chewing. This is common in ulceroproliferative lesions.

4. **Any drooling of saliva:** This should be enquired when you suspect malignancy of the posterior one-third of tongue wherein the patient is not able to swallow (dysphagia). You may see a patient sitting with sputum cup or towel with him and frequently spitting. It suggests carcinoma posterior one-third of tongue.

5. **Can you open the mouth? Inability to open the mouth is called trismus. Trismus** in oral cancers is due to involvement of pterygoid and masseter muscles. This occurs when carcinoma buccal mucosa **extends into the retromolar trigone**. Trismus can also be due to soft tissue fibrosis caused by radiation. **Once perineural lymphatics are involved, spread can occur in the infratemporal fossa resulting in trismus.** Please remember other important causes of trismus are tetanus, temporomandibular joint disorders and severe inflammatory painful conditions of the oral cavity such as acute tonsillitis, peritonsillar abscess, etc. (Fig. 16.10).

6. **Have any of your teeth become loose?** Gingival cancers present as loosening of tooth.

7. **Do you have difficulty in swallowing?** It is a feature of carcinoma posterior one-third of the tongue.

8. **Do you have difficulty in speech-disarticulation?** Disarticulation is a feature of carcinoma tongue wherein effective tongue movements cannot take place. It is also called dysarthria. It occurs due to tumour infiltrating tongue muscles and restricted movements of the tongue. Difficulty in speech can also be due to problem related to cleft lip and palate.

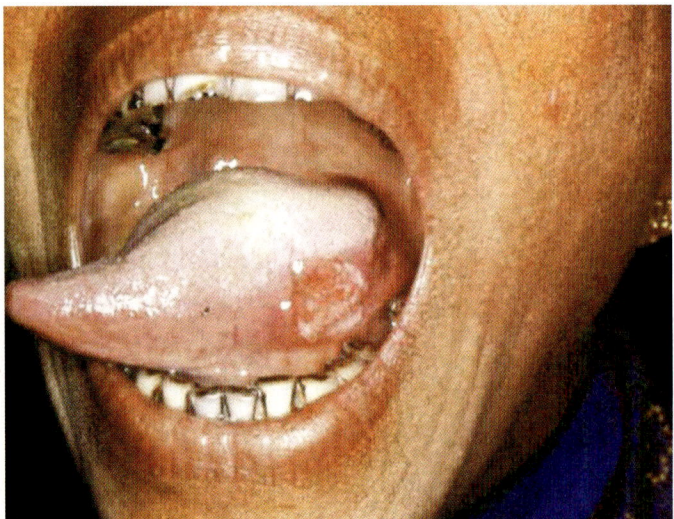

Fig. 16.9: Nonhealing ulcer on the lateral border of tongue due to sharp tooth

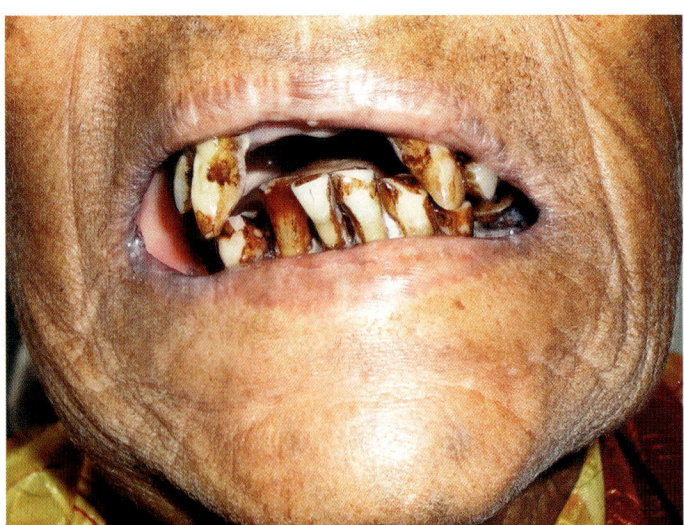

Fig. 16.10: Trismus with tobacco stains

9. *Do you eat pan? Do you smoke, what are your food habits?* **Betel nut** and slaked lime with betel leaf and tobacco (pan) is eaten and usually kept inside the cheek (quid) for many hours. Over the years, it brings about chronic irritation of mucosa of the cheek and causes leukoplakia. Tobacco contains multiple carcinogens including aromatic hydro-carbons. Among all the risk factors for oral cancer, tobacco consumption and quid are the most important causes (Clinical Boxes 16.1 and 16.2).

Clinical Box 16.1 🗝️

Causes of leukoplakia can be remembered as 8 Ss. The causes for leukoplakia are as follows

- **Smoking** results in hyperkeratosis. Nicotine in the form of cigarettes and chewed tobacco produces premalignant changes in the oral cavity. In fact, smoking is one of the important factors responsible for malignancy of the upper aerodigestive tract. Thus, more than one site can be affected by carcinoma of the aerodigestive tract. This is called **field cancerisation.**
- **Spices**
- **Spirits** have synergistic action with smoking
- **Sharp tooth may** cause chronic and constant irritation (for carcinoma tongue)
- **Sepsis, poor oral hygiene**
- **Sunlight**—actinic rays—this is especially for carcinoma lip
- **Syphilis** causes endarteritis obliterans and results in chronic superficial glossitis of the tongue which is a precancerous condition (rare these days—only for academic interest)
- **Susceptibility of a person**

Clinical Box 16.2 🗝️

Chemicals found in the tobacco smoke

- Nicotine
- Lead
- Arsenic
- Formaldehyde
- Nitrosamines
- Benzene
- Polycyclic hydrocarbons, etc.

Cigars. Also have high concentration of nitrates and nitrites. When used, they release tobacco-specific nitrosamines (TSNAs)

---

10. *Halitosis* is very characteristic of carcinoma tongue. Bacteria in the tongue produce malodorous compounds and fatty acids, and account for 80 to 90% of all cases of mouth-related bad breath. Large quantities of naturally occurring bacteria are often found on the posterior *dorsum* of the tongue, where they are relatively undisturbed by normal activity.

11. Advanced cases can present with skin nodules/orocutaneous fistula (Figs 16.11 and 16.12).

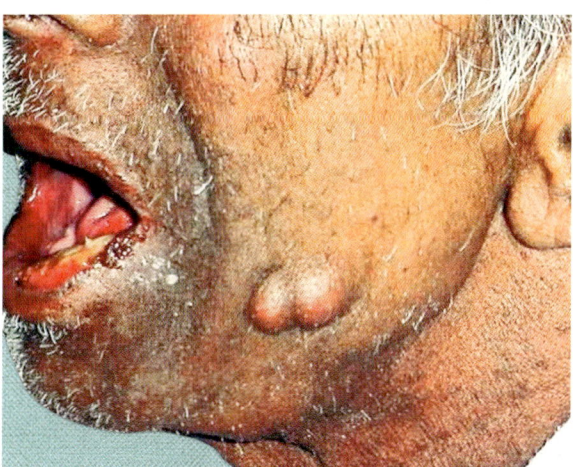

Fig. 16.11: Carcinoma buccal mucosa presenting with cutaneous nodule—warning sign of orocutaneous fistula

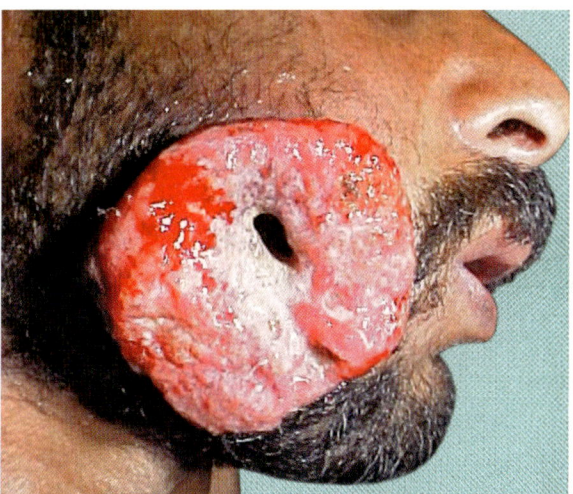

Fig. 16.12: Eight months history of growth of buccal mucosa presenting as orocutaneous fistula

---

Clinical Wisdom

If swelling appears first in the buccal mucosa and then ulcerates, it may be ectopic salivary gland tumour.

Inspection

1. *Appearance, attitude*: Is the patient looking sick? Does he have a nasogastric tube in place? (He may not be able to swallow because of dysphagia or may be receiving radiation causing fibrosis). Has he received radiation? (Radiation skin changes will be seen). Are there any lesions on the outer aspect of cheek? (Orocutaneous fistulas or oedema of the cheek.) Is there any drooling of saliva? (due to dysphagia) (Fig. 16.13)

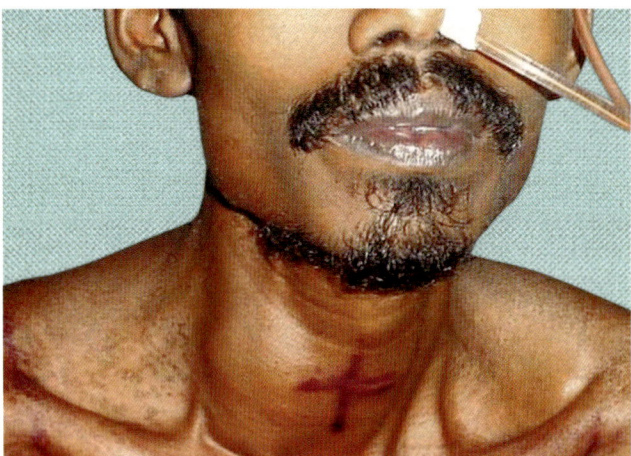

Fig. 16.13: Advanced carcinoma base of the tongue with lymph nodes on both sides of neck receiving radiotherapy

2. ***First ask the patient to open the mouth:*** Inability to open the mouth partially or totally is called trismus. Painful trismus is due to inflammatory conditions.

Trismus (Fig. 16.14): Normal mouth opening ranges from 35 to 45 mm.

Grades of trismus

- *Grade I* : Mouth opening is between 25 and 45 mm.
- *Grade II* : Between 10 and 25 mm.
- *Grade III* : Less than 10 mm.

Common causes of trismus

Tetanus

Retromolar trigone infiltration by carcinoma

Inflammatory cause—tonsillitis, quinsy

Synovitis of temporomandibular joint

Mandibular fractures

Ulcer retromolar trigone

Soft tissue fibrosis due to radiation and **s**ubmucous fibrosis

You can remember as **'TRISMUS'**

- Once you have checked for trismus, oral cavity examination can start (Clinical Box 16.3)

Clinical Box 16.3

Checklist of 'ABCDEFG' of oral cavity examination

A—Anterior two-thirds of tongue, alveolus

B—Base of the tongue

C—Commissure

D—Dental formula, dangerous triangle—retromolar

E—Ectopic salivary tissue—palate/cheek

F—Floor of mouth, fauces, tonsils

G—Gums, gingiva

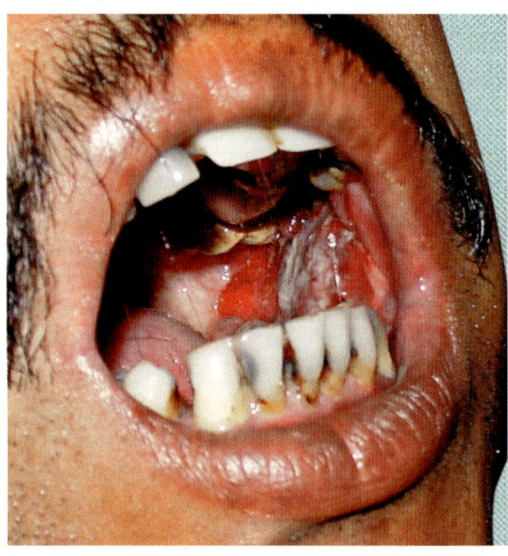

Fig. 16.14: Grade II trismus

- Parts of oral cavity which can be easily missed are alveolar edges, retromolar trigone, posterior one-third (base) of the tongue, floor of the mouth.

3. Ask him to put out his tongue (carefully observe, even if you do not ask this question, many patients voluntarily put out the tongues—observe any restriction in the mobility (ankyloglossia) or any deviation to one side. Deviation occurs to the paralysed side (Fig. 16.15).

- *Ulcer:* Note down the location, size, shape, extension, edge, floor and surrounding area. Carcinomatous lesions are described as ulcer, ulcerative growth or ulceroproliferative growth. ***(Do not describe them as swelling.)***

- *Surface*: Is it normal with papilla or ***bald*** due to ***loss of papilla or anaemia?*** Red tongue can be

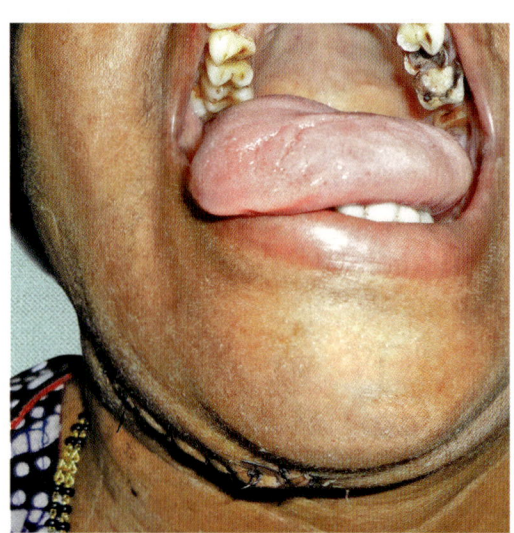

Fig. 16.15: Tongue is deviated to paralysed side

due to glossitis, *white patch* in the tongue can be due to *leukoplakia*. Black colour can be due to malignant melanoma of the tongue.

- Also look at the posterior third more carefully for any growth or ulcer. Foramen caecum is the site of lingual thyroid, and gumma (rare nowadays).

- *Swelling*: Grossly swollen tongue can be due to haemangioma. Surface will have blue colour.

- *Movements*: Restricted movements or inability to protrude the tongue is called **ankyloglossia**. This is one of the important features of malignancy of tongue. It is due to *carcinomatous* infiltration of the *floor of the mouth.* If the tongue is deviated to one side, it could be due to paralysis of the tongue musculature. This can happen due to hypoglossal nerve paralysis. Forward movement, backward movement, elevation and depression and rotating movements have to be checked.

4. If any lesion is found, describe it (use light source):

- *Ulcerative lesions*: Typical nonhealing ulcer with everted edge.

- *Ulceroproliferative lesion—growth*: Here cauliflower-like tissue (proliferative) is more than ulcer.

- *Verrucous*: In this variety, it is more exophytic than ulcerative (Clinical Box 16.4).

- *Excavating ulcers*: These are deep and penetrating into the underlying tissues.

Refer to Clinical Box 16.5 for checklist

Clinical Box 16.4 🗝️

Peculiarities of verrucous carcinoma
- Very slow growing
- Growth is exophytic (than infiltrative)
- Rarely spreads by lymphatics
- It is a well-differentiated carcinoma
- Surgery is the treatment of choice

Clinical Box 16.5 🗝️

Inspection of the tongue—clinical checklist
- Protrusion of the tongue outside
- Any deviation to one side
- Atrophy of the tongue/enlargement
- Chronic superficial glossitis
- Any ulcer or growth

---

5. Typically, these lesions are ulcerative, proliferative or ulceroproliferative. Do not describe it as a swelling. Describe the ulcer or growth in the usual manner of description such as location, size, shape, edge, floor and surrounding area. Proliferative lesions are often verrucous carcinoma. Typical description of an oral cancer is given below.

- An ulcerative growth located in the buccal mucosa measuring about 5 cm, irregular shape with irregular borders. Edges are everted, floor covered with slough. Bleeding spots may be visible.

- Look for any white patches in the surrounding area. These are called leukoplakia (Fig. 16.16).

- Mention dental caries, if any (sepsis—one of the causes of leukoplakia).

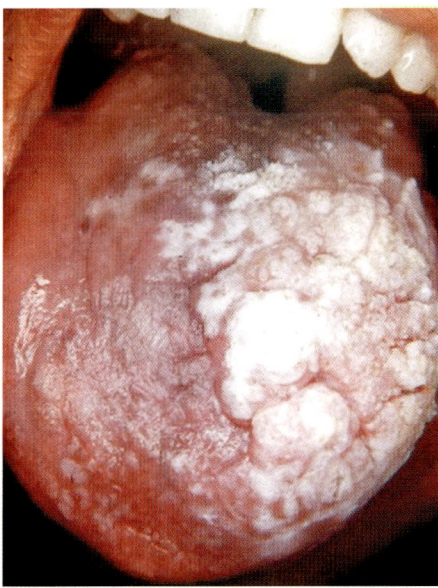

Fig. 16.16: Carcinoma *in situ* arising in leukoplakia patch

6. *Gums and teeth*

- *Gums are normally pink in colour.* In Vincent's angina, it is altered more red and oedematous.

- *Blue-black line* in the free margin of the gums can be due to *chronic lead poisoning* as seen in painters. It is also seen when bismuth treatment is given for leishmaniasis.

- *Red pedunculated* mass is usually an epulis (*refer to page 235*).

- Tenderness over the teeth with an *apical abscess* can be the cause of *median* mental sinus.

- *Recent history of loosening* of the tooth can be due to *carcinoma alveolus* or due to dental cyst.

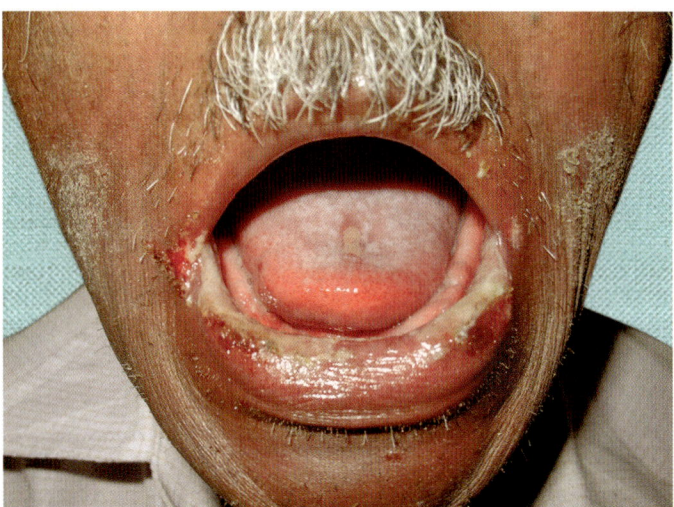

Fig. 16.17: Angular cheilitis, bald tongue

7. Mention any cheilitis or angular stomatitis (Fig. 16.17).

8. *Palate*

   • *Cleft*: Mention, if there is a congenital cleft. If present, describe the extent—has it involved the soft or the hard palate?

   • *Swelling*: If swelling is present, describe the swelling. Swelling in the *palate can be due* to *ectopic salivary gland* tumour or due to carcinoma maxillary antrum which pushes the upper jaw.

   • *Perforation*: Nowadays, it is not due to syphilis. The hole may persist after surgery of cleft palate due to breakdown of suture line.

9. *Floor*: Ask the patient to touch the palate with tongue.

   • *Ulcer or growth*: Is it from carcinoma tongue or has it started there? Describe the growth or ulcer. Typically carcinoma will have everted edge.

   • *Swelling*: **The most common swelling in the floor of the mouth is** a ranula, typically blue in colour and lateral to the midline. Another swelling is sublingual dermoid cyst which is in the midline, opaque with no transillumination.

10. **Wharton's duct opening:** Mention the opening of the submandibular duct on the side of the frenulum. Is it inflamed, is there any discharge of pus or is a stone visible?

11. *Frenulum*: It may be short, a cause of slurred speech in children. Rarely, ulcer in the frenulum of the tongue can be due to whooping cough.

12. Inspect the outer aspect of the cheek and look for any oedema, swelling or any fistula (orocutaneous fistula as in Fig. 16.12).

Palpation

Wear a glove, tell the patient what you are doing and palpate gently. Palpation of the tongue should be done with tongue kept inside the oral cavity (Figs 16.18 and 16.19). There is no need to mention local rise of temperature.

1. *Bleeding:* First sign you may find is the easy friability to touch resulting in bleeding. For the sake of demonstration, do not try to elicit bleeding. Be gentle. Easy friability is one of the features of malignancy.

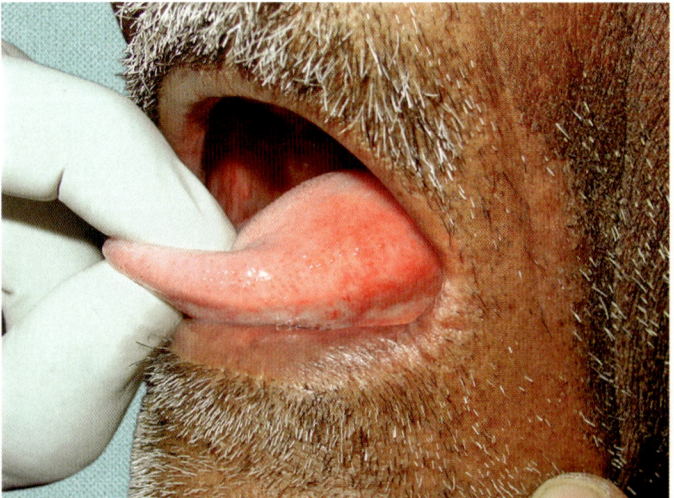

Fig. 16.18: Wrong method of looking for induration with protrusion of the tongue outside

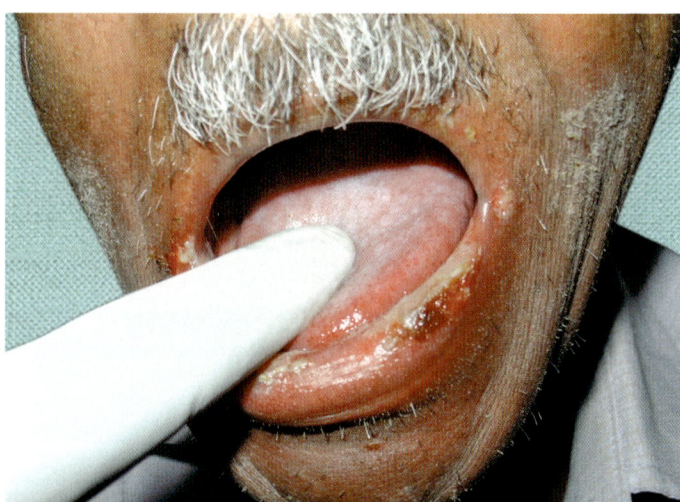

Fig. 16.19: Palpation of the tongue is done with tongue inside oral cavity—correct method

2. *Tenderness*: Quite contrary to conventional teaching that carcinomas are nontender, oral cancers are often tender on palpation because of secondary infection. In advanced cases, tenderness is due to infiltration into the bone and skin.

3. *Size and extent*: Describing extent of the lesion is an important part of the clinical examination because it will decide the type of surgery or even other modality of the treatment. Increased size, retromolar extent, extension into infratemporal fossa may direct the treatment towards chemo-radiation first followed by surgery than vice versa.

4. *Consistency*: Typically ulcers are hard and indurated. It is also important to look for induration beyond the lesions (typically a buccal mucosa lesion going beyond and spreading into retromolar trigone) (Figs 16.19 and 16.20).

5. *Mobility*: Try moving the lesion. Buccal mucosa lesions may show some degree of mobility initially. Later as the lesions advance, they get fixed to cheek muscles such as buccinators.

6. *Fixity*: To the underlying structures such as mandible may be present. *Examples:* Growth in the gingivobuccal sulcus and growth in the floor of the mouth get fixed to mandible.

7. *Palpation of the tongue*
   - Explain to the patient about what you are doing.
   - Two fingers (index and middle) of the left hand are insinuated from outside through cheek between upper and lower jaw (so that he will not bite).
   - Palpate the ulcer—for easy friability and feel the base/edge for induration.

- 'Frozen tongue' is the term given to extensive induration produced by carcinoma tongue.
- Then palpate anterior two-thirds, posterior one-third and gingivolingual sulcus.

8. *Check for movements of the tongue*: More relevant in cases of carcinoma of the floor of the mouth and carcinoma tongue. Ask the patient to move the tongue in all directions and check.
   - **Forward** protrusion—**genioglossus.** This is the muscle commonly involved.
   - **Backward** movement—**styloglossus**
   - **Elevation**—**palatoglossus**
   - **Depression**—**hyoglossus**

Clinical Wisdom

Restriction of tongue movements in carcinoma tongue is usually not due to nerve paralysis but due to fixity of the tongue or due to shortening of the tongue as seen in indurated varieties. All these muscles are supplied by hypoglossal nerve except palatoglossus which is supplied by glossopharyngeal nerve. Hypoglossal nerve paralysis can also be caused by large lymph node mass in the neck.

9. *Examination of the mandible*: Bidigital palpation of mandible is done by examining with index finger on the outer aspect of the mandible and the thumb on the under surface of the mandible. This test should be done on the opposite side first. Only then, the thickening of the mandible can be appreciated (Figs 16.21 to 16.23).

Clinical Wisdom

The mandibular canal is close to occlusive surface in edentulous elderly patients due to decrease in vertical height of horizontal ramus, thus facilitating easy spread.

10. **Look for any loose tooth and examine gingivae carefully** (Clinical Box 16.6)

Clinical Box 16.6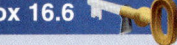

Gingival cancers
- Early cases present as mucosal change in leukoplakia
- Loosening of tooth may be a presenting feature
- Can present with bleeding and pain
- Bone involvement occurs early
- Spread to adjacent structures occurs early

11. Palpate outer aspect of cheek for any induration, tenderness, swelling or orocutaneous fistula. Impending signs of fistula are redness of skin and nodules.

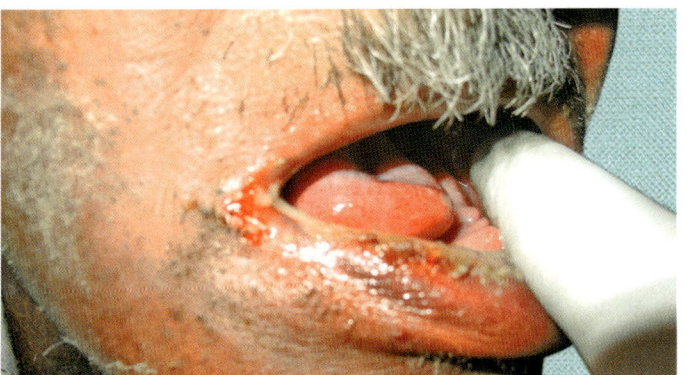

Fig. 16.20: Palpating for gingivobuccal sulcus and advance the finger to palpate retromolar trigone and look for induration

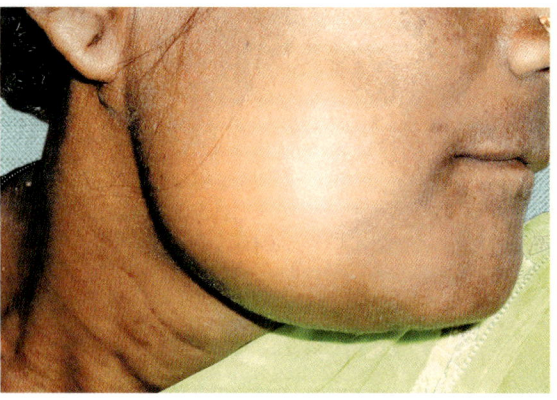

Fig. 16.21: Carcinoma alveolus: Growth had eroded the inner cortex of the mandible

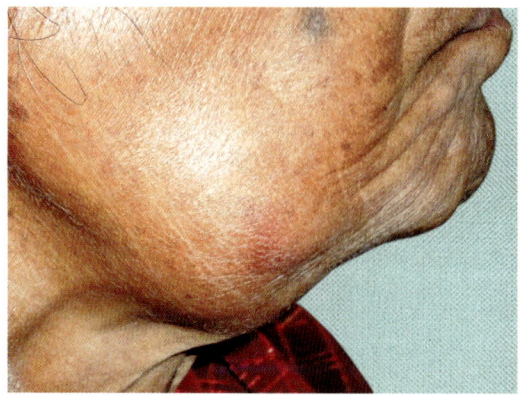

Fig. 16.22: Carcinoma buccal mucosa with infiltration of the mandible

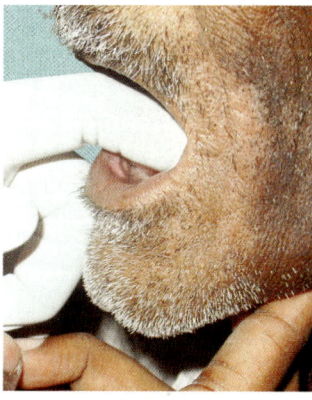

Fig. 16.23: Bidigital palpation of the mandible

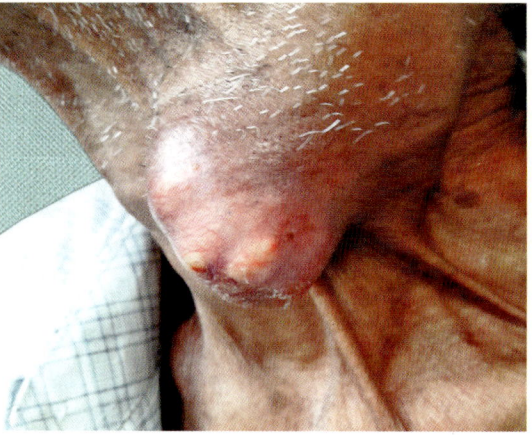

Fig. 16.24: Secondaries in neck with skin infiltration—platysma sign

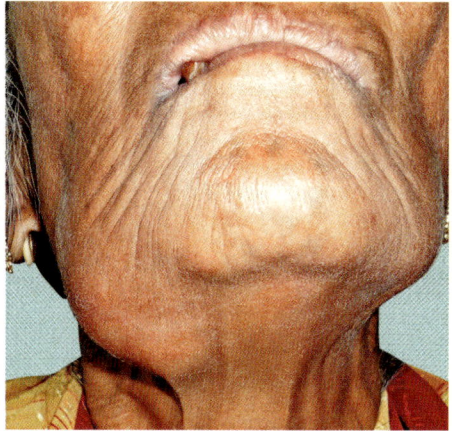

Fig. 16.25: Metastatic submandibular lymph nodes

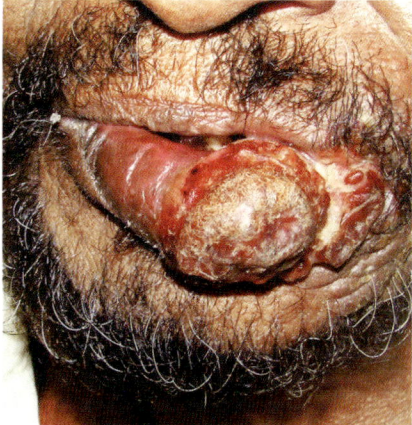

Fig. 16.26: When you see from front with flexion of neck, nothing is visible in the neck

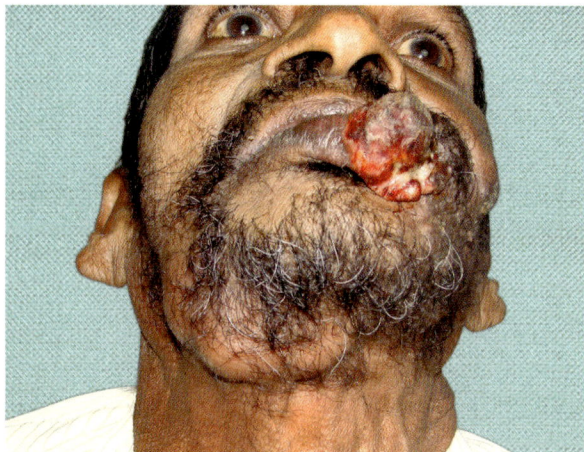

Fig. 16.27: Ask him to extend the neck. Look at the enlarged lymph nodes

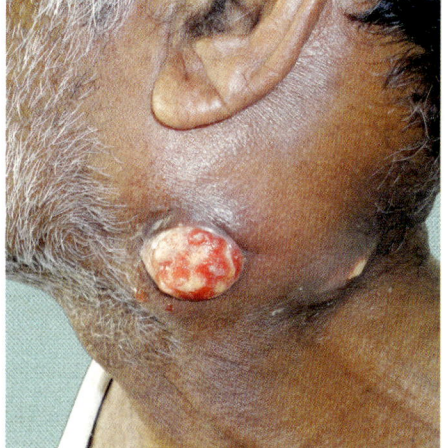

Fig. 16.28: Skin infiltration by malignant submandibular lymph nodes

12. *Examination of lymph nodes* (Figs 16.24 to 16.28): All levels of the nodes (levels 1 to 5) should be examined for enlargement. When do you say they are malignant is the common question asked? Any node which is hard, or fixed or with restricted mobility or a large-sized node more than 2 cm and

a palpable node in presence of a malignant lesion in the neck.

- In a few cases, the lymph node enlargement is due to secondary infection. Such nodes are tender and firm.
- Ulceration is seen in advanced cases.

CLINICAL CHECKLIST

1. Examine the ulcer or growth
2. Examine rest of the oral cavity for leukoplakia
3. Examination of the mandible and chronic hyperplastic candidiasis
4. Examination of the movements of the tongue (Figs 16.29 to 16.31).
5. Examination of the outer aspect of the cheek
6. Examination of the lymph nodes on both sides of the neck
7. Tests for nerves—hypoglossal nerve and cervical sympathetic nerve
8. Systemic examination

   Please note: Clinical Box 16.7 for some special features of carcinoma of the posterior one-third of tongue.

Clinical Box 16.7

Carcinoma posterior one-third
- It presents with dysphagia or with a change in voice
- Easily missed in a clinical examination
- Biopsy should be done under general anaesthesia to avoid aspiration and to assess the spread posteriorly
- Palpation will give the diagnosis—induration
- It is one of the occult primaries for lymph node secondaries in the neck
- Criss-crossing of the lymphatics explain bilateral lymph nodes in the neck
- Blood spread is more common
- Prognosis is bad because well-differentiated carcinoma in this location is rare

DIAGNOSIS

When you give a diagnosis of cancer of the oral cavity, remember the following situations.

1. Is it carcinoma? If so why? Which side?
2. Any benign conditions? Leukoplakia, submucous fibrosis.
3. Is it confined to one region or is it spreading? Example carcinoma buccal mucosa involving lip, carcinoma floor of the mouth infiltrating the tongue.
4. Is it arising from alveolus? Yes, it is fixed to mandible.
5. Are there any significant nodes? If present, describe under *TNM* staging.
6. Is there distant metastasis? Very rare.

TNM STAGING	Oral cancer—American Joint Committee Cancer (AJCC)

Primary Tumour (T)
- T0: No evidence of primary tumour
- Tis: Carcinoma *in situ*
- T1: <2 cm
- T2: >2 cm and <4 cm
- T3: >4 cm
- T4: Any cancer invading adjacent structures such as cartilage, cortical bone, deep (extrinsic) muscles of the tongue, skin or soft tissue of the neck.
  - T4a: Moderately advanced local disease
  - T4b: Very advanced local disease (skull base, pterygoid plate, internal carotid artery, masticator space)

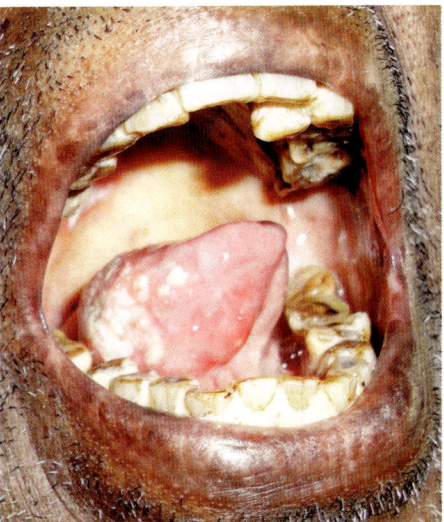

Fig. 16.29: Patient is asked to touch the palate with tongue

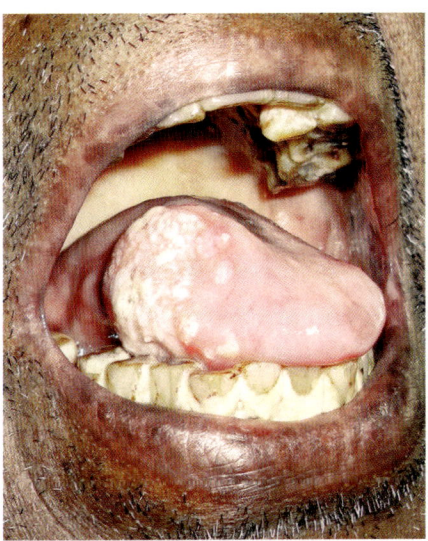

Fig. 16.30: Patient cannot protrude the tongue out

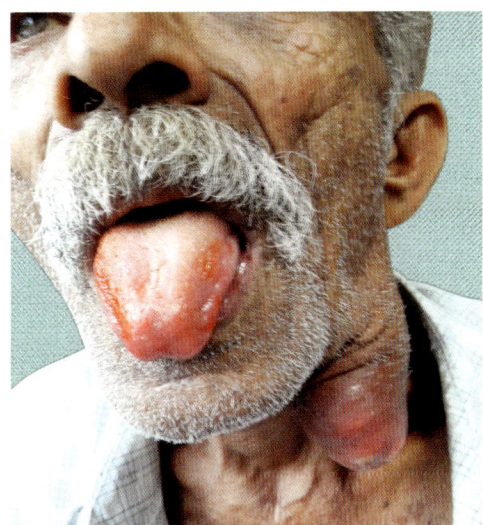

Fig. 16.31: Look for deviation (hypoglossal nerve palsy caused by enlarged lymph nodes)

Regional Lymph Nodes (N)
- Nx: Nodes cannot be assessed
- N0: No lymph node metastasis
- N1: Single positive ipsilateral node less than or equal to 3 cm in greatest dimension
- N2a: Single positive ipsilateral node more than 3 cm but less than or equal to 6 cm
- N2b: Multiple ipsilateral nodes but all less than 6 cm
- N2c: Bilateral or contralateral lymph nodes but all less than 6 cm
- N3: Lymph node more than 6 cm.

Distant Metastasis (M)
- M0: No distant metastasis
- M1: Distant metastasis present

Stage Grouping
Stage I	T1, N0, M0
Stage II	T2, N0, M0
Stage III	T3, N0, M0, T1–3, N1, M0
Stage IV	T4, N0, M0, T, N2–3, M0
	T0, N0, M1

DIFFERENTIAL DIAGNOSIS (DD)

For the sake of DD, you need not offer DD. Classical case of carcinoma having everted edges, induration and hard node has only one diagnosis—that is carcinoma.

However depending upon location of the lesion, let us look at a few D/D.

1. Differential diagnosis of carcinoma buccal mucosa:

a. **Ectopic salivary gland tumours**: Buccal mucosa is a common site. It starts as a swelling and then ulcerates. Induration is much more in cases of carcinoma buccal mucosa.

b. **Leukoplakia**: A slow developing leukoplakia presents as whitish nodule or an ulcer. However, biopsy confirms the diagnosis.

2. Differential diagnosis of carcinoma lip

a. **Keratoacanthoma**
- It is a cutaneous tumour arising from hair follicles on the lips. It is common in white, Western, males between 50 and 70 years of age.
- Sunlight (actinic rays), chemical carcinogen, and viral factors may be responsible for this lesion.
- The central portion of the nodule may ulcerate. The lesion may progress for 6 weeks and may resolve spontaneously within 4–6 months.

b. **Ectopic salivary gland tumour**
- The lip is one of the common sites of malignant salivary gland tumours. This presents with submucous nodules that grow slowly and ulcerate, may mimic squamous cell carcinoma (Fig. 16.32).
- They are also indurated lesions

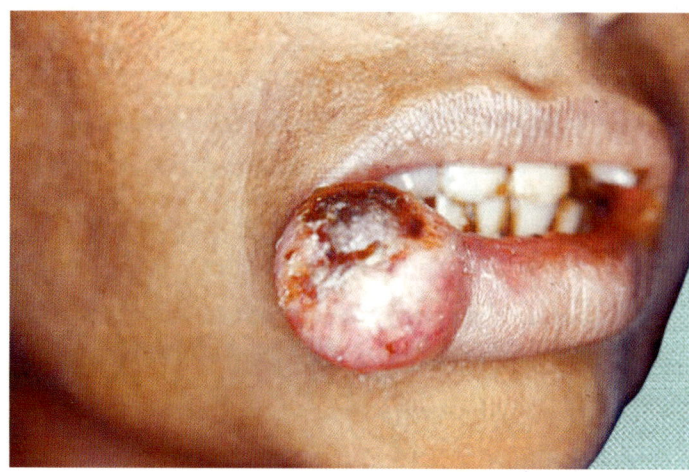

Fig. 16.32: This lesion was diagnosed as carcinoma lip. However, it did not have everted edges. It was indurated. Biopsy reported as ectopic salivary gland tumour. On careful questioning, patient says it started as a swelling not as an ulcer

- However, the characteristic everted edge may not be seen.
- These are adenocarcinomas which are treated by surgery.

3. Differential diagnosis of lesion on the gums:

a. **Pyogenic granuloma** (Fig. 16.33)
- Recurrent infections or trauma produces a polypoidal mass with significant bleeding.
- It is rich in granulation tissue and resembles a polyp.
- It is devoid of epithelium
- Histologically, it is a capillary haemangioma
- Absence of induration gives the diagnosis.

b. **Epulis** (refer to page 235)

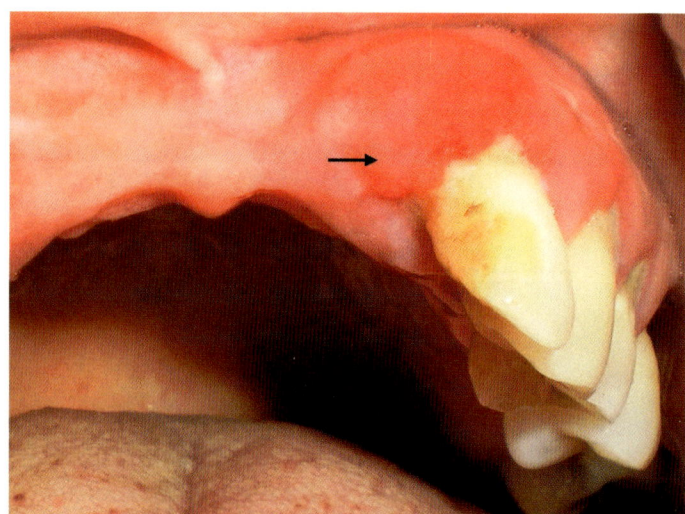

Fig. 16.33: Pyogenic granuloma due to caries tooth (*Courtesy:* Dr Keerthilatha Pai, Head, Department of Oral Medicine, College of Dental Sciences, Manipal)

3. Differential diagnosis of carcinoma tongue (Fig. 16.34)

- When it presents as ulcer, D/D includes ulcer of the tongue, such as dental ulcers, traumatic ulcer, etc.
- The most significant finding of carcinomatous ulcer is induration.

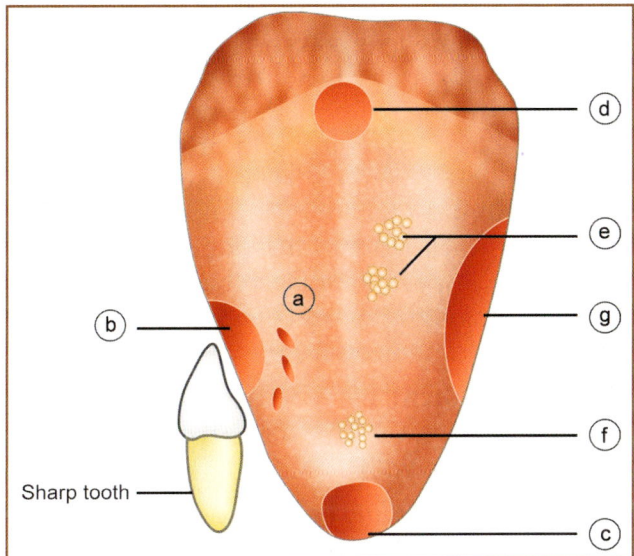

Fig. 16.34: Ulcers of the tongue—*refer* the text

a. Aphthous ulcers

- Small, multiple, very painful ulcers, can occur at any age group. More common in females at the time of menstruation. These are called minor aphthous ulcers.
- When they are larger, deeper and painful, they are called major aphthous ulcers.
- They are due to viral infection. These ulcers are superficial ulcers with erythematous margin.
- They subside within a few days. Temporary relief can be obtained by applying salicylate gel.
- Vitamin B complex is usually given for the satisfaction of the patients.

b. Dental ulcers

- These ulcers occur due to broken tooth, sharp tooth, ill-fitting dentures, prosthesis, etc. They are very painful ulcers.
- Such ulcers are common on the lateral margin and they heal when the tooth is removed. This is an example for traumatic ulcer. It should not be confused with carcinomatous ulcer which commonly occurs on the lateral margin.

c. Tubercular ulcer of tongue

- Tuberculosis affects tip of the tongue. These ulcers are very painful with enlargement of regional nodes.
- It occurs in patients with fulminating pulmonary tuberculosis.
- Ulcers have undermined edges. These ulcers are sometimes multiple with serous discharge.

d. Gummatous ulcer

- Gumma is a complication of tertiary syphilis resulting in a firm swelling in the midline in the anterior two-thirds of the tongue. Induration is absent. Ulcer is nontender. Severe endarteritis obliterans results in the necrosis of gumma giving rise to gummatous ulcer. It has punched out edges and wash leather slough on the floor. Other sites of gumma include testis, palate, clavicle and liver. These ulcers are rare these days.

- ***Primary syphilis:*** Primary chancre that occurs in the tongue is highly contagious. It affects the tip of the tongue. It produces a painful ulcer with large significant enlargement of regional lymph nodes.

- ***Secondary syphilis:*** It produces a white patch in the tongue, lips and on the anterior pillars of fauces. In the tongue, these are multiple which coalesce to form snail track ulcers. The ulcers heal with fine tissue paper scar. In some cases, syphilitic organisms produce a flat, hypertrophied epithelium which is described as condyloma. This is called Hutchinson's wart.

- ***Tertiary syphilis:*** It produces gumma. Syphilis also produces chronic superficial glossitis, which is characterised by bald tongue with loss of papilla and fissured tongue. It is a precancerous condition.

e. Systemic diseases

- Pemphigus
- Systemic lupus erythematosus (SLE)
- Lichen planus

f. Post-pertussis ulcer: It occurs in children due to repeated coughing. Typical location of the ulcer on the under surface of the tongue and on the frenulum clinches the diagnosis.

g. Carcinomatous ulcer (Fig. 16.35)

- Lateral margin
- Nonhealing ulcer
- Everted edge
- Edge and base are indurated
- Bleeds on touch
- Fixity
- Significant lymph nodes in the neck.

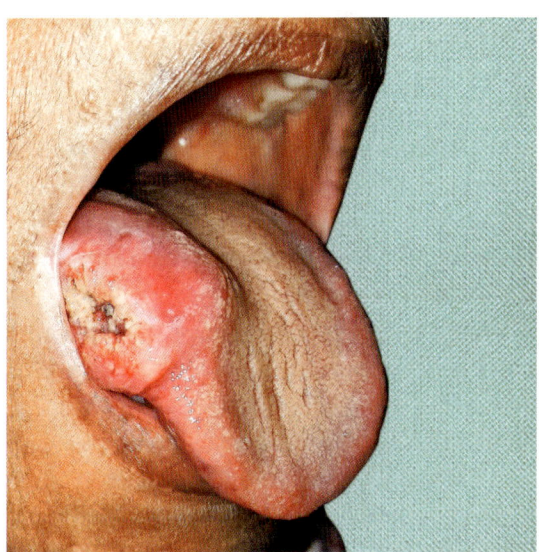

Fig. 16.35: Typical carcinoma lateral border with significant thickening of the surrounding tongue

CARCINOMA MAXILLARY ANTRUM

It is rare in Western countries but common in Asia. The workers in furniture, chromic and nickel industries are more prone for the development of carcinoma maxillary antrum.

Clinical Presentation (Table 16.1)

1. Growth originating on the **floor of antrum** may result in bulge of the hard palate. This results in pain in the teeth and they may become loose.

2. When **medial wall** is involved, nasal obstruction and epiphora occur due to obstruction of the lacrimal duct. Bleeding from the nose can also occur, if there is ulceration.

3. If **anterolateral wall** is involved, asymmetry of the face results in pain in the cheek. Anaesthesia over the skin of the cheek including upper lip occurs due to involvement of infraorbital nerve, a branch of maxillary division of the trigeminal nerve.

4. If the **roof** is invaded, proptosis and diplopia occur.

5. **Posterior extension of the growth** is difficult to assess clinically. When it involves the pterygoid muscles, it results in trismus. Paraesthesia over the cheek, gums, lower lip, and postnasal discharge are the other features of these tumours. They carry poor prognosis because of late presentation.

BENIGN SWELLINGS IN THE TONGUE—MACROGLOSSIA

Diffuse painless enlargement of the tongue is described as macroglossia. It is a rare condition and can occur due to various causes.

1. *Lymphangioma*: In this condition, the tongue diffusely enlarges. Sometimes, it is a localised swelling. It may be associated with lymphangiomas elsewhere in the body such as cheek mucosa, lips, etc. The tongue becomes larger, indurated and gives rise to severe discomfort to the patients. Due to repeated trauma, the surface becomes ulcerated. It is treated by injecting sclerosants such as ethanolamine oleate and hypertonic saline. Partial excision may be necessary in cases of large lymphangioma.

2. *Haemangioma*: Cavernous haemangiomas occur in the tongue, lips, etc. It is present since birth but manifests during childhood. It presents with soft, cystic, fluctuant swelling and at times, pulsatile. Trauma due to teeth or food results in bleeding. Haemangioma of the tongue is treated on the same lines as lymphangioma. It is much more difficult to excise it, especially a large haemangioma. Preoperative angiography and ligation of lingual artery on both sides is necessary (Fig. 16.36).

3. *Neurofibroma*: It may be associated with von Recklinghausen's disease. It is treated by hemiglossectomy.

4. *Muscular macroglossia*: This condition, though rare, is seen in cretins. The tongue is thickened and cannot be held in place. Hence, it protrudes outside. It is treated by partial excision.

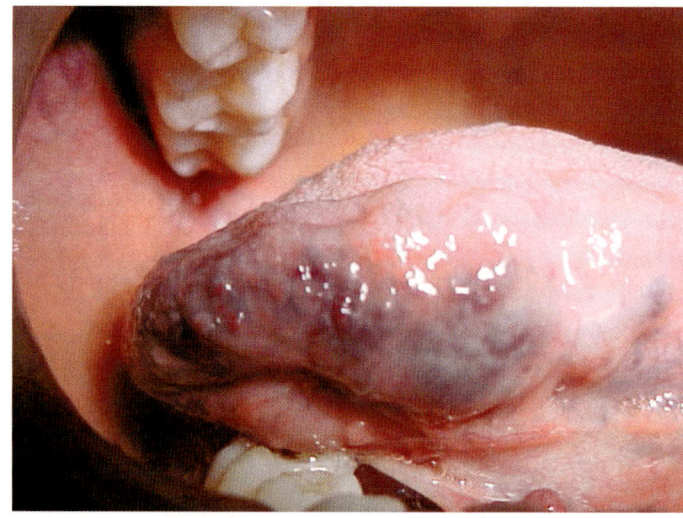

Fig. 16.36: Haemangioma tongue

Table 16.1: Clinical examination of a case of carcinoma maxillary antrum	
• Palatine bulge	Growth in the floor
• Unilateral nasal obstruction (he is asked to breathe, closing the nostrils one by one)	Growth in the medial wall
• Asymmetry of the face	Growth expanding anteriorly, superficial surface
• Change in the level and sharpness of inferior orbital margin, proptosis	Growth on the roof (orbital surface)
• Swelling (indurated) temporal region	Posterior extension into infratemporal region and then into temporal region
• Hard, fixed or mobile submandibular nodes	Metastasis

CLINICAL DISCUSSION

1. **What is p53 gene?**

   It is also called tumour suppressor gene/tumour protein p53 (TP53). It is the gene which prevents mutation. Chemicals in tobacco are known to destabilise this gene.

2. **What are the boundaries of retromolar trigone?**
   - Anteriorly, it is the last molar tooth.
   - Posteriorly, ascending ramus.
   - Apex is at maxillary tuberosity.

3. **Which are low grade tumours in the oral cavity?**

   Carcinoma lip—verrucous variety.

4. **Which are the aggressive tumours in the oral cavity?**

   Carcinoma alveolus, floor of the mouth and carcinoma tongue.

5. **'Indurated' variety of carcinoma is common in which part of oral cavity?**

   Carcinoma posterior one-third of tongue.

6. **Why does trismus follow radiation?**

   It is due to soft tissue fibrosis in and around temporo-mandibular joint.

7. **Which part of the tongue is affected in tuberculosis?**

   Tip of the tongue.

8. **What are the features of oral cancer?**
   - Short duration—rapid growth
   - Nonhealing ulcer
   - Edges are everted (commonly)
   - Ulceroproliferative lesions
   - Induration at the base/edge
   - Fixity
   - Palpable lymph nodes

9. **Do you have any differential diagnoses?**

   In a classical case, no differential diagnosis. Leukoplakia, chronic submucous fibrosis and ectopic salivary gland tumour are the possible differential diagnoses.

10. **Would you consider any other diagnosis in an ulcer in the lateral border of the tongue?**

    Yes, dental/traumatic ulcer.

11. **How do you take a biopsy?**

    In proliferative lesions, punch biopsy and in ulcerative lesions, edge biopsy are taken.

12. **Why edge?**

    It is the site where maximum proliferation of cells occurs.

13. **What is the biopsy report?**

    It is epithelioma or squamous cell carcinoma.

14. **How do you diagnose squamous cell carcinoma?**

    Mitotic figures and epithelial pearls (cell nests).

15. **In what conditions, is it absent?**

    In poorly differentiated carcinoma.

16. **When do you do MRI?**

    Large advanced lesions spreading into intratemporal fossa skull base.

17. **What is the treatment of malignant ulcers in the oral cavity?**

    Wide excision and reconstruction.

18. **What type of reconstruction?**
    - Small lesions can be closed directly.
    - Large lesions need pectoralis major myocutaneous flap.

19. **For stage III and stage IV, what is preferred line of treatment?**

    Initial chemoradiotherapy followed by surgery.

20. **How do they die?**

    Local recurrence, massive bleeding, malignant cachexia and respiratory complications.

MISCELLANEOUS

EPULIS

- Epulis means "**upon the gum**". It refers to solid swelling situated on the gum
- It arises from alveolar margin of the jaw
- Very often patients present with swelling on the gum which is painless.

Types

Granulomatous epulis
- Precipitating factors are caries tooth, dentures, poor oral hygiene.
- It manifests as a mass of granulation tissue around the teeth on the gums. It is soft to firm, fleshy mass and bleeds on touch.
- Pregnancy epulis refers to this variety (gingivitis gravidarum).

Fibrous Epulis
- It is the commonest form. A simple fibroma arising

It may undergo sarcomatous change. It is a firm polypoidal mass, slowly growing and nontender.

Giant cell epulis
- It is an osteoclastoma arising in the jaw. It presents as hyperaemic vascular, oedematous, soft to firm gums with indurated underlying mass due to expansion of the bone. It may ulcerate and result in haemorrhage. X-ray shows bone destruction with ridging of walls (pseudotrabeculation).
- Small tumours are treated by curettage
- Large tumours are treated by radical excision.

Carcinomatous epulis
- This is an epithelioma arising from mucous membrane of the alveolar margin.
- Typically, it presents as a nonhealing, painless ulcer. It slowly infiltrates the bone.
- Hard regional lymph nodes are due to metastasis.
- Treated by wide excision which includes removal

17

Examination of Jaw Swelling

INTRODUCTION

Patients with jaw swellings are short cases kept in undergraduate and postgraduate examinations. Students and practitioners of general surgery should have a broad idea about these cases. Swellings occurring in the jaws have peculiar signs and symptoms. When reference is made regarding the **jaws**, it means both upper and lower jaws. The swellings which arise from the jaws not only tend to involve the bone but also tend to involve the adjacent compartment of periosteum, mucous membrane covering the bone and in advanced cases based on the entity of the lesion they may involve the external skin as well.

Acute infections which cause jaw swellings include acute osteomyelitis, mandibular space infections, infected cysts, malignancy with secondary infection and pericoronitis involving the mandibular third molar tooth.

Chronic infections which cause jaw swellings include chronic osteomyelitis, chronic sclerosing osteomyelitis, tubercular/actinomycotic abscess, osteoradionecrosis, medication associated osteonecrosis and osteopetrosis.

Cysts of the jaw are interesting cases. They are many. Those of surgeon's interest have been discussed here. They are dental cysts, dentigerous cysts, and adamantinomas. Other cysts are: Calcifying odontogenic cyst, radicular cysts, solitary bone cyst, aneurysmal bone cyst, nasopharyngeal cysts, rarely parasitic cysts, etc.

HISTORY AND PHYSICAL EXAMINATION

It is of utmost importance to understand the patient's chief complaint which can be determined *via* a good medical and dental history as well as performing a thorough physical examination.

History of Present Illness

- If the patient complains of pain, the usual questions include nature of pain, character, site where it started and where is it referred to, aggravating and relieving factors. Throbbing pain indicates an abscess (Clinical Box 17.1).

Clinical Box 17.1

A few common entities which may produce facial pain
- Pulpal pain
- Gingival and periodontal diseases
- Maxillary sinus diseases
- Temporomandibular joint diseases
- Neuralgias

- *Swelling*: Usual complaint is a slow-growing swelling in the jaw. Get more details about how it started and how has it progressed.

- If there is any ulceration over the swelling, ask about the duration and progress.

- Enquire about any bleeding.

- Elicit specific history regarding *loose teeth, spontaneous exfoliation of teeth and unerupted teeth* **(in case of dentigerous cyst).**

- History of discharge from the bone (multiple draining sinuses) over the lower jaw may suggest osteomyelitis, faciocervical actinomycosis or tubercular osteomyelitis.

Inspection

It involves visualising the surface tissue and its topography. Points to be considered under inspection are: If the swelling is visible, explain the usual characters such as size, shape, surface, margins, contour, colour, and surface characteristic (examine, if the surface is necrotic, ulcerated or eroded, smooth or glistening, flat or raised).

Palpation

It is considered as third eye to the surgeon, the most useful method or manoeuvre to examine the tissues beneath the surfaces. Details are given in Clinical Box 17.2.

Clinical Box 17.2 🔑

- Unilateral/bilateral
- Anatomic region and planes involved
- Tender or nontender
- Solitary or multiple
- Size and shape
- Surface temperature—local rise
- Induration and fixity
- Mobility
- Extent of the lesion
- Borders of the lesion (malignancies have ill-defined borders)
- Consistency of surrounding tissue
- Thickness of overlying tissue
- Fluctuation (difficult in cysts)

Auscultation

- It is usually done in case of jaw swellings for eliciting bruit or thrill for vascular malformations.
- Temporomandibular joint abnormalities to identify any opening or reciprocal click.

Examination of maxilla: It has five surfaces—orbital, superficial, palatine and nasal surfaces can be examined but posterior surface cannot be reached unless very advanced cases of carcinoma maxilla. Detailed examination is given and discussed in oral cavity chapter (Fig. 17.1).

Examination of neck: This should be done specially in malignancies, for enlargement of lymph nodes.

CLINICAL DISCUSSION

1. **What does the patient experience, if the jaw swelling has eroded the floor of the mandible/corticocancellous junction?**
   Inferior alveolar nerve paraesthesia, anaesthesia (acute osteomyelitis).

2. **When will trismus occur?**
   Trismus is evident if the swelling or the tumour is involving the masticatory apparatus or the infratemporal spaces.

3. **Why do you get loose teeth in the upper jaw?**
   Teeth of the upper jaw (maxilla) can become loose if there is expansion of the alveolus secondary to a cyst or a tumour.

4. **Why is osteomyelitis more commonly seen in mandible than in the maxilla?**
   Because maxilla has far more extensive blood supply.

5. **What are the features when the medial wall of the maxilla is involved?**
   Nasal obstruction and epiphora due to obstruction of the lacrimal duct. Bleeding can occur from the nose, if there is ulceration.

6. **What are the features when the lateral wall of the maxilla is involved?**
   There is resultant asymmetry of the face with pain as well as anaesthesia over the skin of the cheek and the upper lip due to involvement of infraorbital nerve.

7. **What are the features, if the roof of the maxillary sinus (floor of the orbit) is involved?**
   There will be proptosis and diplopia.

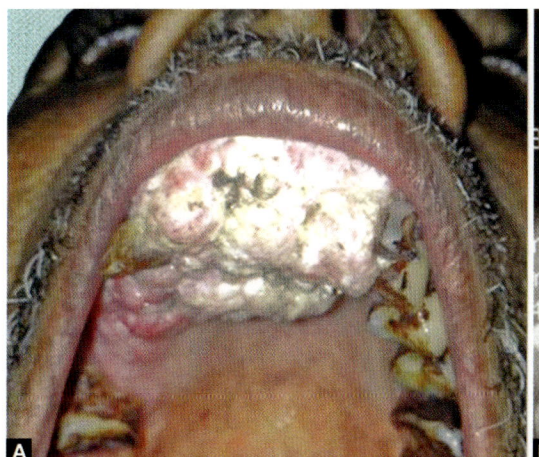 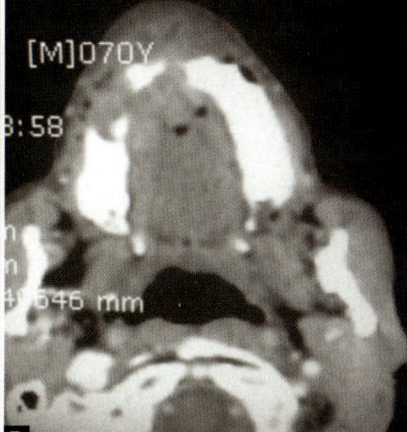 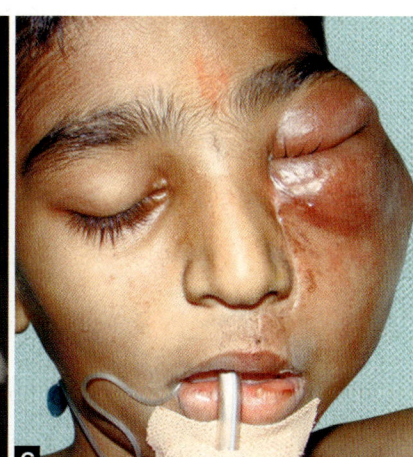

Fig. 17.1: Carcinoma of maxillary sinus (A) Ulceration of hard palate, (B) CT scan image, (C) recurrent carcinoma maxilla

8. **What is the most common type of odontogenic cyst?**
   Radicular cyst which is associated with carious tooth.
9. **What is a cyst associated with an impacted tooth or unerupted tooth called?**
   Dentigerous cyst.
10. **Which cyst has high rate of recurrence and why?**
    Odontogenic keratocyst has a high rate of recurrence attributed to thin lining of the cyst and presence of daughter or satellite cysts as well as due to high mitotic activity. It occurs most commonly in the mandibular ramus region.
11. **What is the most common odontogenic tumour?**
    Ameloblastoma.

DIFFERENTIAL DIAGNOSIS

JAW SWELLING

Radicular cyst or dental cyst: It is the most common of the odontogenic cysts, mainly found around the incisors and canine region of maxilla. Size of the cyst may have variations. It appears as a well-defined unilocular radiolucent lesion in the periapex of the carious tooth (Fig. 17.2). This arises from a normally erupted, chronically infected, pulpless caries tooth. The caries tooth produces a low grade, chronic inflammation which stimulates epithelial debris to proliferate. Later this brings about degeneration of epithelial and mesothelial cells resulting in a cyst within the maxilla. Common in women around 3rd–4th decades. Commonly affects the upper jaw (maxilla). It presents as a slow-growing swelling in the maxillary region resulting in deformity of the face. Features include caries tooth with expansion of maxilla, unilocular cyst in maxilla or orthopantomogram (OPG) showing cyst in the mandible. Aspiration of the cyst demonstrates cholesterol crystals. Excision of the cyst along with its epithelial lining must be done using an intraoral approach. After excision of the epithelium, the cyst wall should be curetted, followed by soft tissue 'push-in' to obliterate dead 'space'.

Dentigerous cyst is a developmental odontogenic cyst commonly seen in the teenage years with a male predilection of **1.6:1**. It is most commonly seen in posterior mandible and

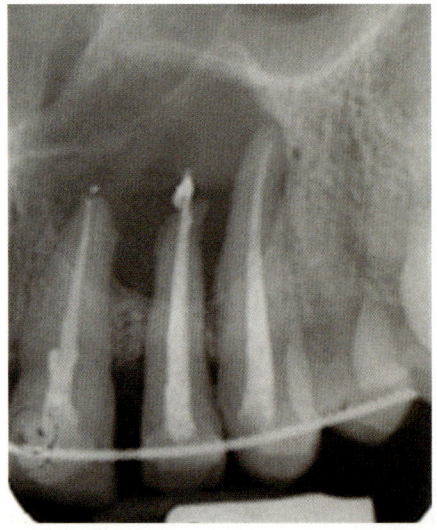

Fig. 17.2: Radiographic presentation of radicular cyst

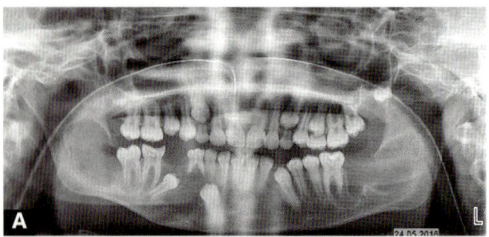

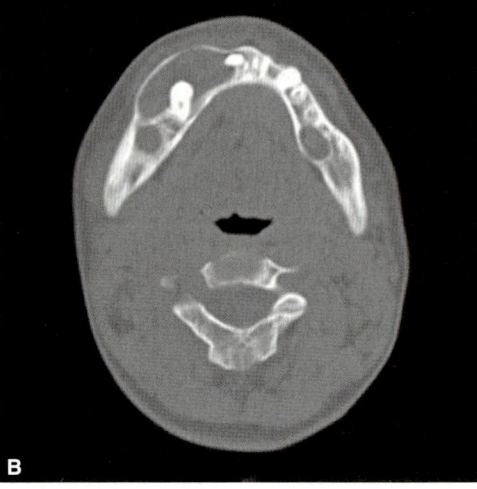

Fig. 17.3: Dentigerous cyst: OPG showing (A) dentigerous cyst, (B) CT scan image

maxilla, associated with unerupted permanent molar tooth. This unerupted tooth constantly irritates the cells, produces degeneration of the cells resulting in a dentigerous cyst. The cyst is lined by squamous epithelium surrounded by connective tissue. Within the cyst, the tooth lies obliquely or sometimes is embedded in the wall of the cyst. As it grows further, the cyst displaces the tooth to which it is attached. Thus, the tooth is displaced deeper and deeper and prevented from eruption. Expansion of mandible, since the inner table of the mandible is strong, mainly occurs in the outer aspect of mandible. The bone gets thinned out resulting in **egg-shell crackling.** Absence of the molar tooth and expansion of the jaws in the buccolingual direction gives a clue to the diagnosis (Fig. 17.3).

X-ray of mandible: It will show tooth in the cyst and soap-bubble appearance due to multiple trabeculations of the bone. It may also show radiolucent well-defined swelling. Small cysts are excised by intraoral approach. Large cysts are managed by marsupialisation.

Odontogenic keratocyst (keratocystic odontogenic tumour): It is the most aggressive of all the odontogenic cysts with a high rate of recurrence. It is most commonly seen in posterior mandibular ramus angle region. It is frequently associated with nevoid basal cell carcinoma syndrome (Gorlin's syndrome), multiple basal cell carcinomas of the skin, multiple odontogenic keratocysts, intracranial calcifications, epidermal cysts of the skin, palmar/plantar pits, enlarged head circumference, hypertelorism, and rib and vertebral anomalies. Prevalence is 1:60,000. The cyst has a tendency to grow in the anteroposterior direction (Fig. 17.4).

Odontoma: Odontomas are hamartomatous lesions rather than a neoplasm. They are diagnosed in the second decade of life. Odontomas are of two types: (a) Compound and (b) Complex

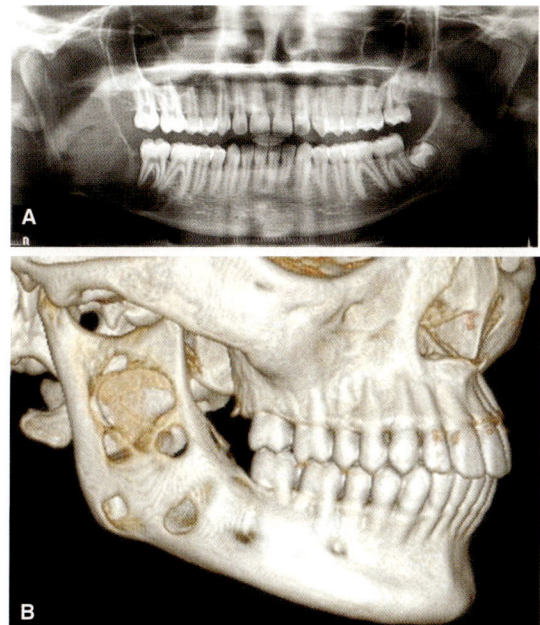

Fig. 17.4: Odontogenic keratocyst. (A) OPG showing odontogenic keratocyst of right side of mandible, (B) CT scan image of same case

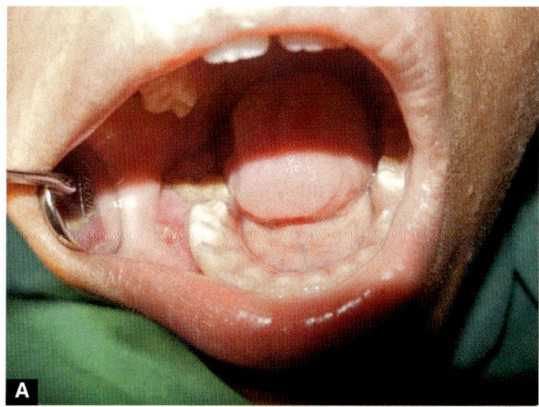

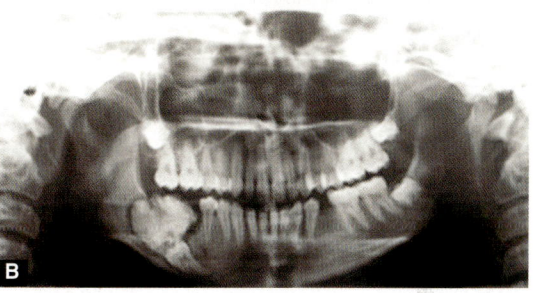

Fig. 17.5: Odontoma. (A) Clinical presentation, (B) OPG showing odontomas

Compound odontomas are composed of *multiple well-formed teeth*. Complex odontomas appear as *irregular calcified tissue* (Fig. 17.5).

Ameloblastoma: It is also called multilocular cystic disease, ameloblastoma, and Eve's disease. This tumour arises from ameloblasts (enamel forming cells). Most common site of occurrence is the ascending ramus and proximal body of the mandible. **Tibia** is the 2nd most common site. It can be explained by inclusion of abnormal embryonic epithelium. **Pituitary** is another common site where adamantinoma can occur. **Both pituitary stalk and enamel arise from oral epithelium.** It is a benign tumour, very slow growing, locally aggressive and destructive, thus compared to basal cell carcinoma. Inadequate treatment results in local recurrence and later metastasis. Ameloblastomas are benign in nature, however, less

than 1% show a malignant behaviour. Resorption of roots of adjacent teeth is a common finding. On radiographic examination, there is marked buccolingual cortical expansion with the presence of multiple internal osseous septa, dividing it into compartments, giving it an appearance of **soap bubble** (Fig. 17.6). Patients in 4th or 5th decade are commonly affected (Clinical Box 17.3).

X-ray: A large cyst and small multiple small cysts due to the trabeculations give it a 'honeycomb' appearance.

Even though it is **benign, simple curettage or enucleation may result in recurrence** and chances of recurrent adamantinoma turning into malignancy are high. Hence, wide

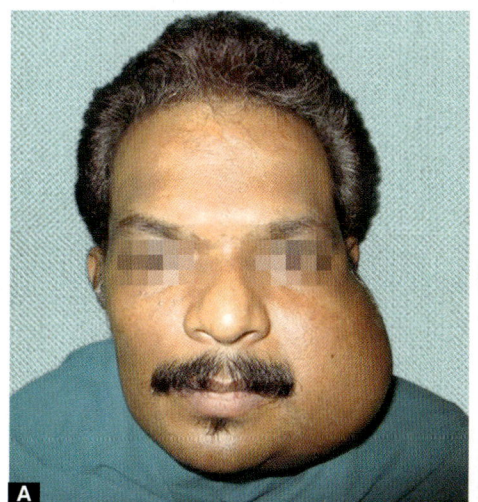

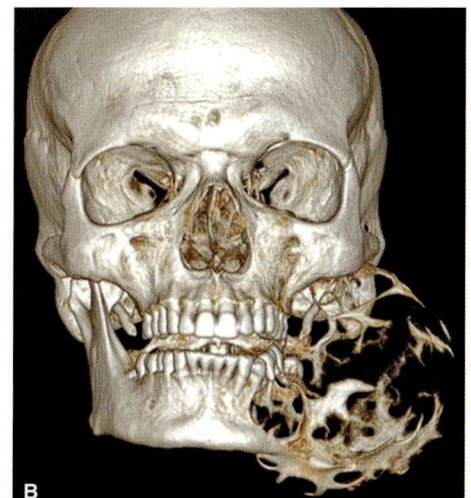

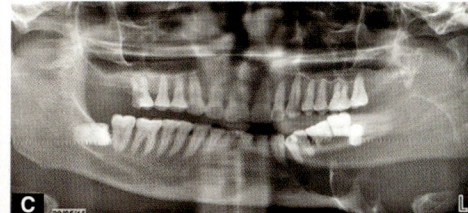

Fig. 17.6: Ameloblastoma. (A) Clinical presentation, (B) CT scan image, (C) OPG

Adamantinoma
- Locally invasive solid tumour
- Nonfunctional, intermittent in growth, unicentric, multilocular
- Spreads within the medullary bone
- Invades soft tissues
- Should not fragment the tumour cells
- Subperiosteal excision should not be done as it may result in recurrence
- Incomplete excision results in recurrence and metastasis to the lung
- Hence, even though it is a benign tumour, it is treated by wide excision or hemimandibulectomy.

excision with 1 cm of healthy normal tissue should be done. It may amount to **segmental excision of the mandible or hemi-mandibulectomy** (refer to Page 241).

Giant celled reparative granuloma (Jaffe tumour): It is a benign tumour which occurs due to haemorrhage within the bone marrow. It affects antral part of maxilla or mandible causing enlargement of the jaw. Stroma is vascular consisting of thin-walled blood vessels, scanty collagen, and connective tissue cells. Microscopic features mimic giant cell epulis or brown tumour of hyperparathyroidism. Unlike an adamantinoma, this tumour affects females in the age group of 10–25 years. Painless enlargement of the jaw is the presenting feature.

X-ray demonstrates radiolucent arteries. Calcitonin 0.5 mg (100 units) daily subcutaneous injection over a period of one year has been recommended as a first-line of treatment. It has shown resolution of the tumour. Curettage is the surgical line of treatment.

SINUSES OF THE JAW

1. ***Acute osteomyelitis*** manifests with fever, malaise, facial cellulitis, trismus and significant leukocytosis. It is a polymicrobial disease with staphylococci, streptococci and bacteroids being the causative organisms. Most periapical and periodontal infections are localised by the production of protective pyogenic membrane or a soft tissue abscess

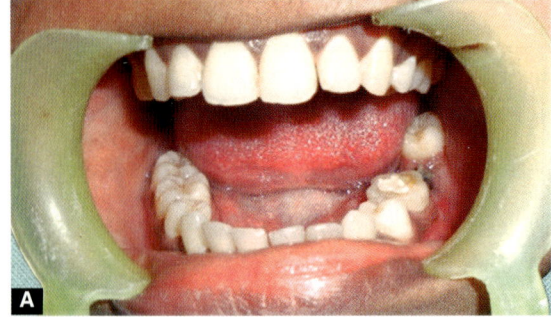
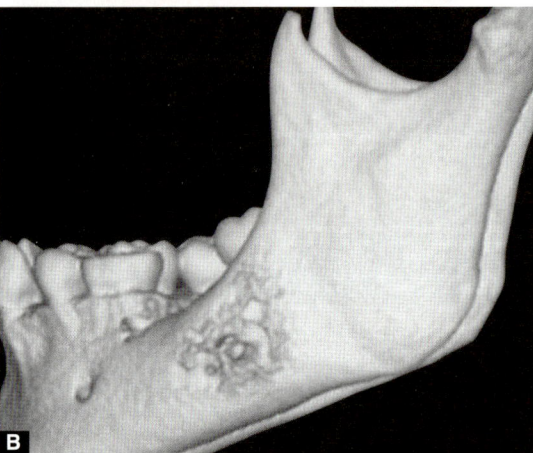

Fig. 17.7. Chronic osteomyelitis: (A) Clinical presentation, (B) CT scan image

wall. If sufficiently virulent, the microorganisms may destroy this barrier leading to osteomyelitis. Untreated cases go for compromised blood supply, necrotic bone, suppuration and later discharging sinuses (Fig. 17.7).

2. ***Tuberculous osteomyelitis*** is almost always haematogenous, originating from a primary focus elsewhere in the body, most likely in the lungs. Mandible may be involved from extension of a tuberculous lesion of the mucous membrane of the oral cavity. The mandible shows a greater predisposition to infection than the maxilla. Presence of ulcers and nodules in the oral cavity, thickening of the mandible, discharging sinuses or nodules will clinch the diagnosis (Fig. 17.8).

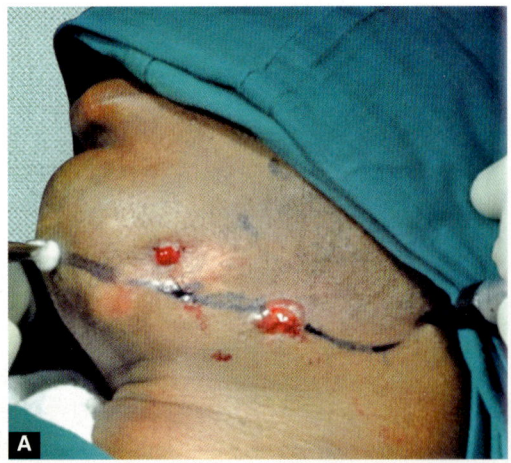
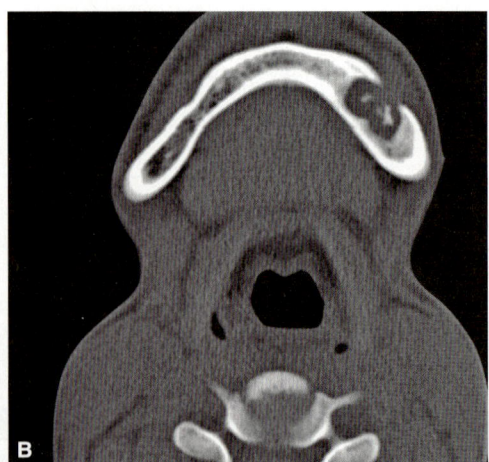

Fig. 17.8. Tubercular osteomyelitis. (A) Clinical presentation of tubercular osteomyelitis. (B) CT scan of the same patient

3. **Faciocervical actinomycosis** is a rare entity caused by *Actinomyces israelii*, which is an anaerobic, gram-positive branching filamentous organism (ray fungus). It is common in patients with poor oral hygiene. The organism produces a subacute or chronic inflammation for many months to years giving an appearance of lumpy jaw. Eventually, the jaws and salivary glands are involved resulting in suppuration as well as extensive induration. There is formation of multiple subcutaneous nodules over the skin of the jaws. The nodules rupture resulting in multiple discharging sinuses. The discharge contains sulphur granules which are gram-positive mycelia surrounded by gram-negative clubs. An important diagnostic point is that **lymph nodes are not involved** (Fig. 17.9).

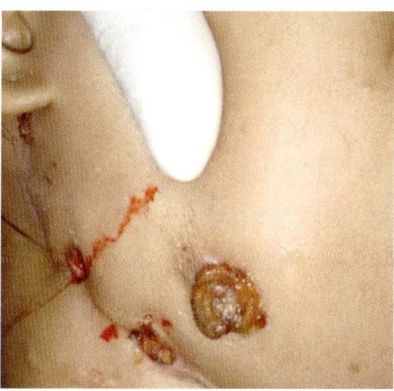

Fig. 17.9: Faciocervical actinomycosis with multiple draining sinuses

MISCELLANEOUS

	Dental cyst	Dentigerous cyst	Adamantinoma
Comparison of three common odontomes			
1. Aetiology	Caries tooth	Unerupted tooth	True neoplasm—ameloblasts
2. Site	Maxilla	Mandible	Mandible
3. Age	30–50 years	20–30 years	40–50 years
4. Palpation	Smooth, thin bone—eggshell crackling	Smooth, expansion of the outer table of mandible	Expansion of mandible in the 3rd molar region, cystic areas
5. X-ray	Radiolucent unilocular cyst	Radiolucent unilocular cyst with unerupted teeth	Large radiolucent area with fine honeycombing
6. Treatment	Subperiosteal excision	Subperiosteal excision	Wide excision hemimandibulectomy even though benign
7. Spread	Does not occur	Does not occur	Local spread, recurrence, late spread to the lung are the features

18

Examination of the Neck Swelling

INTRODUCTION

- Students should understand that examination of any swelling should be in the same order such as location, size, extent, shape, surface, borders (edge), etc. as discussed in detail in the chapter on examination of swelling. Please read this chapter only after reading and understanding the chapter on examination of swellings.

- Neck swellings are one of the most interesting and fascinating cases. In spite of various clinical methods and sometimes even after investigations, diagnosis gets delayed or fails. Final diagnosis is established only after surgical procedure. Developmental anomalies are many resulting in different swellings, e.g. hamartomas, lymphangiomas, vascular malformations. Several important and vital structures are present in the neck **and when diseased, will give rise to peculiar 'surprise' swellings**. To give a few examples: Laryngocoele in trumpet blowers, carotid body tumours in high altitude individuals, etc. Surprises are very well known such as cysticercosis in heavy pork consumers and cystic secondaries from papillary carcinoma thyroid, in young patients.

- Students should learn the art of eliciting symptoms (history) and signs depending upon the site and case. Example: Movement with protrusion of the tongue is a relevant sign for midline swelling, not a lateral swelling. So, if you have a multinodular swelling occupying both sides of the trachea (thyroid), one need not do this test.

Neck examination should also include **extension of neck areas** such as parotid region, retrosternal area, retromandibular region, parapharyngeal spaces and floor of mouth.

- But never forget to examine 'spine' (cervical) for a cystic swelling (cold abscess in the neck), oral cavity for a hard swelling (metastatic nodes), ribs and sternum for carcinoma thyroid and breast for supraclavicular lymphadenopathy.

- Before we discuss the swellings, let us look at a quick review of surgical anatomy of anterior and posterior triangles which will help students in understanding the pathogenesis of the swellings. Figure 18.1 shows the triangles of the neck. It is self explanatory about triangles and boundaries of neck.

Clinical Wisdom

Most common cause of swelling in the neck is from lymph nodes, followed by thyroid swelling. The most common disease of the lymph nodes in the neck is metastasis or secondaries.

TRIANGLES OF NECK

Students are advised to refer anatomy books and get a clear idea about deep fascia of the neck and contents in each triangle of the neck. Very often location of the swelling is so typical that it will tell the diagnosis. Such cases have been included as spotters. Examples: Carotid body tumour in the carotid triangle, branchial cyst in the anterior triangle and thyroglossal cyst in the midline of the neck.

Triangles of the Neck with Two Common Diseases

1. **Submental triangle**

   - Lymph node swelling
   - Submental dermoid swelling

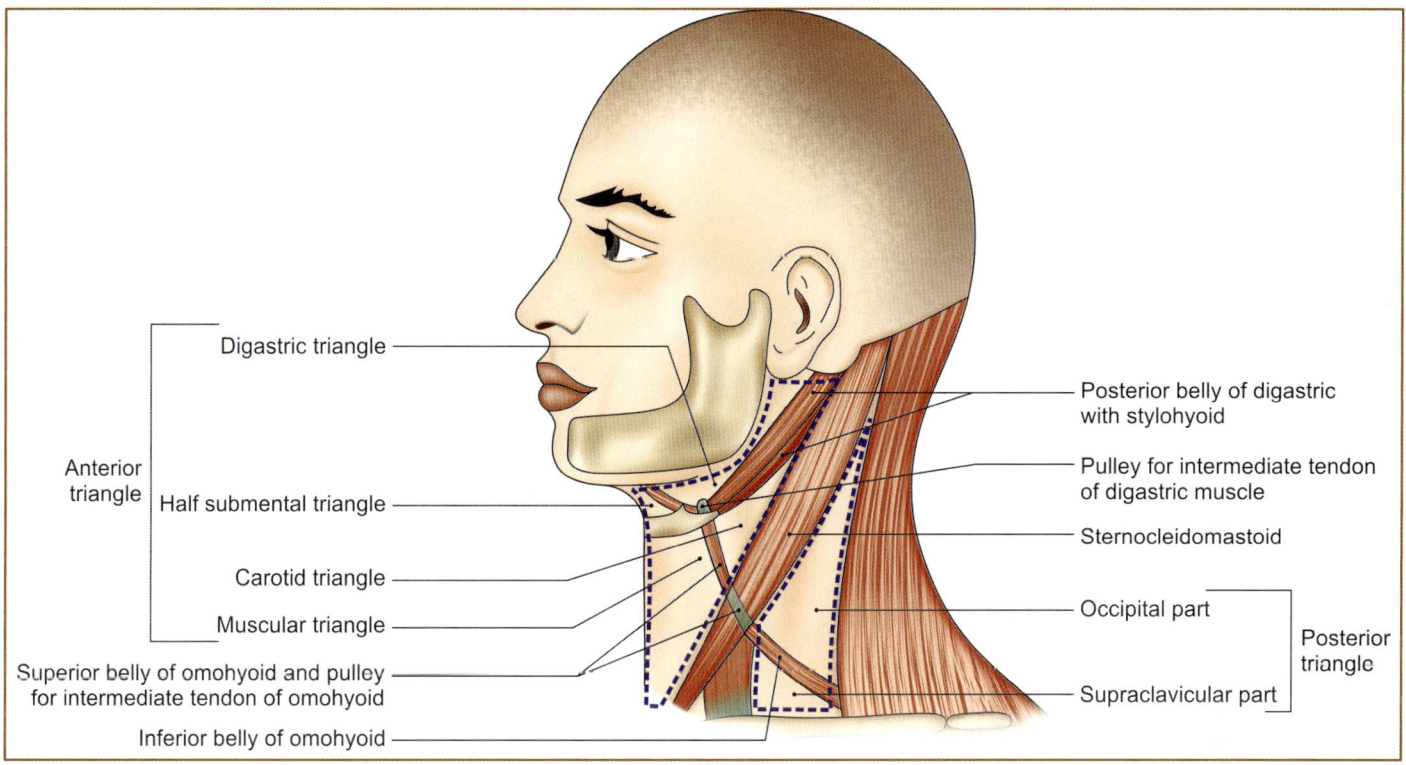

Fig.18.1: The triangles of the neck. The anterior triangle is subdivided by digastrics and superior belly of omohyoid. Posterior triangle is subdivided by inferior belly of omohyoid (*Courtesy*: BD Chaurasia)

2. Submandibular triangle

- Submandibular lymph node
- Submandibular sialoadenitis

3. Anterior triangle

- Branchial cyst
- Cold abscess

4. Carotid triangle

- Carotid body tumour
- Metastatic lymph nodes

5. Muscular triangle

- Metastatic lymph nodes
- Extension of thyroid swellings

6. Posterior triangle

- Neural tumours
- Metastatic lymph nodes

7. Supraclavicular fossa

- Metastatic lymph nodes
- Pancoast tumour—apical bronchogenic carcinoma
- Cervical rib

HISTORY OF PRESENT ILLNESS

- *Age and sex*: A few swellings will occur in young patients. Cystic hygroma and lymphangioma occur in infancy or early childhood (Fig. 18.2). Branchial cyst, and thyroglossal cyst, even though are congenital, they manifest later clinically (Fig. 18.3).

- *What is the duration?* Long duration suggests benign and short duration suggests malignancy (Figs 18.4 and 18.5). Please refer chapter on examination of swellings.

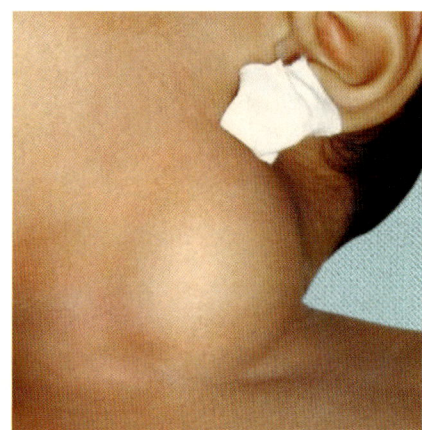

Fig. 18.2: Lymphangioma of the neck (*Courtesy:* Dr Santosh Prabhu, Associate Professor, Department of Paediatrics Surgery, KMC, Manipal)

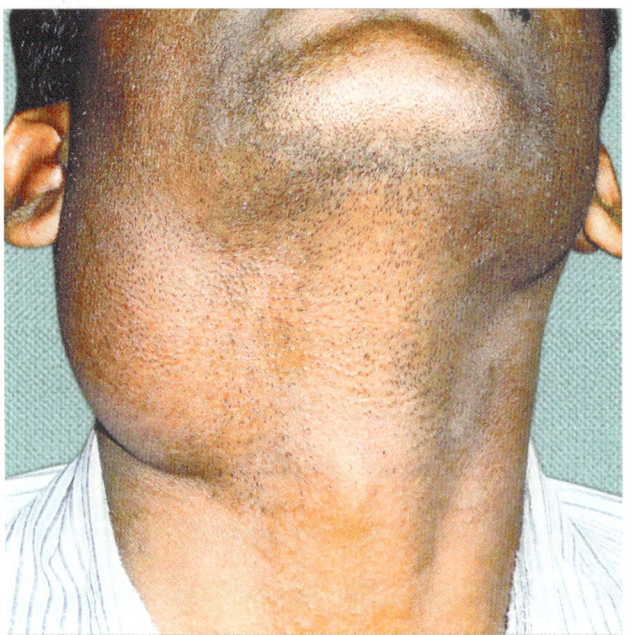

Fig. 18.3: Branchial cyst

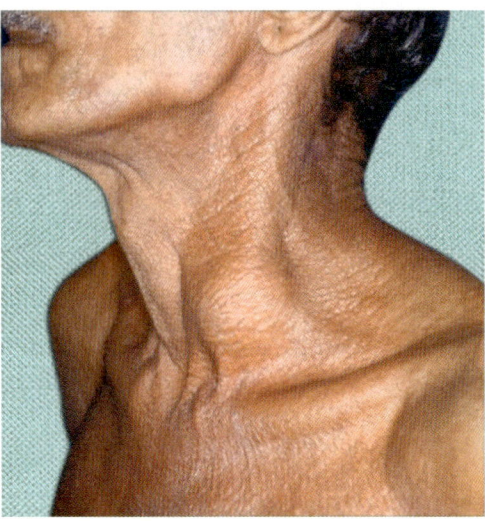

Fig. 18.5: Lower deep cervical nodes in a patient who has carcinoma posterior 1/3rd of the tongue

- *Recent increase or rapid increase:* Classical example is a multinodular goitre, when its starts growing rapidly, suggests malignant change or lipoma turning into liposarcoma (Fig. 18.6).

- *Any pain or fever to start with?* If present, it indicates inflammatory swelling. Example being Ludwig's angina.

- **Swelling first followed by discharge suggests *cold abscess due to tuberculous lymphadenitis.*** Evening rise of temperature will give a clue to the diagnosis. Discharge is due to rupture of the cold abscess into

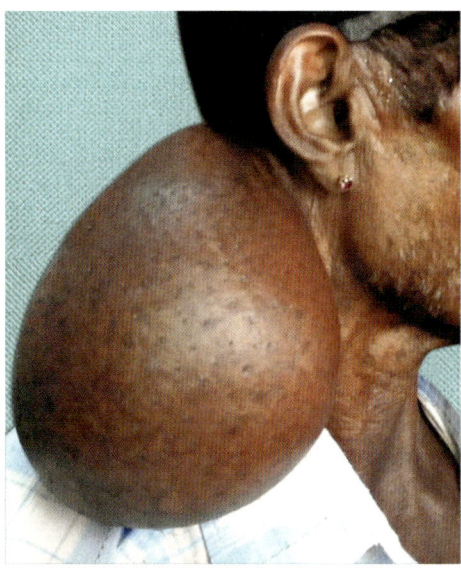

Fig. 18.6: Large lipoma in the nape of the neck since 20 years, rapidly growing since 3 months (*Courtesy:* Dr Mohan SV, Associate Professor, Dept of Surgery, HIMS, Shivamogga)

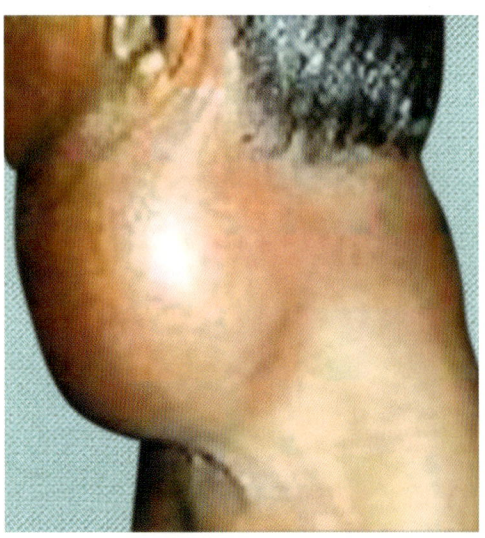

Fig. 18.4: Swelling since 5 years—neural tumour (schwannoma) in the posterior triangle of neck (*Courtesy:* Dr Aditya Patil, Prof Ashok Godhi, Dept of Surgery, JNMC, Belgaum, Karnataka)

the skin resulting in discharge of white cheesy material (Fig. 18.6). Sebaceous cyst (neck is not a common site of sebaceous cyst) also has discharge which is pultaceous or putty in nature.

- History of similar swellings in neck, axilla, and groin suggests possibility of lymphoma.

- History of dysphagia with neck lymph nodes may suggest primary lesion in the posterior one-third of tongue or upper oesophagus.

- History of hoarseness/change in voice—primary may be larynx or thyroid.

- History of nasal bleeding suggests a nasopharyngeal malignancy.
- Elderly man with cough and haemoptysis may be having bronchogenic carcinoma.
- History of loss of appetite and weight loss may suggest malignancy.

  - Before we discuss the clinical examination, students should know the basic classification of cystic swellings—namely congenital, exudative, transudative, degenerative, traumatic, neoplastic and parasitic (page 47).
  - For practical purposes, they can be classified into solid, cystic and pulsatile swellings.
  - Solid swellings are diagnosed by consistency—firm or hard.
  - Cystic swellings are diagnosed by fluctuation.
  - Pulsatile swellings are diagnosed by expansile pulsations.
  - Thus, with the knowledge about the anatomy of the triangles and its contents, pathological diseases along with clinical methods; you should be able to arrive at a correct diagnosis (Clinical Box 18.1).

Clinical Box 18.1

- Complete knowledge
- Complete examination
- Careful examination
- Correlation
- Common sense

LOCAL/REGIONAL EXAMINATION

Inspection

- *Location:* The locations of the swellings are so classical. Many a times, the diagnosis is established, looking at the location of the swelling. Following are a few examples: Nape of the neck is the commonest site of carbuncle. It is also a common site for dermatofibrosarcoma protuberans (Fig. 18.7). Thyroglossal cyst as a midline swelling in the subhyoid position, carotid body tumour in the carotid triangle, branchial cyst in the upper neck partly covered by sternomastoid muscle. Cold abscess also occurs in the same site (hence the differential diagnosis) but it is usually not covered by sternomastoid muscle.

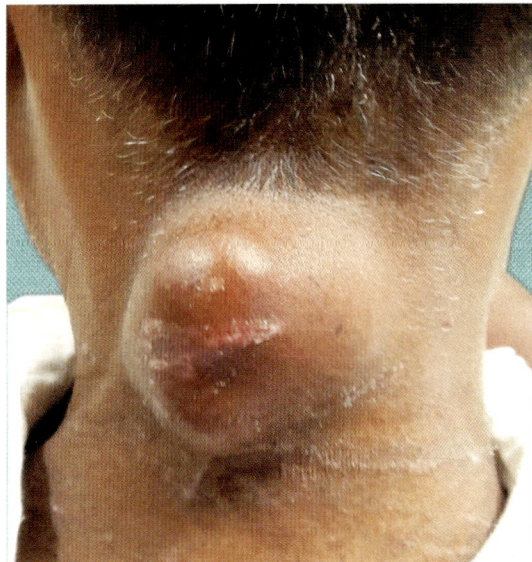

Fig. 18.7: Recurrent dermatofibrosarcoma protuberans in the nape of the neck in a 40-year-old patient

- *Extent:* Intraoral swelling with an extension into the sumandibular triangle is ranula. However big a thyroid swelling is ,its upper extent is always made out since it is confined within pretracheal fascia.

- *Size:* Cystic hygroma and haemangioma attain large size over a period of time. On the other hand, carotid body tumours, and branchial cysts have a size of about 5 cm. Large bulky nodal masses often prove to be Hodgkins's lymphoma.

- *Shape:* Oval swelling in relation to carotid artery may be an aneurysm. Vertically placed midline

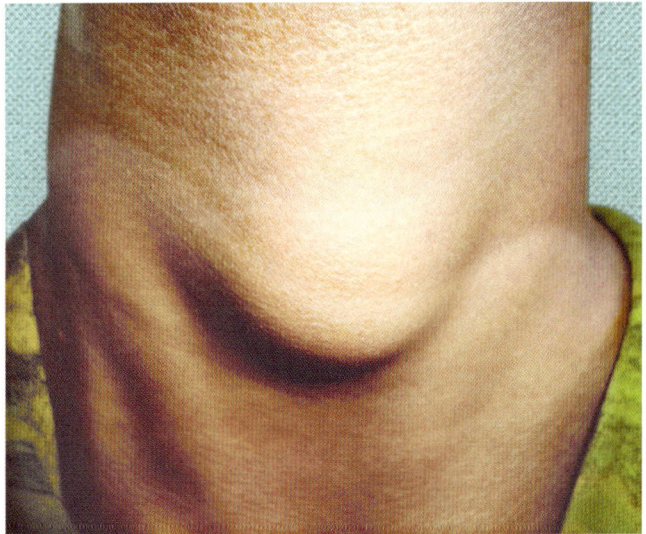

Fig. 18.8: Thyroglossal cyst (*Courtesy*: Dr Satish Deshmukh and Dr Murtaza Akhthar, Professor of Surgery, NKP Salve Institute of Medical Sciences, Nagpur)

swelling is thyroglossal cyst (Fig. 18.8) and horizontally placed oval swelling is subhyoid bursitis. An oval swelling almost like a lobe of the thyroid gland but does not move with deglutition is schwannoma from vagus nerve. Majority of lymph node swellings are oval or round.

- *Surface*: Most of the cystic swellings are smooth, e.g. branchial cyst, thyroglossal cyst, lymphangioma, haemangioma, dermoid cyst, etc.

- *Borders*: Round borders (Fig. 18.9) are typical of benign swellings as in cystic hygroma and irregular borders are seen in malignant lymph nodal masses.

- *Skin over the swelling*: Stretched in large swellings, red and inflamed as in abscess, or secondary infection in a cyst (branchial cyst, thyroglossal cyst). Presence of a punctum indicates sebaceous cyst. Dilated veins represent increased vascularity as in sarcomas. Prominent veins can be due to venous obstruction caused by swellings (Figs 18.10 and 18.11).

- *Platysma sign*: Prominent fold of platysma indicates infiltration of subcutaneous/skin layer.

- *Pulsations*: In areas where a major artery is present, it can give rise to prominent pulsations. In elderly patients, it is due to aneurysmal dilation. Common carotid artery in the carotid triangle is a known site of atherosclerotic aneurysm. Prominent pulsations in posterior triangle may be due to subclavian artery dilatation—often it may turn out to be due to cervical rib (extra rib in the neck).

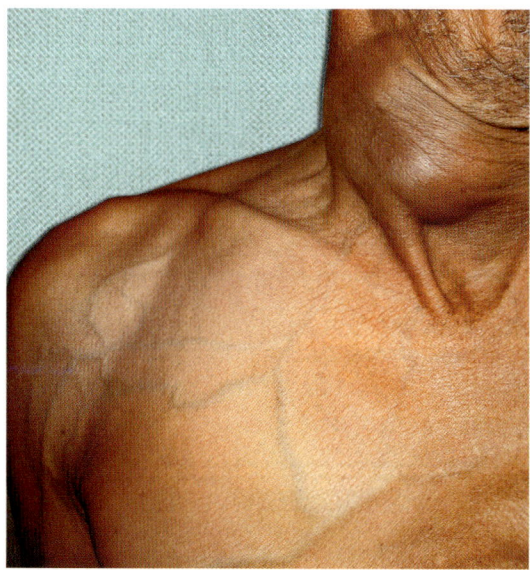

Fig. 18.10: Secondaries in the neck resulting in venous obstruction with dilated veins

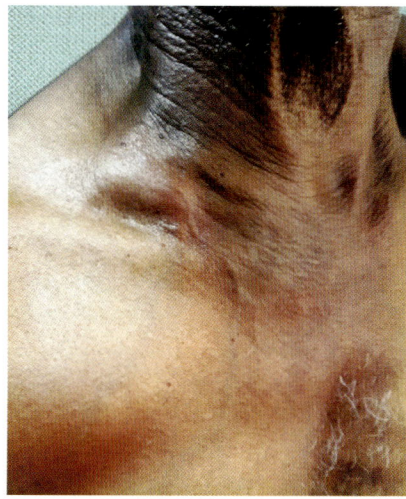

Fig. 18.11: Another case showing prominent veins

- *Pigmentation*: Pigmentation over the swelling and in surrounding area may suggest swelling could be neural (ectodermal) in origin such as neurofibroma, von Recklinghausen's disease (Figs 18.12 and 18.13).

- *Surrounding area*: Oedema is due to inflammation or due to lymphatic obstruction. Atrophy of the muscles and limb oedema are due to compression or infiltration of the neurovascular bundle as in malignant swellings in the posterior triangle.

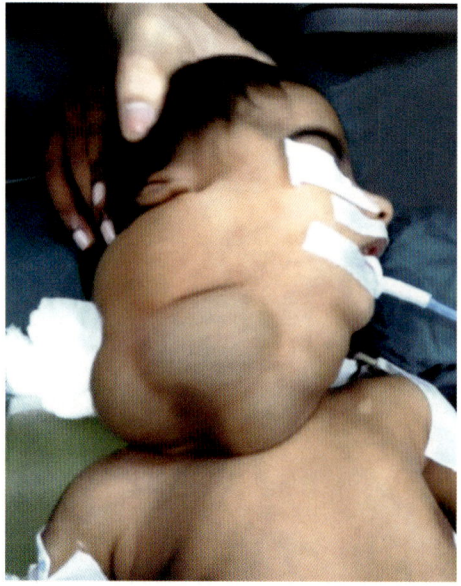

Fig. 18.9: Lymphangioma (cystic hygroma) of the neck. It was very large, child had difficulty in breathing (*Courtesy:* Dr Sandeep PT, Department of Peadiatrics Surgery, KMC, Manipal)

Clinical Wisdom

Do not forget to look for **P**unctum, **P**ulsations, **P**igmentations, **P**latysma sign and **P**uckering of skin, in cases of neck swellings.

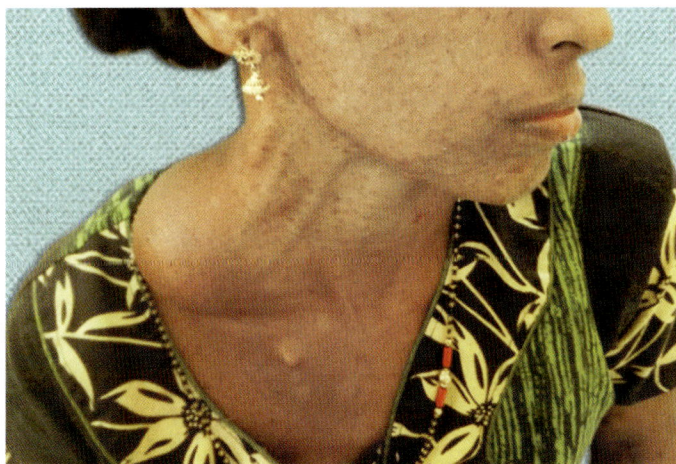

Fig. 18.12: Multiple neurofibromatosis with neurilemmoma in the posterior triangle

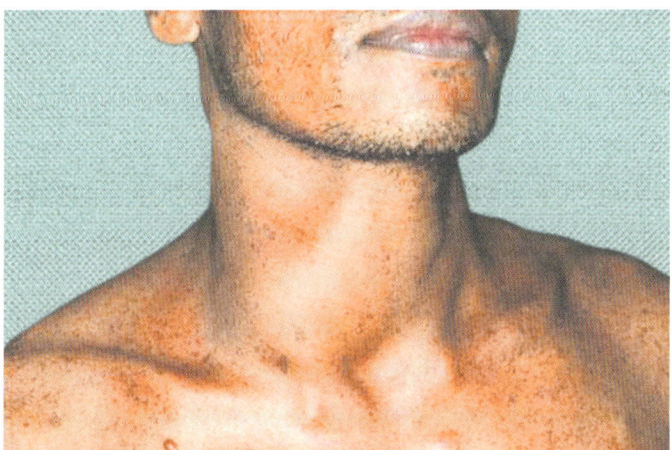

Fig. 18.13: Pigmentation of skin and swelling in the lower neck in the anterior triangle

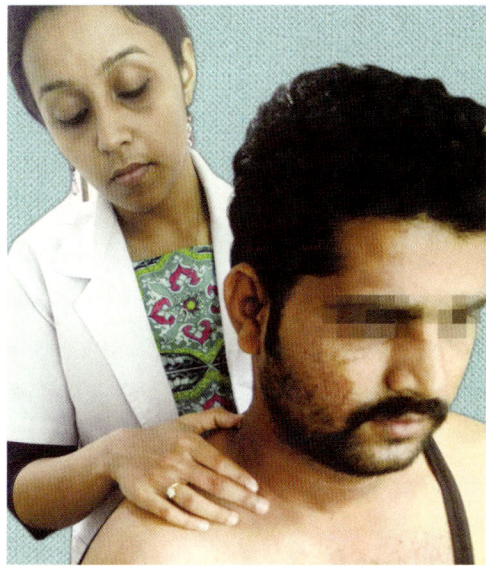

Fig. 18.14: Neck swelling is examined from behind. First find out the location of the swelling

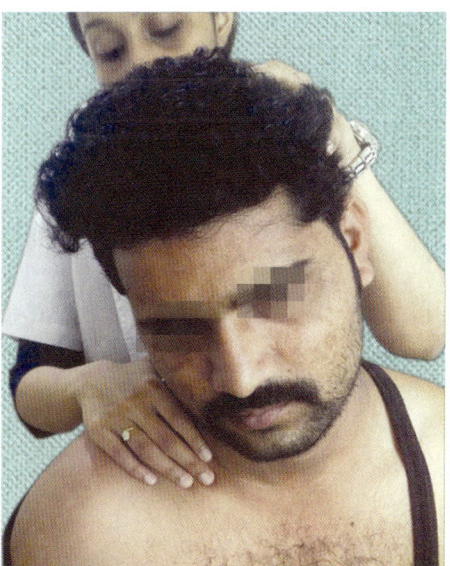

Fig. 18.15: Head is tilted to the same side which relaxes the deep fascia of neck

Palpation

Neck swellings are examined from behind. Head is also tilted to same side which relaxes the deep fascia (Figs 18.14 and 18.15).

1. *Local rise in temperature and tenderness*: Both these findings are typically seen in pyogenic abscesses or in infected cysts. These signs are not seen in cold abscess (name itself tells you why it is cold abscess). If a cold abscess is tender with local rise in temperature, it is due to secondary infection. It is important to realise that in high grade sarcomas such as synovial sarcomas, local rise in temperature may be found but tenderness is usually absent. Arteriovenous malformations also exhibit local rise of temperature.

2. *Size and shape* have to be mentioned.

3. Again confirm **surface** and borders under palpation—smooth, irregular or nodular.

Cauliflower-like appearance of the surface is characteristic of epithelioma—squamous cell carcinoma. Nodular surface is seen in lymph nodal mass/multinodular goitre.

4. *Borders (edge)*

- Round and distinct in benign swellings such as branchial cyst, thyroglossal cyst, and neurofibroma.

- The edge slips under palpating fingers in a case of lipoma. This is pathognomonic sign of lipoma and is called **slip sign**. Lipomas can also occur in the neck (posterior triangle).

5. *Consistency*: This is the most important step under palpation. Your diagnosis should depend upon the finding of consistency, e.g. hard suggests metastasis in lymph nodes or bony swelling as in cervical rib or soft tissue sarcomas.

- *Soft*: Cystic swellings are soft.

- *Firm* in cases of lymph node swellings, neurofibroma.

- *Hard* in metastatic nodes (Fig. 18.16), bony swellings such as cervical rib and malignant swellings. A malignant swelling is not only hard but also indurated. Induration means hardness due to desmoplastic reaction caused by the tumour.

- *Putty consistency*: This is specially described for sebaceous cysts. They have sebum as content. Hence, they have consistency of toothpaste.

- *Variable*: Sometimes, swelling may have variable consistency, where some areas are hard and some, soft or firm. You should be able to explain why there is variable consistency. Variable consistency can be a feature of sarcomas. When they grow rapidly, tumour degeneration or tumour necrosis occurs in a few areas.

- **Rubbery consistency** has been mentioned for lymph nodes in **Hodgkin's lymphoma.**

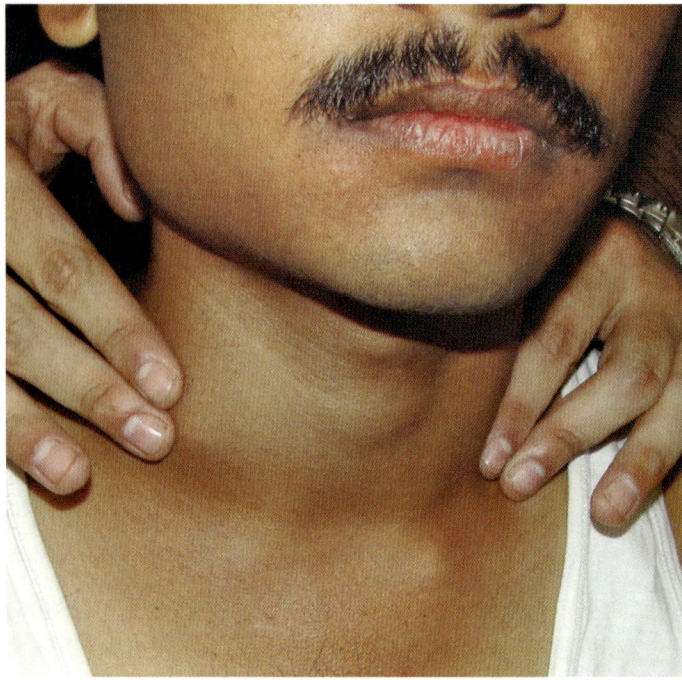

Fig. 18.16: Metastasis in the neck-hard in consistency

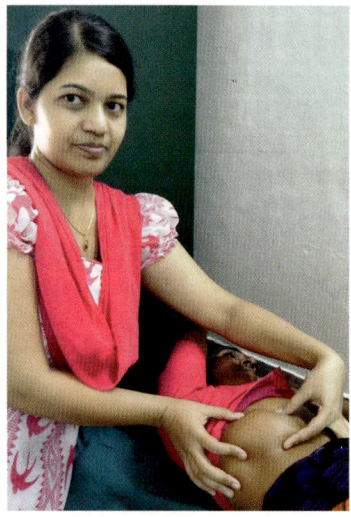

Fig. 18.17: Demonstration of fluctuation test

6. *Fluctuation*: It should be elicited only when swelling is soft—to check whether the swelling contains fluid or not (*refer* to page 23) (Fig. 18.17).

Clinical Wisdom

- If you are wrong in eliciting and interpreting fluctuation test, entire sequence of the remaining tests and diagnosis will be wrong. Hence, do this test carefully.
- Sebaceous cyst does not give rise to fluctuation but yields to pressure and moulds on palpation.

7. *Transillumination test*: Swellings having clear fluid will transilluminate but those with blood (haemorrhage or haematoma) or pus (abscess) or thick contents such as cold abscess (tuberculous) will not. Cystic hygroma and ranula are brilliantly transilluminant swellings in the neck (Figs 18.18).

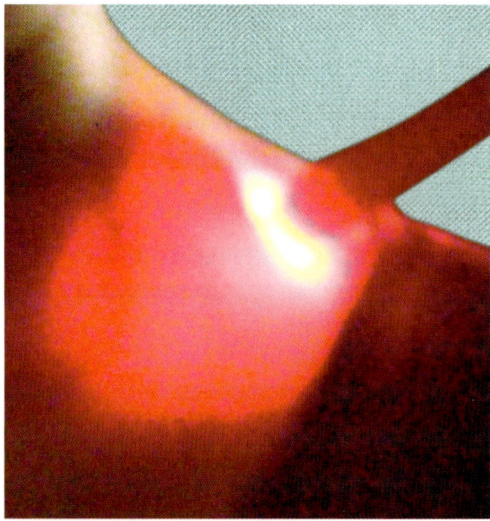

Fig. 18.18: Transillumination positive (*Courtesy*: Dr Vijay Kamath, Professor of Surgery, KIMS, Hubballi, Karnataka)

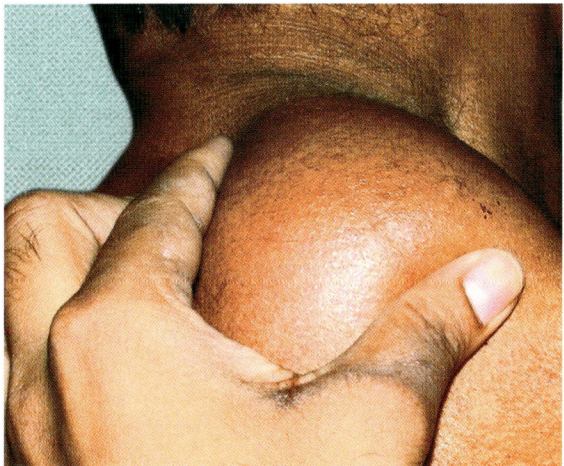

Fig. 18.19: Checking for mobility

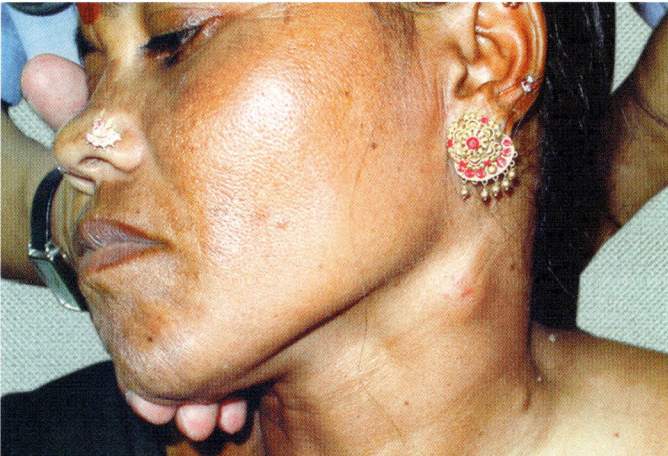

Fig. 18.20: Left sternocleidomastoid contraction test

8. *Intrinsic mobility*

- Hold the swelling and gently move in horizontal and vertical directions. Majority of the subcutaneous swellings—dermoid cysts, neurofibromas, lipoma, etc. have free mobility (Fig. 18.19).

- Restricted mobility is one of the early features of malignant tumours such as soft tissue sarcoma. Malignant lymph node swellings as in metastasis in lymph nodes also may have restricted mobility due to pericapsular spread (transgression).

- Bony swellings are unmistakably immobile, e.g. cervical rib in the posterior triangle.

Clinical Wisdom

- *Branchial cyst*: Restricted mobility is due to its adherence to the sternomastoid muscle.
- *Thyroglossal cyst*: Transverse mobility is absent because the cyst is tethered by remnant of the thyroglossal duct.
- *Metastatic node* has restricted mobility because of infiltration.
- *Mobility of parotid swelling is restricted* because of the tight parotid fascia enclosing it.

---

9. *Plane of the swelling*

- **First lift the skin** and confirm it is not fixed to skin.

- **Move the swelling:** If it moves freely, most often it is a subcutaneous swelling.

- **Contract the muscles:** Subcutaneous swellings become more prominent when the underlying muscles are contracted as in the limbs.

- Almost all swellings in the neck are deep to the deep fascia. Thus, contracting sternomastoid for

laterally placed swellings and bending the chin against resistance for centrally placed swellings must be done to define the plane of swelling (Fig. 18.20). Swellings which are deep to the deep fascia and muscles become less prominent.

- **Immobile swelling:** When one cannot move the swelling at all, two possibilities should be considered. One, it is a swelling arising from the bone or else, it is **fixed to prevertebral fascia** as in anaplastic carcinoma of the thyroid.

10. *Pulsations*: **Expansile pulsations are found in carotid** aneurysms. Transmitted pulsations in the posterior triangle are mostly due to subclavian artery dilatation—commonly due to cervical rib. An enlarged jugulodigastric lymph node may exhibit transmitted pulsations because it is overlying the carotid artery or carotid artery can be pushed anteriorly by jugular lymph nodes (Fig. 18.21).

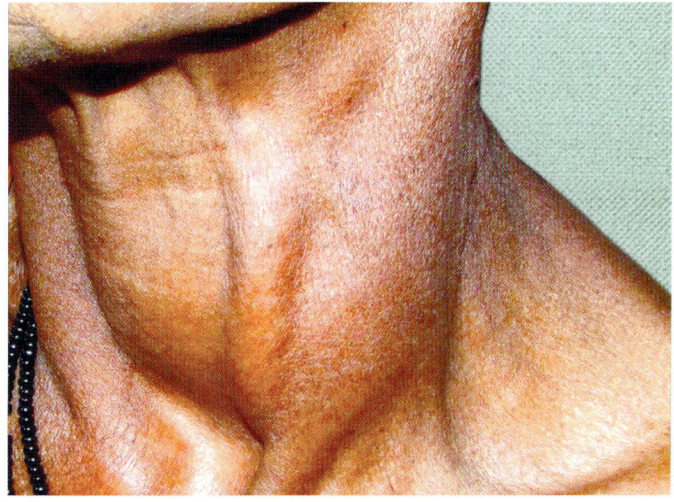

Fig. 18.21: Common carotid artery is pushed anteriorly due to a large jugular chain of lymph nodes

11. *Sign of compressibility*: This test should be done only when swellings are fluctuant. A few swellings elicit compressibility. They are cavernous haemangioma, and lymphangiomas. **C**ompressible swellings reappear when compression is released.

12. *Effects of pressure and paralysis*

    • Distal neurovascular bundle should be checked especially when you suspect malignant swellings such as sarcomas.

    • Large lymph nodal mass can give rise to paralysis of the hypoglossal nerve in the submandibular triangle and paralysis of spinal accessory nerve in the posterior triangle.

    • Look for Horner's syndrome. Hard nodular mass in the lower posterior triangle with pseudoptosis is due to Pancoast tumour—bronchogenic carcinoma arising from apex of the lung.

13. Neck is in-between head and chest. Any hard lymph nodal swelling could be due to metastasis. Thus, examine the oral cavity and breast (in females) for any suspicious lesions (carcinoma)

    • Palpate the abdomen for any mass lesions (specially carcinoma stomach or carcinoma pancreas Fig. 18.22 and Clinical Box 18.2).

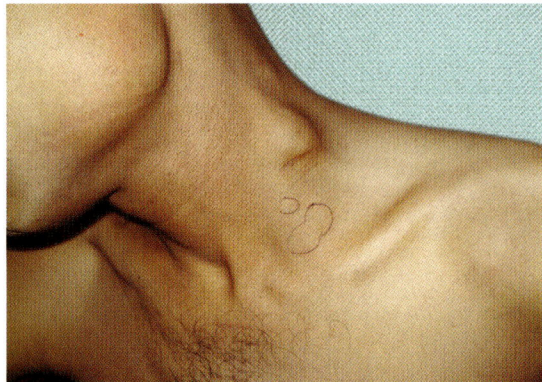

Fig. 18.22: Multiple hard supraclavicular lymph nodes in a case of carcinoma pancreas.

Clinical Box 18.2

• Swelling in upper anterior neck—look for intraoral extensions.
  Example: Submandibular gland enlargement/plunging ranula.

• Swelling in the lower neck—look for retrosternal/intrathoracic extension.
  Example: Schwannomas/lymph cysts within pretracheal fascia.

• If the swelling is a lymph nodal swelling—look for other lymph nodes, liver and spleen.

• If the swelling is metastasis in the lymph nodes, examine for primary sites.

DIFFERENTIAL DIAGNOSIS

DIFFERENTIAL DIAGNOSIS OF MIDLINE SWELLINGS

• Neck swellings can be classified as midline swellings and lateral swellings.

• Lateral swellings are further classified depending upon the triangle in which they arise (details later)

From above downwards

1. Ludwig's angina
2. Sublingual dermoid cyst
3. Enlarged submental lymph nodes
4. Midline dermoid cyst (Fig. 18.23)
5. Subhyoid bursitis
6. Thyroglossal cyst
7. Enlarged isthmus of thyroid gland
8. Pretracheal and prelaryngeal lymph nodes
9. Swelling in the suprasternal space of Burns—lipoma/cold abscess/aneurysm/thymic swellings

1. *Ludwig's angina*: This is an inflammatory oedema of the floor of the mouth spreading to the submandibular region and submental region. Tense, tender, brawny, oedematous swelling in the submental region with putrid halitosis is characteristic of this condition. Broad spectrum antibiotics and drainage play an important role in the treatment of Ludwig's angina.

2. *Enlarged submental lymph nodes*

   A. **Tuberculosis: Matted submental nodes,** firm in consistency, with enlarged upper deep cervical lymph nodes. This is not the common site of tuberculous lymph node enlargement.

   B. **Non-Hodgkin's lymphoma** can present with submental nodes along with other lymph nodes in the horizontal group of nodes such as submandibular, upper deep cervical, preauricular, postauricular and occipital lymph nodes (external Waldeyer's ring). Nodes are *firm or rubbery, discrete without matting.*

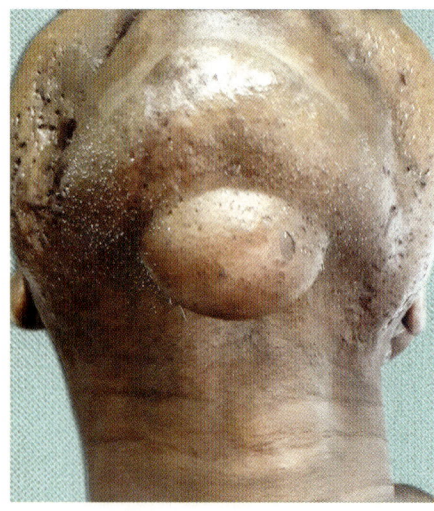

Fig. 18.23: Midline dermoid cyst—submental in position

C. **Secondaries** in the submental lymph nodes can arise from carcinoma of the *tip of the tongue, floor of the mouth, central portion of the lower lip.* The nodes are **hard** in consistency and sometimes, **fixed.**

3. *Sublingual dermoid cyst—midline variety*: It is a type of **sequestration dermoid cyst** which occurs due to sequestration of the surface ectoderm at the site of fusion of the two mandibular arches. Hence, such a cyst occurs in the midline, in the floor of the mouth. Swelling is soft, fluctuant without transillumination. **Bidigital palpation** with one finger over the swelling in the oral cavity and the other finger in the submental region gives a better idea about fluctuation. Differential diagnosis for this condition is a ranula which is brilliantly transilluminant. Other differential diagnosis is thyroglossal cyst in the submental position.

4. *Subhyoid bursitis*
   - The bursa is located below the hyoid bone and in front of thyrohyoid membrane.
   - The swelling is in front of the neck, in the midline below the hyoid bone (Fig. 18.24).
   - The *swelling is oval in the transverse direction.*
   - It moves up with deglutition.

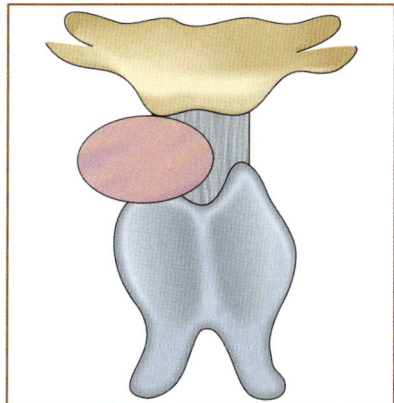

Fig. 18.24: Subhyoid bursitis: Transversely placed oval swelling

- Soft, cystic, fluctuant and transillumination negative swelling **(turbid fluid).**
- The swelling *may be tender* as it contains inflammatory fluid.
- Treated by excision.

5. *Thyroglossal cyst* (Fig. 18.25)
   - It arises from *thyroglossal tract/duct* which extends from **foramen caecum at the base of the tongue to the isthmus of the thyroid gland**. Hence, the thyroglossal cyst can develop anywhere along this duct. Subhyoid position is the most common. (Refer to Clinical Box 18.3).
   - More common in women.
   - Common age of presentation is 15–30 years.
   - It is a painless, midline swelling. However, in the region of thyroid cartilage, the swelling is slightly deviated to the left side.
   - The cyst is soft, cystic, fluctuant, transillumination—negative swelling (very rarely, it can give rise to transillumination) (Figs 18.26 and 18.27).
   - It can be firm if the tension within the cyst is high.

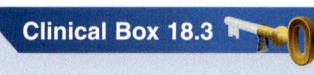

Clinical Box 18.3

Sites of thyroglossal cyst
1. Subhyoid—the most common
2. At the level of thyroid cartilage—2nd common
3. At the level of cricoid cartilage
4. At the foramen caecum (rare)
5. In the floor of the mouth

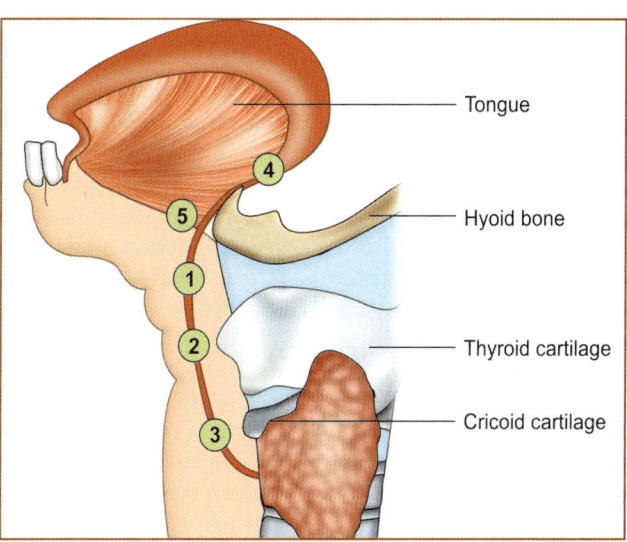

Fig. 18.25: Sites of thyroglossal cyst

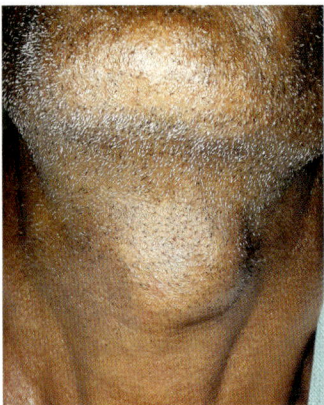
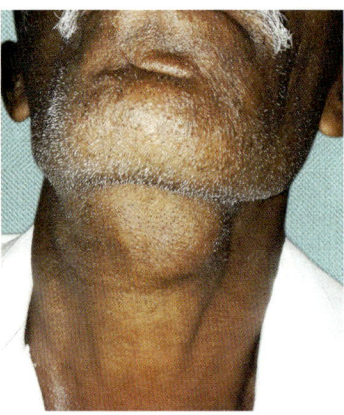

Figs 18.26 and 18.27: Thyroglossal cyst before and after deglutition

- *Mobility*: Thyroglossal cysts **exhibit three types of mobility** which are characteristic of this condition:
  a. The cyst **moves with deglutition.**
  b. **Moves with protrusion of tongue:** Hold the thyroglossal cyst with the finger and thumb and ask the patient to protrude the tongue outside. **The movement of the cyst upwards is described as a tug because of its attachment with the hyoid bone** (Fig. 18.28).
  c. The swelling **moves sideways** but not vertically as it is tethered by the thyroglossal duct.
- You can also extend the neck and watch for movement of the cyst (Fig. 18.29).
- Sometimes you may see a scar of previous surgery. If there is recurrence, it is an incomplete excision (Fig. 18.30).
- **Infected thyroglossal cyst** can be tender, and **inflamed.**

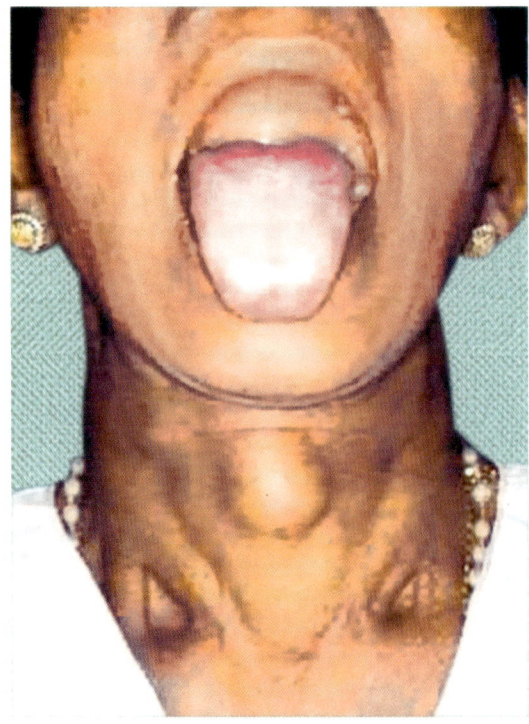

Fig. 18.28: Thyroglossal cyst moves on protrusion of tongue outside

Do not forget to feel the base of the tongue for lingual thyroid/ectopic thyroid. Whenever a patient has one congenital anomaly, examine thoroughly for 'more' associated anomalies.

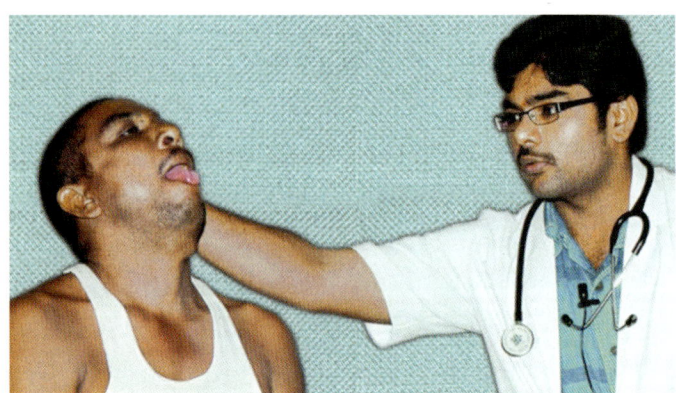

Fig. 18.29: Extend the neck and see carefully for movement on protrusion of the tongue (*Courtesy*: Dr. Challa Srinivas Rao, Professor of Surgery—Undergraduate CME, Konasema Institute of Medical Sciences, Amalapuram, Andhra Pradesh)

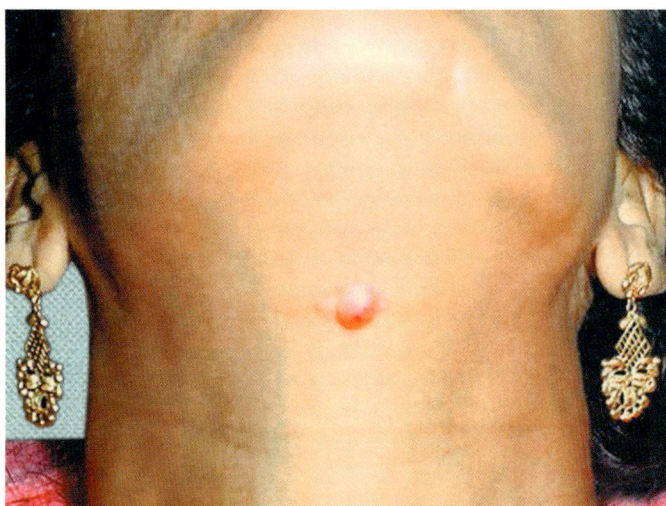

Fig. 18.30: Thyroglossal cyst—you can see the previous operated scar

CLINICAL DISCUSSION

1. **What type of cyst is thyroglossal cyst?**
   It is a tubulo-embryonic type of dermoid cyst
2. **What is the investigation?**
   - Ultrasound can detect cystic nature of the cyst
   - It can also detect normal thyroid gland
3. **What is the treatment?**
   Sistrunk's operations: Excision of the cyst along with thyroglossal duct tract which includes removal of part of hyoid bone also
4. **What are the complications of the thyroglossal cyst?**
   Infection, abscess, fistula. Very rarely carcinoma can arise.

6. Thyroid swellings from isthmus enlargement

- When you cannot feel the tracheal rings—2nd, 3rd and 4th, it means isthmus is enlarged. Smooth enlargement is a part of generalised enlargement as it happens in colloid goitre, pregnancy goitre, primary thyrotoxicosis, etc.
- There can be a solitary nodule also in the isthmus (Fig. 18.31).
- All thyroid swellings move upwards with deglutition (exceptions in page 272).

7. Pretracheal and prelaryngeal lymph nodes:
These lymph nodes produce nodular swelling in the midline. One or two discrete nodes are palpable. They can enlarge due to following conditions:

- **Acute laryngitis:** The nodes are tender, soft.
- **Papillary carcinoma of thyroid:** The nodes are firm without matting, with or without evidence of thyroid nodule (occult primary—**Delphian nodes**).
- **Carcinoma of the larynx:** The nodes are hard in consistency.
- In India, **tuberculosis** should be considered as a possible diagnosis when other diseases are ruled out.

8. Swellings in the suprasternal space of Burns

- **Lipoma:** Soft and lobular, the edge slips under the palpating finger.
- **Cold abscess** *in this location is not uncommon:* It is common in women who present with swelling of a few weeks duration. Typically, it is a fluctuant swelling without transillumination (Fig. 18.32).
- **Sequestration dermoid cyst** is a midline, soft, cystic, fluctuant swelling.
- **Thymic swellings**, *an aneurysm* of innominate artery, (Fig. 18.33), and **gumma** are the other causes.
- Prominent pulsatile swelling in the suprasternal space is due to aneurysmal dilatation of innominate artery. Thrill and bruit are classical features.

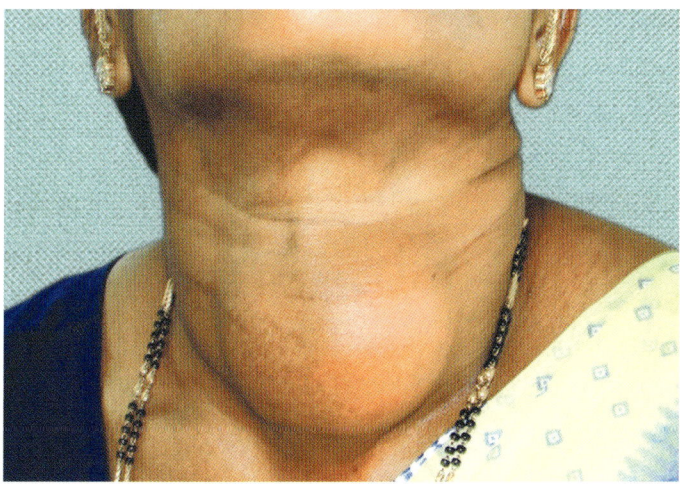

Fig. 18.31: Thyroid swelling

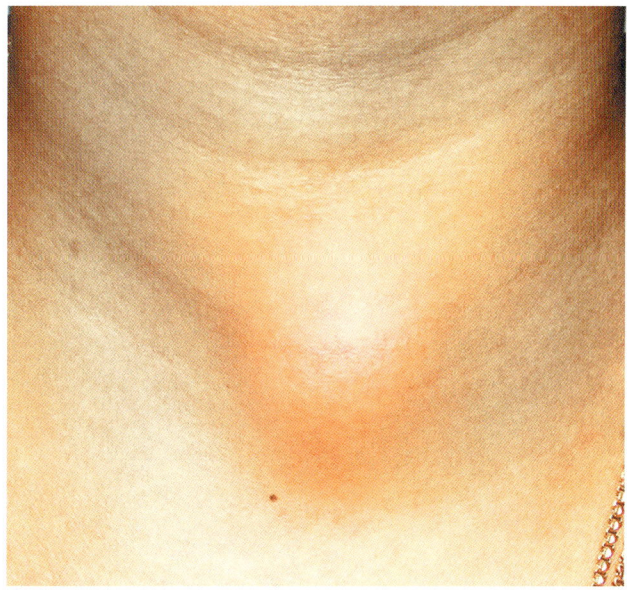

Fig. 18.32: Cold abscess in the suprasternal space of Burns

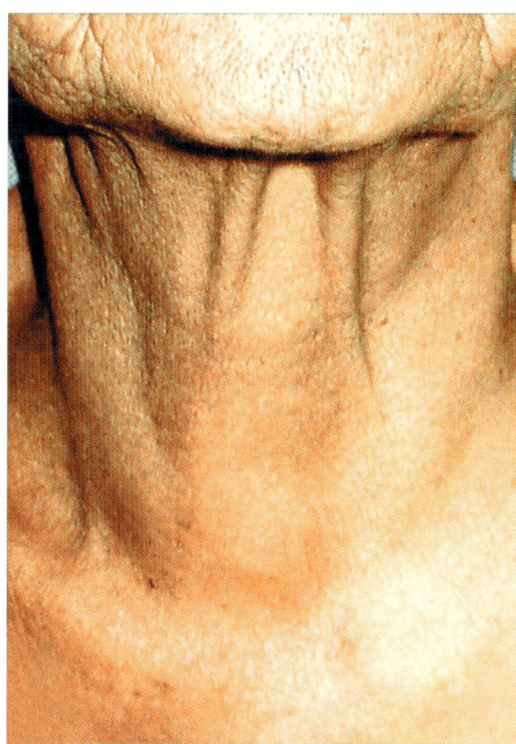

Fig. 18.33: Aneurysm of innominate artery (*Courtesy*: Dr Dilip Amonkar, Govt. Medical College, Goa)

- Since almost all swellings in the midline neck are confined within pretracheal fascia, they do not override sternum. Look at the Fig. 18.34, it is a swelling in the suprasternal space of Burns
- But, it can also go behind the sternum because pretracheal fascia extends below the sternum and gets attached to adventitia of the arch of the aorta. In such cases cough impulse should be tested. It will be positive.

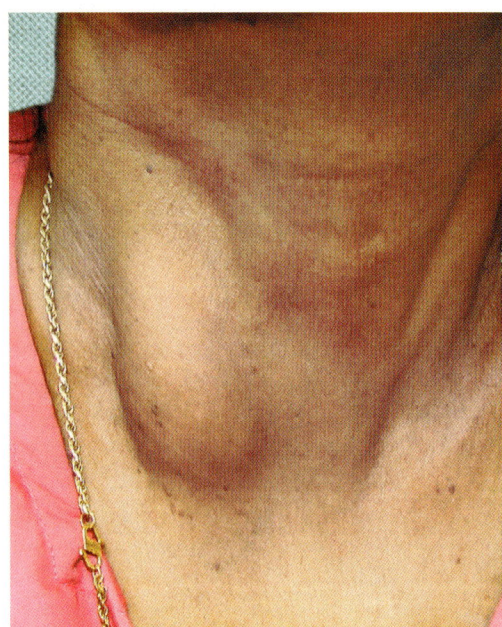

Fig. 18.34: Mediastinal lipoma (*Courtesy:* Dr Salim, Head, Department of Surgery, Trivandrum Medical College, Kerala (PG examination case 2009)

Clinical Wisdom

The swelling was deep to pretracheal fascia and partly substernal. It was soft and lobular—confused for compressible swelling. Impulse on cough was present. Candidate offered haemangioma as diagnosis (Fig. 18.34).

DIFFERENTIAL DIAGNOSIS OF LATERAL SWELLINGS

Each side of the neck is a quadrilateral space subdivided by sternocleidomastoid into anterior and posterior triangles. They are further subdivided as given below. Very interesting swellings occur in this location.

Anterior triangle

1. Submental triangle
2. Digastric (submandibular) triangle
3. Carotid triangle
4. Muscular triangle

Posterior triangle

1. Occipital triangle
2. Supraclavicular triangle

DIFFERENTIAL DIAGNOSIS OF SWELLINGS IN THE ANTERIOR TRIANGLE

Submental Triangle

1. **Enlarged submental lymph nodes**: They form a round swelling (single lymph node) or nodular swelling which is palpable in the midline. The nodes can get enlarged due to following conditions:
   - *Acute lymphadenitis*: Very often, poor oral **hygiene** or a **caries tooth** produces painful, **tender, soft enlargement**

of these lymph nodes. Extraction of the tooth or with improvement of oral hygiene, lymph nodes regress.
   - *Chronic tuberculous lymphadenitis* can affect these nodes along with upper deep cervical nodes. The nodes are firm and matted.
   - *Secondaries* in the submental lymph nodes arise from carcinoma of the tip of the tongue, floor of the mouth and central portion of the upper lip. The nodes are **hard** with or without **fixity**.
   - *Non-Hodgkin's lymphoma* can involve submental lymph nodes along with horizontal group of nodes in the neck. The nodes are **firm** or **rubbery** in consistency.

2. **Congenital**
   - Sublingual dermoid cyst—midline variety (refer to midline swellings)
   - Thyroglossal cyst can present in the submental region—submental variety

3. **Inflammatory** (Ludwig's angina—more of swelling in the floor of the mouth and in the submandibular region.

4. **Malignant**: Carcinoma floor of the mouth can extend into the submental region in neglected cases.

Submandibular Triangle

Surgical Anatomy

- The submandibular triangle is a part of anterior triangle. This is bounded **inferiorly** by anterior and posterior belly of digastric muscles with their tendon, **superiorly** by the attachment of deep fascia to the whole length of mandible. This triangle is covered by deep fascia. The floor is formed by mylohyoid muscle which arises from mylohyoid line of the mandible, thus closing the space.
- **Swellings in the submandibular triangle are**
  1. Enlarged submandibular lymph nodes—common
  2. Submandibular salivary gland enlargement—common
  3. Plunging ranula—not uncommon
  4. Ludwig's angina—not uncommon
  5. Lateral sublingual dermoid cyst—rare
  6. Tumours of the mandible—rare

1. **Enlarged submandibular lymph nodes:** They form a nodular swelling which is deep to the deep fascia. **They are palpable only in the neck (not intraorally)**. The nodes can get enlarged due to following conditions:
   - *Acute lymphadenitis*: Very often, poor oral **hygiene** or a **caries tooth** produces painful, tender, soft enlargement of these lymph nodes. With extraction of the tooth, improvement of oral hygiene, and antibiotics, lymph nodes regress.
   - *Chronic tuberculous lymphadenitis* can affect these nodes along with upper deep cervical nodes. The nodes are multiple, firm and matted.
   - *Secondaries* in the submandibular lymph nodes arise from carcinoma of the buccal mucosa, tongue, palate. The nodes are **hard** with or without **fixity** (Fig. 18.35).
   - *Non-Hodgkin's lymphoma* (Fig. 18.36) can involve submandibular lymph nodes along with horizontal group of nodes in the neck. The nodes are **firm** or **rubbery** in consistency.

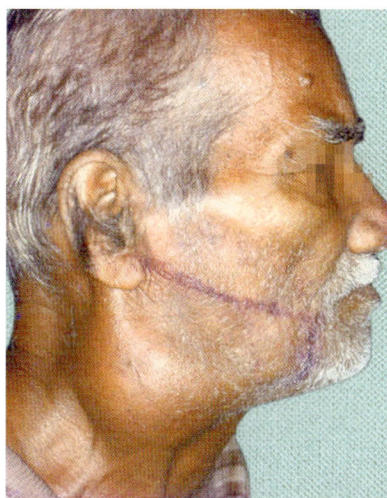

Fig. 18.35: Large metastatic submandibular lymph nodes

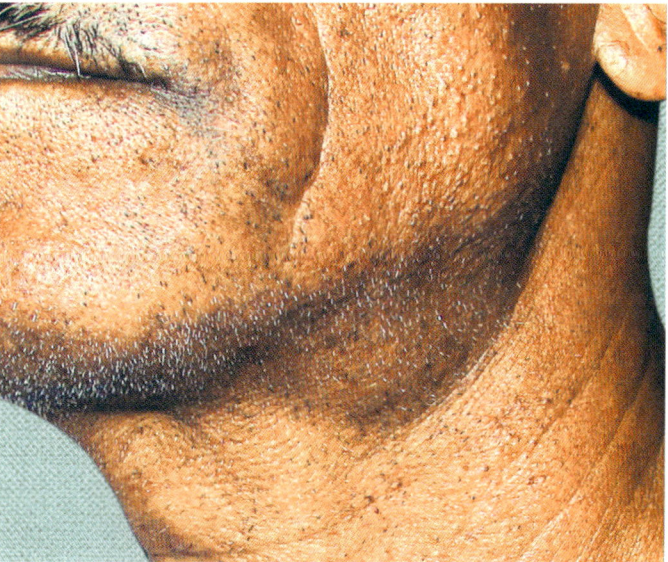

Fig. 18.37: Submandibular sialoadenitis

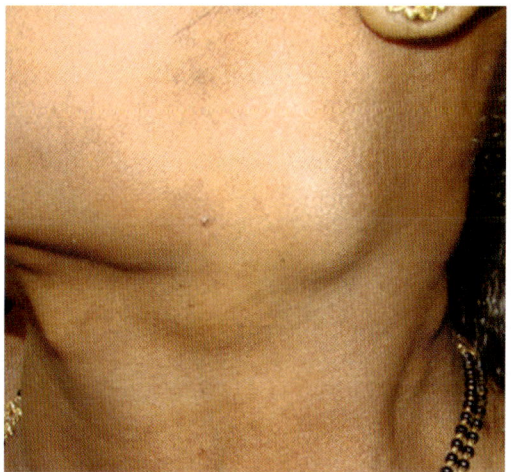

Fig. 18.36: Enlarged submandibular lymph nodes in a case of non-Hodgkin's lymphoma (*Courtesy:* Dr Raghunath Prabhu, Dr Bharath and Dr Adarsh, Dept of Surgery, KMC, Manipal)

2. *Submandibular salivary gland enlargement* (Clinical Box 18.4):

- The common causes are chronic sialoadenitis with or without a stone, tumours of the salivary gland or enlargement due to autoimmune diseases (Fig. 18.37). They form irregular or nodular swelling which is characteristically bidigitally palpable. **Enlarged submandibular gland is bidigitally palpable because the deep lobe is deep to mylohyoid muscle** (Fig. 18.38).
- Mixed tumour can also occur in the submandibular gland (Fig. 18.39).

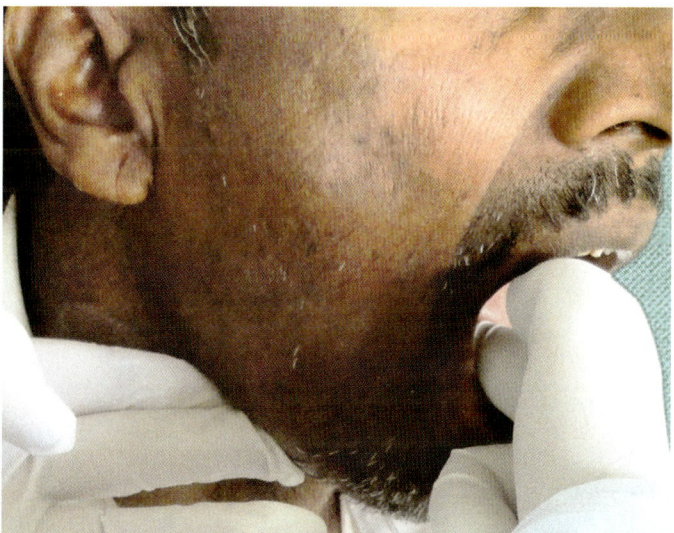

Fig. 18.38: Bidigital palpation of enlarged submandibular gland swelling. Two fingers are placed in the floor of the mouth and the outer fingers over the swelling

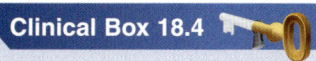

Clinical Box 18.4

Submandibular salivary gland enlargement
- **C**alculus
- **C**hronic sialoadenitis
- **C**ancer—tumour
- **C**hronic diseases: Autoimmune

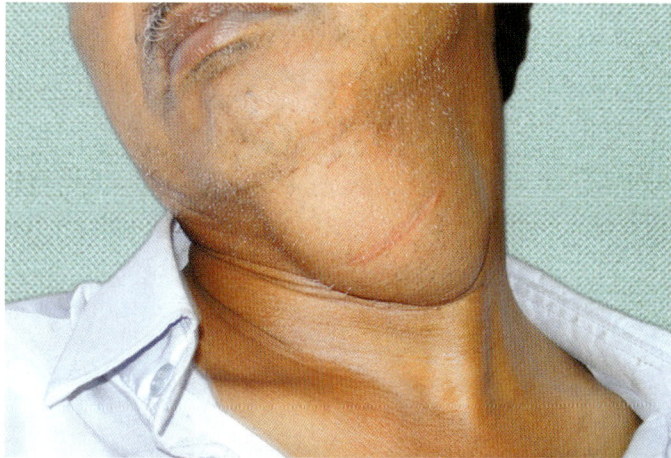

Fig. 18.39: Mixed salivary tumour in a 40-year-old man

3. *Plunging ranula*: Young patient who complains of painless swelling in the floor of mouth of a few days duration. It is soft, fluctuant and brilliant transilluminant swelling. When it extends from the side of the mylohyoid muscle, it forms a swelling in the submandibular region. Both are interconnected which can be demonstrated by cross-fluctuation test.

4. *Sublingual dermoid—lateral variety:* When they arise from **2nd branchial cleft,** they are found lateral to the midline.

5. *Ludwig's angina*

6. *Jaw tumours:* When the horizontal ramus of the mandible expands as in adamantinoma or any other tumour, it will result in a swelling in the sumandibular region also. They are fixed and hard swellings which cannot be separated from the bone.

Clinical Case Capsule

A 35-year-old man presented with pain and swelling in the submandibular region. On examination, it was a very hard swelling which was bidigitally palpable. The surgeon told the relatives that the patient has hard submandibular lymph node and possibly has malignancy in aerodigestive tract. Orthopantomogram/ ultrasound revealed it was a large submandibular stone (Fig. 18.40). Hence a good clinical knowledge is essential.

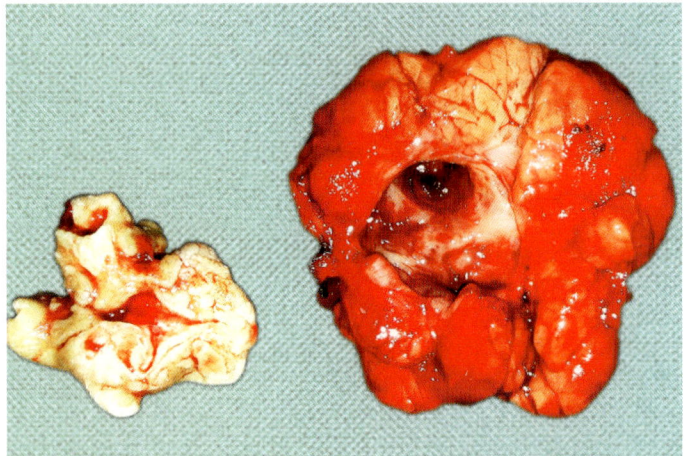

Fig. 18.40: Submandibular sialoadenitis due to stone

Carotid Triangle

The carotid triangle has following boundaries: Laterally by sternomastoid muscle, superomedially by digastric muscle and stylohyoid muscle and inferomedially by omohyoid muscle.

Some important swellings in this triangle are as follows:

1. Branchial cyst
2. Lymph node swelling
3. Aneurysm of carotid artery
4. Carotid body tumour
5. Extension of goitre
6. Schwannoma of the vagus

7. Laryngocoele—rare
8. Sternomastoid tumour—rare

1. *Branchial cyst:* Branchial cyst arises from vestigeal remnants of 2nd branchial arch. Even though congenital, majority of patients are young between the age group 15 and 25 years. The swelling is typically located in the anterior triangle of the neck partly under cover of the upper one-third of anterior border of sternomastoid. This can be explained because of the development of sternomastoid muscle from the myotome in the ridge of second branchial arch (Fig. 18.3). The swelling has smooth surface and round borders. It is soft, cystic, fluctuant and transillumination—negative. The consistency is that of a rubber bag half-filled with water. The swelling is very often firm due to thick inspissated content. In such situations, it is very difficult to elicit fluctuation. The mobility of the swelling is also restricted because of its adherence to the sternomastoid muscle. Sternomastoid contraction test: The swelling becomes less prominent.

2. *Lymph node swelling*

   A. *Tuberculous lymphadenitis:* Multiple, **mobile, matted lymph nodes are characteristic of tuberculosis.** Next stage is stage of cold abscess. It occurs as a result of caseation necrosis of the lymph nodes. This forms a soft, cystic, fluctuant swelling with negative transillumination. Presence of other lymph nodes in the neck or sinuses in the neck gives the clue to the diagnosis. Loss of appetite, weight loss, weakness and evening rise in temperature may be other features (Figs 18.41 to 18.43).

Clinical Box 18.5

Stages of tuberculous lymphadenitis
1. Stage of lymphadenitis
2. Stage of periadenitis or matting
3. Stage of cold abscess
4. Stages of collar—stud abscess
5. Stage of sinus formation

   B. *Metastasis in the level II*: Jugulodigastric lymph node is a common swelling. Classically, the patient is elderly above the age of 50 years, who complains of painless swelling in this location for a few weeks to months duration. On examination, it is round, smooth or nodular, hard and often fixed. Examine the oral cavity, you will find ulcer, growth or indurated lesions may be from tongue, buccal mucosa or tonsil.

   C. *Non-Hodgkin's lymphoma*: These nodes are part of the entire chain of external Waldeyer's ring.

3. *Aneurysm of the common carotid artery:* Atherosclerosis is the most common cause of aneurysm. This weakens the vessel walls uniformly and produces fusiform dilatation of the blood vessel. Typically, elderly aged (above 70) patient who is hypertensive complains of painless swelling in the neck. On examination, it is an oval, pulsatile swelling. Palpation reveals the cystic nature and expansile pulsations. Compressibility is positive. Bruit/thrill is characteristic of this condition.

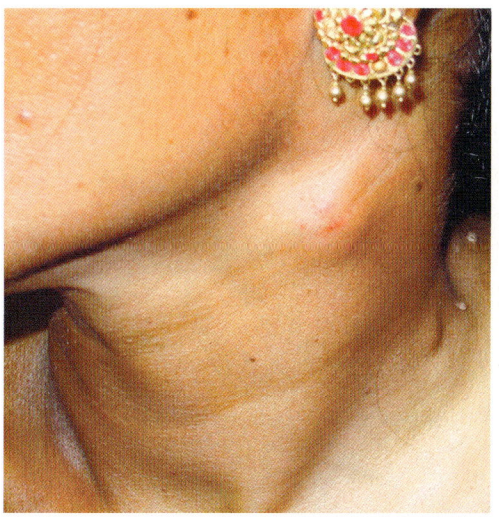
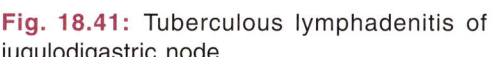

Fig. 18.41: Tuberculous lymphadenitis of jugulodigastric node

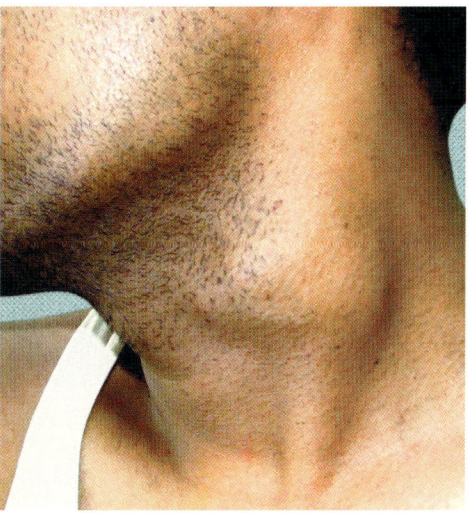

Fig. 18.42: Matted nodes—jugular chain of lymph nodes

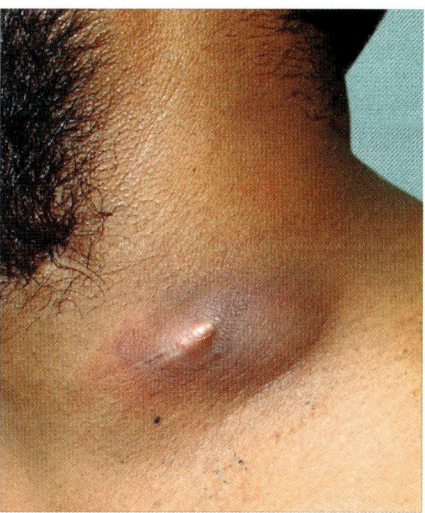

Fig. 18.43: Cold abscess in the posterior triangle

Clinical Wisdom

Classical signs described above may be absent, if thrombus is present within aneurysm.

4. *Carotid body tumour (chemodectoma):* This is a benign tumour arising from chemoreceptors in the carotid body (Figs 18.44 and 18.45). They are situated in the tunica adventitia at the bifurcation of common carotid artery. **Hence, the location is characteristic.** There are several important features of carotid body tumour are given below.

- **Typical location:** In the upper part of the anterior triangle of the neck, at the level of the hyoid bone, beneath the anterior edge of the sternomastoid muscle.
- **Typically, the patient is in fifties,** who presents with slow-growing painless swelling of many years duration.
- **Surface is smooth or lobulated,** borders are round, and **oval, vertically** placed swelling with transverse mobility.
- **Consistency is firm to hard.** Hence, called classical potato tumour.
- **Pressure effects:** Horner's syndrome and unilateral vocal cord paralysis can occur due to involvement of the sympathetic system and recurrent laryngeal nerves, respectively.

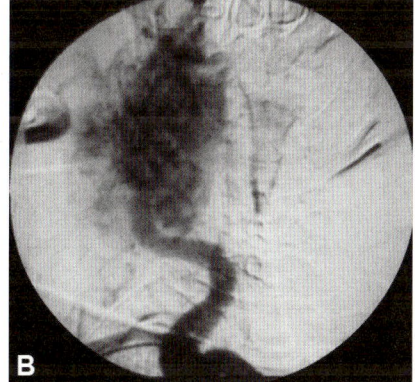

Fig. 18.44B: Carotid angiography—observe tumour blush

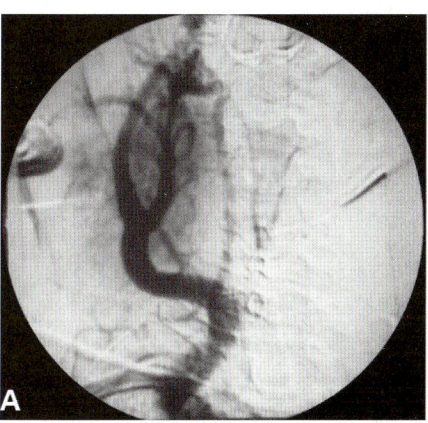

Fig. 18.44A: Carotid angiography—observe separation of internal and external carotid artery by the tumour. (Lyre's sign)

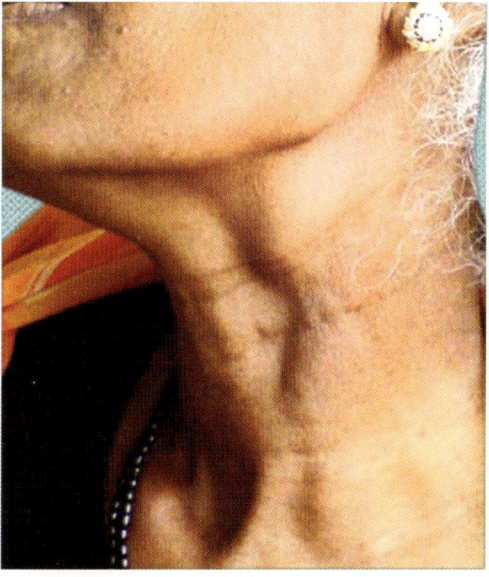

Fig. 18.45: Carotid body tumour in a 45-year-old lady—duration 5 years (*Courtesy:* Dr MR Srivatsa, Prof. and Head, Prof Bagali Babasaheb, Prof Bharathi, Dr Srikar Pai, Department of Surgery, MS Ramaiah Medical College and Hospital, Bangalore)

- **Pressure on the tumour** gives rise to syncopal attack due to decrease in the pulse **rate** (carotid body **syndrome**).
- Carotid artery is stretched over the swelling and so, transmitted pulsations are felt.
- Intraoral examination shows prolapse of ipsilateral tonsil, unless it grows in parapharyngeal space.
- Carotid angiography will demonstrate splaying of the carotid arteries (**Lyre's sign**).

Importance of Intraoral Examination in Neck Swellings

- Prolapse of ipsilateral tonsil in carotid body tumours unless it grows in parapharyngeal space
- Tonsillar shift in deep lobe tumours of the parotid gland
- Source of (primary) hard metastatic lymph nodes may be in the oral cavity
- Enlargement of lingual and palatine tonsils in non-Hodgkin's lymphoma

5. ***Schwannoma of the vagus nerve:*** This condition produces swelling in the carotid triangle in the region of thyroid swelling. It is a vertically placed oval swelling. It is firm to hard in consistency. On pressure over the swelling, dry cough and in some cases bradycardia may occur. Often thyroid nodule is the diagnosis given. However, the swelling does not move with deglutition, thus differentiating from thyroid swellings (Fig. 18.46).

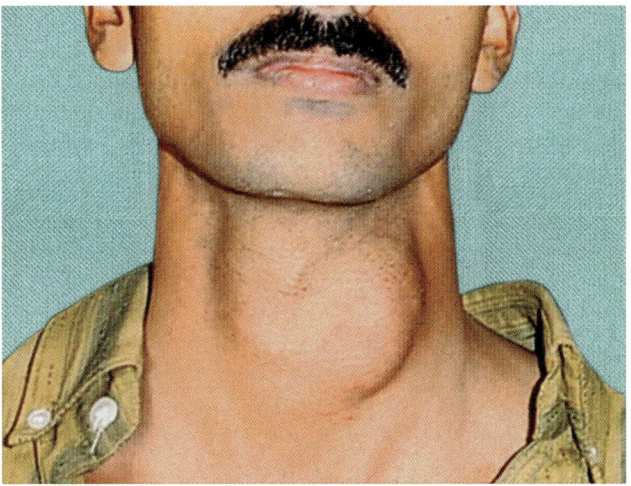

Fig. 18.46: MS examination case—swelling in the region of thyroid (contributed by Prof P Rajan, Prof KK Rajan and Prof Srijayan, Calicut Medical College, Calicut)

6. ***Laryngocoele:*** Two types are recognised.
   1. Occurs due to herniation of the laryngeal mucosa (Figs 18.47 and 18.48)—external laryngocoele.
   2. When it enlarges within the larynx, it may displace vocal cord, produce hoarseness and is called internal laryngocoele.
   - Glass blowers, musicians, wind instruments and trumpet players are commonly affected. Chronic cough may be one of the predisposing factors. It is a smooth, oval, boggy swelling which moves upwards on swallowing, in relation

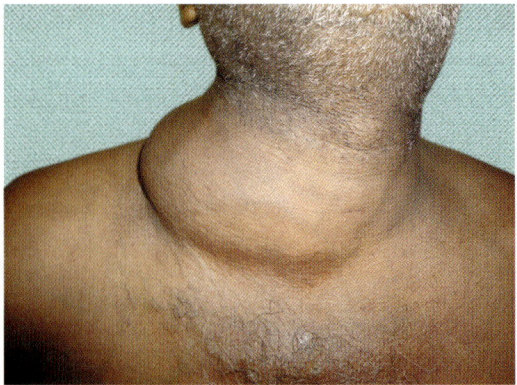

Fig. 18.47: Laryngocoele—cough impulse is positive (Courtesy: Dr Saurabh Agarwal, Dr Kartikeyan, Dr Digvijay Sharma, Department of Surgery, KMC, Manipal)

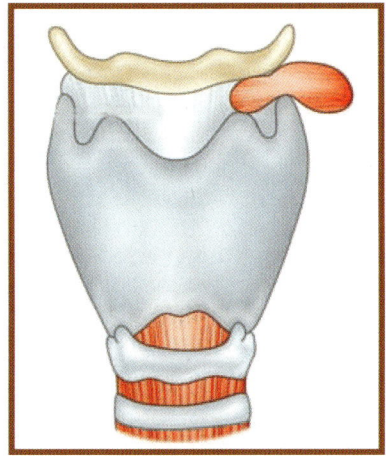

Fig. 18.48: Laryngocoele

to thyrohyoid membrane (subhyoid position). The swelling becomes prominent when the patient is asked to cough or blow (Valsalva manoeuvre). Expansile cough impulse is present. Tympanitic note on percussion (resonant) is classical.

- Other signs of laryngocoele include expansile impulse on cough and tympanitic note on percussion.

7. ***Pharyngeal pouch:*** This occurs due to herniation or protrusion of mucosa of the pharyngeal wall through Killian's dehiscence. Killian's dehiscence is a potential area of weakness in-between the two parts of the inferior constrictor muscle—upper oblique fibres (thyropharyngeus) and lower horizontal fibres (cricopharyngeus).
   - Initially foreign body sensation is present in the throat, later regurgitation of food on turning to one side, sense of suffocation, cough or dysphagia is present.
   - Gurgling sound and aspiration may cause dyspnoea later.
   - It is a soft swelling which can be emptied.

Clinical Wisdom

Laryngocoele is anterior and subhyoid in position. Pharyngeal pouch is posterior and subthyroid in position.

CLINICAL DISCUSSION

Why does pharyngeal diverticulum deviate to one side?

It is a **pulsion diverticulum** and deviates to one side, mostly to the left because of the rigid vertebral column in the midline posteriorly.

Carotid body tumours are common in which group of patients?

Chronic hypoxia can lead to carotid body hyperplasia. Hence, there is a **higher incidence of chemodectoma** in people **living at higher altitudes.**

What is Lyre sign?

Separation of the carotid arteries is called Lyre sign.

Which is the benign swelling having restricted mobility in the neck?

Branchial cyst, because it is adherent to sternocleidomastoid muscle.

In which age group is sternomastoid tumour found?

Newborn babies.

What happens to the distal limb in AV fistulas?

Distal to the AV fistula, ischaemic ulcers may develop due to comparative reduction in the blood supply.

What is Sibson's fascia and what is its clinical significance?

It is suprapleural membrane close to the apex of the lung.

It is the thickened portion of endothoracic fascia. It extends over the cupola of the pleura and reinforces it. It is attached to the **inner border of the first rib and to the transverse process of the seventh cervical vertebra.**

What structure pierces Sibson's facia on the left side?

Thoracic duct.

DIFFERENTIAL DIAGNOSIS OF SWELLING IN THE POSTERIOR TRIANGLE

The posterior triangle (Clinical Boxes 18.6 and 18.7) is an interesting area as far as swellings are concerned. It is the commonest area of metastasis in lymph nodes from occult primary. Lymphangiomas, haemangiomas, cold abscess, and lymphomas commonly occur here. Interesting cases of cervical rib with or without post-stenotic dilatation of subclavian artery, Pancoast tumour, and aneurysms also occur here. It is not surprising when you think of a solid tumour in the posterior triangle, you will bet on a neural tumour because of abundant nerve fibres (C1 to C7). Classify the swellings into cystic, solid and pulsatile swellings.

1. **Haemangioma:** This is a swelling due to congenital mal-formation of blood vessels. It is an example of hamartoma. From clinical point of view, a simple classification such as capillary, cavernous and arterial is enough. For more details *refer* to Manipal Manual of Surgery, 4th edn. Venous haeman-gioma occurs in the neck. Venous haemangioma occurs in place where venous space is abundant, e.g. lip, cheek, tongue, and posterior triangle of the neck. Typically, swelling will be of long duration. History of bleeding is present if there is history of trauma. The swelling is warm and bluish in colour but not pulsatile. It is soft, fluctuant and transillumination negative. Compressibility is present. This sign is also called 'sign of emptying' or 'sign of refilling'. When the swelling is compressed between the fingers, blood diffuses under the vascular spaces and when pressure is released, it slowly fills up. Compressibility is a diagnostic sign of haemangioma.

2. **AV malformation:** Congenital arteriovenous (AV) fistula (arterial haemangioma):
   - An abnormal communication between artery and vein, results in AV fistula.
   - AV fistula can be congenital or acquired.
   - Such AV fistula has got structural and functional effects. **Structurally,** the veins get dilated, tortuous and elongated. This arterialisation of the vein results in secondary varicose veins. Functionally, **due to increased venous pressure and arteriovenous shunt,** physiological effects such as increased pulse rate, **increased cardiac output, and increased pulse pressure occur** (Fig. 18.49).

Clinical Wisdom

Aneurysm of the common carotid artery, cervical rib with post-stenotic dilatation of subclavian artery, and AV fistula are the three differential diagnoses of pulsatile swellings in the neck.

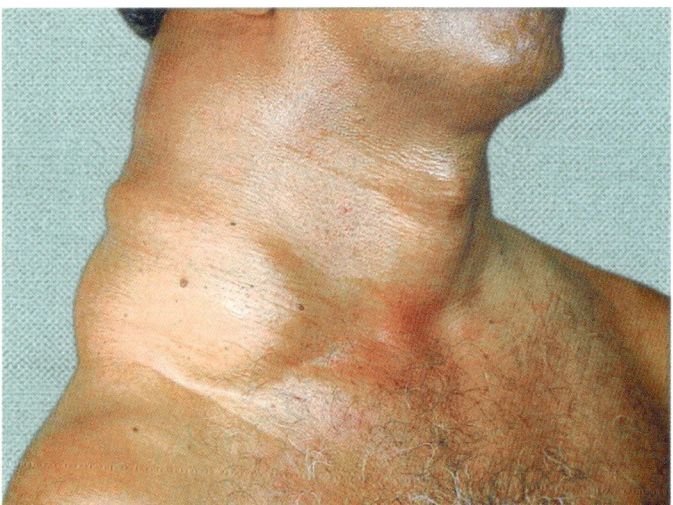

Fig. 18.49: Arteriovenous malformation

Clinical signs

- Soft, cystic, fluctuant, transillumination negative, **pulsatile swelling.**
- A continuous bruit/murmur is characteristic.
- **Nicoladoni sign or Branham sign:** On compressing the feeding artery, the venous return to the heart diminishes, resulting in fall in pulse rate and pulse pressure.
- On compressing feeding artery, pulsation or **continuous murmur** may also disappear and swelling will diminish in size.
- If the AV fistula is big, a **high output cardiac failure** can occur.
- The affected part is swollen (because of high pressure)—**local gigantism.** Thus, overgrowth of the limb or toe can occur, if the AV fistula is in limb—one of the common sites.

3. *Cold abscess in the posterior triangle* (Figs 8.50 and 18.51): Route of infection from **adenoids** or other lymph nodes in the anterior triangle, or infection from **lungs—spread through Sibson's fascia or from tuberculosis of spine (see below for more details).**

Caries Cervical Spine

- Clinically, it presents as pain in the back, cold abscess and neurological signs.
- **Rust's sign:** Child with caries spine will support the head by holding the chin.
- Cold abscess from caries spine can rupture anteriorly or posteriorly.
- A. *Anterior rupture:* It ruptures deep to prevertebral layer of deep cervical fascia. From here, it can take the following routes:
  - *Upper cervical region:* Presents as deep seated abscess in the posterior wall of the pharynx in the **midline.**
  - *Lower cervical region:* Pus will press on oesophagus and trachea anteriorly.
  - *Laterally,* pus passes deep to prevertebral **fascia behind carotid sheath** in the **posterior triangle.**
- B. *Posterior rupture:* Pus may enter spinal canal and then can travel along anterior primary division of the cervical spinal nerves.

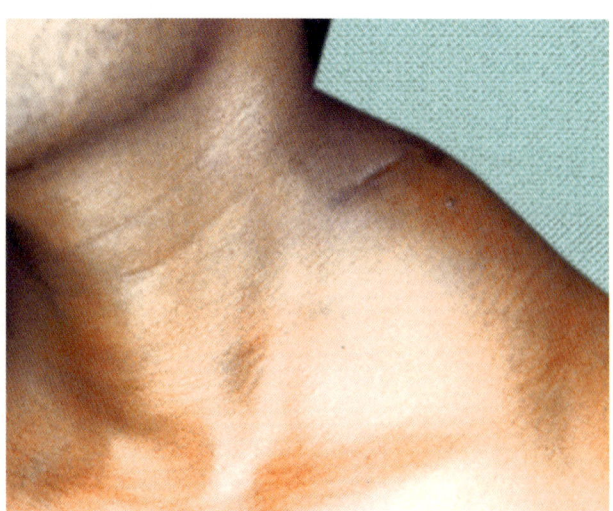

Fig. 18.50: Cold abscess in the posterior triangle

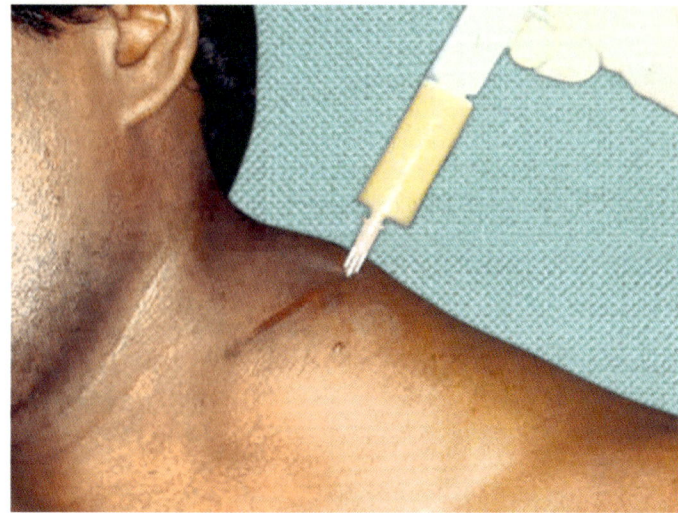

Fig. 18.51: Cold abscess—non-dependent aspiration. Observe the yellow pus due to secondary infection

4. *Lymphangioma:* Posterior triangle is the common site of lymphangioma. Common in children and young adults, typically it is a painless slow-growing swelling. It is soft, cystic and hence, fluctuant with brilliant transillumination. Lymphangioma may also show some degree of compressibility (Figs 18.52 and 18.53). In children, expansile impulse on cough may be elicited because of close approximation of neck structures.

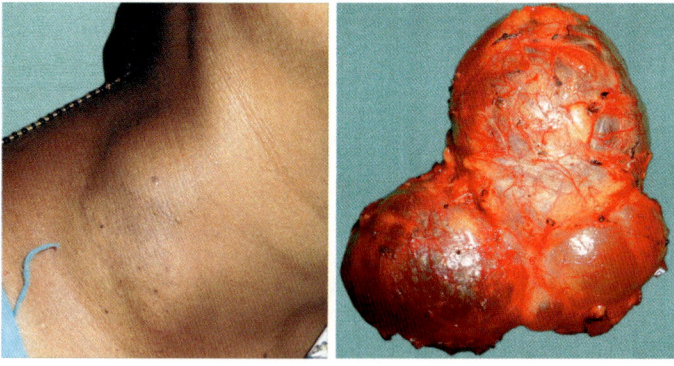

Figs 18.52 and 18.53: Lymphangioma

5. *Metastasis in lymph nodes:* Students are requested to refer and have a correct knowledge about the lateral lymph node classification from Memorial Sloan Kettering Cancer Center (page 264, Manipal Manual of Sugery, 4th edn. The symptoms with which a patient presents to the hospital give the clue to the site of origin of the primary. Some examples are given below (Figs 18.54 and 18.55):

- *Difficulty in swallowing:* Carcinoma posterior one-third tongue, oropharyngeal carcinoma or carcinoma oesophagus
- *Difficulty in breathing:* Laryngeal cancer
- *Hoarseness of voice:* Larynx or thyroid
- *Obvious growth in oral cavity:* Carcinoma cheek, alveolus, tongue, etc.

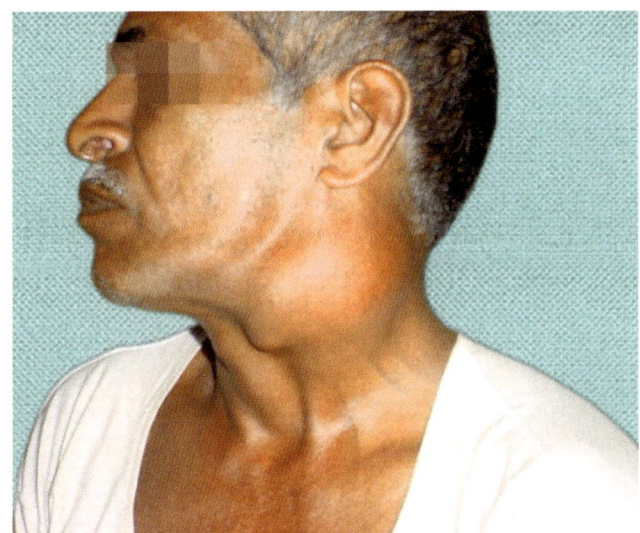

Fig. 18.54: Metastatic lymph nodes in level 2 and 3 due to nasopharyngeal carcinoma

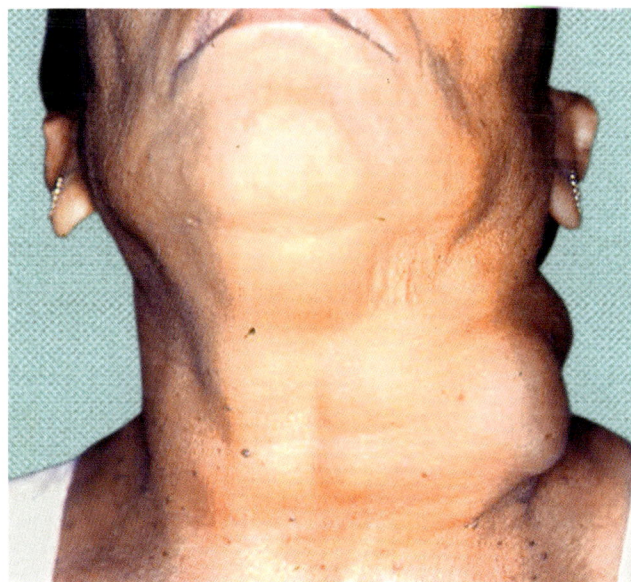

Fig. 18.55: Metastatic lymph nodes in level 2, 3 and 4 due to carcinoma pyriform fossa

- *Haemoptysis, difficulty in breathing*: Bronchogenic carcinoma
- *Epistaxis, ear pain or deafness*: Nasopharyngeal carcinoma (Clinical Box 18.8)

Metastatic nodes are hard, large with or without fixity. Majority of the patients are elderly who present with neck swelling of short duration and it is painless. Fixity to platysma (platysma sign), fixity to the skin, and fixity to sternomastoid muscles are other features. Large nodal mass can infiltrate hypoglossal, accessory and sympathetic nerves resulting in various clinical signs. To find out the primary, examine thyroid, breast in females and oral cavity. The primary malignancy may be evident in the anterior third of tongue, cheek, alveolus, etc.

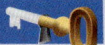

Clinical Box 18.8

Metastatic deposits
- 80% of the lymph nodes in the neck are metastatic deposits.
- Majority of malignant neoplasms are epithelial in origin.
- Nodes in the upper half (levels I and II) can be due to primary in the oral cavity, tongue, oropharynx, and larynx.
- Nodes in the lower half (levels III and IV) can be due to primary in the thyroid, tongue.
- Nodes in the supraclavicular region (level V): Carcinoma from GIT, genitourinary tract, lungs, nasopharynx, breast.
- Nodes in the pretracheal, suprasternal region (level VI): Papillary carcinoma thyroid.

- Posterior one-third of the tongue should be palpated with gloved finger.
- When primary is not detected clinically, it is considered as occult primary site with nodal deposits.

6. **Pancoast's tumour** or superior sulcus tumour is a broncho-genic carcinoma arising from the apex of lung. Typically, the patient is an elderly male around 70 years, **chronic smoker** who presents with cough, weight loss, dyspnoea and chest pain. As the tumour grows, it compresses the **lower roots of brachial plexus C8 and T1** and results in tingling, pain and paraesthesia in the distribution of ulnar nerve. The tumour is felt in the lower part of the posterior triangle. It is **hard in consistency, fixed, irregular** and sometimes tender. The lower border of the mass cannot be appreciated.

The Pancoast's syndrome refers to following components:
1. Pancoast tumour
2. Erosion of the first rib
3. Paralysis of C8 and T1 nerve roots
4. **Horner's syndrome** due to paralysis of cervical sympathetic chain.

The preganglionic sympathetic fibres of the head and neck are given from the 1st and sometimes the 2nd thoracic segments of the spinal cord. These nerve fibres synapse with the cells in the three cervical sympathetic ganglia. They give rise to postganglionic fibres to the head and neck region. Thus, anywhere along this pathway, disruption, damage or infiltration of the nerve roots results in Horner's syndrome. The components of Horner's syndrome are given below in the box.

Components of Horner's syndrome
- *Miosis*: Small pupil
- *Anhidrosis*: Absence of sweating
- *Pseudoptosis*: Drooping of upper eyelid (refer to page 14, Fig. 1.23)
- *Enophthalmos*: Regression of the eyeball
- *Nasal vasodilatation*: Nasal congestion

You can remember as: These patients have
Sinking eyeball, **S**agging upper eyelid, **S**mall pupil, **S**ore nose and **S**weatless face.

7. **Neural tumours in the posterior triangle:** Typically, patients in-between 30 and 50 years old with swelling in the posterior triangle for many years duration. Swelling is firm/hard in consistency which is tender. The patient may also have radiating pain/tingling numbness along the distributions of the involved nerve root (brachial plexus). Also look for café au lait spots, other cutaneous nodules of von Recklinghausen's disease (Figs 18.56 and 18.57).

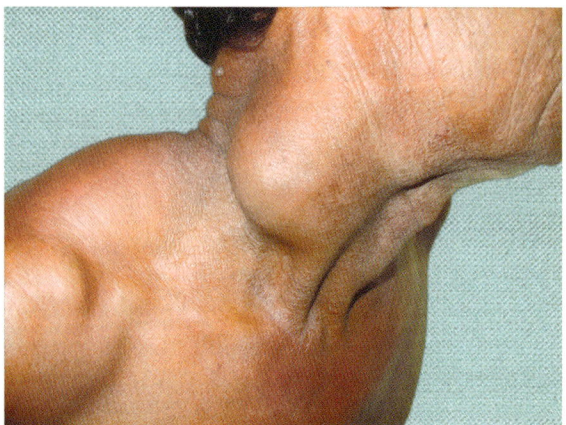

Fig. 18.56: Neurofibroma affecting upper nerve roots of brachial plexus

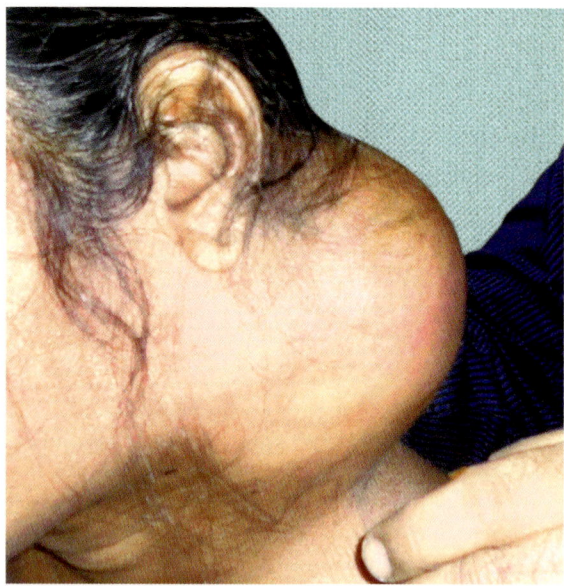

Fig. 18.57: Schwannoma (*Courtesy:* Dr Chella Srnivas Rao, Professor of Surgery and Dr Ravindranath, Postgraduate Student, Konaseema Institute of Medical Sciences, Amalapuram, Andhra Pradesh)

CYSTICERCOSIS AND THE SURGEON

Humans are *T. solium* reservoirs. They are infected by **eating undercooked pork** that contains viable cysticerci. The cysticercus develops into an adult tapeworm in the gut and produces large numbers of eggs which pass out in the faeces. The presence of an adult tapeworm in the gut is reasonably harmless.

Cysticercosis in humans occurs due to the ingestion of tapeworm eggs, either from external sources or from the person's own faeces. The human then becomes an accidental and "dead-end" intermediate host. Pigs, which are the "normal" intermediate host for this parasite, get infected with cysticerci when they ingest human faeces. The incubation period ranges from months to over 10 years. Cysticerci can develop in any voluntary muscle in humans.

Invasion of muscle by cysticerci can cause *myositis*, with fever, *eosinophilia*, and muscular pseudo-hypertrophy, which begin with muscle swelling and later progress to atrophy and fibrosis. In most cases, it is asymptomatic since the cysticerci die and become calcified (Clinical Box 18.9).

Clinical Box 18.9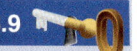

Causes of myositis
1. Autoimmune
2. Pyomyositis: Thigh muscles—skeletal muscles are affected
3. Viral diseases
4. HIV infections
5. Trauma
6. Cysticercosis

---

8. **Sternomastoid tumour**
- This is not a tumour, it is a misnomer. Injury to the sternomastoid during birth causes rupture of a few fibres and haematoma. Later, healing occurs with fibrosis, resulting in a swelling in the middle of sternomastoid muscle.
- This is seen in infants or children. Firm to hard, 1–2 cm swelling in the middle of the sternomastoid muscle. It is tender and mobile sideways.
- Medial and lateral borders of this swelling are distinct but superior and inferior borders are continuous with the muscle. Many cases are associated with torticollis.

9. **Soft tissue Sarcoma**
These are common in young patients. They can arise from nerve, muscles and fibre sheath, synovial tissue, etc. A few important signs and symptoms are given below:
- Sarcomas occur in young patients.
- They are rapidly growing.
- Surface is irregular with irregular margins.
- Dilated veins and redness suggest increased vascularity.
- Shoulder joint/region is one of the common sites of synovial sarcoma.

Clinical Wisdom

A young patient with rapidly growing, painful swelling in the shoulder region: Hard, irregular swelling with dilated veins over the surface occupying posterior triangle and left shoulder region. It is a case of synovial sarcoma (Fig. 18.58).

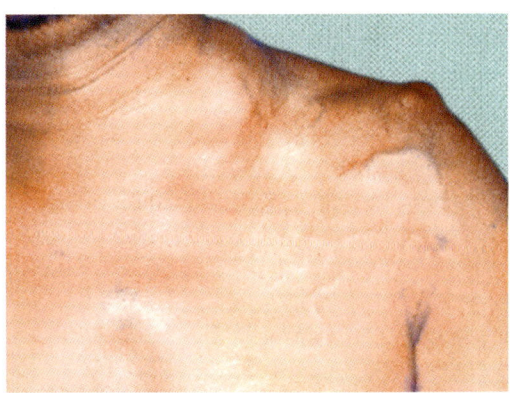

Fig. 18.58: Synovial sarcoma shoulder region, see the secondary varicosity due to pressure effects

10. *Torticollis*

It is a type of deformity wherein head is bent to one side and chin points to other side. Most often it is due to ischaemia of the related muscles—mostly sternomastoid. Any painful condition on one side of neck may also result in torticollis which may be temporary. Most often, the muscles affected are those that are supplied by the accessory nerve (Fig. 18.59).

Causes/Types

1. **Congenital:** It may be related to birth trauma or difficult labour.
2. **Spine related:** It can be seen in TB of cervical spine or fracture dislocation of cervical spine.
3. **Rheumatic:** Sudden exposure to cold.
4. **Inflammatory:** Due to painful enlargement of cervical nodes, retropharyngeal abscess.
5. **Compensatory:** Due to scoliosis or due to defect in the sight.
6. **Neurological:** Cerebellar lesions.

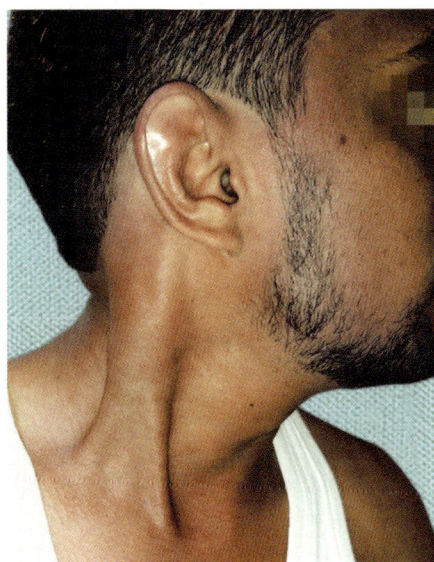

Fig. 18.59: Torticollis

■ **Clinical Case Capsules**

1. A 40-year-old lady presented with swelling in the posterior traingle of the neck of five years duration. On examination, it was soft, lobular and transillumination was negative. It was a case of lipoma in the posterior triangle neck. Supraclavicular region is one of the common sites of lipoma. It is well encapsulated. Make sure it is not neurilemmoma. Make sure it is not a vascular swelling (haemangioma) before incising (Fig 18.60).

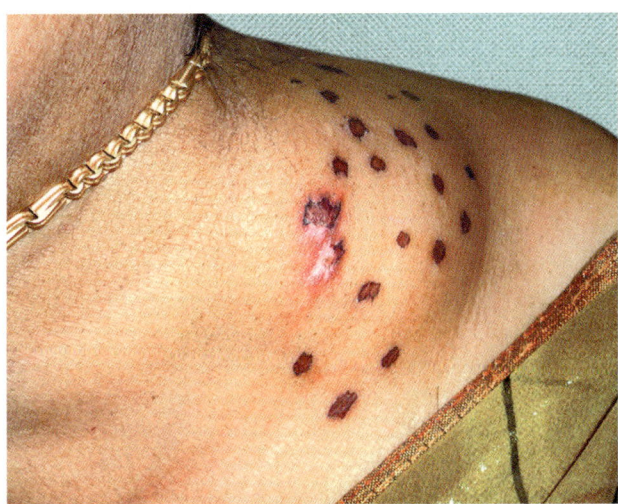

Fig. 18.60: Lipoma in the left supraclavicular region. You can see branding mark on the suface of the swelling

2. A 50-year-old man presented to the hospital with multiple large lymph nodal masses in the anterior and posterior triangle. On examination, lymph nodes were large, bulky, firm to hard in consistency. The diagnosis was Hodgkin's lymphoma (Fig. 18.61).

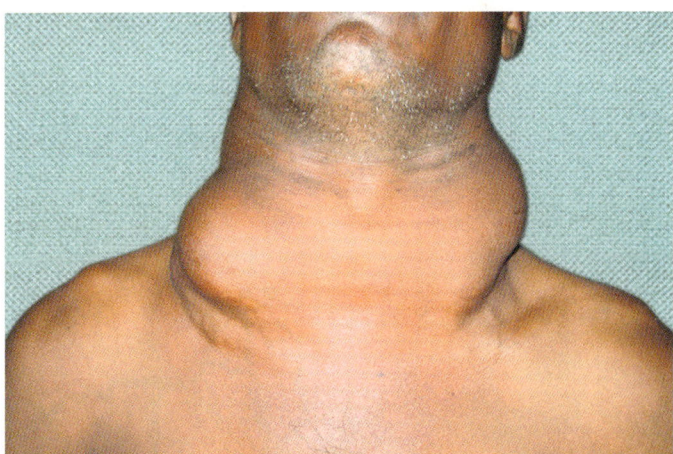

Fig. 18.61: Large bulky nodal mass—bull neck suggestive of Hodgkin's lymphoma

3. A 40-year-old lady presented to the hospital with swelling in the posterior triangle of 2 cm size of 4 months duration. She had no fever or features like that of a lymph node but a tender cord-like structure could be felt above the swelling. That gave

the clue to the diagnosis. It was a case of leprosy. The lymph node-like swelling was nerve abscess and the cord-like structure was posterior-auricular nerve thickening (Fig. 18.62).

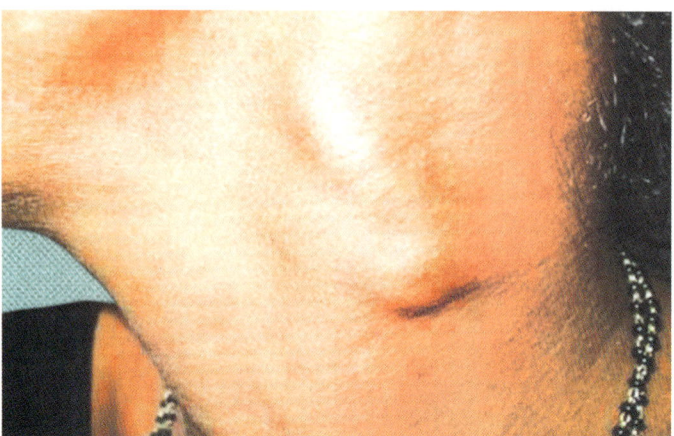

Fig. 18.62: Nerve abscess in the posterior triangle

4. A 26-year-old female, low socioeconomic status, was admitted to the hospital with a swelling in the lower posterior triangle of two years duration. Aspiration of the swelling was done twice which showed brownish-coloured fluid.

On examination: It was soft, fluctuant, transillumination negative swelling close to anterior border of left sternocleidomastoid muscle, not moving with deglutition.

- Analysis of a case of cystic swelling in the posterior triangle in the lower neck close to sternocleidomastoid muscle.

What is the diagnosis?

- The swelling is of 2 years' duration and cystic but transillumination is negative.
- Tuberculous cold abscess is ruled out.
- Thyroid cyst is ruled out because it is not moving with deglutition.
- Lipoma is ruled out because of the history of aspiration of liquid contents.
- Find diagnosis was cystic secondaries from papillary carcinoma thyroid. Patient underwent total thyroidectomy and functional neck dissection (Fig. 18.63).

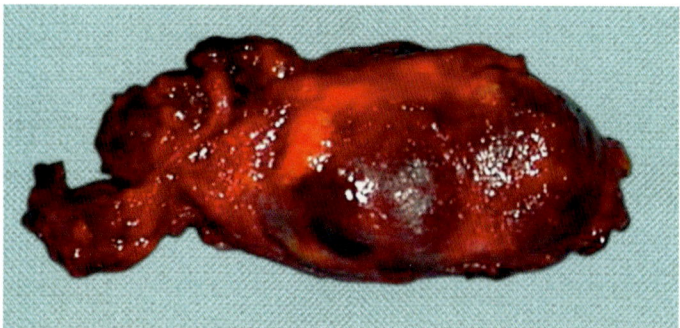

Fig. 18.63: Lymph nodal mass from papillary carcinoma thyroid—bluish black nodes, cystic

A case of swelling in the neck

A 50-year-old man, nonvegetarian and alcoholic presented with a swelling in the right side of the neck of 2–3 months duration. To begin with he had pain in the swelling and now dull aching pain is present. Initially it had progressed to about 5 cm and now it is stationary and he even says the size had decreased by about 1 cm. No other symptoms.

On examination: To summarise the swelling is 5 cm in size, firm, nontender, adherent to sternomastoid muscle—size almost remains same (slightly less than what it was) before and after contraction of the sternomastoid muscle—a possibility of a swelling very close to sternomastoid muscle—in the middle and lower part. Other than this everything else is normal.

Analysis of the case: The first diagnosis as far as anatomical organ is concerned is lymph node swelling, followed by thyroid swelling, non-tumour, etc.

- Firstly malignant swellings—lymph node swellings ruled out because of the decrease in the size and firm consistency.
- Tensely cystic swellings may feel firm and may add confusion to the diagnosis but common cystic swellings such as haemangioma, and lymphangioma are ruled out due to late onset. Branchial cyst is also ruled out due to late onset and the position.
- Is it a cold abscess or tuberculous lymphadenitis? We cannot rule out because it is a common disease and cold abscess from a single node may feel firm.
- What about solid swellings? Consistency is firm. Yes, tuberculous lymphadenitis is possible, we have already considered that possibility.
- What else? The swelling does not move with deglutition and hence, thyroid lobe enlargement is unlikely.
- The swelling started as a slow painful lesion and is unlikely to be a neural tumour.
- What about swelling arising from or close to sternomastoid muscle? Sternomastoid tumour is rare in young and middle-aged people.
- Sarcoma arising from skeletal muscles is very rare in this location.

Opinion from the experts on the stage

- *Examiners*: We accept the diagnosis of tuberculous lymphadenitis, chronic nonspecific lymphadenitis, and Schwannoma arising from vagus nerve
- Ultrasound findings suggest thick-walled cystic swelling.

  At surgery: Swelling was adherent to and arising within muscle fibres of sternomastoid muscle. It was excised. Reported as cysticercosis.

Courtesy: Continuing surgical education—Bangalore Surgical Society, 2012.

AN EXAMPLE OF HOW TO ARRIVE AT THE DIAGNOSIS IN A POSTERIOR TRIANGLE SWELLING

POSTERIOR TRIANGLE SWELLING

SOFT

1. Lipoma:
   - Slip sign positive, lobular
   - Soft, fluctuant

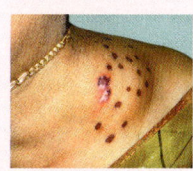

2. Cold abscess:
   - Soft
   - Fluctuant
   - Transillumination negative
   - Lymph nodes may be palpable
3. Lymphangioma: Soft, fluctuant, transilluminant, compressible swelling.

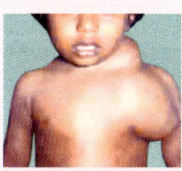

4. Haemangioma: Soft, fluctuant, transillumination negative, non-compressible swelling.

FIRM

1. Lymph nodes:
   - Tuberculous—nodular matted
   - Lymphoma—no matting, rubbery
2. Fibromatosis:
   - Fixed, firm, diffuse lump
   - Something hard
3. Neurofibroma:
   - Slow growing
   - Swelling is firm, irregular, non-tender
   - Tingling and numbness in the distribution of nerve fibres may be present.
4. Soft tissue sarcoma
   - Neurofibrosarcoma and angio-sarcoma are common
   - Firm to hard, irregular
   - Rapidly growing, massive

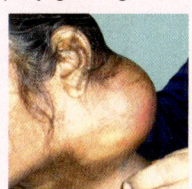

HARD

1. Cervical ribs: Fixed, hard bony mass in young patients may be unilateral. It is bilateral in 10% of cases.
2. The most common hard swelling is secondaries in lymph nodes (metastasis). They are nodular, fixed or without evidence of primary.

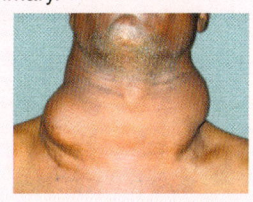

3. Fibromatosis: It presents as a hard and fixed swelling.

PULSATILE

1. Cervical ribs with post-stenotic dilatation is the common cause of pulsatile swelling.
2. AV malformations: Congenital/acquired. AV malformations can present with slow-growing pulsatile swelling.

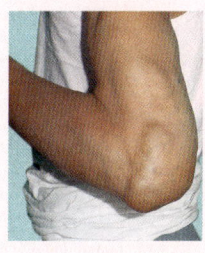

3. Vertebral artery aneurysm with or without rupture can present as pulsatile swelling.

19

Examination of Thyroid Swelling

INTRODUCTION

Diseases of the thyroid gland are very common and thyroid swellings are very often common cases in undergraduate and postgraduate clinical examinations. Enlargement of **thyroid gland is called goitre.** Being an important endocrinal gland, due to fluctuating level of thyroid hormones, it enlarges and nodules develop. Its function may be normal, subnormal or excessive. Malignancies may develop in the gland, even in younger age group. Hence, it is important to study the clinical methods of examination of the thyroid gland in detail, so as to arrive at a proper clinical diagnosis.

PATIENT DATA

Age: They are recorded such as name, age, place, occupation, admitting complaints, etc. A common question is how old are you?

- If the age group is between 10 and 20 years, thyroid swelling could be due to hormone deficiency—**dyshormonogenesis.**
- Goitre at puberty is rightly called puberty goitre.
- Multinodular goitre takes few years for it to establish itself and hence is seen between the age group of 30 and 40 years (Fig. 19.1).
- It is interesting to note that papillary carcinoma is often found in young girls who present to the hospital with thyroid swelling with or without lymph nodes (Clinical Box 19.1).
- Follicular carcinoma occurs in middle-aged women and anaplastic carcinoma occurs in elderly patients.
- Patients with primary thyrotoxicosis are usually young but patients with secondary thyrotoxicosis

are middle-aged because toxicity appears many years after the appearance of a multinodular goitre (Fig. 19.2).
- Anaplastic carcinoma typically occurs after 50 years.

Clinical Box 19.1

Common malignancies in young patients
1. Papillary carcinoma thyroid
2. Testicular tumours
3. Lymphoma
4. Sarcoma
5. Hereditary cancers

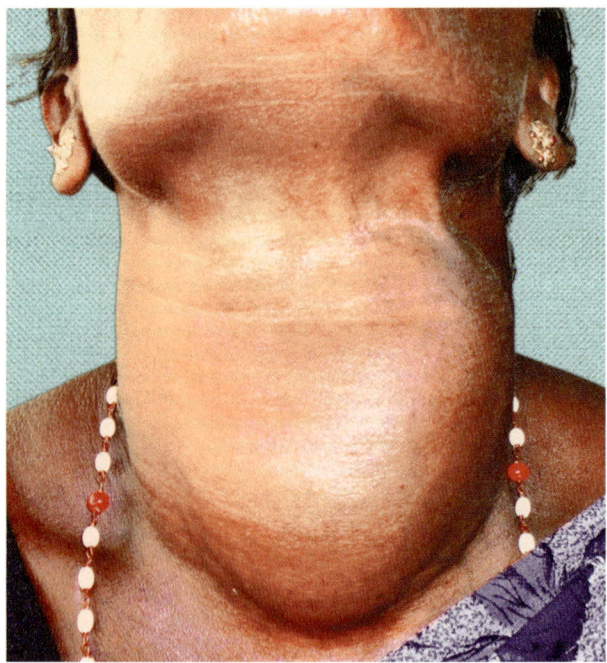

Fig. 19.1: Multinodular goitre

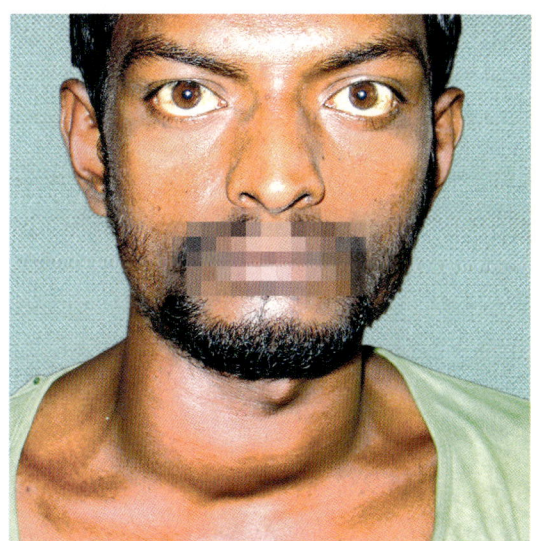

Fig. 19.2: Primary thyrotoxicosis in a 35-year-old man

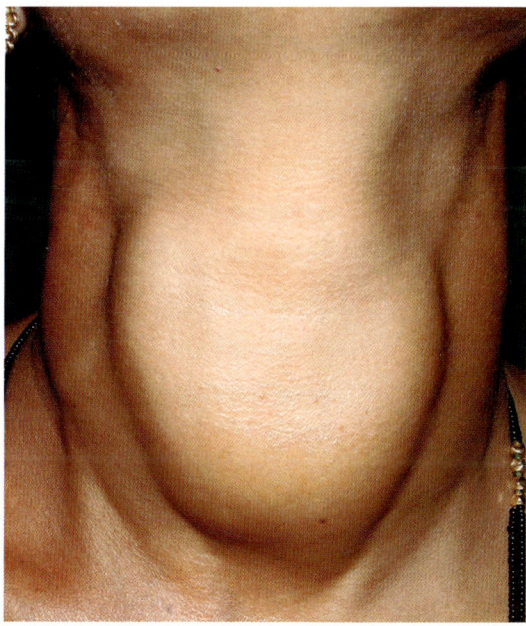

Fig. 19.3: Colloid goitre in a 40-year-old female. The swelling is of 8 years duration

- Colloid goitre or iodine deficiency goitres occur around 35–40 years of age (Fig. 19.3).

Sex: All thyroid disorders are more common in women than in men. Primary thyrotoxicosis is 8 times more common in women than in men. *However, sudden appearance of a thyroid swelling in males should arouse the suspicion of malignancy of the thyroid.*

Occupation: There is no specific correlation between occupation and thyroid swellings.

Residence: Iodine content in the water is low in mountainous areas and some low-lying areas. Iodine deficiency results in decreased production of thyroid

hormones. This in turn causes increased production of TSH which in turn stimulates the thyroid gland producing various forms of goitre. Some examples are given below:

- In Karnataka, incidence is more in districts such as Coorg and South Canara.
- Slopes of Himalayas, Vindhyas, higher reaches of tea estates of Kerala including Wayanad district.
- Certain areas of Australia, including Tasmania and areas along the Great Dividing Range (e.g. the Australian Capital Territory) have low iodine levels in the soil.
- In the ranges of river Struma in Bulgaria (for all practical purposes, so common was the thyroid swelling along the river Struma, Struma is referred to as goitre. **(Struma ovari means goitre of the ovary—thyroid tissue in ovarian teratoma.)**

PRESENTING COMPLAINTS

1. *Swelling and duration:* When did it start and how did it start, are the first questions to be asked. Often, the patient says, 'I did not notice the swelling but it was detected by others'. It means the onset is insidious and slowly progressive. Sometimes, the patient says, 'I had sudden discomfort or pain in the neck and I detected a swelling'. It means there might have been a small nodule which was asymptomatic but suddenly haemorrhage occurred. Please remember haemorrhage is a well-known complication of multinodular goitre or solitary nodule. However, if the nodule is big, breathlessness can also be the complaint following sudden haemorrhage (Clinical Box 19.2).

Clinical Box 19.2

Common causes of haemorrhage within a swelling
1. Thyroid nodule or a cyst
2. Ovarian cyst
3. Omental cyst
4. Pseudocyst of pancreas
5. Polycystic kidney
6. Mesenteric cyst

- Long duration of thyroid swelling indicates benign condition, e.g. multinodular goitre (MNG), colloid goitre, etc. Short duration with rapid growth indicates malignancy such as anaplastic carcinoma. Majority of thyroid swellings do not produce pain. However, in advanced cases of malignancy, due to local infiltration, patients do complain of vague discomfort or pain.

2. Rate of growth

- Usually slow growing in benign disease.

- If it is a rapid growth, it can be **'de novo'** **malignancy** such as anaplastic carcinoma thyroid or malignancy developing in multinodular goitre, e.g. follicular carcinoma in MNG.

3. Pressure symptoms

A. *Dyspnoea*: Difficulty in breathing in a patient with goitre can be due to following reasons:

- Small goitre, rapid growth—anaplastic carcinoma infiltrating the trachea.

- When lower border is not seen, retrosternal goitre (Clinical Box 19.3).

- Hyperthyroidism causing arrhythmias leading to congestive cardiac failure can cause dyspnoea and orthopnoea.

- Long-standing MNG compresses on the tracheal cartilages and produces **pressure atrophy** of tracheal cartilages. This is called **tracheomalacia.**

- Such type of trachea is called **scabbard trachea.**

B. *Dysphagia* is relatively uncommon because oesophagus is a posterior structure, is a muscular

 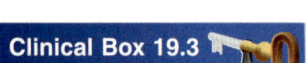
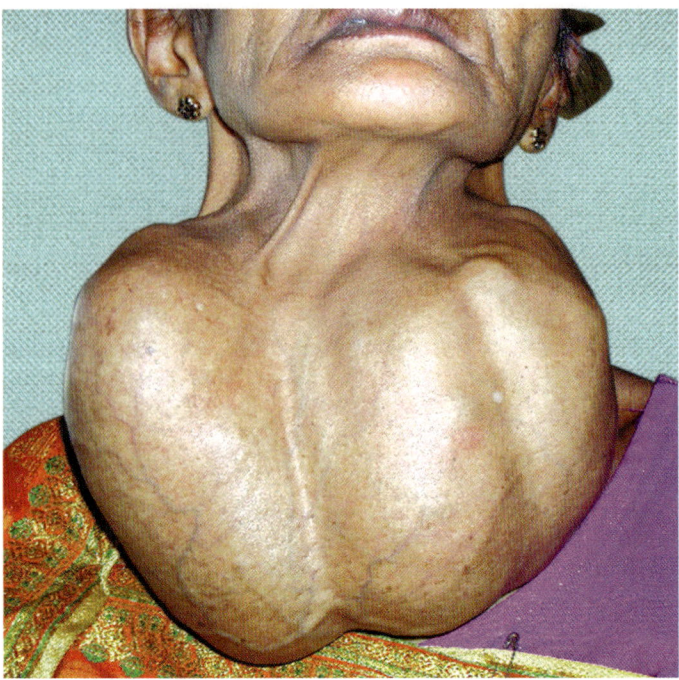

Fig. 19.4: Large MNG (*Courtesy:* Dr Gopinath Pai, Dr Ganapathi Puranik, Dr Chidanand, Professors of Surgery, KVG Medical College, Sullia, South Canara, Karnataka). Gland size was more than 15 cm. The patient did not have change in voice

tube which can be easily stretched and pushed aside. In fact, it is not a true dysphagia but a kind of discomfort during swallowing in cases of goitres (Fig. 19.4).

C. *Hoarseness of voice* indicates malignancy. It always occurs in carcinoma thyroid infiltrating the recurrent laryngeal nerve (Fig. 19.5). It is almost rare for a benign disease of the thyroid, however big it is, to compress the nerve and produce hoarseness.

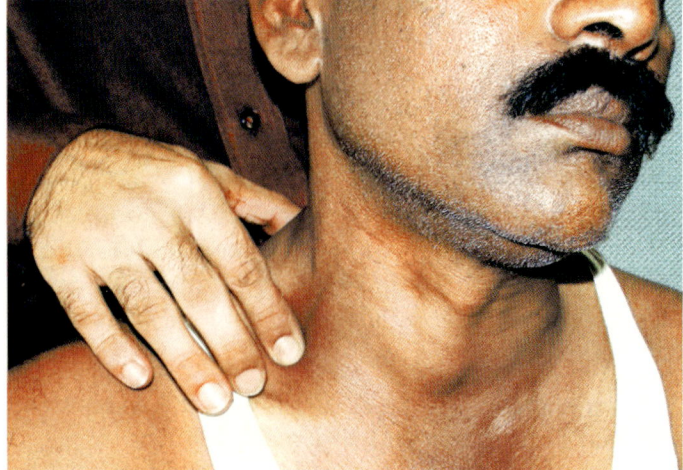

Fig. 19.5: Rapidly growing thyroid malignancy—anaplastic carcinoma. The patient had hoarseness of voice. The gland size was only 3 cm

4. Ask for **toxic features** suggestive of hyperthyroidism. Follow a common order. One example is given below.

A. *CNS symptoms* are predominantly seen in Graves' disease (primary thyrotoxicosis). Common questions are: Do you have?

- Tremors of the hand
- Increased sweating
- Intolerance to heat
- Preference to cold
- Excitability and irritability
- Insomnia
- Did anyone tell you that your eyes have become prominent? (Fig. 19.6) Prominent eyes are observed by other persons. Double vision can also be the complaint.

B. *Cardiovascular symptoms* (CVS) are predominantly seen in secondary thyrotoxicosis. Even though both forms of thyrotoxicosis produce palpitations, it is a significant complaint in multinodular goitre with thyrotoxicosis (secondary thyrotoxicosis). Common questions are, 'do you have any palpitations, precordial chest pain and dyspnoea on exertion'?

C. *GIT symptoms*: Do you have diarrhoea? It is called pseudodiarrhoea. It is due to increased bowel movements. How is your appetite and weight? Do you have any weight loss? **Inspite of good appetite, significant weight loss occurs in Graves' disease.**

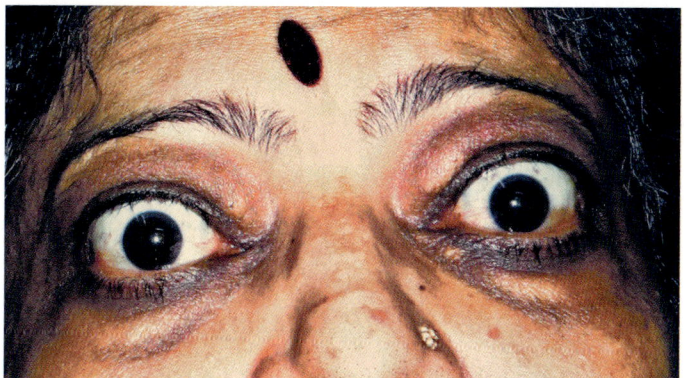

Clinical Wisdom

- Weight gain in hypothyroidism is due to accumulation of fat particularly at the back and shoulder regions.
- Loss of hair on the outer part of eyebrow is one of the features of myxoedema.

Fig. 19.6: Prominent eyes—a feature commonly seen in primary thyrotoxicosis

5. Ask for features of hypothyroidism such as weight gain, constipation, lethargy, intolerance to cold, change in voice, loss of hair, etc.

6. Do you have any other swelling? Swelling in the neck may be due to lymph nodes and swellings in flat bones are due to spread from follicular carcinoma.

7. **Menstrual history must be asked since thyroid disorders are associated with menstrual irregularities.**

- In primary thyrotoxicosis, **free steroid hormone levels decrease.** This results in **ineffective oestrogen** which in turn causes oligomenorrhoea.
- In hypothyroidism, there is menorrhagia.

At the end of the history, students should be able to conclude whether it is a simple or a toxic goitre. Is it a benign or malignant goitre? Hoarseness of the voice and rapid growth are the strong points in the history which suggest malignancy.

PAST HISTORY/TREATMENT HISTORY

- Enquire about any previous treatment taken for thyroid conditions—antithyroid drugs for thyrotoxicosis, thyroxine for hypothyroidism or any surgeries on the thyroid gland such as lobectomy, subtotal thyroidectomy, etc.
- Thyroxine in small doses such as 50/75 µg is given for puberty goitre or even early nodular goitres.
- Drugs which can give rise to goitre are antithyroid drugs, PAS (para-aminosalicylic acid), amiodarone drug used for treatment for arrhythmias.

Personal History

Enquire food habits and type of food. Cabbage, a member of Brassica family, is a known goitrogen.

Family History

- Enzyme deficiency goitre runs in families.
- Endemic goitres are not only seen in family members but also in many others who consume the same water supply.
- Even though rare, medullary carcinoma can run in families specially in Scandinavian countries.

GENERAL PHYSICAL EXAMINATION

- If the patient has a look with a stare, mention it. Detailed examination can be done later.

- *Shake hand*: Warm and moist palms suggest thyrotoxicosis.

- *Facies*: A tense, nervous patient with protruding eyeballs is classical of Graves' disease. A puffy mask-like facies is characteristic of myxoedema.

- *Build and nutrition*: A thin patient, who sweats a lot and has lost significant amount of weight recently suggests thyrotoxicosis.

- *Obvious weight loss*: More so in the face, loss of hair or thinning of hair.

- *Radial pulse*: Tachycardia is an early sign. Various other changes such as extrasystoles, irregular pulse, collapsing pulse. In neglected cases, cardiac failure can also be found.

- *Restlessness*: Patients with Graves' disease are restless, even in bed (Figs 19.7 to 19.10 and Clinical Box 19.4).

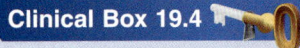

Clinical Box 19.4

- Tremors of tongue
- Tremors of hand
- Tachycardia
- Tense and anxious
- Thin patient—loss of weight

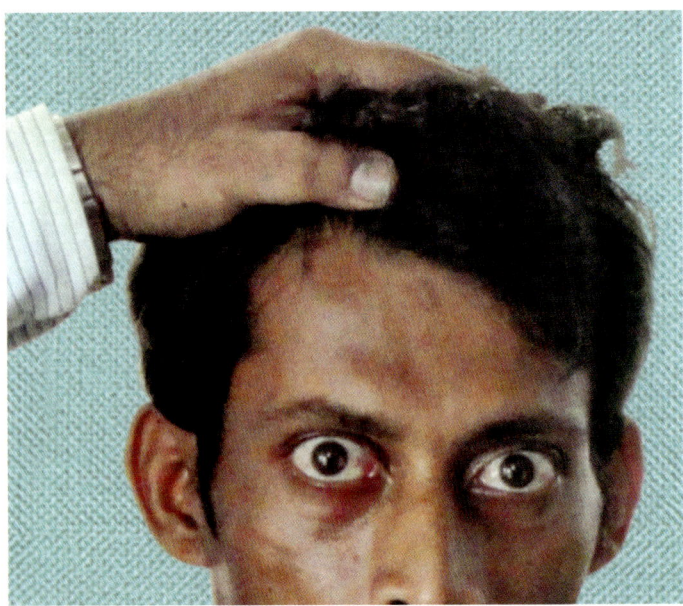

Fig. 19.7: Note the stare-like look in this thin built, 27-year-old man (*Courtesy:* Dr BH Anand Rao, Ex Professor of Surgery, KMC, Manipal)

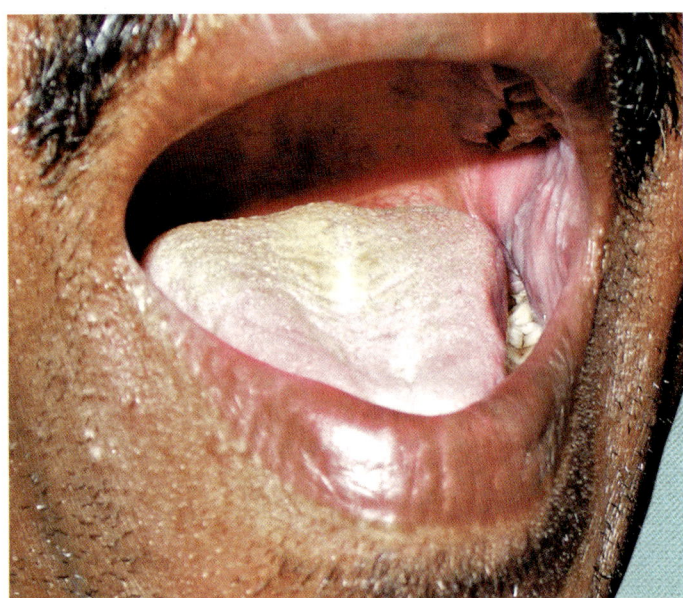

Fig. 19.8: Check for tremors of the tongue with the tongue placed inside the mouth (*Courtesy:* Dr Reetesh Shetty, Assistant Professor, Dept of Surgery, KMC, Manipal)

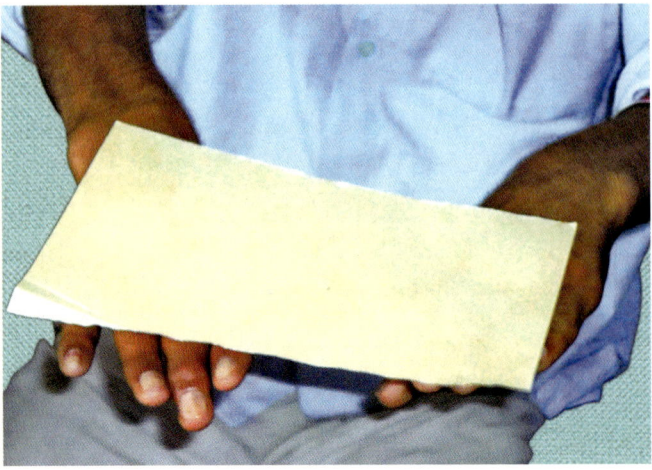

Fig. 19.9: Checking for fine tremors of the fingers

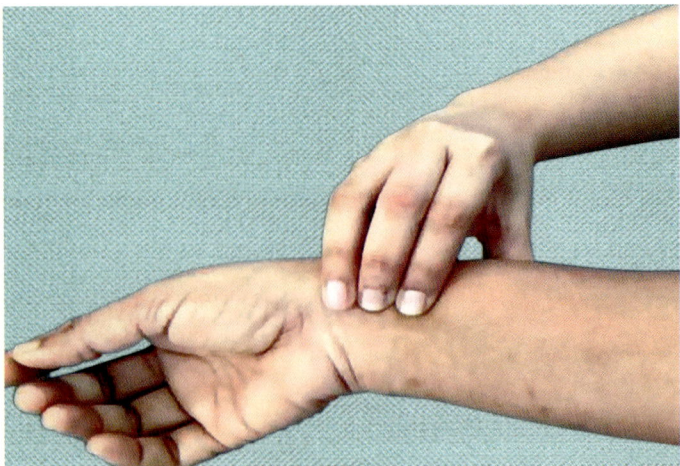

Fig. 19.10: Checking pulse rate—tachycardia

LOCAL EXAMINATION/REGIONAL EXAMINATION

- Examination of thyroid swelling should be done in the usual manner of description of a swelling such as location, size, shape, surface borders (edges), etc. Specific methods and description are given below.

- **Pizzillo's method is indicated in obese patients, especially short-necked individuals.** The patient is asked to clasp hands and press against the occiput with head extended. The thyroid gland becomes more prominent and makes inspection and palpation better (Fig. 19.11).

Inspection

- Inspect from front of the patient. Look for swelling, trachea, common carotid pulsations and anterior and posterior triangle for lymph nodes.

- Ask the patient to extend the neck. Thyroid becomes more prominent and more details can be appreciated. In obese patients with short neck, examine using Pizzillo's method.

- **Give a glass of water and check for movement on deglutition.**

- Classically the swelling is in front of the neck, horizontally extending from one sternomastoid to the other sternomastoid, vertically from suprasternal notch to the thyroid cartilage.

- The size and shape have to be mentioned. Example: approximately measures about 8 cm vertically and 6 cm horizontally.

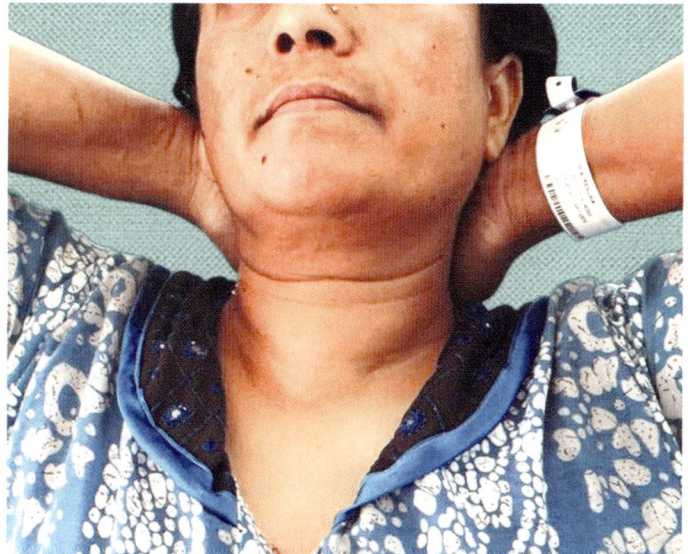

Fig. 19.11: Pizzillo's method (*Courtesy:* Dr Kshama Hegde, Assistant Professor, Department of Surgery, KMC, Manipal)

- *Surface:* Thyroid swellings can have the following types of surfaces:

  a. *Smooth:* Adenoma, puberty goitre, Graves' disease

  b. *Irregular:* Carcinoma of the thyroid

  c. *Nodular:* Multinodular goitre

- *Borders* are usually round and comment on the skin over it—normal or stretched.

Clinical Wisdom

Large or big nodules, all together form the bosselated surface. Polycystic kidney, phyllodes tumour, dermatofibroma protuberans are a few other examples of swelling having bosselated surface (Fig. 19.12). Polycystic disease of the liver and bulky metastasis in the liver also give rise to bosselated surface.

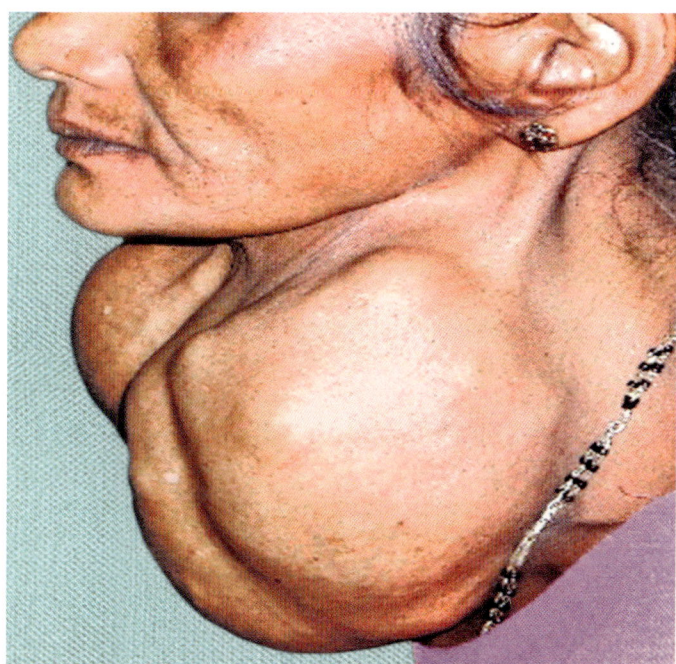

Fig. 19.12 Bosselated surface

1. Prominent subcutaneous veins may be an indication of superior vena caval (SVC) obstruction caused by retrosternal goitre or mediastinal lymph nodes from papillary carcinoma thyroid. If you see these prominent veins then do **Pemberton's test to confirm** (Fig. 19.13).

   - This test is done by asking the patient to raise the hands above the head, and the arms to touch the ears. Keep the same position for a while. Veins become more prominent, if there is obstruction to superior vena cava. When you do not see the lower border of the swelling clearly, it may be retrosternal goitre. Do Pemberton's test.

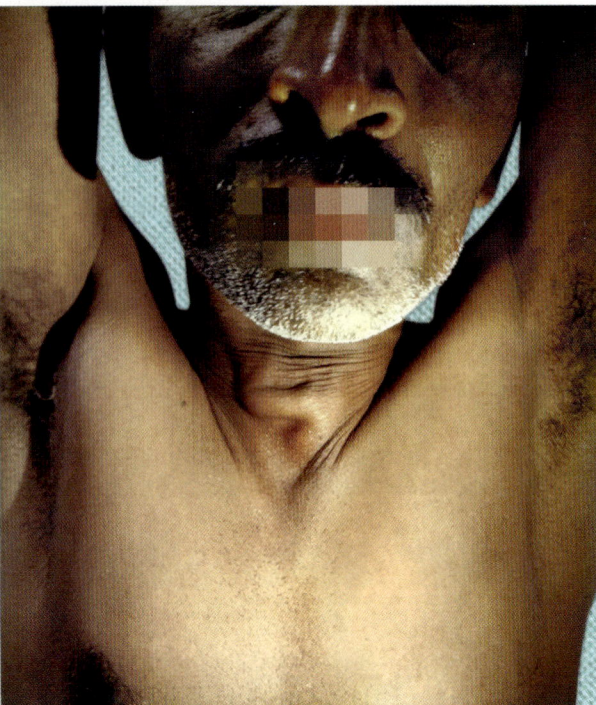

Fig. 19.13: Pemberton test (sign)

- Dilated veins over the chest wall is due to internal jugular vein compression.

2. **Ask the patient to swallow:** Ideally, give the patient a glass of water and then check for movement with deglutition. **Thyroid swelling moves up with deglutition** (Clinical Box 19.5) because of the following reasons:

- Thyroid is enclosed by the pretracheal fascia which is condensed to form a ligament posteromedially called **ligament of Berry**. These are pairs of ligaments attached to cricoid cartilage. During deglutition, the cricoid cartilage moves upwards due to action of inferior constrictors—cricopharyngeal part arises from cricoid cartilage. Thyropharyngeal part of inferior constrictor also arises from thyroid cartilage.

Clinical Box 19.5

Swellings which move upwards with deglutition
- Thyroid swellings
- Subhyoid bursitis
- Pretracheal and prelaryngeal lymph nodes
- Thyroglossal cyst
- Laryngocoele

Inferior Constrictors

- These muscles mainly do the function of swallowing—food enters from pharynx to upper oesophagus.
- It has two parts—thyropharyngeus arises from thyroid cartilage and cricopharyngeus arises from cricoid cartilage.
- When these muscles act, thyroid and cricoid cartilage moves upwards. Thus, thyroid gland also moves upwards.
- Inferior constrictors are supplied by vagus nerve. These are thickest constrictor muscles.

- **If there is restriction of movement, it can be due to**
    - Malignancy with fixity to the trachea
    - Retrosternal goitre
    - Large goitre because of the size
    - Previous surgery
- When the thyroid gland moves upwards, carefully watch the lower border. If it is seen, it is not a case of retrosternal goitre (Figs 19.14A and B).

3. **Ask the patient to protrude the tongue:** Movement of the swelling on protrusion of the tongue suggests thyroglossal cyst (details are given later). This test should be done when there is a nodule or a cyst in the region of isthmus of the thyroid gland (midline swelling). *This test has no relevance in cases of MNG or other lateral thyroid or neck swellings.*

4. **Pulsation:** Prominent pulsations are due to pushing of superior thyroid artery by the enlarged upper pole. Whole gland in primary tyrotoxicosis can be pulsatile.

What else can be pulsatile in thyroid disease? Secondaries from follicular carcinoma thyroid.

Palpation

It should be done from behind. Gently flex the neck to relax the deep fascia and strap muscles which facilitate palpation. Enlargement of lobes, isthmus and neck nodes is better appreciated palpating from behind (Fig. 19.15). Some other tests are better done from front such as intrinsic mobility, finding out the plane of the swelling, etc.

- **Local rise of temperature and tenderness** should be mentioned first, just like in any other swellings. To give an example, if the swelling is tender and local rise of temperature is present, it is probably a case of bacterial thyroiditis. *No doubt it is rare but*

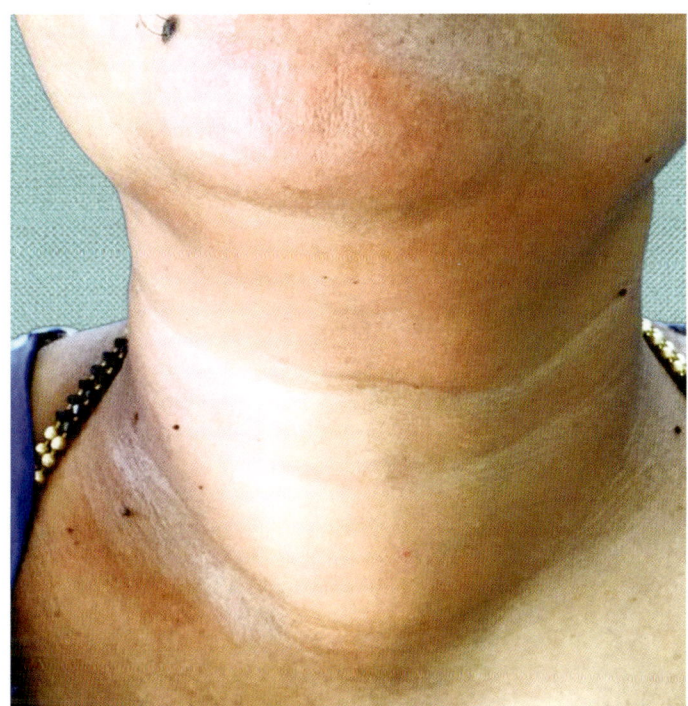

Fig. 19.14A: Thyroid swelling—lower border not seen (before giving water)

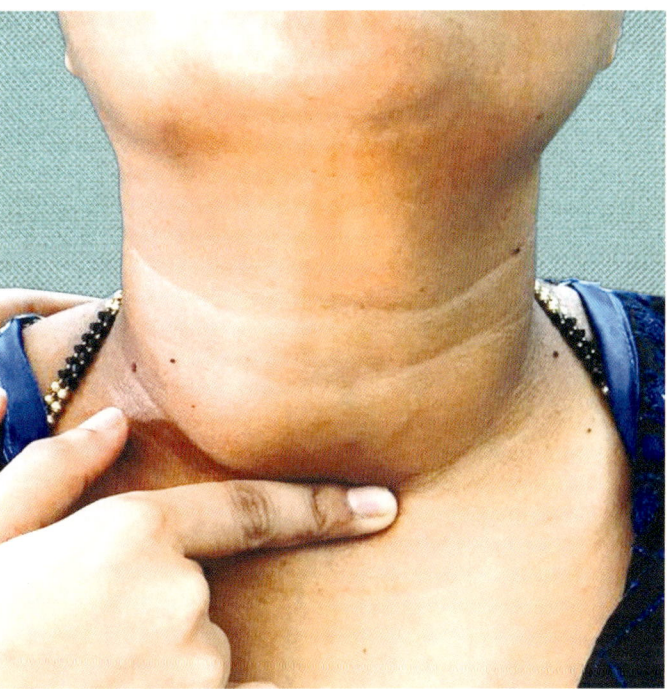

Fig. 19.14B: After giving water—thyroid moves upwards with deglutition. Palpate and also check lower border

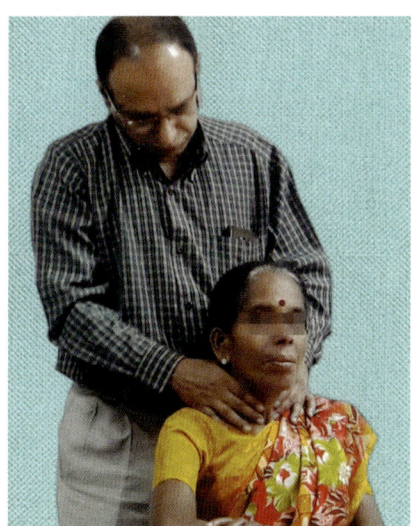

Fig. 19.15: Palpation of the thyroid gland from behind

- Confirm the movement with deglutition by holding the thyroid gland and asking the patient to drink water.

- **Sternocleidomastoid contraction test** is done when one lobe is enlarged. In this situation, the examiner keeps the hand on the side of the chin, opposite side of the lesion and patient is asked to push the hand against resistance. If the gland becomes less prominent (as with thyroid swellings), it indicates the swelling is deep to the sternocleiodomastoid muscle (Fig. 19.16).

bacterial thyroiditis is a very well known entity. More common is tenderness without local rise of temperature as in viral thyroiditis (de Quervain). Then mention size, shape, surface and border. Very large nodular surface is described as bosselated surface.

- Consistency:
  - *Soft:* Graves' disease, colloid goitre
  - *Firm:* Adenoma, multinodular goitre
  - *Hard:* Carcinoma, calcification in the MNG

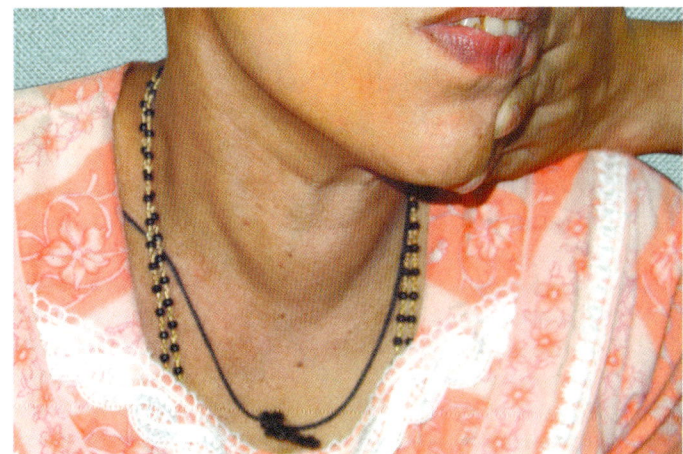

Fig. 19.16: Right sternocleidomastoid contraction test

5. **Chin test (neck flexion test)** is classically done in multinodular goitre, wherein both lobes are enlarged. The patient is asked to bend the chin downwards against resistance. This produces contraction of both sternocleidomastoids and the gland becomes less prominent (Fig. 19.17).

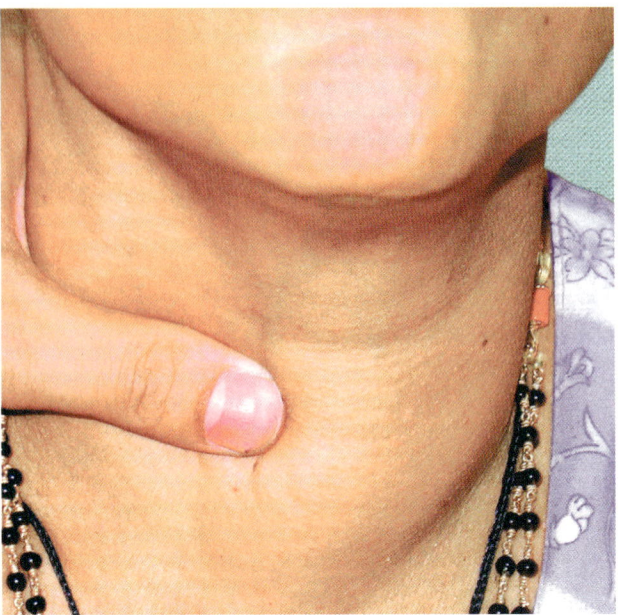

Fig. 19.18: Crile's method

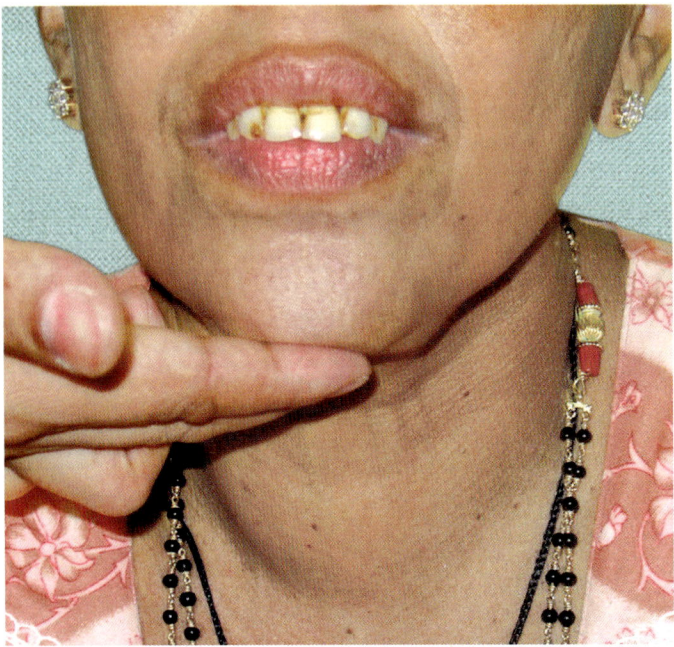

Fig. 19.17: Neck flexion test

6. **Intrinsic mobility** of the gland is very much restricted in carcinoma of the thyroid specially in anaplastic carcinoma because of infiltration into the trachea and pre vertebral muscles. Please understand that the thyroid gland is normally adherent to the larynx. Hence, when you try to move the gland, the whole complex consisting of enlarged thyroid gland, trachea and larynx, moves together.

7. **Special tests** or methods of examination of thyroid gland:

   a. *Crile's method* is indicated when there is a doubtful nodule. Keep the thumb over the suspected area of the nodule and ask the patient to swallow. The nodularity is appreciated better with this test (Fig. 19.18).

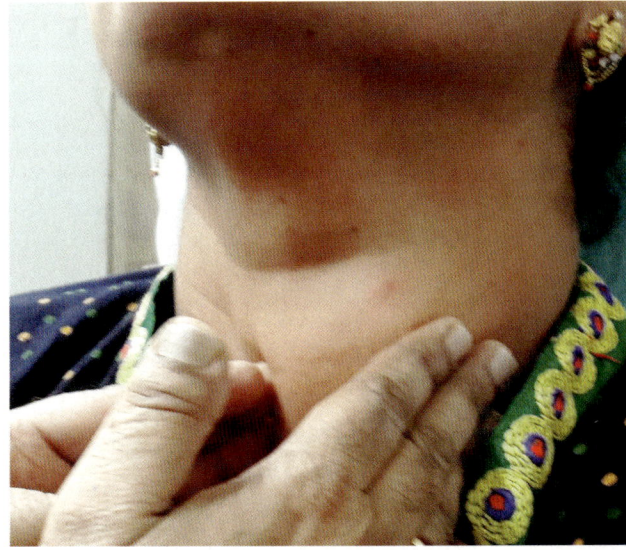

Fig. 19.19: Lahey's method. With the left hand, left lobe is pushed to the left side and right hand is used to palpate for any nodules

   b. *Lahey's method* of examination of thyroid can be done from front as well as behind. In order to palpate the left lobe, push the gland to the left side. The left lobe becomes more prominent and thus palpation becomes easy and nodules are appreciated better (Fig. 19.19).

   c. *Kocher's test*: If gentle compression on lateral lobes produces stridor, it is described as positive. This is due to **scabbard trachea**. Long-standing multinodular goitres causing tracheomalacia (cartilages become soft) and carcinoma with infiltration into trachea are the two common causes (Fig. 19.20).

Clinical Wisdom

- The importance of this test is only in a nodule which is fixed to trachea as in anaplastic carcinoma thyroid. It has no relevance when both lobes are enlarged with isthmus.
- In very advanced cases, there will not be any mobility of the gland. It is due to fixity to prevertebral fascia.

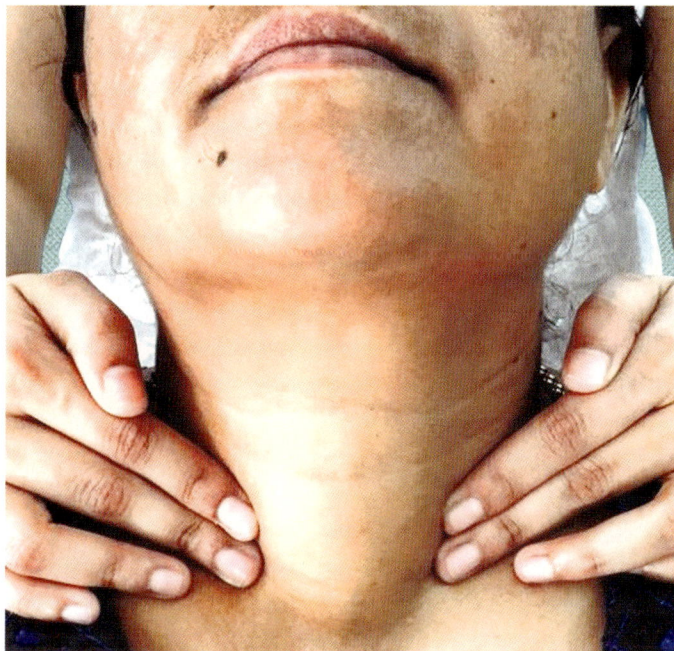

Fig. 19.20: Kocher's test

8. **Position of trachea:** In cases of solitary nodule confined to one lobe, trachea is deviated to the opposite side. However, in cases of multinodular goitres, trachea need not be deviated because of symmetrical enlargement of both lobes. If tracheal position cannot be appreciated because of the large size of the gland, perform the following tests (Fig. 19.21).

- **Feel the Adam's apple** above, which may give some idea about the deviation of the trachea (Fig. 19.22).
- **Trail's sign:** Look at the sternomastoid muscle. If it is prominent on one side, the deviation is to the side of prominence, the reason being both thyroid gland and sternomastoid muscle are enclosed by pretracheal fascia. Hence, when the enlarged thyroid gland pushes the trachea, opposite pretracheal fascia relaxes making sternomastoid muscle becomes more prominent.
- Auscultate above the gland to look for air entry— to localize the trachea.

9. **Palpation of lymph nodes** in the neck. If lymph nodes are palpable, find out which group of nodes are these. Example: Usually level 3 or 4 group of lymph nodes are enlarged. Level 5 and 6 group of nodes must also be checked. Often nodes such as level 1 or 2 may be enlarged. It is not due to thyroid diseases but due to oral cavity infections—common being dental caries and tonsillitis.

- Look for jugular chain of lymph nodes and central nodes (Figs 19.23 and 19.24).

10. **Palpation of common carotid artery:** Draw a line from mastoid process to sternoclavicular joint. Then draw a horizontal line from upper border of thyroid cartilage. The point where these two lines meet is the site of bifurcation of common carotid

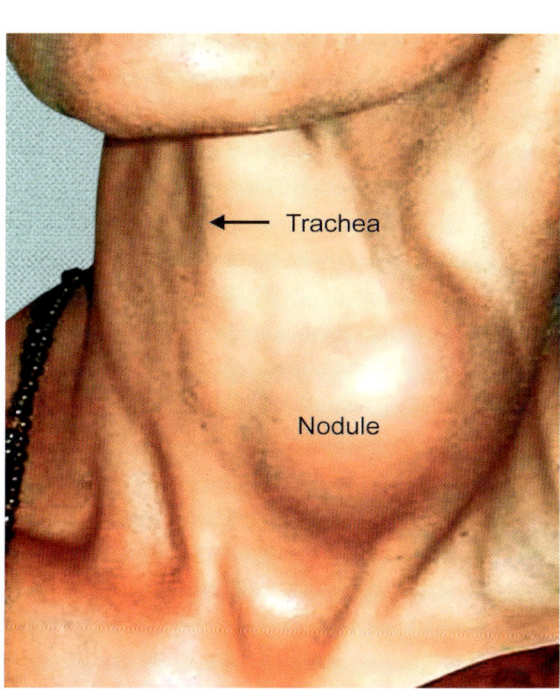

Fig. 19.21: Trachea is deviated to the right side

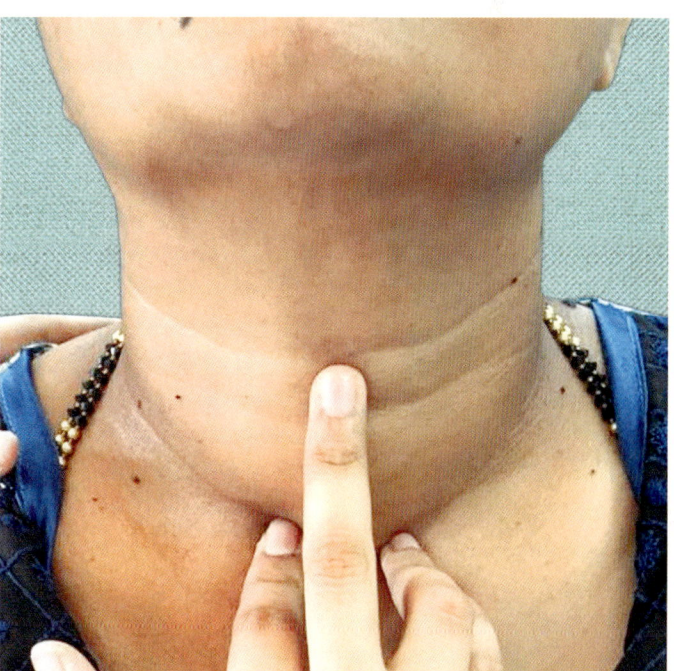

Fig. 19.22: Feeling for the trachea

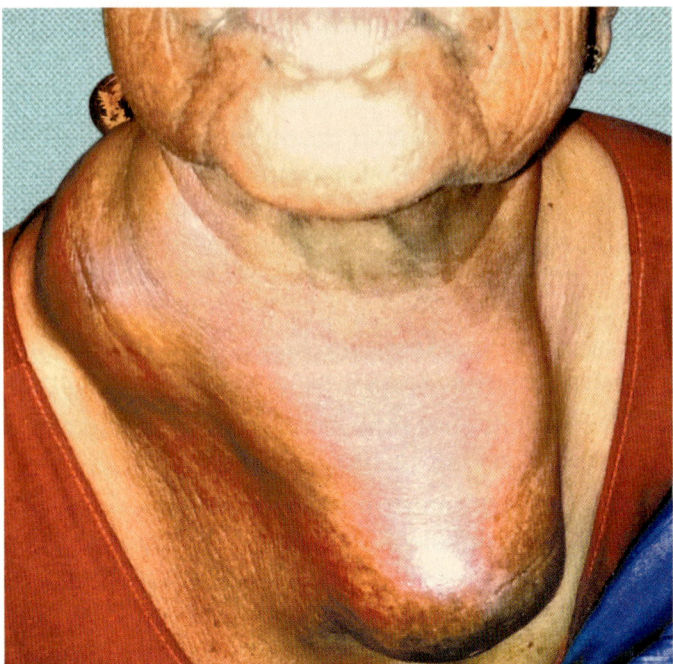

Fig. 19.23: Papillary carcinoma of thyroid with large cystic neck nodes of 7 years duration. It was misdiagnosed as tubercular cold abscess and ATT was given. Biopsy was also done and reported as non specific lymphadenitis. Papillary carcinoma of the thyroid is known to present as cystic secondaries in the lymph nodes of many years duration (*Courtesy:* Dr Geetha Avadani, Dr MA Balakrishna, Dr Dinesh, Dr Ravi Kumar, Dept of Surgery, Mysore Medical College, Mysore)

artery. Just below this point, this artery should be palpated. Artery in this location is palpated against **Chassaignac tubercle—tubercle on the transverse process of the 6th cervical vertebra** (Fig. 19.25).

- In large multinodular goitres, the artery may be pushed backwards and outwards. Hence,

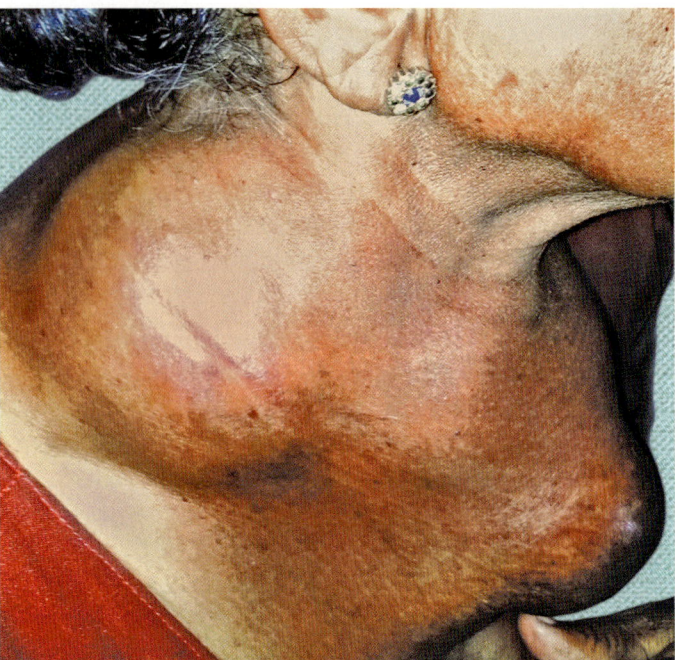

Fig. 19.24: Lateral view of the same patient as in Fig. 19.23 showing large lymph node mass

pulsations are felt behind the posterior edge of the swelling. Carcinoma of the thyroid engulfs the carotid sheath. Consequently, pulsations may be absent. *Absent carotid artery pulsation* is called *Berry sign.* Since the lumen is not narrowed, superficial temporal artery pulsations are felt normally.

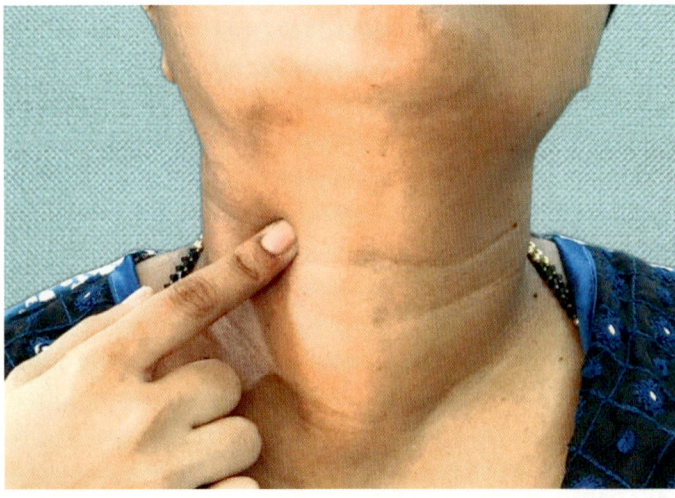

Fig. 19.25A: Normally, common carotid artery pulsations are felt at the upper border of the thyroid cartilage

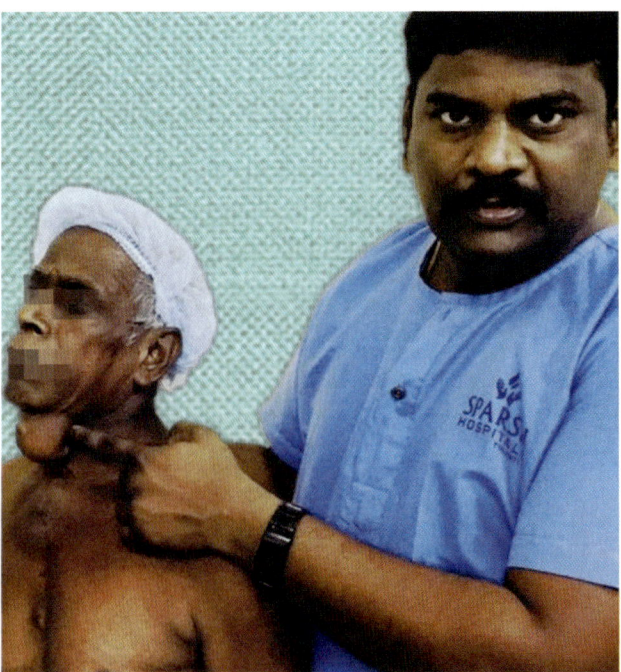

Fig. 19.25B: Common carotid artery is pushed to posterior triangle (*Courtesy:* Dr MA Hari Babu, Department of Surgery, SVMC, Tirupati)

Percussion

Percussion over the sternum gives a resonant note in normal cases. In retrosternal goitres, it gives a dull note.

Auscultation

- It should be done in the upper pole because of the following reasons: Superior thyroid artery is a direct branch of external carotid artery. It is more superficial than inferior thyroid artery (Fig. 19.26).

- Presence of thrill and bruit is the feature of toxic goitre.

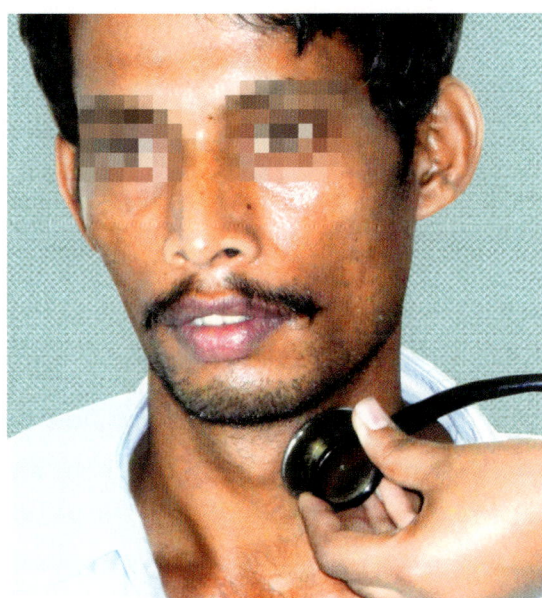

Fig. 19.26: Auscultate upper pole for bruit

SYSTEMIC EXAMINATION

This includes CNS and eye signs, as in Graves' disease, examination of skeletal system to rule out metastasis as in carcinoma of the thyroid, and examination of cardiovascular system in cases of toxic goitre. Deep tendon reflexes also have to be elicited—there is a slow relaxation phase in hypothyroidism.

Examination of Eyes

Thyrotoxic exophthalmopathy is due to several factors and has several components.

Prominent eyeballs or stare look is due to forward protrusion caused by retrobulbar deposition of inflammatory cells and round cells with venous congestion resulting in oedema. This is added by retraction of the eyelid caused by contraction of levator palpebrae superioris muscle. It is innervated by **oculomotor nerve** which also carries sympathetic

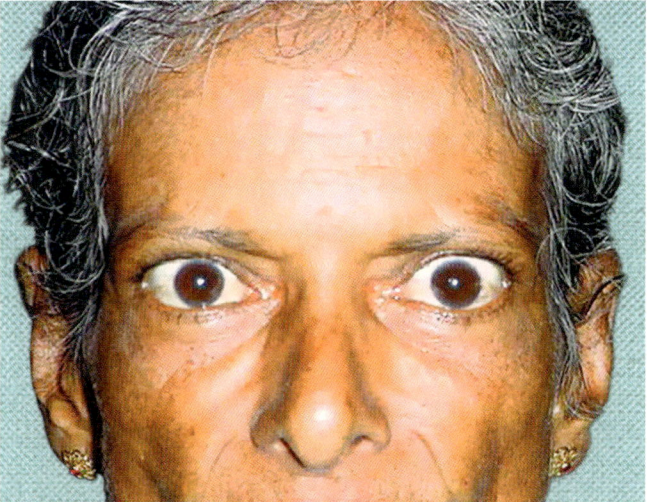

Fig. 19.27: Exophthalmos

fibres derived from cavernous plexus for the smooth muscle part of the levator. Contraction of this muscle produces lid spasm. This is also aided by **spasm of Müller's muscle,** a sympathetic muscle which lies adjoining the levator palpebrae superioris muscle. This is responsible for keeping the eyeball forwards. All these factors together produce a classical stare (Fig. 19.27).

Detailed examination of eye signs is not required in non-toxic goitres. Check for exophthalmos and lid retraction and say that there are no eye signs.

1. *Lid retraction—Dalrymple's sign*: Upper sclera is seen above the limbus (upper margin of the cornea and conjunctiva). This sign is caused by over activity of the involuntary part of the levator palpebrae superioris muscle (Fig. 19.28).

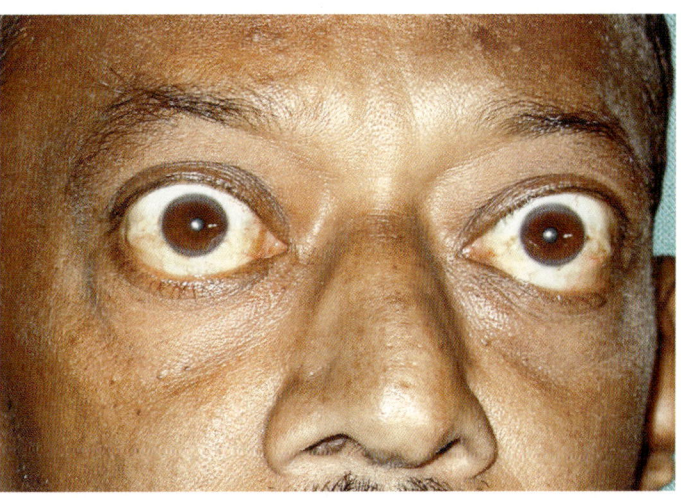

Fig. 19.28: Dalrymple's sign

2. *Assessment of exophthalmos—Naffziger's method*: Stand behind the patient and look at the supraciliary arch, by tilting the patient's head backwards. In normal cases, eyeball is not seen. In cases of exophthalmos, eyeball is protruded outside and hence it is seen (Fig. 19.29).

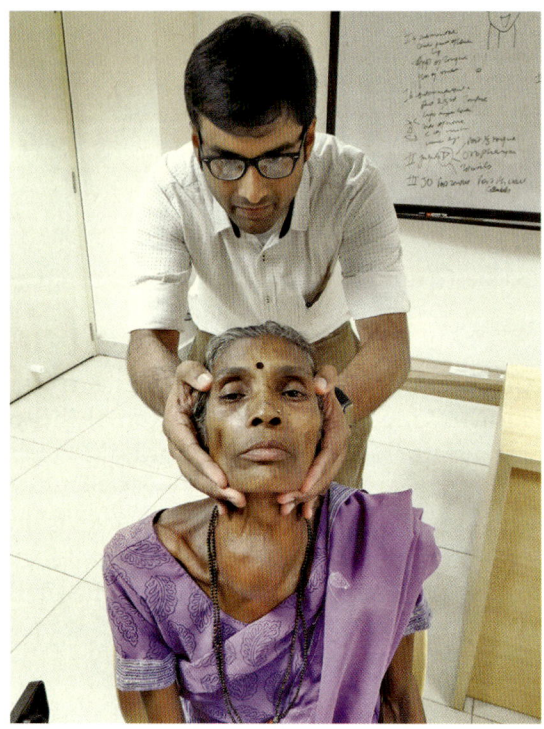

Fig. 19.29: Naffziger's method

3. *Moebius sign*: Loss of convergence of eyeball occurs due to muscle paresis as a part of thyrotoxic ophthalmoplegia. Diplopia is due to weakness of

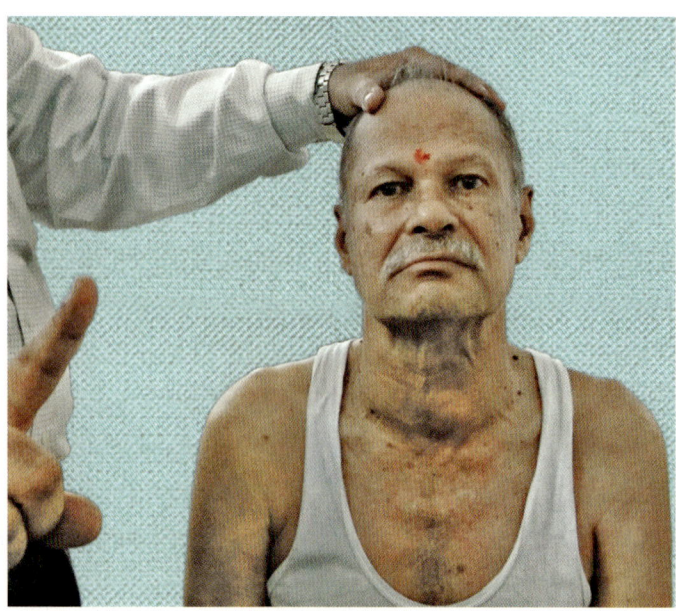

Fig. 19.30A: Moebius sign

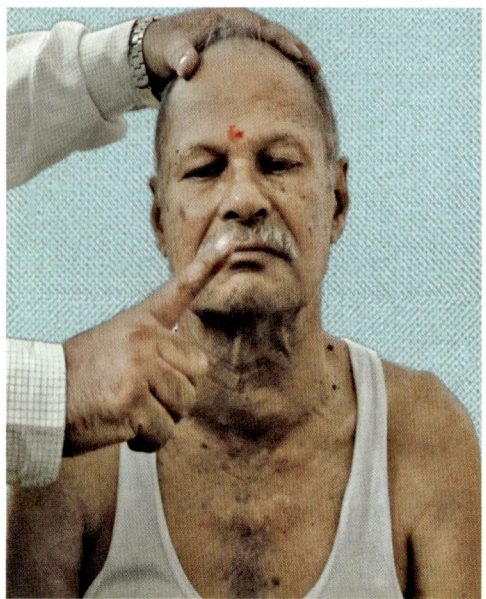

Fig. 19.30B: Convergence of eyeball

extraocular muscles (inferior oblique—elevators). Other muscles involved are superior rectus and lateral rectus (Fig. 19.30).

4. *Stellwag's sign*: Infrequent blinking and widening of palpebral fissure is due to spasm of sympathetic fibres in the levator palpebrae superioris.

5. *Joffroy's sign*: Absence of wrinkling of the forehead when the patient is asked to look upwards. This occurs due to increase in the field of vision due to exophthalmos (Fig. 19.31).

6. *Von Graefe's sign (lid lag sign)*: When the patient is asked to look up and down, upper eyelid cannot cope up with the speed of movement of the finger because of the lid spasm.

7. **Chemosis** is oedema of the conjunctiva.

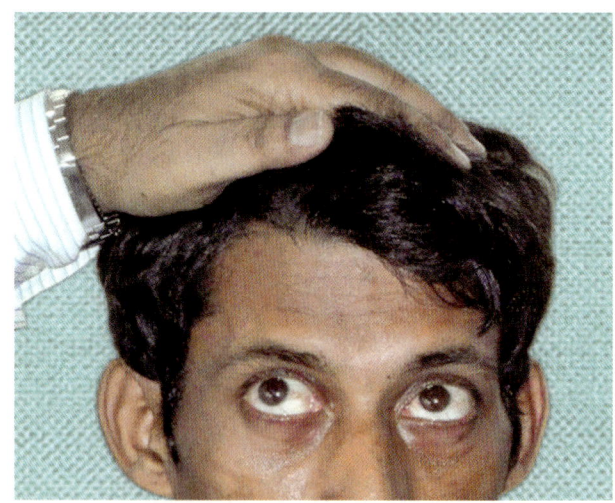

Fig. 19.31: Joffroy's sign

8. In late stages, **optic nerve damage and blindness** can occur.

Examination for Tremors

- **Fine tremors of the tongue** (fibrillations) can be found when the tongue is within the oral cavity. In advanced cases, tremors can be found even when the tongue is protruded out (fasciculations). Keep it outside for half a minute (Fig. 19.32).

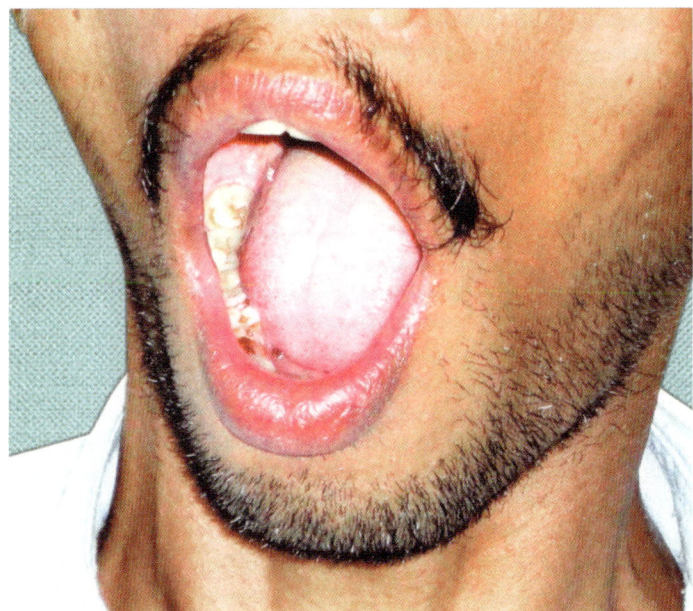

Fig. 19.32: Look for tongue tremors

- **Tremors of the outstretched hands** are characteristic. A piece of paper may be placed on the fingers in doubtful cases for demonstrating the tremors of the hand. Extensor surface of the hand is used because extensors are weak when compared to flexors (Fig. 19.9).

Clinical Wisdom

- If your patient has no toxic features, not even lid retraction, you need not mention that you have checked for chemosis, blindness, etc.
- Sometimes, the gland becomes more visible on extending the neck.
- Some details on palpation can also be obtained from front.

Examination of Skeletal System

- First ask the patient whether she has any swelling or any bony pain. Skull bone, sternum, ribs, etc. are the common sites of skeletal metastasis from follicular carcinoma thyroid (Clinical Box 19.6 and Figs 19.33 to 19.36) hence should be examined.

Clinical Box 19.6

Scalp and surgeon
1. Swelling from follicular carcinoma thyroid and hepatocellular carcinoma
2. Pepper pot in hyperparathyroidism
3. Turban tumours—cylindroma
4. Koch's peculiar tumour (*refer to page 75*)
5. Dermoid cyst, sebaceous cyst, lipoma, exostosis

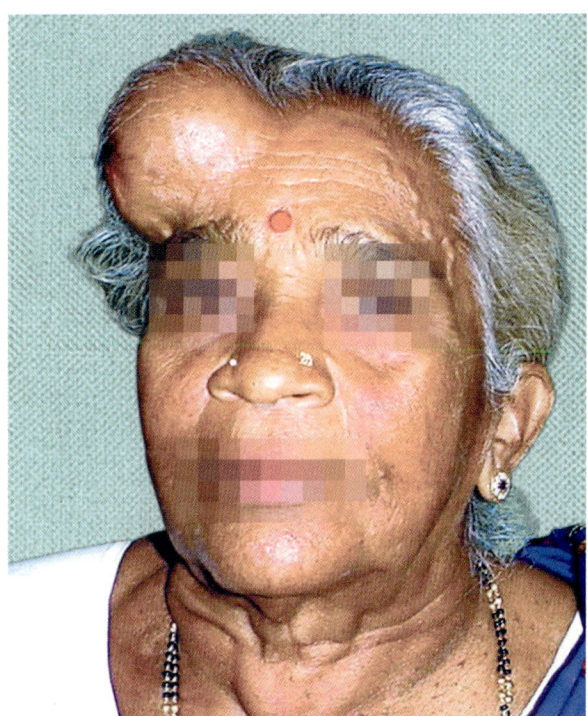

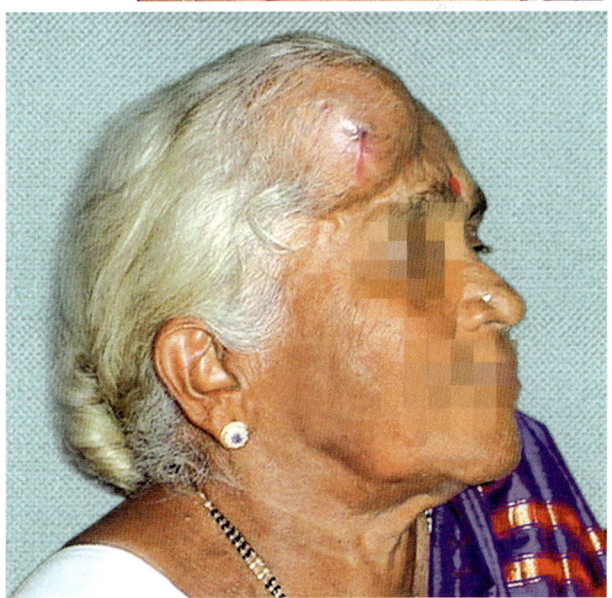

Fig. 19.33A: Follicular carcinoma thyroid with metastasis in the skull bone—tense, tender, pulsatile swelling. **Fig. 19.33B:** Lateral view of the same patient as in Fig. 19.33A showing skin ulceration. (*Courtesy:* Prof. Diwakar Shenoy, Ex-Professor of Surgery, KMC, Manipal)

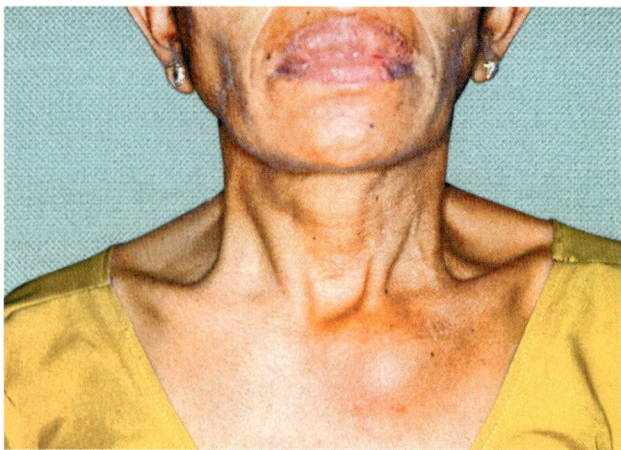

Fig. 19.34: Carcinoma thyroid with metastasis in the second rib

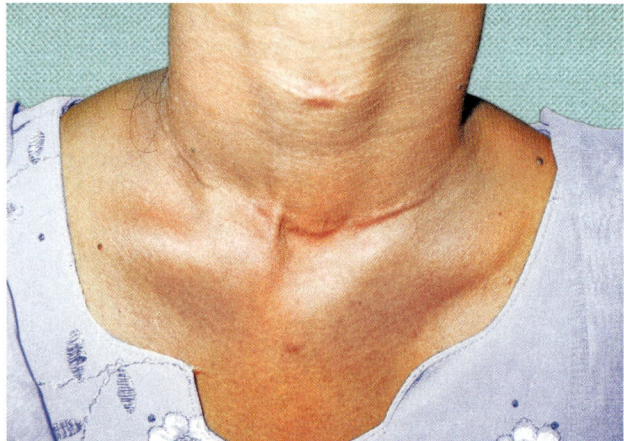

Fig. 19.35: Carefully watch right sternoclavicular joint—it was tender and the swelling had increased temperature

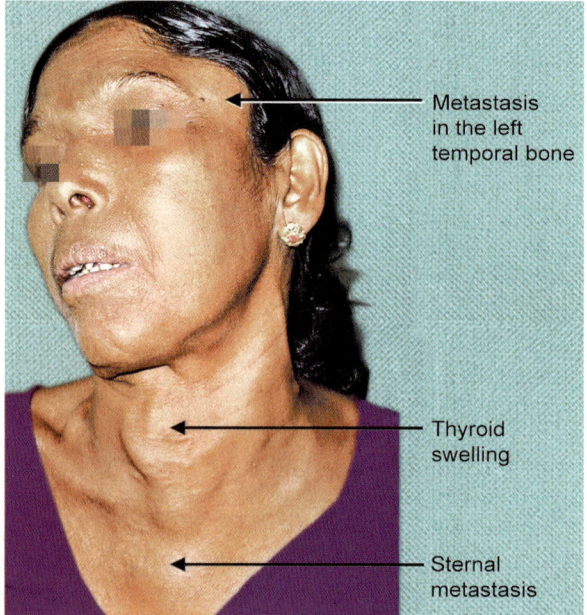

Metastasis in the left temporal bone

Thyroid swelling

Sternal metastasis

Fig. 19.36: A lady with 3 swellings—follicular carcinoma thyroid with metastasis

- If there is a swelling, to call it as a metastasis, it will have following features:
  1. Recent onset
  2. Rapid growth
  3. Local rise in temperature is present.
  4. Pulsations may be present.
  5. Bony erosions may be found.

Examination of Abdomen

- Very advanced cases of follicular carcinoma can spread to liver and produce secondaries resulting in hard and nodular liver.
- Hepatosplenomegaly, if present in cases of goitre, may be Hashimoto's thyroiditis or autoimmune thyroiditis.

CLINICAL DISCUSSION

1. **Why do you think this swelling is arising from thyroid gland?**
   - It is in front of the neck
   - It moves with deglutition
   - When both lobes and isthmus are enlarged, it is butterfly shaped
   - Upper limit (border) is limited to the thyroid cartilage because of the attachment of pretracheal fascia to the oblique line of thyroid cartilage
   - On chin test, swelling becomes less prominent.
2. **Why do you say it is multinodular goitre?**
   - Both lobes are enlarged.
   - Isthmus is enlarged.
   - Many nodules are felt.
   - Nodules are firm in consistency.
   - Borders are round.
3. **When do you suspect malignancy in this case?**
   If nodules are hard, if lymph nodes or bone metastasis are present.
4. **Does hard nodule always indicate malignancy?**
   No. It can be due to calcification.
5. **What type of calcification is this called?**
   Dystrophic calcification. (Other calcification is metastatic calcification.)
6. **Which type of malignancy is commonly seen in MNG?**
   Follicular carcinoma thyroid.
7. **When do you suspect that?**
   When a patient with MNG has pulsatile metastasis in flat bones such as skill, ribs, sternum, etc.
8. **What are the investigations?**
   Ultrasound can pick up a nodule which can be malignant—solid, hypoechoeic and jugular chain of lymph nodes.
9. **What are the indications for surgery in a non-toxic, non-malignant MNG?**
   Symptoms of compression or for cosmetic reasons.
10. **What are the advantages of total thyroidectomy for MNG?**
    - Avoids recurrence—3 to 5%
    - Recurrent goitres are difficult to remove
    - Avoids second surgery, if histopathology of of subtotal thyroidectomy is reported as malignancy

11. **What are the disadvantages of total thyroidectomy?**

Risks of recurrent laryngeal nerve palsy, hypothyroidism (100%), hypocalcaemia.

12. **What is the alternative type of surgery of MNG?**

Total lobectomy on one side and subtotal on the other side.

13. **What are the disadvantages of subtotal thyroidectomy?**

Recurrence and incidental malignancies.

14. **What are the complications of MNG?**

Secondary thyrotoxicosis, follicular carcinoma thyroid, haemorrhage in a nodule causing breathlessness, tracheomalacia and calcification.

15. **What is Dunhill's procedure?**

One side total lobectomy and the other side subtotal lobectomy or excision of diseased nodule is called Dunhill's procedure.

16. **What are the types of retrosternal goitres?**

Substernal, plunging and intrathoracic.

17. **How does multinodular goitre occur and what are the different stages?**

- *Stage I*: Stage of diffuse hypertrophy and hyperplasia of thyroid.
- *Stage II*: Due to fluctuating levels of TSH because of pregnancy, lactation, menstruation, etc. Some areas in thyroid are overstimulated and are converted to active follicles.
- *Stage III*: The active follicle ultimately undergoes necrosis and many such necrosed follicles join to form a nodule. Many such nodules form a multinodular goitre. Nodules contain necrosed tissue, i.e. inactive tissue. The internodular tissue is active.

18. **Why miosis and ptosis may be found?**

It suggests Horner's syndrome. It is also a feature of malignancy of the thyroid infiltrating sympathetic chain.

19. **What is the significance of Lahey's method and Crile's method of palpation?**

To give an example: A patient is diagnosed to have one nodule. Thus, the diagnosis is solitary nodule—the treatment plan would have been lobectomy (in benign conditions). After doing these 2 tests, if some more nodules are felt, it means that it is a multinodular goitre and the treatment is different. However, their relevance is less now because ultrasound will pick up these impalpable or very early nodules.

20. **What test is done to assess the pressure effects on the trachea?**

Kocher's test. Stridor indicates tracheomalacia.

21. **What is malignant exophthalmos?**

This occurs in untreated cases of Graves' disease. Infrequent blinking secondary to exophthalmos results in constant **exposure of the cornea to the atmosphere.** This results in keratitis, corneal ulcer, conjunctivitis, chemosis and may even lead to blindness. This is called malignant exophthalmos.

22. **What are the common primaries which metastasise to skull bone?**

Follicular carcinoma thyroid, hepatoma, carcinoma prostate, carcinoma bronchus and carcinoma kidney.

DIAGNOSIS

Before you give final diagnosis, ask 4 questions to yourself.
1. Is it a normothyroid goitre?
2. Is it a toxic goitre?
3. Is it a malignant goitre?
4. Is it a hypothyroid goitre?
Based on symptoms and signs, it is possible to draw these conclusions.

1. *Normothyroid goitre* : No features of toxicosis and gland is enlarged. Colloid goitre, puberty goitre and iodine deficiency goitre are included, this category.

2. *Toxic goitre*: When CNS symptoms are dominant, the gland is enlarged smoothly, eye signs are present and the patient is young, it is primary thyrotoxicosis. When cardiac symptoms such as palpitation are dominant in middle-aged patients, they are likely to have secondary thyrotoxicosis (Plummer's disease).

3. *Malignant goitre*: Rapidly growing goitre with or without hoarseness of voice is suggestive of malignant goitre. Clinical examination may reveal—hard gland, irregular gland, fixed gland, lymph nodes and bony swellings may be palpable.

4. *Hypothyroid goitre*: Women around middle age, weight gain, excessive fatty deposition in supraclavicular fossae, and slow mental activity may be suggestive of hypothyroidism.

Once you decide on these four categories, you have to further analyse the cases. Read the differential diagnosis, it will help you in getting final diagnosis. Before reading differential diagnosis, let us study relevant investigation.

Commonly asked questions are, 'what do you do in this situation and how do you investigate'?

First study investigations and then read differential diagnosis.

INVESTIGATIONS

1. *Routine blood tests* are normal in most of thyroid surgical patients.

2. *Elevated T4, T3 and low TSH levels* indicate thyrotoxicosis. Even though there may not be any clinical feature of thyrotoxicosis, TSH level must be obtained. A very high TSH levels >100 units are not acceptable. Hence, a small dose of thyroxine (T4) 0.5 mg is given to normalise TSH levels. Then surgery is undertaken.

- Also, there may be subclinical thyrotoxicosis. Hence, T3 and T4 levels are obtained.

  Normal values of T3, T4 and TSH are given below:

  T3 : 0.8–2.0 ng/ml

  T4 : 4.5–12.0 µg/dl

  TSH : 0.3–5.0 µIU/ml

3. *Ultrasound of neck*

  - Firstly, it will show whether it is unilobar enlargement (adenoma) or bilobar enlargement (common example being multinodular goitre).

  - It can also show whether it is a smooth enlargement (colloid goitre, Graves' disease), irregular (carcinoma) or nodular (multinodular goitre).

  - A solitary nodule can be diagnosed with discrete features.

  - More importantly jugular lymphadenopathy (popularly levels 3, 4, 5 and also 2) can be seen, which will help in the diagnosis of papillary carcinoma thyroid.

4. *FNAC (fine needle cytology)* is the chief and diagnostic investigation with adequate cytology. Almost all cases of thyroid diseases can be diagnosed except follicular carcinoma thyroid. The advantage is that it is a simple outpatient procedure. Better results are obtained with ultrasound-guided FNAC.

5. *X-ray neck AP/lateral view* is taken to rule out tracheal compression. It is required especially in long-standing goitres and carcinoma. Tracheomalacia can occur and in the postoperative period, it can result in collapse of tracheal cartilages resulting in stridor.

6. *Videolaryngoscopy/indirect laryngoscopy* is done to rule out vocal cord paralysis. Unilateral vocal cord paralysis can be asymptomatic and it is compensated by the other vocal cord. It is a caution to a surgeon operating on this type of patient.

  In the vast majority of thyroid disorders, these are the investigations done which will help in the diagnosis and management. A few other investigations are done depending upon the nature of the disease.

7. *Radionuclear studies:* I^{131} *scan* is done when you suspect a toxic autonomous nodule. When the scan is done, it will be a hot nodule. Rest of the gland will not take up isotope. In such cases, radioablation can be done. Otherwise, hemithyroidectomy is the treatment of choice after controlling toxicity.

8. *CT scan* is indicated in case of retrosternal goitres, advanced malignancies to know the infiltration into the carotid artery, internal jugular vein, trachea, etc. Infiltration into paravertebral vessels and paravertebral fascia makes it inoperable, as in anaplastic carcinomas.

DIFFERENTIAL DIAGNOSIS

1. *Diffuse hyperplastic goitre, puberty goitre, pregnancy goitre, iodine deficiency goitre*
   - Uniform enlargement of the gland without nodularity.
   - It is seen in young children or girls at puberty or during pregnancy when the metabolic demands are high and the production of T3, T4 is comparatively normal. Due to feedback mechanism, TSH levels increase, which stimulates thyroid gland and causes diffuse hypertrophy and hyperplasia. Goitrogens also will produce goitre due to low levels of thyroid hormone production. This is also called physiological goitre and can be treated by giving tablet thyroxine (T4) 0.2 mg/day to suppress TSH. **Iodine deficiency goitre** is treated with iodised salt (which is used in food) and iodine—containing preparations.
   - Goitre may disappear, if treatment is given in the stage of diffuse hypertrophy.

2. *Colloid goitre*
   - If the iodine deficiency status continues for a long time, it results in accumulation of colloid material in the gland and causes colloid goitre.
   - Patients are between 20 and 40 years depending upon how early or late they come to the hospital. Often, it is symptomless, many may not report at all to the hospital. The whole gland is enlarged, soft or elastic without nodules. No features of pressure or toxicity are present.

3. *Multinodular goitre (MNG)*
   - Typically, the patient is between 30 and 40 years of age who complains of painless swelling in the neck of many years duration. In endemic goitres, swelling appears earlier than sporadic cases. MNG is 6 times more common in females than males. **Both lobes are enlarged and at least 2 nodules should be palpable clinically to give a diagnosis of MNG.** Consistency is usually firm but haemorrhage in a nodule may feel soft and the calcified areas may feel hard. Thus sometimes, variable consistency may be the result. When the size is big, pressure symptoms such as dyspnoea and dysphagia can occur (Fig. 19.37).
   - 20% cases of MNG can develop toxicity which is called secondary thyrotoxicosis. Such patients usually have palpitations and cardiac involvement without tremors and exophthalmos.

4. *Retrosternal goitre:* Usually it is a multinodular goitre when lower border of the swelling is not felt. *Three types of retrosternal goitre are—substernal, plunging and intrathoracic* (Clinical Box 19.7).

6. Solitary nodule (Fig. 19.38)

- It means **only one nodule is felt** and **rest of the gland is not palpable** on clinical examination.
- Very often, the question asked in clinics is, 'what are the possibilities you can consider when you feel only one nodule in the thyroid gland'?
- A. *Multinodular goitre (MNG)* is a diagnosis when a nodule is palpable and the opposite lobe or any other part of the

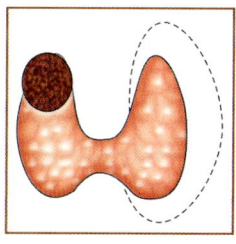
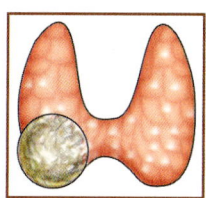

A. Part of MNG   **B. Adenoma**

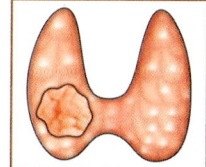
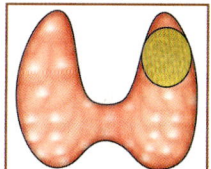

C. Carcinoma   **D. Thyroid cyst**

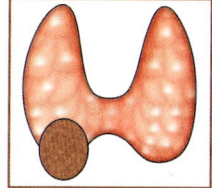

E. Toxic autonomous nodule

Fig. 19.38: Solitary thyroid nodule—differential diagnosis. *Refer to Flowchart 19.1* for treatment algorithm

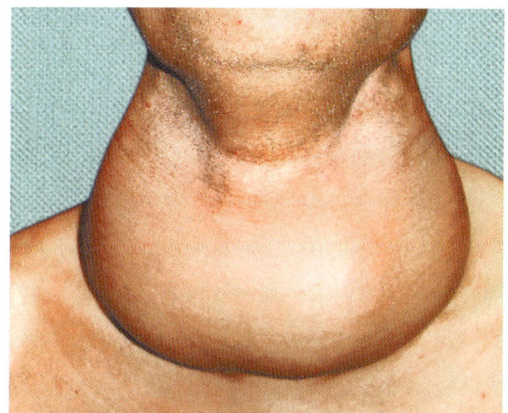

Fig. 19.37: Large MNG in a male. It had areas that were soft, firm and hard

Clinical Box 19.7

Tests to detect retrosternal goitre
A. Cough test: When the patient is asked to cough, lower border may be visible. These goitres are called plunging goitre.
B. Asking the patient to swallow: Lower border is not visible.
C. Pemberton test: Engorged veins over the chest (*see* Fig. 19.13).
D. Dyspnoea on lying to one side.
E. Percussion over the manubrium: Normal resonant note may be replaced by dull note, if there is a retrosternal goitre.

5. Dyshormonogenesis

- Classically, the patient is child/young between 10 and 20 years—mother or the patient complains of painless swelling in the neck of many years duration. It started in early childhood. Otherwise, it will have all other features of MNG. Often, these goitres respond to thyroxine thus avoiding surgery.
- It is an autosomal recessive condition with deficiency of peroxidase or dehalogenase.

Flowchart 19.1

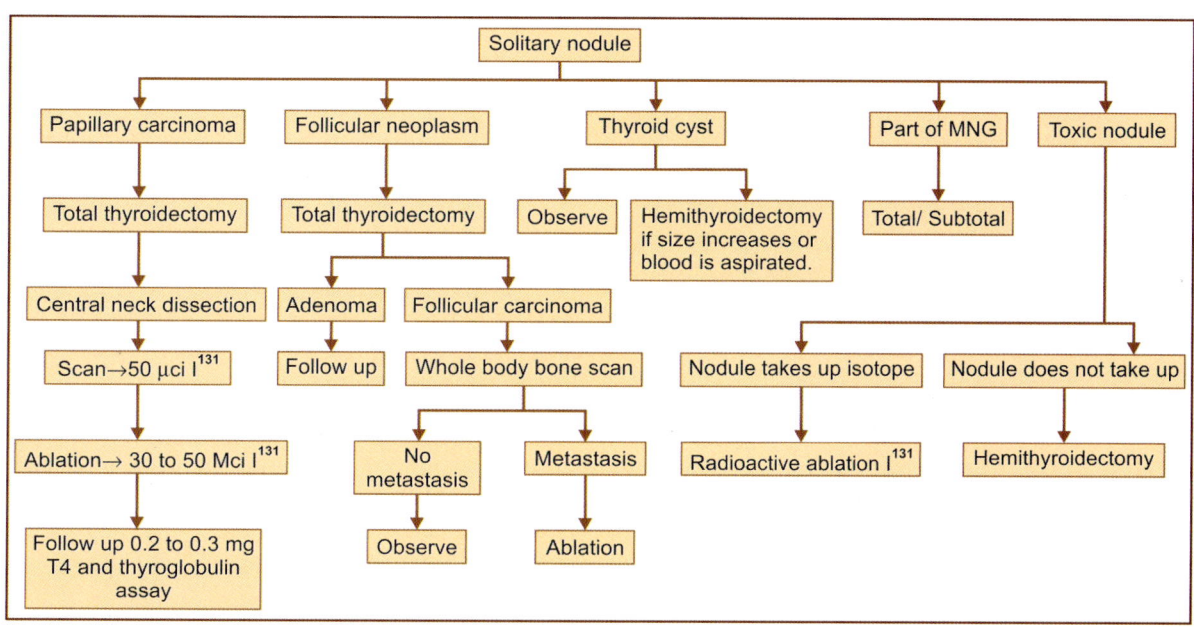

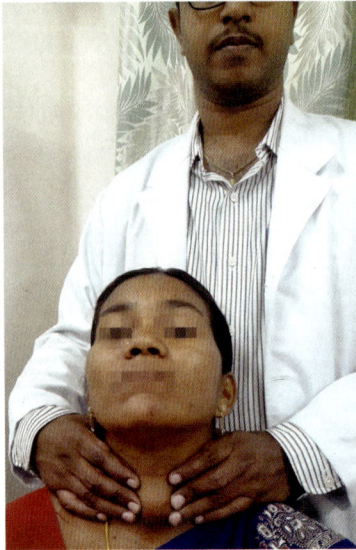

Fig. 19.39: Solitary nodule thyroid gland—FNAC proved to be adenoma (*Courtesy:* Dr Shiva Kumar, PG student, Dr GV Prakash, Dr K Manohar, Professors of Surgery, SVMC, Tirupati)

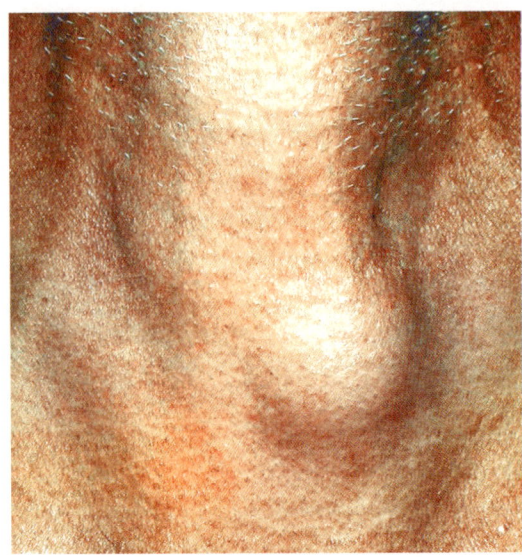

Fig. 19.40: Male patient with a solid solitary nodule. FNAC proved to be papillary carcinoma

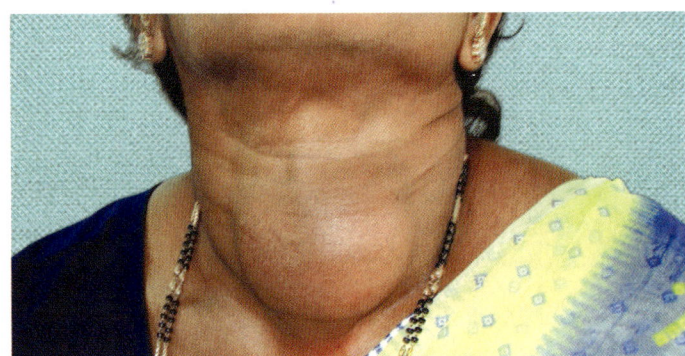

Fig. 19.41: A lady with solitary nodule. It turned out to be thyroid cyst

thyroid is not palpable. Such situation is described as *dominant nodule*. Rest of the nodules are in the process of developing. About 50% of solitary nodules turn out to be multinodular goitre after utrasonography tests.

B. *Adenoma (Fig. 19.39)*: Here whole of one lobe is enlarged with or without isthmus. Opposite lobe is not enlarged.

C. *Carcinoma thyroid*: Papillary carcinoma or follicular carcinoma (common varieties) can present as solitary nodule. Details later (Fig. 19.40).

D. *Thyroid cysts*: These are degenerative cysts which can present as tense (may feel firm or even hard for clinical examination) solitary nodule (Fig. 19.41).

E. *Toxic autonomous nodule*: Usually nodule is firm with features of toxicity. They are autonomous nodules.

> **Please note**: Students are requested to give a diagnosis of solitary nodule. When asked what are the other possibilities, then only give an appropriate answer. *Refer to Clinical Box 19.8* also.

Clinical Box 19.8 🔑

Commonly asked questions about solitary nodule thyroid in clinics

- It is the most common surgical disease of the thyroid gland.
- 15–30% patients of SN have nodule on the other side.
- Solitary solid swelling in a male—risk of malignancy is 48% but it is 12% in females.
- Solitary cystic: Risk of malignancy in males is 24% but in females it is 6%.
- In general, incidence of malignancy is 8–10%.
- Ultrasonography followed by FNAC is the first-line of investigations.
- Which solitary nodule has high risk: Male, solid, solitary nodule.
- About 2 to 3% of solitary nodules are associated with hyperthyroidism.
- Chances of malignancy in a hyperthyroid nodule are very low.

---

7. Primary thyrotoxicosis—Graves' disease

- Symptoms, signs and swelling appear simultaneously.
- Primary thyrotoxicosis is 8 times more common in females than in males, especially in the age group of 15–25 years.
- Very often, young women present with unexplained loss of weight in spite of good appetite. Diarrhoea occurs due to increased smooth muscle activity of small intestines. Intolerance to heat, preference to cold, insomnia, fine tremors, excitability, hyperkinetic movements, and excessive sweating are the other features. *Free steroid hormone levels decrease in Graves' disease. This results in decreased effective oestrogen at the cellular level which in turn causes* **oligomenorrhoea.**

Clinical Wisdom

- It is generally said that one eye sign is mandatory for the diagnosis of primary thyrotoxicosis. In ophthalmoplegia, muscles most often affected are superior rectus and inferior oblique muscles. Hence, upward and outward movement becomes difficult.
- Oligomenorrhoea is seen in primary thyrotoxicosis.
- Menorrhagia is seen in hypothyroidism.

Signs of thyroid gland in Graves' disease
- Uniformly enlarged (mild degree)
- Smooth surface—no nodules (treated cases may have nodularity)
- Gland is soft or firm in consistency
- It is warm and vascular
- Auscultation—a bruit may be heard

- Thyroid gland is uniformly enlarged, without nodularity (Clinical Box 19.9). Tachycardia, tremors, and **exophthalmos** will clinch the diagnosis. Thyrotoxic dermopathy and myopathy, if present, will add onto the diagnosis because they never occur in secondary thyrotoxicosis.

8. **Secondary thyrotoxicosis—toxicosis in a multinodular goitre—Plummer's disease**
   - Swelling appears first and symptoms and signs appear many years later.
   - Patients present with swelling of a few years duration and palpitation of a few months duration. Late cases present with dyspnoea on exertion, pedal oedema, breathlessness suggestive of cardiac failure.
   - The pulse rate is always raised and rapid indicating tachycardia. Depending upon the pulse rate, thyrotoxicosis can be classified as follows: Mild—90–100/minute, moderate—100–110/minute, severe—more than 110/minute (Fig. 19.42).
   - Typically, the gland is firm and nodular, with round borders. Both lobes are enlarged.
   - Eye signs and tremors are extremely rare *(refer to Table 19.1).*

9. **Carcinoma thyroid**: Students can give a clinical diagnosis of carcinoma thyroid, if following features are present.
   - *Hoarseness:* Suggests recurrent laryngeal nerve paralysis which almost always occur in malignant thyroid, not in benign thyroid disorders.
   - *Short duration, rapid growth*—usually anaplastic carcinoma thyroid (Fig. 19.43).

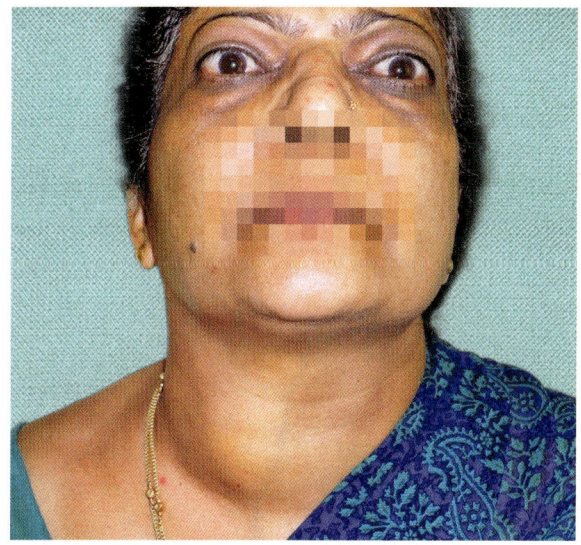

Fig. 19.42: Secondary thyrotoxicosis. Upper sclera is visible. Lid retraction and exophthalmos may also be seen

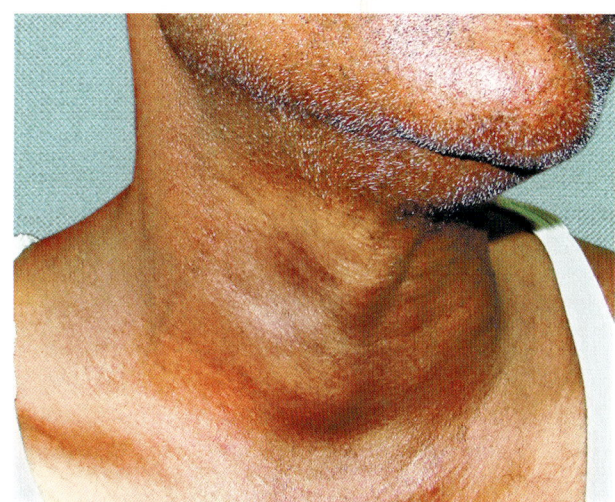

Fig. 19.43: Hard fixed nodule. FNAC proved anaplastic carcinoma thyroid

Table 19.1: Clinical differences between primary thyrotoxicosis and secondary thyrotoxicosis

		Primary thyrotoxicosis	*Secondary thyrotoxicosis*
1.	Age	Young 15 to 30	30 to 40
2.	Symptoms	CNS symptoms—nervousness, sweating, weight loss, prominent eyes	Palpitation
3.	Duration	Short duration of goitre and symptoms	Long duration of goitre and symptoms
4.	Examination of gland	Smooth surface, round borders, soft/firm consistency, bruit may be present	Nodular round firm/hard no bruit
5.	Eye signs	Very predominant lid lag, exophthalmos convergence signs +	Eye signs are not common. Lid retraction may be found
6.	Pretibial myxoedema	May be seen	Never seen
7.	Proximal myopathy	May be seen	Never seen
8.	Progressive exophthalmos	May be seen	Never seen

- *Hard and irregular glands*—anaplastic or other varieties.
- *Restricted mobility due to local infiltration*—Kocher's test may be positive.
- *Lymph nodes* in the lower deep cervical region are involved and thyroid may be palpable (papillary carcinoma). When thyroid gland is not palpable, it is called occult (hidden). However, papillary carcinoma less than 1.5 cm in diameter is also called 'occult' (Fig. 19.44).
- *Berry's sign*: Infiltration of carotid sheath results in absent common carotid artery pulsations. This is described as 'Berry sign positive'. Superficial temporal artery pulsations will be palpable in such cases. It indicates no luminal obstruction but artery is engulfed.
- *Metastasis in the flat bones (skull bones)*: It will be a follicular carcinoma thyroid.
- *Thyroid swelling with mucocutaneous neuromas*: It will be medullary carcinoma of the thyroid (Fig. 19.45).

  Please note: Once you give a diagnosis of carcinoma thyroid, when asked for the type, say papillary or follicular carcinoma thyroid (*see below*).

A. **Papillary carcinoma thyroid:** It is the most common type of carcinoma thyroid (60%). It is common between age group of 20 and 30 years—10 years younger than follicular type. It can present as solitary nodule which is hard or often firm, or can present as nodule with lymph node enlargement, lymph nodes alone without enlargement of thyroid gland (**occult primary site**). Interestingly lymph nodes **need not be hard.** Often they are firm (usually, in malignancies, lymph nodes are hard.) Occasionally, lymph node metastasis presents as **cystic swelling** in the lower neck of many years duration (Figs 19.46 to 19.48).

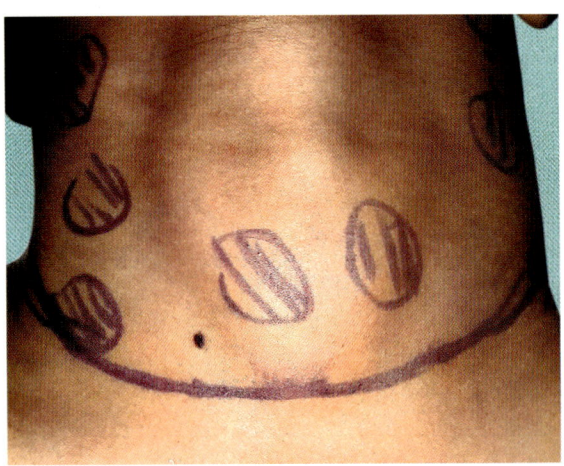

Fig. 19.44: Large jugular chain of lymph nodes from papillary carcinoma thyroid

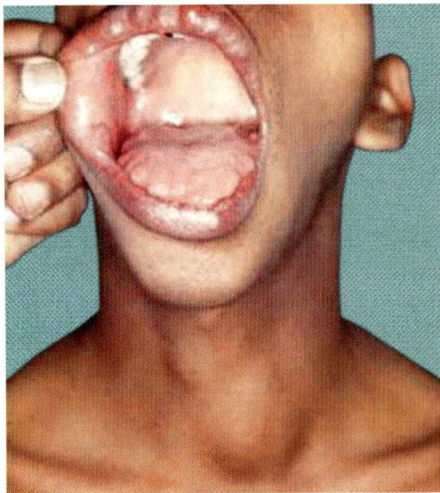

Fig. 19.45: Medullary carcinoma thyroid. See the thyroid swelling and mucocutaneous neuromas. It is a classical example of "what the mind does not know, the eyes cannot see"

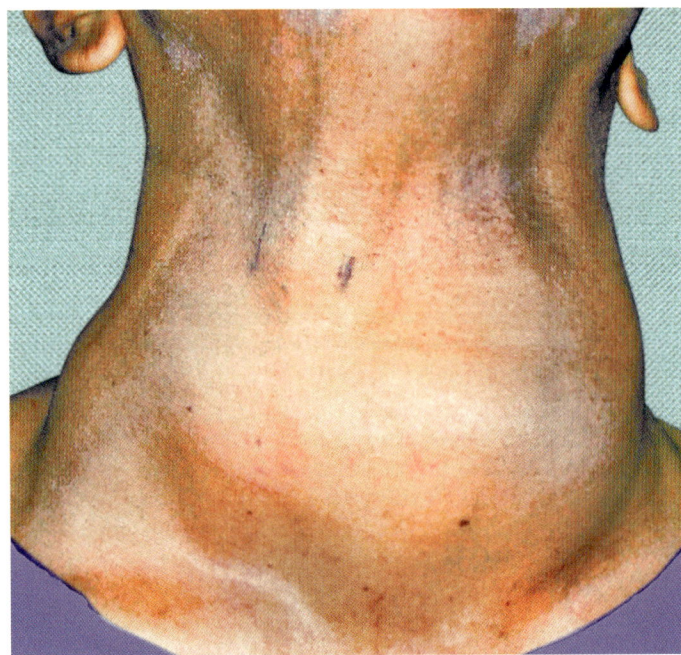

Fig. 19.46: Papillary carcinoma with follicular variant with lymph nodes on the right side

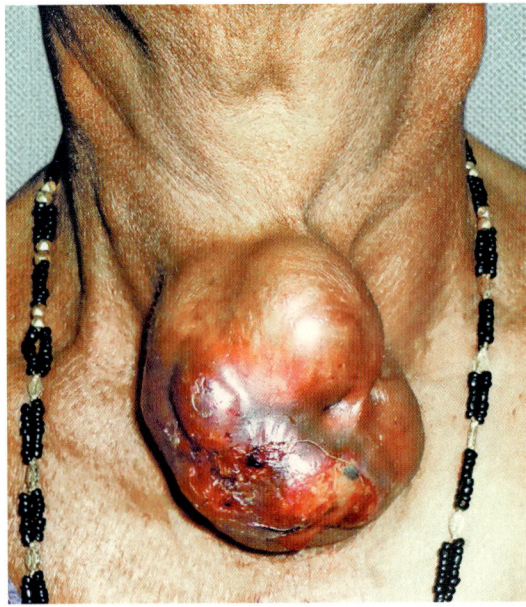

Fig. 19.47: Papillary carcinoma thyroid in elderly patient. A classical example of rapid growth in an elderly patient

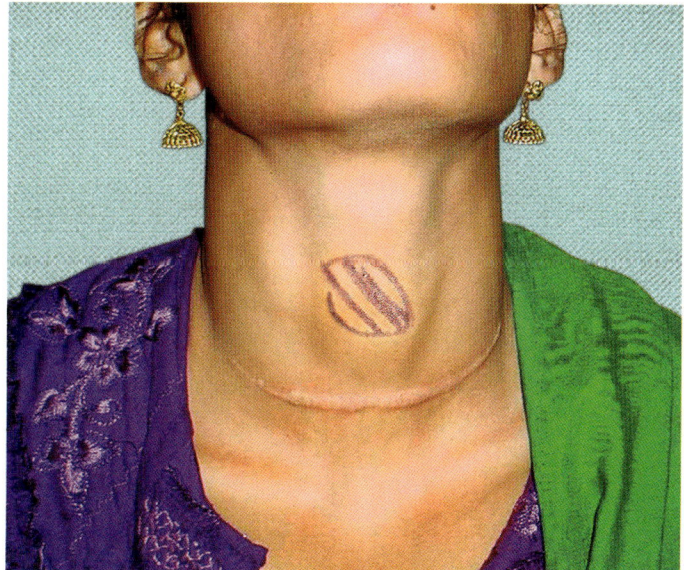

Fig. 19.48: Papillary carcinoma thyroid. Patient presented to the hospital one year later with 2 cm level III lymph node

B. **Follicular carcinoma thyroid:** It is the second common malignancy of the thyroid gland. It is four times more common in females and around 40 years of age. Multinodular goitre more often changes into follicular carcinoma than papillary carcinoma thyroid gland.

- It can also present as solitary nodule. In such cases, clinical diagnosis is solitary nodule—we cannot firmly say it is follicular carcinoma thyroid.

- However, the presentation is a long-standing multinodular goitre. There is a recent history of rapid growth and the gland feels more hard. In this situation also, one can only suspect follicular carcinoma but you cannot be sure.

- The only clinical situation wherein a follicular carcinoma can be considered as the diagnosis is when a patient with a thyroid swelling presents with metastasis in the bone in the form of bony swelling. Commonly, secondaries develop in the flat bones such as skull, ribs, sternum, vertebral column because the flat bones retain red marrow for a longer time. **When bony swelling is obvious and thyroid is not palpable clinically, it is called occult primary.**

Clinical Wisdom

In carcinoma breast with bony metastasis, bony pain (backache) is more common. In follicular carcinoma thyroid, bony swelling—scalp or flat bone is common.

Easy way to remember the spread of follicular carcinoma thyroid: **FBS**

Follicular carcinoma—**B**lood **S**pread
Follicular carcinoma—**B**one **S**pread
Flat **B**one **S**pread

C. **Anaplastic carcinoma thyroid:** This is an uncommon cancer of the thyroid which occurs in elderly patients, above the age of 60 years. This type of tumour presents with dull ache in the swelling and hoarseness of voice. On examination, swelling is hard and irregular with diffuse borders. Because of fixity to trachea and to other structures (pre-vertebral fascia), the gland does not move with deglutition clinching the diagnosis. Prognosis of this tumour is very bad as patients succumb to the disease within a year.

D. **Medullary carcinoma thyroid:** Familial cases present in younger age group with solitary nodule. Diarrhoea which can be present in about 30% cases with mucocutaneous neuromas, high arch palate, if present, will clinch the diagnosis. Sporadic cases present in elderly age group.

Total thyroidectomy and modified radical neck dissection is the treatment. It does not depend on TSH.

- Table 19.2 shows summary of the malignant tumours of thyroid gland.

10. **Lymphoma of the thyroid:** Students should be careful before you make a diagnosis of lymphoma because it is the least common type of malignancy of the thyroid gland. It almost mimics another malignancy such as follicular variety or papillary variety. Definite history of previous thyroid swelling diagnosed as Hashimoto's thyroiditis, palpable lymph nodes in the neck, elderly age group may suggest the diagnosis but it should be given as a second diagnosis, not as first diagnosis.

- Lymphoma of the thyroid may be primary variety or as a part of generalised disease of *non-Hodgkin's lymphoma*.

- Primary lymphoma is an uncommon malignancy of the thyroid, constitutes 5% of all thyroid malignancies and occurs in less than 1% of all non-Hodgkin's lymphomas. Primary thyroid lymphomas occur most commonly in elderly women and are commonly of B cell origin.

- The other subtype is mucosa-associated lymphoid tissue (MALT) lymphomas comprising of approximately 6% to 27% of thyroid lymphomas. These have a relatively indolent course.

11. **Thyroiditis:** These are important to treating physicians and surgeons, not to undergraduate students. Do not offer this diagnosis at the first instance unless asked for. A few types are given below.

- *Hashimoto's thyroiditis:* Typically, she is a perimenopausal woman in the age group of 45–55 years who complains of swelling of the thyroid of a few months duration. On examination, a lobe or the entire gland is enlarged, is usually firm or soft. A few areas may be hard mimicking malignancy. The surface can be smooth or nodular. Initially hyperthyroidism followed by permanent hypothyroidism will occur. Pressure symptoms, such as dysphagia and breathlessness, are common. Being an autoimmune disease, other autoimmune diseases such as rheumatoid arthritis, purpura, sialadenitis, etc. may be present.

- *Subacute thyroiditis—de Quervain's thyroiditis:* Typically, the history is sore throat followed by pain in the gland and fever. Thyroid gland is enlarged, tender on palpation and consistency can be soft to firm. History is short and regression is spontaneous.

- *Riedel's thyroiditis:* Here gland is enlarged and it is hard and irregular. Usually diagnosis of anaplastic carcinoma thyroid is made. This condition is rare.

Table 19.2: Summary of the malignant tumours of thyroid gland

		Papillary	Follicular	Anaplastic	Medullary
1.	Aetiology	Irradiation	Endemic goitre	Unknown	Sporadic or familial
2.	Incidence	60%	17%	13%	6%
3.	Age (years)	20–40	30–50	50 and above	Middle age
4.	Diagnosis	Thyroid swelling with lymph nodes metastasis	Thyroid swelling with bony metastasis	Thyroid swelling, local fixity, stridor	Difficult to diagnose clinically
5.	Microscopy	Orphan Annie eye nuclei, psammoma bodies	Angioinvasion, capsular invasion	Poorly differentiated cells	Amyloid stroma-like carcinoid
6.	Spread	Lymphatic	Blood	Local infiltration	Lymphatic, blood
7.	Investigation	FNAC	Frozen section (±)	FNAC, incision biopsy	FNAC, calcitonin
8.	Treatment of the primary	Total thyroidectomy	Total thyroidectomy	Isthmusectomy, external RT	Total thyroidectomy
9.	Treatment of metastasis	Functional neck dissection	Radioiodine ablation	Palliative external radiotherapy	Radical neck dissection
10.	TSH dependence	Yes	Yes	No	No
11.	Hormone production	Very rare	Very rare	No	Calcitonin, 5-HT, ACTH
12.	Prognosis	Excellent	Good	Worst	Bad

Clinical Wisdom

Perimenopausal thyroiditis is Hashimoto's, hard thyroiditis is Riedel's and tender thyroiditis is de Quervain.

Clinical Case Capsules

1. A 24-year-old lady was diagnosed to have left submandibular sialoadenitis. At exploration, submandibular gland was normal. Excised specimen revealed that it is a case of papillary carcinoma arising from thyroglossal duct tract. Ectopic thyroid tissue is also a differential diagnosis (Fig. 19.49).

2. A 20-year-old girl complains of difficulty in swallowing of 1 year duration. On examination, 5 cm, reddish firm swelling is palpable in the middle of the tongue at the junction of anterior two-thirds and posterior one-third. It is the classical location of lingual thyroid. Rule out other swellings of the tongue—haemangioma, carcinoma (gumma is rare nowadays) (Fig. 19.50).

3. This patient had undergone hemithyroidectomy in a peripheral hospital 15 years back. He did not receive any medication in these years. He presented with ulcerated nodules on the right side of the neck (lymph nodal mass). He successfully underwent completion thyroidectomy with functional neck dissection on the right side. Also observe sebaceous cyst on the right side of the chest wall (Fig. 19.51).

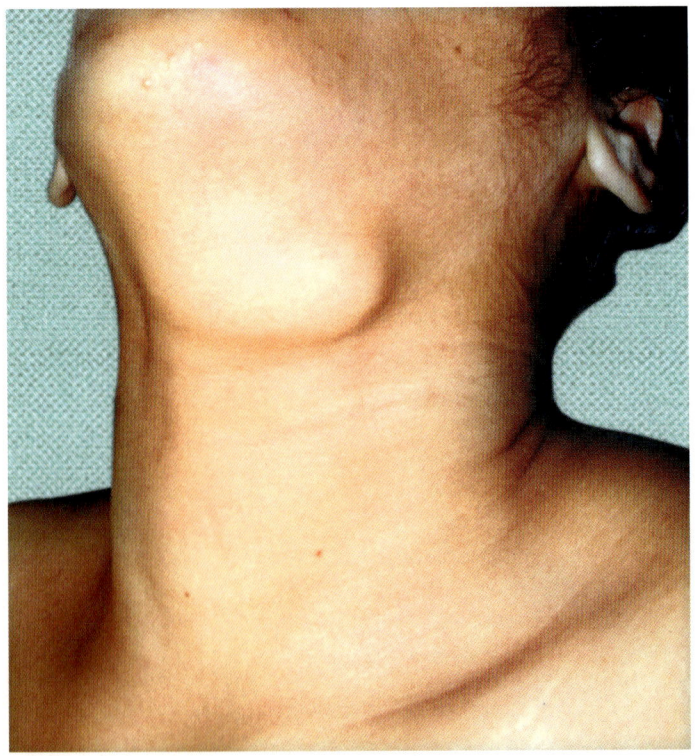

Fig. 19.49: Papillary carcinoma thyroid arising from ectopic thyroglossal duct tract

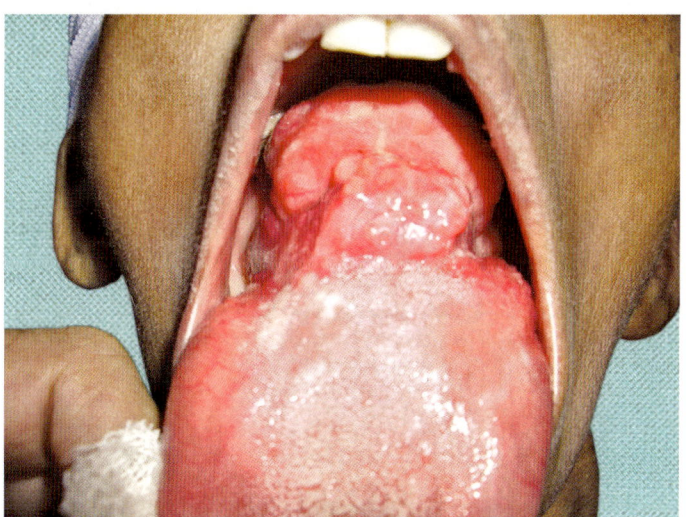

Fig. 19.50: Lingual thyroid

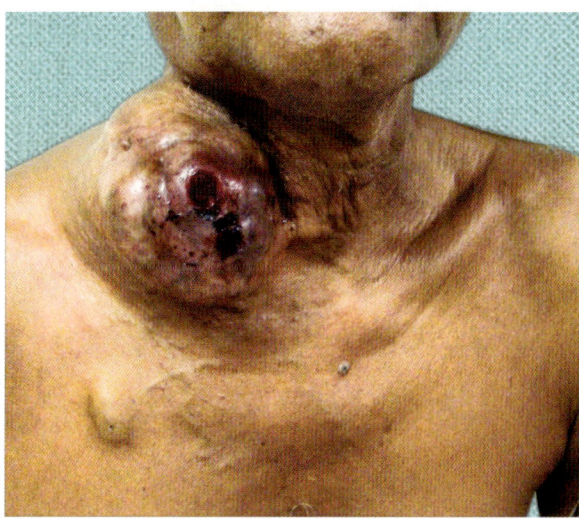

Fig. 19.51: Advanced papillary carcinoma thyroid with fungation—uncommon presentation (also observe two sebaceous cysts)

20

Examination of the Breast

INTRODUCTION

Carcinoma breast and other benign lumps in the breast are common clinical problems encountered in the clinical practice. It is important to conduct a proper clinical examination to arrive at the right diagnosis. They are very important clinical cases in the university examinations also. Hence, detailed evaluation and examination methods have been discussed in this chapter. *Every lump in the breast should be considered as malignant unless proven otherwise.* But equally important are many other benign lumps not only from practice point of view but also from examination point of view.

PATIENT DATA

- Patient's details such as name, age, place, occupation, admitting complaints, etc. are noted.

- Carcinoma breast is common after 40 years of age and is more common there afterwards. Fibroadenoma is common between the age group of 20 and 40 years. Cyclical mastalgia (fibroadenosis) is also common in the same age group—reproductive age group.

- Carcinoma breast is very common in Western world more in Whites, and very rare in Japan and Taiwan.

HISTORY OF PRESENT ILLNESS

1. *Lump:* Common complaint of these patients is palpable lump for which they come to the hospital. Common questions to be asked are: Where is the lump? When did you notice the lump? What is the duration of the lump? Is there any pain? Did you have any trauma? How is the progress? Is it growing rapidly or has it become smaller? *Lump in the breast is the most common presentation of carcinoma breast.* In many cases, the patient points to the site of the lump—commonest site being upper and outer quadrant because breast tissue is more in that quadrant (Fig. 20.1). Carcinomatous lumps begin as painless lumps and grow to about 5 cm size by 2–3 months. Rapid growth indicates mastitis carcinomatosa (Fig. 20.2). Has the lump regressed any time? This history, if present, suggests inflammatory lesion such as bacterial mastitis which responds to antibiotics. Trauma to the breast is not common. In a few cases, trauma may result in a lump which may be hard mimicking carcinoma breast. It is called traumatic fat necrosis. Phyllodes tumour grows very fast—more than malignant tumours.

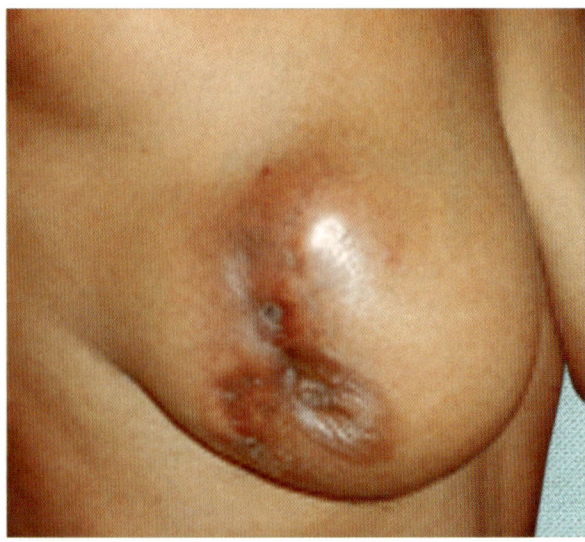

Fig. 20.1: Scirrhous carcinoma—with nipple retraction

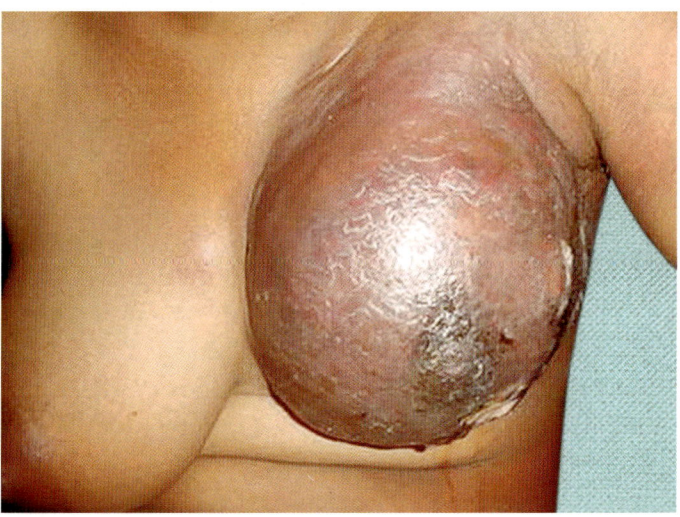

Fig. 20.2: Inflammatory carcinoma—stage T4D—rapidly growing tumour—mastitis carcinomatosa

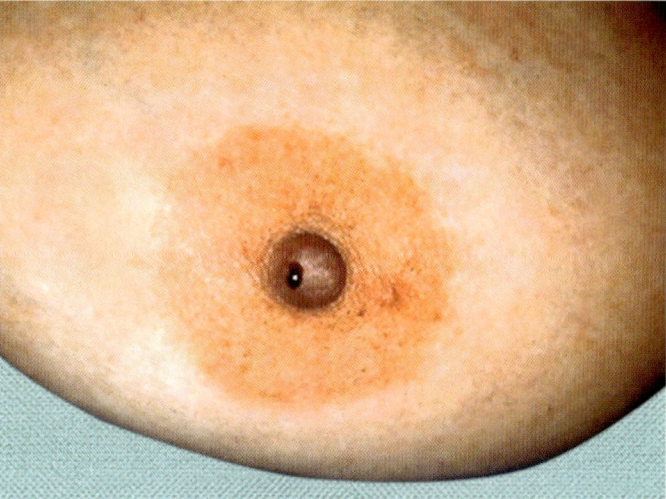

Fig. 20.3: Bleeding nipple

If growth is much more rapid it is not carcinoma but a benign condition—that is phyllodes tumour typically occur in young patients.

2. *Pain*: **Do you have pain in the breast or in the lump? Pain in the breast is known as mastalgia.** Malignant breast lesions are painless to start with. When a patient presents with pain as the leading complaint, it is most likely cyclical mastalgia (fibroadenosis). Pain, fever and lump suggest mastitis and throbbing pain, if present, is a case of breast abscess. Bilateral pain suggests more of benign lesion such as fibroadenosis than mastitis.

- Cyclical mastalgia is uncommon after menopause. Hence, in such patients, pain may be due to periductal mastitis.
- Causes of non-cyclical mastalgia are periductal mastitis, bacterial mastitis, pain from musculo-skeletal structures and advanced cases of carcinoma breast.
- Pain in carcinoma breast can be due to rapidly grow-ing neoplasms such as mastitis carcinomatosa, skin infiltration, nerve infiltration and chest wall infiltration, mainly rib (bony pain).
- Pain/discomfort in *male breast* is due to gynaeco-mastia (male breast enlargement). Often it is tenderness.

3. *Discharge from nipple*: **Did you notice any discharge per nipple?**

- Blood-stained discharge is seen in papilloma (benign condition) and ductal carcinoma (Fig. 20.3).

- Serous or greenish discharge is seen in cyclical mastalgia. Shedding of epithelial cells may result in slight green-coloured fluid.
- Purulent discharge is seen in breast abscess or in periductal mastitis with secondary infection (Fig. 20.4).
- Milky discharge is seen in galactocoele (milk retention during lactation).
- Watery discharge is not pathological but gives anxiety to the patient. It is often seen in cases of hyperprolactinaemia.

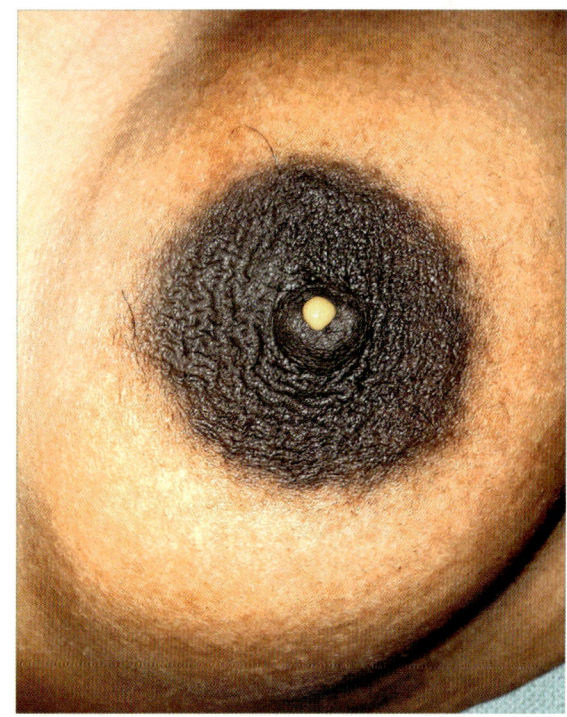

Fig. 20.4: Periductal mastitis with secondary infection

4. *Any change in the nipple*
   - *Recent indrawing of nipple*—retraction is one of the features of carcinoma breast. Very early retraction of nipple and missing nipple is found in Paget's disease of the nipple. (It is a misnomer. It is not a disease of the nipple but intraductal carcinoma close to the nipple–areola complex.)
   - **Remote retraction is due to chronic mastitis or congenital** (Clinical Box 20.1).
   - Slit-like retraction is seen in duct ectasia, periductal mastitis.
   - Ulceration of the nipple, eczema, and discharge may be the complaints in a few other cases.

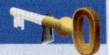

Clinical Box 20.1

Causes of retraction of the nipple—4 Cs
- **C**arcinoma of the breast
- **C**hronic mastitis
- **C**ongenital
- **C**hronic disease—tuberculosis

5. *Have you noticed any lump in the armpit or in the neck?*
   - Lumps in the axilla are due to lymph node metastasis. Lumps in the neck are due to supraclavicular lymph node metastasis.
   - Axillary tail hypertrophy, and lipoma are other swellings in the axilla.

6. *Do you have recent onset bony pains*? Majority of women over 40 years may complain of bony pains due to some form of work they do. Specific question of low backache should be enquired about (Clinical Box 20.2).

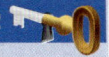

Clinical Box 20.2

Bone metastasis
- Bone metastasis is much more common than primary bone cancers.
- Primary tumours that most often lead to bone metastasis are in the order of incidence: Prostate, breast, kidney, lung, and thyroid cancers.
- Breast cancer is the most common malignant tumour and the main cause of bone metastasis in women.
- Metastasis is usually osteolytic but can also be osteoblastic (mixed).
- Vertebral body is involved before the pedicles but destruction of the pedicles is the most common finding on plain films.
- Cervical spine is the least affected by metastasis from carcinoma breast.

- Bony pains specially backache is a manifestation of carcinoma breast with vertebral metastasis. In order of preference, **Lumbar vertebrae, Femur and Thoracic vertebrae are involved. (You can remember as LFT.)**
- Bone metastasis occurs in a similar fashion. Posterior intercostal veins join paravertebral plexus of vein (Batson's venous plexus). Thus, thoracolumbar vertebrae, femur, and pelvic bones are affected.

7. *Breathlessness*: Carefully watch for difficulty in breathing. Look at the alae nasi or look at accessory muscles. Pleural effusion can cause breathing difficulty.

> Pleural effusion is more common than lung metastasis in carcinoma breast. Explanation given is—cancer spreads from internal mammary nodes by lymphatic communications. Thus, ipsilateral mediastinal nodes and ipsilateral pleural disease resulting in effusion occur. Once cancer cells block the lymphatics, effusion develops.

8. *Loss of weight and loss of appetite*: Interestingly, these two symptoms are not common. However, with advanced fungating lesions, loss of appetite can occur. Loss of weight is a feature with metastasis in the liver.

9. *Do you have any other complaints?* Advanced cases may complain of headache (cerebral metastasis) or abdominal distension due to hepatomegaly or ovarian metastasis.

   (While presenting the case, students often mention that the patient does not have convulsions or jaundice, symptoms that suggest metastasis in the brain or liver. Mention these symptoms only when present.)

Clinical Wisdom

Abdominal distension in a case of carcinoma breast is due to hepatomegaly or ovarian metastasis. In cases of carcinoma stomach, distension is due to ascites and in rectosigmoid strictures, distension is due to intestinal obstruction.

10. If patient has accessory breasts or nipples, patient may show you. Make a note of it.

Past History and Treatment History

- Any previous history of breast surgeries should be enquired. Many of them may not be related such as excision of fibroadenoma or cyst, etc. However, it is not uncommon to find a patient who says that lump has been removed and I do not know what it is. It might have been florid epitheliosis or atypical ductal hyperplasia or carcinomatous lump (Clinical Box 20.3).

- Irradiation in childhood—mostly for Hodgkin's lymphoma increases the risk of breast cancer by 15 to 20%.

Personal History

- Early menarche, late menopause, nulliparous—longer will be the cumulative period of menstruation. Hence, more chances of malignancy. Hence, these questions should be asked.

- Any hormone replacement therapy (HRT)—generally given in premenopausal patients who had undergone bilateral oophorectomy. HRT increases the risk of carcinoma breast.

- Diet—Alcohol, red meat, fatty food

Family History

- Did the patient's mother or sister have carcinoma breast? If yes, it increases the relative risk of carcinoma in the patient by 2–4 times.

- About 10 to 15% patients with carcinoma breast do give history of cancer breast in first degree relatives.

- BRCA-1 and BRCA-2 genes are responsible for 5–10% of breast cancers.

Hereditary breast cancer
- Seen more in younger patients (<40 years)
- It is bilateral
- Can also involve other organs. For example, ovarian malignancy. (Hereditary syndrome—breast and ovarian cancer.)
- Autosomal dominant.

GENERAL PHYSICAL EXAMINATION

- Essentially normal in early carcinoma of breast.
- *Pallor*: Suggests advanced malignancy.
- Icterus may suggest extensive liver involvement.
- Bony tenderness in the lower spine suggests bony metastasis.
- Look for palpable left or right supraclavicular node which gives you the initial clue—details can be mentioned later.

Inspection

- Female nurse mandatory.
- Inspection should be done in *three* positions. With patient in sitting position (Fig. 20.5): 1. Hands by the side, 2. hands raised above the head, and 3. bending forwards.
- Inspection should expose the supraclavicular region to both breasts, axilla, arms and abdomen.
- Reasonably good illumination is required.

I. Hands by the Side of the Patient

1. Nipple

- *Asymmetry*: *Level of the nipples*: The nipple may be elevated and retracted because of fibrosis induced by infilteration of growth along the lactiferous duct. One should carefully look at the level of nipple to detect an early case of carcinoma.

- *Bloody discharge* indicates duct carcinoma or duct papilloma.

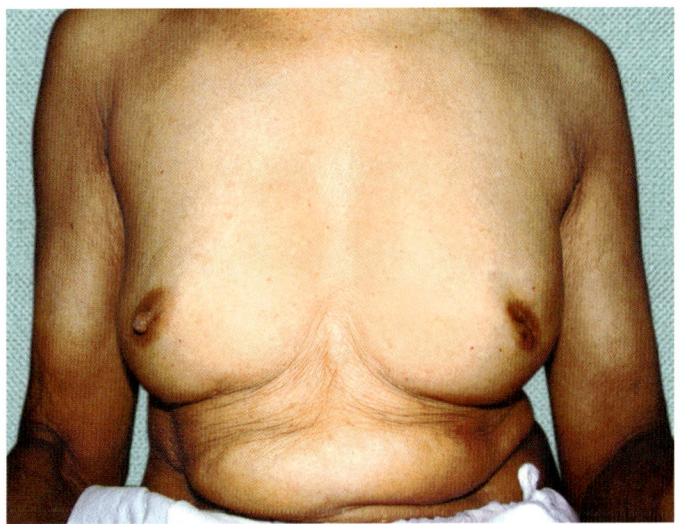

Fig. 20.5: Hands by the side of the patient. Right nipple is elevated compared to the left nipple

- *Centrally (circumferential) retracted nipple*: Circumferential retraction is due to carcinoma. Slit-like retraction is due to duct ectasia or periductal mastitis (Figs 20.6 and 20.7).

- Destruction of the nipple is a feature of Paget's disease of the nipple. Cracks and fissures indicate eczema.

- Elevation of the breast and nipple towards the lesion is due to fibrosis and contraction of the lactiferous duct towards the lesion which classically happens in upper outer quadrant lesions.

- Thus **A**symmetry, **B**leeding nipple, **C**ircumferential retraction, **D**estruction and **E**levation of the nipple are **ABCDE** of nipple changes in carcinoma breast (Fig. 20.8).

2. *Areola*: Presence of *peau d'orange* indicates the tumour infiltrating the areola. It has been compared to the orange skin because of following reasons:

   - The areola becomes thick because of lymphatic obstruction giving rise to lymphoedema.

   - Fixation of hair follicles and sweat glands to the underlying malignancy (Fig. 20.9).

3. *Skin over the breast*: *Puckering or dimpling of skin* is due to thin fibrous bands embedded in the subcutaneous fat. These bands called *ligaments of Cooper* are attached to the skin and are infiltrated by malignancy. Multiple nodules indicate advanced disease (Fig. 20.10).

4. *Lump*: If visible, give details. Typical carcinomatous lump is in the outer quadrant about 4–5 cm in size,

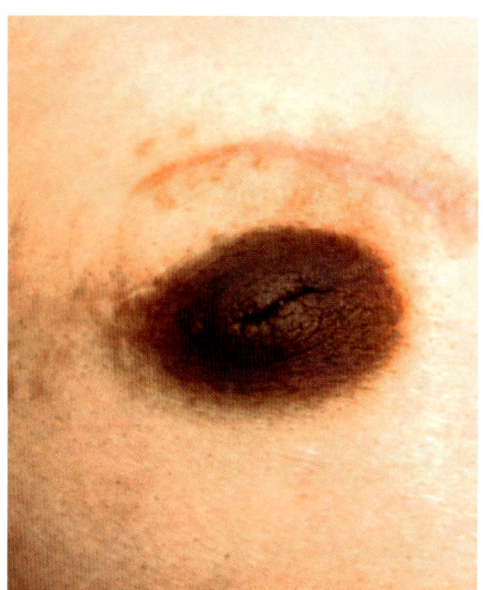

Fig. 20.6: Slit-like retraction

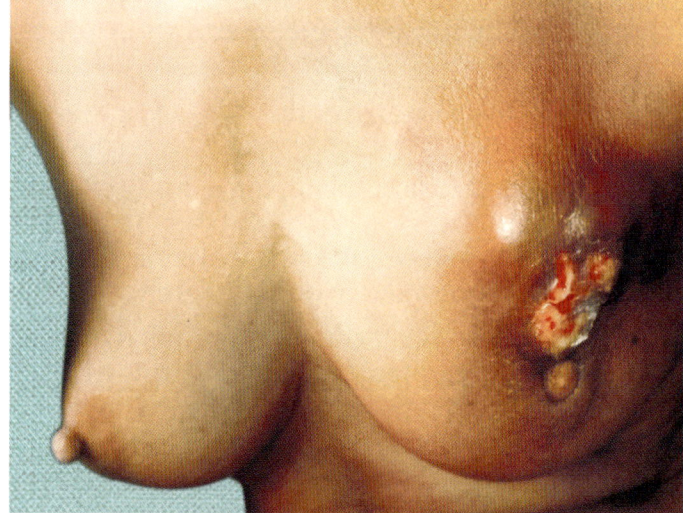

Fig. 20.8: Left nipple is elevated, lump and ulceration are seen (*Courtesy*: Dr Kabali Murthy, Dr Ramesh, Dr Subramanyam, Raja Muttayya Medical College, Chidambaram, Tamil Nadu)

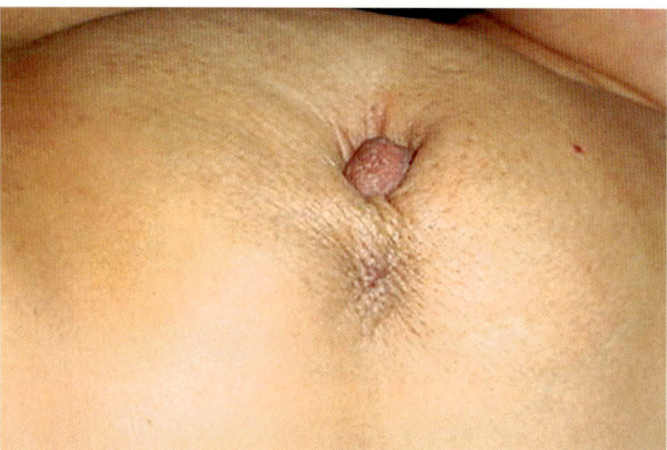

Fig. 20.7: Retraction of the nipple—classical feature of intraductal carcinoma

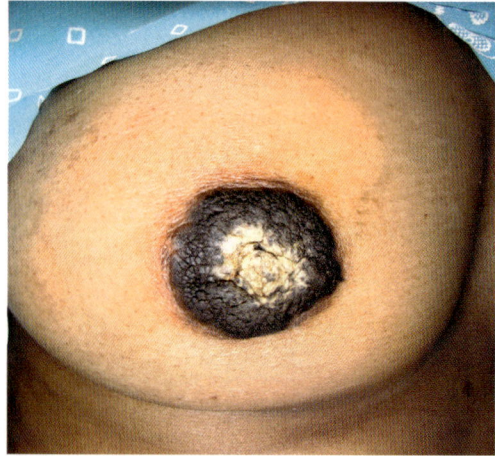

Fig. 20.9: Areola is thickened and nipple is destroyed—Paget's disease of the nipple

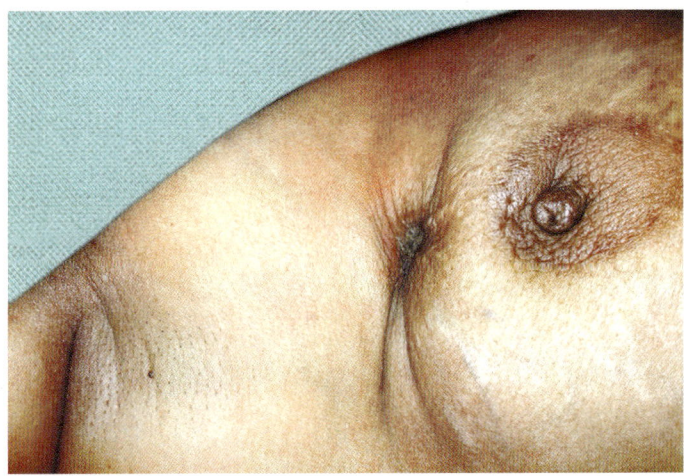

Fig. 20.10: Outer quadrant lump fixed to skin due to infiltration of ligaments of Cooper. (*Courtesy:* Dr Jegan, SR, Dept of Surgery, KMC, Manipal)

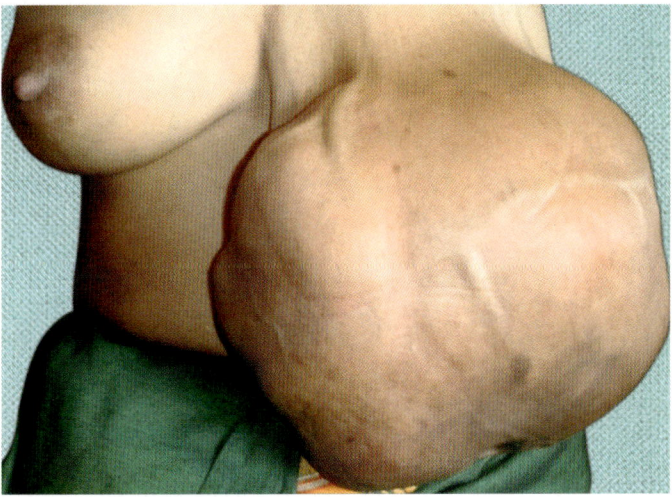

Fig. 20.12: Phyllodes tumour of the left breast in a 50-year-old lady. It was confused for carcinoma breast (*Courtesy:* Prof Srijayan, Prof P Rajan, Calicut Medical College, Calicut)

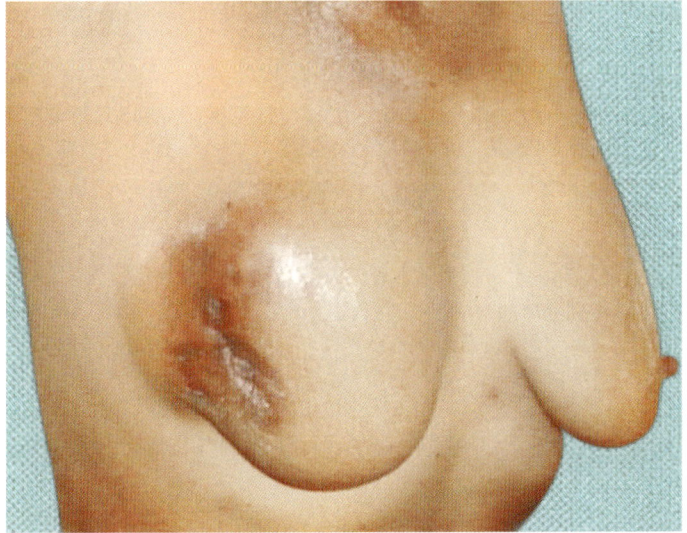

Fig. 20.11: Large lump with skin infiltration, ulceration and bleeding (*Courtesy:* Prof U. Santosh Pai, Ex-Professor of Surgery, KMC, Manipal)

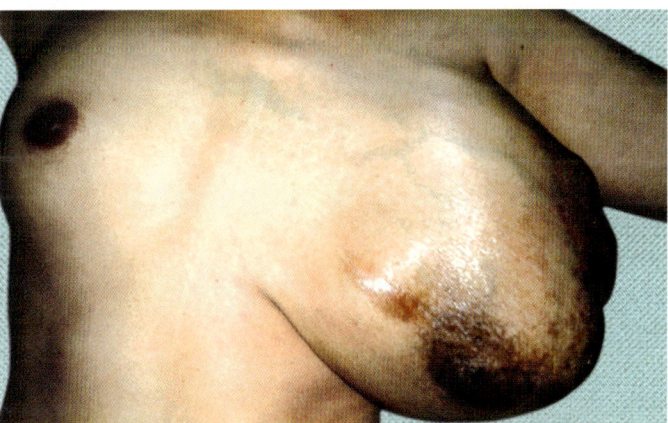

Fig. 20.13: Phyllodes tumour of the left breast

irregular surface with diffuse borders (Fig. 20.11). A few dilated veins may be visible indicating increasing vascularity of the tumour. Large visible lump with nodular surface and visible veins is a typical feature of phyllodes tumour.

5. ***Look at the whole breast:*** Small atrophic breast is seen in scirrhous carcinoma breast. In mastitis carcinomatosa, whole breast is enlarged and engorged (*see* Fig. 20.2) or phyllodes tumour (Figs 20.12 and 20.13).

6. ***Look at the axilla for fullness:*** If present, it suggests enlargement of axillary lymph nodes. Prominent axillary fat is also seen in a few patients (Fig. 20.14).

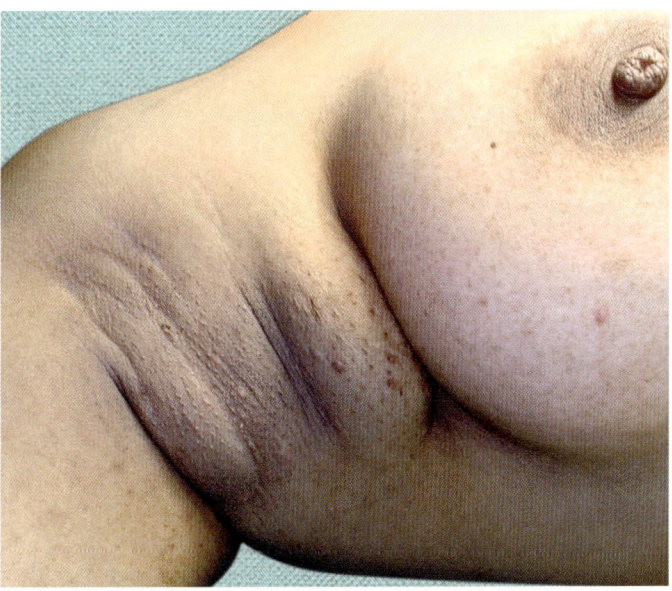

Fig. 20.14: Hypertrophy of axillary fat

7. *Supraclavicular fullness* due to lymph node involvement from carcinoma breast is not common. Significant swelling of supraclavicular region can be due to enlarged lymph nodes as may be seen in testicular tumours, malignant melanoma, carcinoma stomach, and lymphoma.

8. *Oedema* of the arm is due to lymphatic blockage caused by lymph nodes in the axilla.

II. Hands Raised above the Head (Figs 20.15 and 20.16)

• Inferior quadrant of the breast is better seen when the hands are raised above the head. Full view of axilla—for fullness or skin infiltration from the carcinoma tail or fungating lymph nodal mass can be seen.

• Bilateral axillary swellings are often due to axillary tail hypertrophy or lipomas.

• *Peau d'orange* (on elevation of hands) becomes more prominent. (It is best demonstrated by palpation.) By abduction and elevation, skin over the lump is stretched and thus *Peau d'orange* becomes prominent (Fig. 20.17).

III. Bending Forward (Fig. 20.18)

In cases of carcinoma infiltrating the **chest wall**, the breast will not fall forward on bending forwards.

Clinical Wisdom

What is chest wall? Chest wall includes serratus anterior, ribs and intercostal muscles—not pectoralis muscles.

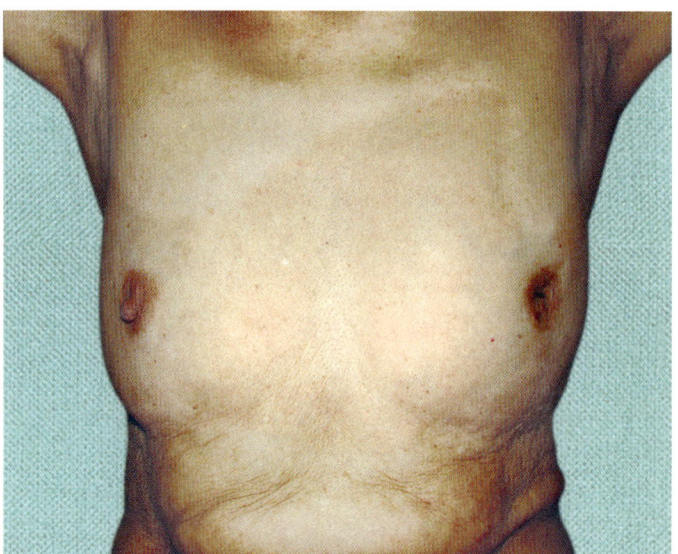

Fig. 20.15: Hands raised above the head

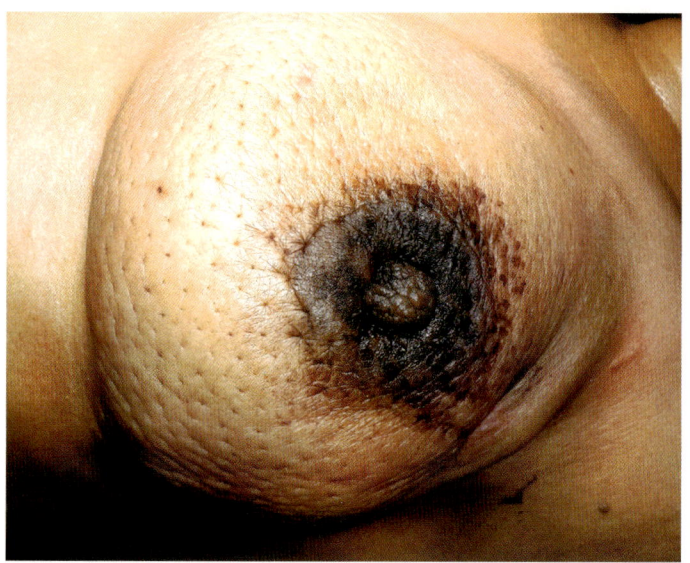

Fig. 20.17: Peau d'orange

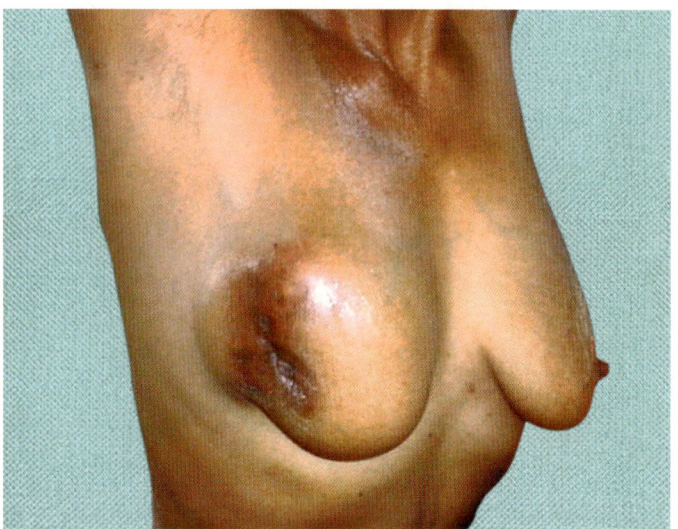

Fig. 20.16: Hands raised above the head, lateral view

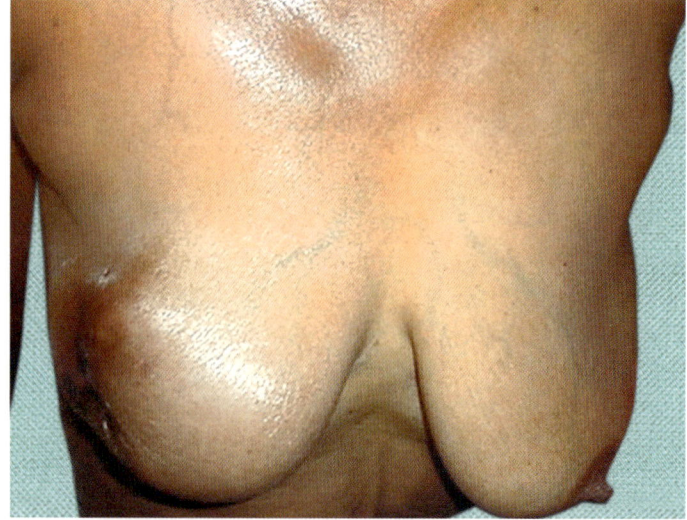

Fig. 20.18: Bending forwards—right breast does not fall forwards

Palpation

- Once inspection is completed, palpation is done in the sitting position, semirecumbent position and recumbent position (Figs 20.19 to 20.21).

- A lump is best palpated with flat of the hand. If a lump is palpable with fingertips, not by flat of the finger, then it is a case of cyclical mastalgia (fibroadenosis), not a case of carcinoma breast.

- Better use the word lump in the breast (not mass in the breasts). Location, extent, size, shape, surface, edges (borders), consistency, mobility, fixity and plane of the lump should be mentioned.

- Of these, mobility, consistency, fixity and plane of the lump are very important.

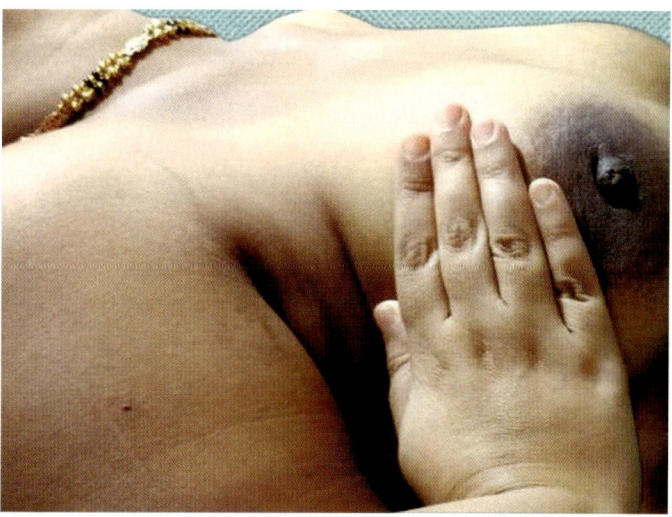

Fig. 20.21: Palpation of various quadrants

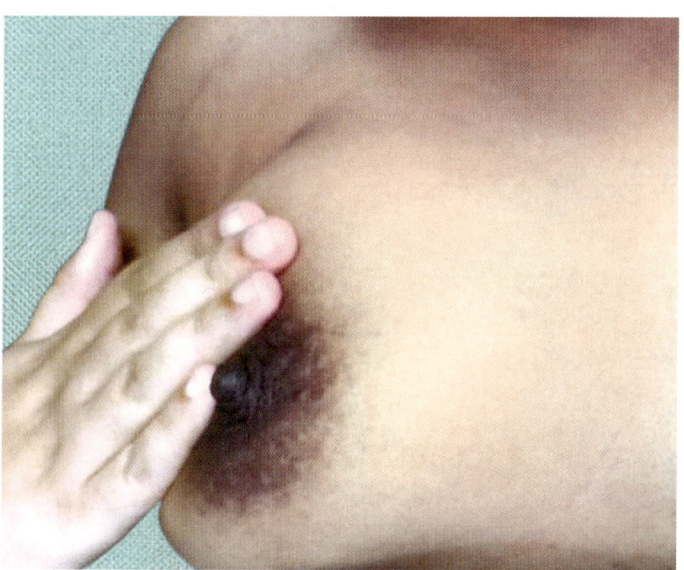

Fig. 20.19: Palpation with flat of the hand, quadrant by quadrant

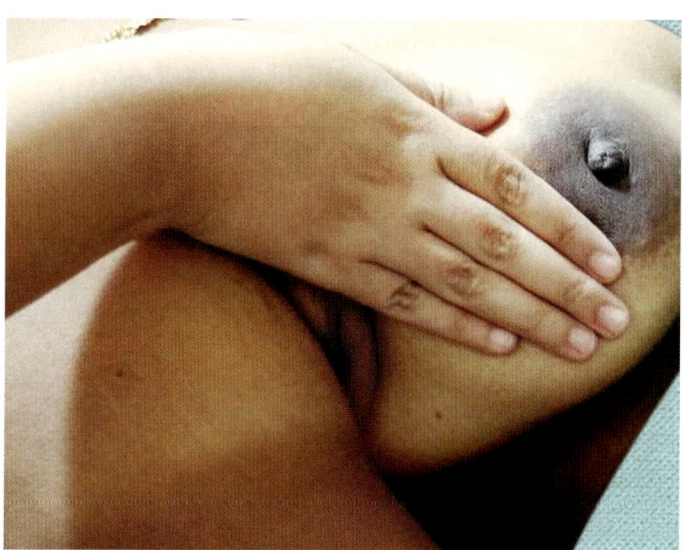

Fig. 20.20: Examination in semirecumbent position

1. *Local rise of temperature and tenderness* **are the features of acute mastitis (with or without breast abscess).** These signs are usually not found in cases of carcinoma of the breast. However, rapidly growing carcinoma and inflammatory carcinomas do exhibit local rise of temperature, redness and tenderness.

2. *Palpation of the nipple and areola complex:* Bloody discharge may reflect duct papilloma.

   - Look for any lump underneath or look at any discharge while pressing the areola.

3. *Describe the lump:* The lump is the commonest presentation of carcinoma of the breast. The upper and outer quadrant is the commonest site of carcinoma of the breast because more breast tissue is present in that quadrant. Typically, malignant lump is nontender, hard and irregular. However, very often carcinoma breast can present as a firm lump. In mastitis carcinomatosa, lump may not be palpable but whole breast will be enlarged. Soft areas may be found due to tumour necrosis (Fig. 20.22).

   - Carcinomatous lumps are single. Fibroadenomas can be multiple and in fibroadenosis, one may feel multiple small lumps.

   - Surface is smooth in fibroadenoma and cysts of the breast. In fibroadenosis, surface feels granular or irregular. Large nodular surface also called bosselated, is typically seen in phyllodes tumour (Figs 20.23 and 20.24).

   - Consistency is typically hard in malignant lumps. However, it should be remembered that tensely cystic swellings and antibiomas may feel

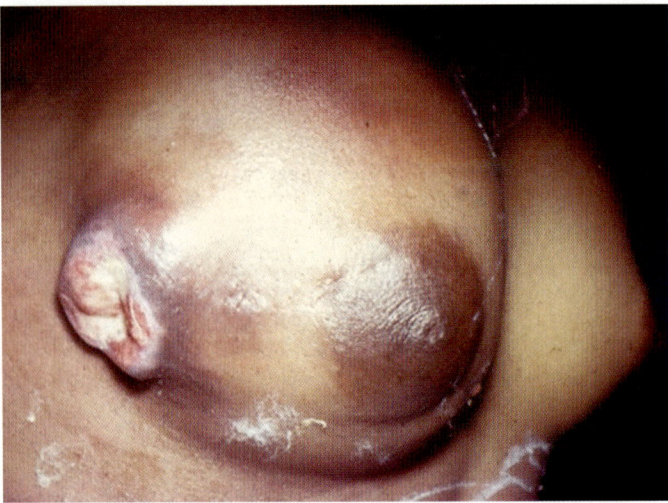

Fig. 20.22: Mastitis carcinomatosa. Whole breast is enlarged, it was diagnosed as breast abscess and incised (blunder)

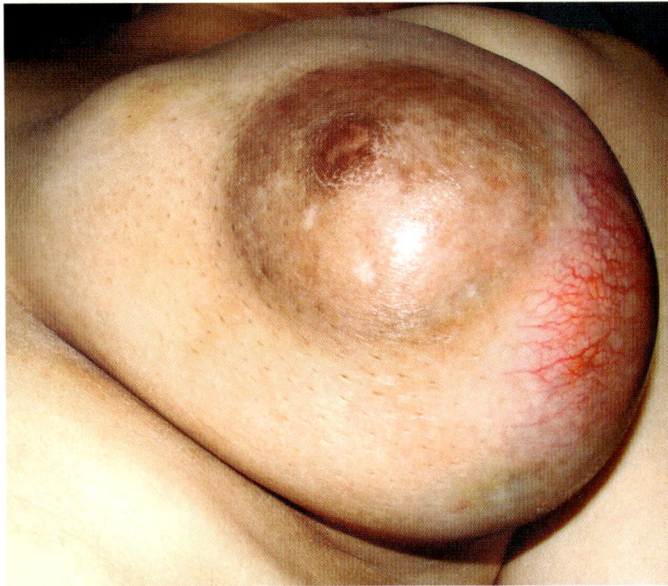

Fig. 20.23: Bosselated surface and dilated veins

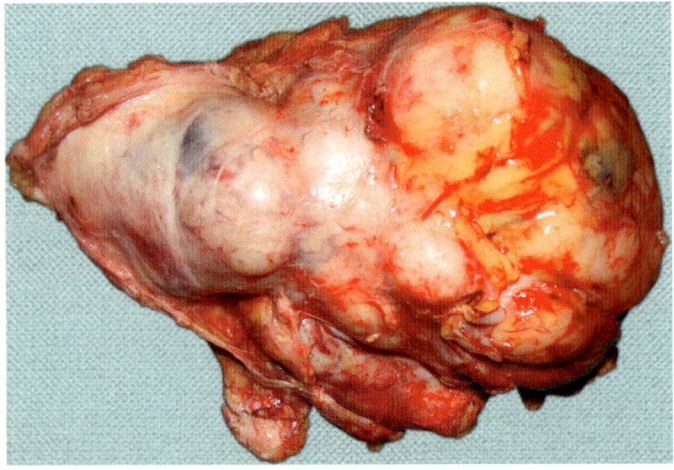

Fig. 20.24: Excised specimen of phyllodes to show the surface

hard. In such situations, other findings, if present, will help in the final diagnosis.

- Lump in gynaecomastia is round, tender with disc-like borders, moves with breast tissues and has smooth surface.
- Rarely sarcoma can occur in the breast. It has variable consistency from soft (due to tumour necrosis), firm to hard, depending on the desmoplastic reaction (better to avoid this diagnosis in clinical cases).

4. *Demonstration of peau d'orange*: When 2 fingers are pressed over the lump and brought together, peau d' orange will be more obvious (Fig. 20.25).

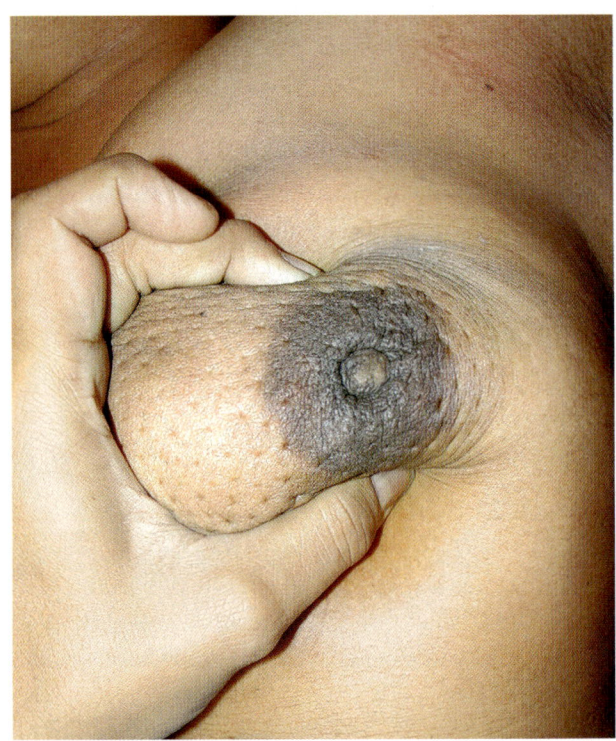

Fig. 20.25: Demonstrating peau d' orange

5. *Intrinsic mobility*: This means to check whether the lump moves or not. Fibroadenoma is a well encapsulated swelling and therefore, moves freely within the breast tissue—called breast mouse. Lumps of carcinoma and fibroadenosis do not have a capsule and hence they move with breast tissue. In advanced cases of carcinoma breast including cancer en cuirasse, lump may not have any mobility due to fixity to chest wall (Figs 20.26 and 20.27).

In phyllodes tumour, intrinsic mobility will be present when the lump is small. However, when the lump is large , the whole breast moves with lump. In periductal mastitis, lump moves with the breast.

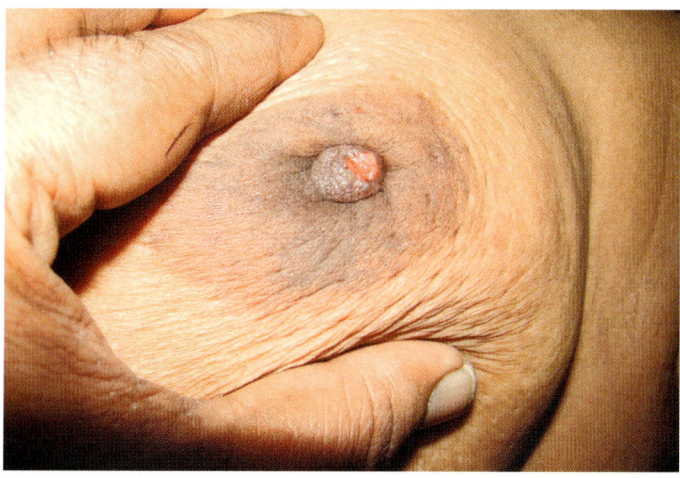

Fig. 20.26: Checking for intrinsic mobility

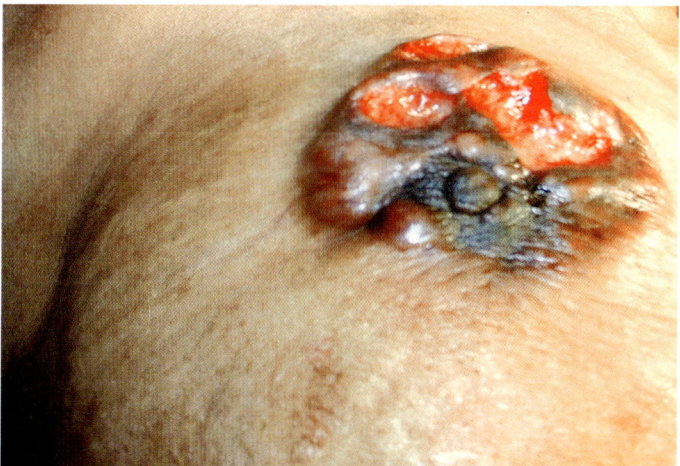

Fig. 20.27: Ulcerated carcinoma breast fixed to the chest wall

Common blunders in surgery

1. Incising testicular tumour through scrotum thinking that it is a epididymo-orchitis or torsion testis.
2. Incising mastitis carcinomatosa thinking that it is a breast abscess.
3. Incising a popliteal aneurysm thinking that it is an abscess.
4. Incising a metastasis of the scalp thinking that it is a lipoma.
5. Incising a swelling around ear lobule thinking it is lymph node (parotid swelling).
6. Excising a parotid swelling thinking it is a lymph node swelling—cause facial nerve palsy.

6. *Plane of the swelling*

- *Lift the skin.* If it is not possible, it indicates the tumour is **fixed** to skin. Try to move the lump. If the lump moves but skin dimpling is found, it means the skin is **tethered** to the lump, but **not fixed** to the lump. Tethering is due to involvement of Cooper's ligaments which are attached to the skin. As you are doing this test, slide the skin over the lump and look for *peau d'orange.*

- *Pectoralis major contraction test:* Ask the patient to keep the hands on the flanks over the iliac bone. Check for mobility of the lump in both directions. Now ask the patient to press against the hip. If the lump cannot be moved after contraction, it indicates fixity to pectoralis major (Figs 20.28 and 20.29).

- *Serratus anterior contraction* test by pressing the hand against the wall. The test has to be done when the tumour is situated in the outer and inferior quadrant.

- *Fixity to the chest wall* is assessed by two methods:
  1. A tumour which is fixed to the chest wall will not be mobile when pectoralis major is relaxed.
  2. Breast will not fall forwards.

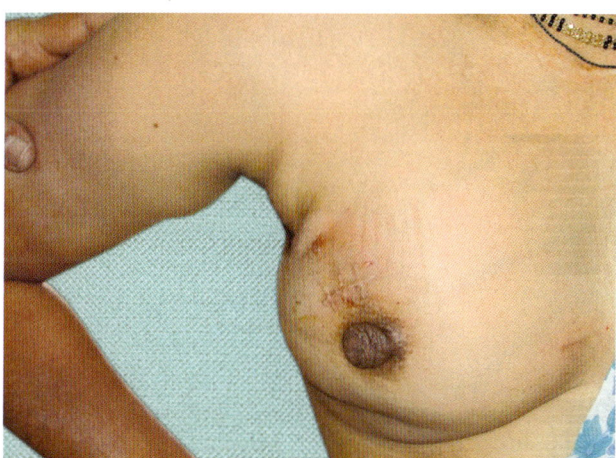

Fig. 20.28: Contracting pectoralis major by pressing hands against hips

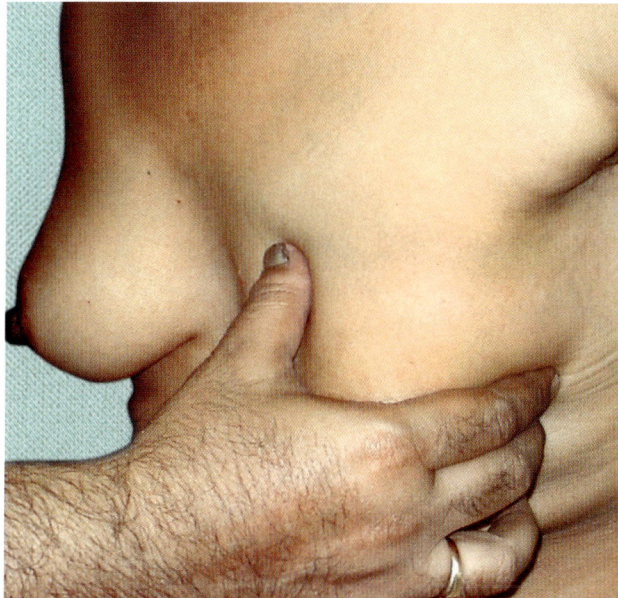

Fig. 20.29: Pectoralis major contracted. Lump is moved in the direction of fibres and perpendicular to them

A FEW ADVANCED CASES OF CARCINOMA BREAST AND THEIR DESCRIPTION

Example 1. Figure 20.30: A large fungating lump is present in the right breast measuring about 15 cm and 8 cm, surface is ulcerated, edges are everted, floor has slough, pigmentation and dilated veins are present. Another large lump is visible in the axilla of the right breast with **nodular surface** and dilated veins. (This is a neglected case of medullary carcinoma breast.)

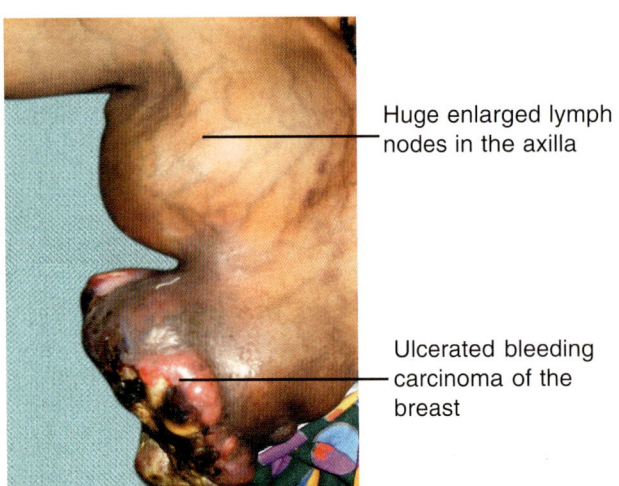

Huge enlarged lymph nodes in the axilla

Ulcerated bleeding carcinoma of the breast

Fig. 20.30: Fungating carcinoma breast with massive enlargement of axillary lymph nodes

Example 2. Figure 20.31: Look at this case. Left breast is not seen indicating post-mastectomy/lumpectomy status. Two scars are seen, one at the mastectomy site and another at the axilla.

A large nodular lump is seen in the region of left breast extending medially from midline to anterior axillary line, vertically extending from inframammary line to about 5 cm above. Surface is nodular, and ulcerations are found on the medial side with slough.

Most important signs under palpation are consistency, mobility, fixity, and plane of the swelling. This swelling is hard, fixed (absolutely no mobility) to skin as well as chest wall. Chest wall fixity was assessed by asking the patient to bend forwards. No significant lymph nodes were found in the axilla.

Two scars are present: First scar is a case of local wide excision and 2nd scar is axillary clearance scar. Local recurrence has taken place and patient has not taken any treatment.

Axillary Lymph Nodes Examination

- There are 5 groups of nodes in the axilla which need to be checked. Apical group of lymph nodes are very difficult to feel. Students are requested not to mention that they felt apical nodes. They are located very high in the axilla. Most of such nodes are central group of lymph nodes.

- First abduct the shoulder to about 30° degrees. Place 4 fingers (thumb excluded) into the hollow of the axilla and gently palpate, moving in circumferential manner (Fig. 20.32).

- Central group of nodes are in the centre of the axilla.

- Rotate the fingers and feel behind the pectoral muscles which form anterior fold of axilla with the thumb kept over the skin of anterior fold of axilla. Pectoral nodes are best felt in this manner (Fig. 20.33).

- Standing in front of the patient and feel for the brachial or lateral group (Fig. 20.34).

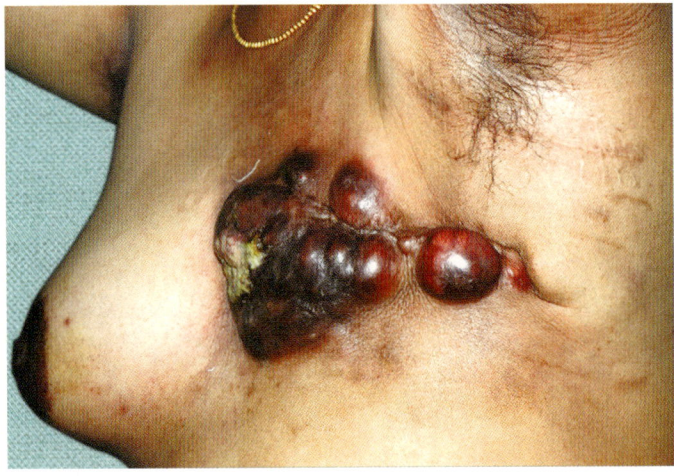

Fig. 20.31: Recurrent advanced carcinoma breast

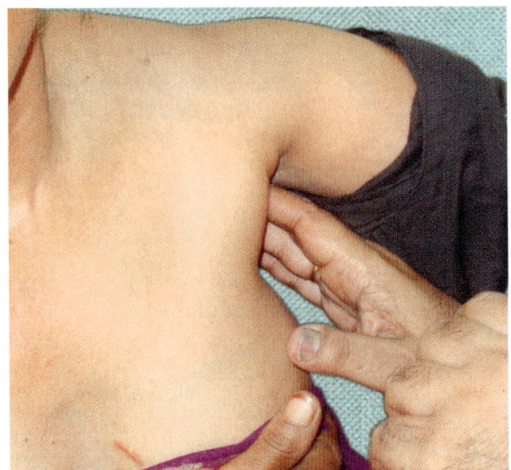

Fig. 20.32: Examination of central group of nodes

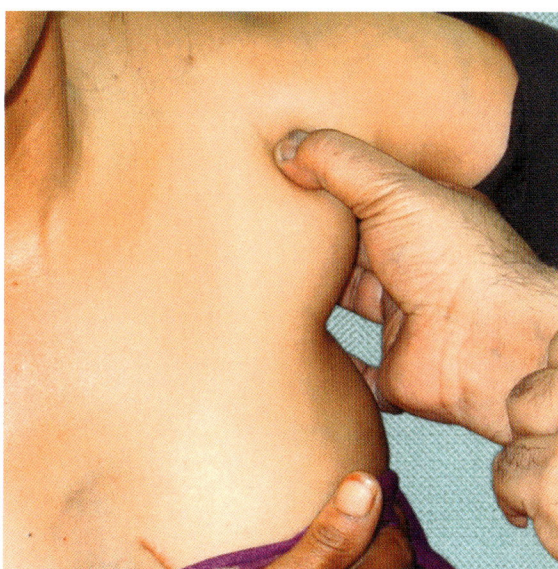

Fig. 20.33: Examination of pectoral or anterior group of nodes

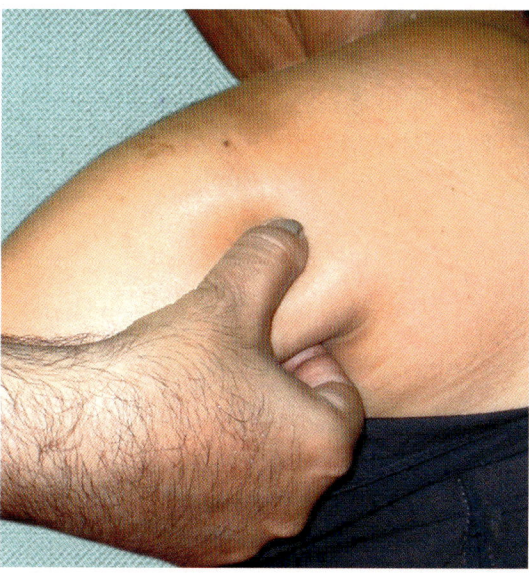

Fig. 20.35: Examination of subscapular (posterior) group of lymph nodes

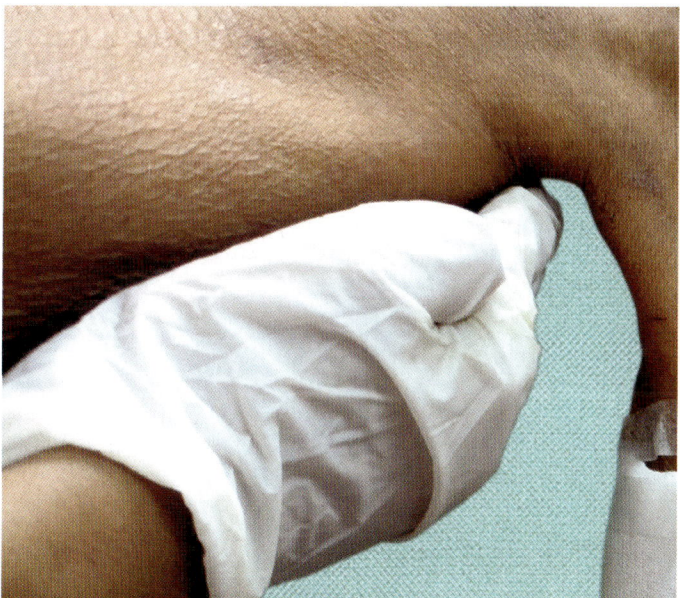

Fig. 20.34: Brachial group or lateral group

Clinical Wisdom

Often breast lump may be firm and clinician may be thinking of benign lesion but axillary nodes may be enlarged and hard which gives the clue. Also, patient may present to the hospital with axillary nodes or carcinoma arising from axillary tail of the breast (Fig. 20.36). It is important to examine the breast and you may find a primary in the breast. If you do not find a primary then search for lesions in the upper limb. Think of lymphoma also.

- Stand behind the patient and feel for posterior group or subscapular group underneath the posterior axillary fold (Fig. 20.35).
- If the *axillary nodes* are firm or *hard*, with or without *fixity*, they are significant.
- Soft to firm, tender nodes need not be malignant. Tenderness can be due to secondary infection because of fungating, ulcerating growth.
- However, in oncological principles, when a node is palpable in the drainage area of the malignant tumour, it is considered as significant.

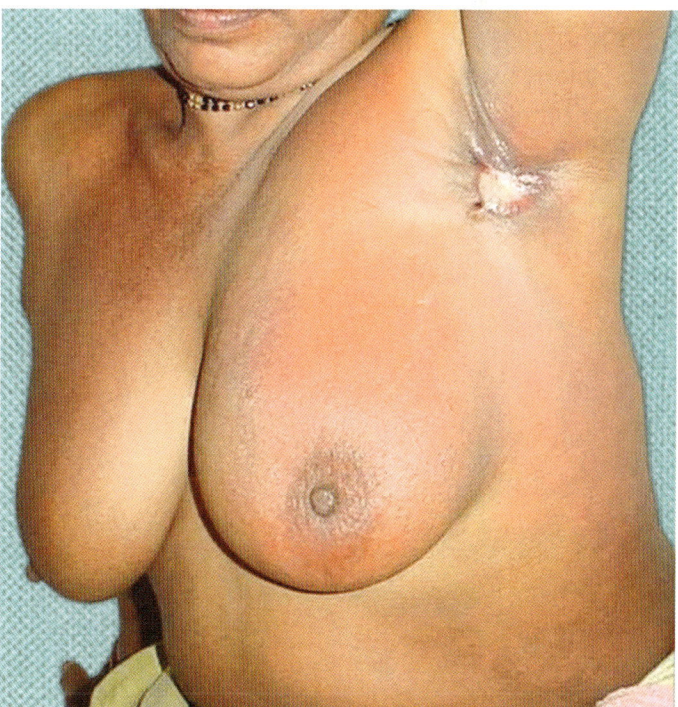

Fig. 20.36: Carcinoma axillary tail of Spence with fungation. You can also see extensive lymphangitis of the breast

Supraclavicular Lymph Nodes Examination

- Palpable supraclavicular nodes irrespective of their size and consistency are considered as clinically positive for malignancy. Presence of lymph nodes indicates advanced disease.

- They are better palpated from behind with slight bending of neck and tilting the neck towards the same side (Fig. 20.37).

Clinical Wisdom

- Supraclavicular node in a 70-year-old smoker—suspect bronchogenic carcinoma
- Supraclavicular node in a 50-year-old man—suspect gastric carcinoma
- Supraclavicular node in a 50-year-old lady—suspect breast carcinoma
- Supraclavicular node in a 20-year-old boy—suspect seminoma testis

Contralateral Axilla and Contralateral Breast

- Please examine the contralateral breast and axilla in the usual manner of inspection and palpation. 6–8% of cases of carcinoma breast can be bilateral.

- There can be spread across the midline resulting in a nodule as shown in Fig. 20.38.

- Opposite axillary nodes can get enlarged in carcinoma breast due to following reasons:
  - Lymphatic spread through **subareolar plexus of Sappey** of one side across the other side.
  - Haematogenous spread
  - Another carcinoma in the contralateral breast (case of bilateral breast carcinoma)

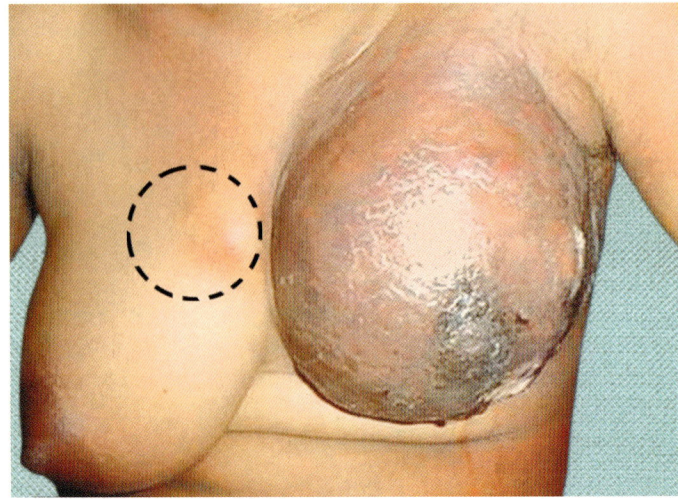

Fig. 20.38: Mastitis carcinomatosa—inflammatory carcinoma. Whole breast is enlarged and a nodule is present on the contralateral breast

Examination for Distant Metastasis

1. *Abdominal examination*: What to look for in the abdominal examination?

   - Secondaries in the liver which present as nodular liver (Fig. 20.39).

   - Ascites—demonstrated by shifting dullness.

   - Krukenberg's tumour—lower abdominal masses. Bilateral bulky ovarian metastasis in menopausal patients.

Clinical Wisdom

Why abdominal examination? The usual answer by the students is to find out hepatosplenomegaly….? Why mention spleen here? Talk about your case and what is relevant?

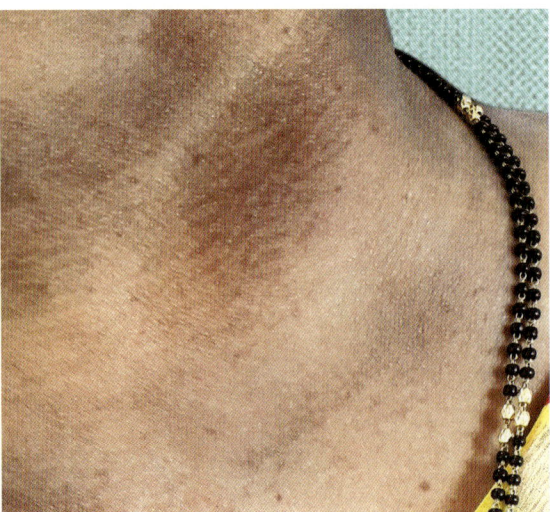

Fig. 20.37: Supraclavicular lymph nodes in a 50-year-old lady after 5 years of surgery for carcinoma of the breast

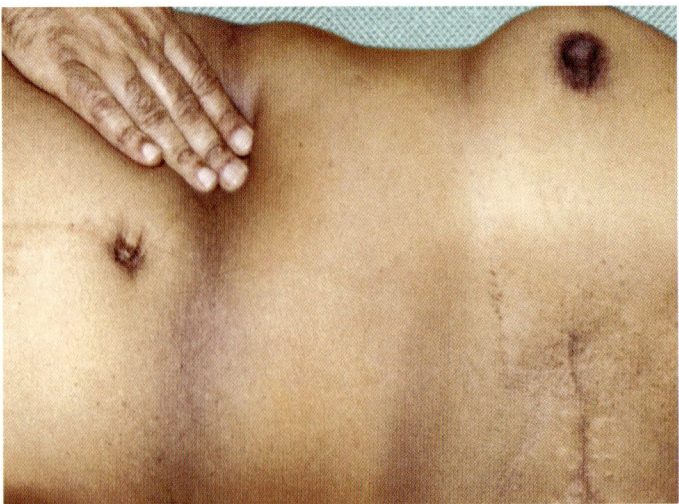

Fig. 20.39: Look for nodular liver—carcinoma breast 2 years follow up. Watch the mastectomy scar on the left side

2. *Vaginal and rectal examination*: Look for nodular deposits in rectouterine pouch—nontender lumps with intact mucosa. They indicate peritoneal disease reflecting transcoelomic spread.

3. *Respiratory system examination*: Look for pleural effusion. Tracheal shift and dullness on percussion are the features.

4. *Skeletal system examination*: Bony tenderness should be looked for in the spine, long bones, skull, etc.

5. *CNS examination*: Reflexes and power.

Diagnosis

Give a complete diagnosis. A few examples are given below:

- Carcinoma right breast, with lymph node metastasis in the axilla—T2 N1 M0. Under what category is it included? It is **early breast carcinoma.**
- Advanced carcinoma left breast with fixed axillary nodes—T4 N2 M0. Under what category is it included? It is **locally advanced breast carcinoma (LABC).**
- Carcinoma right breast with metastasis in the liver—T3 N1 M+. Under what category is it included? It is **metastatic breast carcinoma.**

CLINICAL DISCUSSION

1. **What way is trauma important in the history?**
   Trauma can give rise to traumatic fat necrosis which may feel hard. It is uncommon.
2. **Which malignant tumour of breast grows very rapidly?**
   Mastitis carcinomatosa—inflammatory carcinoma.
3. **Which tumours occur more rapidly than carcinoma?**
   Phyllodes tumour.
4. **Which lumps may regress in size?**
   Inflammatory such as breast abscess.
5. **Why is there nipple retraction seen in carcinoma breast?**
   Due to extension of growth along lactiferous ducts and fibrosis.
6. **When you feel a hard lump, what possibilities come into your mind?**
   Carcinoma, chronic mastitis, traumatic fat necrosis, and antibioma.
7. **Which type of carcinoma breast is hard?**
   Infiltrating scirrhous variety because it evokes a lot of desmoplastic reaction.
8. **How does carcinoma breast spread to ovary?**
   Lymphatic spread from the inner quadrant via penetration of posterior rectus sheath into peritoneal cavity resulting in ascites. The cells then drop into ovary resulting in ovarian metastasis called Krukenberg tumours.
9. **How does metastasis in vertebrae and pelvic bones occur?**
   Posterior intercostal veins join the azygos and then to the paravertebral plexus of veins called Batson's venous plexus.

These are large valveless veins which receive blood from vertebrae and thoracic cavity. Spread occurs through these veins.

10. **What are common bones affected in carcinoma breast?**
    Lumbar vertebrae, femur and thoracic vertebrae in that order **(you can remember as LFT).**
11. **How do you elicit tenderness of spine?**
    It is not pressing on the spine but by using thumb, press on the paraspinal region and do a rotationary movement. In this way, it presses on body and pedicle of the vertebrae which are affected.
12. **How does Krukenberg tumour occur?**
    Transcoelomic spread.
13. **What are the investigations in carcinoma breast?**
    FNAC is the first investigation because it is easy and can give histological diagnosis
14. **Any other better investigation to get histopathology report?**
    Tru-cut biopsy
15. **What is the advantage of tru cut biopsy?**
    We can do the receptor studies and thus can plan treatment accordingly
16. **What receptors?**
    ER, PR, Her2 neu
17. **What are the investigations for metastasis?**
    Chest X-ray to rule out cannonball metastasis, ultrasound abdomen to rule out Krukenberg metastasis and liver metastasis, and bone scan in all symptomatic bony pain cases and locally advanced carcinoma breast cases.
18. **Let us say it is an early breast cancer. What are the treatment options?**
    Classical case of an outer and upper quadrant tumour is treated by local wide excision, axillary dissection, radiotherapy to the breast and chemotherapy depending upon the receptor studies. Tamoxifen is given for 5 years in premenopausal patients. Other option is to go for modified radical mastectomy (MRM)
19. **If it is LABC, what will you do?**
    Neoadjuvant chemotherapy is given for 4 to 6 cycles. It will downstage the tumour, then either local wide excision and axillary clearance or MRM depending upon size of tumour or patient's choice is done.
20. **What are the advantages of neoadjuvant chemotherapy?**
    It will downstage the tumour, we can see the response of tumour decreasing *in vivo*, more importantly it will target the micro-metastasis.

DIFFERENTIAL DIAGNOSIS OF BREAST LUMP

1. *Carcinoma breast*: Typically, a middle-aged woman complains of slow progressing breast lump of 3–6 months duration. She may also complain of bleeding per nipple which is an uncommon symptom. Clinical examination reveals a hard lump which moves with breast tissue with or without axillary nodes. Nipple retraction, skin puckering and peau d' orange, if present the diagnosis is almost certain. Many times the symptoms and signs are so classical, when asked for the differential diagnosis, students can always say that there is no differential diagnosis. However, doubtful lesions without lymph nodes and other signs, if present, one has to consider differential diagnosis. Given below are some histological types. You can tell them only when asked.

Invasive Carcinomas

A. *Scirrhous carcinoma*

- It is the most common form seen in about 60–75% of patients. In this variety, there is increased fibrotic reaction and less cellular reaction. It presents as a hard lump. Hence the name, scirrhous carcinoma. It produces grating sound when cut. Cut surfaces are concave. The chalky white necrosis and calcification may be visible occasionally. This is the type of lesion which produces retraction of the nipple, infiltration of the skin and fixity to the chest wall.

- Atrophic scirrhous is an infiltrating duct carcinoma seen in elderly patients when there is atrophy of the breast (Fig. 20.40).

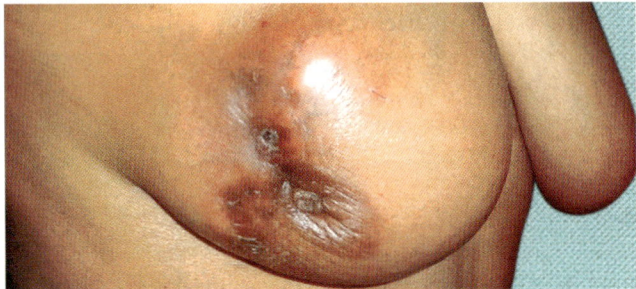

Fig. 20.40: Scirrhous carcinoma with nipple retraction

B. *Medullary carcinoma of the breast:*
It is seen in around 15% of cases. It tends to occur in **well-formed breasts** (in the reproductive age group) and it feels more firm than hard. In addition to undifferentiated cells, occasionally well differentiated gland formation is present. Hence the name, medullary adenocarcinoma. Presence of lymphatic infiltration is thought to represent a good host response, thus indicating a good prognosis (Fig. 20.41).

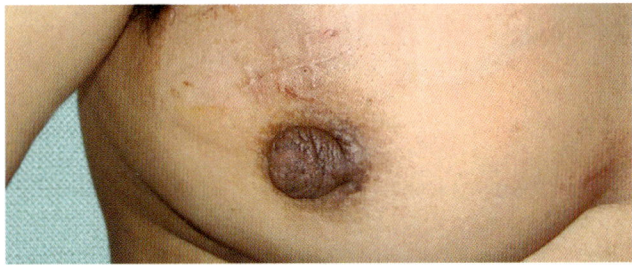

Fig. 20.41: Medullary carcinoma breast in a 35-year-old lady. You can see incision biopsy mark

C. *Inflammatory carcinoma*

- It constitutes less than 1% of all cases of carcinoma breast. **Dermal lymphatic invasion is characteristic.**
- Predominantly seen during pregnancy and lactation.
- Malignancy grows so rapidly that it invades more than half of the breast tissue. It comes under locally advanced breast cancer (LABC).
- Redness, pain and sudden enlargement appear so suddenly that it is diagnosed as breast abscess. Hence the name, *mastitis carcinomatosa*. It is differentiated from breast abscess by absence of fever and presence of gross *peau d'orange* due to blockage of subdermal lymphatics.

- High angiogenic and angioinvasive capability.
- Most of them are ER negative.
- It comes under stage T4D.

> **Clinical Wisdom**
>
> Mastitis carcinomatosa often causes enlargement of the whole breast without a lump, engorged, enlarged breast with dilated veins, redness and skin changes. Breast looks erythematous and oedematous.

D. *Paget's disease of the nipple*

- It is a misnomer. It is **not a disease of the nipple** but an **intraductal carcinoma** involving excretory ducts that infiltrates nipple and areola, early (Fig. 20.42).
- Nipple can be ulcerated, fissured and cracked. Oozing is present.
- In advanced cases, entire nipple is destroyed (ulcerated) (Fig. 20.43).
- Lump appears much later than changes in the nipple (Fig. 20.44).
- Microscopically, large **hyperchromatic cells** with clear cytoplasm or *clear halo* are seen.
- It is due to intracellular accumulation of **mucopolysaccharides**. These cells are called **Paget's cells**.
- It is differentiated from eczema as follows:
  Eczema is bilateral—carcinoma breast is unilateral.
  Eczema gives rise to itching—carcinoma does not.
  Eczema responds to symptomatic treatment—carcinoma does not.

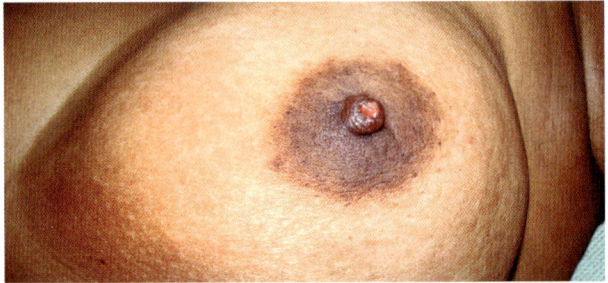

Fig. 20.42: Paget's disease of the nipple. Indurated small lump was palpable beneath nipple–areolar complex

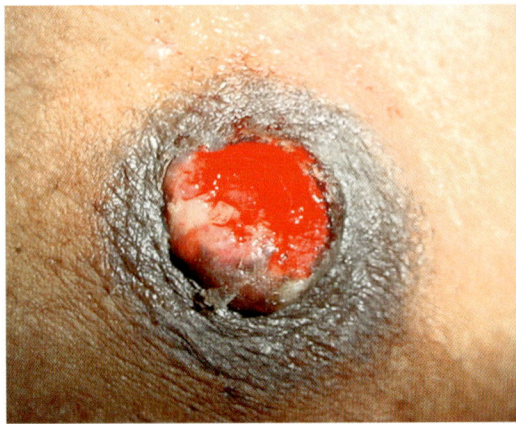

Fig. 20.43: Paget's disease of the nipple—totally destroyed nipple

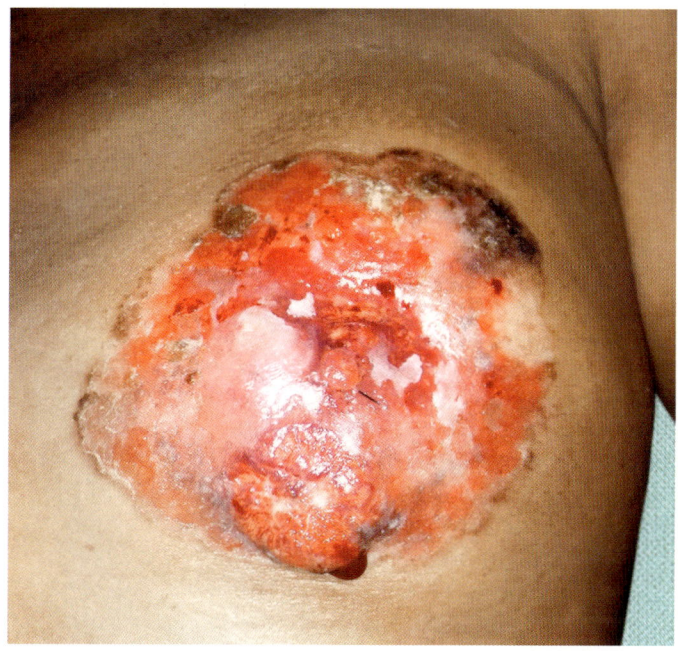

Fig. 20.44: Paget's disease treated as eczema for 3 months—it is not an uncommon mistake

E. Colloid carcinoma
- It is diagnosed because of production of mucin, intracellularly and extracellularly.
- Prognosis of this variety of carcinoma breast is better than other infiltrating duct carcinomas.

Non-infiltrative Lesions

A. Carcinoma in situ
- It can be ductal—ductal carcinoma *in situ* (DCIS)
- Lobular—lobular carcinoma *in situ* (LCIS)

This is a type of **cancer without infiltrating** epithelial basement membrane.
- Lobular carcinoma refers to a lesion developing from the acini or terminal ductules of the lobule.
- More *in situ* carcinomas are diagnosed because of mammography and most of the breast conserving surgery is done in this group of patients.

Clinical Wisdom

Lobular carcinoma is more dangerous because it is multifocal and bilateral.

B. Comedocarcinoma of breast: Comedos means cast or plug. It is a peripheral carcinoma wherein the tumour cells block the ductules by forming a case or plug producing a small cystic lesion. It is an example for intracystic carcinoma.

2. Fibroadenoma: It is common in young patients between 20–40 years of age group. Classically patient complains of a lump in the breast which is very slowly growing and has free mobility within the breast tissue. **It is painless and commonly affects only one breast.** (Fibroadenosis affects both breasts and is painful—called cyclical mastalgia.)

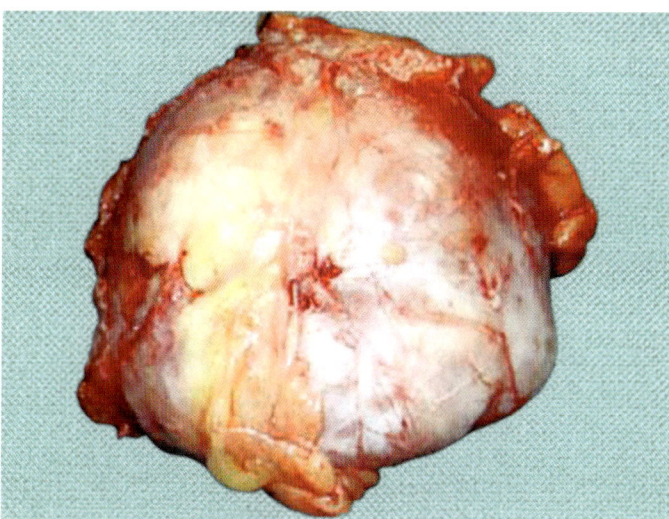

Fig. 20.45: Fibroadenoma

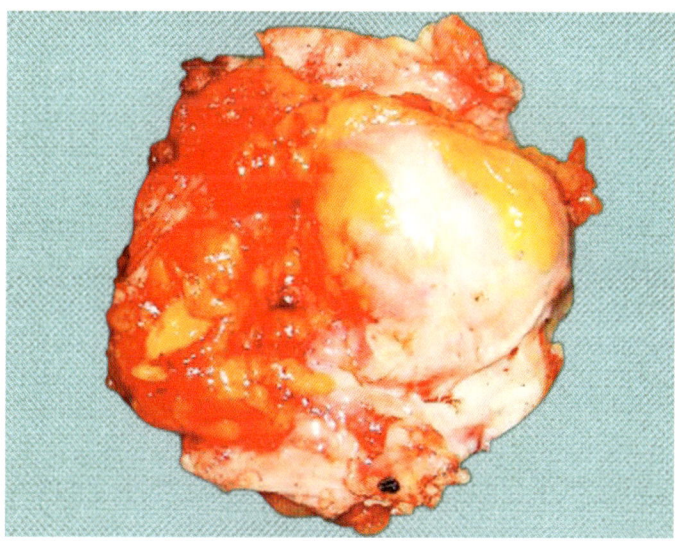

Fig. 20.46: Excised specimen

Sometimes they can be multiple. Free mobility within the breast is the diagnostic feature of fibroadenoma
- Single, freely mobile swelling
- Smooth surface and round borders
- Nontender
- Not fixed to any structure
- No lymph nodes in the axilla
- Large fibroadenoma should be excised (Figs 20.45 and 20.46).

3. Fibroadenosis: *Cyclical mastalgia with nodularity*—a spinster or a nun or a lady in the reproductive age group complains of bilateral breast pain which is often related to menstruation. On examination, granular or irregular small lumps are palpable. They are tender and firm in consistency. Lumps move with breast tissue (Fig. 20.47).
- Single or multiple swellings
- Tender, smooth or irregular surface
- Moves with breast tissue

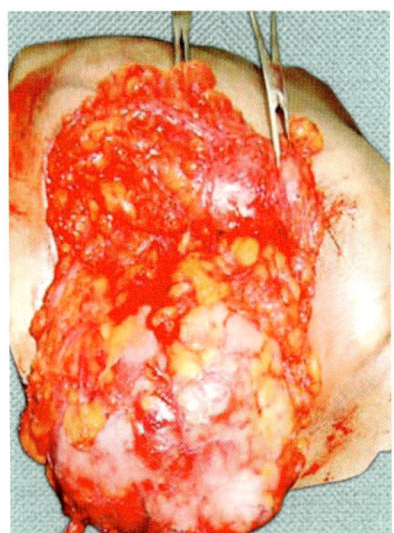

Fig. 20.47: Cyclical mastalgia with nodularity (*Courtesy:* Dr Kshama Hegde, Assistant Professor, Dept of Surgery, KMC, Manipal)

- No lymph nodes in the axilla
- Reassurance, support to the breast, and evening primrose oil (1000 mg) two times/day for 1 to 2 months are the treatment available.
- Excision is last resort.

Clinical Wisdom

- Small fibroadenomas (1 cm in size or less) are considered normal.
- Larger fibroadenomas (up to 3 cm) are disorders.
- Giant fibroadenomas (more than 3 cm) are *disease*.

4. Phyllodes tumour (cystosarcoma phyllodes): It is common in young patients between 20 and 40 years age group. Classically patient says her breast has become big or she noticed a lump just a few days back and now it has become very big. It is painless and commonly affects only one breast (Fig. 20.48).

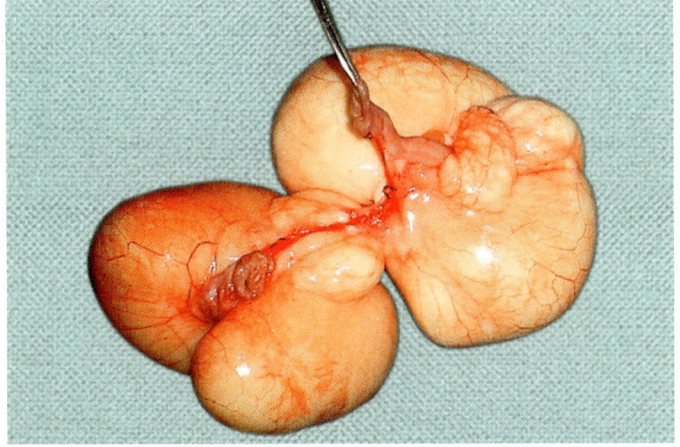

Fig. 20.48: Excised specimen of phyllodes. Malignancy is decided by mitotic figures

Diagnostic features of phyllodes tumour are:

- Rapid growth
- Stretched, shiny skin
- Red, dilated veins over surface, warm to touch
- Bosselated surface (big nodules), a few cystic areas.
- Variable consistency—firm or even soft areas due to tumour necrosis

CLINICAL DISCUSSION

1. **Why it is called phyllodes tumour?**
   Histologically, the tumour cells have a branching pattern, penetrating the cystic cavity (*phyllus* means leaf-like pattern). Fibrous stromal proliferation is a feature.

2. **Why is it not a carcinoma?**
   a. No fixity to the skin
   b. No fixity to the pectoralis major
   c. Lymph nodes will not be involved
   d. No nipple retraction.

3. **What are the swellings that have bosselated surface?**
   a. Phyllodes tumour
   b. Polycystic kidney
   c. Polycystic liver
   d. Large nodular goitre

4. **Can phyllodes tumours have skin infiltration?**
   No. Skin may undergo necrosis due to rapid growth. In such cases, edge of the skin will not be everted. In carcinoma breast, when skin is infiltrated, edge of the ulcer will be everted.

5. **What is the treatment of phyllodes tumour?**
   Lumpectomy. Very large cases are treated by subcutaneous mastectomy or even simple mastectomy.

5. *Breast abscess:* Lactational breast abscess is common. Cracks/fissures in the nipple will allow *Staphylococcus aureus* to enter and proliferate intraductally, causing clotting of milk. Initial stage is cellulitic stage which may revert back to normal if promptly treated. Untreated cases will go for abscess formation (Fig. 20.49). High grade fever, tense indurated

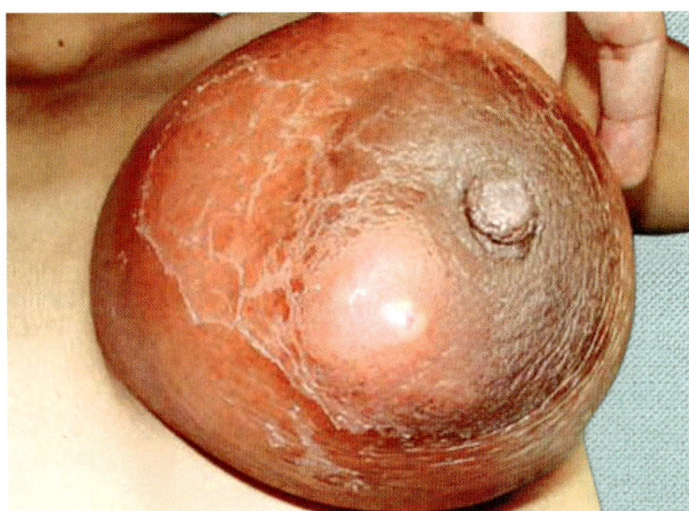

Fig. 20.49: Acute lactational breast abscess (*Courtesy:* Dr Geetha B, Ex-Assistant Professor, KMC, Manipal)

breast, and throbbing pain are the features. Fluctuation is a late feature. Ultrasound helps in the diagnosis. Ultrasound-guided aspiration is the treatment of choice. Recurrent abscess, and multiple abscesses are indication for incision and drainage. Drug of choice is cloxacillin. MRSA (methicillin resistant *Staphylococcus aureus*) responds to vancomycin 1.5 gm/12 hourly for 7–10 days of treatment.

6. **Antibioma**: It means antibiotic-induced. 'Oma' = Tumour (swelling).
   - When an abscess occurs in the breast and antibiotics are given, without draining it, the abscess cavity may become fibrous and form a **firm to hard lump** in the breast. It gives rise to vague **ill health of the patient**. This hard lump can be confused for *malignancy*. It is treated by excision.
   - Such patients are young and will not have any other features of malignancy such as skin fixation, pectoral fixation, hard nodes in the axilla, etc.
   - A few common sites of antibioma are breast, gluteal region, and pyaemic abscess in the thigh.

7. **Periductal mastitis**: It results due to primary dilatation in one of the lactiferous ducts.
   - A few other organs wherein such dilatation can occur are lungs—bronchiectasis, salivary glands—sialectasis, cutaneous blood vessels—telangiectasis. It is common in middle-aged women.
   - **Mild low-grade infection:** Anaerobic bacteria have been considered as one of the factors.
   - Increased incidence in **smokers**: Smoking increases the **virulence** of commensal bacteria.
   - Due to dilatation, the contents tend to undergo stasis. The epithelial debris, and serous fluid collectively form a thick paste-like material which is rich in lipid. It may cause discharge per nipple which is classically paste-like. Nipple retraction can occur due to periductal fibrosis.
   - A few important points to differentiate from carcinoma breast are given in Table 20.1.

8. **Macrocysts**: They occur due to excessive secretion of thin fluid within the lobules which enlarge to produce a cyst. Clinically, they present as firm swelling in the breast. They are common in the reproductive age group. They can be single or multiple. One of them can have huge dimensions with a thin bluish capsule—blue domed cyst of Bloodgood (Fig. 20.50 and Clinical Box 20.4).

Clinical Box 20.4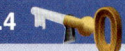

Breast cysts
- Maximum incidence is between 40 and 50 years of age.
- Smooth and tense—hence, firm on palpation
- One-third of the patients may have more than one cyst in the breast.
- Diagnosis is by clinical examination
- If you suspect cyst, the investigation of choice is ultra-sonography.
- Increased incidences of benign breast lumps including cysts have been reported with prolonged use of hormone replacement therapy.

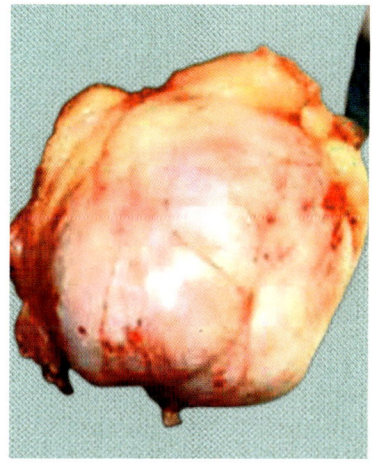

Fig. 20.50: Macrocyst (*Courtesy:* Prof. Santhosh Pai, Professor and Head, MMMC, Manipal)

Clinical Wisdom

Tensely cystic swellings in the breast, thyroid, neck, testis and scrotum may feel hard and even cause a clinical worry. Only when one does ultrasound or aspiration of fluid as in breast and thyroid, the diagnosis will be certain.

9. **Galactocoele**: It is a solitary, subareolar retention cyst filled with milk. It occurs in the lactational age group. It occurs due to inadequate drainage of the milk added by epithelial debris which block the lactiferous duct. Once the duct is

Table 20.1: Periductal mastitis and carcinoma breast

Periductal mastitis	Carcinoma breast
• Middle-aged woman	• More common in middle and elderly age
• History of recurrent abscess is common	• No previous history of recurrent abscess
• Paste-like discharge per nipple	• Blood-stained discharge may be found
• Lump can be felt, ill-defined, firm	• Lump is the most common complaint and it is usually hard, with or without fixity to skin
• Bilateral slit-like retraction of nipple of long duration	• Nipple retraction is present (not slit-like but circumferential)
• Axillary nodes, if present, are firm or soft and tender	• Axillary nodes, if present, are firm or hard and nontender
• Other features of metastasis are not found	• Other features of spread such as supraclavicular lymph nodes, bony tenderness, enlarged nodular liver, Krukenberg tumours, if present, clinch the diagnosis

blocked, proximally, the milky fluid accumulates resulting in a huge enlargement of breast. Rarely, they undergo calcification. It is treated by repeated aspirations. Excision is the last choice.

10. *Gynaecomastia*: This is a painful, unphysiological *enlargement of the male breast due* to increase in the ductal and connective tissue element.

- **Idiopathic** type is the most common cause of gynaecomastia. A **disc-like tender lump** is palpable. Surface is smooth. Gynaecomastia following oestrogen therapy is usually of soft variety and it is bilateral. In idiopathic variety, it is hard and bilateral. In other cases, it may be unilateral (Figs 20.51 and 20.52).

- Examination should also include palpation of the testis and looking for signs of liver cell failure.

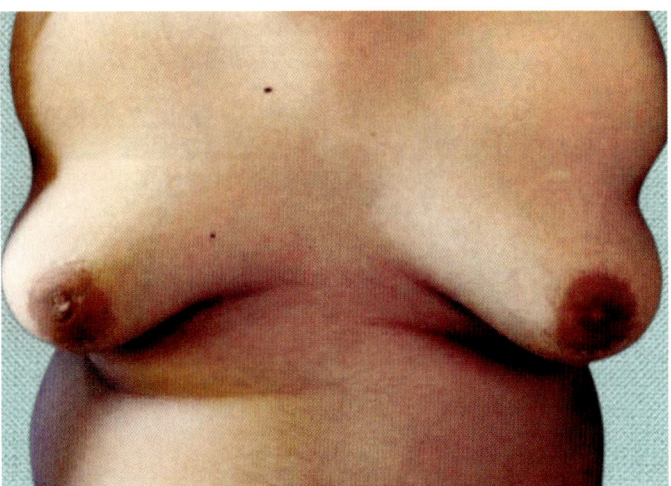

Fig. 20.51: Bilateral gynaecomastia (*Courtesy:* Dr Satish Deshmukh and Dr Murtaza Akhthar, NKP Salve Institute of Medical Sciences, Nagpur)

- **Disc-like lump which is tender in a male is gynaecomastia.**

There are many other causes of gynaecomastia which can be summarised as **MASTIA**.

- **M**alignant tumour: Teratoma, bronchogenic carcinoma
- **A**norchism: Absent testis
- **S**ex chromosome anomaly: Klinefelter syndrome (XXY)
- **T**ablets: Cimetidine, stilboestrol, digitalis, spironolactone
- **I**diopathic: No cause is found
- **A**trophy of the testis: Liver cell failure, leprosy, etc.

Clinical classification of gynaecomastia

Grade I: Mild enlargement

Grade IIa: Moderate enlargement

Grade IIb: Moderate enlargement with skin redundancy

Grade III: Marked enlargement with skin redundancy and ptosis (simulates a female breast)

Treatment: Lumpectomy or mastectomy with preservation of nipple and areola (subcutaneous mastectomy).

Complications: Rarely, gynaecomastia can predispose to male breast carcinoma.

11. *Carcinoma male breast*

- It is less common but more aggressive and more locally infiltrative (Fig. 20.53).
- Chest wall infiltration occurs fast because of less subcutaneous tissue.
- Fungation occurs early for the same reason.

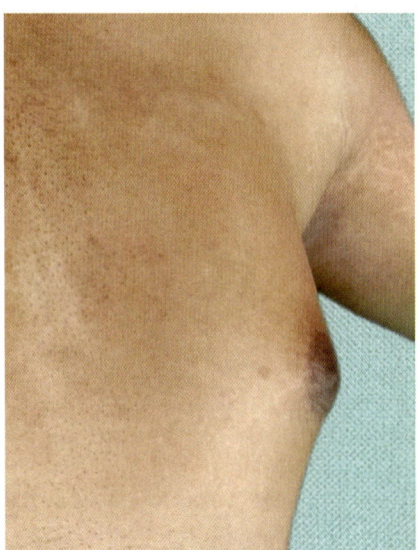

Fig. 20.52: Unilateral gynaecomastia (*Courtesy:* Dr Joseph Thomas, Assistant Professor, Department of Plastic Surgery, KMC, Manipal)

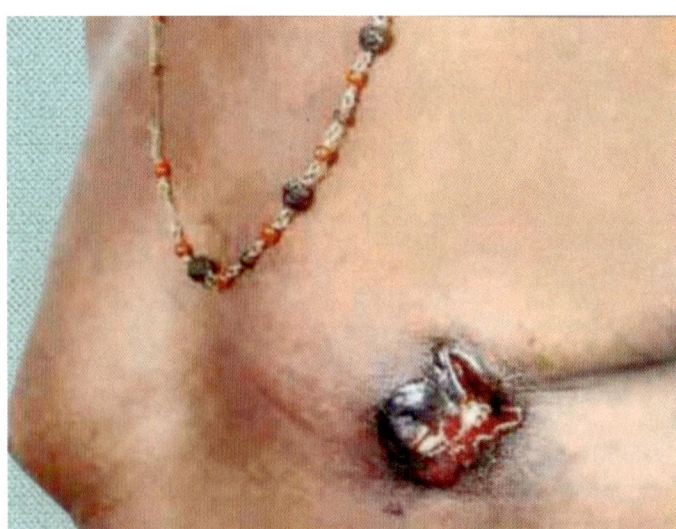

Fig. 20.53: Male breast carcinoma—tends to ulcerate and infiltrate chest wall early (*Courtesy:* Dr Surya Prakash Saxena, District Surgeon, Durg, Chhattisgarh)

DIAGRAMMATIC REPRESENTATION OF COMMON BREAST LESIONS (Figs 20.54 to 20.60)

1. *Carcinoma breast*: Hard, irregular, fixed, lymph nodes in the axilla. Evidence of metastasis may be present.

2. *Fibroadenoma*: Round, single or multiple, freely mobile (breast mouse). Firm consistency.

3. *Cyclical mastalgia with nodularity (ANDI)*: Fibroadenosis. Tender, bilateral, granular, vague lumps which move with breast tissue.

4. *Periductal mastitis*: Vague lump—firm consistency, history of recurrent abscess, nipple retraction may be present.

5. *Phyllodes tumour*: Bosselated, large lump dilated veins, nipple and areola normal, skin is free and no lymph nodes.

6. *Macrocysts*: Tensely cystic lump, nontender, feels firm, smooth and round, nipple areola normal.

7. *Galactocoele*: Large lump in lactating women, smooth surface and round borders.

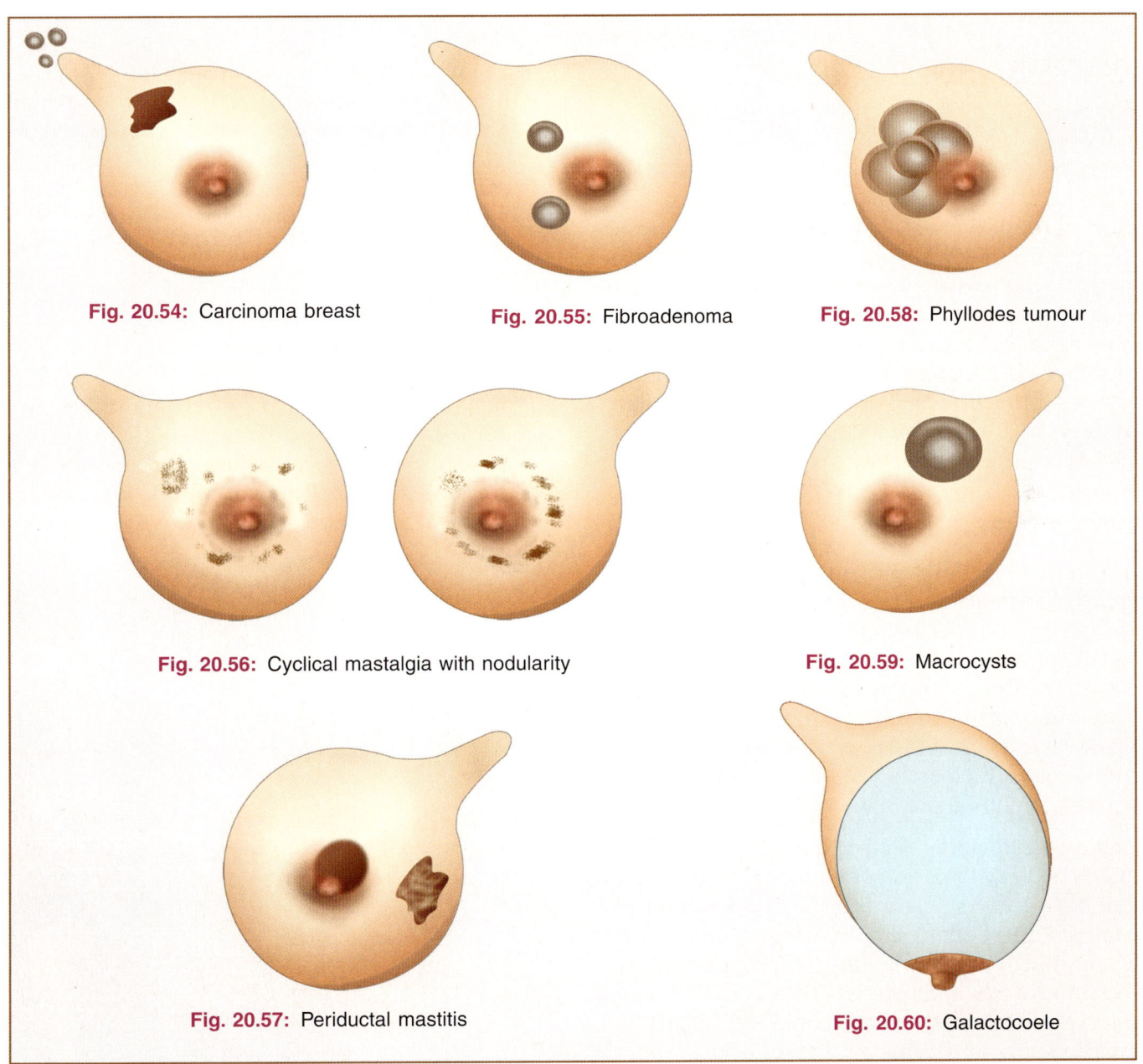

Fig. 20.54: Carcinoma breast

Fig. 20.55: Fibroadenoma

Fig. 20.58: Phyllodes tumour

Fig. 20.56: Cyclical mastalgia with nodularity

Fig. 20.59: Macrocysts

Fig. 20.57: Periductal mastitis

Fig. 20.60: Galactocoele

21

Examination of a Case of Dysphagia

INTRODUCTION

Dysphagia (difficulty in swallowing) is a common problem encountered by physicians and surgeons. Dysphagia generally reflects a disease of pharynx and oesophagus. Odynophagia means painful swallowing. It reflects oropharyngeal diseases of inflammatory pathology such as pharyngitis, tonsillitis, etc. There are many causes of dysphagia which are given in this chapter. Common causes being carcinoma oesophagus, achalasia cardia, mediastinal tumours or masses. Detailed history adds to the diagnosis in many cases. Clinical examination may help in a small percentage of cases. Endoscopy, CECT (contrast enhanced) scan help in a vast majority of the cases.

HISTORY OF PRESENT ILLNESS

1. *Age and sex*: Elderly patient between 50 and 70 years old, emaciated may be having carcinoma oesophagus (Fig. 21.1). Between 30 and 40 years of age, benign diseases are more common. They are achalasia cardia, Plummer-Vinson syndrome, etc. Carcinoma is more common in men. Plummer-Vinson syndrome affects exclusively in females. Achalasia cardia occurs both in men and women equally, slightly more in women, than men.

2. *Acute dysphagia*: Is it of sudden onset or has it developed over a period of time? Is it painful? Do you have any change in voice? These are the few common questions. In children, foreign bodies are a common cause of acute dysphagia. Acute dysphagia with pain suggests tonsillitis or pharyngitis. Sudden onset painless difficulty in swallowing with change in voice may be a manifestation of a vertebrobasilar insufficiency.

- History of ingestion of caustics either suicidal or accidental should be enquired when patient presents with acute onset severe pain and inability to swallow. Late cases present as stricture. Detergents, toilet cleaning agents and batteries contain sulphuric acid (caustic).

3. *Chronic and progressive dysphagia*: Stricture, achalasia, Plummer-Vinson syndrome and carcinomas produce chronic dysphagia. The increasing difficulty to swallow, first to solids and

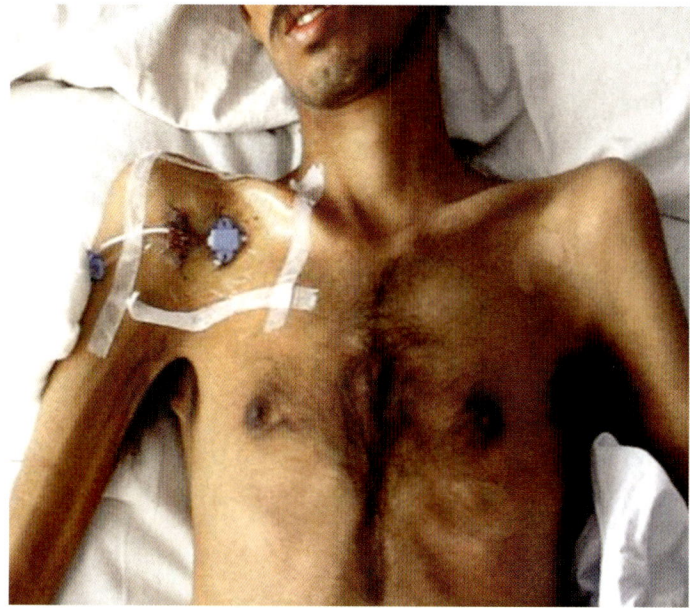

Fig. 21.1: Carcinoma oesophagus—emaciated patient

later to liquids is typical of carcinoma oesophagus. (In achalasia cardia, it is reverse.) It is because in cases of achalasia cardia, there is spasm of the lower end of the oesophagus. Food bolus, because of the weight, opens the lower end of oesophagus and hence there is no dysphagia to solids. Periods of remission in between are common in spastic lesions such as Plummer-Vinson syndrome and Schatzki's rings.

4. *Change in voice* or even hoarseness with dysphagia suggests advanced laryngeal carcinoma.

   • Advanced cases of carcinoma oesophagus infiltrating vagus and anaplastic carcinoma of thyroid produces change in voice or hoarseness of voice.

5. *Regurgitation*: It is the symptom of oesophageal disorders and vomiting is a symptom of stomach disorders. In cases of achalasia cardia and carcinoma lower end of oesophagus, typically, when significant contents accumulate in the lower oesophagus, it results in regurgitation. The contents may have a foul odour also. If blood stains are present, it may be carcinoma oesophagus.

6. *Vomitus*: Enquire about the frequency, contents and blood in vomitus. Postprandial vomiting also occurs in large paraoesophageal hernia. Streaks of blood may be found in carcinoma oesophagus.

7. *Chest pain*: It is a vague discomfort felt deep inside the chest—behind the sternum. Dilated oesophagus in achalasia also can present as chest pain. Severe pain or backache indicates advanced carcinoma oesophagus which is inoperable. Coeliac nodes may be enlarged in such cases.

   Retrosternal pain: It is burning in nature and becomes worse on lying down. The pain reduces in the sitting position. The pain is described as *heart burn and can be confused for angina pectoris*. It is relieved on taking antacids. **Heart burn** is otherwise called **pyrosis**.

8. *Cough*: Cough is not a common symptom. Mediastinal masses can irritate bronchus and can give rise to cough. Regurgitation may be followed by cough. It is due to food contents entering into trachea as in cases of achalasia or even pharyngeal pouch cases.

9. *Sensation of a substernal lump*: A few patients may complain of a lump behind the sternum. It is called globus. When this occurs during fasting, it is termed 'globus hystericus'. It is a neurotic symptom in patients with emotional instability.

10. *Loss of appetite and weight loss*: Both are typical of carcinoma oesophagus. However, in achalasia cardia, loss of weight is obvious but appetite is good. Weakness is due to anaemia.

Clinical Wisdom

It is not uncommon to find a few patients with severe reflux oesophagitis. Gastro Esophageal Reflux Disease (GERD) and frequent aspirations are diagnosed and treated as bronchitis and asthma.

Past History

• Previous **history of irradiation** suggests that it may be a case of carcinoma oesophagus and patient has developed stricture subsequently.

• Previous **laparoscopic surgery** may be laparoscopic fundoplication. Too tight a wrap causes dysphagia.

• Patients may have dysphagia post-sclerotherapy for oesophageal varices.

• Previous history of **hospitalisation/regular dilatation** in case of corrosive strictures.

• History of **fungal infections**—moniliasis may be found in cancer, diabetic and immunocompromised patients (suspect AIDS).

• *History of tuberculosis*: Tubercular masses of lymph nodes may compress on oesophagus or even ulcerate into the oesophagus and can present as dysphagia.

GENERAL PHYSICAL EXAMINATION/ REGIONAL EXAMINATION

• Thin, cachectic, emaciated patient presenting with dysphagia typically has carcinoma oesophagus.

• Anaemia or pallor may indicate carcinoma oesophagus.

• Bald tongue, angular cheilitis, pallor together may indicate Plummer-Vinson syndrome with or without hypopharyngeal carcinoma (Figs 21.2A and B).

• Cervical lymphadenopathy, if present, gives the clue for a possibility of a mediastinal lymph nodal mass as typically happens in Hodgkin's lymphoma.

• Palpable left supraclavicular lymph node—may suggest carcinoma oesophagus.

• Look for thyroid swelling (Fig. 21.3).

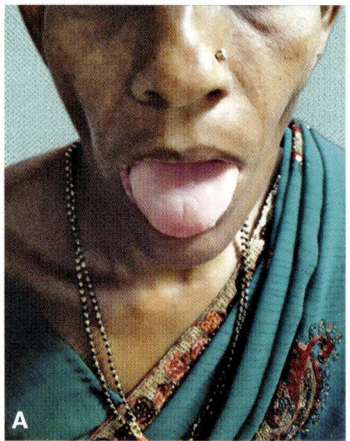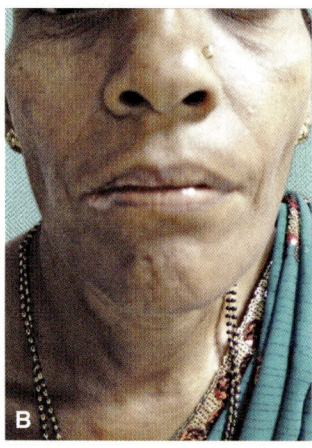

Figs 21.2: (A) Bald tongue, severe pallor, (B) angular cheilitis (*Courtesy*: Dr Kshama Hegde, Assistant Professor, KMC, Manipal)

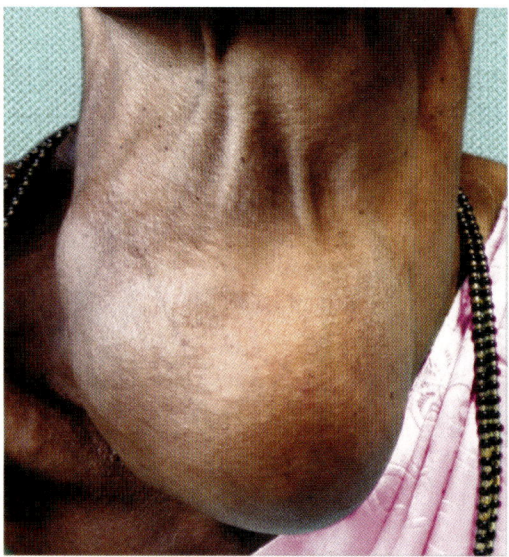

Fig. 21.3: Large multinodular goitre of 8 years duration. Patient presented to the hospital for dysphagia

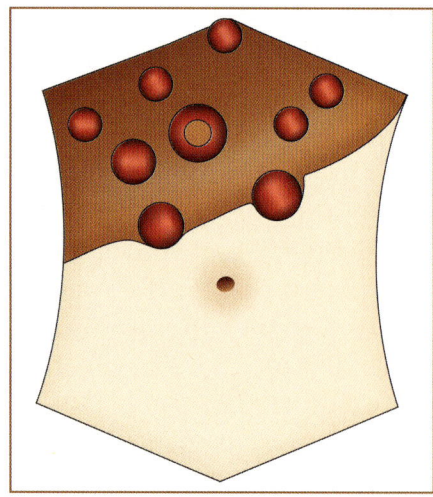

Fig. 21.4: Secondaries in the liver

Abdominal Examination

- Most often, in all 'benign' diseases, it is normal. Exceptionally, spleen may be palpable, if any 'autoimmune' aetiology is detected as a cause for dysphagia.
- Palpable nodular liver (Fig. 21.4) is due to secondaries in the liver. Primary may be in the oesophagus. Look for ascites and para-aortic lymph nodes.
- As a rule, carcinoma lower end oesophagus and Gastro-oesophageal junction tumours are not palpable unless very advanced (Fig. 21.5).

CAUSES

I. Causes from Outside Oesophagus (Extraluminal)

- Thyroid swellings
- Cardiomegaly
- Aortic aneurysm
- *Mediastinal nodes*: Tuberculosis, lymphoma or secondaries
- Rolling hiatus hernia

II. Causes in the Wall of Oesophagus (Luminal)

1. Oesophageal stricture
   - Corrosive acid poisoning
   - Tuberculous stricture
   - Barrett's oesophagus
2. Carcinoma oesophagus (Fig. 21.6)
3. Oesophageal diverticulum

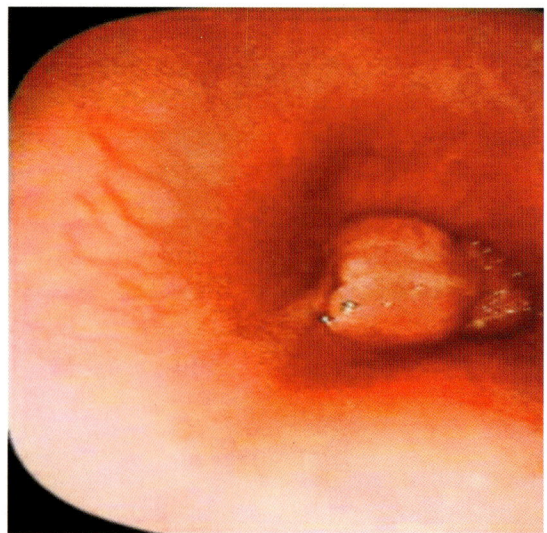

Fig. 21.5: Carcinoma GE junction in Barrett's oesophagus

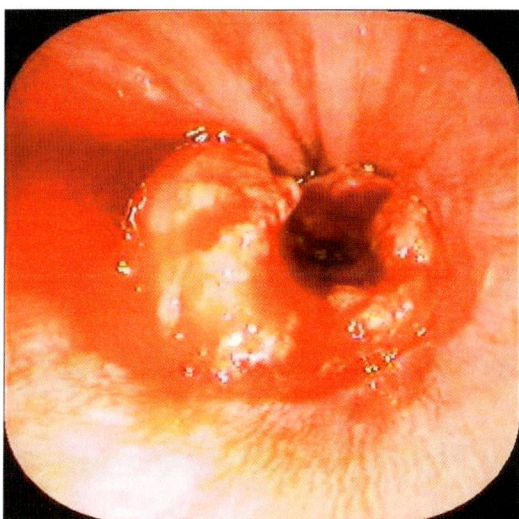

Fig. 21.6: Advanced carcinoma of GE junction

4. *Muscular spasm*: Plummer-Vinson syndrome and achalasia cardia.

5. Tetanus

III. Causes in the Lumen of Oesophagus

Foreign body: Dentures, coins, chicken bone, etc.

DIFFERENTIAL DIAGNOSIS

1. Carcinoma oesophagus: Typically, a male about 50–60 years old, emaciated who complains of dysphagia first to solids and later for liquids. It is progressive and painless. He frequently may be spitting in the outpatient department. He may complain of constipation. On examination, he has lost weight, thin built. Skin wrinkles are present. Left supraclavicular node, and palpable liver which is nodular, are typical findings indicating advanced nature of the disease. As a rule, growth is not palpable per abdomen. Oesophagoscopy followed by biopsy will clinch the diagnosis. It is treated by surgery (for adenocarcinoma), radio-therapy (for squamous cell carcinoma) and both in a few selected patients. Prognosis is poor (Figs 21.7 to 21.9). Neo-adjuvant chemoradiation is given in Stage III disease wherein serosa is involved with lymph nodes. This is followed by oesophagectomy.

2. Achalasia cardia: Typically, a young patient who complains of dysphagia for liquids than solids of many months to years duration. Patient has significant weight loss in the recent times. Recurrent aspirations, mouthful regurgitation is common. Barium swallow shows a large dilated oesophagus. Oesophagoscopy shows dilated oesophagus with fluid contents. Biopsy is required because achalasia can give rise to carcinoma oesophagus. Balloon dilatation/Heller's cardiomyotomy/Lap Heller's myotomy are the treatment options available as per the expertise of the treating surgeon. Antireflux procedure can be added (Fig. 21.10).

3. Paterson-Kelly syndrome: It is also called Plummer-Vinson syndrome. It is a precancerous condition in which there is a severe spasm of circular muscle fibres at the cricopharyngeal sphincter level or pharyngo-oesophageal junction, and it is

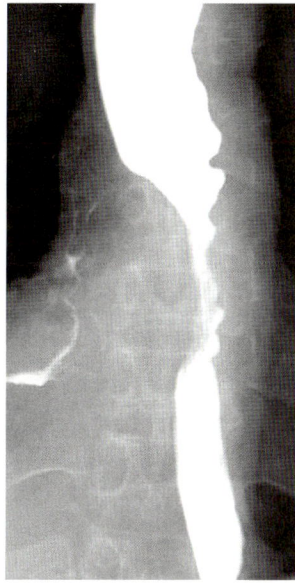

Fig. 21.7: Barium swallow—carcinoma middle oesophagus

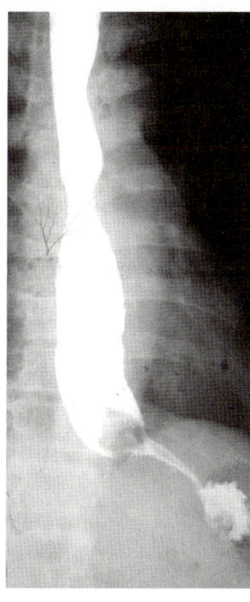

Fig. 21.8: Carcinoma lower end of the oesophagus. Observe proximal shouldering

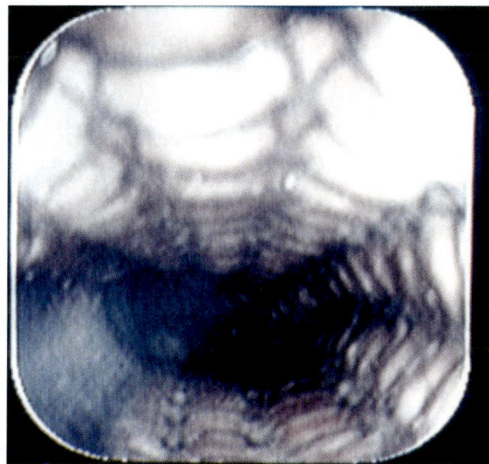

Fig. 21.9: Expandable stent as palliative treatment

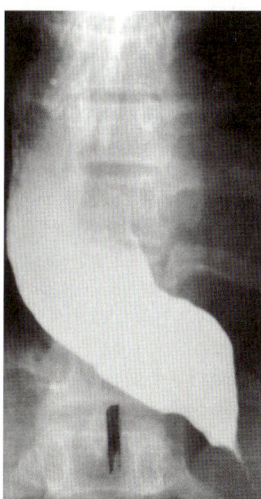

Fig. 21.10: Barium swallow showing sigmoid oesophagus

associated with **development of postcricoid web.** Women in the middle age group are affected. Worries and anxiety may precipitate the condition.

As a result of the spasm and web, dysplasia occurs and leads to features of anaemia later. The proximal mucosa is constantly irritated due to stasis. It undergoes hypertrophy, hyperkeratosis and desquamation. This, over a period of years, predisposes to carcinoma oesophagus (carcinoma oropharynx). They have increasing **dysphagia** for solids and liquids due to spasm. Features of **anaemia** such as pallor, stomatitis, ulcerations, bald tongue (without papillae), koilonychia, splenomegaly and microcytic hypochromic anaemia are also present. As a result of obstruction, the fluid tends to spillover into the larynx giving rise to recurrent aspiration, respiratory tract infection, cyanosis or choking. It is treated by reassurance, improving anaemia with iron tablets or blood transfusion and correction of nutritional deficiencies. Regular dilatation by using gum elastic bougies has to be done. Women in the middle age group are affected.

4. *Corrosive strictures*: Very often patients are young between 20 and 40 years of age who have consumed corrosive acids and alkalis. The agents are sodium hydroxide, sulphuric acid, and household bleach. In acute cases, severe pain, drooling of saliva, inability to swallow, retrosternal burning, abdominal guarding and rigidity can occur. Other features include hoarseness, stridor, and laryngeal oedema, if there is laryngeal injury. Dysphagia occurs later due to stricture. Diagnosis is established by endoscopy and, if necessary, biopsy. Treatment is by dilatation and later oesophagectomy and gastric pull up (Fig. 21.11).

5. *Gastro-oesophageal reflux disease (GORD/GERD)*: Patients are middle aged who complain of regurgitation, heartburn, retrosternal burning, etc. Sliding hernias produce dysphagia due to lower oesophageal ulcers as a result of recurrent reflux disease. GORD can also produce dysphagia due to lower oesophageal strictures (Fig. 21.12) and carcinoma. Barrett's oesophagus is a columnar lined lower oesophagus due to reflux disease (Fig. 21.13). It is a precancerous condition. *Paraoesophageal type of hiatus hernia can produce dysphagia due to extraluminal compression by the hernial sac on the oesophagus.* Treatment of GORD is complicated—change in lifestyle, proton pump inhibitors, and laparoscopic fundoplication are the choices available. (More details are given in the Manipal Manual of Surgery, 4th edition).

6. *Rare causes (rings, slings and webs)*

   A. **Oesophageal ring: Schatzki's ring:** It is located at the squamocolumnar junction with oesophageal squamous epithelium above and columnar epithelium below. There is a concentric symmetrical narrowing with restricted distensibility of lower oesophagus. It presents as *dysphagia and episodic aphagia*. Diagnosis is by barium oesophagography. It is treated by repeated bougie dilatation. The *cause is obscure* but there is *strong association* with *reflux disease*. Many rings are incidental findings in radiology. They do not have any symptoms.

   B. **Vascular slings and pulmonary artery slings:** It is also called **dysphagia lusoria.** It occurs due to developmental anomalies of great vessels causing dysphagia. More common is aortic arch anomaly wherein the right subclavian artery arising from the descending aorta travels

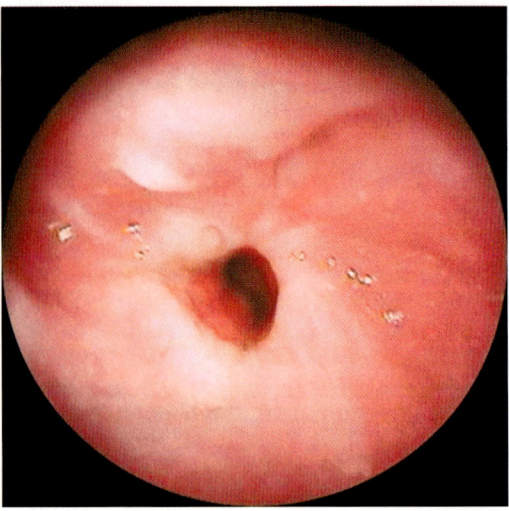

Fig. 21.11: Oesophageal narrowing of lower end

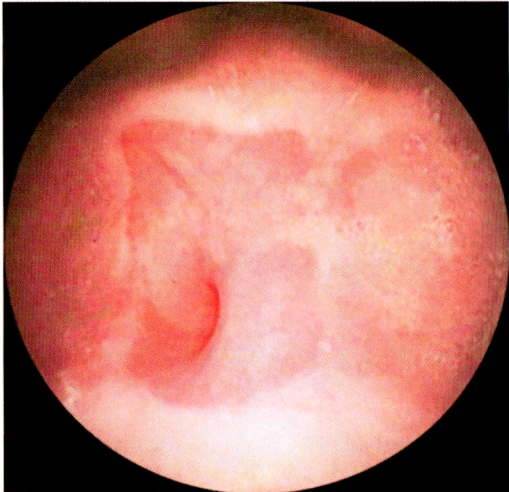

Fig. 21.12: Barrett's oesophagus with stricture

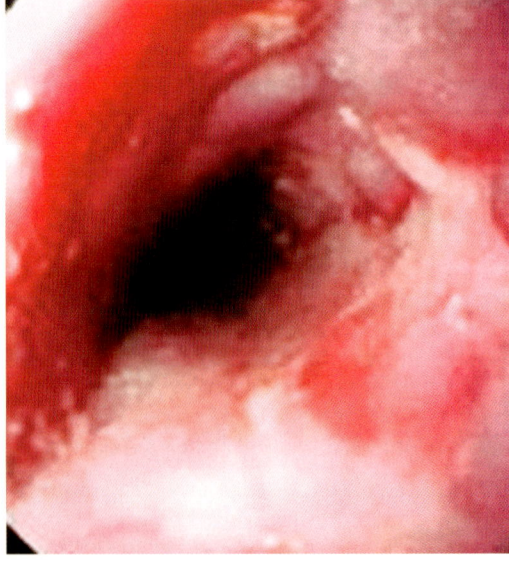

Fig. 21.13: Endoscopic view of reflux oesophagitis

behind oesophagus creating an incomplete vascular ring (to complete the course). Pulmonary artery sling is due to left pulmonary artery arising from right pulmonary artery causing anterior compression of oesophagus.

C. *Webs*: Oesophageal webs are uncommon causes of dysphagia. They are treated by oesophageal dilatation.

7. *Oesophageal atresia*: The diagnosis is established at birth when a child has abundance of saliva in the mouth which bubbles out from the mouth. Atresia of the oesophagus with tracheo-oesophageal fistula (TOF) at the lower end is the commonest anomaly. Newborn baby regurgitates all feeds. Aspiration, cough and cyanosis are other features. It is commonly associated with maternal hydramnios (50%). TOF should be recognised and diagnosed within 24 hours of birth—by introducing a red rubber catheter. It is managed by right thoracotomy, ligation of TOF and primary anastomosis of oesophageal ends.

> ***Associated anomalies—remember as VACTER***
>
> **V**: Vertebral defects
> **A**: Anorectal malformation
> **C**: Cardiac defect (PDA/VSD)
> **TE**: Tracheo-oesophageal fistula
> **R**: Radial hypoplasia and renal agenesis

8. *Zenker's diverticulum*: Pharyngeal pouch is the other name. It is a cervical diverticulum proximal to the upper oesophageal sphincter. It is the commonest type of diverticulum. In this condition, protrusion of oesophageal mucosa between cricopharyngeus muscle inferiorly and thyropharyngeus muscle superiorly occurs. It is also called pulsion diverticulum. It is acquired diverticulum, more common in men between the age group of 40 and 50 years. As the pouch enlarges, it will compress on oesophagus and give rise to dysphagia. When patient is asked to take food, mainly liquids, pouch may show enlargement with some gurgling noise. It can present with regurgitation of meals, aspiration of food contents into the lungs, suffocation or recurrent respiratory tract infections. Regurgitation of food particles may occur after turning to one side and it is a typical symptom. It is treated by excision of the sac and repair of the defect along with cricopharyngeal myotomy—posterior midline.

9. *Nut cracker oesophagus*: Aetiology is not known. Chest pain is the most common symptom followed by dysphagia. Barium swallow is usually normal. An epinephric diverticulum is usually present. Majority of the patients have normal propagation of peristaltic waves. However, in the distal oesophagus, peristaltic waves have **very high amplitude (>180 mmHg)** and duration (>6 seconds). Dilatation, myotomy, proton pump inhibitors, and calcium channel blockers are used with limited success.

10. *Scleroderma*: In this condition, due to fibrous replacement of the oesophagus, oesophagus loses the tone of the muscles and motor disturbances occur resulting in dysphagia. It is a chronic *systemic autoimmune disease* characterised by hardening (*sclero*) of the skin (*derma*). Strong associations with certain mutations in *HLA* genes have been identified. CREST syndrome refer to calcinosis cutis, Raynaud's phenomenon, oesophageal dysfunction, sclerodactyly and telangiectasis.

MEDIASTINAL MASSES

These are also the unusual causes of dysphagia in surgical wards (Figs 21.14 to 21.16). They can be thymoma, lymphoma (mediastinal), and neural tumours. In a plain X-ray, the mediastinal mass can be seen as **'pseudotumours'**. Aortic aneurysm, cold abscess (paravertebral), and scoliosis are a few pseudotumours seen on chest X-ray.

- In case of mediastinal lymphoma, mediastinal mass ratio (MMR) is calculated.

- MMR is defined as the ratio of maximum transverse diameter of mediastinal mass to the maximum transverse intrathoracic diameter. MMR greater than 0.33 by chest X-ray or 0.35 by CT scan predicts a bad prognosis.

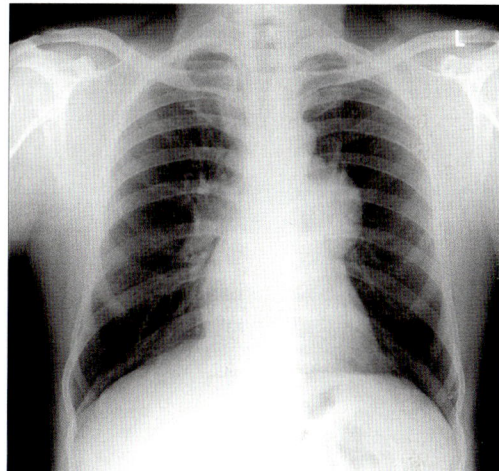

Fig. 21.14: Chest X-ray pseudotumour

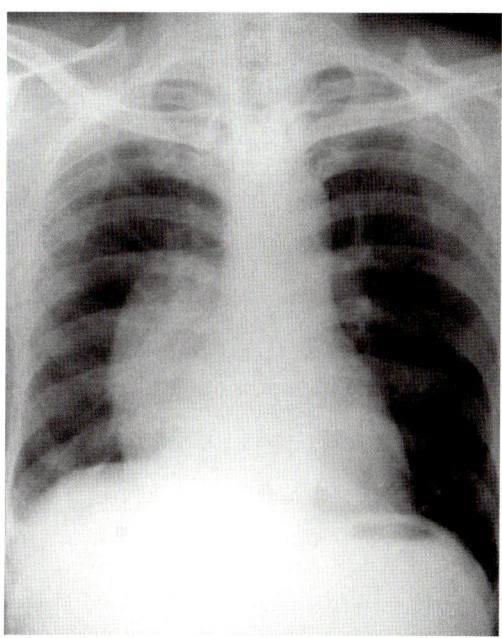

Fig. 21.15: Mediastinal mass—thymoma

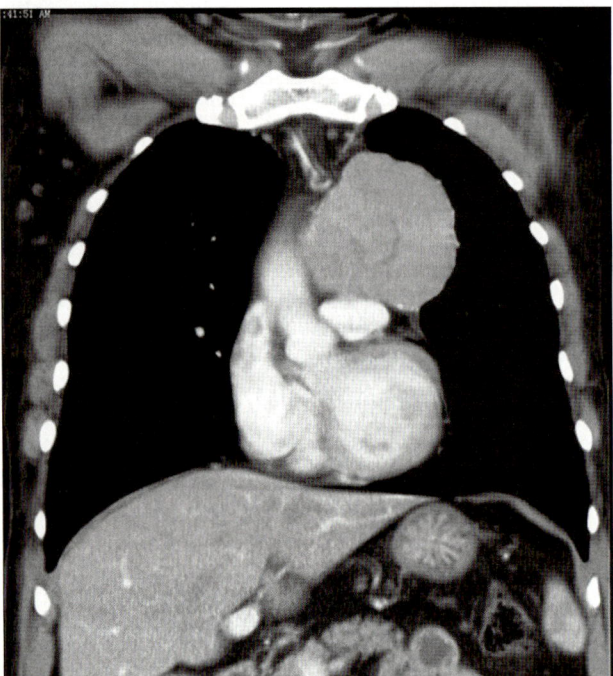

Fig. 21.16: Thymoma CT scan findings

Clinical Case Capsule

1. *Interesting case of dysphagia*: A 45-year-old lady complained of backache of 30 days duration. It was low backache and various causes of backache were investigated. X-ray thoracolumbar spine was normal. It was treated with analgesics and local application of ointments. However, after a few days, she complained of dysphagia which worsened to odynophagia within 10 days. Gastroenterologist did the gastroscopy and he saw a few ulcers in the oesophagus. He took biopsy and asked for CT thorax. CT thorax revealed a few lymph nodes compressing the oesophagus. Incidentally, it showed destruction of thoracic 9th and 10th vertebrae. Biopsy of the oesophageal ulcers was reported as granulomas. ESR was asked for. It was 110. Diagnosis of tuberculosis was made. With antituberculous treatment, all symptoms disappeared and patient was back to normal activities.

2. A 60-year-old agriculturist was referred to the department of ENT for dysphagia of 3–4 days duration. A registrar who saw the case did rigid oesophagoscopy under GA. The findings were normal. Later in the evening, he was called to see this patient who had rigid abdomen. A general surgeon was consulted. He suspected a perforation. An X-ray abdomen (erect), however, was normal. A senior faculty surgeon was consulted who examined the case properly and gave a correct diagnosis. It was a case of tetanus with mild trismus. The patient had injured his left thumb a few days back. The anaesthesiologist acknowledged later that there was some difficulty in opening the patient's mouth during endotracheal intubation. Occasionally, patients undergo gastroscopy for dysphagia which will be normal only to realise later that what he is having is a stroke.

3. A 55-year-old lady presented to the hospital with a history of dysphagia of 30 days duration. Clinical examination of the neck revealed large lymph nodes. It was a case of Hodgkin's lymphoma. The dysphagia was due to enlargement of mediastinal lymph nodes (Fig. 21.17).

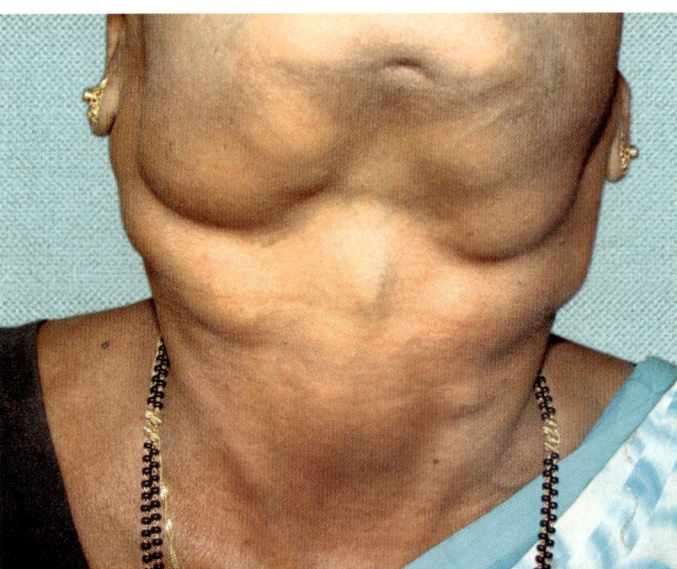

Fig. 21.17: Hodgkin's lymphoma with cervical lymph nodes and she also had large mediastinal lymph nodes

Examination of an Acute Abdomen

Happy is he who has no serious consequences of his erroneous diagnosis to regret.

—*Marsh*

INTRODUCTION

Acute abdomen can be defined as an emergency condition of the abdomen which presents as acute severe abdominal pain which lasts for 6–12 hours. It often requires emergency intervention in the form of surgery or medical management. It is one of the most common surgical emergencies a surgeon encounters. It is often first seen by a family physician who refers the patient to hospital. Vast majority of the causes are benign—hence curable.

However, the diagnosis is challenging and requires thorough knowledge and clinical acumen. Early cases can be managed successfully with reduced mortality and morbidity. Late cases have up to 8–10% mortality and carry significant morbidity. Pain is the most common symptom for which patient rushes to hospital.

Diagnosis is established by laboratory investigations and imaging. With advances in the investigations, majority of the cases can be diagnosed and treated properly.

Clinical Wisdom

Acute abdomen and sudden collapse (haemodynamic instability)
- Acute pancreatitis
- Aortic dissection
- Acute mesenteric ischaemia
- Ruptured ectopic gestation

■ **Clinical Case Capsule**

An 18-year-old boy who had severe pain in the right iliac fossa and tenderness over the McBurney point was diagnosed to have acute appendicitis. He was operated upon and the appendix was removed. The boy continued to have severe pain which prompted the surgeon to get an ultrasound of the abdomen which revealed torsion in an undescended testis. Nobody had examined the testis. This one case report depicts several pitfalls by the surgeon in the clinical examination of an acute abdomen such as history was not taken properly—no checklist was used, no analytical power, did not use common sense, did not use the most common, useful and non invasive test—ultrasound and no clinical wisdom. He has not examined the 10th quadrant of the abdomen (testis).

PATIENT'S DATA

Age: Neonatal intestinal obstruction is a known entity and the causes are many. Examples: Imperforate anus, Hirschsprung's disease, atresia, bands and adhesions, volvulus and malrotation of the gut. Younger children may present with ileal obstruction due to roundworm bolus obstruction. School going boys may have Meckel's diverticulum with a band, and adult patients may be having acute appendicitis. Perforation of duodenal ulcer is common between the age group 20 and 40 years. Gallbladder diseases are common after 40 years of age.

Mesenteric ischaemia, sigmoid volvulus, and carcinoma colon occur after 40–50 years of age.

Sex: Perforated duodenal ulcer and acute pancreatitis are common in men. On the other hand, acute cholecystitis and adhesions are common in women. Some important conditions that present as acute abdomen in women are ruptured ectopic pregnancy, severe pelvic peritonitis, bilateral salpingo-oophoritis, and twisted/torsion of ovarian cyst.

Place/native: In Punjab, acute cholecystitis and volvulus are common. Peptic ulcer perforations are common in Southern India. Chronic pancreatitis is common in the South Indian state Kerala (consumption of tapioca). In Nigeria, intussusception is common and remember haemolytic crisis and sickle cell anaemia in Blacks.

Occupation: People working in paint and watch industries are vulnerable for lead poisoning—lead colic.

COMPLAINTS—HISTORY OF PRESENT ILLNESS

1. *Abdominal pain*: When did it start and how is it now? Is it sudden in onset? Is it more or less or increasing now? What is the type? Is it unbearable? Show the site of pain (Fig. 22.1). Do you have any other symptoms such as vomiting or fever? These are the common questions to be asked. Interestingly abdominal pain cannot be measured unlike temperature and pressure but the severity, radiation and referral to a distant region, past experience, extent of suffering will help in the diagnosis. There may be variations in the descriptions given by the patient. *Example*: Cutting is the word used by a few patients who describe the pain of pancreatitis. What they mean is that it is a severe and sharp pain.

   - Sudden onset of pain occurs in perforation, volvulus, torsion. Slowly developing pain in young patients and presenting in the early morning suggests colic due to appendicitis. Severe abdominal pain in a fatty lady which

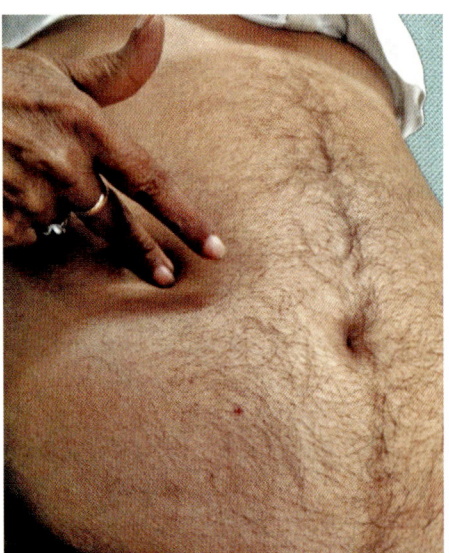

Fig. 22.1: Patient shows the exact site of pain

started after lying down can be due to acute cholecystitis.

- Ask him to show the site of pain. He will show the site. It can be typical as in acute appendicitis wherein he will point at McBurney point. Pointing at right hypochondrium may suggest acute cholecystitis or amoebic liver abscess. Pointing in the epigastric region suggests pancreatitis or gastric perforations.

- How is it now compared to yesterday or to begin with? Colicky pain of intestinal obstruction will become burning when there is strangulation. Pain may diminish to some extent after vomiting as in cases of obstruction but it restarts again later.

- Does it become worse on any posture? Pain of pancreatitis and to some extent mesenteric ischaemia become better with bending forward (Fig. 22.2).

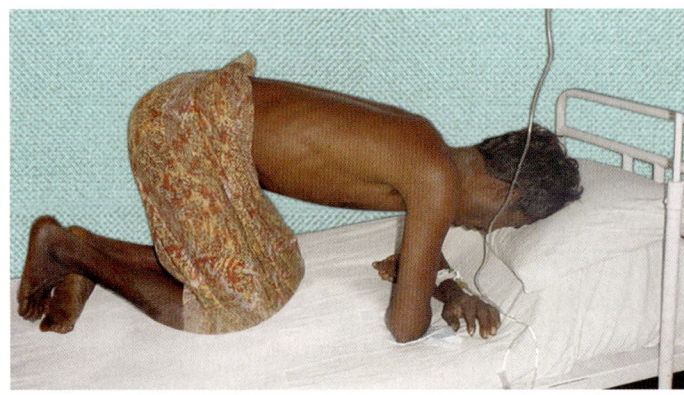

Fig. 22.2: Posture of the patient. He had mesenteric ischaemia

- Any movement of the abdomen will worsen the pain of peritonitis. Such patients prefer to lie down flat. *Examples*: Perforated duodenal ulcer, gastric ulcer or appendicular perforation with peritonitis, etc.

- On the other hand, patients with ureteric colic can never lie down. The intensity of pain is so severe that these patients keep on moving here and there and they just do not know what to do.

- Different types of pain are given in Clinical Box 22.1.

A. **Dull aching pain:** It suggests a solid organ enlargement. It is a continuous pain felt in the anatomical location of the swelling. Patients often describe it as a discomfort rather than pain. *Examples:*

Clinical Box 22.1

Different types of pain
- Colicky — Hollow viscus
- Dull ache — Solid organs
- Referred — Dermatomes
- Radiating — Along the nerve
- Postprandial — Abdominal angina
- Shifting — Hollow viscus (colicky) to parietal peritoneum

- *Liver enlargement*: They have pain in the right hypochondrium. It occurs due to stretching of parietal capsule (Glisson) (Fig. 22.3A). In cases of amoebic liver abscess or hepatoma, there will be dull aching pain in the right hypochondrium. Typically, pain is aggravated on movements such as jumping or jolting.

- *Renal enlargement*: Pain in the back and costal region is called costovertebral pain (Fig. 22.3B). Patients with ureteric colic with hydronephrosis have this complaint in addition to the severe loin to groin pain.

B. Colicky pain suggests hollow viscus obstruction. It is sudden and severe and often unbearable. This pain is due to hyperperistalsis. It is severe and intermittent (comes and goes). Each attack may last for 5–10 minutes. The patient bends on himself, holds the abdomen and puts pressure on the abdomen which gives some kind of relief. Being visceral type of pain, it is not very well localised. Following are a few examples:

- Intestinal obstruction is the most common example. Pain is centrally located in small intestinal obstruction and peripherally located in large bowel obstruction.

- Ureteric colic and biliary colic (Fig. 22.3C) are severe colics with typical characteristics.

C. Referred pain: Is the pain referred to any other site? The pain originates in one area and manifests in a different area. This is because of the same segmental nerve supply of these two organs/anatomical locations. Tuberculosis of spine (Pott's spine) is a common problem in India. Often patients present with iliopsoas abscess. Patients complain of referred pain in the lower abdomen (Fig. 22.4). The referred pain is due to the irritation of the corresponding nerve root by the collapse of the vertebrae. On the right side, it can mimic acute appendicitis and many appendices have been removed erroneously. When diaphragm is irritated by exudate (peritonitis fluid, acute cholecystitis), blood (haemoperitoneum), pus (subphrenic abscess), or bile (biliary peritonitis), pain is referred to the shoulder region. This is because the diaphragm is supplied by phrenic nerve (cervical—C3, 4 and 5—main nerve supply comes from C4) and shoulder region is supplied by supraclavicular nerves (cervical 3 and 4 cutaneous nerves). In ureteric colic, typically pain is felt in the loin and it is referred to the groin and genitalia—testis in males and labia in females. It is due to irritation of the genitofemoral nerve (root value—lumbar L1 and L2).

D. Radiating pain: Acute pancreatitis and carcinoma pancreas present often as pain radiating to the back. It is due to retroperitoneal nerve plexus irritation in acute pancreatitis and due to infiltration of the nerve plexus by carcinoma pancreas. Typically the pain has been described

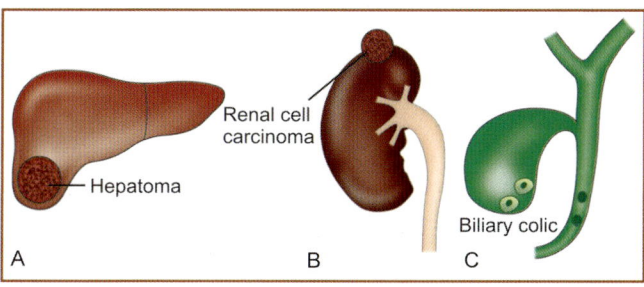

Figs 22.3A to C: Source of the pain

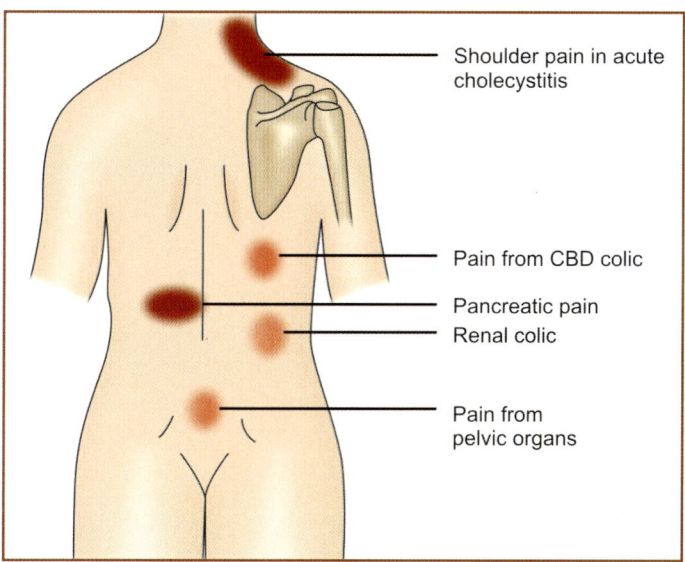

Fig. 22.4: Referred pain (posterior view)

as illimitable agony. Patient bends forward and attains a flexion position.

E. Postprandial pain: It is characteristic of mesenteric ischaemia. It is also called **abdominal angina.** Mesenteric ischaemia is one condition which presents as severe abdominal pain with haemodynamic instability very early, within a few hours of the presentation. **There may not be any abdominal findings.** They may give history of postprandial pain which appears after a few hours of food. Within a few hours, patients can develop septic shock and acidosis.

F. Shifting pain: This is characteristic of acute appendicitis. Pain is severe, colicky type, initially felt in the umbilical region and it is due to distension of appendix. This is a visceral pain. After a few hours, the pain localises to the right iliac fossa. It is a somatic pain which is due to inflammation of parietal peritoneum. This is called shifting pain of acute appendicitis (Fig. 22.5). This is also called **migratory pain—** most reliable symptom of acute appendicitis.

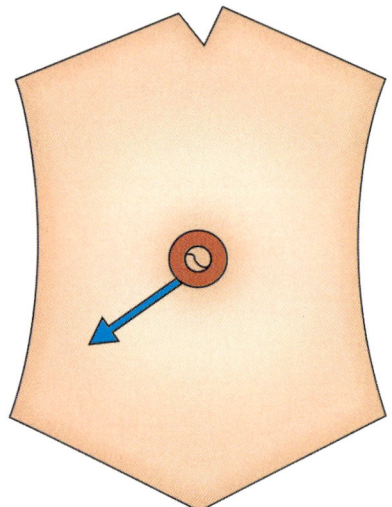

Fig. 22.5: Shifting pain (migratory pain)—most reliable symptom of acute appendicitis

2. *Vomiting:* In almost all cases of acute abdomen, vomiting is a feature. It occurs due to reflex pylorospasm. One or two vomiting episodes is a feature of acute appendicitis, acute cholecystitis and ureteric colic. Frequent and persistent vomiting is a feature of acute intestinal obstruction.

- Persistent, profuse, projectile, bilious vomiting indicates obstruction below the level of ampulla of Vater. For example, intestinal obstruction due to ileocaecal tuberculosis, stricture of the small bowel, adhesions (pain is severe and colicky). Vomiting of bilious contents with no pain or mild pain indicates high jejunal or duodenal obstruction.

- Faeculent vomiting is characteristic feature of terminal ileal obstruction. **Faeculent does not mean faecal matter.** It is terminal ileal contents which have been degraded due to **stasis and bacteria resulting in smell of faecal matter.**

- Coffee ground vomitus and peritonitis is suggestive of perforated duodenal ulcer.

3. *Fever:* Fever suggests inflammatory condition. Acute appendicitis, acute diverticulitis, and acute cholecystitis are a few examples. Low grade fever indicates inflammation. High grade fever indicates sepsis, e.g. gangrenous bowel or pancreatic necrosis. High grade fever with chills and rigors indicates urinary tract infection—common in women. High grade fever with jaundice indicates cholangitis (inflammation of the biliary radicles). Amoebic liver abscess is another example of acute abdomen with fever associated with chills and rigors.

Clinical Wisdom

Pain first, followed by vomiting and then by fever is called Murphy's triad of symptoms of acute appendicitis (Murphy's syndrome).

---

4. *Abdominal distension:* This is a common symptom in all cases of acute abdomen. Distension is what patient tells you "Doctor, my tummy is tight now". This is how abdominal distension can be differentiated from protuberant abdomen. Distension may be significant in cases of intestinal obstruction. Distension is due to accumulation of normal contents of the gastrointestinal tract, due to swallowing of lot of air or due to paralytic ileus as in cases of perforation or gangrene of bowel. In perforation peritonitis, significant fluid accumulates in the peritoneal cavity (3rd space loss) resulting in abdominal distension in addition to the factors mentioned above (Fig. 22.6).

Clinical Wisdom

If fever has started first and then acute abdomen (may be tenderness and guarding), it may be a medical problem. Medical causes of an acute abdomen should be ruled out.

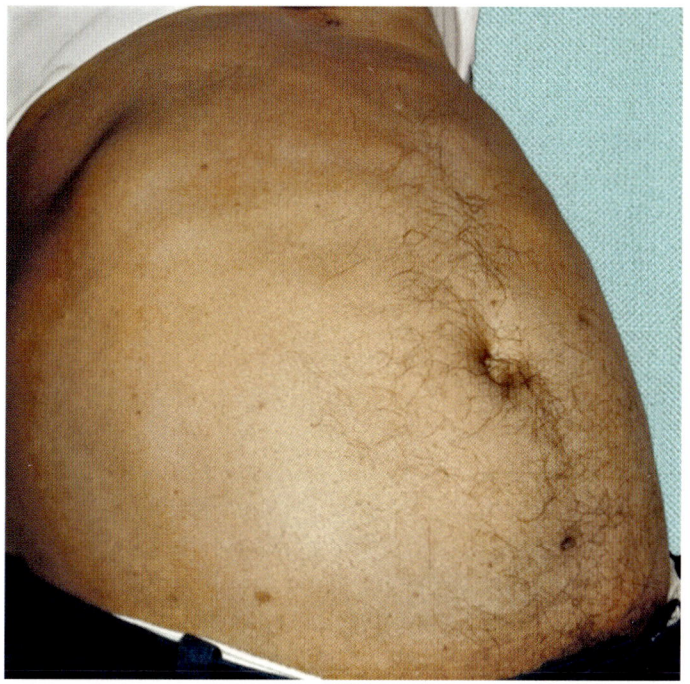

Fig. 22.6: Case of acute pancreatitis—36 hours following abdominal pain. You can see distension of the abdomen

5. *Constipation:* Failure to pass stools is a feature in cases of intestinal obstruction. Initially only stool may be passed but later neither stools nor flatus is passed. Failure to pass stools and flatus has been described as obstipation. Paralytic ileus also adds to constipation and distension of the abdomen. **Rectosigmoid growths are notorious in presenting as intestinal obstruction.**

6. *Bleeding per rectum/loose stools*

   • Acute abdomen with bleeding per rectum indicates a few conditions such as mesenteric ischaemia, ischaemic colitis, ulcerative colitis with toxic megacolon, etc.

   • In cases of mesenteric ischaemia with gangrene, there will be bleeding with putrid stools.

   • Significant blood loss can occur in cases of ischaemic colitis and inflammatory bowel diseases.

   • Blood and mucus with acute abdomen in a child is due to acute ileocolic intussusception.

   • Loose stools before acute abdomen can occur in intestinal tuberculosis. Mucus discharge is also a feature. Patients with amoebic liver abscess may give history of loose stools with blood (dysentery).

   • Patients with enteric ulcers with or without perforation can have bleeding per rectum.

7. *Jaundice:* Intermittent pain, intermittent fever and intermittent jaundice have been called Charcot's triad. It suggests stone in the common bile duct. If above three symptoms are associated with shock and altered mental status, it is called **Reynold's pentad**.

8. *Anorexia:* How is your appetite? Anorexia is an important feature in cases of acute appendicitis.

9. *Micturition:* What is the colour of the urine? Do you have burning micturition? What is the frequency? Ureteric colic is associated with passage of frank red blood in the urine. More details are given in examination of urinary case. However, passage of faecal matter or air (pneumaturia) suggests hollow viscus fistula as in Crohn's disease.

10. *Weight loss:* Significant weight loss in patients who present with acute abdomen suggests underlying diseases such as malignancy, tuberculosis or lymphoma. Acute abdominal pain, vomiting, low grade fever and weight loss in young patients are classical features of intestinal tuberculosis. On the other hand, in middle-aged or elderly patients, such symptoms with or without fever may be due to carcinoma caecum or lymphoma.

> Carcinoma colon and carcinoma stomach can present with acute abdomen due to perforation.

Personal History

Habits, such as smoking and hypertension, may be a factor for mesenteric ischaemia. Missed periods in a woman may suggest ruptured ectopic pregnancy presenting as abdominal pain, hypotension and shock.

Past History

• *History of recurrent upper abdominal pain* in a fatty woman may be due to gallstone pancreatitis and in alcoholic male patients, due to alcoholic pancreatitis.

• *History of surgery:* Specially lower abdominal—cases of hysterectomy, caesarean sections, and pelvic peritonitis are more prone for adhesions and intestinal obstruction.

• Recurrent colicky abdominal pain and vomiting suggest **stones, strictures or chronic intussusception.**

GENERAL PHYSICAL EXAMINATION (GPE)

- Look for Hippocratic facies (Clinical Box 22.2).
- Examine the entire patient and you may get the clue to the diagnosis (Clinical Box 22.3).
- Is he anxious? Is he drowsy? Is he in agony? Is he breathing rapidly?
- They will have an anxious look in peritonitis.
- The patient lies flat without any movement, e.g. peritonitis.
- They are drowsy in septic shock.

Clinical Box 22.2

Hippocratic facies
- Hollow, bright eyes
- Pale and pinched face
- Cold perspiration in the head and brows
- Blue lips
- Dry, cracked tongue

Clinical Box 22.3

GPE and acute abdomen (Figs 22.7 to 22.14)
- *Coated tongue*: Acute appendicitis, acute pancreatitis
- *Anaemia, malnutrition*: Chronic illness, blood loss, colonic cancer
- *Melanin spots*: Peutz-Jeghers syndrome and adult intussusception
- *Jaundice*: Acute pancreatitis, stones in the CBD
- *Arthritis, purpuric spots*: Henoch's purpura, intussusception
- *Blue line on gum*: Lead colic
- *Hypertension*: Ruptured aneurysm, SMA thrombosis
- *Irregular pulse*: SMA thrombosis
- *Hypotension, collapse*: Ruptured ectopic pregnancy, dissection of aorta, massive gangrene with septic shock
- *Cervical lymph nodes*: Tuberculosis, lymphoma
- *Spine tenderness, deformity*: Pott's spine (Tb spine)
- Preherpetic vesicles–can be confused for acute cholecystitis

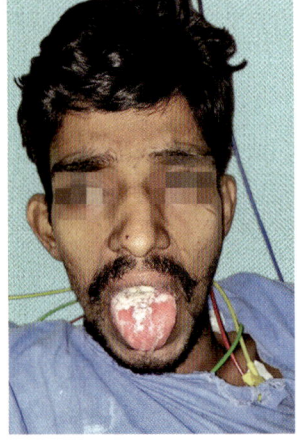

Fig. 22.7: Dry coated tongue in perforated appendicitis

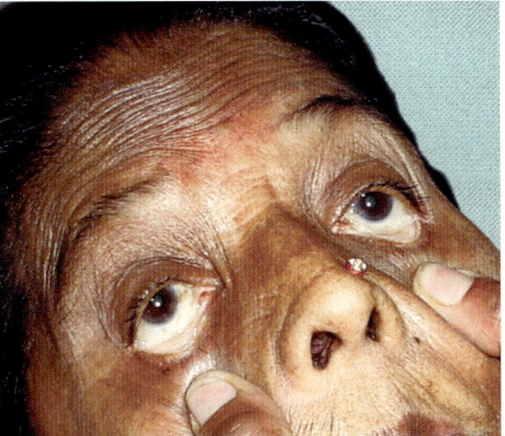

Fig. 22.8: Gross pallor in a 60-year-old lady. Examination revealed a mass in the right iliac fossa. It was proved later by colonoscopy as carcinoma caecum

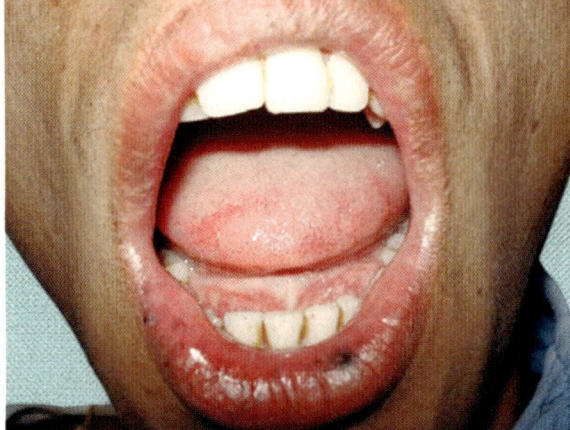

Fig: 22.9: Melanin pigment spots in the lips. This patient had presented with acute abdominal pain and a mass due to intussusception—case of Peutz-Jeghers syndrome

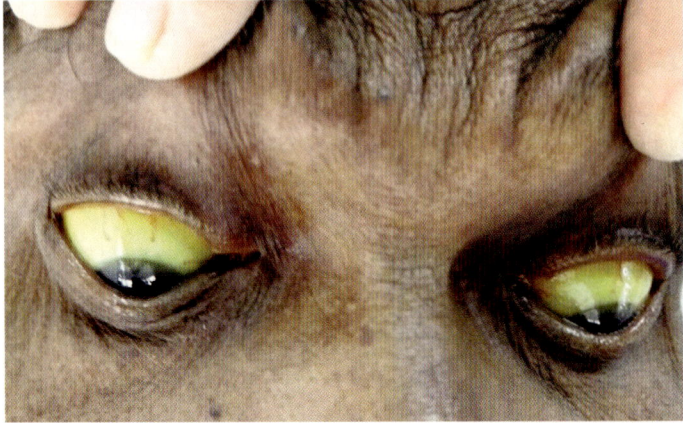

Fig. 22.10: Deep jaundice in a 65-year-old man who presented with cholangitis due to periampullary carcinoma

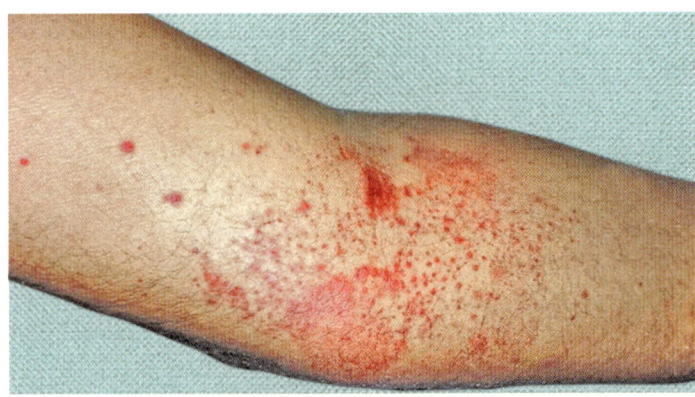

Fig: 22.11: A 32-year-old man with acute abdominal pain secondary to Henoch-Schönlein purpura

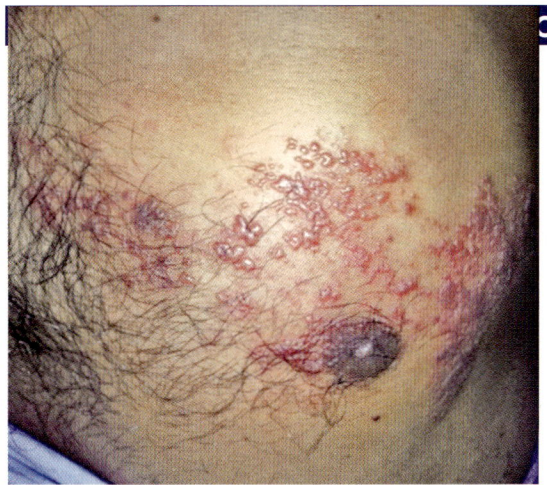

Fig: 22.12: Herpes zoster—preherpetic neuralgia causing lower chest and upper abdominal pain. Before the days of ultrasound, these cases were diagnosed as acute cholecystitis and even operated upon

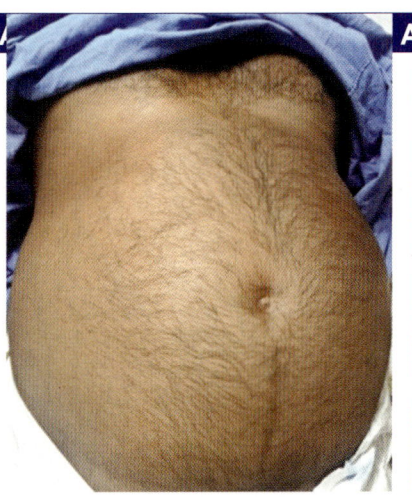

Fig: 22.13: Abdominal distension secondary to cervical spine fracture. Distension is due to paralytic ileus

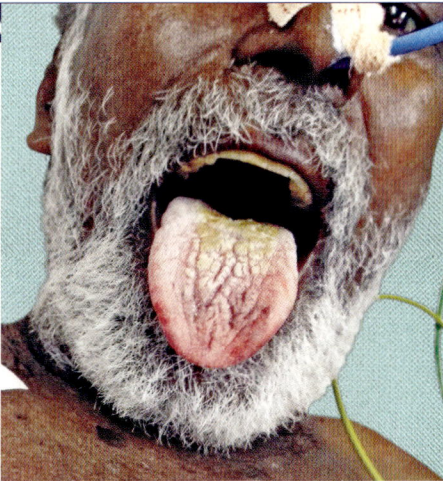

Fig: 22.14: Dry coated tongue of acute pancreatitis. Severe hypovolaemia and dehydration are the chief factors

ABDOMINAL EXAMINATION—PER ABDOMEN

Inspection

Spend a few minutes and watch the abdomen for movement, distension, peristalsis, scars, deformed umbilicus and hernial orifices.

- In cases of peritonitis, there will not be movement of abdominal wall. The patient is quiet, prefers to just lie down and breathe slowly. Classical example of this is a perforated duodenal ulcer.

- Distension of the abdomen occurs within a few hours of peritonitis/intestinal obstruction due to accumulation of fluid and paralytic ileus (Figs 22.15 and 22.16). Gross localised distension of abdomen is a feature of sigmoid volvulus.

- Look for scars of previous laparotomy or laparoscopy. Such patients may be having intestinal obstruction (Fig. 22.17).

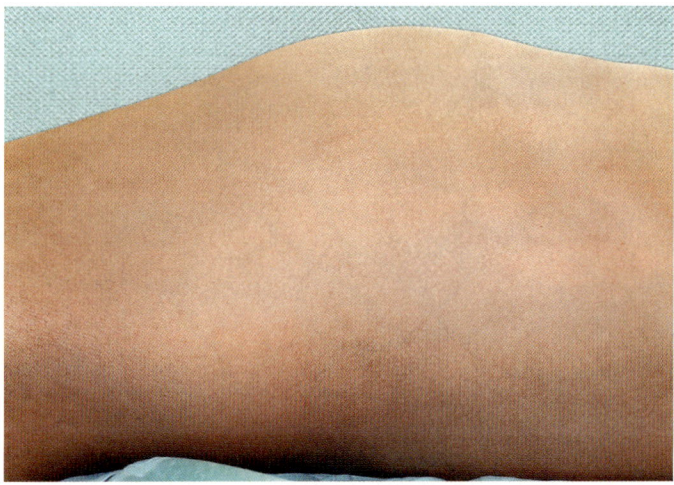

Fig. 22.16: Upper abdominal distension following acute pancreatitis

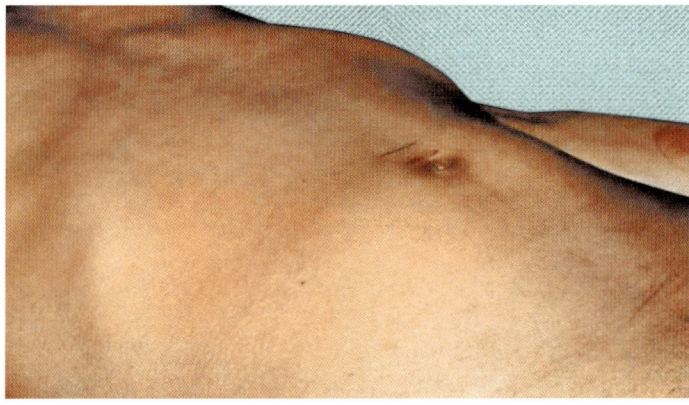

Fig. 22.15: Carefully look at central abdomen, watch for distension, prominent loop of intestines and peristalsis

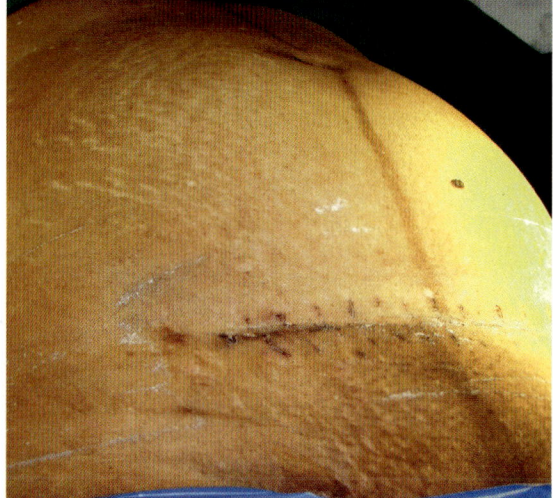

Fig. 22.17: Intestinal obstruction due to adhesions. You can see a transverse scar

- *Look for peristalsis*: Step-ladder peristalsis is seen in terminal ileal obstruction (Fig. 22.18). Right to left colonic peristalsis is seen in left-sided colonic obstruction, classically rectosigmoid obstructions. Visible gastric peristalsis indicates gastric outlet obstruction.

- Look at the hernial orifices, especially for a femoral and incisional hernia in females, inguinal hernia in males and other hernial sites such as Spigelian hernia, umbilical hernia or iliac bone graft sites (Figs 22.19 to 22.24).

- *Ask the patient to cough*: See if it hurts him. Cough tenderness indicates parietal peritoneal inflammation. On the right side, this is very reliable test to differentiate acute appendicitis from ureteric colic (Dunphy's sign) (Fig. 22.25).

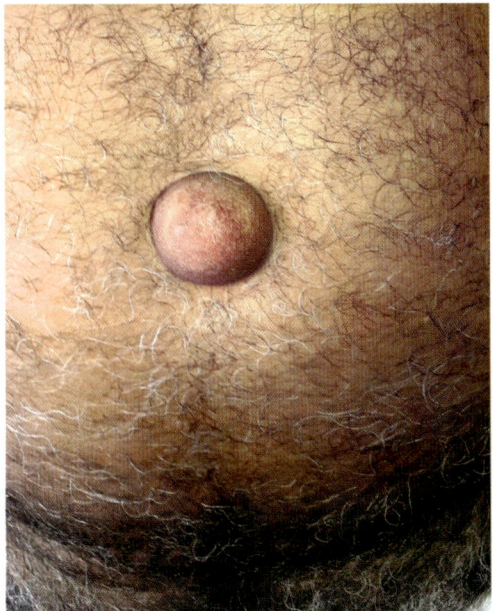

Fig. 22.19B: Obstructed umbilical hernia

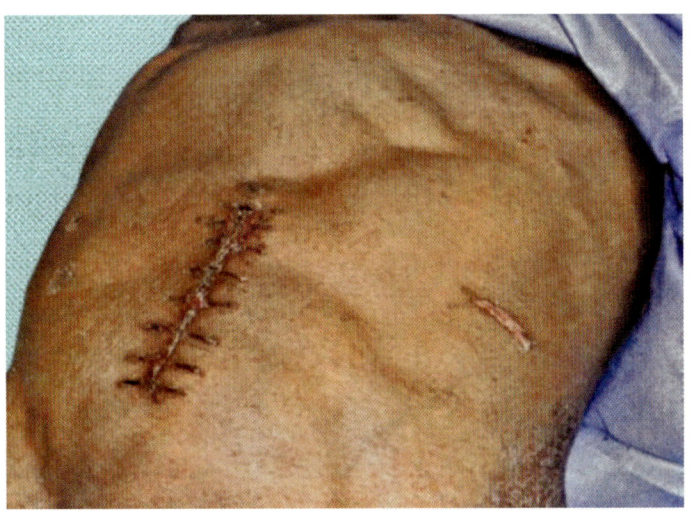

Fig. 22.18: Step-ladder peristalsis due to terminal ileal obstruction. Patient was misdiagnosed as acute appendicitis and appendicectomy was done—a case of ileocaecal tuberculosis

Palpation (Cinical Box 22.4) /Percussion

Look for specific tender spots which help clinch the diagnosis of acute abdominal pain

- *Murphy's point:* Just beneath the tip of the 9th costal cartilage in cases of acute cholecystitis (Fig. 22.26).

- *McBurney's point:* Junction of lateral one-third and medial two-thirds of spinoumbilical line (Fig. 22.27).

- Tenderness between 5th and 8th intercostal spaces—amoebic liver abscess (Figs 22.28A to C).

- Tenderness in the corresponding McBurney's point on the left side **Sir Philip Manson-Bahr amoebic point of tenderness** in acute amoebic dysentery (Fig. 22.29).

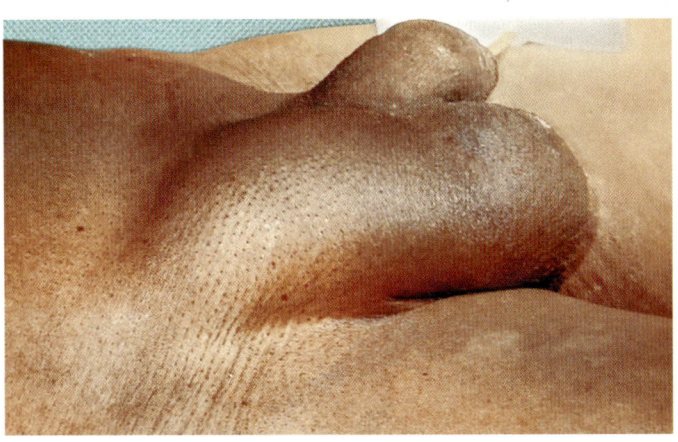

Fig. 22.19A: Obstructed inguinal hernia

Clinical Box 22.4

A few tips for palpation
- Ask the patient to show the maximum area of pain and start away from this region.
- Tell him what you are doing and tell him that you will not cause pain.
- Ask him to breathe well and relax the abdomen.
- Be gentle always.
- Palpate all 9 regions, look at hernial orifices including femoral hernia.
- Palpate testis—12th region.
- Palpate both loins for tenderness and bulge—10th and 11th regions.
- **Remember to examine 12 regions in the abdomen, not 9.**

LOOK FOR HERNIAL SITES

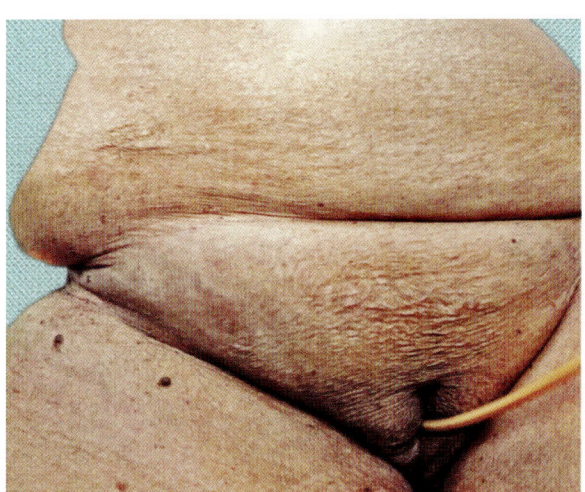

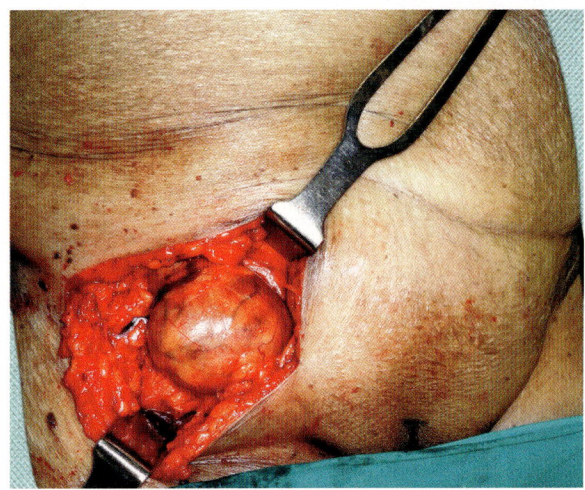

Fig. 22.20: Obstructed inguinal hernia **Fig. 22.21:** Hernial sac after opening (*Courtesy:* Dr Naveen, Associate Professor, KSHEMA, Mangalore)

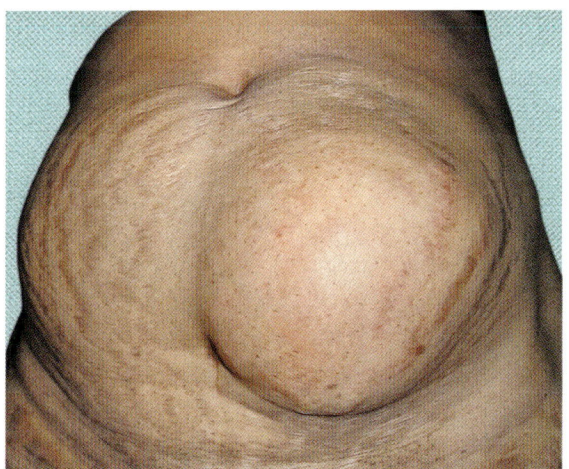

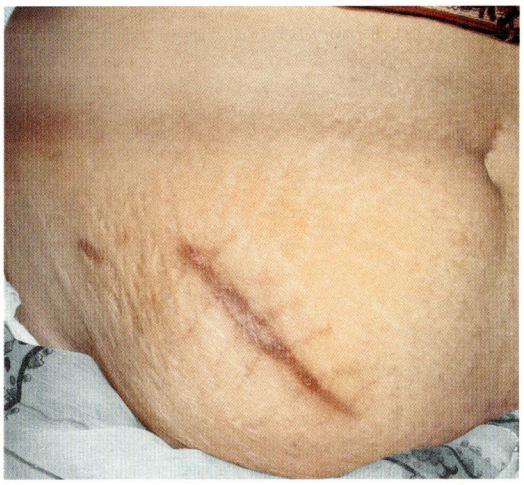

Fig. 22.22: Obstructed Spigelian hernia (*Courtesy:* Prof MG Shenoy, Ex-Professor of Surgery, KMC, Manipal)

Fig. 22.23: Obstructed incisional hernia through appendicectomy scar

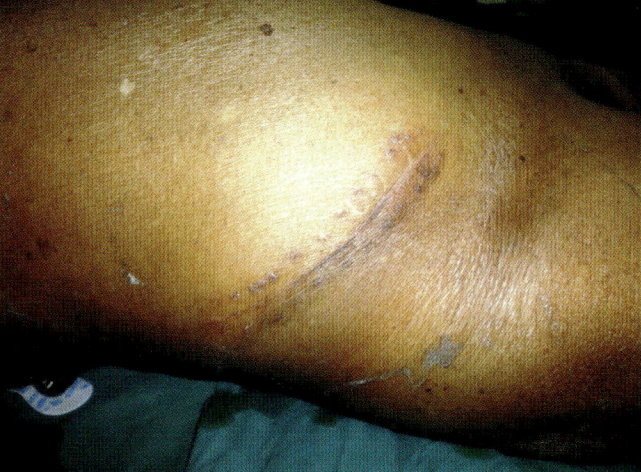

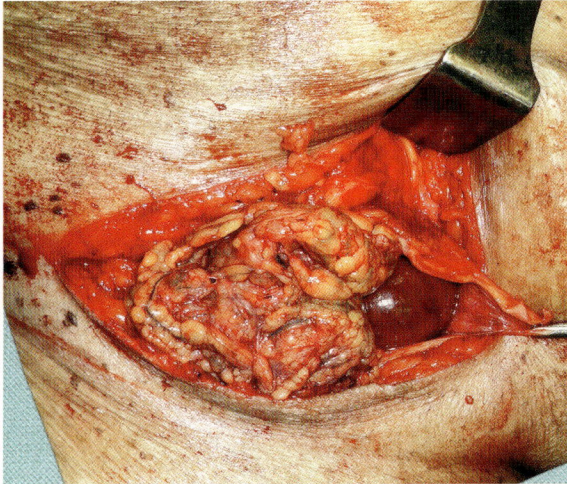

Figs 22.24A and B: First picture shows the iliac graft site—bone graft was taken for the treatment of fracture humerus. Second picture shows greater omentum and caecum. They were reduced and a mesh repair was done (*Courtesy:* Dr Prashanth Tubachi, Dr Pramod, Dr Raghunath Prabhu, KMC, Manipal)

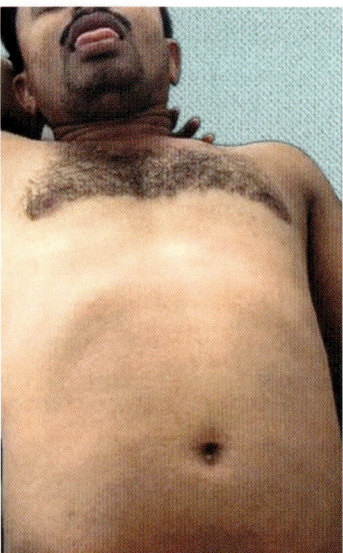

Fig. 22.25: On asking the patient to cough, he says there is pain in the appendicular point—cough tenderness or Dunphy's sign positive

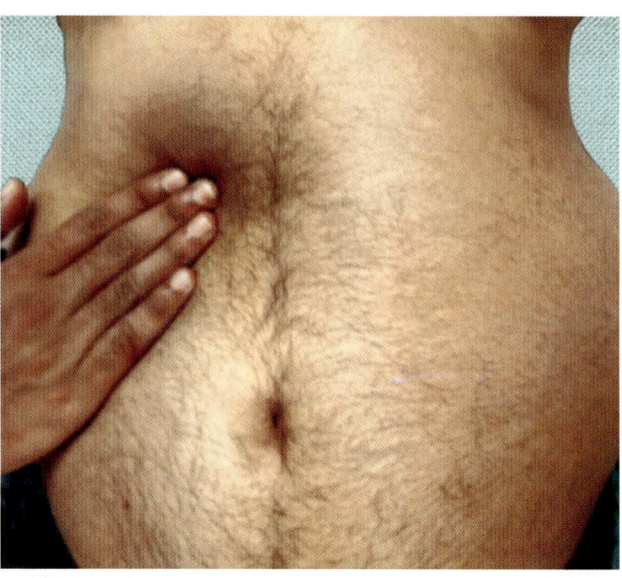

Fig. 22.26: Murphy's point—just lateral to the lateral border of rectus abdominis and just below the ninth costal cartilage. Murphy's point will change in position when the liver is enlarged

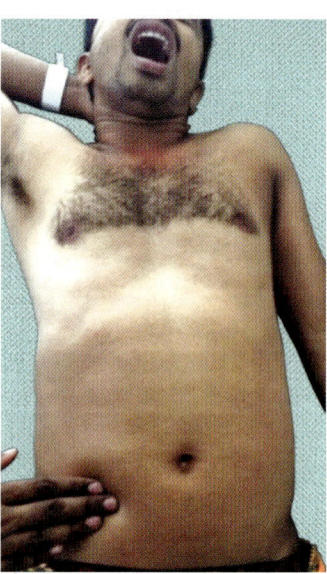

Fig. 22.27: Tenderness at the McBurney's point is typical of acute appendicitis in vast majority of the cases

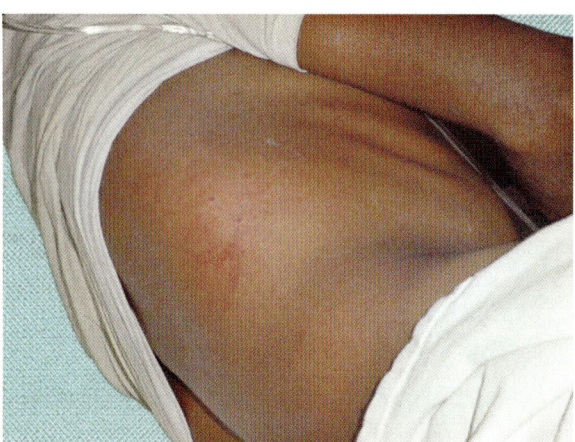

Fig. 22.28A: Intercostal bulge

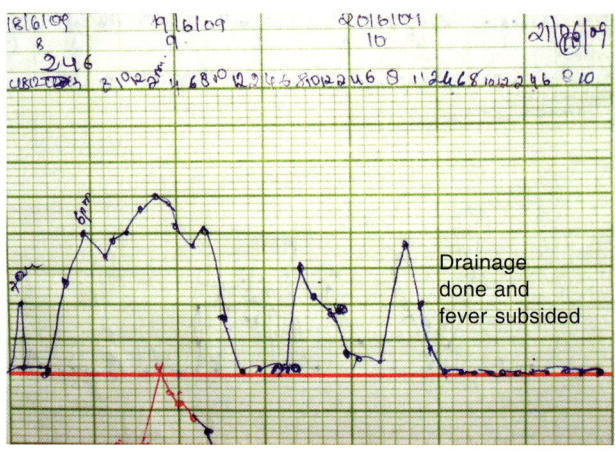

Fig. 22.28B: Temperature pattern of amoebic liver abscess

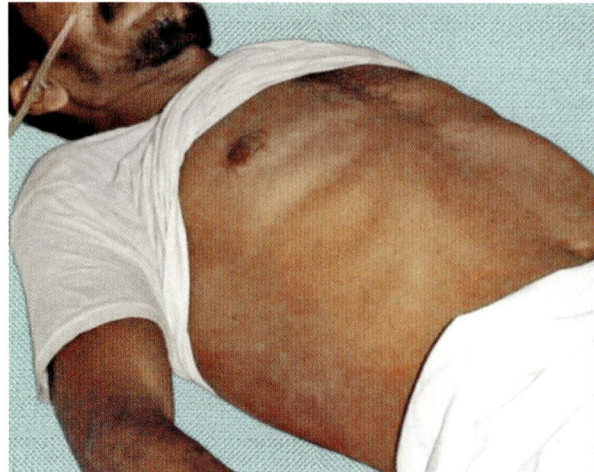

Fig. 22.28C: Ruptured liver abscess—bulge in the right lateral side of abdomen

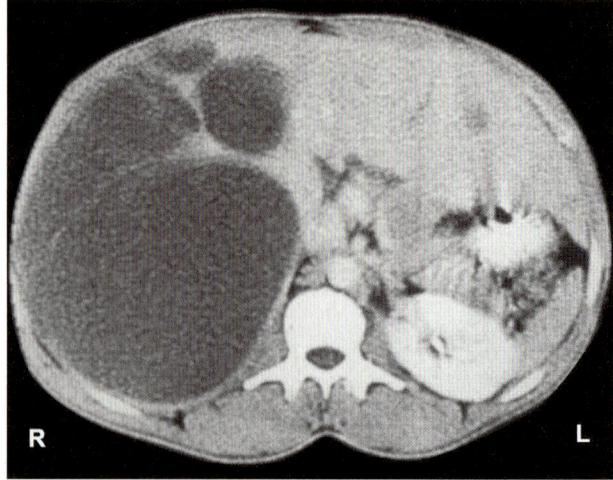

Fig. 22.28D: CT scan showing multiple liver abscesses proved to be due to amoebiasis

- *Rovsing sign*: Pressure on the left iliac fossa results in pain in the right iliac fossa due to impingement of bowel on the appendix (Fig. 22.30).

- *Murphy's kidney punch test*: Tenderness over the loin below the 12th rib lateral to erector spinae (Fig. 22.31).

- *Cope's psoas extension test*: The patient is turned to the left and hyperextend the hip slowly. Since there is spasm in retrocaecal appendicitis, the patient complains of pain (Fig. 22.32).

Look for evidence of localised peritonitis

- *Acute cholecystitis*: In this condition, tenderness is confined to the right hypochondrium. Ask the patient to take a deep breath. At the height of inspiration, if the patient experiences sudden catch during inspiration, it suggests that the inflamed gallbladder is underneath the palpating fingers. This sign has been described as Murphy's sign.

- *Acute appendicitis*: Tenderness at McBurney's point, localised guarding and rigidity in the right iliac fossa.

- *Acute pancreatitis*: Tenderness in the epigastric region, upper abdominal guarding and rigidity.

- *Acute diverticulitis*: Tenderness in the left iliac fossa, vague mass and localised peritonitis in sigmoid diverticular perforation.

- *Acute perforation of ileum in enteric fever*: There will be tenderness , guarding and rigidity in the

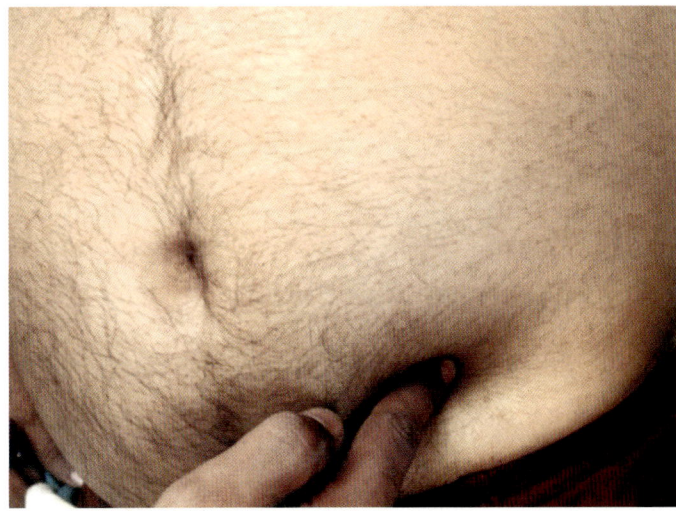

Fig. 22.29: Sir Philip Manson-Bahr amoebic point of tenderness in acute amoebic dysentery

subumbilical region and an inflammatory mass can also be palpated.

Look for evidence of generalised peritonitis

- *Abdominal tenderness* is elicited in all quadrants of the abdomen in generalised peritonitis. This is very reliable and must be carefully elicited. Abdomen is tender in cases of mesenteric ischaemia.

- *Rebound tenderness (Blumberg's sign)*: Abdomen is pressed for a few seconds. The patient experiences pain. Sudden release of pressure causes severe pain.

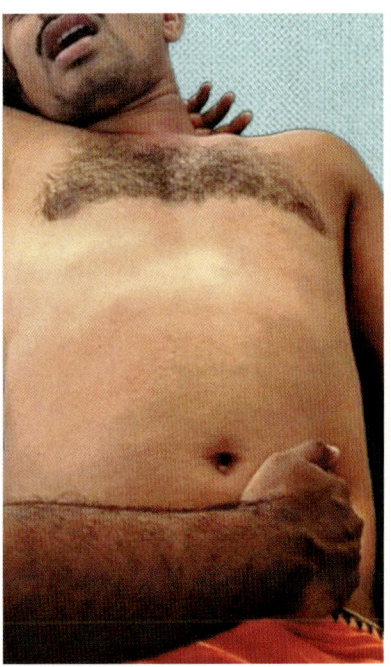

Fig. 22.30: Rovsing sign

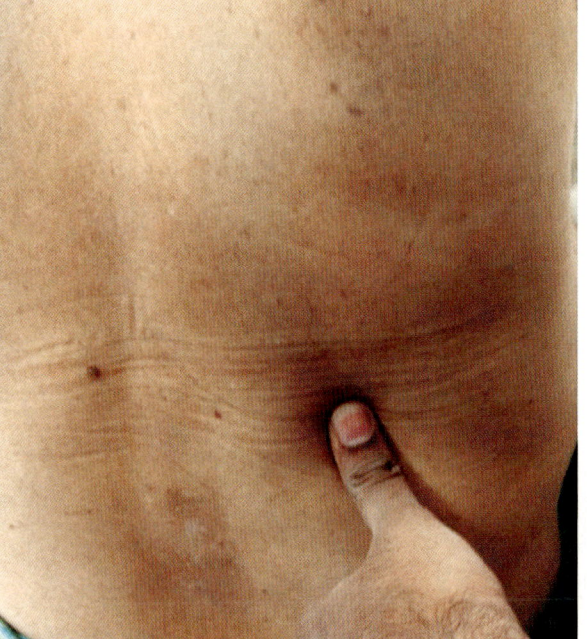

Fig. 22.31: Murphy's kidney punch test

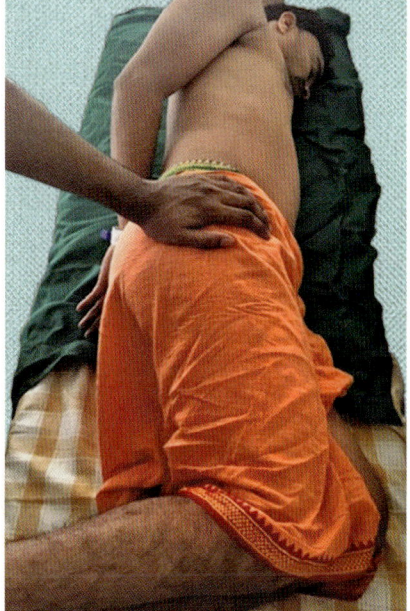

Fig. 22.32: Cope's psoas extension test

It is due to sudden movement of the sensitive parietal peritoneum (Fig. 22.33).

- *Guarding* and *rigidity* of abdominal wall.
- *Liver dullness is obliterated* in hollow viscus perforation. Shifting dullness can be elicited when significant fluid accumulates in the peritoneal cavity (Fig. 22.34).
- Bowel sounds are absent.

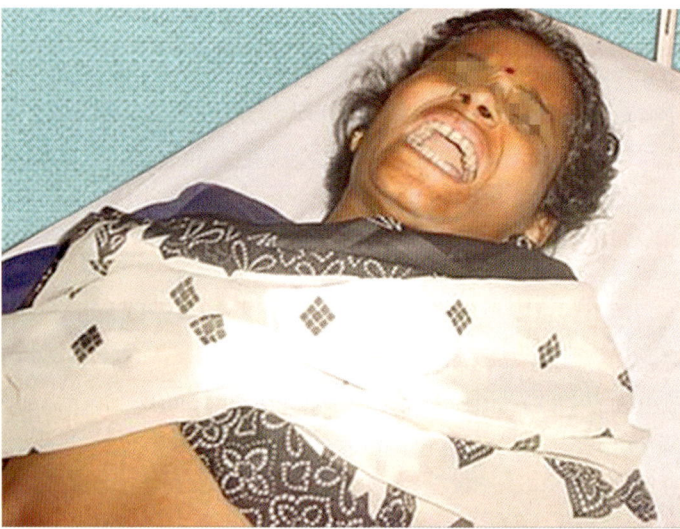

Fig. 22.33: Rebound tenderness is the diagnostic sign of peritonitis

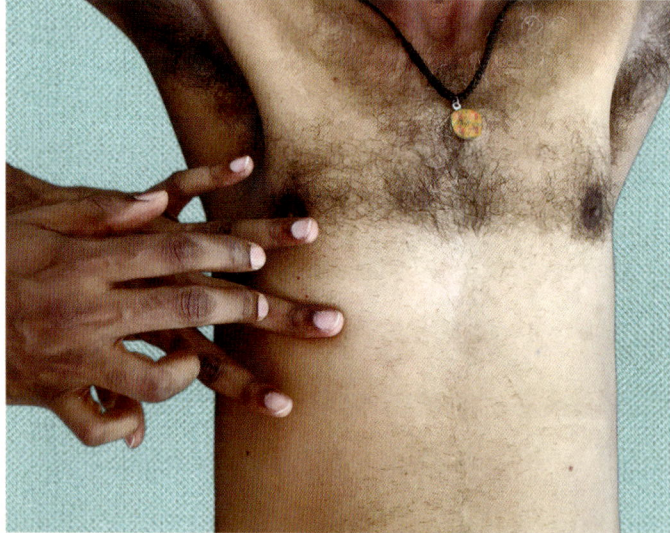

Fig. 22.34: Percussion to look for liver dullness which gets obliterated in cases of perforation

Look for evidence of specific causes of pain—intestinal obstruction

- *Distended bowel loops* can be seen and palpated. Tender, tense (distended), tympanitic loop on the left side is due to sigmoid volvulus.

- *Peristalsis is seen.* Keep the hand over the loops and check for any contractions during hyperperistalsis. Classically, it is described for **intussusception in children.** The mother is asked to feed the child while the examiner keeps the palmar aspect of his hand over the baby's abdomen. A contracting mass is felt near the umbilicus. This is typical of intussusception. It is usually of the ileocolic variety and the right iliac fossa is empty (**signe de Dance**).
- **Doughy abdomen, rolled up omentum, ascites** or **loculated ascites,** mass in the right iliac fossa or lumbar region may be seen in a case of tuberculous abdomen.
- Mass in the right iliac fossa—carcinoma caecum with obstruction.
- Look at hernial orifices for obstructed inguinal or femoral hernia.

Auscultation

- Loud, noisy intestinal sounds can be heard by auscultating in the right iliac fossa. They are called **borborygmi.** They suggest distal ileal obstruction.
- *Silent abdomen*: Absent bowel sounds are found in perforation peritonitis which causes paralytic ileus. However, a few tinkling sounds can be heard due to shift of fluid from one coil of bowel to other (Fig. 22.35).
- Normal bowel sounds occur once in 20 seconds. (thus 3 per minute).

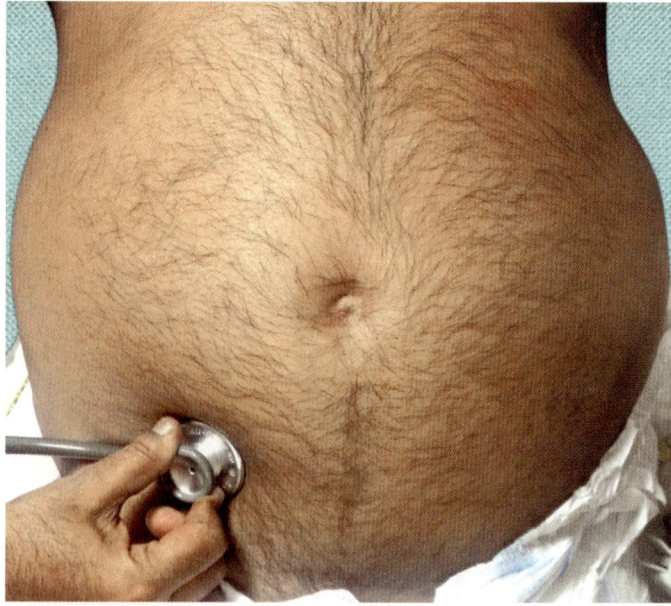

Fig. 22.35: Auscultation to hear for bowel sounds. It is done in the right iliac fossa

Rectal Examination

- In small bowel obstruction, rectum is empty and is often ballooned out.

- Carcinomatous growth with or without stools can be felt. The finger may be stained with blood (Fig. 22.36).

- In **acute appendicitis,** there may be right-sided tenderness. It has been described as **differential tenderness.** This sign will be present in cases of pelvic appendicitis.

- Foul putrid odour, green stools and altered blood may suggest **gangrene of the bowel** as in **mesenteric ischaemia.**

- Red **currant jelly stools** are diagnostic of intussusception.

- Hard **impacted stools** may be the cause of intestinal obstruction.

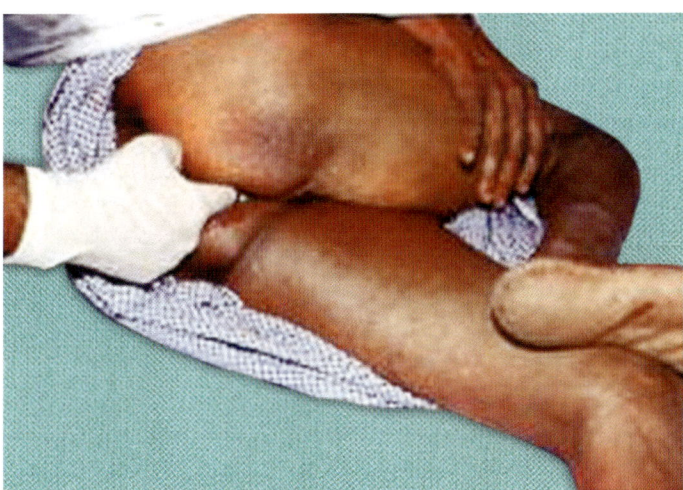

Fig. 22.36: Rectal examination

Vaginal Examination

- Tenderness in the fornices suggests salpingo-oophoritis.

- Gentle movement of the cervix causing severe pain suggests ruptured ectopic pregnancy.

- Ovarian mass can be felt—ovarian torsion may be the cause.

DIFFERENTIAL DIAGNOSIS

I. *Medical causes of acute abdominal pain*: This is important knowledge because one can avoid a blunder laparotomy. Read the clinical notes below—a case of post-appendicectomy death (*refer* to Clinical Box 22.5 and Clinical Case Capsule).

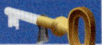

Clinical Box 22.5

10 Ps of non-surgical causes of acute abdomen
- **P**leurisy
- **P**neumonia
- **P**reherpetic neuralgia
- **P**urpura
- **P**ott's spine
- **P**orphyria
- **P**haeochromocytoma
- **P**lumbum (lead colic)
- **P**ancreatitis
- **P**olyserositis syndromes

In all patients presenting with acute abdomen, especially those who present with fever, think of these causes.

Clinical Case Capsule

A 23-year-old construction worker presented to the hospital with features of acute appendicitis such as severe pain in the right iliac fossa, vomiting and fever. Tenderness at McBurney point was present including rebound tenderness. Total count was elevated. Ultrasound reported as probe tenderness and minimum fluid in the abdomen. He underwent laparoscopic appendicectomy. Postoperatively within 48 hours, his saturation dropped and chest X-ray revealed ARDS features. He succumbed within 4 days even after providing him ventilator support, antibiotics, etc. On retrospection, the patient's symptoms had started with fever a few days back. This history could not be elicited initially rather it was missed or ignored by the surgeon. Probably it was a case of dengue fever. The cause of abdominal pain was due to peritoneal inflammation as a part of polyserositis syndrome.

II. *Conditions which can be managed without surgery most of the time* (localised peritonitis):

1. ***Amoebic liver abscess/hepatitis***: Male alcoholics are commonly affected. There may be history of dysentery. Typically, after 7–10 days following desentery or diarrhoea, patient complains of severe pain in the right hypochondrium which gets aggravated on taking deep inspiration. Abdominal pain, high grade fever, chills and rigors, tender hepatomegaly and intercostal tenderness clinch the diagnosis. Many of cases are in the stage of hepatitis which can be managed conservatively with antiamoebic treatment. Ultrasound is the key investigation. However, once pus is confirmed, it is better to drain by pigtail catheter insertion, laparoscopic method or open method depending upon expertise and facilities available. With effective treatment, amoebiasis cutis is rarely found after drainage nowadays.

2. ***Acute cholecystitis*** (Fig 22.37): Typically, a fatty female in forties presents with severe pain abdomen in the upper region, with vomiting and low grade fever. On examination, **Murphy's sign is positive.** Tenderness, guarding and rigidity in the upper abdomen are common. Previous history of abdominal pain may be present. Ultrasound will clinch the diagnosis.

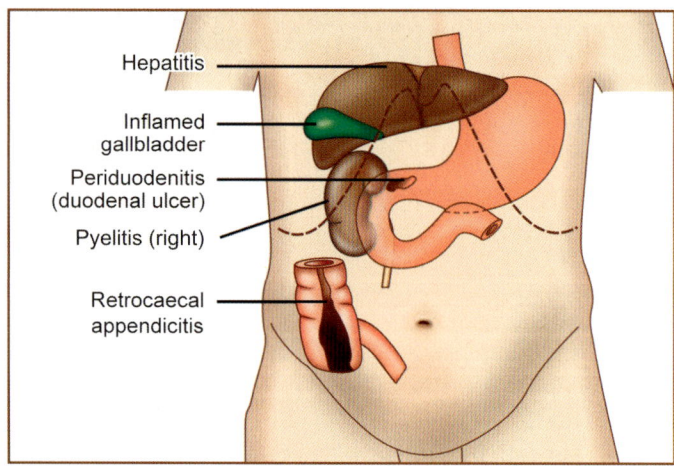

Fig. 22.37: The differential diagnosis of acute cholecystitis

Managed by conservative line of treatment in the form of antibiotics, rest to the part by allowing nil per oral and IV fluids. Again early cholecystectomy can be done within 48 hours, if experience of surgeon is good. Otherwise elective cholecystectomy is done after 6–8 weeks.

3. **Acute pancreatitis:** Typically, he is an alcoholic male around middle age group. He complains of severe upper abdominal pain radiating to the back. Pain is continuous and severe. Typically patient prefers to lie on his abdomen and prefers to bend forwards. Vomiting and abdominal distension are the usual features. Tachycardia, tachypnoea, and hypotension are other features. Recurrent attacks are common. Epigastric tenderness is a feature. **Cullen's sign and Grey Turner's sign** are bluish discolouration around the umbilicus and flank respectively. Serum amylase, and serum lipase are elevated. Ultrasound will help in the diagnosis in vast majority of the cases. CECT scan is generally obtained after a week, if patient does not show improvement, possibly because of necrosis. Immediate resuscitation with intravenous fluids, analgesics and rest to pancreas is the treatment of choice. **More than 80% cases can be managed without surgery at the initial admission.** However, if gallstones are the cause of pancreatitis by obstructing the lower CBD, sphincterotomy and extraction

■ Clinical Case Capsule

Acute pancreatitis

A 30-year-old patient complained of severe abdominal pain in the centre and right side of abdomen since two days.
The surgeon who examined the patient, found maximum tenderness in the right iliac fossa. Ultrasound could detect fluid and probe tenderness in the right iliac fossa. With diagnosis of acute appendicitis (with no mass), he underwent appendicectomy. Fluid was sent for analysis. It showed high amylase count. It was a case of acute pancreatitis. Fluid which gravitates in the right paracolic space can be confused for acute appendicitis. Duodenal ulcer perforation also results in severe right upper abdominal pain and later rebound tenderness can occur in right iliac fossa confusing it for acute appendicitis (Valentino appendix).

of the stones should be done immediately, followed by laparoscopic cholecystectomy.
- Sterile necrosis is managed without surgery. Injection Imipenem may be required.
- Infected necrosis is treated by necrosectomy which is done after 6 weeks.

4. **Adhesive obstruction:** Postoperative adhesions are the most common cause of intestinal obstruction in middle-aged and elderly patients. Pelvic surgery in females and surgery done for peritonitis such as appendicular perforation or gangrene of intestines are the chief factors. Other than these, ischaemia is one strong factor for adhesions. As the old saying goes, 'once adhesions, always adhesions'. A typical patient is in his/her thirties or forties, and has undergone previous abdominal surgery. *Example:* Abdominal hysterectomy or appendicectomy, presents with colicky abdominal pain and vomiting. Scar of laparotomy gives the clue. Conservative line of treatment in the form of nasogastric aspiration and intravenous supplementation is successful in majority of cases. Generally by 2–4 days, obstruction settles down. Careful monitoring is required to check for development of gangrene or perforation.

5. **Faecal impaction:** This can give rise to acute on chronic obstruction in elderly patients. Poor nutrition, less consumption of liquids and fibre diet, and hot climatic conditions may precipitate large bowel obstruction. Other factors which can precipitate are some drugs such as clonidine, opiate analgesics, and tricyclic antidepressants. Narcotics increase the tone in intestinal smooth muscle, reduce propulsion and the strength of contractions. Tricyclic antidepressants also have powerful anticholinergic effects and these can cause severe constipation. This type of obstruction has been described as pseudo-obstruction. Withdrawal of drugs causing constipation, hydration, stool softening agents, repeated enemas or manual evacuation of hard stools is the treatment of choice.

6. **Acute mesenteric lymphadenitis:** This is common in children. It is viral aetiology. It is self-limiting. Another bacterial infection in children is *Yersinia enterocolitica*. It is the most common cause of mesenteric lymphadenitis in children. The presentation is with severe abdominal pain mimicking acute appendicitis. In adults, it can be confused for Crohn's disease. However, pain is non-shifting and rebound tenderness is absent. In thin patients, tender swollen lymph nodes can be palpated along the line of mesentery.

7. **Mittelschmerz syndrome:** Mid-menstrual syndrome: Rupture of lutein cyst or follicular cyst occurs in the mid-menstrual period. It causes lower abdominal pain, sometimes bilateral. On the right side, it is the differential diagnosis of appendicitis. However, in appendicitis, pain is shifting in nature (migratory pain). It is important to rule out all other causes such as torsion of the ovarian cyst and ruptured ectopic before considering rupture of lutein cyst.

8. **Acute appendicitis:** In early cases of mild appendicitis, it can be managed with antibiotics and liquid diet. In these cases, tenderness is only limited to McBurney's point and

usually there will not be guarding and rigidity. WBC counts are within 10,000 cells/mm³. Ultrasound examination neither show faecolith nor perforation.

III. *Conditions which should be managed with surgery*

Perforation peritonitis causes
- Acute peptic ulcers: Drug induced, stress ulcers
- Chronic peptic ulcers: Chronic gastric ulcer
                            Chronic duodenal ulcer
- Acute appendicitis with perforation
- Carcinoma stomach
- Tubercular ulcers in the ileum
- Enteric ulcers in the ileum
- Meckel's diverticulitis with perforation
- Acute jejunal diverticulitis
- Carcinoma colon
- Sigmoid diverticular perforation

1. **Perforation peritonitis**: Severe abdominal pain, which is cutting in nature, becomes worse on movement of the abdominal wall. Hence, the patient lies still on the bed. Persistent vomiting is due to irritation of parietal peritoneum. High-grade fever with chills and rigors indicates a septicaemic process.

   - *The pulse rate is increased.* An increase in the pulse rate may be an early indication of peritonitis, in cases of gangrene of the bowel or peritonitis following perforation of bowel.

   - *Cough tenderness* indicates **parietal peritoneal inflammation.** Abdominal tenderness is elicited in all quadrants of the abdomen.

   - *Rebound tenderness (Blumberg's sign)*: Abdomen is pressed for a few seconds. The patient experiences pain. Sudden release of pressure causes severe pain. It is due to sudden movement of the sensitive parietal peritoneum.

   - Guarding and rigidity of abdominal wall.

   - *Percussion*: Liver dullness is obliterated.

   - Bowel sounds are absent. Distension of the abdomen occurs within a few hours due to accumulation of fluid and paralytic ileus.

   - *End-stage disease*: Hippocratic facies.

Investigations
- Except appendicular perforation, vast majority of perforations can be diagnosed by free gas under the right dome of the diaphragm in plain X-ray chest PA view.
- If patient cannot stand, left lateral decubitus films are taken. (Fig. 22.38).
- To know the exact site of perforation (so as to plan on incision—upper abdomen, lower abdomen or mid-abdomen), CECT is done.

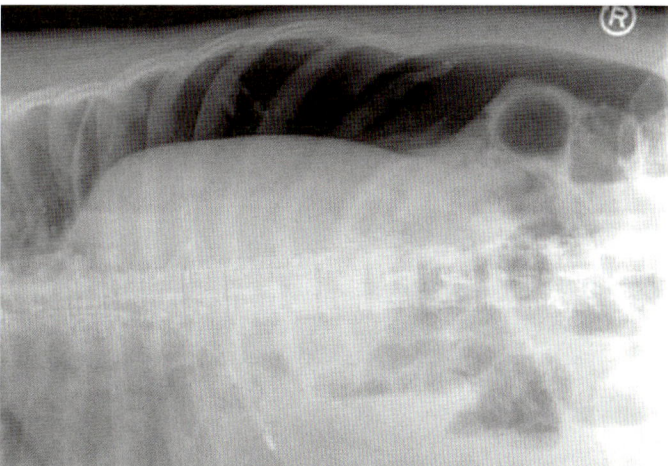

Fig. 22.38: Case of duodenal perforation resulting in collection of free gas under the abdominal wall—lateral decubitus X-ray

Management principles of perforation peritonitis

*****ABCDEF** are the basic principles of management of acute abdomen

A. *Aspiration*: Nasogastric aspiration to prevent contamination, to prevent aspiration/vomiting.

B. *Bowel care*: No purgatives, no enema. Blood may have to be arranged. Purgatives can increase peristalsis and can result in more contamination.

C. *Charts*: Pulse rate, temperature, respiration, intake/output chart, abdominal girth—increase in all these parameters suggests peritonitis/sepsis/shock.

D. *Drugs*: Cephalosporins, amikacin and metronidazole are used against gram-positive, gram-negative and anaerobic organisms.

E. *Exploratory laparotomy* (Fig. 22.39) is done. The perforation site is identified, closed by suturing with nonabsorbable silk sutures (2-0 sutures). Care is not taken to narrow the lumen. In a few cases, intestinal resection may have to be done, especially when multiple perforations have been identified. Thorough peritoneal wash/toilet is given. Laparotomy wound is closed. Skin sutures can be left open and can be tied after 48 hours to prevent wound infection.

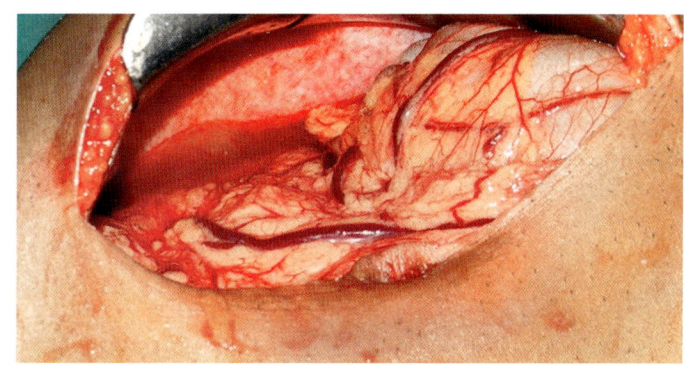

Fig. 22.39: Collection of blood-stained bile just below the liver. A case of acute duodenal perforation due to NSAIDs (non-steroidal anti-inflammatory drugs)

Few examples:

1. *Chronic gastric ulcer:* Distal gastrectomy.

2. *Chronic duodenal ulcer:* Closure with omental patch.

3. *Perforation of enteric/tubercular ulcer:* Resection anastomosis or even a simple closure.

4. *Meckel's diverticulum with perforation:* Excision of Meckel's diverticulum with adjacent normal intestine.

5. *Appendicular perforation:* Appendicectomy, drainage of pus and drain the peritoneal cavity.

6. *Colonic ulcer/cancer perforation:* Resection and anastomosis with or without diversion ileostomy / colostomy.

F. *Fluid and electrolytes:* The patients are severely dehydrated, toxic and septic. Severe electrolyte imbalance and acidosis are the features. Immediate replacement of fluids and electrolytes must be done to treat shock and third space loss. Ringer lactate and dextrose normal saline are commonly used solutions.

Various causes of perforation—details

a. **Peptic ulcer perforation:** Usually young patients between 30 and 40 years, who used to complain of dyspepsia, hunger pain (duodenal ulcer) and burning pain which increases after food (gastric ulcer) suddenly present with severe upper abdominal pain which is cutting in nature.

- In middle-aged and elderly, perforation is often drug induced—nonsteroidal anti-inflammatory drugs (NSAIDs). Often patients say that something has given way. On examination, patient is anxious. Tachycardia and tachypnoea are present. Abdominal examination reveals board-like rigidity and guarding. Bowel sounds are absent. **X-ray chest reveals free air under the right dome of the diaphragm.** Emergency laparotomy, closure of perforation in duodenal ulcers, closure or sometimes a distal gastrectomy may be necessary in gastric ulcers.

- Anterior ulcer perforates, posterior ulcer bleeds.

Clinical Wisdom

In elderly patients, gastric ulcer which perforates can also be due to malignancy. Hence, a biopsy from suspicious area is required.

b. **Enteric ulcer perforation:** Perforations occur in the terminal ileum. It can be single in more than 80% of cases. An oval, vertical, perforation results in peritonitis. Enteric perforation need not give rise to all signs of peritonitis. Guarding and rigidity can be minimal because of poor, immunocompromised nature of the diseases and due to Zenker's degeneration of abdominal wall muscles. Perforation is situated in the antimesenteric border of the terminal ileum. Typically, it occurs in the third week of enteric fever. Bradycardia, dehydration, and toxicity are the other features.

- Diagnosis of perforation is based clinically on the acute abdominal pain, bleeding per rectum with/without guarding and rigidity. **High-grade fever—step-ladder type, early toxicity and bradycardia** are other features that help in the diagnosis.

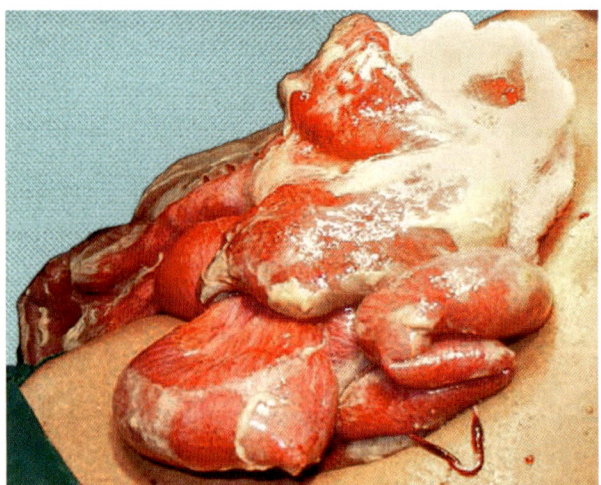

Fig. 22.40: Enteric perforation which is 4 days old—very friable edges. Re-leak after suturing is common

- Plain X-ray abdomen may reveal gas under the diaphragm. If perforation is small and sealed off, gas need not be present.

- The most useful investigation is CECT scan which can reveal not only pneumoperitoneum but also pericolic collection, which can be missed by ultrasound (Fig. 22.40).

  - Treated by third generation cephalosporins, emergency laparotomy, resection of bowel and end-to-end anastomosis or closure of the perforation by using non-absorbable sutures. Abdomen is closed with a tube drain.

  - If bowel is very oedematous or not healthy, another option is small bowel exteriorisation. **Relaparotomy is done after 8 weeks and closure of ileostomy is done.**

Clinical Wisdom

- **Suspect enteric perforation**
- When you suspect peritonitis, no guarding and no rigidity
- When you suspect toxicity, no tachycardia but bradycardia

c. **Tubercular stricture/ulcer perforation:** Many patients are young, emaciated with or without low grade fever. Abdominal pain is the most common symptom. It can be a dull, vague pain or colicky pain (stricture) which increases after taking food or relieved by vomiting. Diarrhoea is watery, small in quantity and abnormally foul smelling. Non-specific symptoms, such as flatulence, noisy sounds in the abdomen (borborygmi), are not uncommon. Abdominal distension is due to ascites and subacute intestinal obstruction. Weight loss is very common. **Anorexia, tiredness, and pallor may be the presenting features.**

Signs

- Typically, patients are malnourished and pale.
- Visible intestinal peristalsis may be seen.
- Distended bowel loops can be palpated.
- Doughy abdomen in case of peritoneal involvement.
- Features of peritonitis such as guarding and rigidity are found in cases of perforation.

Investigations

- Chest X-ray to look for gas under the diaphragm. It may also show evidence of pulmonary tuberculosis.
- Ultrasound and CT scan to confirm the perforation.

Surgery: Laparotomy, closure of perforation with or without resection anastomosis or exteriorisation are the treatment of choice.

d. **Acute appendicitis with perforation**

- Incidence is about 6–12% of all cases of perforation peritonitis.
- Factors which favour perforations are faecolith and severe inflammation. Elderly patients are more vulnerable for gangrene and perforation due to decreased blood supply. In children, perforation spreads easily and causes peritonitis due to small omentum. Clinical features include tachycardia, tenderness in the McBurney's point, guarding, rigidity and signs of septic shock. Ultrasound can demonstrate several distended bowel loops and fluid in the abdomen. CECT can diagnose a perforation in about 80–85% of cases. Laparoscopy/laparotomy and drainage of pus, appendicectomy, peritoneal wash and drain tube are the treatment of choice. Up to 5% mortality has been described (Fig. 22.41).

e. **Amoebic perforation of caecum** or sigmoid can occur resulting in acute abdomen. Incidence is less now due to the effective treatment for amoebiasis. History of diarrhoea, blood and mucus in the stools gives the clue to the diagnosis. Tenderness over McBurney point on the right side and Manson-Bahr amoebic point on the left side will help in the diagnosis. Plain X-ray abdomen and CT scan will clinch the diagnosis. Treatment includes antiamoebic medication, urgent laparotomy, closure of the perforation, peritoneal toilet followed by closure of the abdomen.

f. **Meckel's diverticulitis with perforation**: Often patients are young who might have had previous episodes of abdominal pain—often confused for appendicitis. It is a diagnosis at laparotomy. Resection of Meckel's diverticulum with adjacent intestine followed by anastomosis and thorough peritoneal toilet is the treatment of choice (Fig. 22.42).

Rule of 2 for Meckel's diverticulum

- Incidence: 2%
- Location: 2 feet proximal to ileocaecal junction
- Length: 2 inches long
- Ectopic tissue: 2 types—gastric and pancreatic
- Presentation: 2 years or below 2 years is the most common age
- Male:female ratio—1:2

g. **Crohn's disease**: The disease is often insidious, slowly progressive with a protracted course and commonly affects young adults in the second or third decade of life. Intermittent colicky lower abdominal pain, diarrhoea and weight loss are common. It may be associated with fever. Presence of pain and tenderness in the right iliac fossa mimics appendicitis. If there is a mass, it may be confused for an appendicular mass. Perforation presents with more severe abdominal pain and rectal bleeding. Laparotomy and closure of perforation

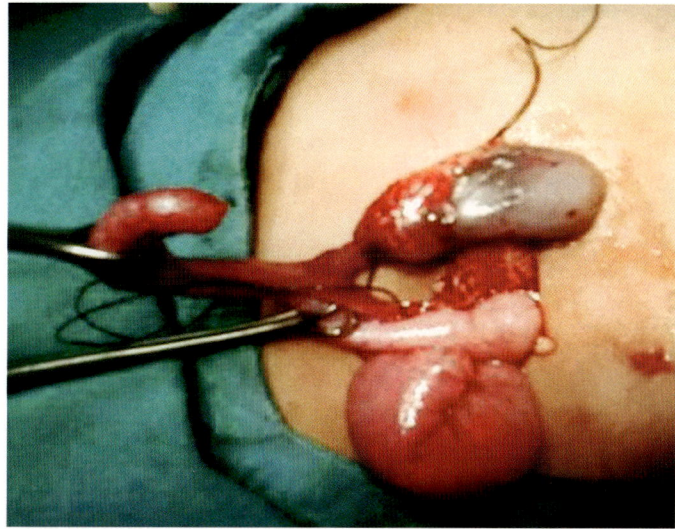

Fig. 22.41: Acute appendicitis

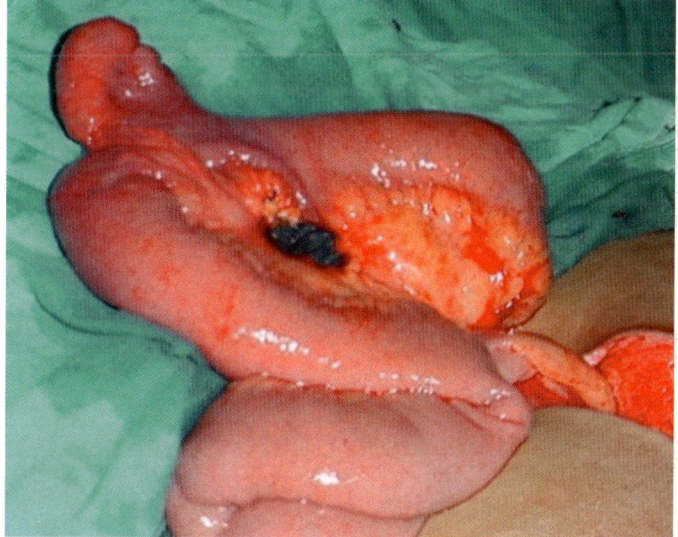

Fig. 22.42: Meckel's diverticulum at surgery

is ideal. However, some cases need resection. Please note that the aim of treating Crohn's disease is to save as much bowel as possible and try resection.

h. **Colonic diverticulitis with perforation**: Usually elderly patients above 60–70 years of age are affected. Patients have lower abdominal distension, heaviness, flatulence, etc. Vague abdominal pain is also felt in the left iliac fossa. Left-sided lower abdominal pain, moderate to severe pain is associated with passage of loose stools, fever, tenderness and a vague mass suggest diverticulitis with or without perforation (Figs 22.43 to 22.45).

- More often diverticular perforation produces localised peritonitis (abscess) than generalised peritonitis.
- Bleeding per rectum can be the presenting feature. Sometimes, it can be massive.
- It is managed conservatively with antibiotics and rest to the part.

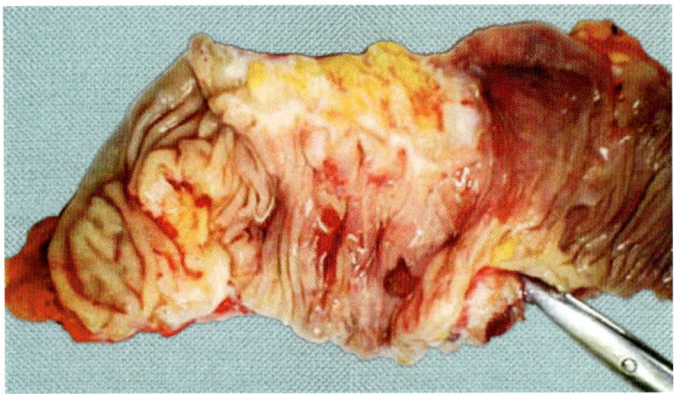

Fig. 22.43: Sigmoid diverticular perforation

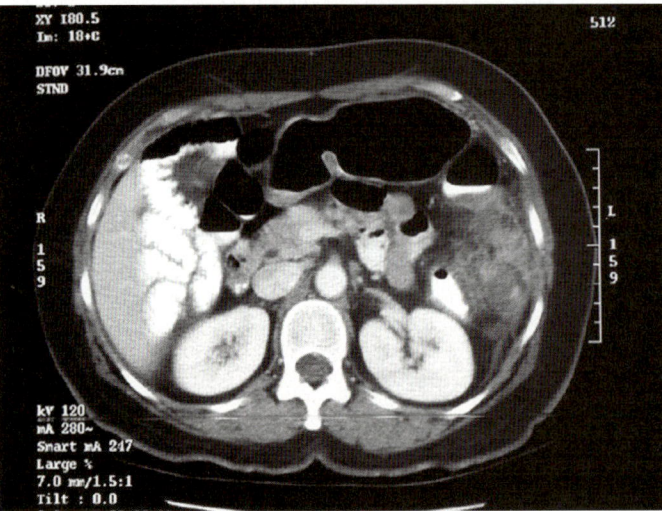

Fig. 22.44: CECT scan showing pericolic abscess on the left side due to diverticular perforation

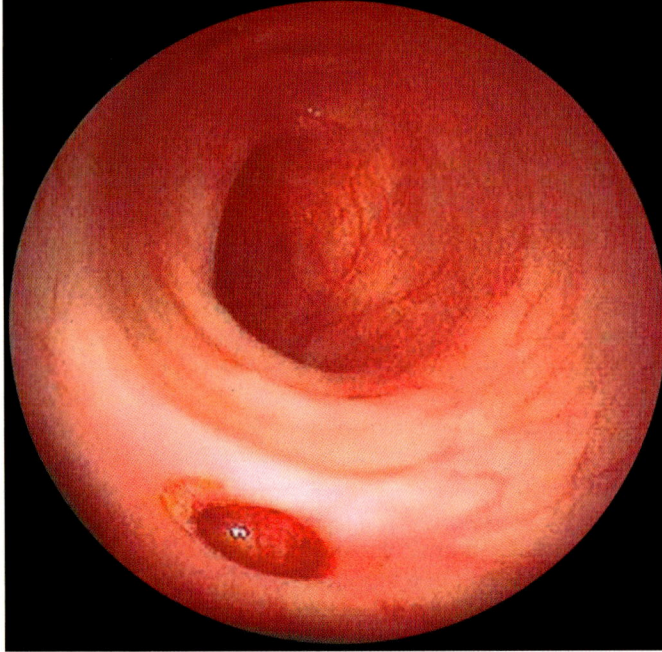

Fig. 22.45: Colonoscopy showing opening of diverticulum (*Courtesy:* Dr Rajesh Sisodia, Ex-Associate Professor, KMC, Manipal)

- Localised abscess can be treated with ultrasound-guided pigtail insertion. A few weeks later, when inflammation settles down, resection is done.

- Generalised peritonitis requires laparotomy, resection anastomosis with or without diversion colostomy.

2. **Acute intestinal obstruction:** This is a common emergency encountered in the casualty. Young or old, male or female present with sudden crampy or colicky abdominal pain. The pain lasts for about a few seconds, subsides and starts again. The pain is very severe and pressure on the abdomen relieves pain a little bit. Vomiting is more frequent in small bowel obstruction. Vomitus contains food particles and bile in small bowel obstruction. Faeculent (no faecal matter but vomitus with faecal smell) vomiting is characteristic of terminal ileal obstruction. **Abdominal distension follows soon and constipation is common.** Large bowel obstruction causes more of constipation and distension than vomiting. It is usually caused by carcinoma at rectosigmoid junction or sigmoid volvulus. Previous history of constipation and bleeding per rectum are found in carcinoma rectum. As a rule, left-sided growth is not palpable because it is constrictive (typical rectosigmoid carcinoma). Sigmoid volvulus is an acute emergency seen in elderly patients. Severe abdominal pain, and uneven gross distension, hypovolaemic shock are early features. A prominent distended sigmoid loop which is tympanitic is seen when inspected (Figs 22.46 to 22.54).

There are several causes of intestinal obstruction which have been discussed in great detail in Manipal Manual of Surgery, 4th edition. A few details are given below. A broad idea of following details should be known to all residents. Is it obstruction? At what level? What may be the cause? Does this require immediate surgery? Can we wait for a few hours? Can we manage without surgery?

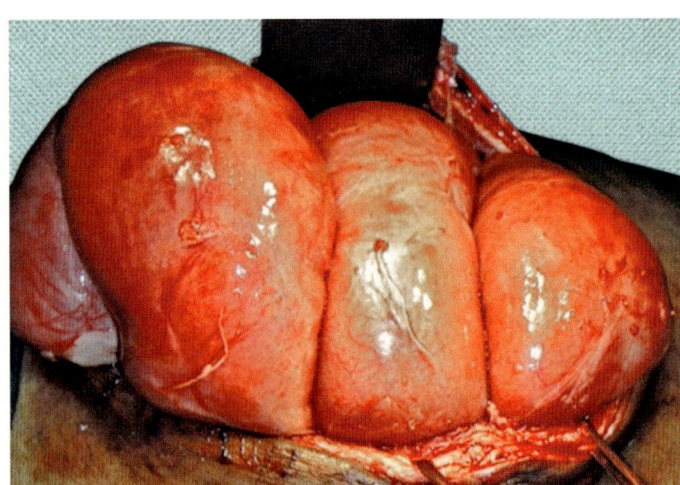

Fig. 22.46: Gross distension of the bowel in acute intestinal obstruction due to stricture terminal ileum

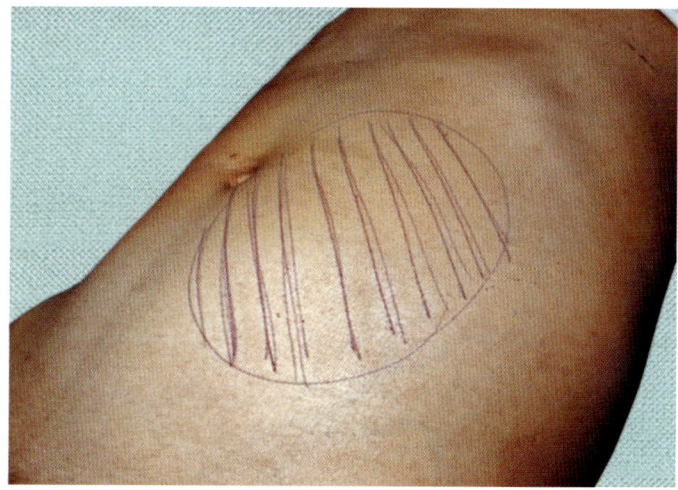

Fig. 22.47: Caecal volvulus: Distended caecum in the left hypochondrium

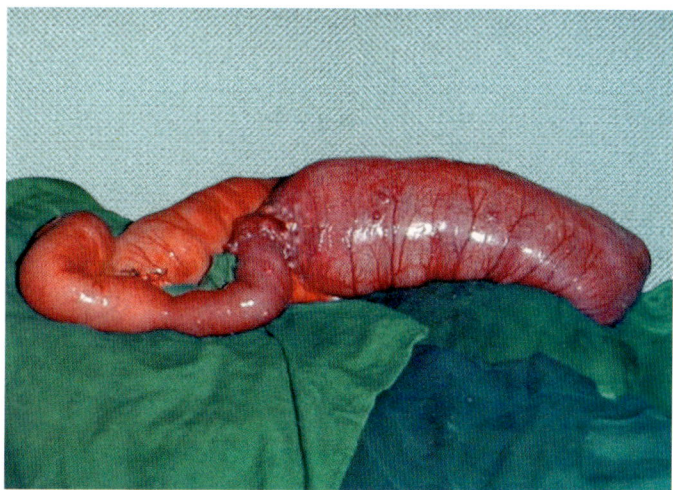

Fig. 22.50: Tubercular ileal stricture causing intestinal obstruction

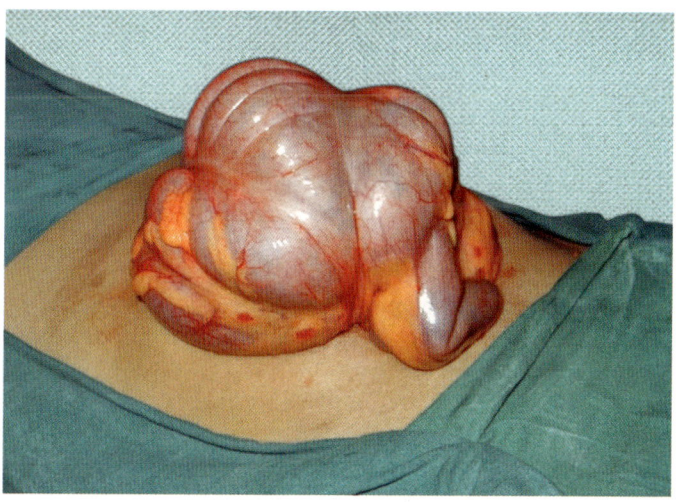

Fig. 22.48: Caecal volvulus: Distended caecum in the left hypochondrium at surgery

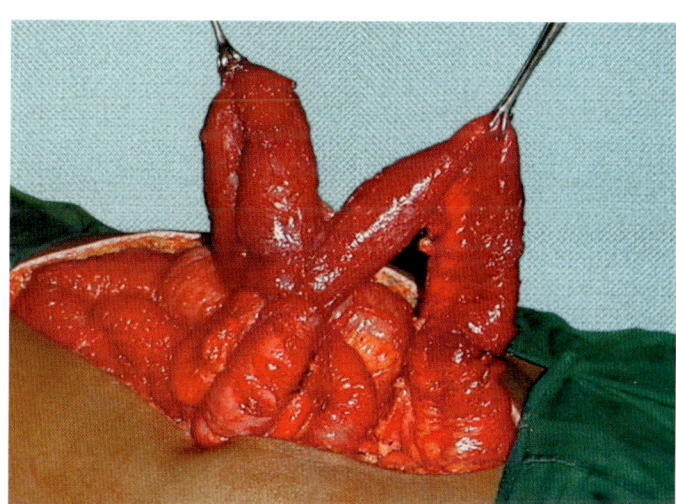

Fig. 22.51: Extensive tubercular peritonitis with adhesions, matting of the loops resulting in intestinal obstruction

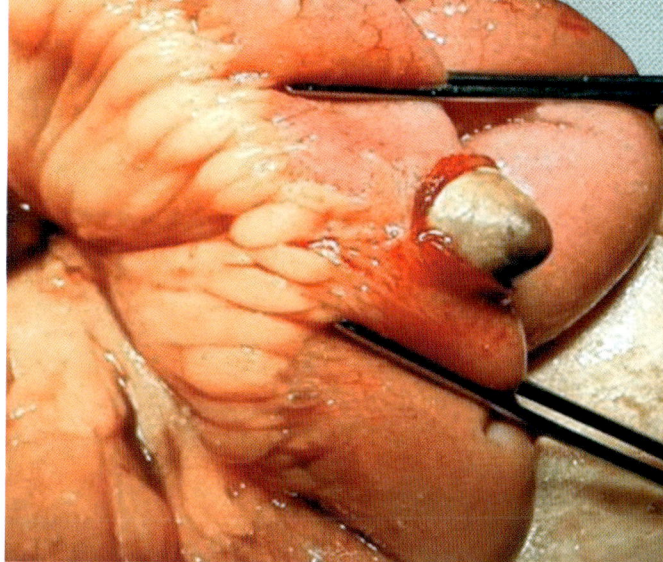

Fig. 22.49: Gallstone ileus: Stone is removed by an enterotomy

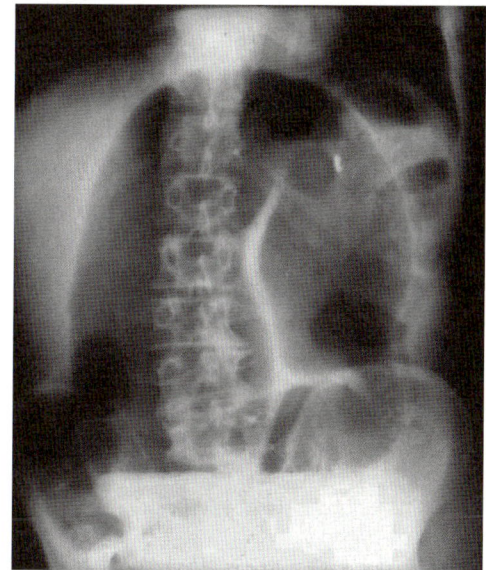

Fig. 22.52: Sigmoid volvulus showing large distended bowel loop

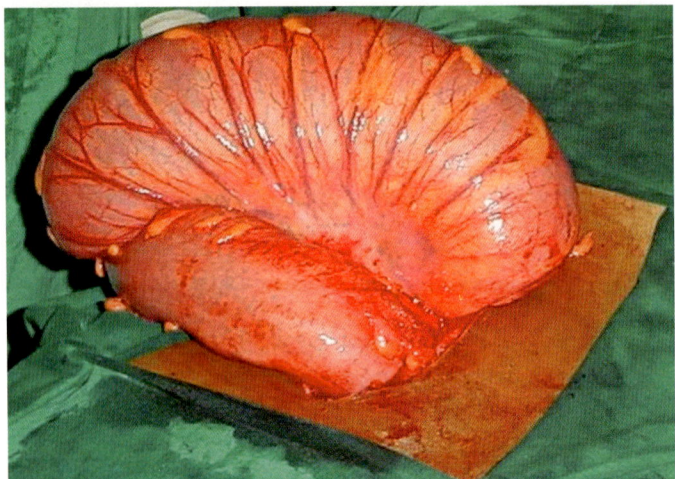

Fig. 22.53: Plain X-ray abdomen showing a hugely dilated sigmoid loop. A case of sigmoid volvulus at surgery

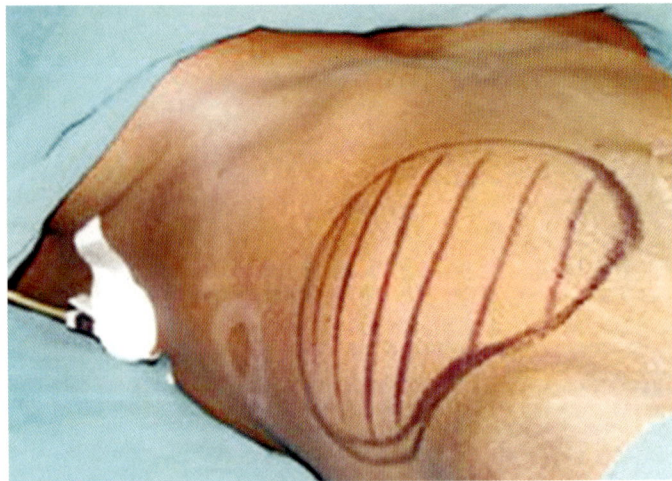

Fig. 22.55: Carcinoma caecum in a 65-year-old lady with mass in the right iliac fossa and intestinal obstruction

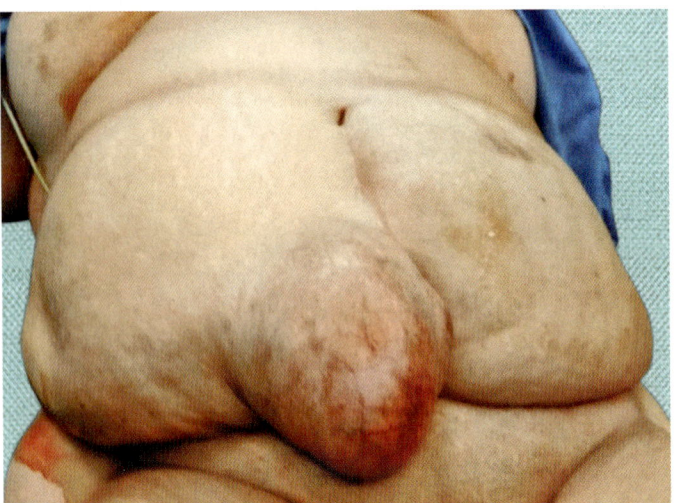

Fig. 22.54: Obstructed incisional hernia

- **In neonates and children**: Imperforate anus, meconium ileus, atresia, Hirschsprung disease, and worm ball obstruction are a few causes. The first three causes are seen in the neonatal period and diagnosis is not difficult. Hirschsprung disease also causes obstruction in young children. Intussusception in children is classical with a contracting mass in the umbilical region with its concavity towards umbilicus. **Look at the deformed umbilicus in a young child—it may be a Meckel's diverticulitis or vitello-intestinal anomaly.** *Ascaris lumbricoides*—roundworms form a worm ball and cause terminal ileal obstruction.

- **In adults and middle age**: Important and common causes are adhesions, obstructed hernia including incisional hernia, volvulus, tuberculous abdomen, etc. Adhesive obstruction—scar especially in the lower abdomen or post- appendicectomy scar gives the clue. Always look at the hernial orifices—obstructed inguinal hernia is still a common cause. In females, it is important also to look into the femoral hernia site—below and lateral to pubic tubercle. It may be hidden under the fatty belly. Feel for a mass in the right iliac fossa in a young patient

who may possibly give history of evening rise in temperature. It may be ileocaecal tuberculosis. Contracting mass under palpating finger with circumoral pigmentation may be a case of Peutz-Jeghers syndrome and the mass is due to intussusception. Middle-aged female with previous history of cholecystitis or with ultrasound diagnosis of gall stones may have gall stone ileus—stones obstructing the terminal ileum, narrowest portion of the intestines.

- ***In elderly age group—5th decade onwards***: Carcinoma colon (Fig. 22.55) or rectum is an important cause which requires surgery. Volvulus, diverticular strictures, and ischaemic strictures can also present with features of obstruction and require surgery.

Clinical Wisdom

In cases of intestinal obstruction—look for scars, hernias, deformities, glands, stones, masses, melanin spots and search for cancer.

3. **Acute mesenteric ischaemia** (Fig. 22.56): This is one of the important causes of severe acute abdominal pain. Typically patients are 50–60 years old, known hypertensives, atherosclerotic complaining of severe abdominal pain. Recurrent attack of postprandial pain is present. **Pain is disproportionate to the signs and symptoms not relieved even by narcotics.** Abdomen is usually soft and mildly distended without any guarding or rigidity but tachycardia, tachypnoea and hypotension occur fast and give clue to the diagnosis. Tenderness all over the abdomen indicates gangrene and it warrants early laparotomy and resection of gangrene bowel.

4. **Torsion of undescended testis**: A young boy presents with severe abdominal pain on the right or left iliac fossa with or without vomiting. Pain is very severe and continuous. The diagnosis will be obvious, if there is **empty scrotum**. Mistakes do happen, especially if the pain is on the right side, confusing it for appendicular or intestinal pathology. Fever and elevated

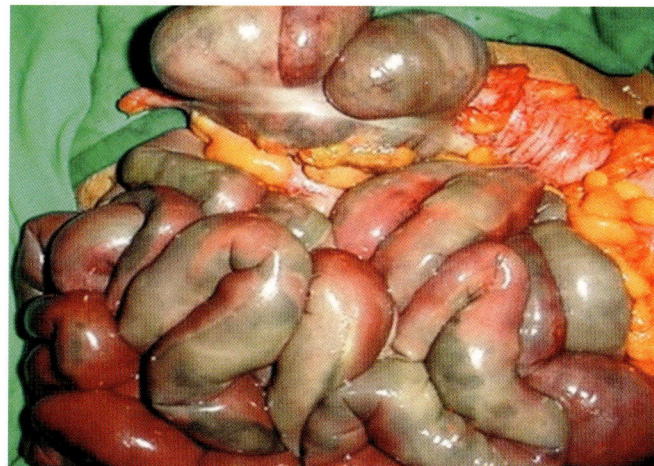

Fig. 22.56: Superior mesenteric ischaemia resulting in massive gangrene. (*Courtesy:* Prof U Santhosh Pai, Professor of Surgery, MMMC, Manipal)

leucocyte count is a late feature differentiating it from acute appendicitis. Ultrasound clinches the diagnosis. Removal or excision is the treatment of choice. Remember to examine opposite testis and if required, correct any anomaly.

5. *In women*
   a. **Torsion of ovarian cyst:** Any lower abdominal severe pain in a woman is presumably due to ovarian or tube pathology. Torsion of the ovarian cyst produces severe lower abdominal pain and vomiting. Small cysts will not be palpable in the abdomen but large cysts are palpated in the abdomen. Mild guarding may be present in the lower abdomen. Ultrasound is the investigation of choice. It is important to realise that dermoid cysts of the ovary are bilateral. While treating dermoid cysts of ovary, also look into opposite side and enucleate the opposite cyst also.

   b. **Ruptured ectopic gestation:** Any female patient in the reproductive age group presenting with severe lower abdominal pain and collapse—features of shock, pallor, hypotension—ruptured ectopic gestation should be considered first. History of missed periods will suggest pregnancy. It is typically seen after 4–6 weeks of pregnancy. The lower abdominal pain is severe and may radiate backwards. As blood accumulates in the entire peritoneal cavity, shoulder tip pain and distension are seen. One rare physical finding is bluish discolouration of the umbilical region. Abdominal distension, rebound tenderness, and rigidity can also be found. Per vaginal examination reveals cervix softer than normal, extreme tenderness on gentle movement of the cervix, all fornices are tender.

   c. **Iatrogenic acute abdomen:** These can be summarised as complications of 'OBG' cases post-hysterectomy, post-caesarean section. Patients who recover well for one or two days are referred to the surgeon as they are not doing well or not had bowel movements. Careful examination reveals tenderness in the lower abdomen, tachycardia, and tachypnoea. CT is the investigation of choice and may reveal pneumoperitoneum and perforation which is 'missed' during first surgery.

AN INTERESTING CASE OF ACUTE ABDOMEN

Clinical Case Capsule

A 32 year old male, was admitted with severe upper abdominal pain and breathing difficulty of 1 day duration following a large meal. There was no history of alcohol intake preceding the event. He had 3 episodes of vomiting food particles. Similar episode was present 6 months back which was relieved with medication. On examination, he was tachypnoeic and tachycardic. Tracheal and mediastinal shift to the right were present . Decreased air entry was noted in the left lower zones of lungs on auscultation. Chest X-ray (Fig. 22.57) revealed intestines inside the thoracic cavity. CECT (Fig. 22.58) confirmed the diagnosis of diaphragmatic hernia. He underwent emergency laparotomy. The caecum, ileocaecal junction, ascending colon, part of jejunum, ileum and stomach were present in the left hemithorax. An 8 x 6 cm oval shaped defect in the left hemidiaphragm was noted extending on to central tendon. There was no hernial sac. The contents were reduced. A 15 x 10 cm prolene mesh was placed and sutured to the structures available in the surrounding area. **The final diagnosis was adult Bochdalek's hernia.** It usually presents in neonates as emergency – it is a congenital posterolateral hernia of the diaphragm and is rare in adults.

(*Courtesy:* Professor B. Srinivas Pai, SDM Medical College, Dharwar, Karnataka).

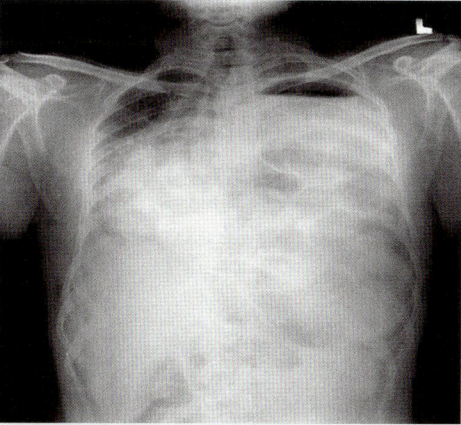

Fig. 22.57: Chest X-ray showing gas filled loops of intestines within thoracic cavity and gross deviation of trachea and mediastinum to the right side

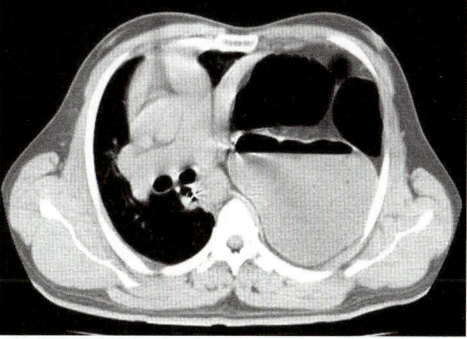

Fig. 22.58: Contrast enhanced CT scan showing gas filled loops of intestines in the thoracic cavity

23

Examination of Chronic Abdomen

INTRODUCTION

Once a challenging task of diagnosing chronic abdomen based only on clinical examination, it has become relatively easy now with investigations such as ultrasound, CT scan, endoscopies, etc. However, since many of the problems have a unique history and findings, attempt has been made here to simplify the presentations and the clinical diagnosis. It helps the students in the outpatient department to arrive at proper diagnosis, in patients who have chronic abdominal complaints.

HISTORY OF PRESENT ILLNESS

1. *Abdominal pain*: This is the most common complaint for which patient approaches a surgeon. What type of pain? How many months duration? Is it decreasing or increasing now? When did you notice it first? Is it severe sometimes? Show the site of pain. Do you have any other symptoms such as vomiting or fever? These are the common questions to be asked. Ask him to show the site of pain. He will show the site. This will give some idea about the anatomical organ involvement. *Example*: Right hypochondriac pain is due to liver enlargement, gallbladder stone disease or gallbladder carcinoma, etc. Dull aching pain is due to enlargement of solid organs such as hepatoma or hydatid cyst of the liver. In the same fashion, pain in the left upper abdomen is due to splenomegaly. Pain in the loin is caused by renal enlargement. Common surgical causes of renal enlargement are renal cell carcinoma, hydronephrosis and polycystic disease. Colicky pain is due to hollow viscus obstruction partial or total. Typically, it is

intermittent and more severe. Small intestinal pathology results in central abdominal pain and large intestinal pathology causes peripheral colicky pain. Classically duodenal ulcer patients present with pain which appears after 2–3 hours of meal what has been called hunger pain. On the other hand, in gastric ulcer, food causes pain due to direct irritation of ulcer and after 1–2 hours, pain will subside. Recurrent attacks of epigastric pain radiating to back is a feature of chronic pancreatitis. Abdominal pain or discomfort after fatty meals can occur in chronic cholecystitis. It has been described as **flatulent dyspepsia**.

2. *Vomiting*: Vomiting is a feature of upper gastrointestinal pathology. Enquire about nature of contents, frequency, blood stains, relation to food, a foul odour. Common cause of nausea, vomiting in elderly/middle-aged men is carcinoma stomach. In cases of chronic **gastric ulcer, patient puts his fingers in the posterior third of the tongue and induces vomiting to relieve pain.** Persistent, profuse, projectile, non-bilious vomiting is typical of pyloric stenosis (gastric outlet obstruction) caused by cicatrized chronic duodenal ulcer. **Often patients describe this as a ball rolling sensation in the abdomen.** Duodenal ulcer patients do not vomit unless there is pyloric stenosis. Even though it is described as painless, at height of peristalsis, patients do complain of upper abdominal pain. Nausea preceding vomiting occurs in carcinoma stomach, recurrent appendicitis and chronic pancreatitis. **Chronic or subacute** intestinal obstruction due to ileocaecal tuberculosis, stricture of the small bowel, and adhesions (pain is severe and colicky), patients

have vomiting which is more after having a good meal. Typically, it occurs after 6–8 hours.

3. *Haematemesis/melaena*: Haematemesis is vomiting of blood. Massive haematemesis can occur due to rupture of oesophageal varices caused by portal hypertension. Streaks of blood along with vomitus may suggest carcinoma stomach also. Haematemesis is also a feature of chronic gastric ulcer. Melaena is tarry altered blood which is sticky and with foul odour. It is a feature of upper gastrointestinal tract bleeding. Common causes being chronic duodenal ulcer, chronic gastric ulcer, erosive gastritis, etc.

4. *Early satiety/fullness after meals*: This is a feature of carcinoma stomach. Also any large upper abdominal mass may compress on the stomach and give rise to this history. In carcinoma stomach, as the growth infiltrates the muscle layers, **receptive relaxation cannot take place**. Hence fullness after meals or early satiety is seen.

5. *Abdominal distension*: Upper abdominal fullness or distension occurs in pyloric stenosis, pseudocyst of pancreas, and large abdominal masses. Ascites can be the cause of distension. In surgical wards, it is due to tubercular peritonitis or due to advanced malignancies such as carcinoma stomach or colon or pancreas.

Clinical Wisdom

Sudden abdominal distension without pain in middle-aged/old-aged female is due to ascites caused by malignant ovarian tumour.

6. *Jaundice*: Again same questions such as the duration, progress of jaundice, colour of urine and colour of stools, should be enquired. Short duration of progressive jaundice occurs in carcinoma of pancreas or periampullary region. Long duration suggests stones in the common bile duct. Postoperative (postlaparoscopic cholecystectomy) stricture is more common now as more laparoscopic cholecystectomy is being done. Intermittent pain, intermittent fever and intermittent jaundice have been called **Charcot's triad.** It suggests stone in the common bile duct. Pain radiates to the right back in between shoulder blades in these cases. Even though progressive, sloughing of tumour takes place in periampullary carcinoma resulting fluctuating jaundice. All such surgical jaundice cases are associated with pruritus, high coloured urine and clay-coloured stools. Faint lemon yellow

jaundice with splenomegaly occurs in hereditary spherocytosis. This type of jaundice occurs due to haemolysis. It is called haemolytic jaundice. It is not associated with clay-coloured stools and pruritus.

7. *Fever*: Fever suggests inflammatory condition. Chronic amoebic liver abscess, infected hydatid cyst, and infected pseudocyst are a few examples. However, a few tumours can present as low grade fever, notably hepatocellular carcinoma and renal cell carcinoma. These are missed unless clinician carefully analyses the symptoms. **High grade fever with chills and rigors** with jaundice indicates cholangitis (inflammation of the biliary radicle) with or without stone disease. **Evening rise of temperature** is typically seen in abdominal tuberculosis. It should not be confused for abdominal lymphoma which gives rise to remittent bouts of intermittent fever.

8. *Bowel habits*: Altered bowel habits for a few months are a feature of carcinoma colon. Increasing constipation in case of left-sided tumours and blood and mucus in stools in right-sided tumours are common. Gaseous distension, incomplete evacuation, and gas colics are also other complaints in obstructed colon. Steatorrhoea (fatty stools) are seen in chronic pancreatitis when exocrine deficiency occurs. Blood and mucus in stools are features of inflammatory bowel diseases such as ulcerative colitis and Crohn's disease, and carcinoma rectum.

9. *Loss of appetite and loss of weight*: Both are very important symptoms of carcinoma stomach and carcinoma pancreas. Appetite loss is a dominant symptom of carcinoma stomach and weight loss is a dominant symptom of carcinoma pancreas. All other gastrointestinal tract malignancies also produce these symptoms.

10. *Haematuria, urgency, frequency, hesitancy (more details are given in Chapter 26)*: Intermittent haematuria in an elderly man could be due to renal cell carcinoma. Other three features are due to benign prostatic hyperplasia.

11. In female patients, history should be elicited to rule out uterine/ovarian pathology. Lower abdominal discomfort, distension, dull aching pain can be caused by uterine fibroids/ovarian tumours. Subserosal fibroids may not give rise to menorrhagia. Sudden abdominal distension, and weight loss can be caused by malignant ovarian tumours.

Past History

History of tuberculosis, history of surgery, history of family members having cancers should be enquired.

Personal History

Smoking and tobacco chewing are factors not only for cancers but they can be the cause for postprandial pain due to superior mesenteric ischaemia. Spicy food habits may contribute to peptic ulcer disease. Chronic alcohol intake can be associated with cirrhosis of the liver resulting in portal hypertension.

Family History

Colonic cancers can run in families. Ask whether any member of the family is affected and treated for colonic cancers.

GENERAL PHYSICAL EXAMINATION

- *Pallor*: Carcinoma stomach, carcinoma pancreas, colonic cancer
- *Icterus*: Periampullary carcinoma, carcinoma head of pancreas
- *Clubbing*: Chronic lung diseases
- *Lymph nodes*: Lymphoma, tuberculosis
- *Left supraclavicular node (Virchow node)*: Gastrointestinal tract malignancy
- *Oedema feet*: Large liver masses, advanced malignancies, deep vein thrombosis (DVT) (Fig. 23.1) tuberculosis
- *Tenderness spine (paraspinal)*: Tuberculosis
- *Melanin spots*: Peutz-Jeghers syndrome
- *Hypertension*: Aneurysm, SMA thrombosis

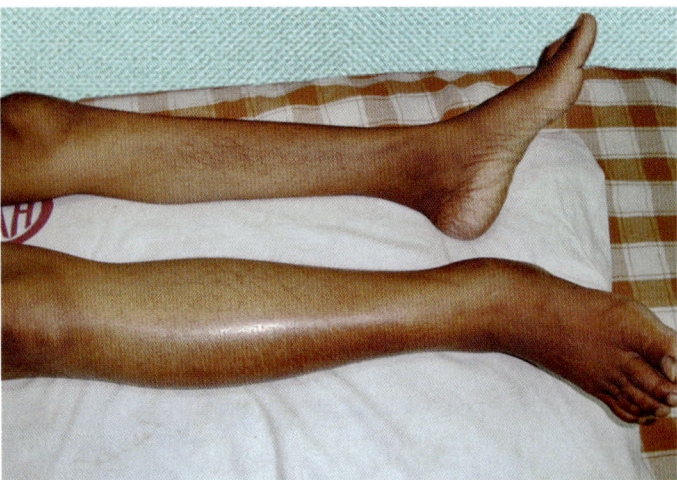

Fig. 23.1: DVT right leg caused by carcinoma pancreas resulting in oedema

ABDOMINAL EXAMINATION

Inspection

Spend a few minutes carefully watching the abdomen for shape, umbilicus, distension and flank fullness, peristalsis, pulsations, dilated veins, scars and nodules. These careful observations will help to some extent in the final diagnosis.

1. *Shape*: Normal abdomen is flat or concave (Fig. 23.2), protuberant in fatty individuals. Convexity is also due to a large mass in the abdomen.

2. *Distension*: Uniform distension occurs in gross ascites. Look at the flanks. It is easy to observe this. In ascites, distance between xiphoid process and umbilicus is more than between umbilicus and pubic symphysis. **It is called Tanyol sign** (Fig. 23.3). Mention whether flanks seem full or not. Fullness can also be found in large pericardial effusion. It has been called **Auenbrugger's sign.**

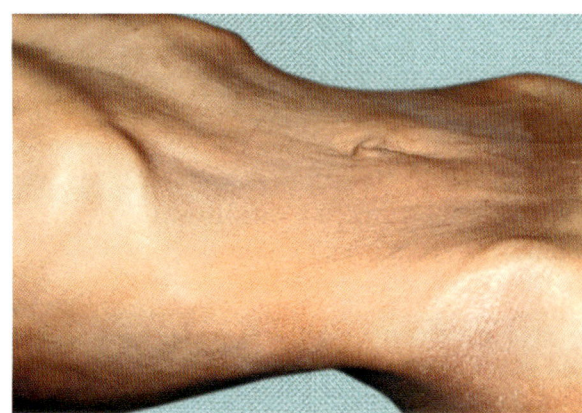

Fig. 23.2: Concave abdomen of pyloric stenosis due to repeated persistent vomiting, resulting in weight loss

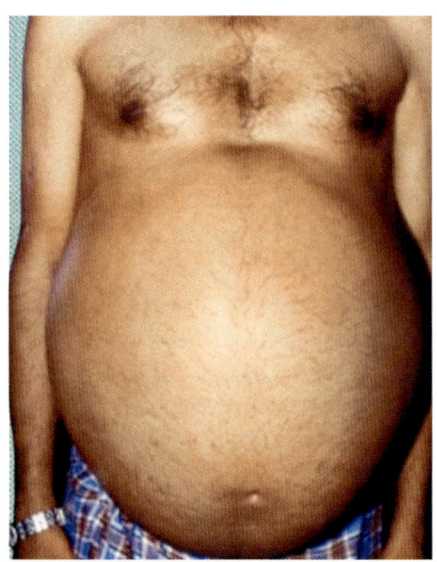

Fig. 23.3: Tanyol's sign

The most common cause of generalised distension of abdomen is ascites. Localised upper abdominal distension more on the right side is usually due to an enlarged liver. Epigastric fullness/distension is often caused by pseudocyst (Fig. 23.4). Lower abdominal central/lateral distension is caused by a large ovarian tumour. Suprapubic fullness presenting as a tense cystic mass is due to a distended bladder secondary to benign prostatic hypertrophy (BPH). Any large cystic masses in the abdomen such as mesenteric cyst, omental cyst, ovarian cyst and a large hydronephrosis can give rise to distension of the abdomen.

Clinical Wisdom

Remember common causes of distension are fluid, fat, flatus (intestinal obstruction), faeces (pseudo-obstruction) and foetus.

3. **Umbilicus**: Large pelvic tumours can displace umbilicus upwards. Normal umbilicus is inverted. It is everted in cases of ascites. Deformed umbilicus may be the clue for vitellointestinal duct anomaly with a band. One of the them is Raspberry tumour which gives rise to recurrent attacks of pain and discharge from the umbilicus. It is also called as umbilical granuloma. If any nodule is seen within or adjacent to the umbilicus, with or without ulceration, mention that (Sister Mary Joseph nodule) (Figs 23.5 to 23.8).

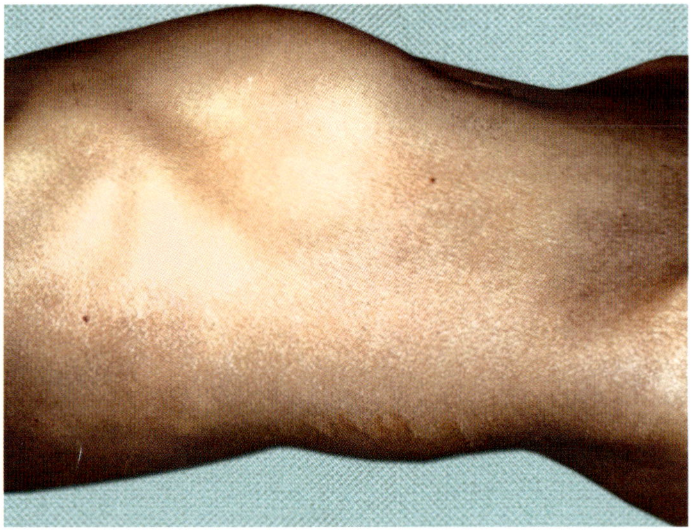

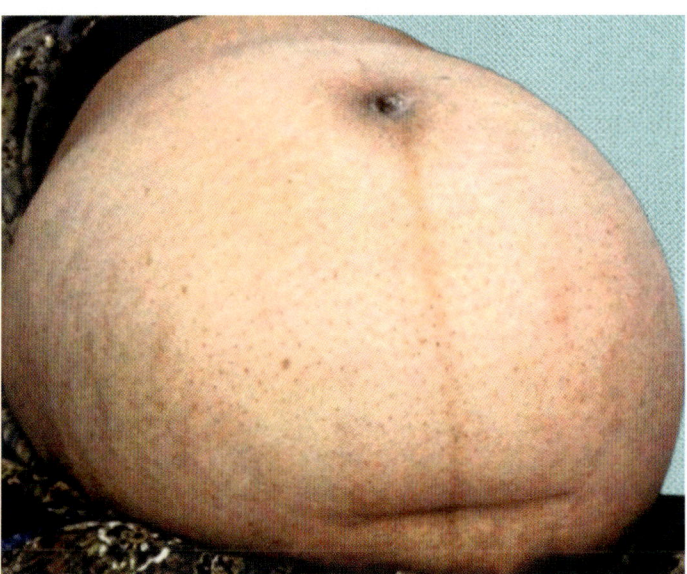

Fig. 23.4: Large epigastric mass/distension caused by pseudocyst of pancreas (a complication of acute pancreatitis)

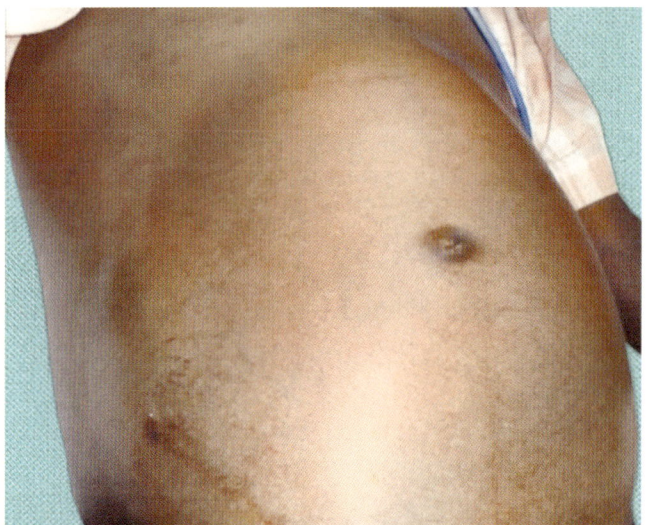

Fig. 23.5: Tense ascites resulting in everted umbilicus

Fig. 23.6: Large ovarian tumour displacing umbilicus upwards

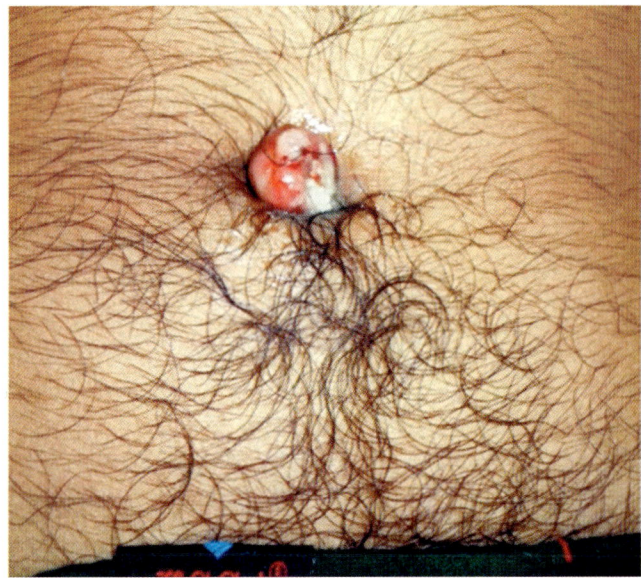

Fig. 23.7: Raspberry tumour of the umbilicus—due to patent umbilical end of vitellointestinal duct

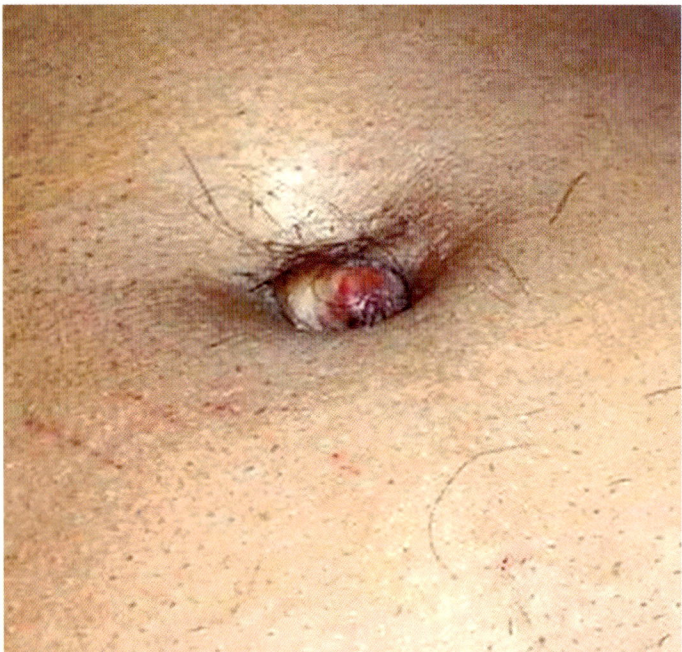

Fig. 23.8: Sister Mary Joseph nodule in the umbilicus. It indicates advanced gastrointestinal malignancies. Nodule was indurated, hard and ulcerated

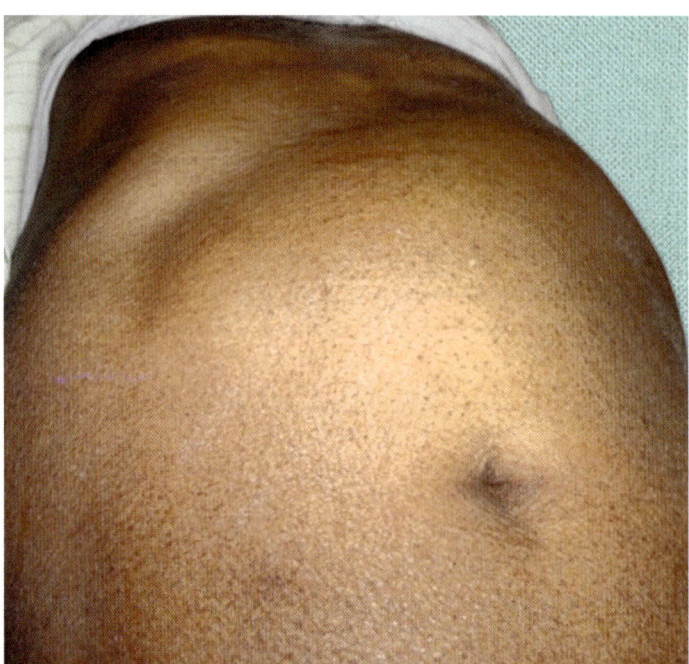

Fig. 23.9: Large stomach wave rolling across umbilicus to reach right side (VGP) (*Courtesy:* Prof. SS Prasad, Department of Surgery, KMC, Manipal)

Sister Mary Joseph Nodule or Sister Mary Joseph Sign

- This refers to a metastatic hard umbilical nodule from gastrointestinal malignancies commonly carcinoma stomach, pancreatic carcinoma, colonic carcinoma and ovarian carcinoma.

- Method of spread mostly is direct transperitoneal route or through lymphatics which run along obliterated umbilical vein.

- Significance is that it indicates poor prognosis.

- Sister Mary Joseph (1856-1939) was assistant to William H Mayo, St. Mary Hospital–Rochester.

- She discovered the nodule, brought to the notice of William J Mayo.

4. *Peristalsis*: Three types of peristalsis have been described in the abdomen (Fig. 23.10).

- *Visible gastric peristalsis (VGP)*: When you suspect pyloric stenosis, ask the patient to drink water till he feels full (may be more than 500 to 1000 ml) and observe for wave of stomach moving from left hypochondrium across umbilicus to the right hypochondrium (left to right). Please wait for 1 or 2 minutes and watch the abdomen. Carcinoma pyloric antrum can also give rise to VGP. Only other condition which can give rise to something similar to VGP is

duodenal obstruction (Wilkie's disease or carcinoma head of pancreas with duodenal obstruction) (Figs 23.9 and 23.10—1).

Clinical Wisdom

Visible Gastric Peristalsis (VGP)

- Classically, it is seen in idiopathic, hypertrophic pyloric, stenosis in infants and in chronic duodenal ulcer with cicatrisation. In chronic duodenal ulcer, enough time will be present for stomach to undergo distension and dilatation.

- It is seen sometimes in carcinoma pyloric antrum. When growth infiltrates the body, stomach loses the capacity to distend and one may not see VGP. Also it is a shorter period of obstruction and hence dilatation is not much.

- *Step-ladder peristalsis*: It is seen in terminal ileal obstruction, common causes of this being ileo-caecal tuberculosis or carcinoma caecum. Often these patients have bilious vomiting. Step-ladder peristalsis coincides with patient experiencing abdominal colic (Fig. 23.10—2).

- *Right to left peristalsis*: This is found in left colonic obstructions specially splenic flexure growth. Since the diameter of the colon is large and in some cases ileocaecal valve is competent it is not easy to find this peristalsis. One may find distended loops or prominent loops in the right hypochondrium or in the right iliac fossa (distended caecum) (Fig. 23.10—3).

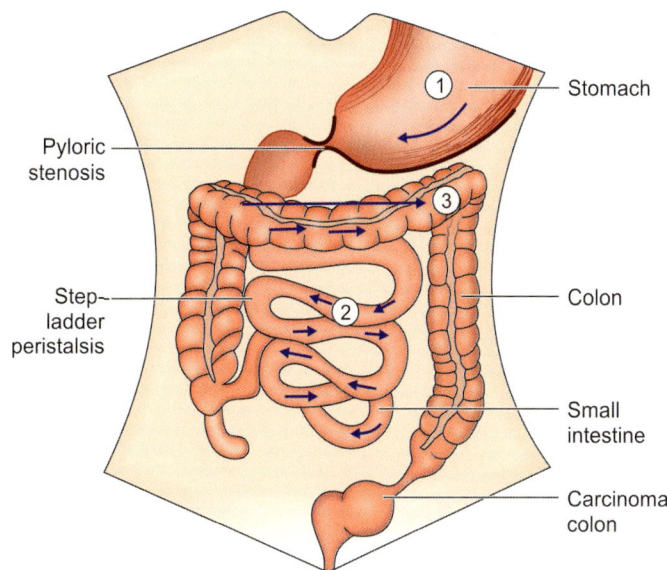

Fig. 23.10: Three types of peristalsis

5. *Pulsations*: Carefully watch the abdomen. Prominent pulsations in the upper abdomen in a thin patient can be normal (transmitted from the heart) or due to aortic aneurysm. Again aortic pulsations can be transmitted by a large pseudocyst of pancreas in the epigastrium.

6. *Dilated veins* (Figs 23.11 to 23.13):

   • *Central abdominal veins around umbilicus* are called caput medusae. They represent portal hypertension. Portal component in these veins are veins which run in the falciform ligament and systemic component being branches of superior and inferior epigastric veins. It is not common to get caput medusa because in vast majority of cases umbilical veins which run in the falciform ligament are obliterated.

   • *Flank veins*: These veins run from the inguinal region towards the axilla. These have been called inguinoaxillary veins. They are found in cases of inferior vena caval obstruction.

7. *Scars* (Fig. 23.14): These are previous laparotomy scars. Common clinical scenario will be incisional hernia presenting as abdominal swelling, carcinoma stomach arising from previous gastrojejunostomy done 15–20 years back, or previous laparoscopic cholecystectomy and obstructive jaundice now (bile duct stricture).

Clinical Wisdom

If you see a upper midline scar and the epigastric mass is palpable—think of stump carcinoma. (Mostly surgery done is vagotomy + GJ.)

8. *Nodules/lumps*: These are part of generalized diseases such as multiple lipoma/neurofibroma. Typically, they are of long duration. Recent development of nodules suggests malignancies such as lymphoma and disseminated melanoma.

9. If any mass is visible, mention it (more details in the next chapter).

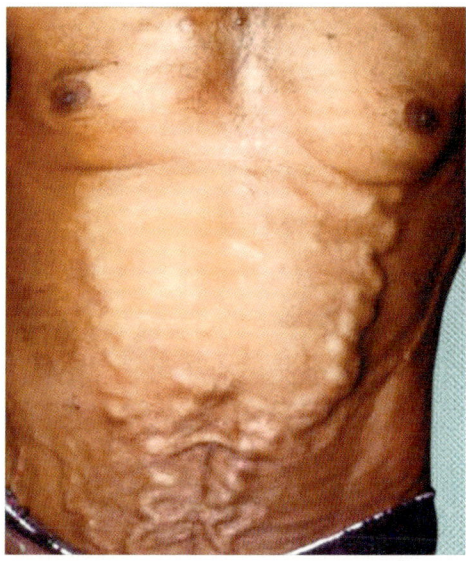

Fig. 23.11: Caput medusae and the direction of flow is away from umbilicus

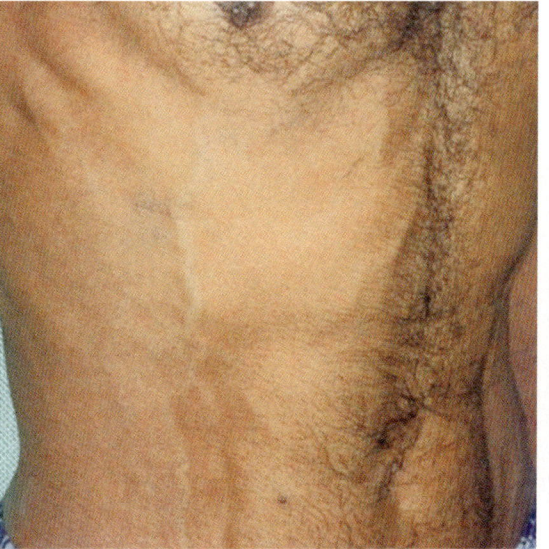

Fig. 23.12: Inguinoaxillary veins: Veins on the lateral abdominal wall suggestive of inferior vena caval obstruction

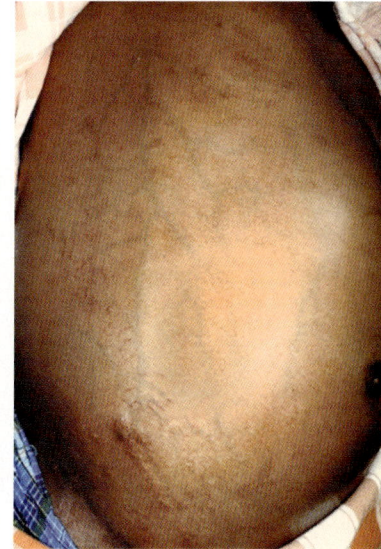

Fig. 23.13: Budd-Chiari syndrome: Tense ascites, inguinoaxillary veins

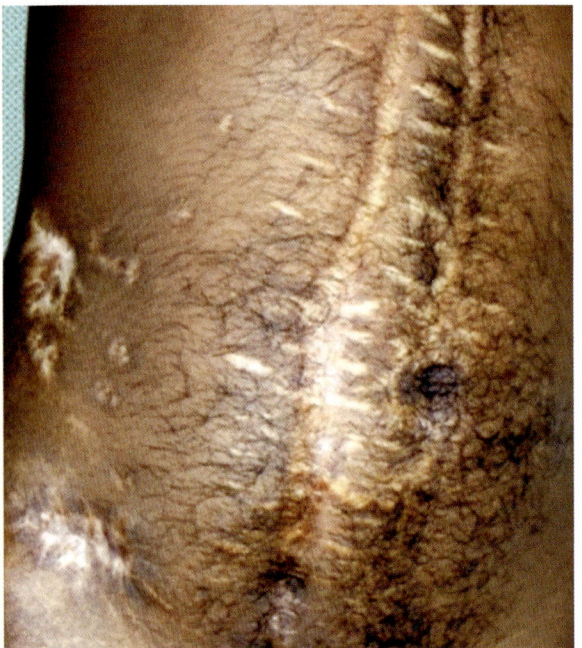

Fig. 23.14: Case of duodenal ulcer perforation—opened and sutured, leaked again, reexplored. Healed after 6 weeks

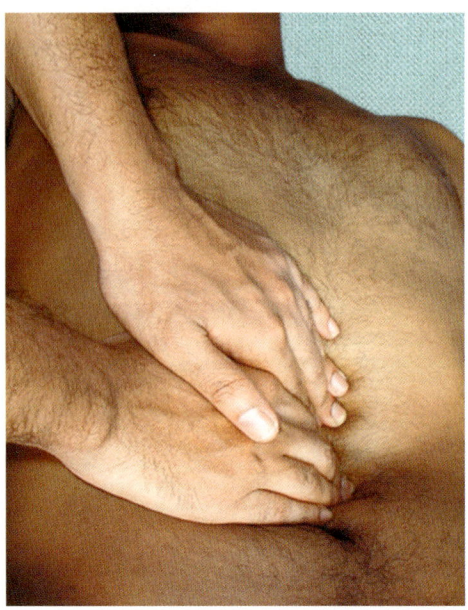

Fig. 23.16: Two-hand method of palpation in obese patients. One above the other—it also helps in deep palpation

Palpation (Figs 23.15 to 23.19)

- Ask the patient to lie down on the examination table. He has to fold the legs and breathe well so that abdominal palpation becomes easy (*refer* to Clinical Box 23.1).

Methods of Palpation

Superficial palpation *to detect abdominal wall swellings such as lipomas, nodules, hernias, etc.* ***Deep palpation*** *region by region, to look for tenderness, any mass which is felt and to know the details about the mass.* ***Dipping method*** (Fig. 23.17) *is done in cases of ascites.* ***Nicolson's method of palpation:*** *This is applied when patient holds the abdomen tight (voluntary guarding). With both hands one above the other, pressure is applied over lower chest near the xiphisternum, abdominal wall relaxes and palpation becomes easy* (Fig. 23.18).

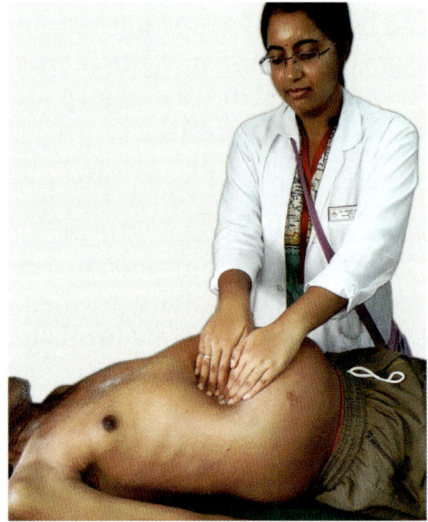

Fig. 23.17: Dipping method in cases of tense ascites

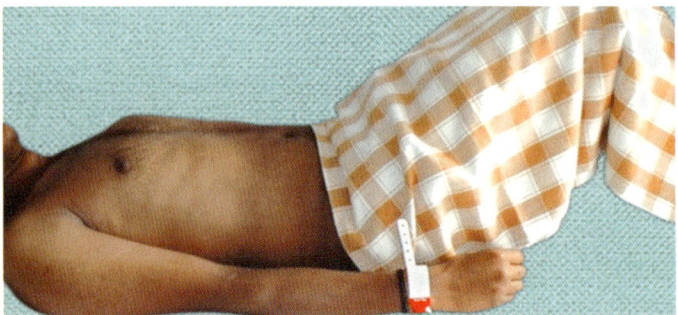

Fig. 23.15: Ask the patient to lie down supine, breathe well, relax and bend the knees to relax the abdominal muscles

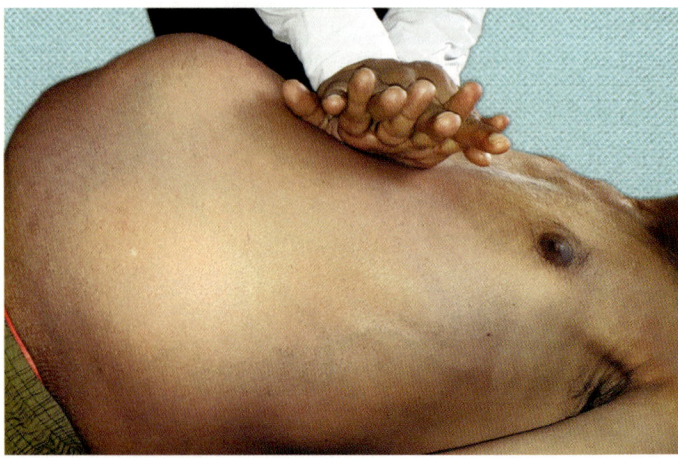

Fig. 23.18: Nicolson's method

Palpation Tips

- Take the patient into confidence.
- Tell him what you are doing.
- Turn the face to opposite side.
- Flex the leg. This will relax the abdominal wall. Palpation becomes easy.
- Palpation should be gentle, region by region by rolling the fingers.
- Ask him to breathe well, relax the abdomen. Palpate deep when breathing is in expiration.
- The most important factor which limits palpation is guarding and rigidity which can be minimised, if you follow the guidelines mentioned above.

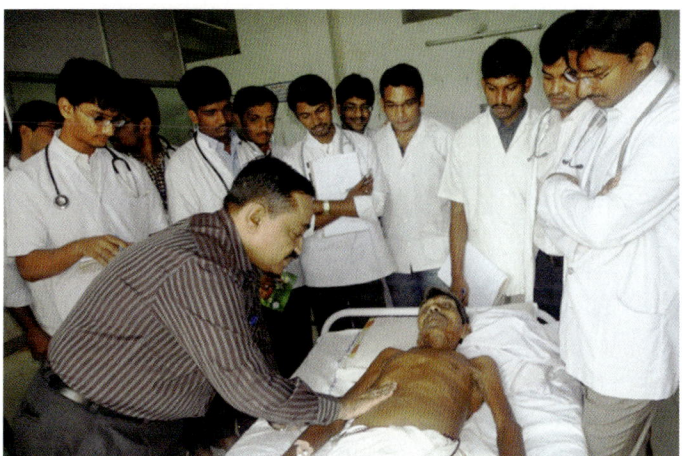

Fig. 23.19: Region by region, palpate 9 regions in the abdomen gently by flat of the hand and check for any specific areas of tenderness or any palpable mass (*Courtesy*: Dr Ravindranath, Dr Challa Srinivas Rao, FRCS, KIMS, Professor of Surgery, KIMS—Amalapuram, AP)

1. *Feel of the abdomen*: Normal abdomen is soft without any guarding and rigidity. Doughy is the term described for the feel of abdomen in tuberculous peritonitis. Guarding and rigidity indicates peritoneal inflammation resulting in contraction of underlying muscles. *Example*: Upper abdominal guarding and rigidity in cases of acute cholecystitis, or acute pancreatitis, perforated duodenal ulcer (initial hours).

2. *Tenderness*: The site of tenderness will help in deciding which organ is involved. Following picture is self explanatory (Fig. 23.20).

3. *Palpating the abdominal organs*

   a. *Enlarged liver* is palpable in the right hypochondrium (normal liver is not palpable in adults). Since the liver enlarges in the downward direction up to the right iliac fossa, better to start palpating in the right iliac fossa and then slowly go up. As the patient takes a deep breath, the lower border comes and touches the palpating fingers. To detect the upper border, percuss from the 4th or 5th intercostal space downwards in the midclavicular line and find out the dullness (Fig. 23.21).

   b. *Gallbladder*: It is felt when enlarged in the Murphy's point below the tip of the 9th costal cartilage as a smooth globular mass. Just like the palpation of the liver, start palpating from right iliac fossa and go above, this globular mass can be felt a step deep to the enlarged liver—a point to differentiate from the liver itself. More details

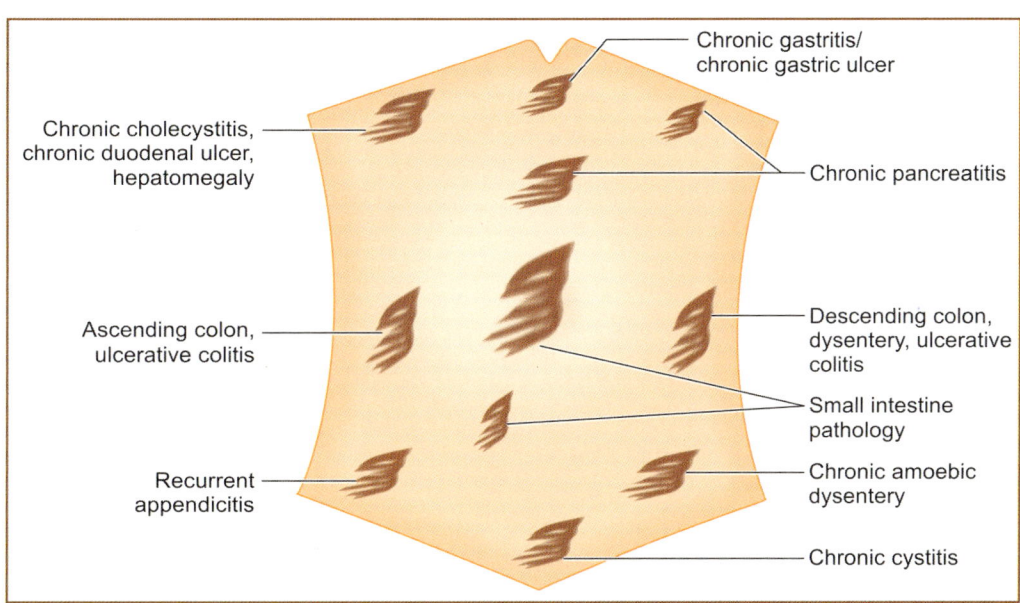

Fig. 23.20: Tender areas on palpation

Chronic gastritis/chronic gastric ulcer

Chronic cholecystitis, chronic duodenal ulcer, hepatomegaly

Chronic pancreatitis

Ascending colon, ulcerative colitis

Descending colon, dysentery, ulcerative colitis

Small intestine pathology

Recurrent appendicitis

Chronic amoebic dysentery

Chronic cystitis

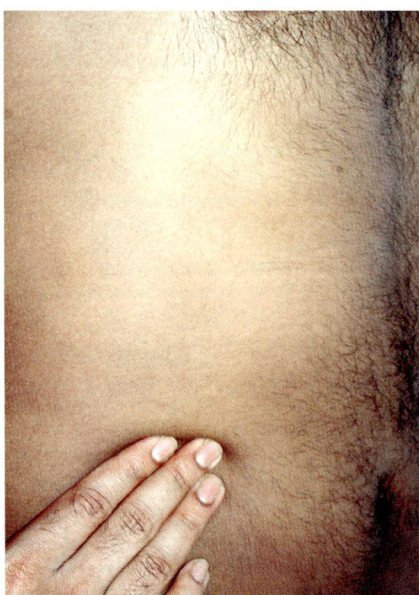

Fig. 23.21: Palpation of the liver. Liver should be palpated not only in the right hypochondrium but also in the epigastrium and also in the left hypochondrium. It has a characteristic lower border (*Courtesy:* Dr Sunilkrishna, Associate Prof, KMC, Manipal)

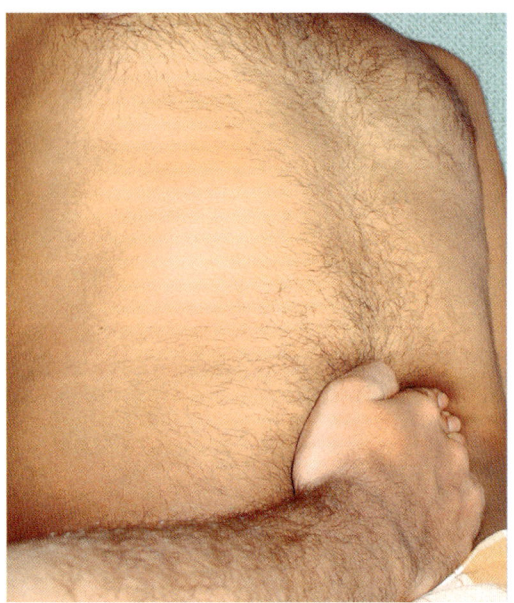

Fig. 23.22: Various causes of splenomegaly result in vague pain/discomfort. It is a common mistake to palpate the spleen medially. In mild cases of splenomegaly, spleen has to be felt more laterally in the left hypochondrium (*Courtesy:* Dr Sunilkrishna, Associate Professor, KMC, Manipal)

are given in Chapter 24 on mass abdomen. For all practical purposes, enlarged gallbladder and jaundice mean periampullary/carcinoma head of pancreas.

In chronic cholecystitis, gallbladder is not palpable but tenderness on deep palpation may be present.

c. *Enlarged diseased stomach* is felt as a mass in the epigastrium. Details are given in Chapter 24. Both upper and lower borders can be palpated. Start palpating near umbilical region and slowly go up. At the height of deep inspiration, the lower border can be felt. In vast majority, the small mass is due to carcinoma stomach and large mass is caused by gastrointestinal stromal tumour (GIST).

d. *Spleen*: Since it enlarges in the downward and its axial direction up to the right iliac fossa, depending upon the size of the spleen, one can palpate from the umbilical region or from the right iliac fossa and go towards the left hypochondrium (standing from the right side of the abdomen). At the height of inspiration, lower border comes and touches the palpating fingers. When splenomegaly is grade 1, it can be missed, specially in obese patients. There are a few tips

in such situations. Turn the patient to the right lateral position by about 30 degrees. Palpate standing on the left side of the patient and insinuate behind the left costal margin for mass or for lower border and confirm movement with respiration. Often a mistake is done by trying to feel the spleen more medially and telling that spleen is not palpable. However, it should be noted that spleen is felt under the 10th rib not under 9th costal cartilage (Fig. 23.22).

Clinical Wisdom

Splenic notch, if felt on the anterior border, is diagnostic of a splenic mass.

e. *Pancreas*: It is a deep-seated and retroperitoneal organ and hence is not palpable easily. Tenderness in the epigastrium is suggestive of acute pancreatitis. In majority of cases of chronic pancreatitis, no signs are elicited because pancreas is not enlarged but it is atrophic and fibrosed. However, with an attack of acute on chronic pancreatitis, a sign called **Mallet-Guy sign** (Fig. 23.23) is elicited. The patient is asked to roll to the right lateral decubitus position and examiner palpates in the epigastrium and left deep hypochondrium. Tenderness, if elicited, the sign is said to be positive.

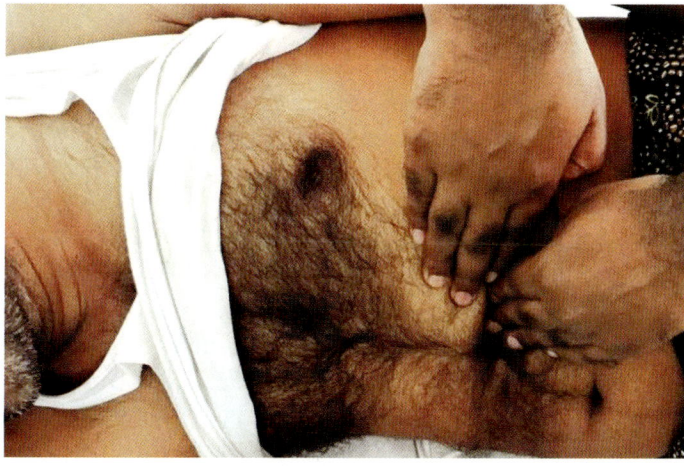

Fig. 23.23: Palpation of pancreas—Mallet-Guy sign. Patient is in the right lateral position

f. *Kidneys* are palpable in the loin both—anteriorly under costal margin and posteriorly in the para-vertebral space. More details are given in the renal chapter. Kidneys can be palpable in thin patients (without enlargement).

g. *Colon*: Palpate the entire length of colon from right iliac fossa (caecum) till sigmoid colon (Fig. 23.24). Go in the vertical direction towards right hypochondrium, then feel for transverse colon till left hypochondrium and then palpate vertically downwards from left hypochondrium to left lumbar region and left iliac fossa. Loaded colon in elderly patients or patients with chronic constipation have confused many a great teacher in their diagnosis. Except splenic flexure growth

(deep and high location) and rectosigmoid (stricture), all other growths can be palpable.

h. *Small bowel and mesentery* are not palpable but the lesions arising from them are palpated in the centre of the abdomen (details in the next chapter).

Percussion

• Liver and spleen are solid organs and no other organs can enlarge over these and hence, they are dull to percuss.

• Retroperitoneal organs when they enlarge, intestines are spread over the tumour and a resonant note is elicited. However, when the tumour displaces the intestines to the periphery, note is dull in the centre but resonant in the periphery.

• Shifting dullness suggests fluid—tuberculous ascites, and malignant ascites are two common conditions in the surgical ward.

• In women, large ovarian cysts are common. This should not be confused for ascites. In ovarian cysts, dullness is over the cyst—anteriorly and resonance is in the side-flanks. It is vice versa in cases of ascites.

Auscultation (Fig. 23.25)

• Bowel sounds are better heard in the right iliac fossa. In ileocaecal tuberculosis, with obstruction, loud noisy sounds can be heard (borborygmi).

• Bruit can be heard in over vascular tumours such as hepatocellular carcinoma.

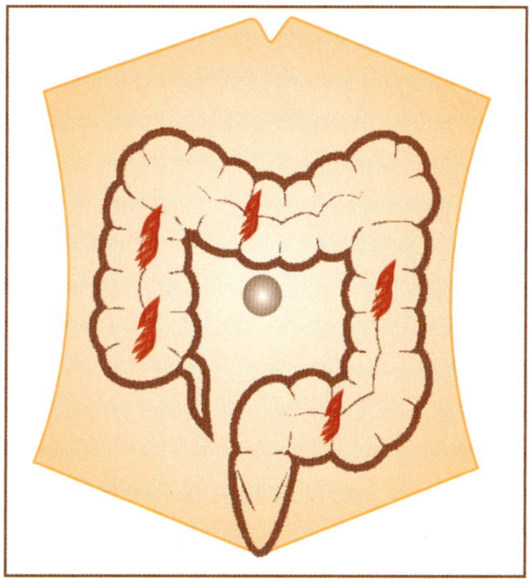

Fig. 23.24: Multiple tender areas—a case of ulcerative colitis—acute exacerbation

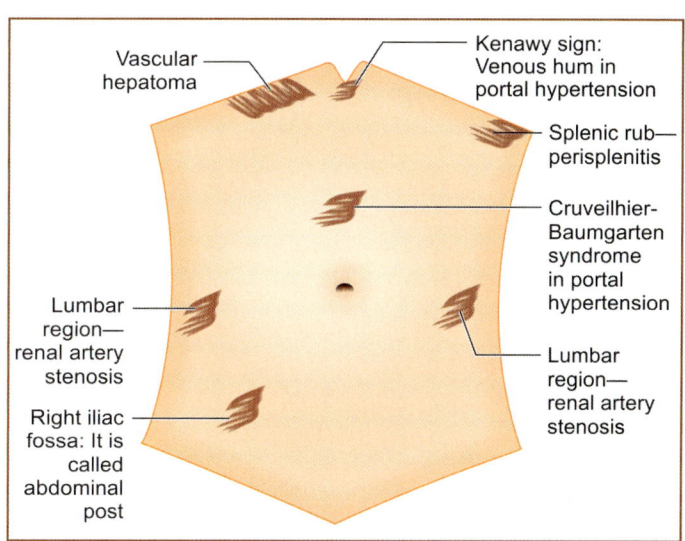

Fig. 23.25: Importance of auscultation for surgeon

- Bruit can be heard in the lumbar region in cases of renal artery stenosis.

- *Splenic rub* can be heard in cases of splenic infarction due to perisplenitis (sickle cell anaemia).

- *Kenawy's sign*: Venous hum can be heard in the epigastrium just beneath xiphoid process in cases of portal hypertension. Hum is caused by dilated splenic veins. When the spleen gets compressed during deep inspiration, venous flow increases and a hum can be heard.

- *Cruveilhier-Baumgarten syndrome*: It is a venous hum heard between umbilicus and epigastrium. It is heard in portal hypertension and is due to patent umbilical vein joining portal vein.

- *Ausculto-percussion test or ausculto-scraping test*: This is done when you suspect pyloric stenosis. Stomach gets dilated in cases of pyloric obstruction and large amount of fluid gets accumulated. Lower border is often below the umbilicus.

  Clinically, dilated stomach can be detected by this test. Keep the bell of the stethoscope in the upper umbilical region and percuss away from the bell of the stethoscope or scrape downwards at different points as shown in Figs 23.26A and B. When the dull note (fluid) is replaced by resonant note it indicates the limit of greater curvature. When a line is made with such many points it indicates the greater curvature of the stomach. This was the test done by clinicians in cases of pyloric stenosis caused by cicatrised duodenal ulcer patients to find out the distended stomach and greater curvature of the stomach

EXAMINATION OF THE LEFT SUPRACLAVICULAR NODE—VIRCHOW'S NODE

- Thoracic duct drains into left subclavian vein at a point where it is joined by innominate vein. This is the place where classical supraclavicular node is palpable when enlarged. The position may vary a few centimetres left or right side. The reason why it gets enlarged is not known. However, a few theories have been postulated. One theory is that, **the tumour cells block the thoracic duct at the junction and come out of thoracic duct and get enlarged.** Another postulate is that one of the supraclavicular nodes corresponds to the end node along the thoracic duct and hence the enlargement. Enlargement of left supraclavicular node in visceral malignancies has been described as **Troisier's sign** (Fig. 23.27).

- Originally, German pathologist Rudolf Virchow described this node for carcinoma stomach. It is involved in visceral malignancies such as colon, pancreas, liver, etc. testicular tumours.

- Stand behind the patient. Bend the neck of the patient to the left side. Gently feel the posterior triangle of the neck just above the clavicle. Start lateral to the lower end of sternocleidomastoid muscle and go laterally.

- Irrespective of the size palpable, supraclavicular lymph node must be considered as significant.

PER RECTAL EXAMINATION AND PER VAGINAL EXAMINATION

- Finding of a growth in the rectum—blood stains on rectal examination suggest carcinoma or inflammatory bowel diseases. Anteriorly recto-vesical pouch deposits can be felt as a shelf-like projection. These are called Blumer shelf deposits. It occurs due to tumour cells that gravitate down

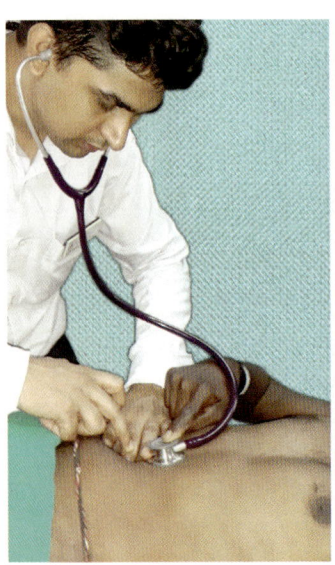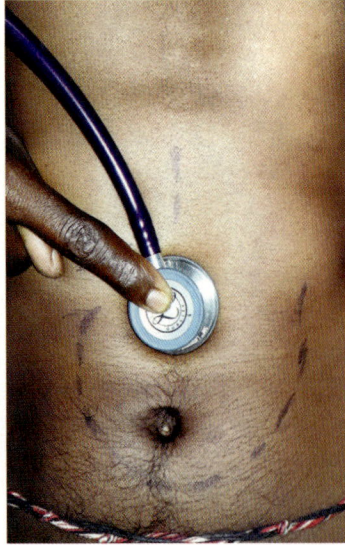

Figs 23.26A and B: Auscultopercussion test

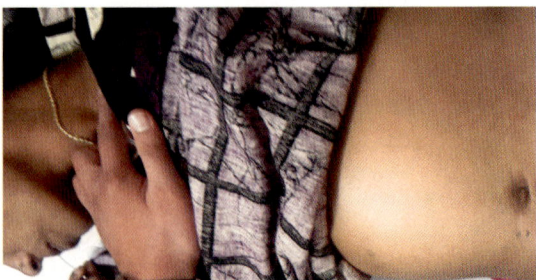

Fig. 23.27: Looking for left supraclavicular lymph node in case of carcinoma stomach—also observe distended stomach due to pyloric obstruction caused by carcinoma pyloric antrum. Patient was sick with wide spread metastasis

and settle down in the rectovesical or rectouterine pouch and grow. They indicate advanced inoperable nature of the disease (cure is not possible). Spread is by transcoelomic route.

- In women, vaginal examination is done to detect malignant deposits in the pouch of Douglas. Ovarian tumours can be felt as a part of bimanual examination.

DIFFERENTIAL DIAGNOSIS

1. *Chronic peptic ulcer*: Typically, patients are between 20 and 40 years of age who have burning in the epigastrium with food pain relationship. Symptoms are of many years duration. They are exaggerated on empty stomach in duodenal ulcer and on eating food in gastric ulcer. Other differences are given in Table 23.1. Tenderness is the only physical finding. Endoscopy (Oesophago gastro duodenoscopy (OGD)) is the key investigation followed by medical line of management (Figs 23.28 to 23.30). Pantoprazole is widely used drug which cures the problem in vast majority of the cases. Refractory cases need to undergo antral biopsies to detect the presence of *Helicobacter pylori* infections. If present, it has to be treated by triple therapy. Rarely a gastrin secreting tumour may be present in the pancreas called gastrinoma which can be diagnosed by CT scan and measuring gastrin levels. Triggering factors such as smoking alcohol, spicy food and drugs such as NSAID to be avoided or minimized.

2. *Gastric outlet obstruction*: Earlier it was called pyloric stenosis. However, gastric outlet obstruction is a better word. Chronic cicatrisation of a duodenal ulcer or juxtapyloric ulcer results in narrowing of pyloric antrum which is described as pyloric stenosis. Stenosis is very often found in the first part of duodenum. In India, pyloric stenosis is more common in South Indian patients, who usually present with a long history of duodenal ulcer and a recent history of vomiting. Classical hunger pain of duodenal ulcer disappears. It may be replaced by a dull aching pain because of gastric distension. Colicky pain is due to hyperperistalsis of stomach. Vomiting is

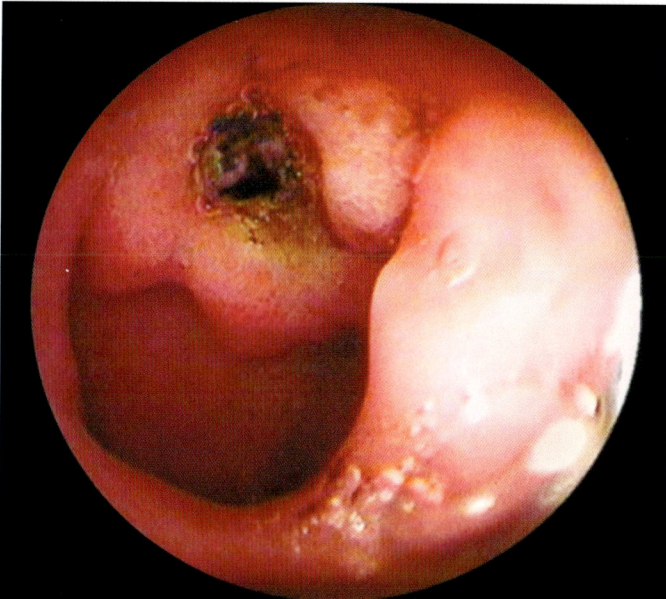
Fig. 23.29: OGD showing bleeding duodenal ulcer

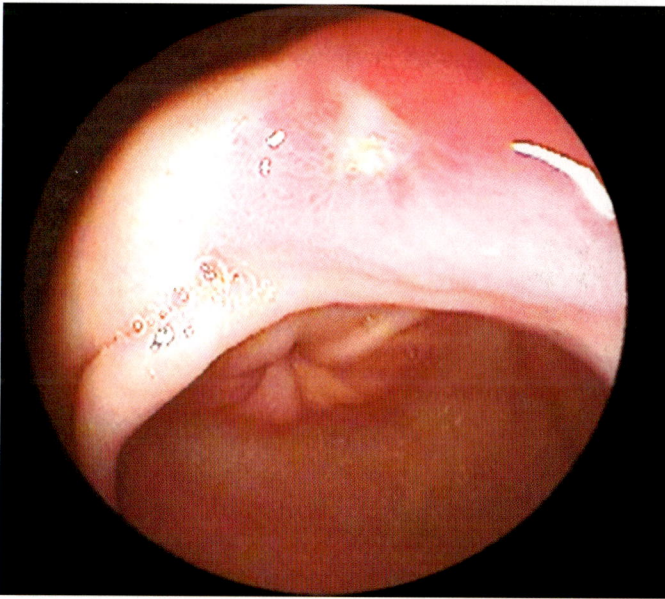
Fig. 23.30: OGD showing chronic gastric ulcer

profuse, projectile, persistent, foul-smelling (because of stasis) and nonbilious. There may be distension of upper abdomen with epigastric fullness. Visible gastric peristalsis (VGP) is found which can be made more obvious by asking the patient to drink about a litre of water. When stomach contracts, not only one can see the stomach but the contractions can also be felt. In pyloric stenosis, there is always residual fluid in the stomach, which gives a splashing sound that can be heard with/without stethoscope. Stomach mass is not palpable. However, when pyloric obstruction occurs due to carcinoma pyloric antrum, a pyloric mass will be palpable in the right hypochondrium or epigastrium. Gastroscopy will detect large amount of residual fluid. Hence, one should do endoscopy after inserting a nasogastric tube and emptying the stomach.

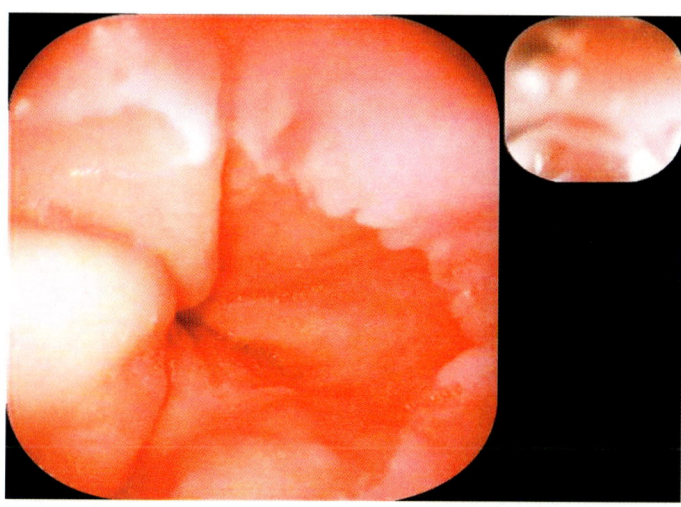
Fig. 23.28: Normal squamocolumnar junction—Z-line

Table 23.1: Comparison of clinical features

	Chronic duodenal ulcer	*Chronic gastric ulcer*
1. Incidence	Common	Less common
2. Site	1st inch of 1st part of duodenum	The lesser curvature or prepyloric region
3. Pain	It is due to the acid irritating the ulcer (hunger pain). It is relieved on taking food. After 1–2 hours of food, the pain becomes severe. It is burning in nature with retrosternal radiation (heart burn) and increased salivation (water brash)	Pain occurs on taking food and it is relieved by induced vomiting. Pain is of burning nature as in duodenal ulcer
4. Vomiting	Never occurs in duodenal ulcer till the patient develops pyloric stenosis	Frequent and it occurs immediately after consumption of food
5. Weight	Weight gain	Weight loss
6. Periodicity	Common	Less
7. Haematemesis : melaena ratio	40 : 60	60 : 40
8. On examination	Tenderness in the right hypochondrium	Tenderness in the epigastrium
9. Incidence of malignancy	Never becomes malignant	0.5–5% (2%)

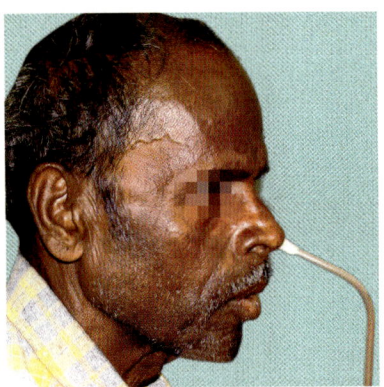

Fig. 23.31: Persistent vomiting and hiccoughs. Nasogastric tube inserted. Endoscopy revealed pyloric stenosis

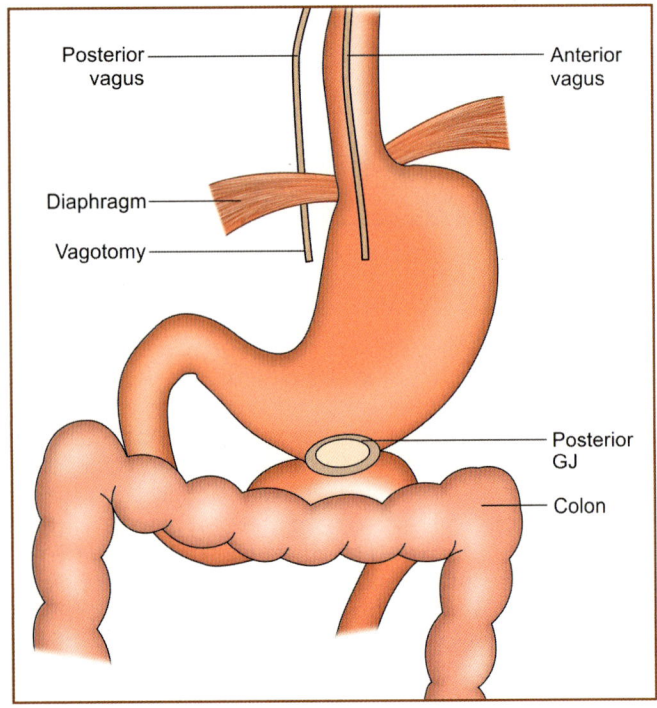

Fig. 23.32: Posterior GJ (Mayo) with total truncal vagotomy

Gastroscopy is done to rule out carcinoma stomach. Total truncal vagotomy and posterior gastrojejunostomy (GJ) are the treatment of choice (Figs 23.31 to 23,33).

Clinical Wisdom

- Stomach which is seen, felt and heard is diagnostic of pyloric stenosis.
- Signs of pyloric stenosis:
  1. Visible gastric peristalsis
  2. Succussion splash
  3. Ausculto-percussion test—dilated stomach

3. **Carcinoma stomach**: Very often patients would have vague symptoms—early satiety, flatulence, discomfort, pain in the upper abdomen. Early satiety is due to decreased distensibility of the stomach. Iron is absorbed in ferrous form in the duodenum. Anaemia is an important feature of carcinoma stomach. It is due to several factors such as nutritional or due to ulcerating lesion. But major cause is achlorhydria resulting in failure of conversion of ferric ions to ferrous ions. Following 5 groups have been identified, you can remember as **SOLID** (Figs 23.33 to 23.38).

- **S S**ilent: Growth is silent but manifests with secondaries in the liver, ascites, Virchow's node, rectovesical deposits, (Blumer's shelf), umbilical nodule (Sister Mary Joseph nodule), left axillary nodes (Irish nodes), and palpable ovarian mass (Krukenberg tumour).

- **O O**bstruction at pylorus (pyloric antrum) producing pyloric obstruction with features of vomiting with/without blood. Visible gastric peristalsis can also be present. Obstruction at cardio-oesophageal junction produces dysphagia.

- **L L**ump in the abdomen which is hard and irregular having altered tympanic resonant note.

- **I I**nsidious in onset: **Anaemia, anorexia and asthenia of short duration.**

- **D** **D**yspepsia in a man over the age of 40: Carcinoma stomach should be ruled out. Early gastric cancer presents as dyspepsia.

Gastroscopy is done and biopsy taken to confirm the diagnosis of adenocarcinoma. CT scan is done to find out the resectability. Treatment is radical gastrectomy followed by chemoradiotherapy. Prognosis is poor when patients present with a palpable mass and with metastasis.

D1– Gastrectomy refers to gastrectomy with removal of perigastric nodes.

D2– Gastrectomy with removal of perigastric lymph nodes and lymph nodes at the origin of major arteries—left gastric, hepatic, coeliac etc.

- Also see endoscopic and operative pictures in the next page, Figs 23.39 to 23.41.

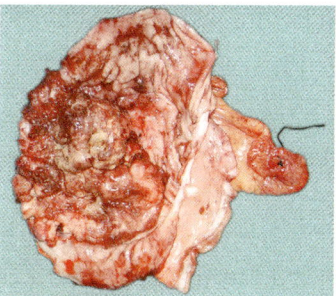
Fig. 23.35: Carcinoma stomach—large ulcerative lesion with involvement of serosa

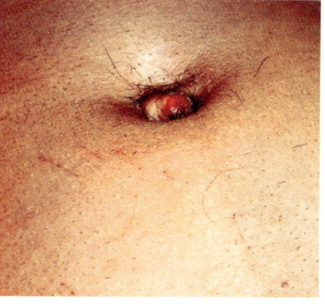
Fig. 23.36: Umbilical nodule—popularly called Sister Mary Joseph nodule

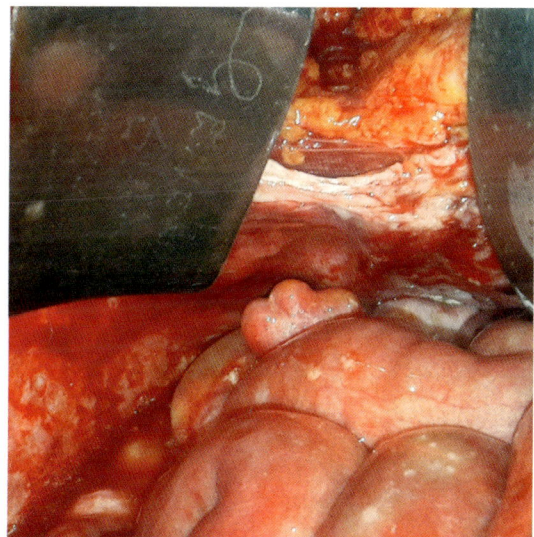
Fig. 23.33: Advanced carcinoma stomach with peritoneal nodules. Inoperable disease. Laparotomy was done because of perforated growth (*Courtesy:* Dr Chitra Bhat, Assistant Prof, KMC Manipal)

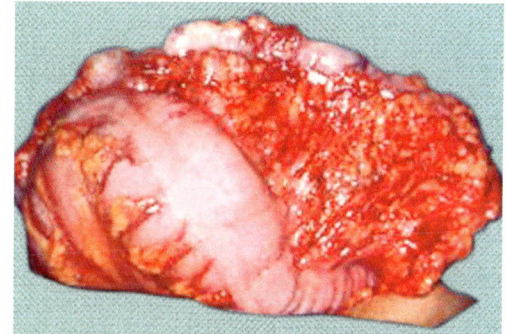
Fig. 23.37: Carcinoma stomach with nodules in the greater omentum

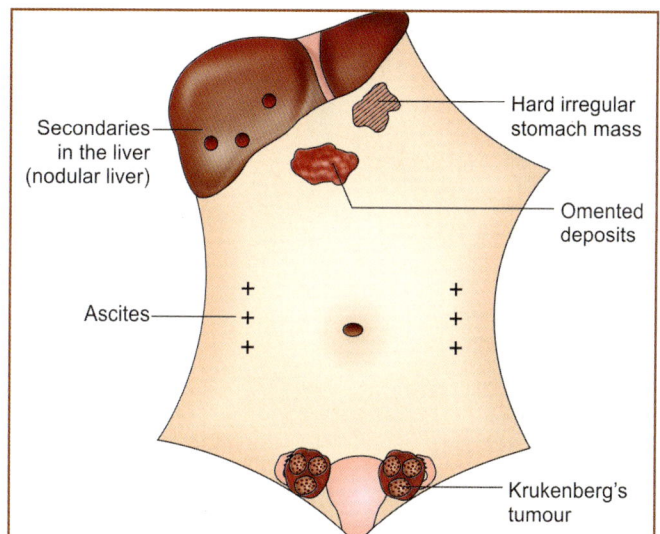
Fig. 23.38: Diagrammatic representation of secondaries from carcinoma stomach

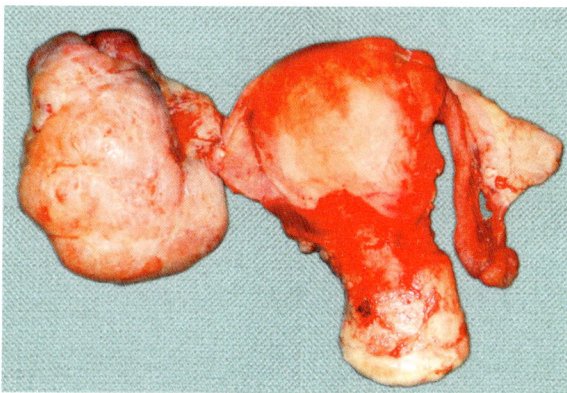
Fig. 23.34: Krukenberg tumours

4. ***Chronic cholecystitis***: Flatulent dyspepsia is a common presentation. If an obese woman (fatty, fertile, flatulent, female in forties) complains of gaseous distension, intolerance to fatty food and discomfort in the abdomen, heartburn and belching, she probably has gallstones. They can also present with severe abdominal pain called gallstone colic. Pain may last for a few minutes to a few hours. It usually occurs at night wherein a stone tends to block the cystic duct or neck of gallbladder in the supine position. It is a severe colicky upper abdominal pain felt in the right hypochondrium, may shoot to the back or between shoulder blades. The pain is continuous and lasts for a few hours. Pain may radiate to the chest also. It is associated with vomiting, restlessness and sweating. There is tenderness in the right hypochondrium. No

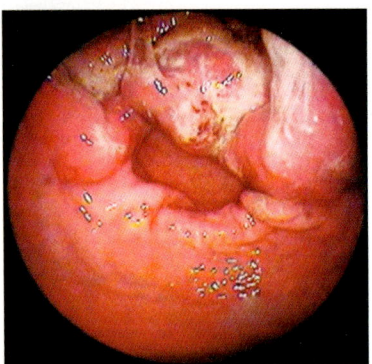

Fig. 23.39: Endoscopy—carcinoma stomach

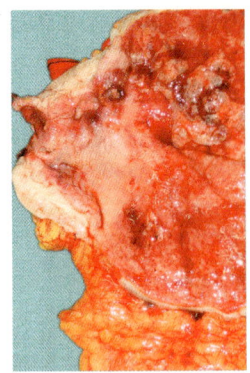

Fig. 23.40: Linitis plastica—Localised variety

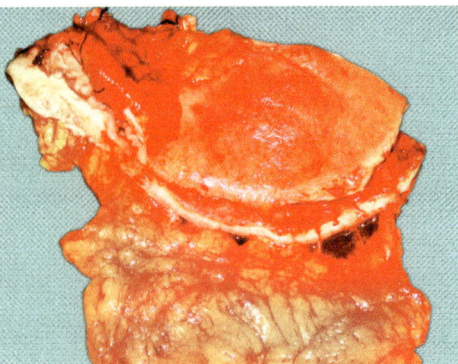

Fig. 23.41: Linitis plastica—Diffuse variety

(*Courtesy:* Prof U Santhosh Pai, Professor of Surgery, MMMC, Manipal)

mass is palpable in the right hypochondrium unless mucocoele of the gallbladder develops due to a stone blocking the cystic duct. Ultrasound clinchés the diagnosis in more than 98% patients. Laparoscopic cholecystectomy is the treatment of choice. In 3–5% patients, gall bladder will be shrunken and contracted due to chronic cholecystitis (Fig.23.42) due to fibrosis and adhesions, laparoscopic surgery, for that matter even open surgery may be difficult. In such cases, better to do partial cholecystectomy specially if the anatomy of the Calot's triangle is not clear.

diagnosis. As per Courvoisier's law—in a jaundiced patient, if gallbladder is palpable and enlarged, it is not due to stones because in case of stones previous inflammation would have resulted in fibrosed and contracted gallbladder hence not palpable. Early diagnosis by imaging, endoscopy, ERCP, MRCP is possible. It is treated by extraction of the stones by endoscopic basketing followed by laparoscopic chole-cystectomy (Figs 23.43 and 23.44). It should be done early to prevent complications such as cholangitis, liver abscesses, septicaemia, renal failure and even death (Table 23.2).

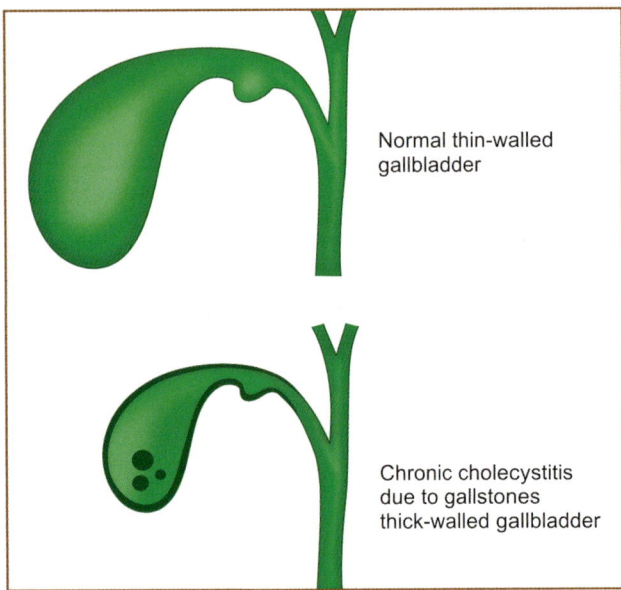

Normal thin-walled gallbladder

Chronic cholecystitis due to gallstones thick-walled gallbladder

Fig. 23.42: You can see normal gallbladder and contracted gall-bladder due to stone

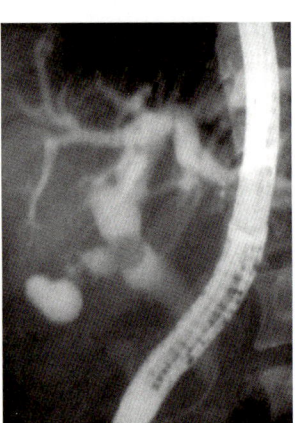

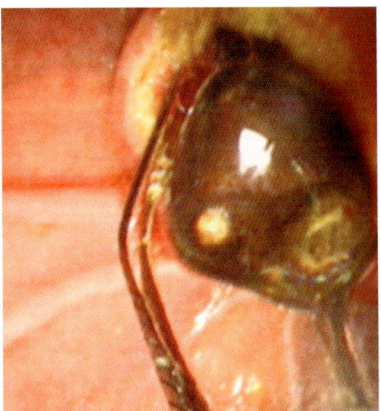

Fig. 23.43: ERCP showing stones in the CBD and contracted gallbladder (*Courtesy:* Dr Ganesh Pai, Prof and HOD of Medical Gastroenterology, KMC, Manipal)

Fig. 23.44: Stone was removed through endoscopic papillotomy followed by basketing. There is a small risk of perforation and pancreatitis in these patients (*Courtesy:* Dr Ganesh Pai, Prof and HOD of Medical Gastroenterology, KMC, Manipal)

5. **Choledocholithiasis:** Stones in the common bile duct or choledocholithiasis is an important cause of obstructive jaundice. Typically, patients are middle aged with history suggestive of gallstones or they may come to the hospital with the ultrasound report (done earlier) of gallstones. Presence of jaundice, high-coloured urine, clay-coloured stools and itching gives the clue to the diagnosis. Three symptoms—pain, fever and jaundice can be intermittent—called Charcot's triad. It suggests a partial obstruction of the CBD. Palpable liver, without palpable gallbladder supports the

6. **Chronic pancreatitis:** Typically, patients are emaciated, young alcoholic males or a young female present with recurrent central abdominal pain radiating to the back. Pain is often severe disturbing the work and sleep. Significant weight loss, steatorrhoea, and diabetes are the other presentations. Recent history of diabetes in a patient with abdominal pain suggests chronic pancreatitis. State of Kerala has high incidence of chronic pancreatitis supposedly due to consumption of tapioca. **Presence of a mass in a patient with chronic pancreatitis suggests carcinoma pancreas.**

Table 23.2: Differences between stone in the CBD and periampullary carcinoma (Ca)/Ca head of pancreas

		Stone in the CBD	*Periampullary carcinoma /carcinoma head of pancreas*
1.	**Age**	30–50 years	50–70 years
2.	**Sex**	More common in females	Equally common in both sexes
3.	**Duration of symptoms**	Long duration	Short duration (1–3 months)
4.	**Symptoms**		
	Pain	It is due to a stone blocking the CBD resulting in spasm of CBD. It is severe colicky pain like gallstone colic.	There may be some discomfort in abdomen but colicky pain is not a feature. Pain is relatively rare in carcinoma head of the pancreas
	Fever	As a result of obstruction, multiplication of organisms results in fever.	When obstruction becomes severe, there is bile stasis. Cholangitis, fever with chills and rigors can occur
	Jaundice	Occurs due to obstruction. Once inflammation subsides all these three symptoms are relieved partly but they occur after sometime. Hence, intermittent pain, intermittent fever, intermittent jaundice are classical of stone in CBD—**Charcot's triad**	As a result of slow developing obstruction in periampullary region, jaundice is **persistent, progressive, painless, pruritic**. In 5% of cases, growth may ulcerate into the duodenum. It can cause melaena and jaundice may temporarily subside.
	Stools	Since the obstruction is never complete, clay-coloured stools are not commonly seen	Clay-coloured stools are common and when mixed with blood, it is called **silvery stools** or aluminium paint stools.
	Pruritus	May be present but mild	Severe—due to bile salts in the circulation.
	Loss of appetite	No	Significant
	Loss of weight	No	Significant
5.	**Signs**		
	Jaundice	Deep yellow	Sometimes, greenish yellow
	Anaemia	Absent	It is usually present
6.	**Per abdomen**	Liver can be enlarged due to back pressure. It is smooth, with round border, firm in consistency.	Liver can be enlarged due to back pressure. If it is nodular, with sharp border, hard in consistency, it is due to secondaries in the liver.
7.	**Gallbladder**	As a rule, gallbladder is not palpable	Gallbladder is palpable in 70–75% cases.
8.	**Metastasis**	No	Left supraclavicular node, ascites, etc. may be seen.

Plain X-ray shows calcification of pancreas. Ultrasound, CT scan is done to know the diameter of the duct. Pain is the chief indication for surgery. Drainage (longitudinal pancreaticojejunostomy) and resection are the two types of commonly done surgery when medical line of treatment fails (Figs 23.45 and 23.46).

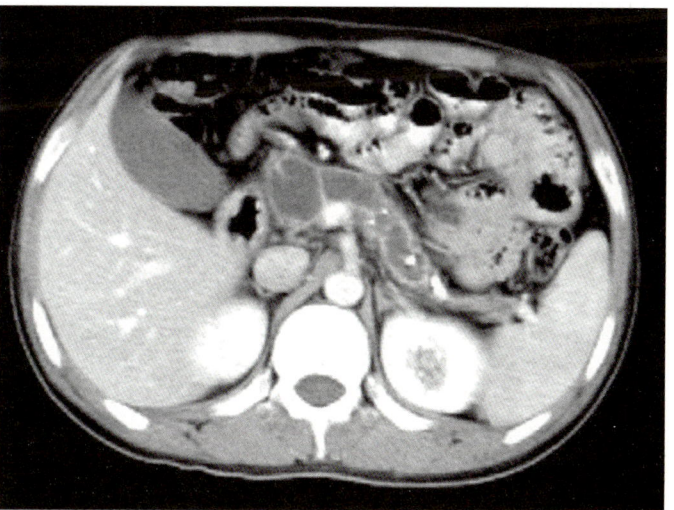

Fig. 23.46: CT shows dilated pancreatic duct of 10 mm in size with stones. ERCP is not required in such patients. This patient underwent LPJ

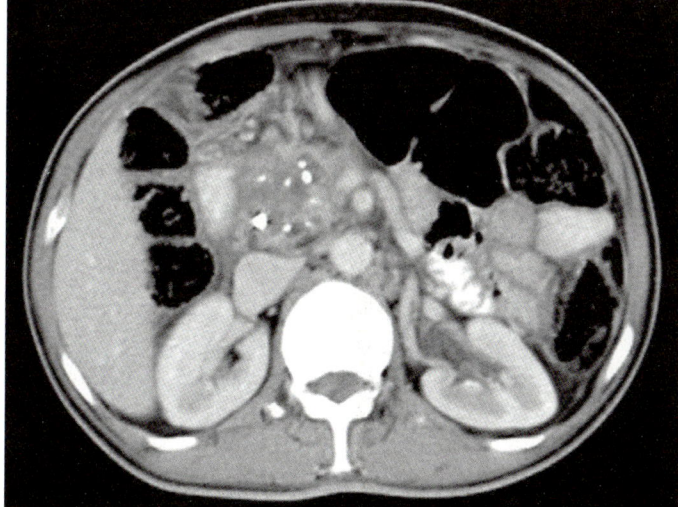

Fig. 23.45: CT scan showing chronic pancreatitis with head mass. This case should be treated with **head-coring** operation. Body and tail of pancreas are not enlarged

7. ***Pseudopancreatic cyst*** (Figs 23.47 to 23.49): Typically, a young or a middle-aged patient who after a bout of alcohol develops pancreatitis. After 2–3 weeks, he complains of abdominal distension. Examination reveals a tense cystic mass which feels firm, in the epigastrium. Its upper border can be made out. It does not usually move with respiration.

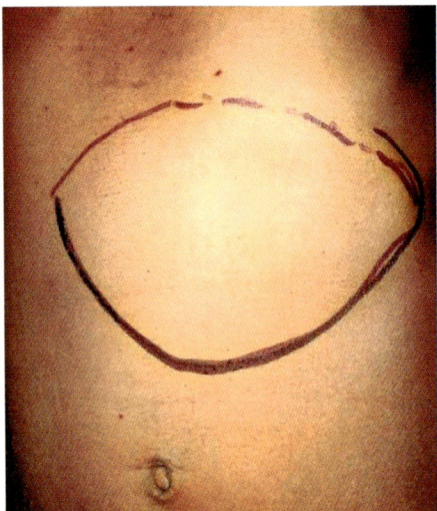

Fig. 23.47: Large pseudocyst of pancreas (*Courtesy:* Dr Prashath Tubachi, Associate Professor, SDM Medical College, Dharwad)

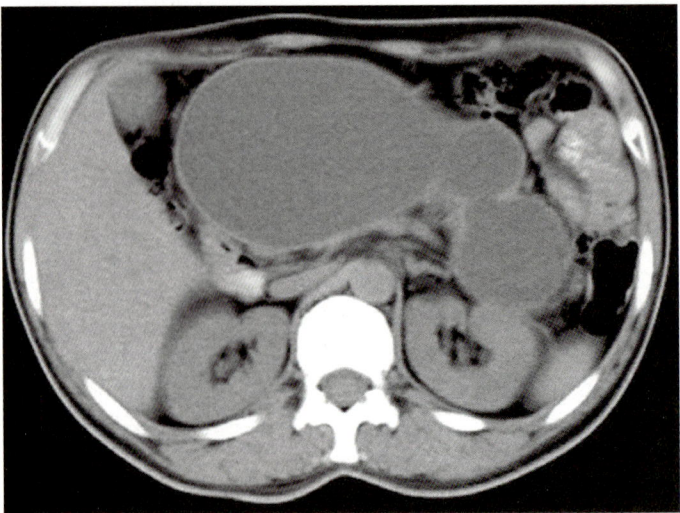

Fig. 23.48: CT scan showing large pseudocyst with multiple pockets. Cystojejunostomy can also be done

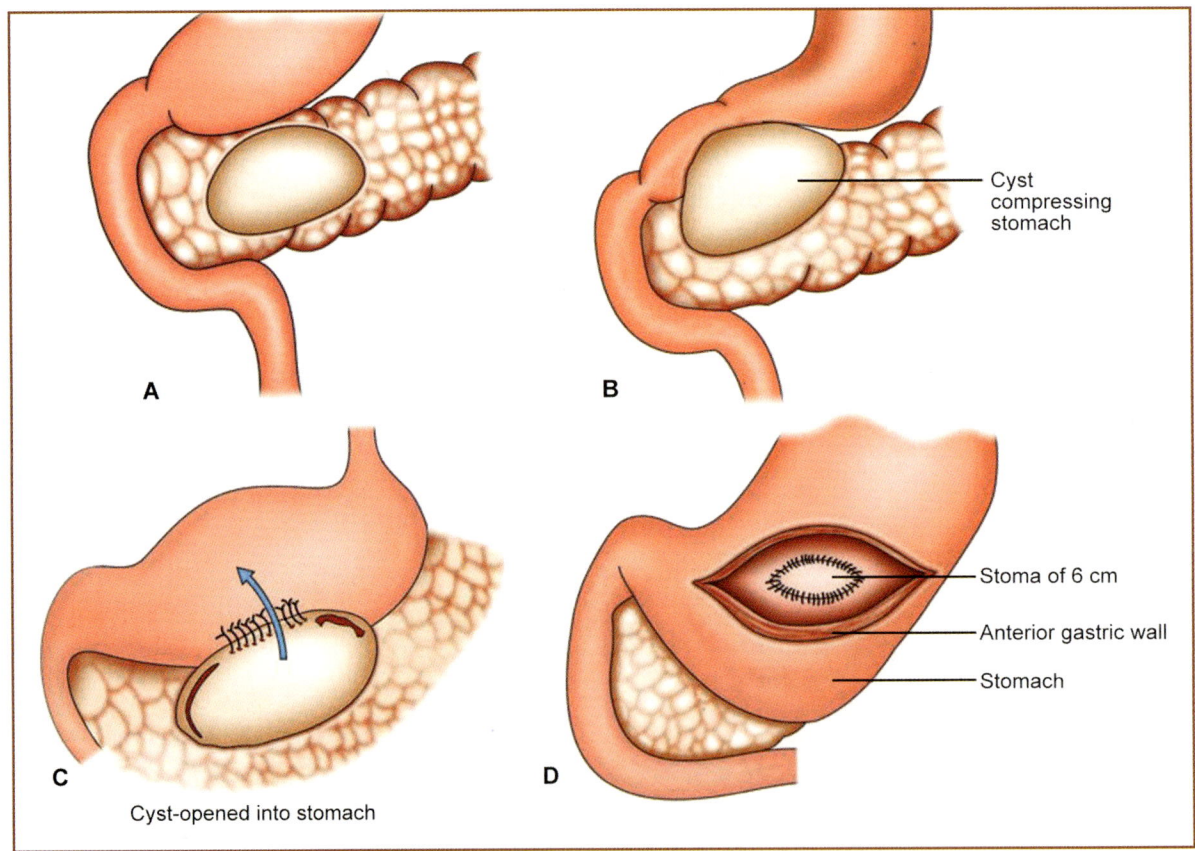

A

B — Cyst compressing stomach

C — Cyst-opened into stomach

D — Stoma of 6 cm — Anterior gastric wall — Stomach

Figs 23.49A to D: Steps of cystogastrostomy (contributed by Miss Vidushi, MBBS student, 2015, KMC, Manipal)

It has smooth surface and round borders. Pulsations over the mass (transmitted) suggest that it is a mass close to the aorta. In such a case, it is a pseudocyst. Gurgle heard anteriorly suggests distended stomach. Acute pancreatitis is the commonest cause, other cause being blunt abdominal trauma. Ultrasound and CT scan help in the diagnosis and localization. Majority of pseudocyst will resolve spontaneously over 2 months. Symptomatic pseudocysts persisting after 2–3 months need a drainage procedure—the most popular and commonly performed one is cystogastrostomy.

8. **Cystadenoma:** Cystadenomas of pancreas are benign and can attain huge sizes. It can present as a mass in the epigastrium, left hypochondrium or umbilical region. Vague abdominal pain and distension of the abdomen are the features. They exhibit what is described as 'tree top mobility'. Typically, it is a retroperitoneal mass which does not move

with respiration, firm and mobile. Females are affected more than men. Cystadenoma should be differentiated from pseudocyst by thick wall, rich mucin content and epithelium in the wall. Ultrasound and CT scan are the investigations. Mucinous cystadenomas have malignant potential needs to be removed. Asymptomatic serous cystadenoma can be observed (Fig. 23.50). Other tumours of the pancreas are uncommon such as endocrine tumours (Figs 23.51 and 23.52) and pseudopapillary tumour of the pancreas (Fig. 23.53). Clinical presentations of these tumours can be asymptomatic, backache and weight loss. Ultrasound, CT scan or endosono-guided FNAC helps in the diagnosis. Treatment is primarily surgery. Chemotherapy and radiotherapy can also be used.

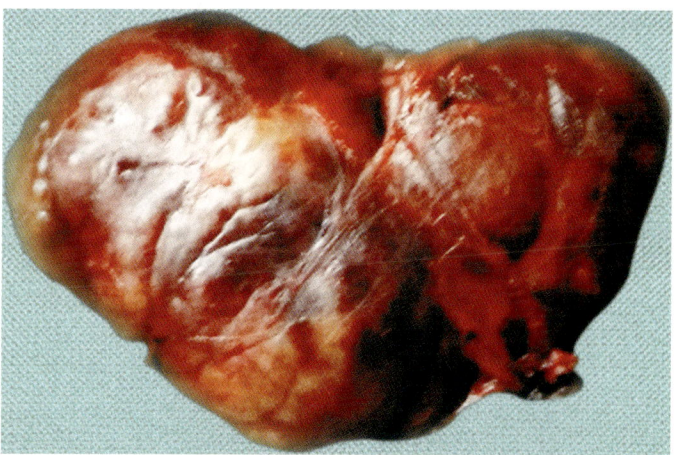

Fig. 23.52: Specimen of endocrine tumour of the pancreas

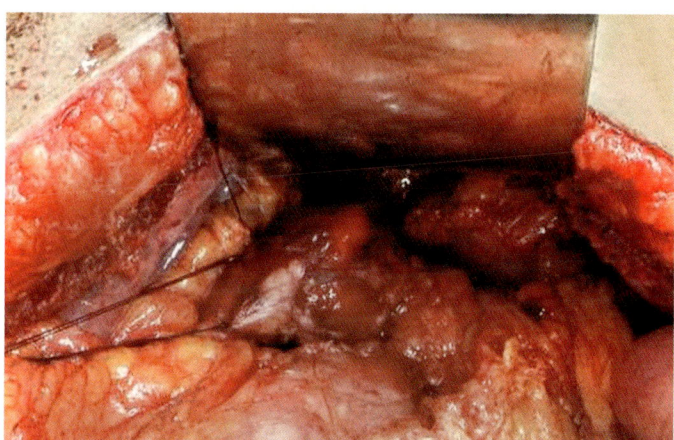

Fig. 23.53: Pseudopapillary tumour of the pancreas (*Courtesy:* Dr Sunilkrishna, Dr Ranjani, Dr Keerthan Upadhya, Department of Surgery, KMC, Manipal)

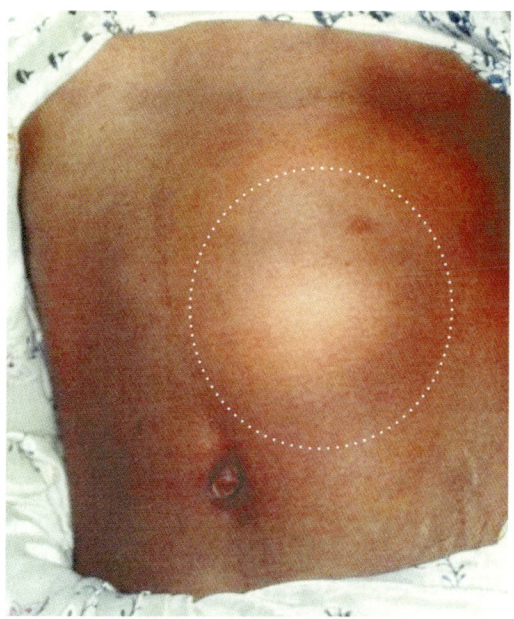

Fig. 23.50: Cystadenoma of the pancreas

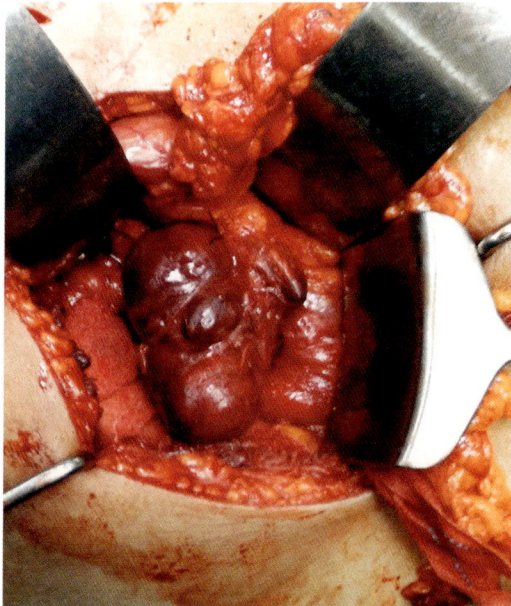

Fig. 23.51: Endocrine tumour of the pancreas

9. **Carcinoma body of pancreas** can present as a mass in the lower part of epigastrium or upper umbilical region. Typically seen after 60 years of age. Male smokers are commonly affected. Initial presentation is backache, flatulence, weight loss, indigestion, etc. By 3 months of time, significant weight loss occurs and mass can be palpable. The mass is hard, irregular, fixed and does not move with respiration. Presence of severe backache and loss of weight are important features. Majority of them are inoperable by the time of presentation. Gemcitabine-based chemotherapy followed by resection or radiotherapy are various modalities of treatment. However, prognosis is very poor.

10. **Portal hypertension:** The most common clinical situation which can be encountered by a surgeon with splenomegaly is due to portal hypertension. Majority of them are due to prehepatic portal hypertension with palpable spleen without ascites and features of liver cell failure. Many of them come to the hospital due to haematemesis. Liver function is normal. Patients are young, present with dull aching pain in the left hypochondrium. Anaemia is not only due to haematemesis but can also be due to hypersplenism. Upper gastrointestinal endoscopy will reveal oesophageal and fundal varices. Treatment of portal hypertension is complicated. Vast majority of the cases are managed today

by injection sclerotherapy or banding and with propranolol. Minority of cases require shunt surgery. Life-saving devascularisation procedures can also be done depending upon surgeon's experience, if all measures fail including Sengstaken Blakemore tube.

11. **Haemolytic anaemias:** After a thorough workup by physician, cases which require splenectomy are referred to a surgeon. Often history is long, may be in months or years. Hereditary spherocytosis and immune thrombocytopaenic purpura are two common examples. In hereditary spherocytosis, the symptoms of abdominal pain and faint jaundice are usually from childhood. Spleen is enlarged to moderate extent (5 cm in size). Eyes will reveal a faint lemon yellow jaundice. Liver is usually not palpable. They can also develop gallstones. Ultrasound is done to look for gallstones and rule out other causes of splenomegaly. Normal red cell haemolysis occurs in 0.47% saline solution. Here, it occurs at 0.6% or even weaker solution. This is called osmotic fragility test positive. Splenectomy is the treatment of choice.

12. **Tuberculous abdomen** (Figs 23.54 to 23.57): Tuberculosis of the abdomen can affect intestines (ileocaecal tuberculosis), peritoneum (peritoneal tuberculosis) and mesenteric lymph nodes (tuberculous mesenteric lymphadenitis). These are common. Young to middle-aged patients between 20 and 50 years of age group are affected. Low grade fever, weight loss and ill health, weakness, loose stools, emaciation may be present. Intestinal tuberculosis is of 2 types—ulcerative and hyperplastic. Ulcerative presents as increased frequency of stools, blood and mucus in stools, emaciation, etc. Hyperplastic variety affects ileocaecal region. It results in mass in the right iliac fossa. Colicky pain, vomiting, distension are the features. It suggests intestinal obstruction. Mass is felt in right iliac fossa, which is mobile,

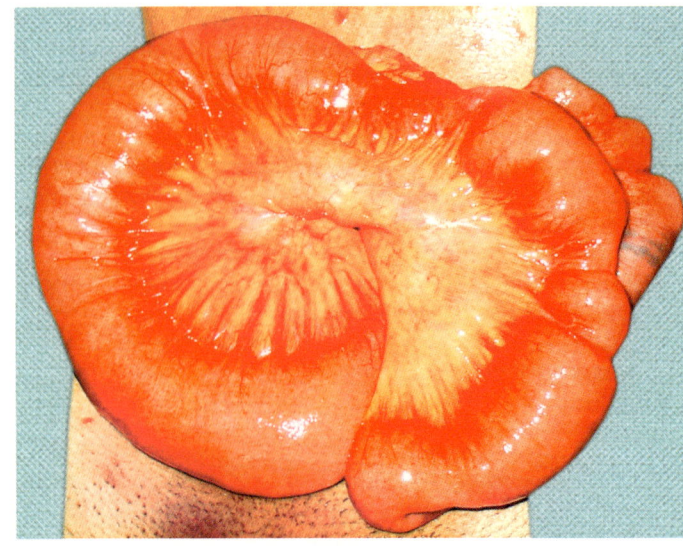

Fig. 23.55: Stricture of the ileum due to tuberculosis

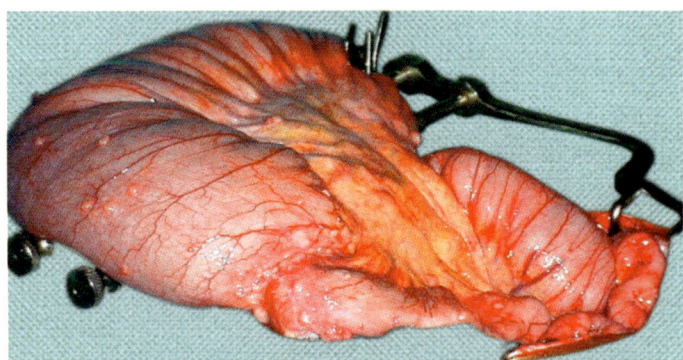

Fig. 23.56: Intestinal obstruction due to abdominal tuberculosis with ileal stricture. You can also see tubercles on the intestinal surface

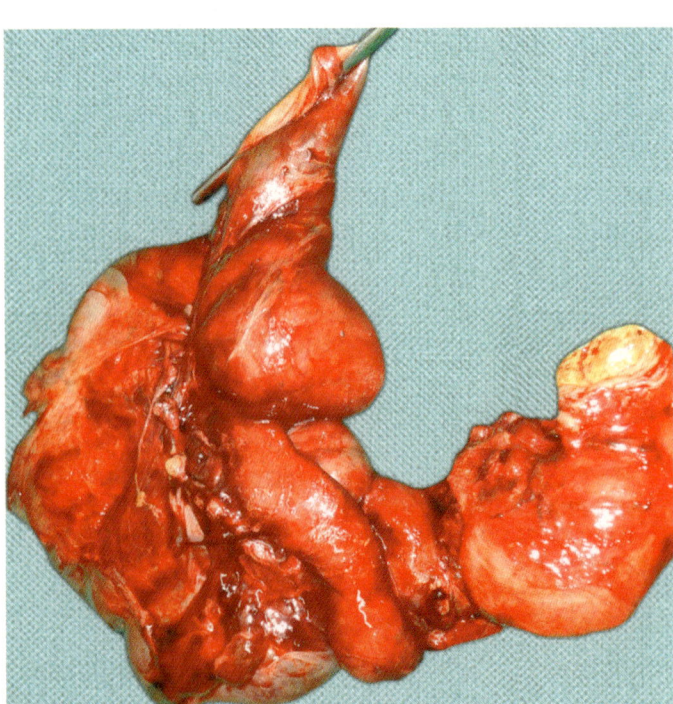

Fig. 23.54: Ileocaecal tuberculosis—limited colectomy specimen

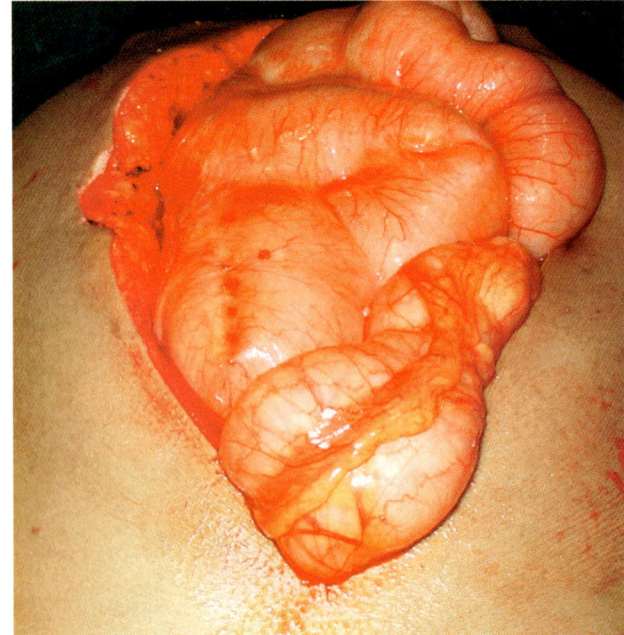

Fig. 23.57: Matted bowel loops due to abdominal tuberculosis (*Courtesy:* Dr Satyanarayan N, Consultant Surgeon, Mangaluru)

located high up and firm. Tuberculosis of the peritoneum can present with ascites detected by shifting dullness. Rolled up omentum may be felt in the upper abdomen specially in children. Other presentation is as a localised mass due to loculated ascites. Sometimes on deep palpation, mesenteric lymph nodes and rarely para-aortic lymph nodes may also be felt. Colonoscopic biopsy of caecal ulcers or terminal ileal lesions can detect tuberculous pathology. Diagnostic laparoscopy and biopsy of tubercles/lymph nodes from peritoneal surface is the investigation in cases of tuberculous peritonitis and tuberculous lymphadenitis. Antituberculous treatment is given to all cases for a minimum of 6 months. Limited ileocolectomy is done in cases of obstruction due to strictures or a hyperplastic mass from ileocaecal tuberculosis, with obstruction (refer to page 401 also).

13. **Inflammatory bowel diseases:** Ulcerative colitis and Crohn's disease are two common inflammatory bowel diseases. Both are common in young patients between 20 and 40 years of age. Both will present as loose stools, blood and mucus in stools dysentery, weight loss, abdominal cramps. Remissions and relapses are common. Ulcerative colitis starts as small ulcers (pinpoint ulcers) in the rectum and gradually can affect the whole colon and terminal ileum. Progression of the disease results in pseudopolyps and pipestem colon. Anus is never involved. Stools may vary from 15 to 20 per day resulting in severe dehydration, nutritional disturbances, anaemia, hypoproteinaemia. Dangerous complications (Figs 23.58 to 23.60) include toxic megacolon and perforation—both require emergency colectomy and massive bleeding. Long-term complications are carcinoma colon, recurrent perianal abscess and perianal fistula. Ideal surgical procedure is total proctocolectomy with a pouch restoring the gastrointestinal continuity. Crohn's disease starts in the terminal ileum and can affect not only small and large intestines but oesophagus also. Aphthoid ulcers, skin lesions, cobblestone reticulations, and transmural inflammation are characteristic of Crohn's disease. Initial stage of ileocolitis eventually leads to narrowing of terminal

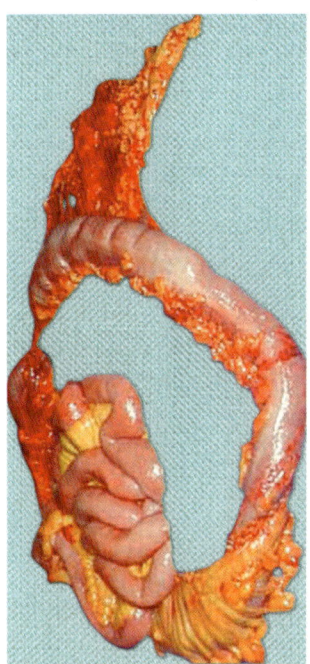

Fig. 23.59: Total colectomy for synchronous carcinoma due to ulcerative colitis (*Courtesy:* Dr Satyanarayan N, Consultant Surgeon, Mangaluru)

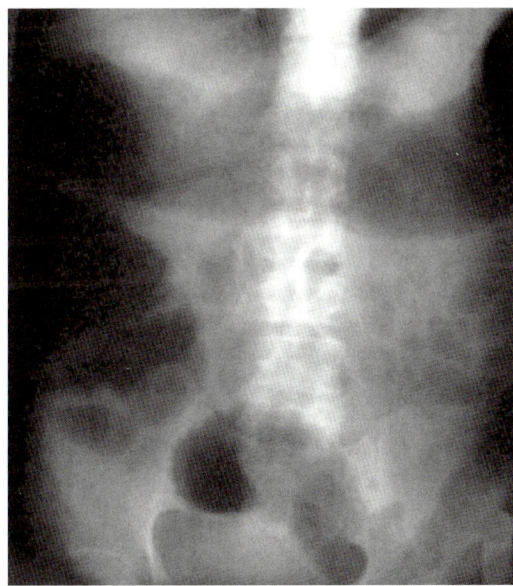

Fig. 23.60: Toxic megacolon

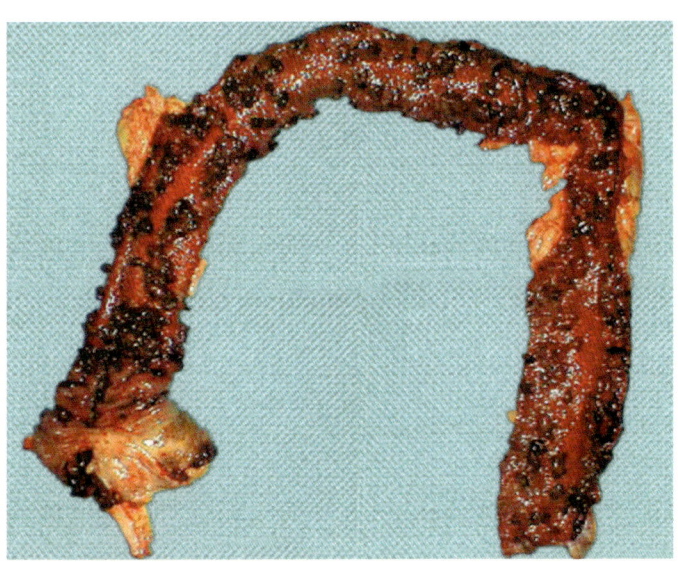

Fig. 23.58: Total colectomy done for massive bleeding due to ulcerative colitis

ileum (**string sign of Kantor** in barium studies) resulting in intestinal obstruction. Two other characteristics of Crohn's disease are various internal and external fistula formation—ileocolic, ileovesical, ileovaginal, etc. and ulcers, fistulae, abscesses in the anorectum. Treatment of Crohn's disease needs expertise—aim is to conserve the intestines as much as possible. Steroids are mainstay of medical treatment. Strictures need to be resected, internal fistulae need to be disconnected, anorectal abscesses should be drained and anorectal fistulae should be treated by fistulectomy.

14. ***Diverticular disease of the colon** (Figs 23.61 and 23.62)*:
It is an acquired condition, in which colonic mucosa herniates through the circular muscle fibres at weak points, where blood vessels penetrate the colonic wall. Since it is acquired, it lacks the muscle coat. They are thin, more prone for infections and perforation. The disease is common in Western population wherein diet is very **poor in fibres** because of refining of sugar and flour. In Africans and Indians, the disease is rare because of high fibre content of the diet. The disease starts after the age of 40. Any stress or emotional disorders may add to the constipation already caused by dietary factors and result in diverticular formation. **90% of them affect sigmoid colon**. Rectum is spared in majority. Diverticulae project between antimesenteric and mesenteric borders with taenia but they never penetrate taenia. Diverticulae refer to presence of diverticulosis without much symptoms. But on careful questioning, patients do have lower abdominal distension, heaviness, flatulence, etc. Vague abdominal pain is also felt in the left iliac fossa. Diverticulitis: Left-sided lower abdominal pain, moderate to severe is associated with passage of loose stools. The pain is partially relieved on passing flatus. Bleeding per rectum can be the presenting feature, sometimes it can be massive. Low grade fever, tenderness, rigidity and even mass may be present in the left iliac fossa (like left-sided appendicitis). The mass is thickened, inflamed, tender and sigmoid. Such attacks result in abscess which rupture into hollow organs and give rise to fistulae. Other causes of internal fistulae include carcinoma of colon, Crohn's disease, radiation and tuberculosis. Diagnosis is by colonoscopy and CT scan. Asymptomatic diverticulae need to be observed. Patient is advised to take high fibre diet and stool softening agents. Resection and anastomosis is the surgical treatment of symptomatic disease. Pericolic abscess is treated with ultrasound-guided aspiration and followed 6–8 weeks later by elective treatment.

15. ***Carcinoma colon** (Figs 23.63 and 23.64)*: Details have been given in Chapter 24 (mass abdomen). However, typically patients are 40–50 years and above who have lower gastrointestinal tract symptoms such as increasing constipation from left-sided colonic cancers specially from rectosigmoid growths, bleeding per rectum and mucus from rectal carcinomas and altered blood, mucus and sometimes diarrhoea from right-sided lesions. Differences between right colonic and left colonic malignancies are given in Table 23.3. Colonoscopy followed by radical resection and with or without chemotherapy is the treatment of choice. In advanced lesions, palliative bypass or colostomy is done to relieve obstruction.

• Rectosigmoid growths are constrictive lesions and difficult to feel. However, dilated sigmoid colon above loaded with faecal matter may be felt as a mass. In advanced cases, right to left peristalsis can be visible (colonic).

• Right-sided lesions can be felt—typically an irregular hard mass in the right iliac fossa for caecal carcinoma and lumbar or hypochondriac mass for ascending colonic carcinomas. In hepatic flexure growths, it will result in a closed loop obstruction when ileocaecal junction is competent and caecum will be distended which can be made out by eliciting tympanic note over the caecum.

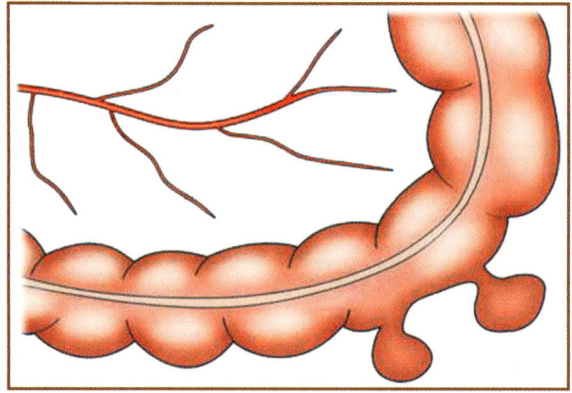

Fig. 23.61: Sigmoid diverticuli

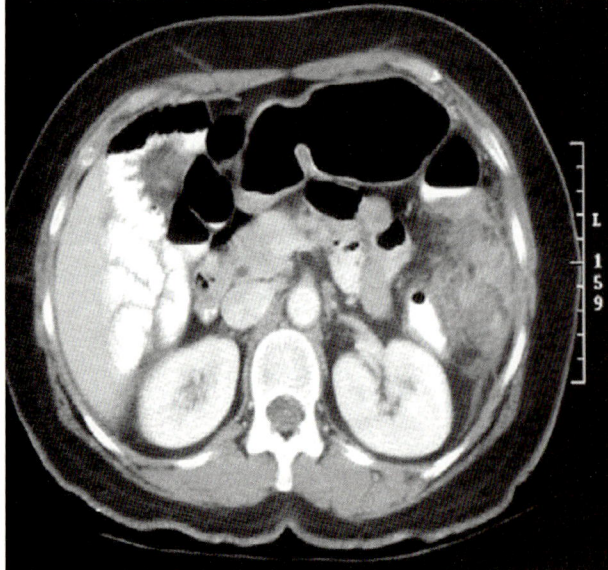

Fig. 23.62: CECT scan showing an abscess in the left paracolic space due to perforated diverticulitis

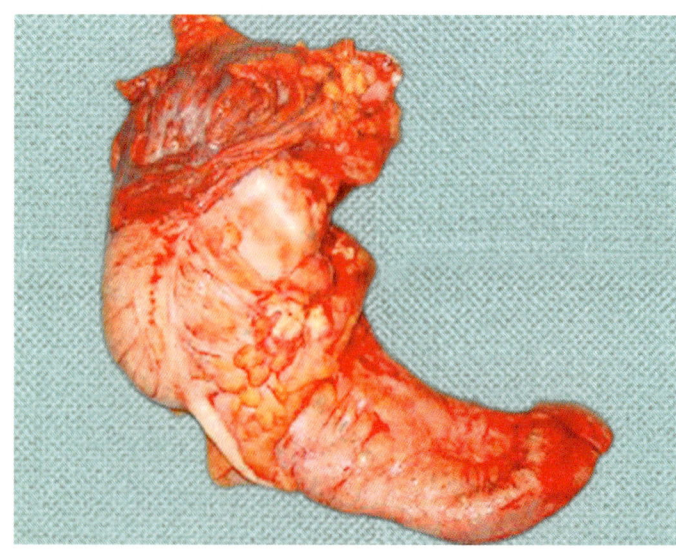

Fig. 23.63: Right hemicolectomy for carcinoma caecum

Table 23.3: Comparison between carcinoma right colon and carcinoma left colon

	Carcinoma right colon	Carcinoma left colon
• Presentation	Unexplained weakness, anaemia	Change in bowel habits
• Bleeding	Occult blood in stools	Gross blood in stools
• Abdominal discomfort	Right side and dyspeptic symptoms also	Constipation and obstruction
• Incidence	More common in women	More common in men
• Frequency	About 10–20%	About 60–70% (including rectum)
• Pathology	Ulcerative/proliferative lesion	Strictures (rectosigmoid)
• Investigation	Colonoscopy	Flexible sigmoidoscopy
• Complication	Obstruction—less common	Obstruction, perforation, pericolic abscess—common

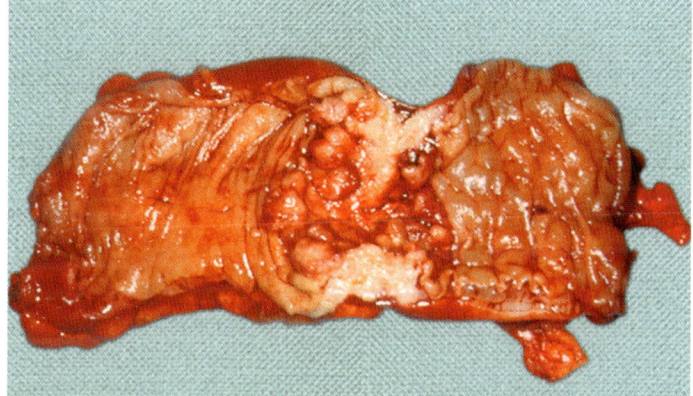

Fig. 23.64: Sigmoid colectomy—specimen opened showing ulceroproliferative lesion with luminal narrowing

- Transverse colonic carcinoma is felt in the umbilical region as an irregular or nodular hard mass having vertical mobility but not transverse mobility.
- As a rule, splenic flexure carcinomas are not palpable (hidden), present with obstruction and a careful palpation at laparotomy will reveal splenic flexure growth. Hence, they are easily missed, if someone is not careful enough to find it (also refer to Table 23.3 for comparison of carcinoma right colon and carcinoma left colon).

Clinical Case Capsule

- A 60-year-old man was admitted to the hospital with large bowel obstruction. Previous history of 2 months of increasing constipation could be elicited. Plain X-ray abdomen revealed large bowel obstruction. Ultrasound could detect a mass in the sigmoid colon and dilated loops. Contrast CT was not done as creatinine was 2.4 mg%. Per rectal examination and proctoscopy were normal. With clinical diagnosis of large bowel obstruction, laparotomy was done. Findings at laparotomy was 4 cm obstructing lesion in the sigmoid colon. Sigmoid colectomy was done. Postoperatively the patient continued to have obstruction for 6 days and was treated as paralytic ileus. However, a CT contrast was done on 7th day to detect any anastomotic leak. There was no extravasation of contrast into peritoneal cavity to suggest leak but revealed a second primary in the splenic flexure. Patient underwent 2nd laparotomy—left hemicolectomy. It was uneventful. What are the lessons learnt from this?
- Surgeon who saw the sigmoid lesion resected it but did not examine the rest of the large intestines.
- In carcinoma colon, synchronous lesions are very well-known.
- CT scan could have detected the second primary. If CT could not be done, one could also do MRI scan.

24

Examination of Abdominal Mass

INTRODUCTION

The abdomen is like Pandora's box. However, a student who is examining a case of abdomen is like an investigating CBI (Central Bureau of Investigations) officer. He has to collect information at every level of examination, i.e. age, history, past history, treatment history, general examination, abdominal examination and other systemic examination. An attempt has been done here to highlight the importance of history and clinical examination. *Ten points* in the history, if taken and analysed properly, may give a definite *clue* in majority of cases. After getting this *clue*, clinical examination of the mass may become easy.

When you palpate the mass, two important points must be considered. Firstly, what is the likely anatomical structure from which this mass is arising? Think of 5 points to prove this. Second point is what is the probable pathology and reasoning behind the diagnosis? To prove this again think of 3–5 points. Then think of a few differential diagnoses. It may be one, two or more (Clinical Box 24.1).

CLINICAL EXAMINATION OF ABDOMINAL MASS

Regions in the Abdomen

- *Abdomen is divided into nine regions by two horizontal lines and two vertical lines.*

- *Upper horizontal line (transpyloric line) is midway between xiphisternum and umbilicus.*

- *Lower hoizontal line (transtubercular line) is the line joining iliac crest tubercles of each side, about 5 cm behind the anterior superior iliac spine.*

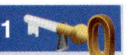

Clinical Box 24.1

Abdominal mass
- Which anatomical structure is this mass arising from?
- What is the probable pathological diagnosis?
- What is the final diagnosis?
- What is the differential diagnosis?
- What are the most important key points in the history and examination that help clinch the diagnosis?

- The vertical lines are drawn on either side through the midpoint between anterior superior iliac spine and symphysis pubis. Following are the nine regions of the abdomen (Figs 24.1 and 24.2):

  1. Right hypochondrium   2. Epigastrium
  3. Left hypochondrium   4. Right lumbar region
  5. Umbilical region   6. Left lumbar region
  7. Right iliac fossa   8. Hypogastrium
  9. Left iliac fossa

Special note: It is important to realise that both renal angles/regions must be included under examination of the abdomen so that one will not miss a renal mass. Thus, it becomes 11 regions. Then comes the most important region to examine in male patients, that is testis. Missing a testicular tumour presenting as mass abdomen (para-aortic nodes) and left supraclavicular node can be avoided, if you include examination of testis. Hence, remember to examine 12 regions in males (Fig. 24.3) and 11 regions in females.

HISTORY OF PRESENT ILLNESS

1. *Abdominal pain:* It is present in most of the cases of abdominal mass. Do you have pain abdomen? This is the first question you have to ask. Abdominal pain can be of the following types:

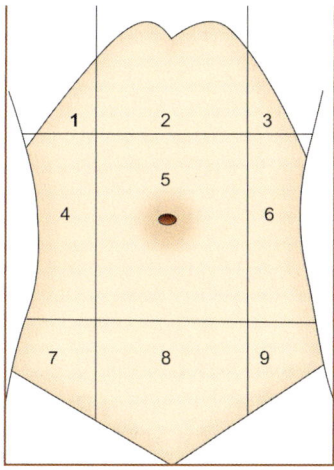

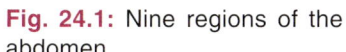

Fig. 24.1: Nine regions of the abdomen

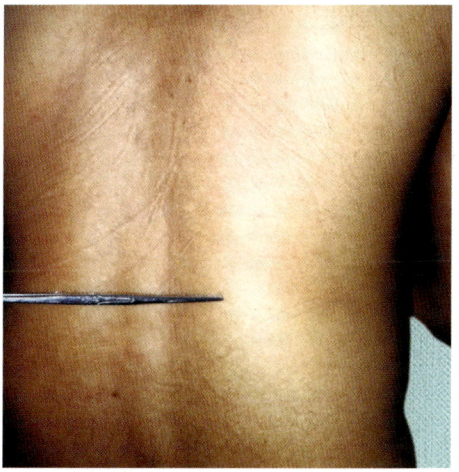

Fig. 24.2: Showing the loin

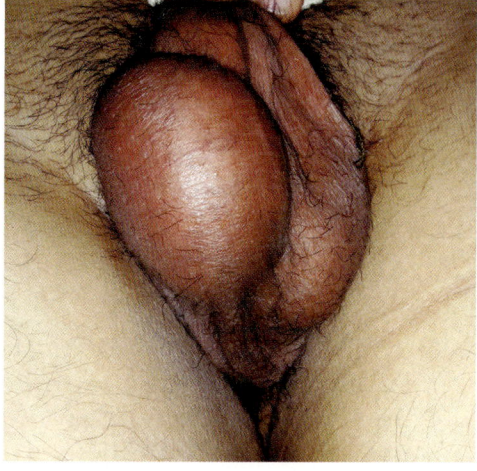

Fig. 24.3: Rapidly enlarging testicular swelling in a 22-year-old boy

A. Dull aching pain: It suggests a solid organ enlargement. It is a continuous pain felt in the anatomical location of the swelling. Patients often describe it as a discomfort rather than pain. A few examples are given below:

- *Liver enlargement*: Pain in the right hypochondrium. It occurs due to stretching of parietal capsule (Glisson) (Fig. 24.4A). Examples are hepatocellular carcinoma, secondaries in the liver, hydatid cyst, etc.

- *Splenic enlargement*: Pain in the left hypochondrium. Examples are splenomegaly in cases of portal hypertension, hereditary spherocytosis or lymphoma, etc.

- *Renal enlargement*: Pain in the back and costal region is called costovertebral pain (Fig. 24.4B).

Hydronephrosis, renal cell carcinoma and polycystic kidney are a few examples.

- *Enlarged lymph nodes (para-aortic), pancreatic tumours*: Dull backache is common. It is due to infiltration or encasement of coeliac plexus by the tumour or due to enlarged lymph nodes. A common cause of enlarged para-aortic nodes is lymphoma.

B. Colicky pain (Figs 24.4C and D) suggests hollow viscus obstruction. This pain is due to hyperperistalsis. It is severe and intermittent (comes and goes). Each attack may last for 5–10 minutes. The patient bends on himself, holds the abdomen and puts pressure on the abdomen which gives some kind of relief. Being visceral type of pain, it is not very well localised. Following are a few examples:

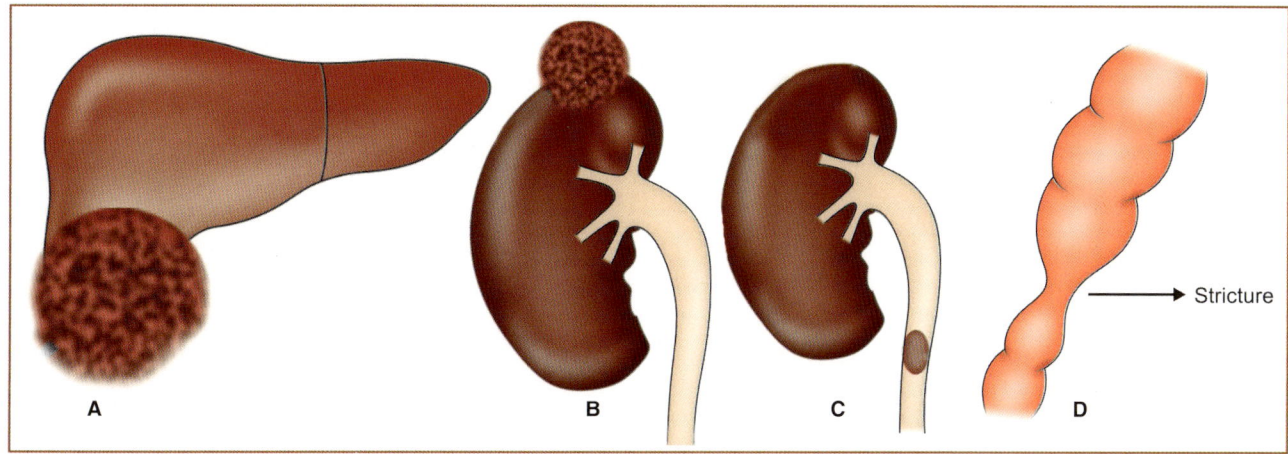

Fig. 24.4: Different pathology and causes of pain. (A) Hepatoma; (B) Renal cell carcinoma; (C) Renal colic due to stone; (D) Intestinal colic caused by tubercular stricture

- Mass in the right iliac fossa (carcinoma caecum or ileocaecal tuberculosis). Initially there may be a vague discomfort. However, when partial obstruction occurs, it results in a colicky abdominal pain which is centrally located and sometimes unbearable.

- Chronic intussusception is another example of a mass with intermittent colicky abdominal pain.

C. **Referred pain:** Here, pain originates in one area and manifests in a different area. This is because of the same segmental nerve supply of these 2 organs/anatomical locations. Tuberculosis of spine is a common problem in India. Often patients present with iliopsoas abscess. Patients can complain of referred pain in the lower abdomen. The referred pain is due to the **collapsed vertebrae pressing on the dorsal nerve roots.**

> **Clinical Wisdom**
>
> Recent backache in elderly male may be due to carcinoma prostate and in females may be due to carcinoma breast.

- When diaphragm is irritated by exudate (peritonitis fluid, acute cholecystitis), blood (haemoperitoneum), pus (subphrenic abscess), or bile (biliary peritonitis), pain is referred to the shoulder region. This is because diaphragm is supplied by phrenic nerve (cervical—C3, C4 and C5, mainly C4) and shoulder region is supplied by supraclavicular nerves (C3 and C4 cutaneous nerves). In the similar fashion, **a large hepatoma or advanced liver tumour can present with hiccoughs and shoulder pain. It is due to irritation of phrenic nerve.**

D. **Radiating pain:** Carcinoma pancreas present often as pain radiating to the back. It is due to retroperitoneal nerve plexus infiltration or due to enlarged coeliac lymph nodes.

2. *Vomiting*

- Persistent, profuse, projectile and nonbilious vomiting of undigested food particles—foul contents suggest pyloric stenosis. Cicatrised chronic duodenal ulcer and carcinoma stomach are the common causes of pyloric obstruction (pain is absent/negligible).

- Persistent, profuse, projectile, painful bilious vomiting indicate obstruction below the level of ampulla of Vater, e.g. ileocaecal tuberculosis,

stricture of the small bowel, and adhesions. (Pain is severe and colicky.)

- Vomiting of bilious contents with no pain or mild pain indicates high jejunal or duodenal obstruction in the third part (Wilkie's disease).

3. *Haematemesis:*

- Epigastric mass with haematemesis suggests carcinoma stomach in elderly patients (typically a man above 40 years). However, a **large epigastric mass with haematemesis in a young patient with no features of loss of appetite and weight loss suggests a gastrointestinal stromal tumour (GIST). Stomach is the most common site of GIST.**

- Haematemesis with splenomegaly is an indication of portal hypertension (Fig. 24.5).

> **Clinical Wisdom**
>
> History of gastrojejunostomy and vagotomy done a few years back presenting with severe pain abdomen, epigastric mass and haematemesis could be due to retrograde jejunogastric intussusception.

4. *Sensation of fullness/early satiety:*

- Typically these symptoms are seen in cases of carcinoma of the stomach. In cases of pyloric obstruction, stasis of the food is a feature resulting in feeling of fullness. Also hepatoma, large pseudocyst of pancreas or large pancreatic tumours can cause extraluminal (extrinsic) compression on the stomach resulting in sensation of fullness in the abdomen.

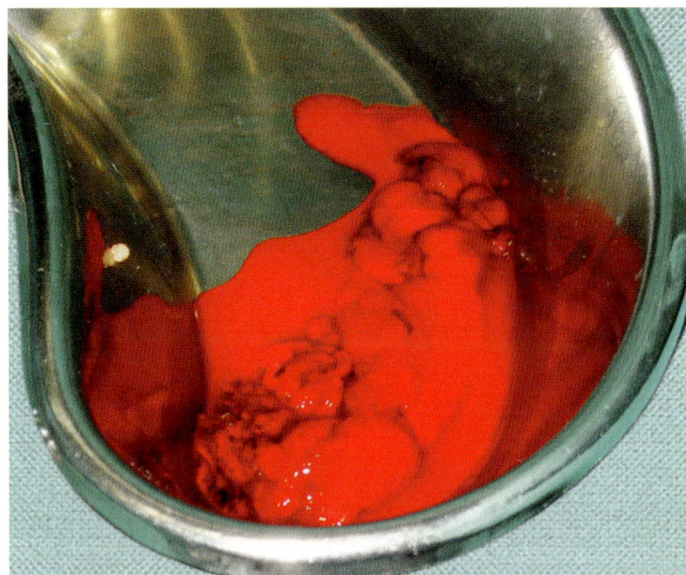

Fig. 24.5: Haematemesis due to portal hypertension

- Early satiety is due to **loss of receptive relaxation of stomach due to malignant infiltration** of muscle layer in cases of carcinoma stomach.

5. *Bleeding per rectum*:

- Fresh blood per rectum with a mass in the left iliac fossa suggests carcinoma sigmoid colon and mass in the right iliac fossa suggests carcinoma caecum. Fresh blood per rectum with mass in the liver (mostly nodular liver) suggests secondaries in the liver from carcinoma rectum. Rectal growths are rarely palpable per abdomen and are known for liver metastasis.

- Melaena or altered blood together with a mass suggests carcinoma stomach, portal hypertension, GIST, small bowel tumours, etc.

- Altered blood mixed with mucus with a mass in the right iliac fossa suggests carcinoma caecum and ileocaecal tuberculosis.

6. *Loss of appetite and loss of weight*

- These are common symptoms of GI malignancies. Please note that these two symptoms are seen not only in intra-abdominal malignancies but also in many diseases such as tuberculosis. However, it should be noted that one of the earliest symptoms of carcinoma stomach is loss of appetite. Severe weight loss is an early and important feature of carcinoma body of the pancreas.

- Significant weight loss refers to unintentional loss of 10% of body weight or more in the last 6 months.

7. *Bowel habits*: *Fresh bleeding per rectum* with or without mucus suggests carcinoma rectum. *Alternating constipation and diarrhoea* is one of the features of carcinoma colon. Constipation is due to partial obstruction. Mucus accumulates in the proximal colon which is passed out as mucus diarrhoea. Increasing constipation suggests left-sided tumours specially carcinoma rectosigmoid junction.

8. *Jaundice*

- *Progressive, persistent, pruritic jaundice* is seen in periampullary carcinoma or carcinoma head of pancreas. However, in periampullary carcinoma, fluctuation can occur, if growth ulcerates. This will manifest as slight improvement in jaundice and passage of clay-coloured stools mixed with the blood—what has been described as aluminium paint stools by Sir Ogilvie.

- *Mild recurrent jaundice*: Haemolytic anaemia

- *Intermittent jaundice, pain, fever*: Charcot's triad—stone in the common bile duct.

9. *Haematuria*: Fresh bleeding/clots in the elderly may be due to renal cell carcinoma. Fresh bleeding in middle age may be polycystic disease of the kidney. Fresh painless bleeding with suprapubic discomfort is seen in carcinoma bladder.

10. *Fever*

- *High-grade fever with chills and rigors*: Stone in common bile duct (cholangitis).

- *Low-grade fever*: Hepatoma, renal cell carcinoma, lymphoma are a few examples. Fever is due to some pyrogens released into circulation by the tumour or due to tumour necrosis. In a tropical country like India, **hepatomas with fever are often diagnosed as amoebic liver abscess and mistreated.**

11. *Abdominal distension*: The only chief complaint can be abdominal distension, most often due to ascites. In surgical wards, the common cause of ascites in young patients is tuberculous ascites, in middle-aged men is due to cirrhosis (alcohol is the most common cause) and in elderly patients, malignancy. Large pseudocysts, retroperitoneal tumours, and in females ovarian tumours can present with abdominal distension. In the absence of any of these, distension can be caused by retroperitoneal tumours.

Clinical Wisdom

- After taking all this history, when nothing is pointing towards any specific site of involvement of intra-abdominal organs, think of retroperitoneum.
- Distension is what patient says, protuberant is what the patient's abdomen can be.

Past History (Relevant to the Mass Abdomen)

- History of blood transfusions in the past and jaundice (hepatitis-B and hepatitis C)—hepatocellular carcinoma.

- History of pulmonary or lymphatic tuberculosis—ileocaecal tuberculosis.

- *History of surgery*

  a. **Hemicolectomy, gastrectomy or mastectomy** and patient has a palpable liver mass suggest secondaries in the liver.

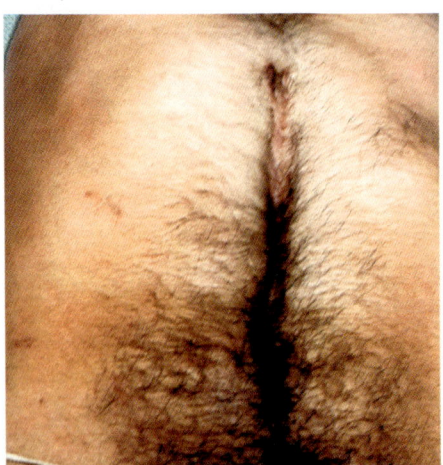

Fig. 24.6: Laparotomy scar—done for GJ and vagotomy

b. **Gastrojejunostomy** done 20 years back and now a stomach mass suggests carcinoma stomach (stump carcinoma) (Fig. 24.6).

c. **Mastectomy for carcinoma breast:** Large pelvic masses can be bilateral ovarian masses called Krukenberg tumours.

d. **Disarticulation** of the toe or toes, wide excision of malignant skin tumours, amputation of the limb and patient has nodular liver mass suggest malignant melanoma.

Family History

Polycystic kidney, colonic cancers, and breast cancers can run in families.

Personal History

- Appetite is poor in gastrointestinal malignancies. Weight loss is an important feature of carcinoma pancreas, stomach and oesophagus.
- Smoking also predisposes to carcinoma pancreas and urinary bladder.
- Too much consumption of red meat is a factor for carcinoma colon.
- Recent changes in bowel habits suggest carcinoma colon.

GENERAL PHYSICAL EXAMINATION

The aim is to assess general condition of the patient— Is he sick? Is he emaciated? Is he cachexic? Is he dehydrated? Also to find any clue to the abdominal mass.

- **Pallor** signifies bleeding or malignancies— examples, bleeding tumours such as carcinoma

stomach or GIST, carcinoma caecum, and advanced malignancies. Also keep in mind renal pathology.

- **Jaundice** suggests a liver mass or periampullary carcinoma / carcinoma head of the pancreas — and a palpable mass could be gallbladder.
- **Supraclavicular fullness** or palpable node— mostly carcinoma stomach, carcinoma pancreas, and testicular tumours.
- **Palpable lymph nodes** in the neck—multiple, matted, mobile lymph nodes may give a clue that abdominal mass could be of tubercular aetiology such as intestinal tuberculosis or encysted ascites (loculated ascites).
- **Multiple discrete nodes** may suggest lymphoma as a cause of abdominal mass, e.g., hepato-splenomegaly, para-aortic nodes.
- **Pigmentation** in the oral cavity and a contracting abdominal mass can be intussusception and it is a case of Peutz-Jeghers syndrome.
- **Bilateral pedal oedema** with flank veins suggests inferior vena caval obstruction and mass could be from the liver—hepatoma or metastasis in the liver. Flank veins are called inguinoaxillary veins.
- **Spine tenderness/collapse** is due to tuberculosis and the mass (flank or iliac fossa) is due to psoas abscess.

ABDOMINAL EXAMINATION—REGIONAL EXAMINATION

Inspection

- The patient is asked to breathe well, face turned to other side, legs flexed, with mouth open.
- Students should spend a few minutes watching the abdomen carefully.

1. *Shape of the abdomen*
   - Scaphoid in normal cases (Fig. 24.7).
   - Protuberant in fatty abdomen (Fig. 24.8).
   - Generalised distension with fullness in the flanks is usually due to ascites.
   - Localised distension can be due to a mass.

2. *Movements of the regions or quadrants*: Restricted movement of any one region of the abdomen indicates an inflammatory pathology (difficult to appreciate). In cases of amoebic liver abscess or acute cholecystitis, the right hypochondrium may not move like other regions.

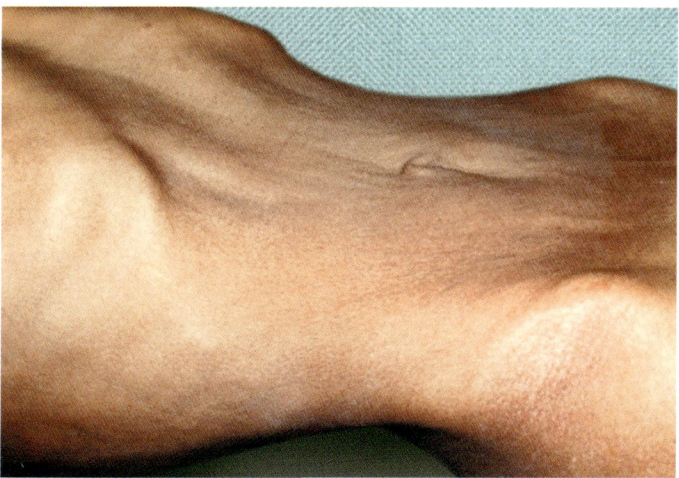

Fig. 24.7: Normal scaphoid abdomen

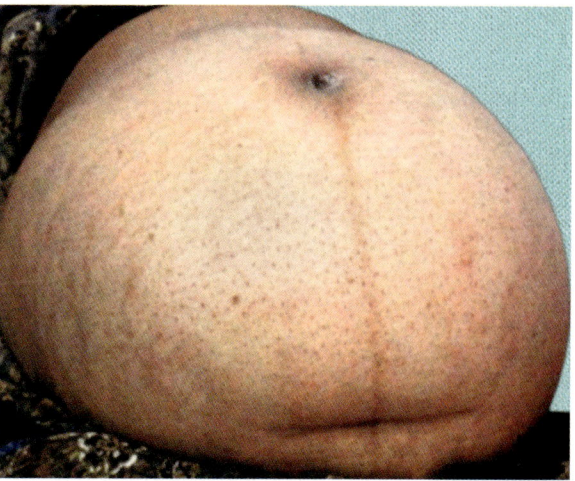

Fig. 24.9: Displacement of umbilicus upwards in a large ovarian tumour

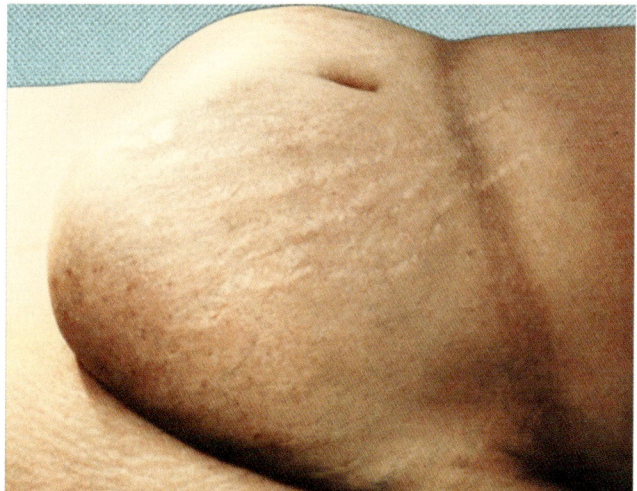

Fig. 24.8: Protuberant abdomen due to central obesity

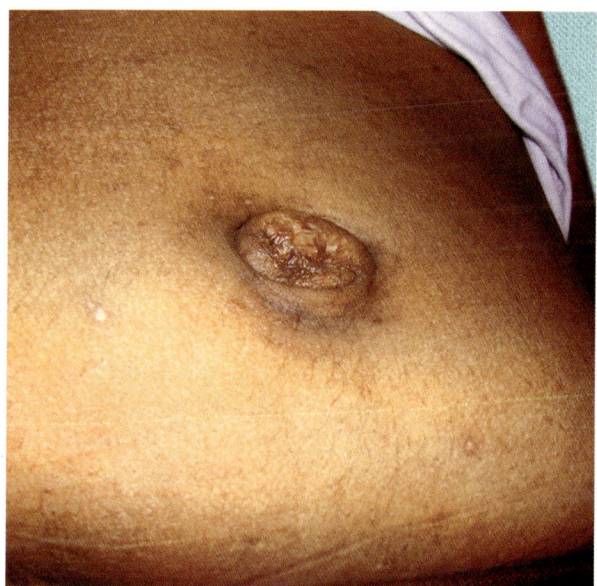

Fig. 24.10: Umbilical hernia

3. *Umbilicus*

  a. Displacement of umbilicus occurs in large ovarian tumours (Fig. 24.9).

  b. Umbilicus is everted in cases of raised intra abdominal pressure as in cases of ascites.

  c. Umbilical nodule (Sister Joseph) indicates intra-abdominal malignancy (carcinoma of stomach, colon, pancreas).

  d. Ask the patient to cough and look for umbilical hernia (Fig. 24.10).

4. *Details about the mass* such as location, extent, size, shape, surface, borders, and movement with respiration have to be mentioned if mass is visible. If the details about the mass cannot be appreciated (Fig. 24.11) or if mass is not clear on inspection, it is better to say "there is fullness" rather than trying to manipulate the details about the mass. **Fullness has no dimensions and no descriptions.**

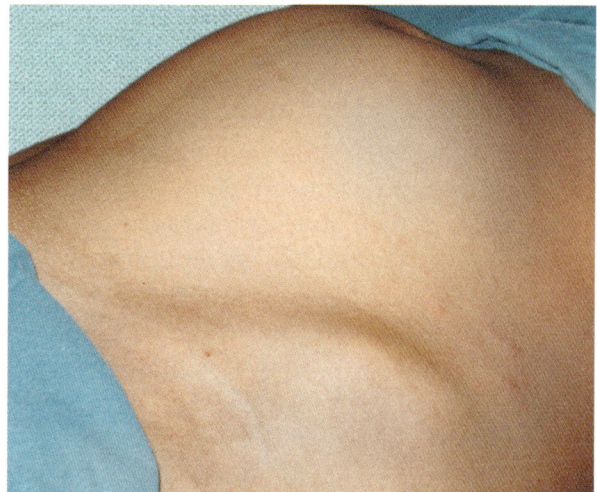

Fig. 24.11: Mass is obvious. Give details—smooth surface, round borders, lower border not made out

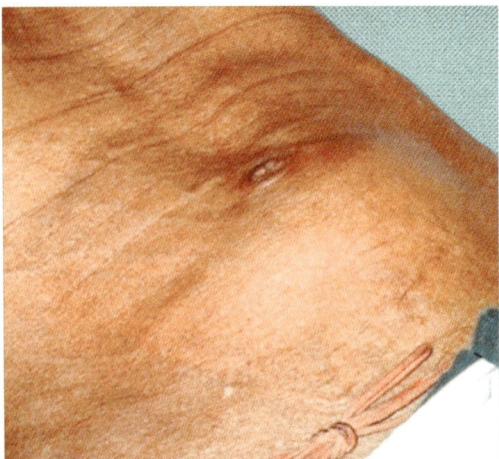

Fig. 24.12: Visible gastric peristalsis (VGP)—prominent wave below the umbilicus (dilated stomach)

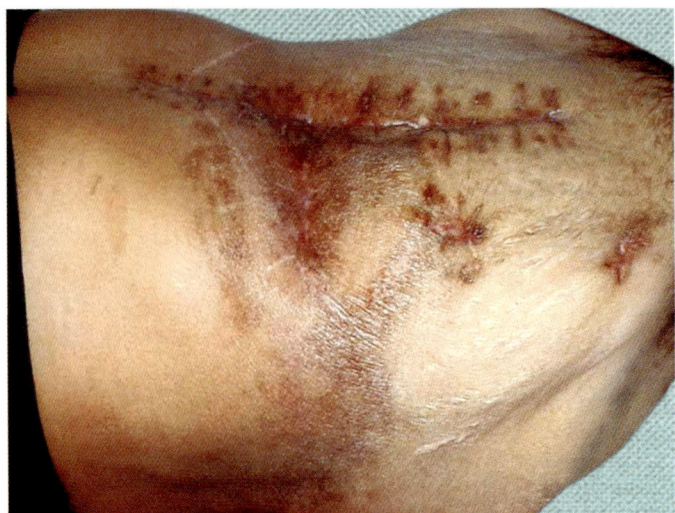

Fig. 24.13: Operated for gangrene bowel. Resection anastomosis was done. You can see ragged scar and drain marks

5. *Peristalsis*: Three types of peristalsis are seen in the abdomen.

  a. Presence of step-ladder peristalsis indicates small bowel obstruction. It may be a case of ileocaecal tuberculosis or carcinoma caecum.

  b. Visible gastric peristalsis (VGP) from left to right indicates pyloric stenosis. VGP is seen in pyloric stenosis due to cicatrised duodenal ulcer and sometimes in carcinoma pyloric antrum. In case of the former, stomach is normal and obstruction occurs slowly over a period of time, it dilates well. In carcinoma, it is of a short duration and some infiltration of the stomach musculature is always present restricting the distension (Fig. 24.12).

  c. Right to left peristalsis indicates left colonic obstruction—mass may be of transverse colon or left colon.

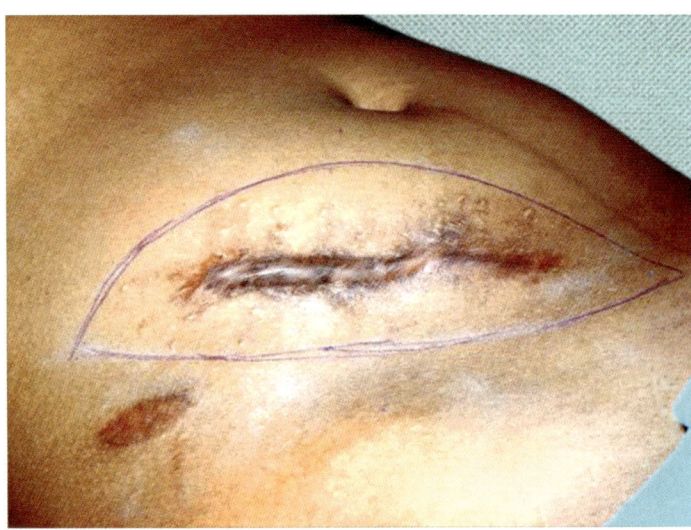

Fig. 24.14: Desmoid tumour in the anterior abdominal wall

6. *Scars*: Scars represent previous surgery. Look at the site of scar and get following details.

  • *Site of the scar*: Examples—upper midline surgery done 20 years back mostly for gastrojejunostomy and vagotomy. If you find a mass now, it could be carcinoma stomach. Similarly, scar in the upper abdomen and surgery done one year ago for carcinoma stomach, presenting with palpable liver can be due to secondaries in the liver.

  • *Healing*: A clean scar indicates healing with primary intention (without infection). Ragged scar indicates wound infection. Such patients are vulnerable for development of incisional hernia (Fig. 24.13).

  • *Any nodule over the scar*: Mention about the details. Desmoid tumour is one possibility

(Fig. 24.14). They may suggest intra-abdominal malignancy. **In women, scar endometriosis is a differential diagnosis.**

  • *Drain mark*: Any major surgical procedure, e.g. resection and anastomosis, surgeons usually favour inserting a drain tube. Example: After gastrectomy, you can see a drain mark in the lumbar region.

  Common question: Is it vagotomy GJ, or is it gastrectomy? No drain is placed after vagotomy GJ, whereas it is placed after gastrectomy.

7. *Inspection of groin and male genitalia*: If scrotum is empty, it could be a case of undescended testis. Look also for phimosis. Retention of urine can present as suprapubic mass. Look for impulse on cough and rule out hernia.

Recent development of left-sided hernia in elderly males may suggest carcinoma left colon. Carefully take the history of constipation and examine for a mass high up.

Palpation

Following are the methods of palpation available to the clinician depending upon the merits of the case:

A. *Superficial palpation*: Superficial palpation is done with the flat of the hand or fingers. Gentle superficial palpation of the abdomen gains confidence of the patient. It can detect superficial lesion of the abdominal wall such as lipomatosis, neurofibromas, endometriosis, stage 4 lymphoma with cutaneous deposits. It can also detect an area of tenderness, so that clinician is careful while doing deeper palpation (Fig. 24.15).

B. *Deep palpation*: These are important requirements for deeper palpation:

- Patient should be told what you are doing. He should be well-relaxed, with flexion of the knee by about 45°.
- With the patient's face turned to the opposite side, ask him to breathe comfortably with the mouth open.
- Deep palpation (Fig. 24.16) should be started from the region situated diagonally opposite to the site of pain.
- Palpation should cover not only the 9 quadrants region of the abdomen, but also two more quadrants region, i.e. two renal angles and 12th quadrant region—external genitalia in males.
- Deep palpation is carried out with the palmar surface of the fingers and some degree of angulation depending upon the depth of palpation.

C. *Dipping method*: Significant ascites is the hindering factor for palpation of the abdominal masses. In such cases, dipping method by using fingertips or palmar surface, mass can be appreciated. Examples are stomach mass, colonic mass or tuberculous omentum in children.

- Once mass is felt, following details have to be documented. If you cannot feel a mass in the supine postion, change the posture of the patient

Draw a simple diagram of the abdomen and sketch of the mass. Look carefully at your diagram. Location and shape will give the diagnosis often.

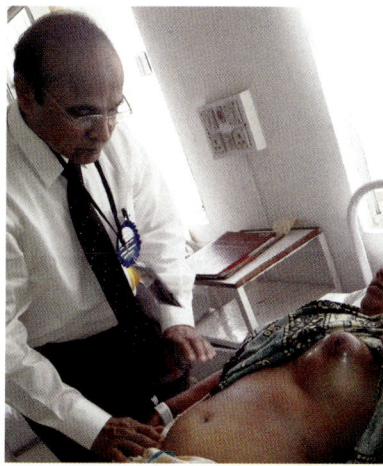

Fig. 24.15: Abdominal palpation should be gentle. Palpate region by region with flat of the fingers. Flexion of the hip and knee joint will also help. This is a case of carcinoma breast and the surgeon is looking for enlargement of liver or Krukenberg tumours

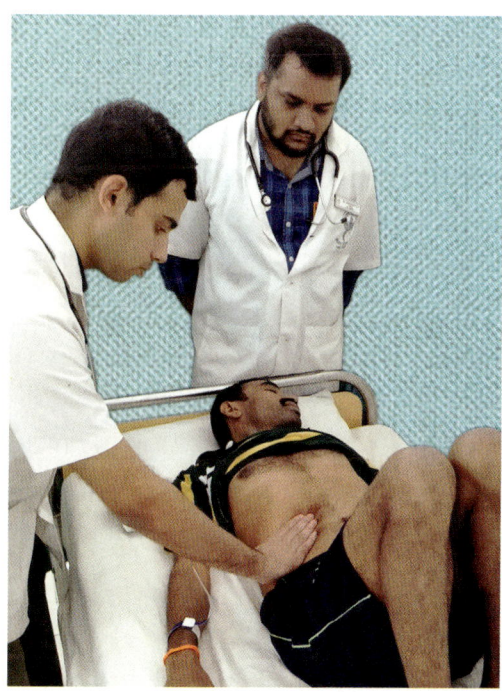

Fig. 24.16: Deep palpation of the abdomen. (*Courtesy:* Dr Navneeth S Kamath, Dr Kaustabh KP, interns, KMC, Manipal)

to right or left lateral, sitting or even prone—read the Clinical Case Capsule given on the next page (Fig. 24.17).

D. *Nicolson's method of palpation* (page 345)

- It is done only when abdominal palpation becomes difficult due to upper abdominal guarding.
- Left palm is kept over the lower end of sternum and pressed firmly with the base of the left palm.
- Abdomen relaxes and palpation becomes easy.

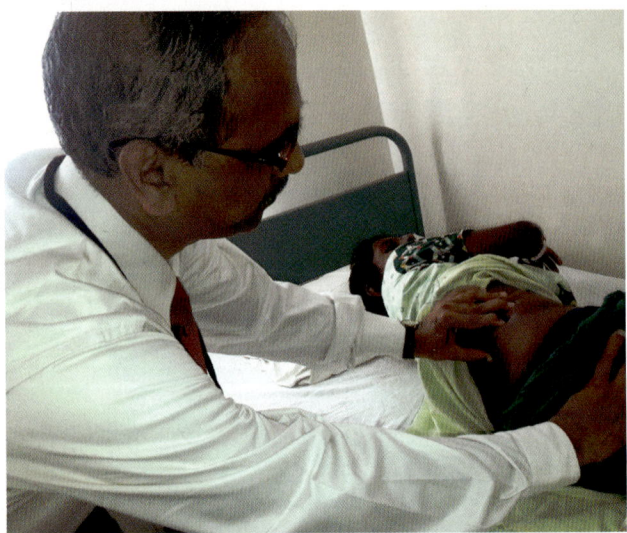

Fig. 24.17: Examination in the lateral position. Also read the clinical case capsule below

---

Clinical Case Capsule

MS Exams, Calicut 2008

A 28-year-old lady was admitted with history of abdominal pain since 3 months. It was dull aching pain which was radiating to the back. No other symptoms.

Examination in supine position did not reveal any mass. It was a surprise to examiners also. Interestingly, the patient herself said she could feel something when she turned to one side. Yes, in the left lateral position, a mass was felt as a smooth round firm mobile swelling. It was a case of pedunculated cystadenoma pancreas. It was easily palpable in the prone position

---

• Depending upon the location of the mass, the patient can be turned to right or left lateral position or even prone position and palpate the mass.

1. *Location and extent:* The mass may start in one region but extension into the other regions have to be mentioned. In the differential diagnosis section, you will get information about what anatomical structures are present in the respective regions and what pathology can occur in that region. A few examples are given below: Carcinoma body of the stomach is felt as a mass in the epigastrium and may extend to umbilical region. If the entire stomach is involved, the mass can be felt not only in the epigastrium but also in the hypochondrium. Thus, a large liver is not only felt in the right hypochondrium and epigastrium but also in right lumbar region, umbilical region and sometimes even in the right iliac fossa.

2. *Size and shape:* Larger the tumour, lesser are the chances of malignancy (carcinoma). A few

examples of large masses are hydronephrosis, omental cysts, gastrointestinal stromal tumours, retroperitoneal tumours, large pseudocysts, etc.

Measure the size with the tape (Figs 24.18A and B). Different shapes of the masses will give anatomical diagnosis often. Examples are given below. Mention the size.

a. An egg-shaped mass or globular mass suggests gallbladder lesion (Fig. 24.19A).
b. A horseshoe shape may indicate a horseshoe kidney (Fig. 24.19B) with pathology, e.g. hydronephrosis.
c. Reniform shape suggests a renal swelling (Fig. 24.19C).
d. Globular swelling in the hypogastrium could be due to distended urinary bladder (Fig. 24.19D).

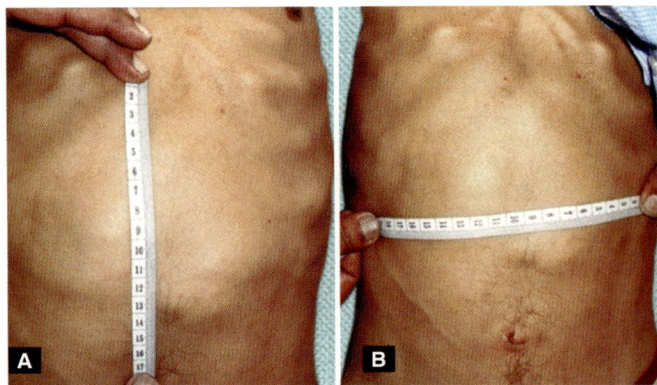

Figs 24.18A and B: Vertical and horizontal measurements

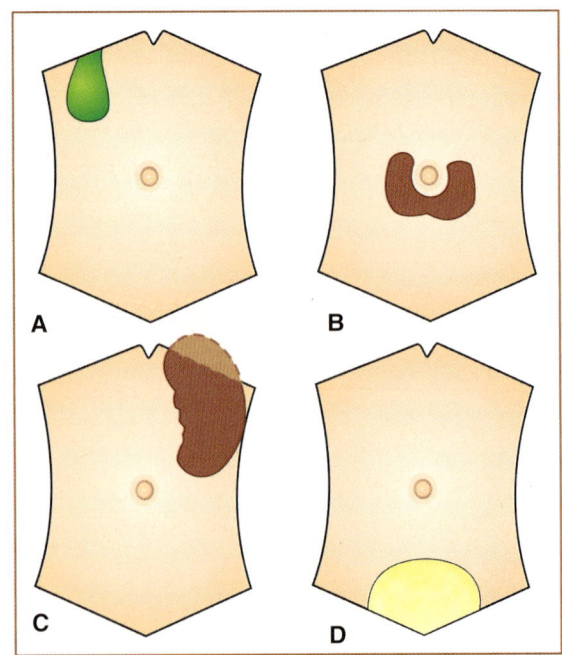

Figs 24.19A to D: Shapes of the intra-abdominal mass

e. Round right iliac fossa swelling in a female is usually an ovarian cyst.

f. Dome-shaped epigastric swelling is usually pseudocyst of pancreas.

Clinical Wisdom

Tensely cystic swellings may feel firm. *Examples*: Tense distended gallbladder in cases of obstructive jaundice due to periampullary carcinoma.

3. *Surface*: Carefully palpate the surface with palmar aspect of or flat of the fingers. For all practical purposes, mention whether it is smooth, irregular or nodular. **Smooth surface** usually indicates a benign lesion. For example splenomegaly, hydronephrosis, ovarian cyst, and gallbladder masses have smooth surface. **Irregular surface** is an important feature of malignancy such as carcinoma of the stomach, carcinoma caecum or hepatoma. **Nodular surface** is seen in secondaries in the liver, ileocaecal tuberculosis, carcinoma caecum or carcinoma stomach, etc. When the size of the nodule is more than 1 cm, it can be described as large nodular or **bosselated surface. Look at the Fig. 24.20. Examples of swelling with bosselated surface are given under clinical wisdom.**

* **The term lobular surface is not to be used for abdominal masses**

Clinical Wisdom

- Polycystic kidney
- Polycystic disease of the liver
- Secondaries in the liver
- Large para-aortic lymph nodes
- Phyllodes tumour of the breast
- Large multinodular goitre

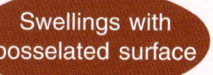
Swellings with bosselated surface

4. *Margins or borders*: Feel the borders of the mass all around. In a deep mass arising from retroperitoneal structures, it is difficult to feel all borders. When you cannot appreciate the borders, say diffuse.

- **Upper border** cannot be made out in liver, splenic and renal swellings. When you are able to feel it mention in relationship to a bony mark or umbilicus (Fig. 24.21).

- **Lower border** can be **sharp** as in liver masses (Fig. 24.2). Lower border is not appreciated in pelvic masses, e.g. uterine fibroid, ovarian cyst (Fig. 24.3).

- A **characteristic notch** is felt in the anterior border of splenic swelling.

When you cannot appreciate the upper border or lower border of the masses, do the next test as given below.

- All borders (edge) can be made out in stomach masses, mesenteric masses, pancreatic masses and a few colonic masses (Fig. 24.24).

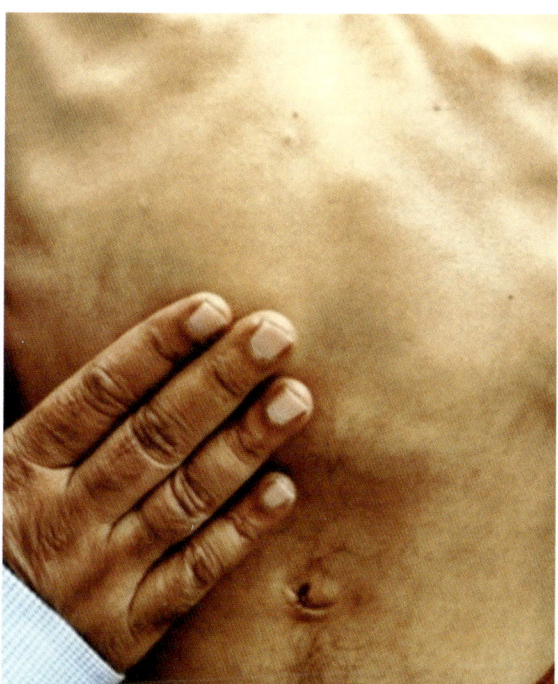

Fig. 24.20: Secondaries in the liver (nodular liver)

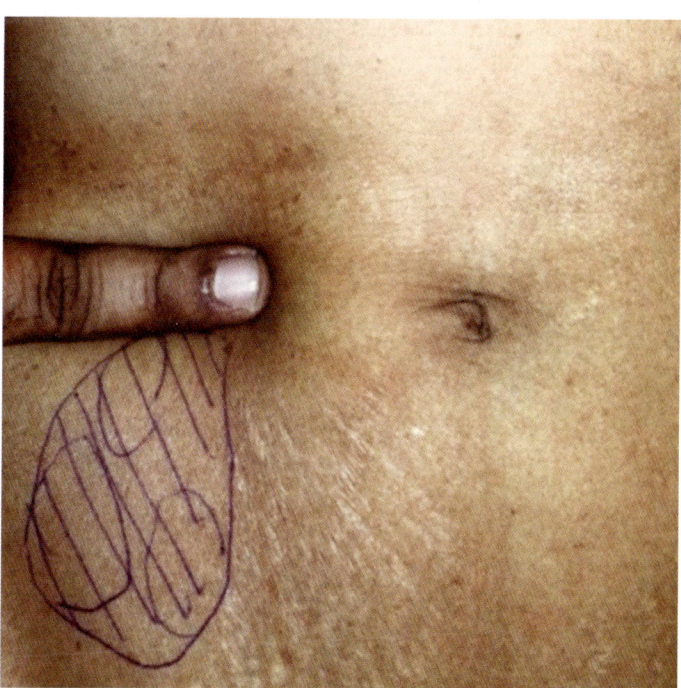

Fig. 24.21: Upper border of the mass at the level of umbilicus

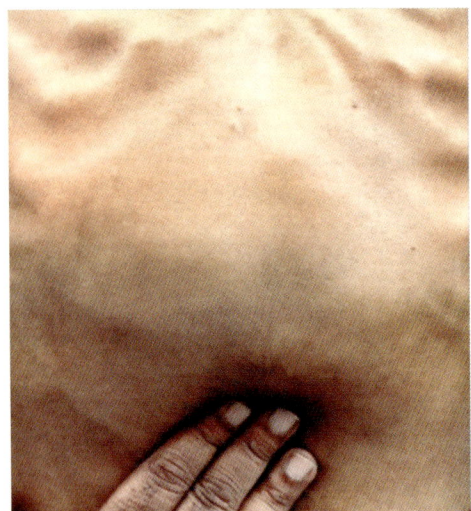

Fig. 24.22: Lower border is sharp in liver masses

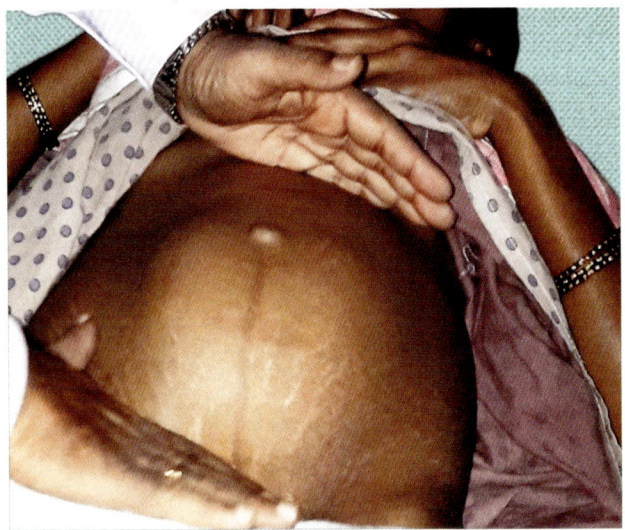

Fig. 24.23: Upper border is clearly defined. Lower border not felt. Finger insinuation was not possible. A case of ovarian cyst

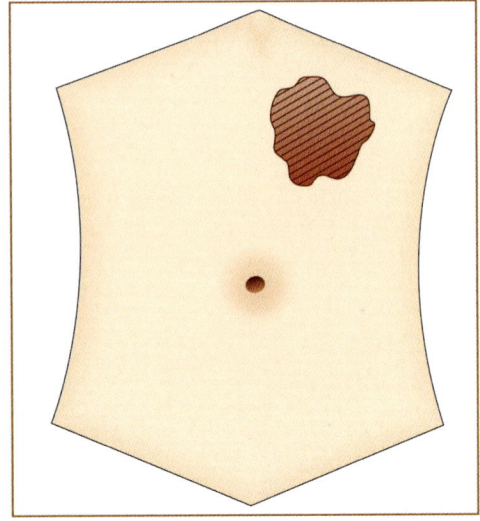

Fig. 24.24: Stomach mass in the left hypochondrium, all borders could be made out

5. *Finger insinuation test—getting above the mass and getting below the mass* (Fig. 24.25):

- This test has relevance in upper and lower abdominal masses. Liver and spleen are under right and left costal margins, respectively. Hence, it is not possible to get the upper margin or upper border of these organs. An attempt to invaginate between the costal margin and these masses is not possible. On the other hand, finger invagination under the costal margin is possible in a stomach mass. This is one of the tests to differentiate liver mass from stomach mass.

- **Large pseudocyst:** Difficult to get the upper margin of the mass and it is possible to get above the mass in retroperitoneal masses (Fig. 24.26).

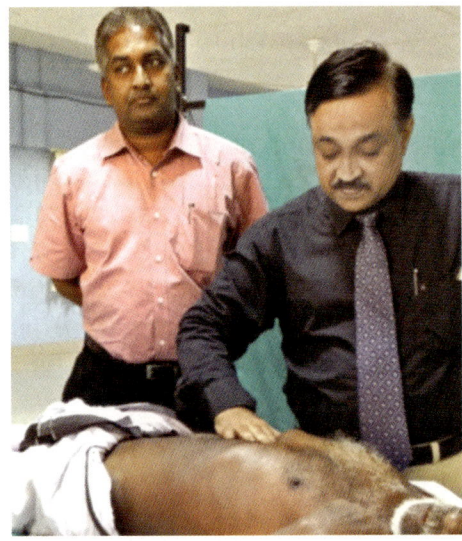

Fig. 24.25: Checking for finger insinuation test (CME, Calicut Medical College, 2014)

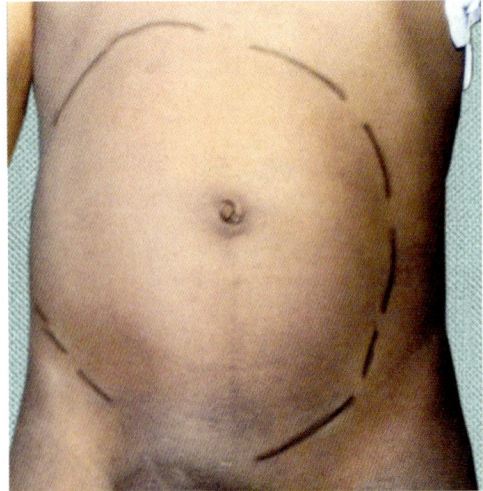

Fig. 24.26: Retroperitoneal cyst—upper border could be easily made out (*Courtesy:* Dr Chetan, Professor of Surgery, KMC, Manipal)

- In the same fashion, in a mass arising from uterus, ovary and urinary bladder (pelvic masses), it is not possible to get the lower border. However, when ovary comes out of pelvis with free mobility, it is possible to get the lower border as in large ovarian cysts (Figs 24.27 and 24.28). This is also helpful to differentiate carcinoma caecum (common in females) from carcinoma of the ovary. It is possible to get the lower border in carcinoma caecum but not in ovarian malignancies.

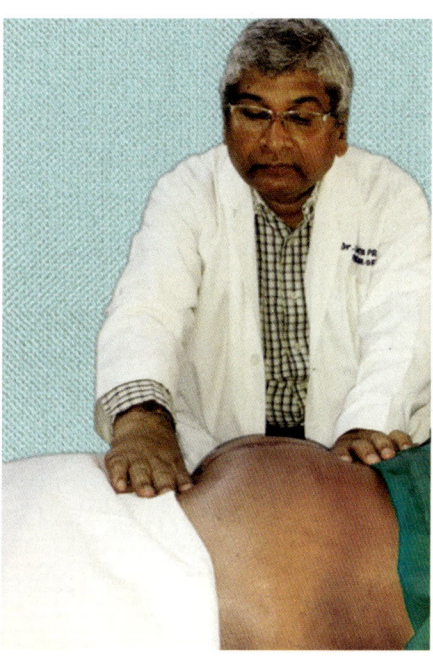

Fig. 24.27: Defining upper and lower borders of the mass (*Courtesy:* Dr Prakash GV, Head, Department of Surgery, SVMC, Tirupati)

6. *Consistency*

- **Hardness** is a feature of malignant lump. Thus, hepatoma, carcinoma stomach, pancreatic carcinoma, and colonic carcinoma present as hard lump. However, it should be remembered that often the malignant lump is firm and not hard. A portion of rapidly growing tumour, such as hepatoma, may feel firm (rarely soft) due to tumour degeneration or tumour necrosis.

- **Firm** consistency is found in ileocaecal tuberculosis, nodes of lymphoma.

- A peculiar **doughy** feel is described for tuberculous abdomen.

- It is difficult to elicit fluctuation test for intra-abdominal swellings, and often tensely cystic swellings feel firm on palpation, e.g. pseudocyst

of pancreas, hydronephrosis, tense gallbladder as in periampullary carcinoma.

- Indentation or pitting on pressure can be found in a colon loaded with faeces.

7. *Movement with respiration*: This test is done by placing the fingers over the lower border of the swelling and the patient is asked to take a deep breath. Movement with respiration is positive when there is "up and down" movements—not anteroposterior movement. Any structure in contact with diaphragm moves with respiration (Clinical Box 24.2). For example, liver, stomach, spleen, and gallbladder move very well with respiration. Splenic flexure growth due to contact with the lower pole of the spleen and hepatic flexure growth due to contact with liver move with respiration. Renal swelling moves with respiration because kidney is enclosed by fascia of Gerota which is attached to the diaphragm above. As it moves down with inspiration, it can be held and pushed back to the renal pouch.

Clinical Wisdom

- A large pseudocyst of pancreas may move with respiration due to contact with diaphragm. What it means is that diagnosis is not made based on one physical finding. It is the conglomeration of all physical findings which help in the diagnosis.
- It should be remembered that a swelling or the mass which moves with respiration is obviously an intra-abdominal mass.

Clinical Box 24.2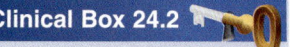

Movement with respiration
- Liver, spleen and stomach masses move freely with respiration
- Gall bladder mass also moves freely with respiration because of its proximity to liver
- Mass arising from hepatic flexure and splenic flexure of colon also has some mobility because it is in contact with liver and spleen
- Renal masses exhibit minor degree of movement with respiration because of indirect attachment to diaphragm

---

8. *Intrinsic mobility test* (Figs 24.28 to 24.30): An intra-abdominal mass can be mobile, if it has loose attachments or if it is not within the bony cage. Thus, liver, spleen, and uterine masses are not mobile because of their location within bony cage. Following masses exhibit intrinsic mobility. Hold the mass with hand between fingers and try moving them in both horizontal and vertical direc-

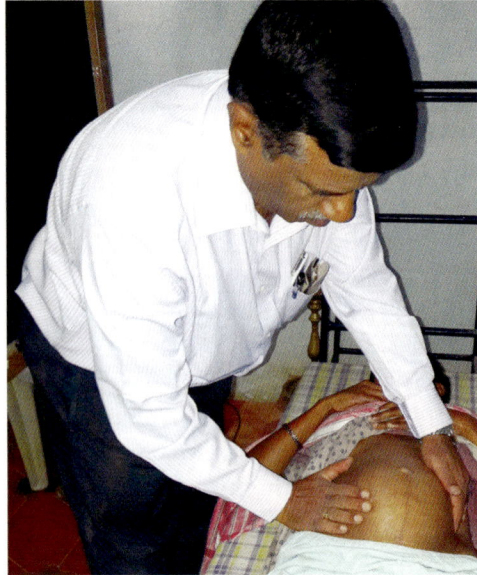

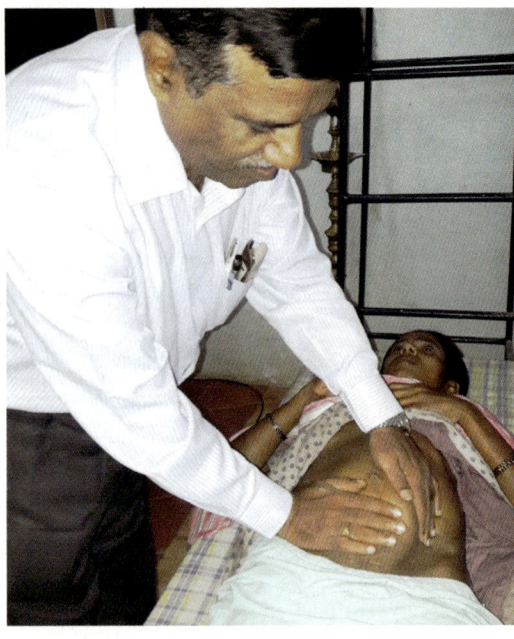

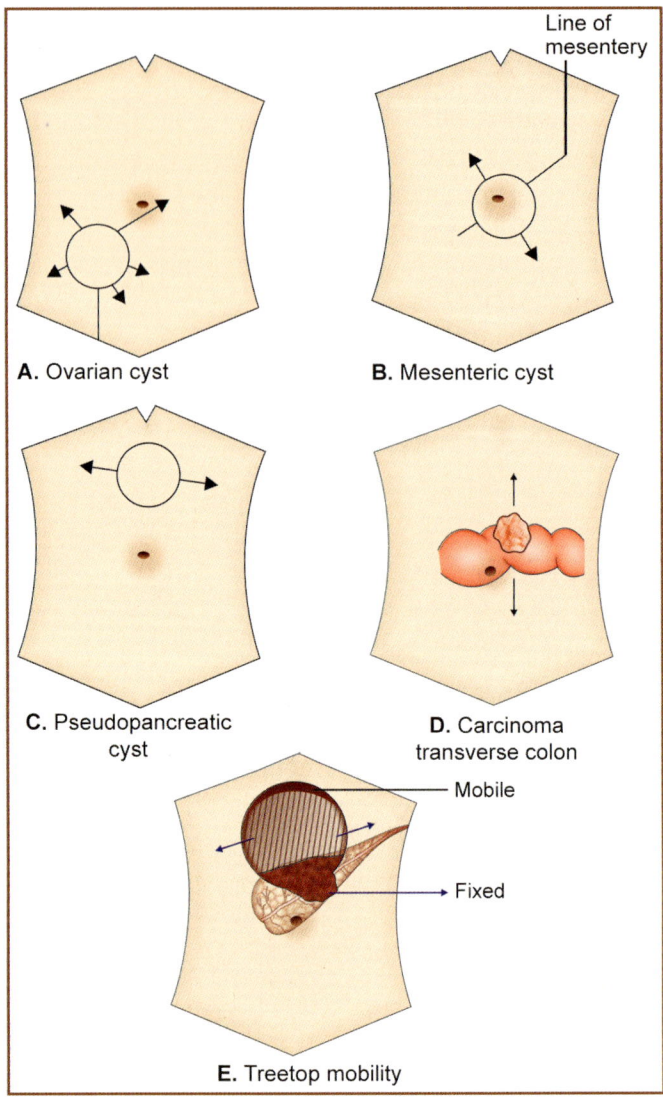

Figs 24.30A to E: Different types of intrinsic mobility

Figs 24.28 and 24.29: Dr Vidyadhar Kinhal, Head, Department of Surgery, VIMS, Ballary, examining mass abdomen. Observe left hand of examiner and he is trying to move the mass. Mass has been moved to right side in Fig. 24.29 (*Courtesy:* Dr Sangeetha Kalabhairav, Dr Madhu B.S. Dr M.A. Balakrishna, Dept of Surgery, CME, Mysore Medical College, Mysore 2017)

Clinical Box 24.3

Intrinsic mobility—mass

• Side to side	— Gallbladder
• Vertical	— Transverse colon
• All directions	— Ovarian cyst
• Right angle to the direction of mesentery	— Mesenteric cyst
• Push back to renal	— Kidney pouch
• Treetop mobility	— Pancreatic cystadenoma

---

tions. And record the mobility. Unique features of some mobile swellings have been given here.

a. Ovarian cyst is a freely mobile swelling once it comes out of pelvis and it can be moved in all directions.

b. Mesenteric cyst moves at right angles to the direction of the line of mesentery.

c. Carcinoma transverse colon has vertical mobility unless it is advanced.

d. *Pancreatic masses* (Fig. 24.31): Even though they do not exhibit mobility, a cystadenoma of the pancreas because of the size and a narrow base, will exhibit **treetop mobility**. Any big mass abutting the under surface of the diaphragm also moves with respiration.

e. Interesting case of mesocolic cyst has been described in Figs 24.32 to 24.35.

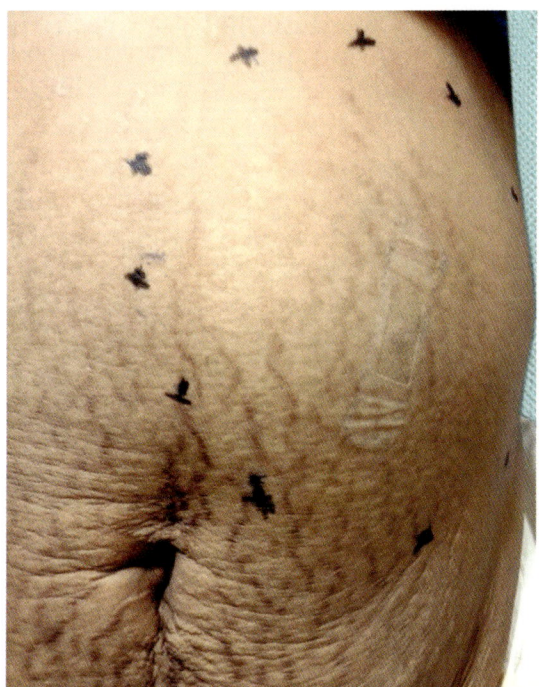

Fig. 24.31: A large cystadenoma of pancreas

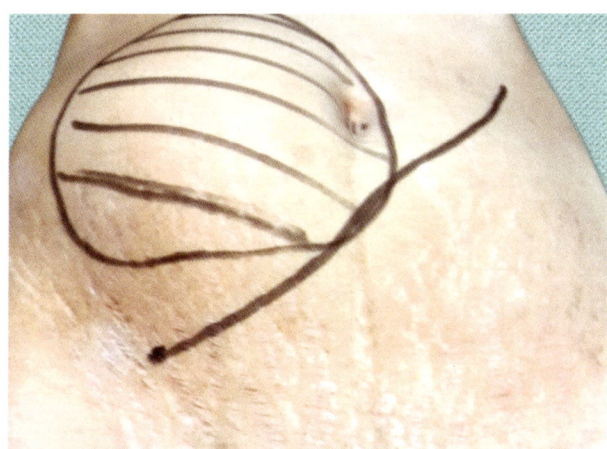

Fig. 24.32: Large cystic mass being marked. Almost like mesenteric cyst, more towards right side

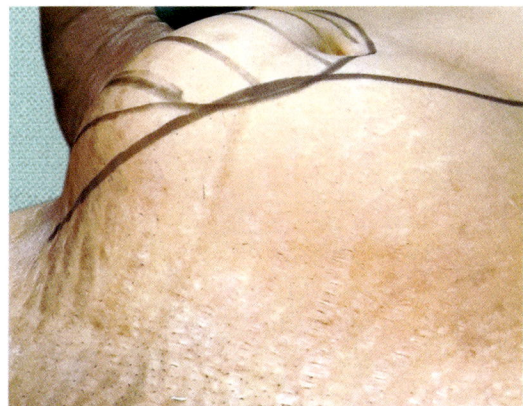

Fig. 24.33: The mass could be pushed down but not into the pelvis. Lower border easily made out

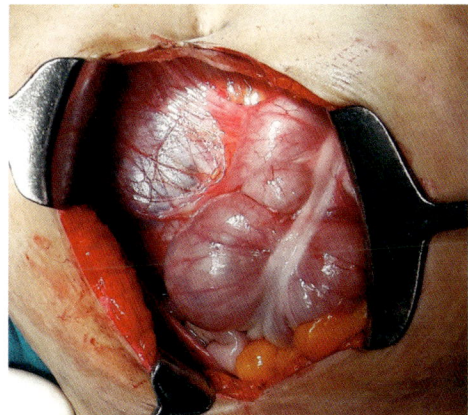

Fig. 24.34: Ascending colon was anterior to the cyst which was shown in Fig. 24.32

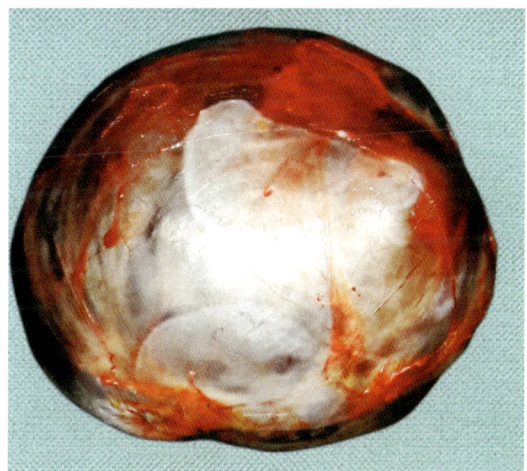

Fig. 24.35: 14 cm sized cyst was excised

9. *Plane of the swelling*

   a. *Leg raising test (Carnett's test) or head raising test:*

- The purpose of this test is to contract rectus abdominis muscles (also other abdominal wall muscles). Intra-abdominal swellings become less prominent. On the other hand, abdominal wall swellings become more prominent, e.g. neuro-fibroma, or lipoma in the abdominal wall, abdominal wall hernias including umbilical, incisional epigastric, Spigelian.

- This test is done by asking the patient to raise his legs without bending at the knee (extended legs) or by raising the shoulders from the bed with arm folded over the chest (Fig. 24.36).

b. *Nose blowing test or straining test*

- This test can be done by asking the patient to blow through the nose with mouth closed. **The lateral abdominal muscles are more contracted with this test.**

- This test is ideal for mass in the region of flanks.
- During head raising test, umbilical hernia, and epigastric hernia become more prominent. Rectus gets contracted and divarication of rectus can be better appreciated (Fig. 24.37).

c. *Knee-elbow test*

- This test differentiates an intraperitoneal mass from retroperitoneal mass. It is more useful when there is a **mass in the centre of the abdomen— more so in the upper abdomen.** To give a few examples, stomach mass or omental mass will

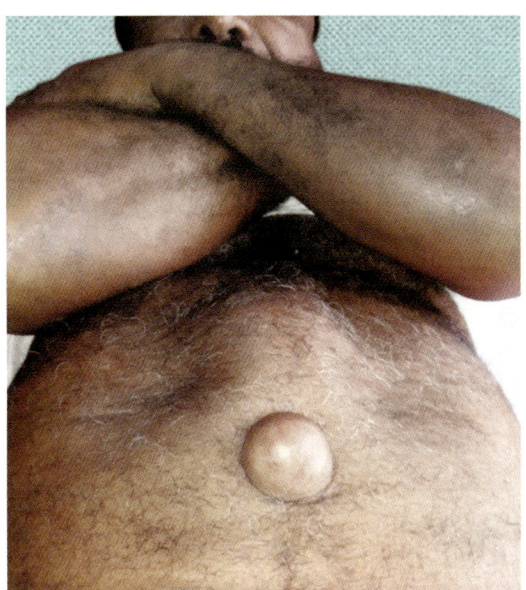

Fig. 24.36: Divarication with umbilical hernia

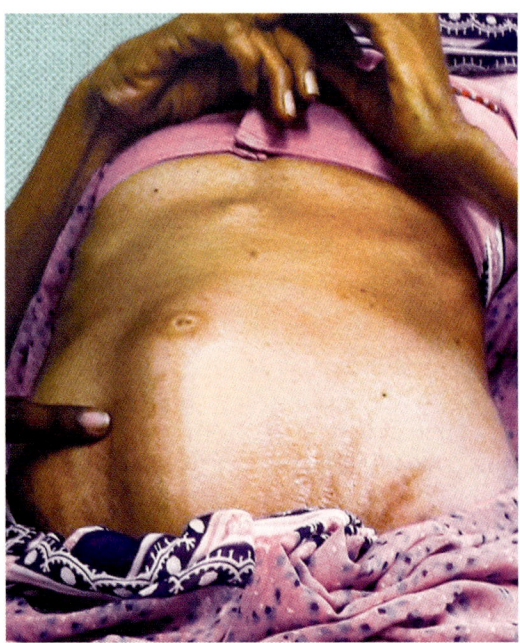

Fig. 24.37: Defining lateral border of rectus abdominis

fall forwards because they are intraperitoneal. On the other hand, pancreatic mass or a lymph node mass will not fall forward. **The test has significance only in 'selected' cases.**

- However, knee-elbow test helps to differentiate expansile pulsation from transmitted pulsation. *Examples:* A pseudocyst of pancreas will have transmitted pulsations because it overlies aorta. In the knee-elbow position, pulsation disappears as it gets separated from the aorta. On the other hand, aneurysms exhibit expansile pulsations.

10. *Bimanual palpation and ballotability:* **These tests should be done for peripherally located swellings.** Grossly enlarged swellings and peripheral swellings may be bimanually palpable such as liver, spleen, ascending and descending colonic masses and renal masses. Only kidney is ballotable. What is ballotability? (Fig. 24.38) 'Ballot' means to toss about. To ballot, the swelling should be bimanually palpable and there should be a gap or space between hands which are kept anterior and posterior to the mass. Typically, renal swellings are **ballotable because it enlarges more posteriorly, it is placed peripherally, it has a pedicle and perirenal pad of fat.** This test is done when the patient is in supine position, by keeping one hand anteriorly in the lumbar region over the swelling and the other hand posteriorly in the renal angle. A gentle push is given from behind and the swelling

Renal Ballotability
- **P**osterior enlargement is more—thus space for movement anteriorly
- **P**laced peripheral—thus can be felt by both hands
- **P**edicled organ—free movement possible
- **P**erirenal pad of fat—thus cushion effect
4 Ps to remember

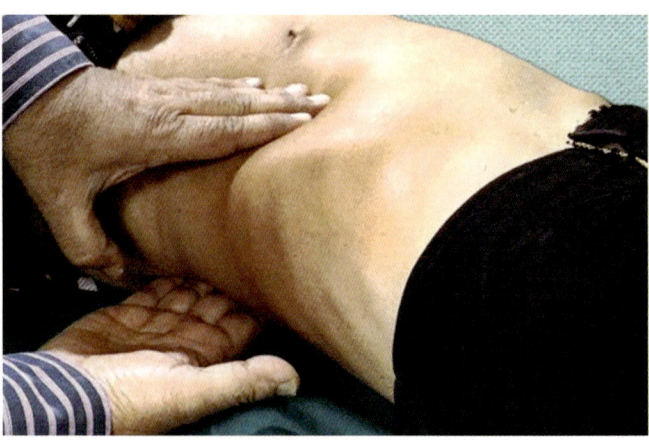

Fig. 24.38: Bimanual palpation and ballotability

touches the hand which is placed anteriorly and it goes back (also read ballotability in Chapter 4 and ovarian ballottement).

Percussion

1. *Detect fluid in the abdomen*

A. Puddle sign: To demonstrate mild ascites (about 200 ml), the patient is put in a knee-elbow position and percussion is done around umbilicus. It gives a dull note, if minimal fluid is present. (Normally, area around the umbilicus is resonant.)

B. Shifting dullness: Significant or moderate amount of fluid (more than 500 ml) in the abdomen is demonstrated by percussion of the centre and flanks of the abdomen in the lying down position, and in the left or right lateral position. In the supine position, flanks give a dull note due to fluid. However, in the lateral position, fluid shifts down and coils of bowel float up.

C. Fluid thrill: In tense ascites, this method is followed. An assistant keeps the edge of his hand and gently presses the centre of the abdomen. Then abdominal wall on one side is flicked and thrill is felt by another hand which is kept in the flank on the other side (Fig. 24.39).

2. *Liver dullness*: Normal liver dullness is elicited in the 5th intercostal space. Make a note of this and start percussing from above downwards. If it is a liver mass, dull note is continuous with that of the mass. If it is not a liver mass, example stomach mass in the epigastrium, dull note will change into tympanitic or impaired resonant note. Upward enlargement of the liver also can be defined by

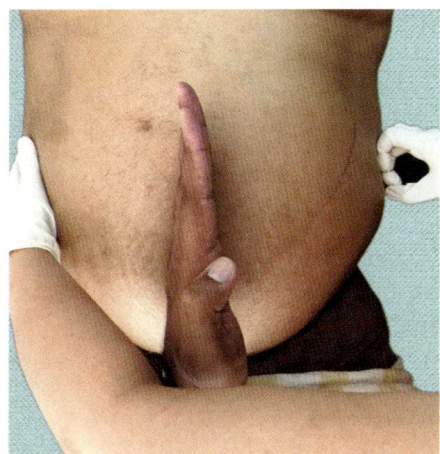

Fig. 24.39: Checking for fluid thrill in cases of tense ascites

percussion and finding the upper limit where dull note is obtained. Thus, the distance between upper border and lower border or margin has been described as liver span.

Clinical Wisdom

Any painless suprapubic swelling (mass) in elderly males should be considered as enlarged urinary bladder due to benign hypertrophy of prostate (BPH) unless proved otherwise.

3. *Splenic dullness*: It is elicited in the 9th intercostal space in the left midaxillary line and it is continuous with splenic mass.

Traube's space is a semilunar space between the lower edge of the left lung, the anterior border of the spleen, the left costal margin and the inferior margin of the left lobe of the liver. Anatomically superiorly bounded by left sixth rib, laterally by the left midaxillary line and inferiorly by left costal margin. Stomach which is posterior to this space hence gives tympanitic note normally but gives dull note when spleen is enlarged.

4. *Percussion over the mass* (Clinical Box 24.4)

- Splenic and liver masses classically are **dull** to percuss.
- Retroperitoneal masses may give **resonant** note because of intestines anterior to it. However, when they attain large size, e.g. retroperitoneal liposarcomas, they push the bowel to one side and hence, they are dull to percuss.
- Stomach mass may give **impaired resonant** note because of solid growth and due to the presence of air in the stomach.
- *Renal angle percussion*: In cases of enlargement of kidney, there will be a band of resonance anteriorly due to the colon but posteriorly it gives a dull note.
- *Hydatid thrill*: It is demonstrated by placing 3 fingers over the swelling and percussing the middle finger. Due to the fluid in the cyst, the fluid thrill (after-thrill) is felt by the other two fingers. **This clinical sign is rarely demonstrable.**

Clinical Box 24.4

Percussion
- Dull note—liver, spleen, urinary bladder, renal angle
- Resonant—bowel anterior to the mass (e.g. retroperitoneal mass)
- Impaired—stomach mass
- Shifting dullness—ascites

Auscultation (Fig. 24.40)

1. **Loud noisy sounds (borborygmi)** with or without peristalsis may indicate subacute obstruction. Such patients may be having ileocaecal tuberculosis or carcinoma caecum. Auscultation should be done at right iliac fossa to listen to bowel sounds.

2. Auscultation over the **liver mass** may reveal a **bruit** as in a rapidly growing hepatoma.

3. **Succussion splash** is a splashing sound in cases of pyloric obstruction either due to carcinoma or due to cicatrised chronic duodenal ulcer.

4. Perisplenitis and perihepatitis give rise to **friction rub** as in sickle cell anaemia due to repeated infarction and adhesions.

5. Aortic aneurysm will give a **continuous murmur** in the upper abdomen.

6. **Auscultopercussion** or auscultoscraping test is done to assess lower border of the stomach or greater curvature of the stomach.

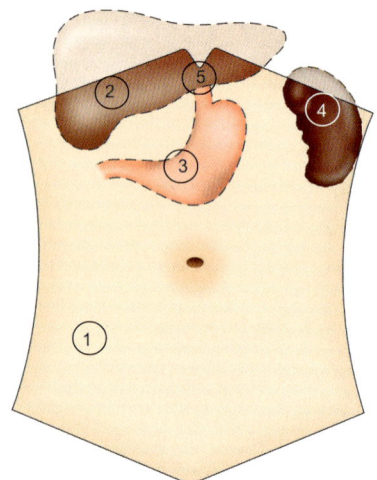

Fig. 24.40: Auscultation sites: 1–5 (*see* text)

Examination of all Hernial Orifices

Recent development of epigastric hernia/umbilical hernia may be manifestation of raised intra-abdominal pressure including tumours (Fig. 24.41)

Rectal Examination (Fig. 24.42)

It should be done in a case of intra-abdominal mass. Blood stains on a gloved finger suggest rectal bleeding.

1. It can detect a carcinoma or a growth in the rectum in a case of secondaries in the liver.

2. It can detect secondaries in the rectovesical pouch. **Blumer's shelf**—as hard, nodular mass and rectal mucosa is free during digital examination.

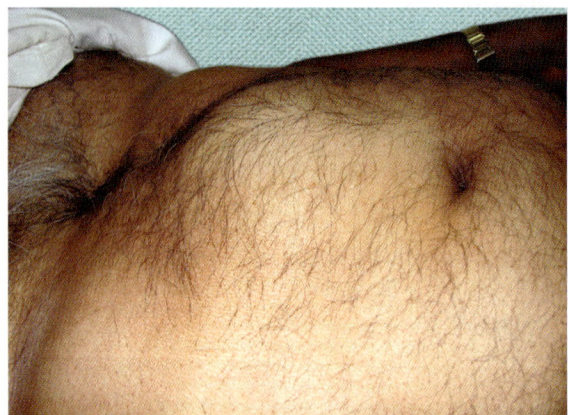

Fig. 24.41: Pancreatic neoplasm presenting as epigastric hernia

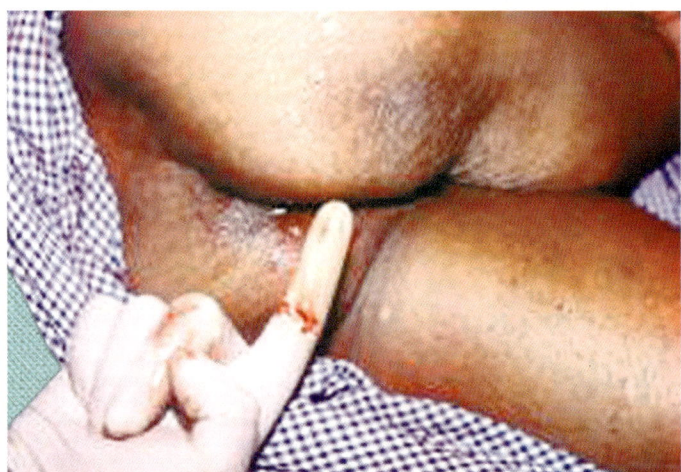

Fig. 24.42: Per rectal examination: Glove stained with blood

3. An ovarian mass can be felt in one of the fornices.

4. Enlarged prostate can be felt in chronic retention of urine.

Vaginal Examination

It should be done to rule out carcinoma cervix or to detect lymph nodes in the pouch of Douglas. Ovarian masses may be palpable through fornices.

Bimanual Examination

This should be done in cases of pelvic masses. One hand (left) is placed over the mass in the hypogastrium and right index finger or fingers inserted in the vagina (or rectum in virgin females). The left hand is pressed downwards and backwards above the pubic symphysis. By this manoeuvre, details of the pelvic mass, whether solid or cystic, uterine or ovarian and the mass is free or fixed can be made out.

Examination of Lymph Nodes

• In cases of abdominal masses arising from lymph nodes, a thorough search of the body should be done to rule out other group of lymph nodes such as axillary, iliac, inguinal, neck nodes (lymphoma).

- **Left supraclavicular nodes** (Virchow) are enlarged very often in visceral malignancies mainly from gastrointestinal tract. It indicates "inoperable" nature of the disease. Entire gastrointestinal lymph drains into the thoracic duct which joins the point of confluence of internal jugular vein and subclavian vein on the left side. This explains the significance of enlargement of Virchow's node. In 20% of cases, thoracic duct is single and 10–15% of cases, it is double.

- **Significance of right supraclavicular node:** The lymphatics from the right mediastinal lymph trunk, and from the posterior right thoracic wall which form the right upper lymph trunk drain into the commencement of the right brachiocephalic vein.

Systemic Examination

Systemic examination should include respiratory system and cardiovascular system. Evidence of tuberculosis of the chest gives a clue about the mass in the abdomen, which may be a tubercular mass.

DIFFERENTIAL DIAGNOSIS

MASS IN THE RIGHT HYPOCHONDRIUM (Fig. 24.43)

I. Parietal

On head raising test, the lump becomes more prominent.

a. *Lipoma and neurofibroma*: They can be part of multiple lipomatosis or multiple neurofibromatosis. If pain and pigmentation are present, it is neurofibroma.

b. A hard nodule in the parietal wall can be due to:
   - Secondary deposit in the skin/subcutaneous tissue specially when skin is infiltrated and ulcerated. Common

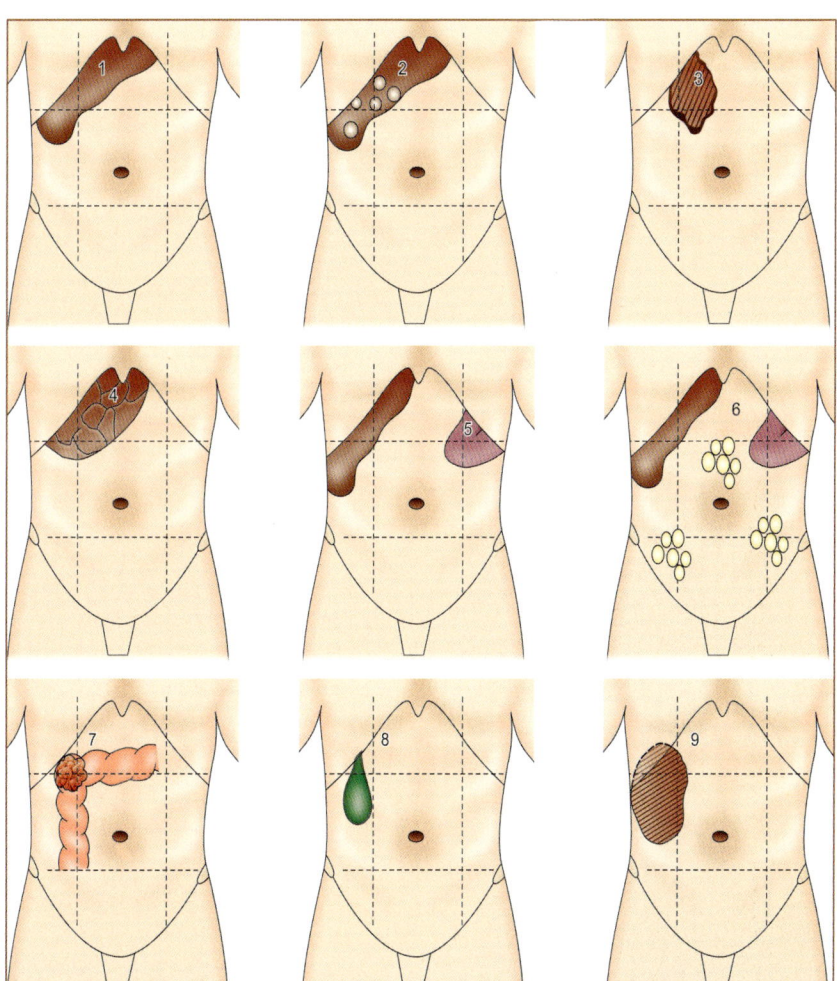

Fig. 24.43: Differential diagnosis of mass in the right hypochondrium. (1) Smooth hepatomegaly in lymphoma or due to medical causes, (2) secondaries in the liver—hard and nodular, (3) hepatoma—irregular, hard or firm, (4) polycystic disease of the liver—firm and nodular with round borders, (5) hepatomegaly with splenomegaly—could be portal hypertension, (6) hepatomegaly, splenomegaly, para-aortic lymph nodes and iliac nodes—Hodgkin's lymphoma, (7) carcinoma ascending colon—hard irregular mass, (8) palpable gallbladder—smooth, round borders, and (9) renal mass

primaries are malignant melanoma, bronchogenic carcinoma, hepatoma.

- *Non-Hodgkin's lymphoma*: 'T' cell type.

c. *Cold abscess*: Spine tenderness with or without history of tuberculosis gives the clue to the diagnosis.

II. Intra-abdominal Swellings

On head raising test, the lump becomes less prominent.

1. ***Mass arising from the liver*** (only chronic masses are discussed):

   a. Secondaries in liver (Fig. 24.44)

   - Entire liver is enlarged (both lobes)
   - Nodular surface
   - Sharp border
   - Hard in consistency
   - *Rare umbilication sign*: Softening in the centre of the nodule (due to necrosis)

   Typically, a patient is elderly male or female, who mostly has primary malignancy of the stomach, colon or pancreas for which he or she was operated, presents with emaciation, poor health, loss of appetite and loss of weight. Jaundice is rare in cases of metastasis. Many times, secondaries in the liver is the first manifestation of a hidden or occult primary. Again look for the common primary sites, not only from GIT but also from breast, bronchus, kidney, etc. Massive enlargement due to secondaries can occur in cases of colloid carcinoma rectum and malignant melanoma. One should look for clues such as vomiting for carcinoma stomach, dysphagia for carcinoma oesophagus, backache for carcinoma pancreas, cough for bronchogenic carcinoma and previous surgery. In majority of the cases of secondaries of liver, treatment is difficult and not worthy other than to give palliation. However, secondaries from carcinoid and

neuroendocrine tumours have good prognosis after resecting the tumours and treatment with chemotherapy/ imatinib. Hence histological proof is a must before starting any treatment.

   b. Hepatoma (Clinical Box 24.5, Figs 24.45 and 24.46): Typically a male alcoholic or patient with hepatitis-B or C presents with dull-aching pain in the right hypochondrium, weight loss and low grade fever and rapidly growing lump abdomen. On examination, liver is palpable, hard with irregular borders. Evidence of chronic liver disease such as viral hepatitis or cirrhosis is usually present. Diagnosis is done after ultrasound, CT scan and CT angiogram. Alfa fetoprotein levels are grossly elevated. Hepatoma can also spread within the liver giving rise to multiple secondaries in the liver. Also metastasis by blood spread can result in skeletal secondaries (Figs 24.47 and 24.48). Tissue biopsy is not mandatory in operable cases. Some form of hepatectomy is the treatment of choice. Quickly to summarise, the clinical points which suggest hepatoma are:

   - One lobe enlargement
   - Firm to hard, irregular mass
   - Tender mass
   - Bruit/thrill may be present
   - No other mass

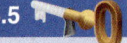

Clinical Box 24.5

Tender liver mass
- Hepatoma
- Amoebic liver abscess
- Suppurative pylephlebitis
- Congestive cardiac failure
- Infected hydatid cyst

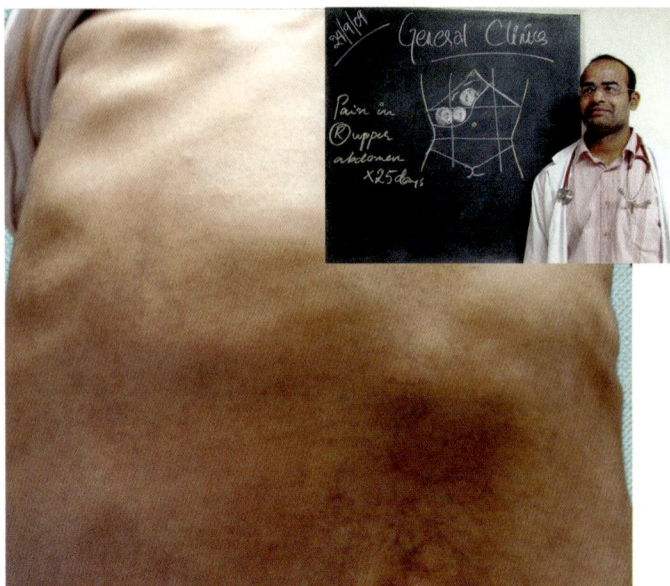

Fig. 24.44: Secondaries in the liver. On inspection, you can make out the nodularity of the surface (*Courtesy:* Dr Pavan Addala, PG 2009, KMC, Manipal)

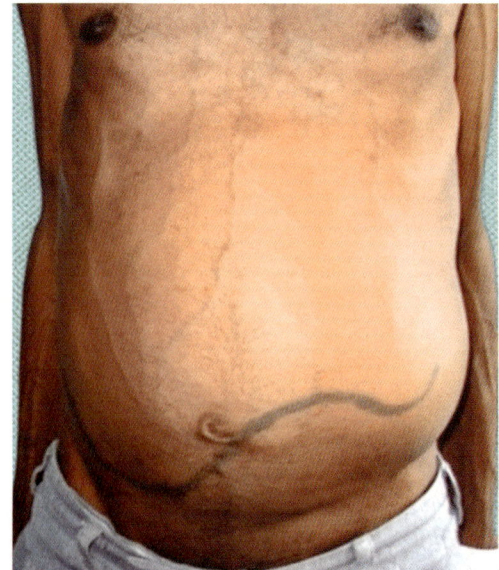

Fig. 24.45: Large hepatoma with dilated veins. Right inguino-axillary veins are prominent suggesting inferior vena caval obstruction

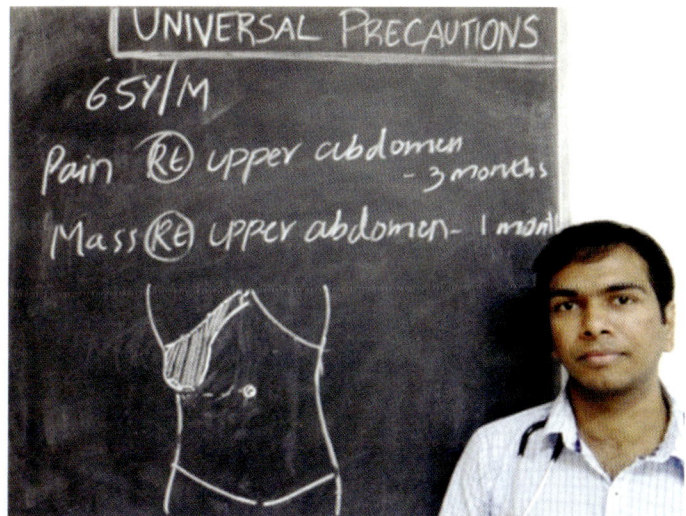

Fig. 24.46: Hepatoma in a hepatitis-B patient (*Courtesy*: Dr Nikil Shellagi, Postgraduate in General Surgery, KMC, Manipal)

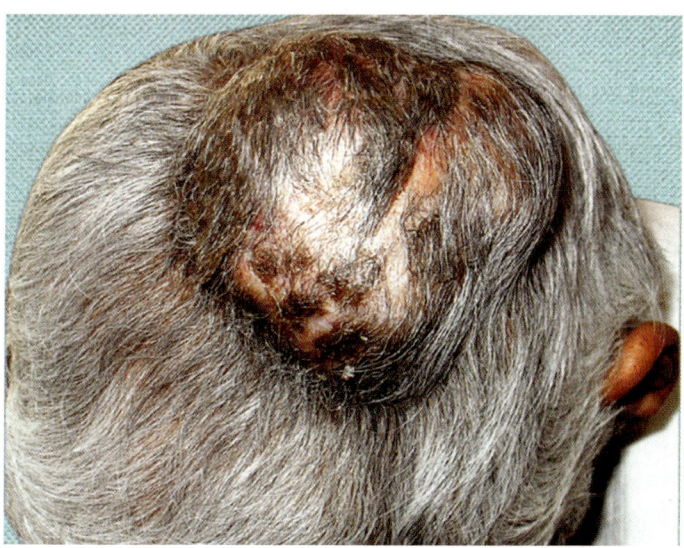

Fig. 24.47: Metastasis from HCC

Clinical Case Capsule

Manipal Clinifest 2014 (Fig. 24.47)

A 65-year-old man was admitted with complaints of rapidly growing scalp swelling of 4 months duration. Clinical examination revealed an ulcerative swelling with everted edges, indurated and fixed. Case of metastasis of scalp was diagnosed. Other diagnosis was epithelioma or even a sarcoma was considered. Abdominal examination revealed a hard irregular 8 × 3 cm mass suggestive of a hepatic origin. The patient never complained of any pain abdomen. He says he used to have dull abdominal pain. Ultrasound was suggestive of hepatocellular carcinoma. Alpha fetoprotein was elevated. Edge biopsy report was hepatocellular carcinoma.

c. **Polycystic disease of the liver** (Fig. 24.49): The patient would have presented to the hospital with pain due to haemorrhage in a cyst. Typically, they are young between 20 and 30 years. Majority are asymptomatic and are detected during a routine ultrasound examination done for some other condition. This disease is easily confused for secondaries in the liver. Clinical points and clinical case capsule (given below) will give you more details.

Clinical Case Capsule

A 30-year-old lady with no comorbidities was brought to the hospital with pain in the right hypochondrium and ultrasound diagnosed as secondaries in the liver. The treating surgeon called the relatives and told them that this case is advanced. She may not survive for 6 months. Patient went home against medical advice. After 10 years, I saw this patient, to my surprise, hale and healthy. She had not taken any treatment. It was a case of polycystic disease of the liver. Moral of the story is prognosis of the patient must be explained only after histological proof of a malignancy and staging of the disease. Also look at the age of the patient. She was 30 years. She was healthy with no loss of weight or appetite. In younger patients, think of congenital diseases also.

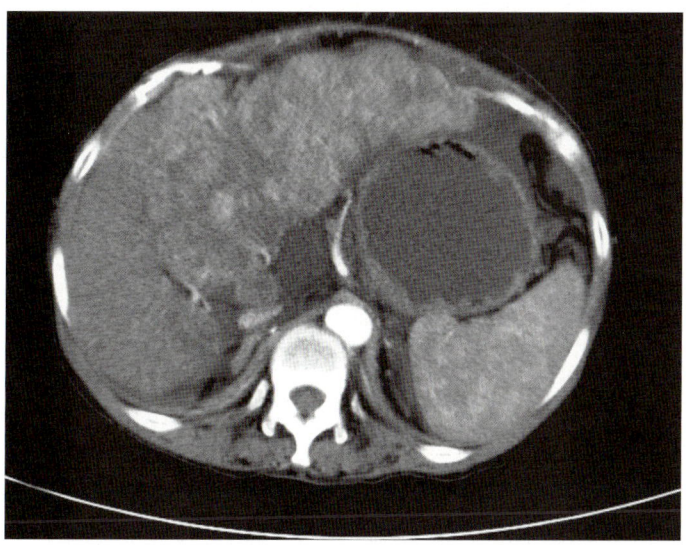

Fig. 24.48: Hepatoma with secondaries in liver

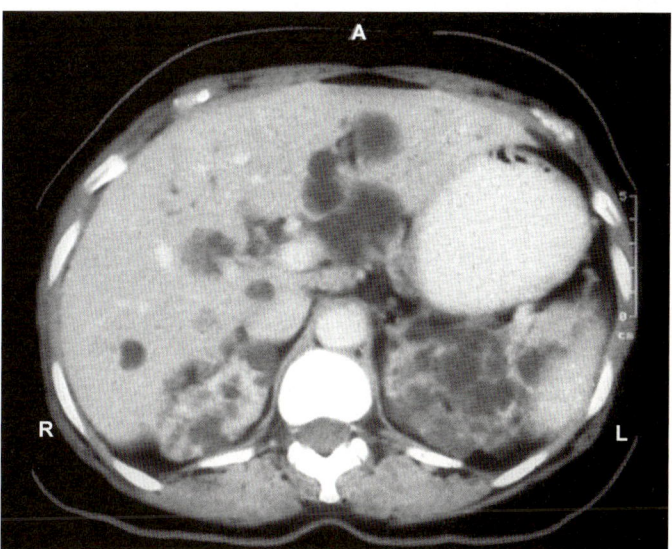

Fig. 24.49: Polycystic liver and kidney

Clinical Features

- Both lobes are enlarged
- Nodular
- Nontender
- Round borders
- General health is good

d. **Hydatid cyst** (Figs 24.50 to 24.53): Typically, a middle-aged patient presents with vague dull-aching pain in the hypochondrium or epigastrium. Very often, it is asymptomatic and detected when ultrasound examination is asked for abdominal pain for some other condition. History of contact with dogs may be present. The disease is caused by *Echinococcous granulosus*. Some patients can present with severe abdominal pain and high grade fever with chills and rigors also. This is due to secondary infection of the hydatid cyst or due to rupture of the cyst into one of the biliary radicles. It is also associated with jaundice. Liver is tender in such cases. Diagnosis is made by ultrasound and CT scan. CT scan

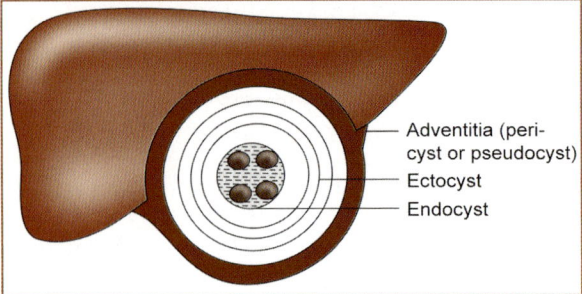

Fig. 24.51: Layers of the hydatid cyst

Adventitia (peri-cyst or pseudocyst)
Ectocyst
Endocyst

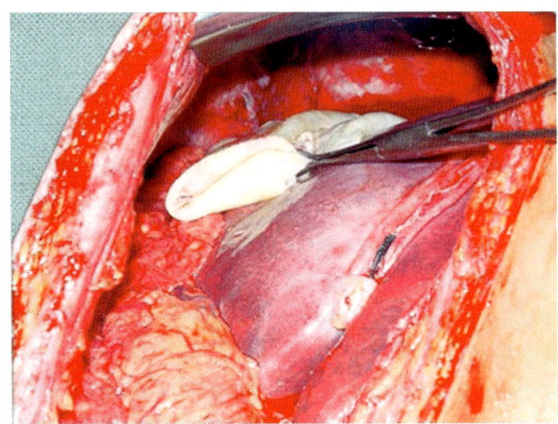

Fig. 24.52: Laminated membrane removed at surgery with sponge-holding forceps

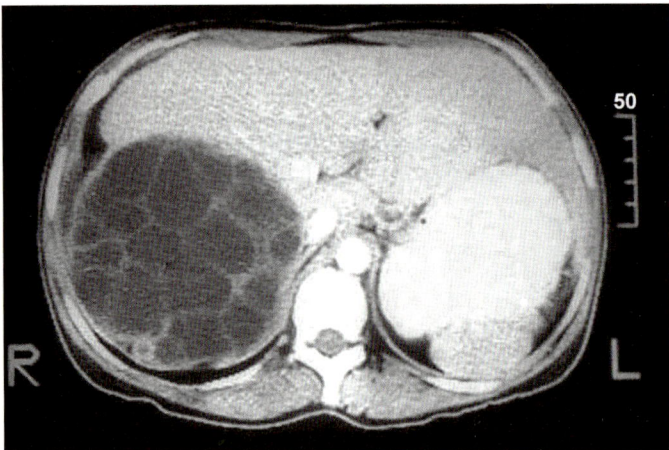

Fig. 24.50: Cart wheel appearance in a case of hydatid cyst of the liver

shows classical cart wheel appearance. Albendazole should be given before and after surgery. Surgery is in the form of excision. Infected cases require excision followed by careful visualisation of the cyst cavity and suturing any bile leak if visible. If bile leak, persists after surgery, common bile duct stenting should be done. Clinical features are summarised as follows.

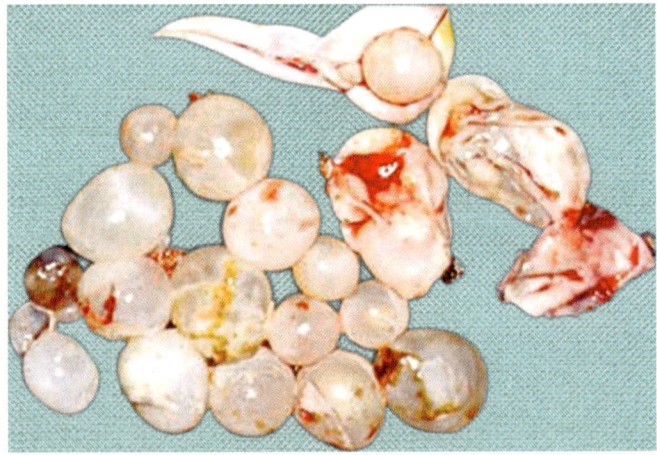

Fig. 24.53: Daughter cysts—it is important to clear all these to prevent recurrence

Clinical Wisdom

- One or both lobes are enlarged
- Smooth or nodular surface
- Round borders, nontender
- General condition of the patient is good
- Hydatid thrill—rare 'physical sign' may be present

e. **Cirrhosis of liver:** Alcohol is the most common cause for cirrhosis of the liver, another cause being hepatitis B. Liver may be enlarged, firm and irregular in pre-cirrhotic cases. Splenomegaly, and ascites will help in the diagnosis. Other

features of liver cell failure such as gynaecomastia, spider naevi, palmar erythema may be present. Pain in the hypochondrium is due to enlarged liver. Treatment is medical. Liver transplantation is the best solution when medical treatment fails.

Clinical Wisdom

When impalpable liver becomes palpable or sudden deterioration of health develops in patients with cirrhosis of liver think of hepatoma.

f. **Lymphoma:** Liver is palpable, one or two finger—breadths, firm or hard, smooth or irregular, nontender. Splenomegaly and lymphadenopathy will help in the diagnosis. In Hodgkin's lymphoma with stage IV, typically, cervical, axillary and para-aortic lymph nodes are enlarged. Patients are in the middle age group who present with painless enlargement of lymph nodes. Nodes are discrete, mobile and rubbery in consistency. Lymph node biopsy will show cellular pleomorphism and Reed-Sternberg cells. Treatment is by chemotherapy.

g. **Congenital Riedel's lobe:** It is a tongue-shaped projection from the inferior border of liver. It is on the right side, can be mistaken for gallbladder. Sometimes it can be so big so as to reach right iliac fossa. It is considered to be congenital in origin and occurs due to anatomical variation. Incidence is equal in both sexes, it is prevalent in both sexes. Its palpability is dependent on age-related changes in liver size and skeletal shape. It is one of the differential diagnosis of a palpable liver in an otherwise healthy person.

2. **Gallbladder mass:** To say anatomically that the mass is from gallbladder, it should have the following features:

   - It is in the right hypochondrium
   - It moves with respiration
   - It is typically oval shaped (egg shaped)
   - Felt just beneath the abdominal wall
   - It is felt just a step below (posterior) to the inferior border—edge of the liver.
   - May have slight side-to-side mobility.

Causes of gallbladder enlargement

- *Back pressure:* Distal obstruction as in periampullary carcinoma or carcinoma head of the pancreas. Such gallbladder is **firm (tensely cystic), smooth, oval shaped** and associated with jaundice. Classically an elderly patient presents with jaundice, itching, clay-coloured stools and high-coloured urine. The patients also say loss of appetite and loss of weight. On examination, palpable gallbladder will be the only important clinical finding. Thus one should look for gallbladder carefully. If ascites is present or in an obese patient, it is difficult to feel. Also in one-third of patients, obstruction need not be total and hence gallbladder may not be palpable (Figs 24.54 to 24.56).

- *Carcinoma gall bladder:* It is hard, irregular, fixed and not so common in the southern states but is common in the northern states along the Ganges belt. The patient presents with pain in the right hypochondrium, loss of weight and jaundice. Jaundice indicates infiltration into the common hepatic duct or common bile duct. Spread occurs very fast by local spread, lymphatic spread and blood spread. Metastasis to the liver is common. CT scan is the investigation of choice. Treatment is extended cholecystectomy, removal of the involved segment of the liver with removal of lymph nodes.

- *Acute cholecystitis:* It is usually a tender, vague, well-defined mass. Like appendicular mass, following an attack of cholecystitis, a mass can develop in the region of the gallbladder within 2–3 days. It is distended, tender gallbladder and surrounded by omentum, duodenum and colon. Local guarding and rigidity may be a feature also. Sometimes the mass can also be due to perforation of gallbladder which is sealed off. Conservative management is successful in majority of the cases. Elective cholecystectomy is done after 8–10 weeks.

- *Mucocoele:* It is a nontender, palpable gallbladder without jaundice: A stone blocking the neck of the gallbladder results in closure of both ends of the gallbladder. All the bile within the gallbladder is absorbed and mucus is secreted within the gallbladder. This results in enlargement of the gallbladder. This is called as mucocoele of the gallbladder. The tense, nont-tender gallbladder is palpable in the right hypochondrium and sometimes it can attain huge size. Diagnosis is by ultrasound and the treatment is cholecystectomy.

- *Empyema:* Very tender gallbladder mass with fever. Infected mucocoeles can result in purulent fluid in the gallbladder. This is called empyema of the gallbladder. Diabetic patients are more vulnerable. Tender gallbladder with toxic features are present. Urgent drainage of the pus

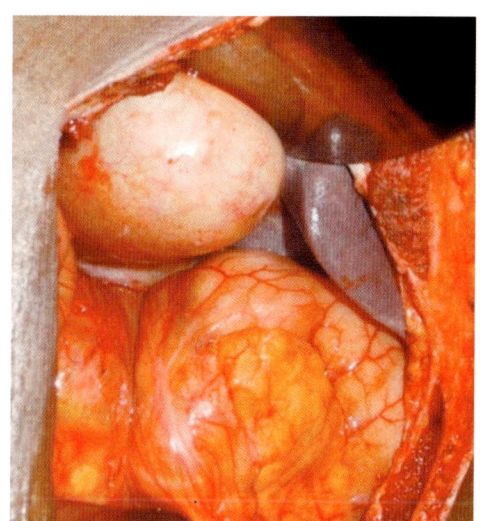

Fig. 24.54: Large distended gallbladder at surgery

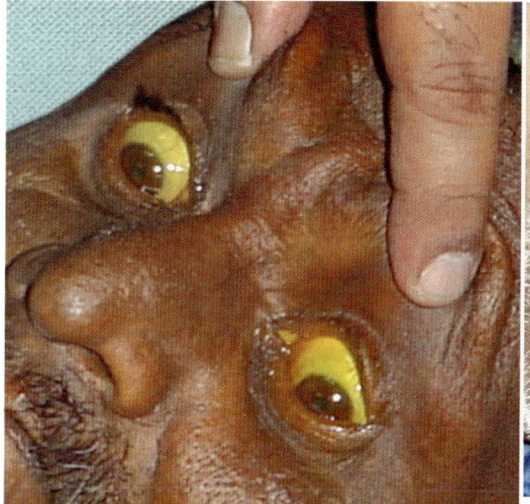

Fig. 24.55: Greenish hue (due to biliverdin) of deep jaundice—a case of obstructive jaundice

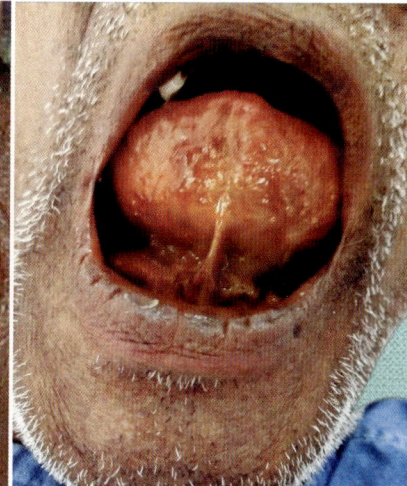

Fig. 24.56: Look for jaundice on the undersurface of the tongue also

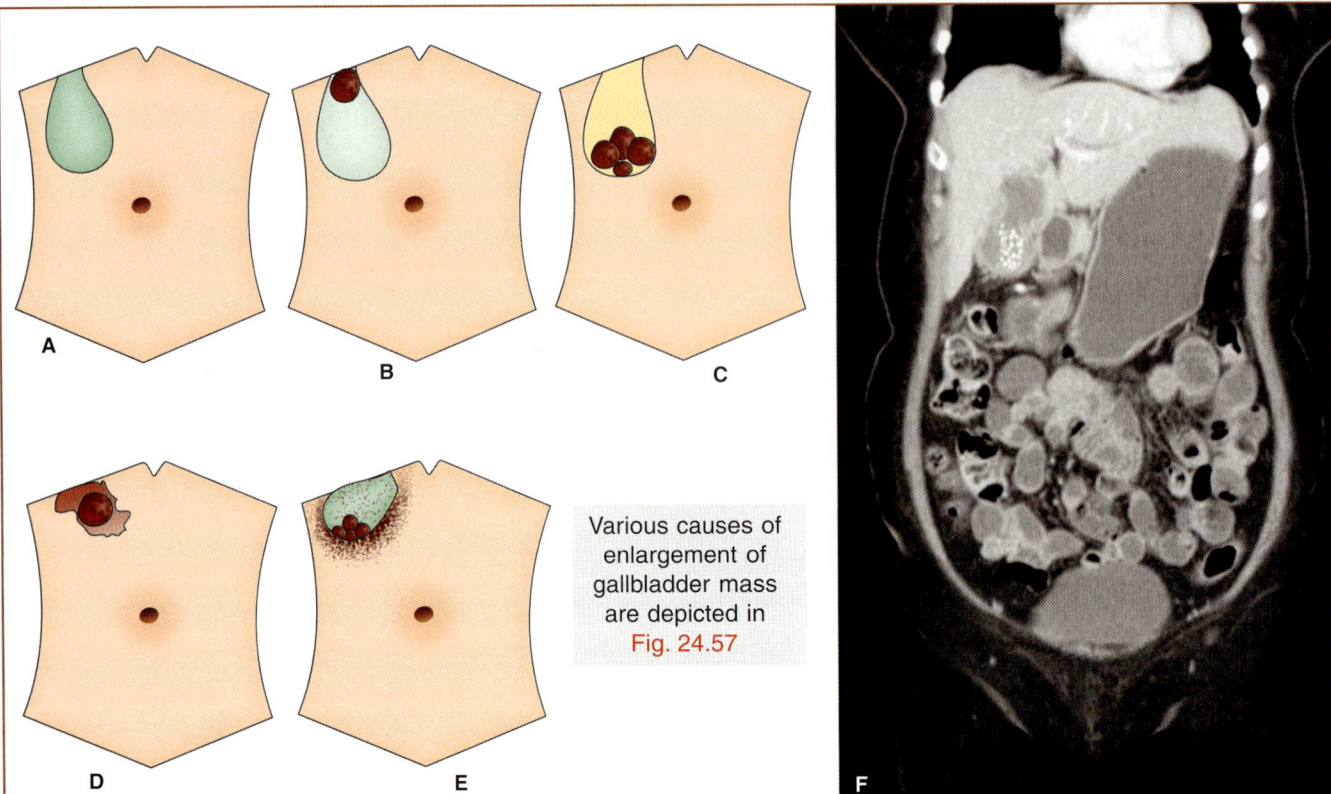

Various causes of enlargement of gallbladder mass are depicted in Fig. 24.57

Fig. 24.57: (A) Case of carcinoma head of pancreas. Enlarged gallbladder mass, jaundice is present; (B) Mucocoele of the gallbladder; (C) Empyema of the gall bladder—tender gall bladder, toxic, tachypnoeic patient; (D) Irregular hard fixed mass—carcinoma gallbladder; (E) Inflamed tender mass of acute cholecystitis; (F) Advanced carcinoma gallbladder with extension into the liver, lymph nodes and ascites. It was inoperable. The patient was 52-year-old and a known case of gall stones since 10 years

by cholecystostomy in high-risk patients, cholecystectomy when anatomy of the Calot's triangle can be well-defined and partial cholecystectomy when anatomy of the Calot's triangle cannot be well-defined are the various options available.

3. Colonic mass

a. *Carcinoma hepatic flexure* (Fig. 24.58): This is more common in men. (Carcinoma caecum is more common in women.) Typically, presents as constipation and sometimes loose stools (mucus) what has been described as alternating constipation and diarrhoea. Loss of appetite and loss of weight occur late. Very often there is a delay in diagnosis of right-sided tumours including carcinoma caecum. A high index of suspicion is necessary. The mass will be palpable on careful examination because it is situated higher in position and deeper in location. Gurgling may be present. Colonoscopy is done to prove the diagnosis and take a biopsy. Ultrasound of the abdomen is obtained to know the spread of the disease. Extended right hemicolectomy is the treatment of choice. A typical mass has the following features:

- Firm to hard irregular mass
- Restricted mobility
- Moves with respiration because of its contact with liver
- Resonant or impaired resonant note on percussion.
- Caecum may be distended, if there is obstruction (Fig. 24.59).

4. *Renal mass*: Importantly renal mass is palpable mainly in the lumbar region, loin and then extends into the right

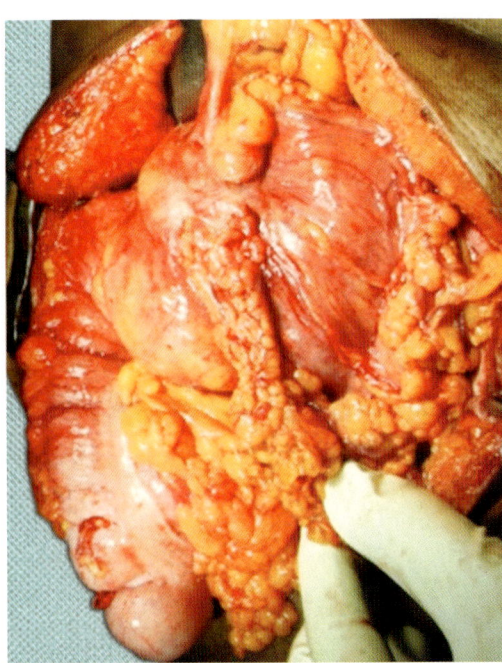

Fig. 24.58: Carcinoma hepatic flexure—can present as a mass in the right hypochondrium. Often these patients have features of intestinal obstruction

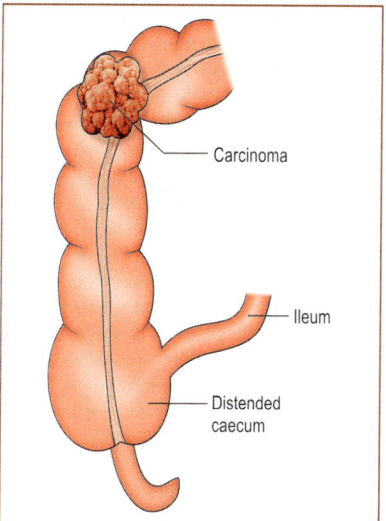

Fig. 24.59: Carcinoma hepatic flexure—Diagrammatic representation. This eventually results in closed loop obstruction. Distended caecum will give rise to tympanitic note on percussion

hypochondrium. All three important diseases of the kidney which cause enlargement can present as a mass here. They are renal cell carcinoma, hydronephrosis and polycystic disease of the kidney. They are discussed in detail in the mass in the lumbar region.

5. **Suprarenal mass:** Students are hereby requested not to offer the diagnosis of suprarenal mass as first diagnosis. It is better to give them after exclusion. Suprarenal glands are situated under the lower ribs and cartilages, and hence small masses are not palpable. However, when symptoms and signs suggest a suprarenal mass, one can consider the diagnosis. A few examples: Cushing's syndrome: Moon face, abrupt onset of obesity, purple striae, distension of abdomen, hypertension, fear and palpitations in young patients (*refer* to Clinical Case Capsule given in the next page). Clinically they all have features of a renal mass and because their position in the abdomen is high, they can be confused for liver mass. Interestingly, they can attain huge size also. Adenomyolipoma of adrenal glands is a benign tumour which can attain huge size. The lesion arising from adrenal cortex can be a benign adenoma. When it secretes excess cortisol, it is Cushing's syndrome. Excess of aldosterone causes aldosteronism (Figs 24.60 to 24.62).

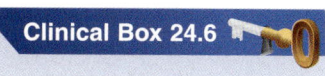

Clinical Box 24.6

Adrenal swellings of surgeons' interest
1. Cushing's syndrome—moon face, abrupt obesity
2. Phaeochromocytoma—hypertension, palpitation
3. Adenomyolipoma—mass abdomen

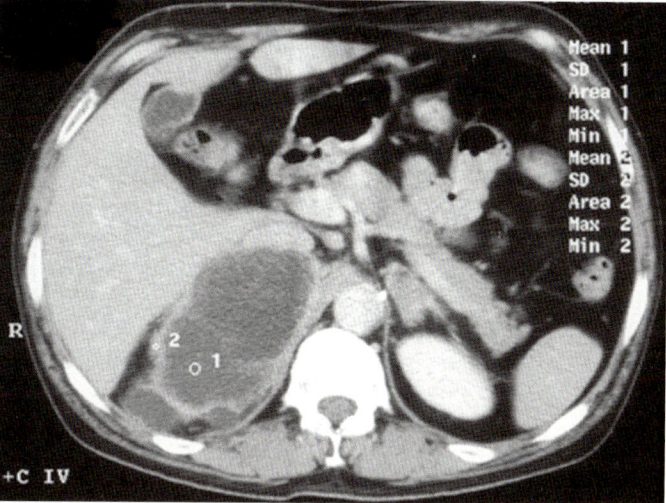

Fig. 24.60: Large adrenal cyst, mass confused for liver cyst clinically

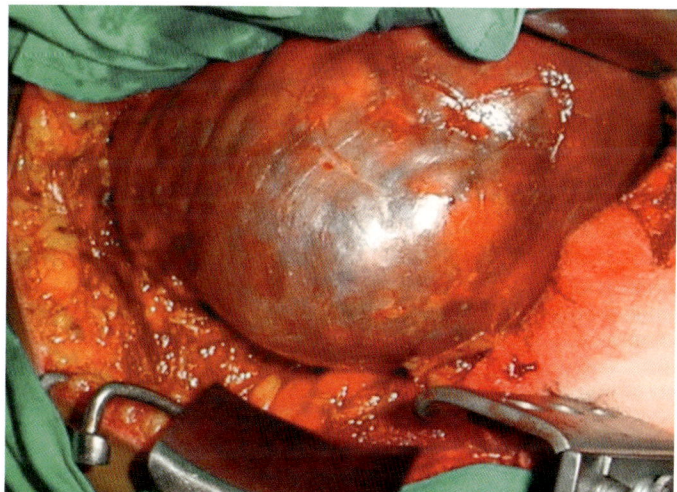

Fig. 24.61: Adenomyolipoma, very close to inferior margin of the liver

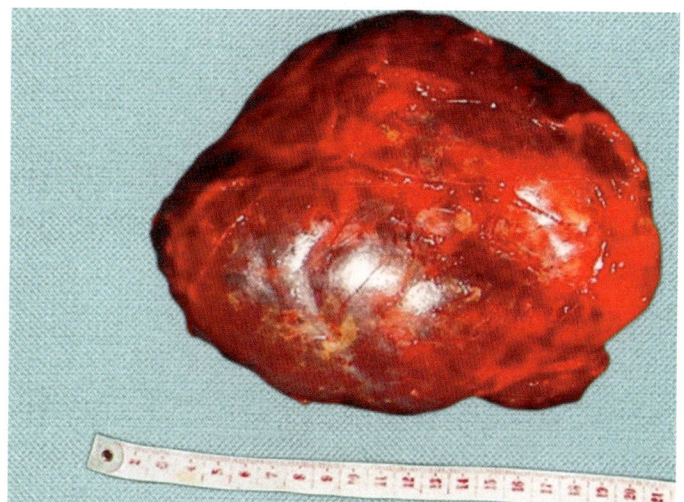

Fig. 24.62: Large adenomyolipoma of the adrenal removed

MASS IN THE EPIGASTRIUM

Mass in the epigastrium is one of the common long cases kept in the examination. Students should consider mass arising from liver, stomach and pancreas first. Other possibilities must be considered later by exclusion.

Classification

I. Mass Arising from Abdominal Wall

- First do the head raising test. If the mass becomes more prominent, it is extra-peritoneal (abdominal wall) (Fig 24.63).
- Lipoma, neurofibroma or desmoid tumour arising from the rectus sheath can present as a mass in the epigastrium. Since desmoid tumour arises from fascio-aponeurotic layer, it becomes immobile on contracting the rectus abdominis.
- Also note that epigastric hernia occurs in this region. It is a hernia, not a mass.
- Tumour recurrence in the abdominal wall can occur from GI malignancies.

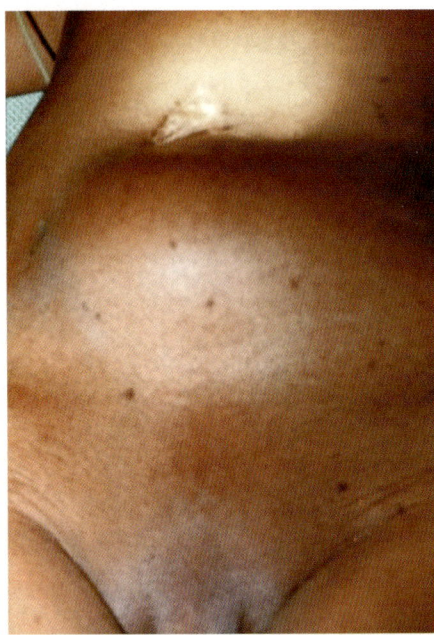

Fig. 24.63: Abdominal wall swelling—recurrence from carcinoma colon

II. Intraperitoneal Mass

1. **Mass arising from the liver** (Fig. 24.64):
   a. **Hepatoma:** Liver is enlarged, hard, irregular, and nontender. However, rapidly growing hepatomas are tender, firm and even a bruit is heard over the swelling. Rapid deterioration of health in a cirrhotic patient is usually due to the development of a hepatoma.
   b. **Secondaries in the liver** (Fig. 24.65): Usually both lobes are enlarged and have a nodular surface without a bruit. Jaundice is a late feature in secondaries of the liver. The primary may be obvious as a colonic mass, a stomach mass or a testicular tumour, etc.
   c. **Hydatid cyst** (Fig. 24.66): It is a benign swelling. History of contact with a dog is usually present. Epigastric swelling is due to enlarged liver which is smooth or irregular, nontender with rounded borders. Classical hydatid fremitus and thrill are rarely elicited. General health of the patient is usually good.
   d. **Simple cyst** (Fig. 24.67): It is not a clinical diagnosis but is mentioned here only for discussion. It is a serous cyst. A single big cyst can also be a part of polycystic disease of the liver.

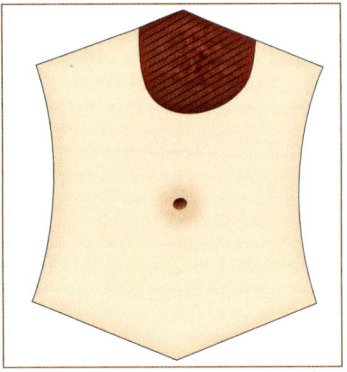 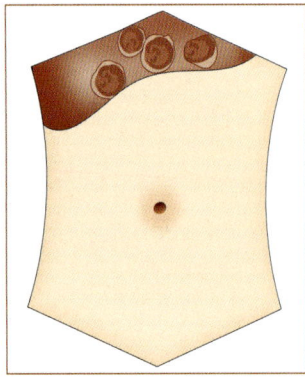

Fig. 24.64: Hepatoma   **Fig. 24.65:** Secondaries in the liver

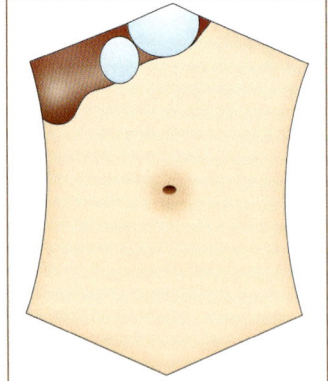 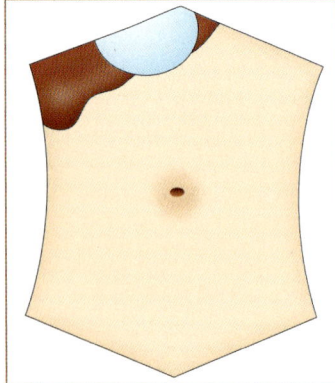

Fig. 24.66: Hydatid cyst   **Fig. 24.67:** Simple cyst

2. **Mass arising from the stomach**
   a. **Carcinoma stomach** (Figs 24.68 to 24.73): For all practical purposes, the only mass arising from the stomach in the epigastrium is carcinoma stomach. It is hard, irregular and moves with respiration with minimal intrinsic mobility.

- *Please Note*: Kindly refer Table 24.1 to differentiate stomach mass, liver mass and pancreatic mass.
- Usually the patient is a male around 40–50 years of age, with loss of appetite and weight. Early satiety and vomiting are other important features. If there is a growth in the pyloric antrum, visible gastric peristalsis (VGP) can be seen in the epigastrium. It is a wave of peristalsis starting from left hypochondrium across umbilicus towards right hypochondrium. VGP will not be classical as seen in pyloric stenosis due to chronic cicatrised duodenal ulcer because some amount of stomach wall is infiltrated in carcinoma stomach. That portion may not distend.
- Endoscopy is done to visualise the growth to assess level of growth and obstruction. It also helps in biopsy. Ultrasound is done to detect metastasis in the liver, para-aortic lymph nodes, ascites, etc. CECT scan is done to know the local spread and thus to assess resectibility.
- Subtotal gastrectomy for distal lesions and total gastrectomy for more proximal lesions are the treatment of choices. Palliation can be done in the form of anterior GJ in cases of antral carcinoma which are advanced or with metastasis. The benefit may last for only a few months after doing anterior GJ.

- *Please note*: These are guidelines. Clinical signs vary from case to case. It is an overall consideration of the symptoms and signs together that clinches the diagnosis. Example, carcinoma stomach with infiltration into pancreas, the mass may not move with respiration. Carcinoma pancreas which infiltrates posterior stomach wall may show some movement with respiration.

Clinical Clue

Look for the following sites for metastasis from carcinoma stomach:
- Left supraclavicular lymph node—Troisier's sign
- Left axillary lymph nodes—Irish nodes
- Umbilical nodule—Sister Mary Joseph's nodule
- Secondaries in the liver—nodular liver
- Para-aortic lymph nodes—nodular mass in the epigastrium
- Ascites
- Krukenberg tumour—bilateral bulky ovarian masses due to metastasis
- PR: Blumer shelf deposits

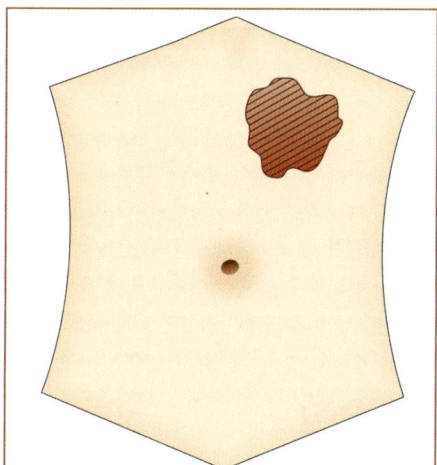

Fig. 24.68: Carcinoma of the stomach arising from body of the stomach. All borders are made out

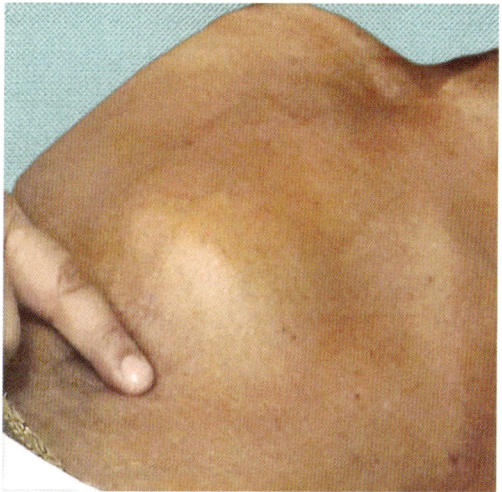

Fig. 24.69: Lower border is clearly made out

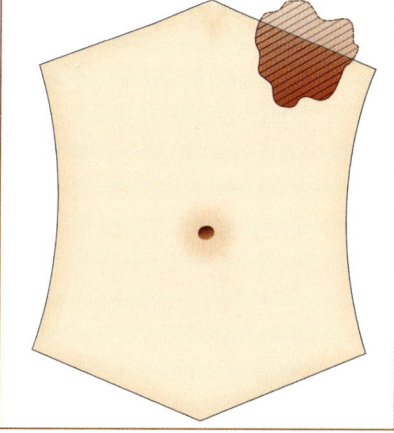

Fig. 24.70: Carcinoma of the stomach arising from fundus of the stomach. In such cases, it is difficut to get above the mass

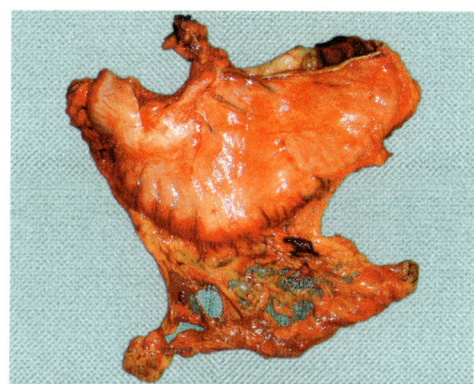

Fig. 24.71: Total gastrectomy for carcinoma stomach

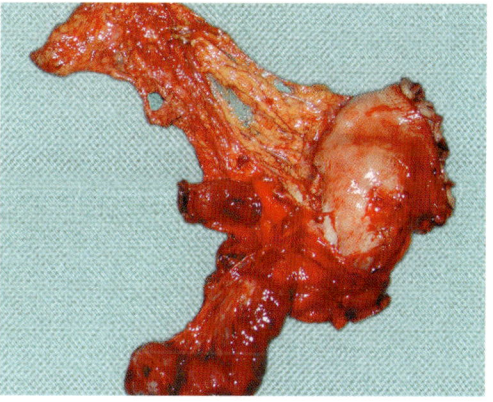

Fig. 24.72: Total gastrectomy for stump carcinoma stomach. (You can see the previous GJ)

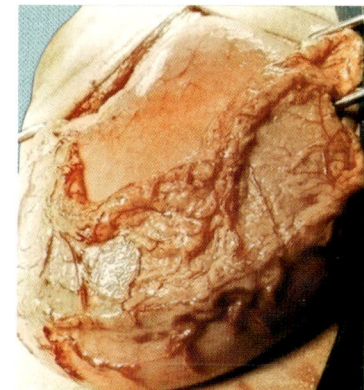

Fig. 24.73: Dilated stomach at surgery—carcinoma pyloric antrum

b. **Gastrointestinal stromal tumour (GIST):** Stomach is the most common site of GIST. These tumours arise from interstitial cells of Cajal. Typically, the patients are young and asymptomatic. They present with a large mass in the epigastrium or with bleeding. Appetite is good. On examination, the mass is **large, mobile,** with nodular or even bosselated surface which moves with respiration. Bleeding/haematemesis occurs when tumour ulcerates into the gastric mucosa. Resection/partial/total gastrectomy is the treatment of choice. Malignancy depends upon greater mitotic figures. Immuno-histochemistry is mandatory for the diagnosis—C kit gene amplification. It is the tumour marker of the GIST (Figs 24.74 to 24.78).

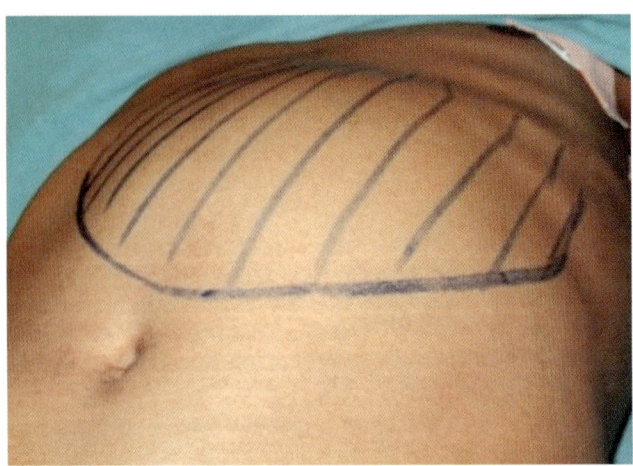

Fig. 24.76: Look carefully the extent and upper border. It was possible to get above the mass (*Courtesy*: Late Dr Srinivasan, Surgery postgraduate student, KMC, Manipal, Year 2010)

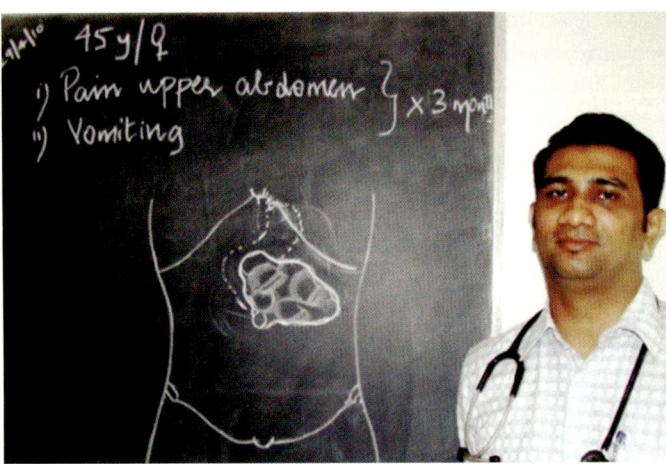

Fig. 24.74: Blackboard sketch of the stomach mass

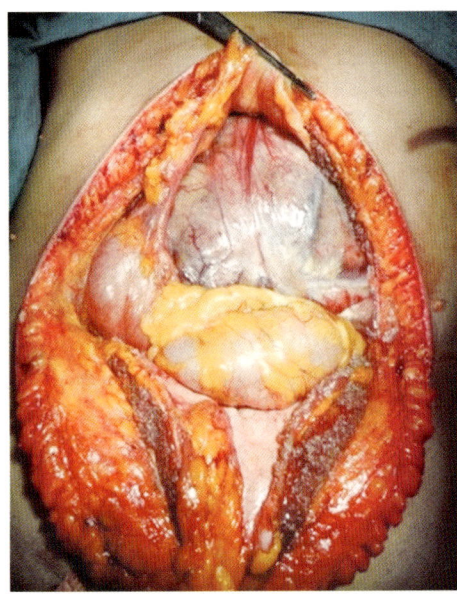

Fig. 24.77: At exploration, the mass was arising from the stomach. It was mobilised by dividing greater omentum

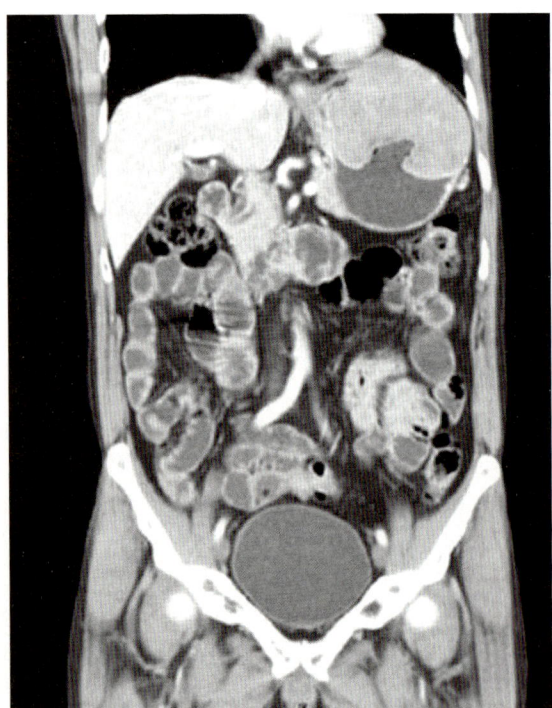

Fig. 24.75: CT scan picture of the mass confirming a GIST from the greater curvature of the stomach

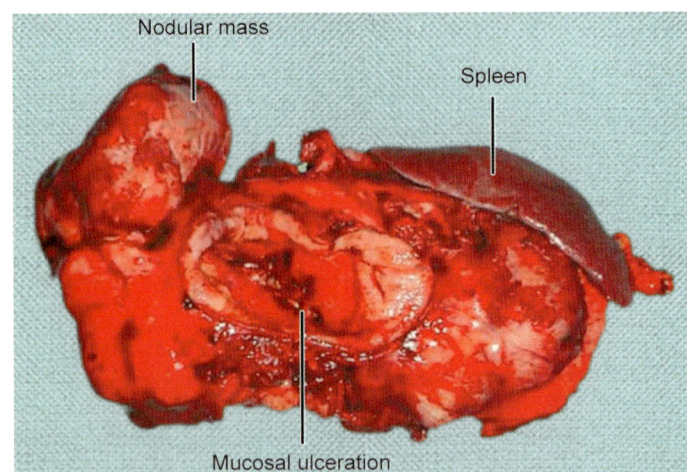

Fig. 24.78: Resected specimen with spleen. Large gastrointestinal stromal tumour (GIST) arising from the stomach

Table 24.1: Clinical points to differentiate stomach mass, liver mass and pancreatic mass

	Carcinoma stomach	*Hepatoma*	*Carcinoma pancreas*
Movement with respiration	Yes	Yes	No
Upper border	Can be made out	Cannot be made out	Can be made out
Percussion note	Impaired note	Dull note	Resonant
Nature of the mass	Irregular, hard, restricted	Irregular, firm to hard	Nodular or irregular
Finger insinuation	May be possible	Not possible	Possible
Intrinsic mobility	Minimal	No	No (except cystadenoma)
Knee elbow test	Falls forward	Not relevant test	Does not fall forward

Clinical Wisdom

In cases of carcinoma stomach with a large nodule in the epigastrium close to xiphoid process, it is difficult to insinuate fingers between the mass and costal margin. In the same fashion, it is true for a large pseudocyst, large stomal tumour also.

c. **Lymphoma of the stomach** (Fig. 24.79)**:** It is better to avoid giving a clinical diagnosis of lymphoma of the stomach. It is an exclusion diagnosis. It is a primary gastric lymphoma. They are B-cell derived from mucosa associated lymphoid tissue **(MALT)—MALTOMA (Diffuse large B-cell lymphoma).** Pain is an important feature. (Carcinoma stomach will not begin as pain.) Weight loss, and bleeding are common presentations. **6th decade** is the common age group. Endoscopic features are not specific but diffuse thickening with or without ulcerations may be seen. It is important to rule out **generalised process of lymphoma** by CT, ultrasound, and bone marrow aspirate. Gastrectomy is the best treatment. Chemotherapy is better for systemic disease.

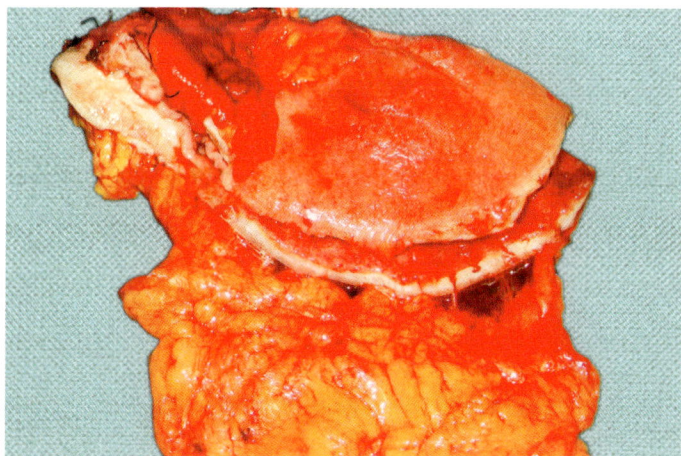

Fig. 24.79: Lymphoma of the stomach

3. **Omental mass:** Structure attached to stomach and colon is greater omentum. Greater omentum is a rich vascular and lymphatic organ and hence, gets involved in various diseases such as tuberculosis and malignancy. In tuberculosis, omentum gets involved as a firm, **granular rolled up mass.** Ascites is common when omentum is involved. In secondaries from intra-abdominal malignancies, omentum can be felt also as a hard, nodular mass (Fig. 24.80). Rarely, omental

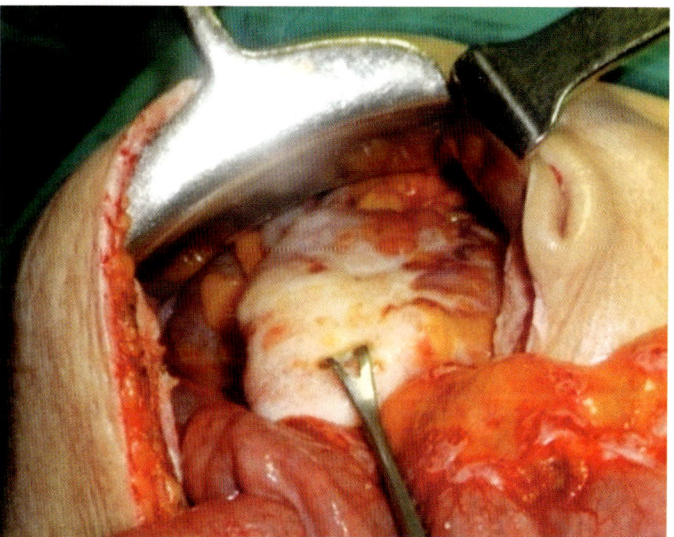

Fig. 24.80: Omental cake in advanced carcinoma stomach

cyst can present as a tensely cystic mass in the epigastrium. **Mass arising from omentum moves with respiration.**

III. Retroperitoneal Mass

1. **Pseudopancreatic cyst—pseudocyst of the pancreas** (Figs 24.81 and 24.82)**:** Typically, the patient is a 30–40 years old, male alcoholic who presents with severe abdominal pain,

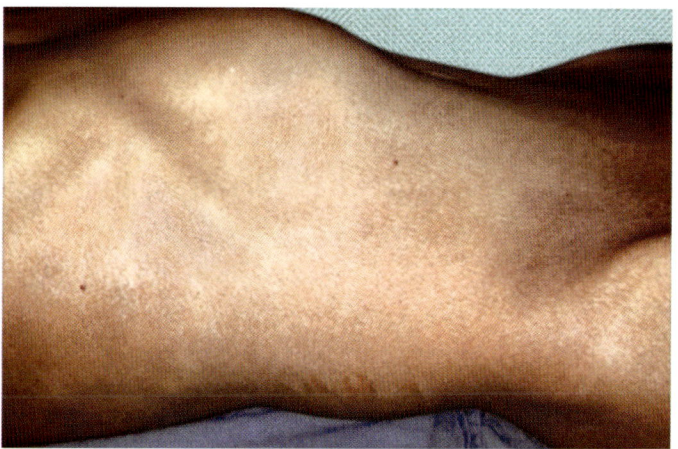

Fig. 24.81: Large pseudocyst of pancreas after 8 weeks of pancreatitis—lateral view

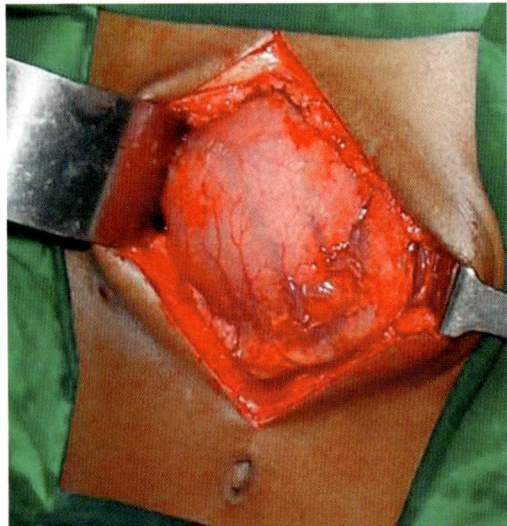

Fig. 24.82: At surgery, stomach is pushed anteriorly. Ideal case for cystogastrostomy

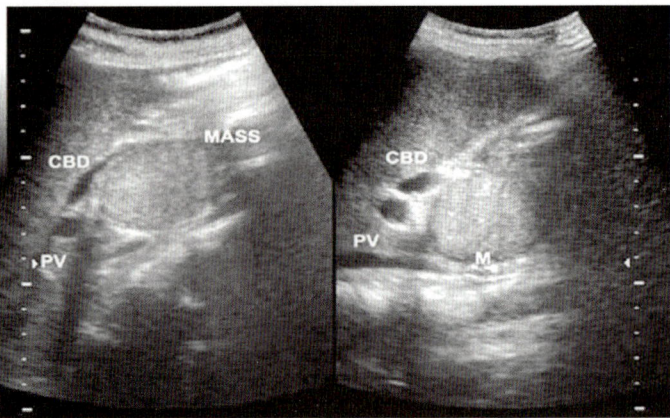

Fig. 24.83: Ultrasound showing a large cyst

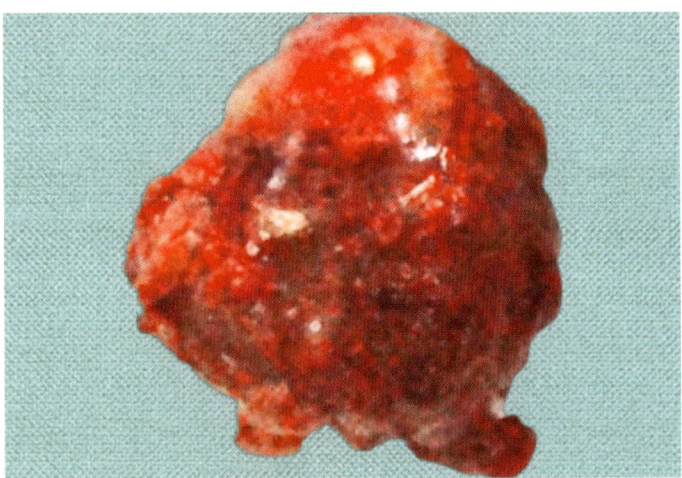

Fig. 24.84: Resected cystadenoma pancreas

and diagnosed to have acute pancreatitis and was treated. Another cause is blunt abdominal trauma followed by a mass in the abdomen after a few weeks. After 20–30 days of acute pancreatitis, he presents to the hospital with swelling in the abdomen and inability to eat properly. On examination, a tense, cystic mass is felt as firm mass in the epigastrium. It has a smooth surface and round borders. The upper border of the mass can be made out unless it is large. It does not usually move with respiration but a large cyst may exhibit some movement with respiration when it is in contact with the diaphragm. History of acute pancreatitis or blunt injury to the abdomen is usually present. **Pulsations over the mass (transmitted) suggest that it is a mass close to the aorta. This is an important point which differentiates this mass from liver mass. Liver mass will not exhibit transmitted pulsations.** Gurgle heard anteriorly suggests distended stomach. Ultrasound and CECT are the investigations. Most of the pseudocysts will resolve over 3–6 weeks. Persistent, symptomatic cyst is treated by cystogastrostomy.

Rule of 6: When the cyst wall is mature (usually it takes 6 weeks) cystogastrostomy (size of stoma 6 cm) is done. 6 weeks time is also given because majority of the fluid collection will resolve or disappear by that time.

2. **Cystadenoma pancreas:** Cystadenomas of pancreas are benign and can attain huge sizes. It can present as a mass in the epigastrium, left hypochondrium or umbilical region. They exhibit what is described as 'tree top mobility'. More common in middle-aged women. Pedunculated tumours exhibit free mobility and sometime become obvious in different postures such as supine, prone, lateral, standing, etc. Two major types are mucous and serous cystadenomas. Details are given in (Figs 24.83, 24.84 and Table 24.2).

3. **Carcinoma body of pancreas** can present as a mass in the lower part of epigastrium or upper umbilical region. The mass is hard, irregular, fixed and does not move with respiration. Presence of severe backache and loss of weight

Table 24.2: Cystic neoplasms (*refer* to Clinical Box 24.7)

	Serous	*Mucinous*
• Gender	• No predilection	• More common in women
• Nature	• Multiple cysts are present	• More often multilocular
• Cut surface	• Microcystic adenomas with cut surface appearance of a sponge	• Macrocystic adenomas with smooth lining with papillary projections
• CT scan	• CT may show cysts with calcification	• Septal on CT scan are characteristic
• Nature of fluid	• Cystic spaces contain serous fluid	• Cystic spaces contain mucus
• Lining epithelium	• Lining is by cuboidal epithelium	• Lining is tall columnar and goblet cells
• Malignant potential	• No malignant potential	• Most of them turn into cystadenocarcinoma

True cystic pancreatic neoplasms (CPN)

A. Serous cystadenoma: Benign
- Common in women, located in head of pancreas. They account for 30% of all CPN. They can be observed if asymptomatic.

B. Mucinous cystic neoplasms (MCN)
- More common in women
- More often found in body and tail
- More incidence than serous cystadenoma (40%)
- Considered premalignant
- Do not communicate with ductal system
- Lesions if more than 2 cm need resection

C. Intraductal papillary mucinous tumours (IPMTs)
- Slightly more common in males
- Communicate with duct
- Incidence is about 25%
- High malignant potential
- More common in head involving ampulla of Vater
- Treated by Whipple's resection

are important features. Typically, a man, smoker in his 60–70s is affected. The first complaint is backache which is confused for musculoskeletal in origin. This will be followed by severe weight loss within 2–3 months. By the time diagnosis is established, mass becomes advanced and fixed to retroperitoneal structures. Infiltration of coeliac plexus results in backache. Symptoms of vomiting suggest duodenal obstruction. **Trousseau's sign** (thrombophlebitis migrans): Migrating thrombophlebitis of the legs can occur in visceral malignancies particularly from carcinoma of pancreas, rarely carcinoma stomach, colon, etc. It is supposedly due to sluggish blood flow resulting in thrombus formation. It is superficial and affects the leg veins such as long saphenous vein. ***Sudden development of diabetes mellitus is an early manifestation in 25% of patients.*** **Anaemia** may be present as in any other malignancy. **Jaundice** is not a feature. Left supraclavicular node may be palpable. Anatomical features of pancreatic mass have been already discussed. (Refer to the Clinical Discussion given below).

CLINICAL DISCUSSION—CARCINOMA PANCREAS

1. **What are the features that suggest malignancy?**
   Hard, irregular, fixed lump.
2. **What are the evidences of metastasis?**
   - Secondaries in the liver, supraclavicular node, para-aortic nodes, ascites
3. **What is Trousseau's sign?**
   - Migratory superficial thrombophlebitis.
4. **What is a common cause of pain abdomen and diabetes, other than carcinoma pancreas?**
   - Chronic pancreatitis
5. **When does carcinoma of the body of pancreas produce jaundice?**
   - When portal lymph nodes are enlarged.

4. ***Abdominal aortic aneurysm (AAA):*** An elderly patient, usually a hypertensive, presents with features of abdominal pain, swelling or features of ischaemia of the lower limb. On examination, tender swelling in the epigastrium with a characteristic expansile pulsation is present. Knee-elbow test will help to differentiate it from transmitted pulsations. Presence of a bruit and weak or absent lower limb pulses (due to thrombus) also helps in establishing the diagnosis. Aneurysms greater than 6 cm in size have very high chances of rupture. CT angiogram followed by reconstruction is the treatment of choice.

5. ***Lymph node mass:*** Lower epigastrium and upper umbilical region are the sites of para-aortic nodes. When para-aortic nodes are enlarged, the following diagnosis must be considered (Fig. 24.85).
   - *Lymphoma*: Clue—other groups of lymph nodes, hepatosplenomegaly, involvement of bones. Fever, and weight loss are other features.
   - *Testicular tumours*: Enlargement of the testis in young males could be due to seminoma testis. Testis will be hard and irregular in case of testicular tumours.
   - *Carcinoma stomach or carcinoma colon*: Clue—evidence of primary tumour—mass
   - *Tuberculosis*—not common—low grade fever, ascites, abdominal distension, etc. (Figs 24.85 and 24.86)

Anatomical points that suggest para-aortic lymph node mass are
- Located in the upper umbilical and lower epigastrium
- Does not move with respiration
- Nodular mass
- Fixed
- Transmitted pulsation may be present.

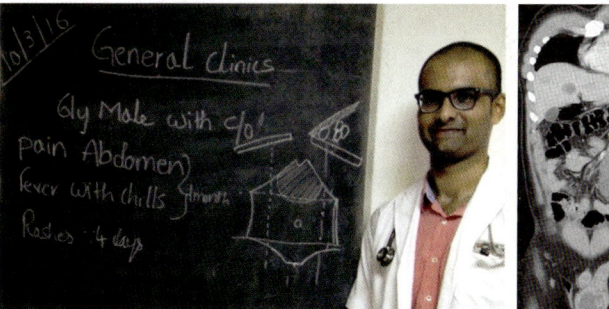

Fig. 24.85: It shows lymph node in the neck and para-aortic lymph nodes. **Fig. 24.86:** Testicular tumour with para-aortic lymph nodes (*Courtesy*: Dr Naveen Lella, postgraduate, KMC, Manipal)

MASS IN THE LEFT HYPOCHONDRIUM

Most important organ in the left hypochondrium is the spleen. There are several causes of splenic enlargement (read medicine books for more details). Only surgically important causes have been given below. Splenic mass can be confused for left renal mass. A few details are given below.

1. ***Splenic mass:*** Clinical points to say it is spleen are:
   - Located in the left hypochondrium
   - Moves with respiration

- Enlarges obliquely towards right iliac fossa—renal swellings enlarge upwards and downwards directions.
- **Splenic notch, if present, is characteristic of spleen.** It is in the anterior border of the spleen. You can bet on this point in the university examination.
- Finger insinuation between the left costal margin and the splenic mass is not possible.
- Dull on percussion and the dullness is continuous with splenic dullness.
- Refer to Table 24.3 for points to differentiate splenic mass from renal mass

Examination methods

a. *Supine with one hand palpation.* Remember spleen is felt very lateral and actually in the left hypochondrium. If you do a casual examination, you will most likely miss the mass because hypochondrium is the smallest quadrant in the abdomen (Fig. 24.87).

b. *Supine with two-hand palpation with right lateral tilt position:* Left hand is placed behind the lower ribs posteriorly and help in giving a push anteriorly, thus palpation of a mild enlargement of the spleen can be made out (Fig. 24.88).

Differential diagnosis of a splenic mass

a. *Portal hypertension*: One important cause is extrahepatic or prehepatic portal hypertension. The exact cause is not known but it may be the result of umbilical sepsis resulting in portal vein thrombosis or splenic vein thrombosis. Congenital absence of portal vein or portal vein agenesis is also

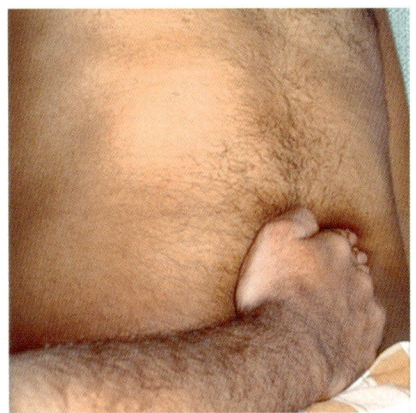

Fig. 24.87: Examination of the spleen by using one hand

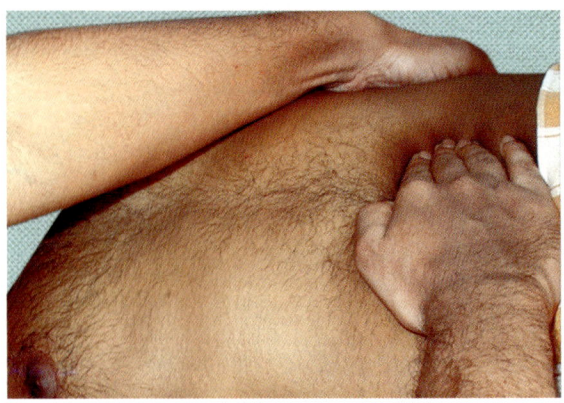

Fig. 24.88: Both hands are used, left hand behind the costal margin applying gentle pressure

responsible for this. Typically, the patient is a child or young adult who presents with haematemesis. Haematemesis is due to bleeding from oesophageal varices. On examination, spleen is palpable. Spleen is moderate in size. It is nontender, smooth and firm in consistency. It is congestive splenomegaly. Liver function is normal and hence, ascites, jaundice and other features of cirrhosis are absent. Diagnosis is by ultrasound of the abdomen followed by gastroscopy to confirm varices. Peripheral smear may show evidence of pancytopaenia which is also an indication of hypersplenism. Varices are treated with sclerotherapy or variceal banding followed by pharmacotherapy with the beta-blocker propranolol. With advances in the field of endotherapy, shunt surgery has become rare. Left-sided portal hypertension caused by splenic vein thrombosis causes massive enlargement of spleen. It is not only due to congenital cause but can also be due to carcinoma pancreas. This type of portal hypertension is curable by splenectomy. When the mass is very big, renal mass is the differential diagnosis. (*Refer to Table 24.3* for differences between splenic mass and renal mass.)

b. *Haemolytic anaemias*: Two varieties have been recognised: Congenital and acquired. Hereditary spherocytosis is an example of hereditary or congenital variety. In this condition, RBCs are spherical in shape and are broken down in the splenic pulp because of increased permeability of the membrane to sodium. In the splenic pulp, there is deficiency of both glucose and oxygen. As a result, bilirubin is released. Due to the overload, **most of the bilirubin remains**

Table 24.3: Large mass: Spleen or kidney?		
	Splenic mass	*Renal mass*
• Enlargement	Usually towards right iliac fossa	Usually towards left iliac fossa
• Direction	Left hypochondrium to umbilical to right iliac fossa	Left lumbar region above to left hypochondrium below to left iliac fossa
• Notch	Notch is felt anteriorly	No notch is felt
• Moves with respiration	Very free	Very limited
• Bimanual palpation	Uncommon	Common finding
• Ballotability	Not found	Ballotable
• Loin bulge	No	Can be present

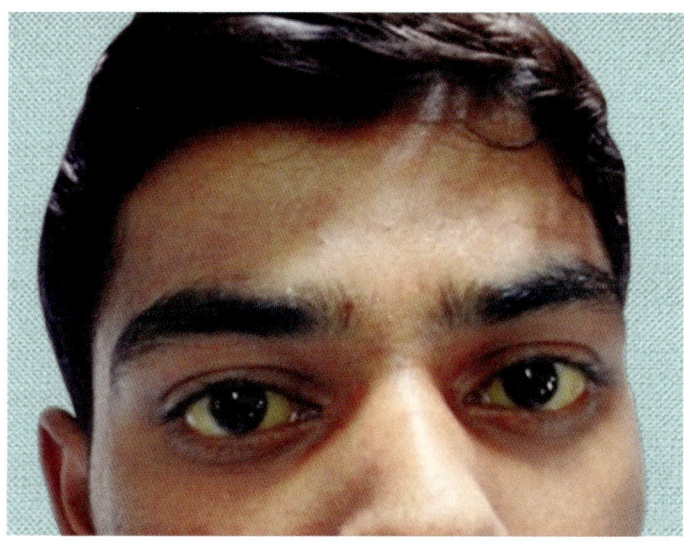

Fig. 24.89: Haemolytic anaemia: Light yellow discolouration of skin and sclera

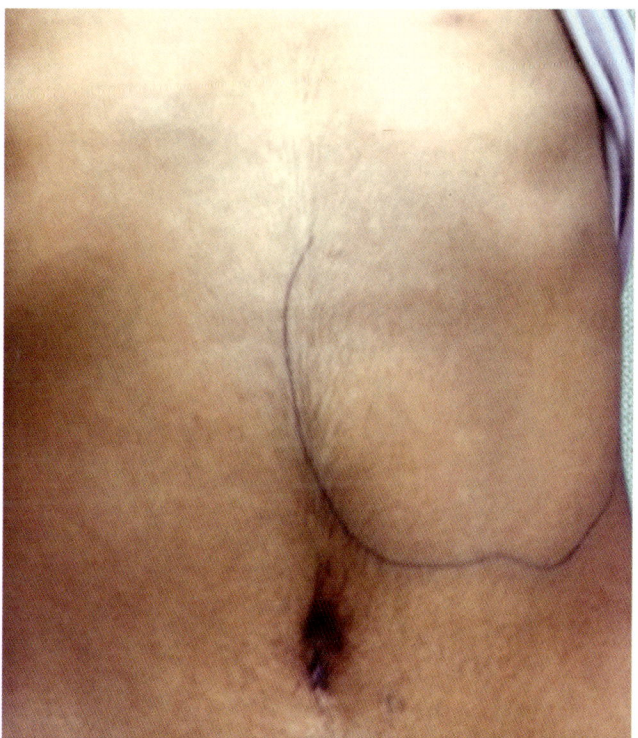

Fig. 24.90: Enlarged spleen. A case of haemolytic jaundice

unconjugated. **It is called acholuric jaundice. Anaemia, faint jaundice (lemon yellow) and splenomegaly constitute the triad of haemolytic jaundice.** Severe abdominal pain can be due to haemolytic crisis (Figs 24.89 and 24.90).

Acquired haemolytic anaemias: This occurs due to production of autoantibodies and desolution of RBCs. Coombs' test is usually positive. Family history is absent. Spleen is palpable in 50% cases; liver and lymph nodes may also be palpable. **Splenectomy is beneficial in almost every case of congenital spherocytosis but in only half the cases of the acquired defect.**

c. *Lymphoma:* Isolated splenic enlargement is not common in lymphoma. Usually, it is enlarged along with lymph nodes in the neck. One has to examine for all group of lymph nodes, liver, spleen and skeletal system in such cases.

d. *Idiopathic thrombocytopaenic purpura (ITP):* This condition occurs due to development of autoantibodies against patient's own platelets. Normal levels of platelets are between 1,50,000 and 4,00,000 cells per cumm. The spleen is probably responsible for sequestration of platelets and for production of antibodies. **Type 1:** Acute—children: Follows an acute infection and resolves spontaneously in about two months. **Type 2:** Chronic—adults: Longer than six months. No cause is identified. Spleen is just palpable. This condition is common in females, F:M :: 3:1. **Purpuric patches** (ecchymosis refers to skin discolouration due to extravasation

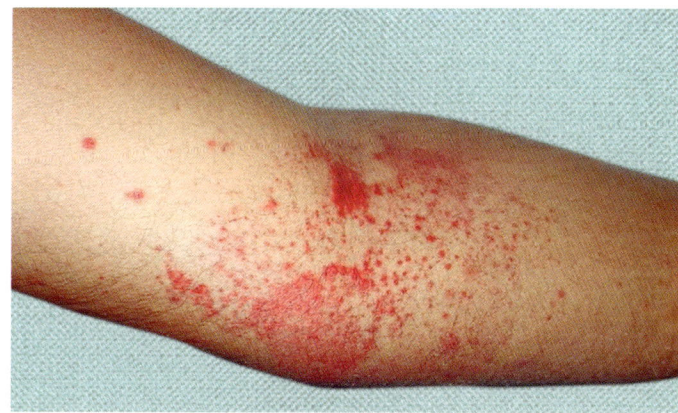

Fig. 24.91: Purpuric spots in the forearm

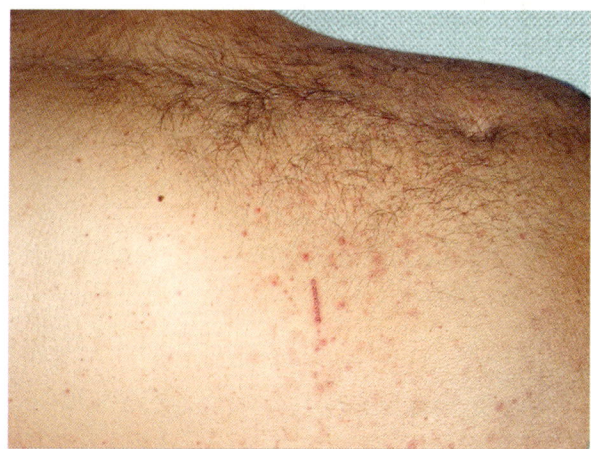

Fig. 24.92: Purpuric spots on the abdomen

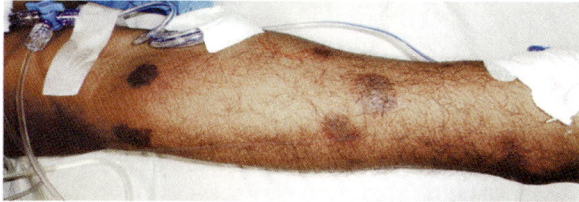

Fig. 24.93: Severe sepsis with thrombocytopenia

of blood) are found on the buttocks and petechial haemorrhages (spots) are found on the limbs. These are **dependent areas** having high intravascular pressure (Figs 24.91 to 24.93).

- All types of haemorrhages are common and can be mild to moderate. Intracranial haemorrhage is found in 1–2% of patients but it may be the cause of death.

- In 25% of cases, the spleen is just palpable (small size). **Hess's tourniquet test: More than 20 petechiae in a circle of 3 cm diameter in cubital fossa suggests purpura.** Bleeding time is prolonged in purpura. Clotting and prothrombin times are normal. Platelet count is reduced. Bone marrow biopsy: Precursor of platelets (megakaryocytes) is increased. In children, spontaneous regression occurs in majority of cases. Short course of corticosteroids is beneficial. Tablet predinsolone 10 mg/day is given over a period of 6 weeks. In adults, **splenectomy** is indicated **when ITP has presented for more than 6–9 months and ITP has relapsed in spite of steroids,** e.g. prednisolone 1 mg/kg/day. Platelet count rises within 7 days of starting steroids, after which splenectomy can be done.

e. *Other uncommon causes:* Splenic cysts, splenic dermoid cysts, splenic tuberculosis, splenic hydatid cyst, pseudocyst of spleen, lymphoma involving only spleen and hairy cell leukaemia are a few examples (Figs 24.94 to 24.97).

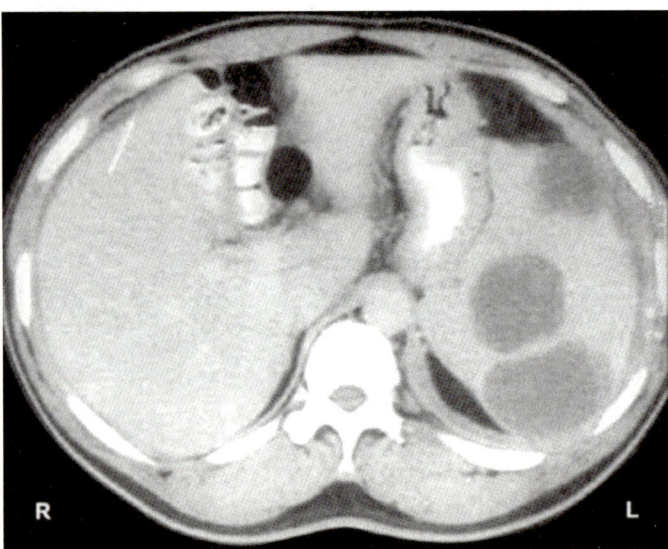

Fig. 24.94: Splenic tuberculosis: CT showing abscesses

2. *Mass arising from tail of pancreas*

a. Carcinoma tail of the pancreas can present as a mass in the left hypochondrium. By the time it is palpable, it is sufficiently big. Often the patient goes from specialist to specialist with backache. It may be detected during ultrasound or CT scan and the patient is referred to the surgeon. The patient would have lost 5 to 10 kg weight in 2–3 months. On examination, a hard, irregular mass is palpable on deep palpation, appreciated better with right lateral position. It may exhibit movement with respiration because of the close attachment to the spleen. However, classical notch is absent. It may be possible to insinuate fingers between costal margin and the pancreatic mass.

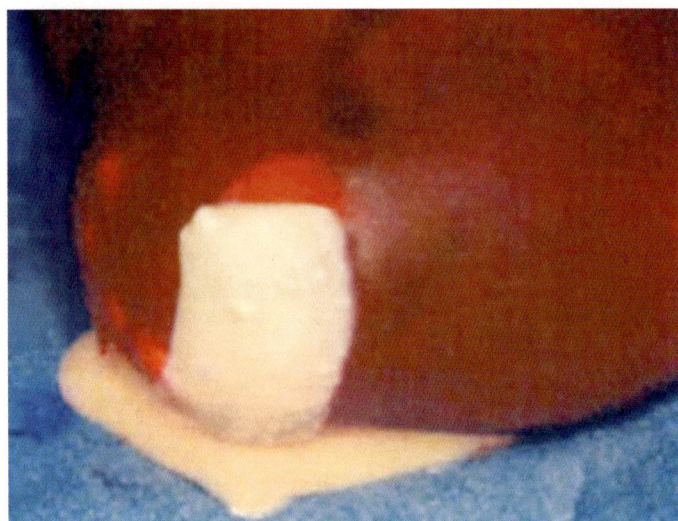

Fig. 24.95: At exploration pus, coming out. Splenectomy was done which proved tuberculosis

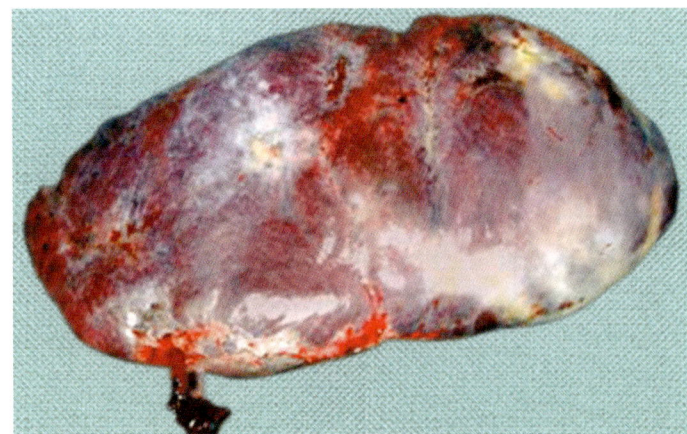

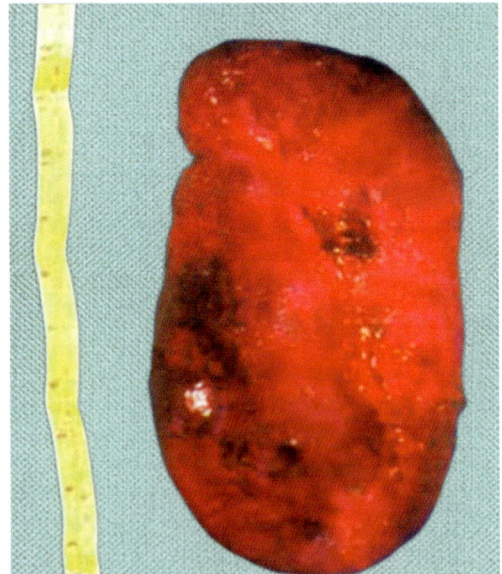

Figs 24.96 and 24.97: Hodgkin's lymphoma and hairy cell leukaemia presented as fever and splenomegaly. After routine investigations when the diagnosis could not be established, splenectomy was done which proved the diagnosis

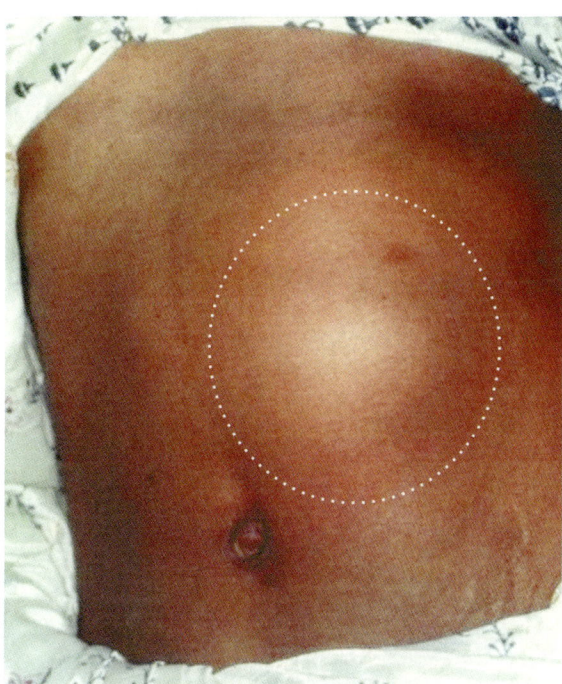

Fig. 24.98: Cystadenoma pancreas

Backache and diabetes may be present. CA 19–9 helps in the diagnosis. CT-guided FNAC will confirm the diagnosis. Resection is the only best option. Every attempt should be aimed at resection. Resection may include spleen, two-thirds of pancreas, colon or even kidney (total or partial). Gemcitabine-based chemotherapy can be given in large and fixed lesions. Reassess after 2–3 months and go for resection. Results are not very good even after resection and chemotherapy.

b. *Cystadenoma pancreas* (Fig. 24. 98): There are two types: Serous and mucus cystadenomas. Cystadenomas are known to attain large size and they are mobile having smooth surface. Their mobility has been described as tree-top mobility. They have been discussed under mass in the epigastrium.

3. **Colonic mass:** Carcinoma splenic flexure—splenic flexure is the deepest part of the colon and easily missed at laparotomy. Such growths are usually not palpable in the abdomen. It has a male predominance, many patients are diagnosed at a younger age with a high incidence of mucinous adenocarcinoma and obstruction as compared to the patients with colon cancer at other sites. Often patients present with increasing constipation and obstruction. The mass is firm to hard and irregular with restricted mobility. It moves with respiration because of its contact with spleen. It has a resonant or impaired note on percussion. (Liver is dull on percussion.) Caecum may be distended, if there is obstruction.

4. **Renal mass:** Importantly renal mass is palpable mainly in the lumbar region extending into left hypochondrium. Three masses which have been discussed later under mass in the lumbar region. Upper border is usually not palpable—it is under cover of the 12th rib. The three renal masses are renal cell carcinoma, hydronephrosis and polycystic kidney.

5. **Suprarenal mass:** Clinically, suprarenal masses have all the features of a renal mass. These are similar to the ones in the right hypochondrium.

MASS IN THE RIGHT LUMBAR REGION

1. **Renal mass** (Figs 24.99 and 24.100): Renal masses are the most common masses in the lumbar region followed by colonic masses. Kidney is present in the loin and it is a posterior structure. Hence, in majority of the cases, enlargement is more obvious posteriorly. However, uniform enlargement causes the kidney to enlarge anteriorly thus making it bimanually palpable. One characteristic feature of a renal mass is ballotability. Kidney ballots because it has a pedicle and a cushion of perirenal pad of fat surrounding it. Ballotability is demonstrated by the following method. One hand is kept posteriorly close to the abdominal wall and the other hand anteriorly. A push (ballot means to toss) is given with posterior hand. The mass tosses and touches hand, anteriorly placed and goes back. Thus, following features of a kidney help to say that mass is arising from kidney.

   • Kidney is present in the lumbar region and it has reniform shape.
   • It enlarges in superoinferior direction.
   • It moves with respiration because it is enclosed by fascia of Gerota which blends with diaphragm above.
   • It is bimanually palpable and ballotable.
   • It is possible to insinuate the fingers between the upper border of the mass and the costal margin.
   • Normal resonant note posteriorly in the loin (colonic) gets obliterated because as the kidney enlarges, it displaces the colon.

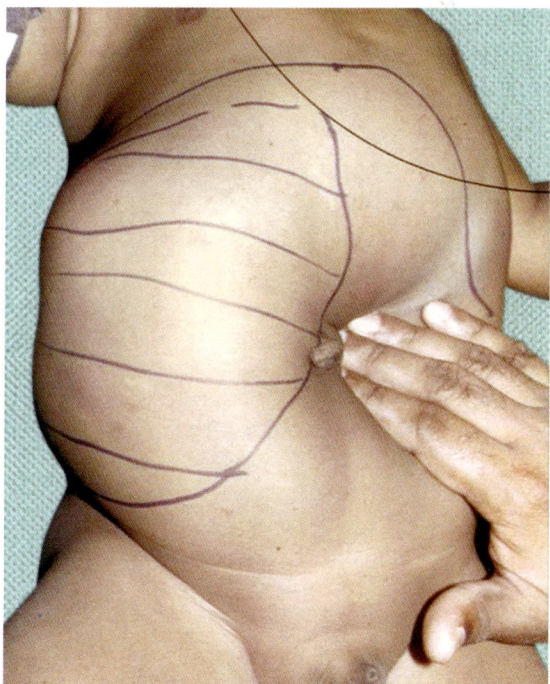

Fig. 24.99: Wilm's tumour in a two-year-old child (*Courtesy:* Dr Vijay Kumar, Dr Sandeep PT, Department of Paediatrics Surgery, KMC, Manipal)

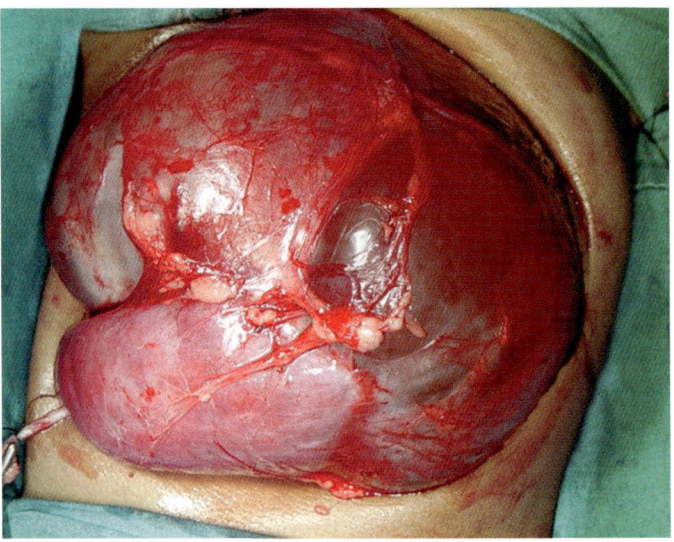

Fig. 24.100: Renal cell carcinoma

CECT scan is the most common useful investigation to differenciate renal masses (Figs 24.101 and 24.102). The most common renal masses which are palpable in the lumbar region—renal cell carcinoma, polycystic disease and hydronephrosis have been compared in Table 24.4.

Various causes of hydronephrosis have been given in Fig. 24.103.

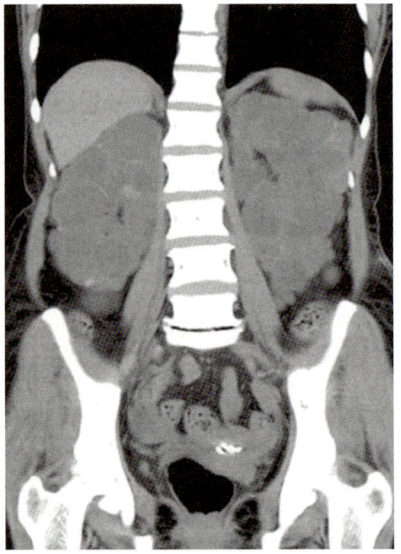

Fig. 24.101: CT scan showing cysts

2. **Liver mass:** A large liver mass is easily palpable in the lumbar region. In these cases, you have to present the case as a mass is felt in the right hypochondrium and it extends into lumbar region. Once you confirm it is liver, common differential diagnoses include hepatoma, secondaries in the liver, hydatid disease of the liver, etc.

3. **Gallbladder mass:** A large gallbladder mass is palpable in the lumbar region but it starts from the right hypochondrium, Shape is oval with smooth surface and tensely cystic. The usual cause is mucocoele. Mucocoele of the gallbladder is

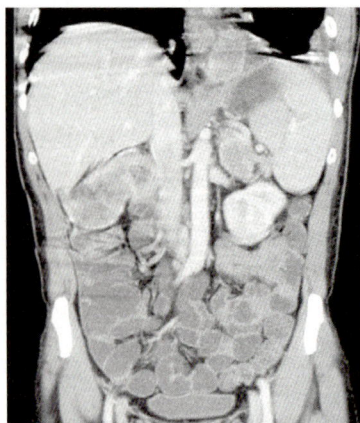

Fig. 24.102: CT scan—renal cell carcinoma affecting the upper pole of the right kidney

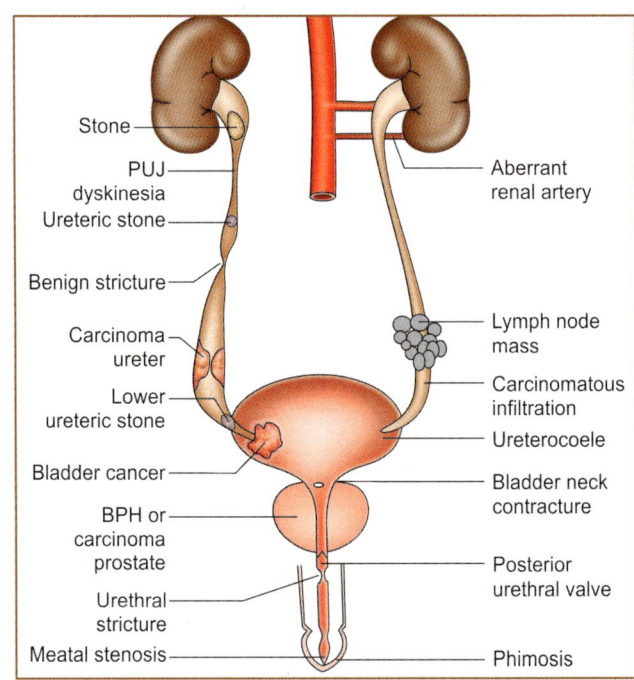

Fig. 24.103: Diagrammatic representation of hydronephrosis

due to a stone blocking the cystic duct and causing massive enlargement of the gallbladder. These patients do not have jaundice. Other causes of enlargement have been already discussed.

4. **Ascending colonic mass**
   a. **Ileocaecal tuberculosis** is felt as an irregular or nodular firm mass in the right iliac fossa and in the lumbar region. The mass is due to thickened caecum and ascending colon. **The caecum is higher in position because it is pulled up. Younger age of the patient, fever, weight loss, loose stools and colicky abdominal pain are the symptoms. (More details under mass in the right iliac fossa).**

   b. **Carcinoma ascending colon:** Typically, a patient is around 50–60 years of age who presents with change in bowel habits—mucus in the stools and bleeding per rectum. Anaemia, loss of weight and weakness are the features.

Table 24.4: Three common masses arising from kidney

Feature	Polycystic kidney disease	Hydronephrosis	Renal cell carcinoma
Age	30–40 years	**Congenital—young 20–30 years Acquired—elderly**	40–60 years
Incidence	Females > Males	Females > Males	Males > Females

Clinical features Renal mass
 	
Upper border cannot be made out when the kidney is enlarged
	• **Mass per abdomen**
	  – Bilateral
	
	  – Massive enlargement
	  – Nodular/Bosselated surface
	  – Firm to hard, sometimes cystic
	  – Not fixed, nontender
		• **Mass per abdomen**
		  – Unilateral/bilateral enlarged kidney(s)
		  – Smooth surface
		  – Firm, tensely cystic
		  – Not fixed, nontender
			• **Mass per abdomen**
			  – Unilateral enlarged kidney
			
			  – Irregular, nodular surface
			  – Hard, ballotable, bimanually palpable
			  – Fixity +/–, nontender

Other features	• Dull aching pain in loins—dragging pain
	• Micro-/macroscopic haematuria
	• Hypertension
	• Features of renal failure: Thirst, vomiting, abdominal distension, anuria, uremic smell, coated tongue, anaemia
	• Infection—pyelonephritis
	• Acute pain: If there is haemorrhage into or infection of a cyst; colicky pain—due to blood clot in ureter
	• Urea, creatinine: Rule out renal failure
	• Plain X-ray KUB: Enlarged kidney
	• Abdominal USG/CT scan: Confirm Dx; multiple hypodense areas without enhancement
	• IVU—spider leg deformity of calyces
		• May be asymptomatic, or
		• Abdominal distension
		• Abdominal pain-dull aching pain in loin
		• Previous history of calculus disease in the ureter and symptoms—colicky radiating abdominal pain, hematuria
		• Elderly male—it is BPH, hence history of hesitancy and frequency of micturition
		
		• Urea, creatinine: Rule out renal failure
		• Plain X-ray KUB: Enlarged kidney, stones
		• Abdominal USG: Detect enlarged kidney and the cause. CT scan: investigation of choice; dilated pelvicalyceal system with uniform filling of contrast
			Triad of RCC
			1. Pain-dragging/intermittent
			2. Intermittent haematuria
			3. Palpable mass
			   Other features
			   • Pathological fractures
			   • Anaemia
			   • Fever
			   • Hypertension
			   • Liver dysfunction
			
			• Urine exam: Look for malignant cells if haematuria is present
			• Plain X-ray KUB: Enlarged kidney
			• Abdominal USG: Enlarged kidney, locate tumour, size, extent
			• CECT scan: Investigation of choice for staging
			• IVU: Irregular calyces

Investigations	Biopsy is not done—no role for FNAC	• IVU: Gross dilation of pelvicalyceal system—not done if we do contrast CT No role for biopsy or FNAC	
Treatment	1. Asymptomatic: Regular follow up 2. Symptomatic, dialysis plus renal transplantation if uncontrolled hypertension or renal failure is present	Congenital: Anderson Hyne's pyeloplasty Acquired: Treat the cause, example: BPH with hydronephrosis = TURP	Radical nephrectomy with or without other treatment

On examination, the mass is palpable in the lumbar region which is firm to hard, irregular with restricted mobility. Gurgling is elicited due to presence of air in the lumen, thus it differentiates from solid organ enlargement. **Large tumours can be bimanually palpable** but they are not ballotable. Colonoscopy to confirm the diagnosis followed by ultrasound and CT scan to know the metastasis and resectibility are the investigations. Right radical hemicolectomy or extended hemicolectomy depends upon

whether the hepatic flexure is involved or not is the treatment of choice (Fig. 24.104).

c. GIST: Patients with gastro-intestinal stromal tumour are between 20 and 50 years of age. These tumours attain a large size. They grow outside the lumen and hence do not produce obstruction. However, a mucosal ulceration results in bleeding. The stomach is the commonest site of GIST. GIST arising from intestines can present in the lumbar region. This should be the exclusion diagnosis. If you

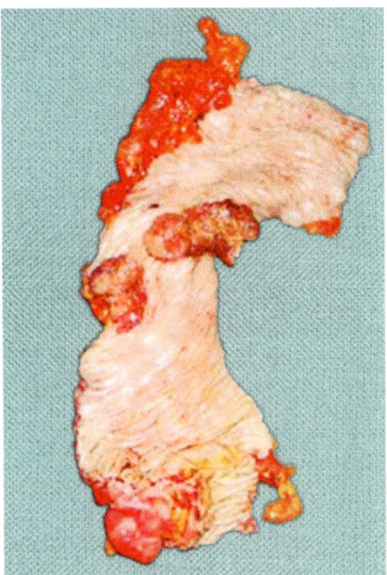

Fig. 24.104: Carcinoma ascending colon

suspect a bowel mass think of colonic malignancy first, followed by tuberculosis as second and chronic intussusception as third. When all 3 are ruled out, if features of GIST are present, then offer the diagnosis of GIST.

d. Chronic intussusception: It is usually a firm gurgling mass with regular borders which may contract during palpation. Recurrent or intermittent abdominal pain for one or two years may be present. Chronic intussusception is non tender. When the intussusception reduces, all symptoms will disappear. Percussion will reveal a resonant note. Most of the patients are young. If intussusception is the diagnosis in elderly, it is usually ileocolic or colo-colic and invariably a colonic malignancy is the cause. These intussusceptions are called secondary intussusceptions. The common causes of secondary intussusception or chronic intussusception are polyps, purpura, submucosal lipoma, Meckel's diverticulum, carcinoma, carcinoid, etc. Ultrasound followed by CECT scan is done to confirm the diagnosis followed by resection of the bowel and anastomosis.

5. Retroperitoneal mass: Typically retroperitoneal masses are liposarcomas. They occur in young patients. They can attain huge size before they become clinically palpable. They present with painless, progressive, massive enlargement of the abdomen. Compression on the iliac veins will result in unilateral limb oedema. Inferior vena caval obstruction may cause bilateral limb oedema and dilated veins in the flank (inguino-axillary veins). Examination will reveal a large, firm, irregular mass with all borders felt and with restricted mobility. On percussion a resonant note is felt because of intestines over the surface of the mass. Liposarcoma is the commonest retroperitoneal sarcomas followed by fibrosarcoma or epithelioid sarcomas. CT scan is done to locate the tumour and to find out the vascular invasions and to find out the infiltration of the surrounding structures. Resection of the tumour is the best form of treatment. All other modalities such as chemotherapy and radiotherapy are palliative.

MASS IN THE UMBILICAL REGION

Masses in this region are from transverse colon, stomach, pancreatic mass, lymph nodes omentum, mesentery, retroperitoneal structures including aorta.

1. **Colonic carcinoma:** Middle aged patients are affected who present with altered bowel habits and abdominal pain. Pain is due to partial obstruction. Loss of appetite and loss of weight are other features. On examination, a hard nodular mass is palpable in the umbilical region which has vertical mobility but not transverse. Mass does not move with respiration. If it is loaded with faecal matter, it is dull on percussion. Otherwise a resonant note can be elicited due to the presence of air within the lumen of the colon. **Transverse colonic carcinoma is known to produce intussusception.** A mass which is palpable can be due to the growth itself (hard and irregular), lymph nodes (hard and nodular), omental mass (deposits— moves with respiration), faecal matter (indentable) and due to intussusception—contracting mass. In cases of total obstruction, right to left peristalsis may be seen or at least prominent loops are seen. Caecum may be distended with tympanitic note over. Diagnosis is by ultrasound and CT scan of the abdomen. Colonoscopy is done to establish the diagnosis. Biopsy may not be possible in cases of total obstruction. Laparotomy and colectomy are done followed by colo-colic anastomosis.

Carcinoma transverse colon mass can be due to
1. Growth
2. Faecal matter
3. Omental deposits
4. Intussusception
5. Pericolic lymph nodes

2. **Omental mass**
   a. **Malignancy** of the stomach and colon is a common disease, hence metastatic deposits in the omentum are often from these primaries. As a rule, the condition is fairly advanced in these cases. The patient will have ascites, colonic or stomach mass and with or without secondaries in the liver. Typically, an omental mass is nodular, thickened and hence firm to hard in consistency and moves with respiration.
   b. **Omental mass in children or young adults is usually due to tuberculosis** of the peritoneum resulting in granularity and rolled up omentum. Typically, child's abdomen is protuberant due to ascites. Rolled up omentum is felt. In adults, **tuberculosis** is usually a more serious disease with involvement of intestines, peritoneum and omentum.
   c. **Omental cake:** It means abnormal thickened omentum, usually caused by metastatic deposits in the omentum. Often it is a part of extensive peritoneal carcinomatosa— disseminated, usually from stomach, colon, pancreas or ovary. Multiple nodularity can be felt in the abdomen. Patients are very thin cachectic and emaciated. Other unusual causes of omental cake are lymphoma and tuberculous peritonitis.

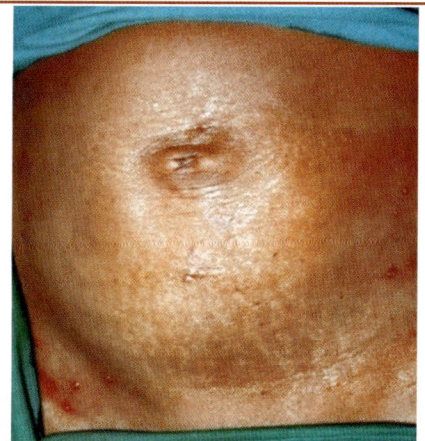

Fig. 24.105: Mass in the umbilical region

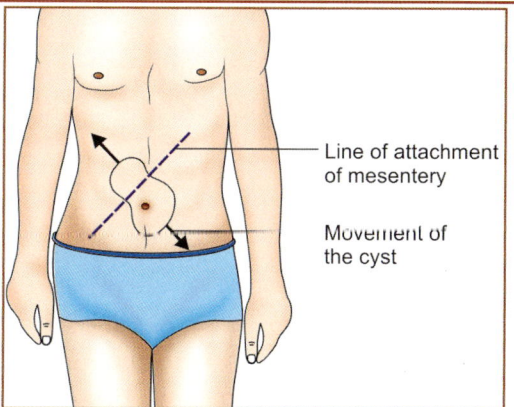

Line of attachment of mesentery

Movement of the cyst

Fig. 24.106: Line of mesentery and classical movement of mesenteric cyst

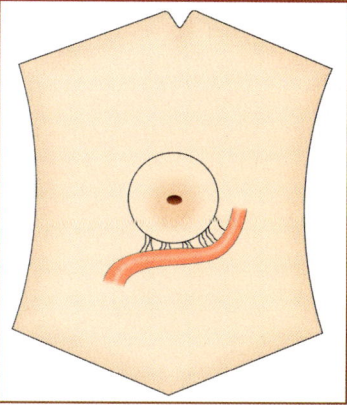

Fig. 24.107: Chylolymphatic cyst—simple excision is the treatment

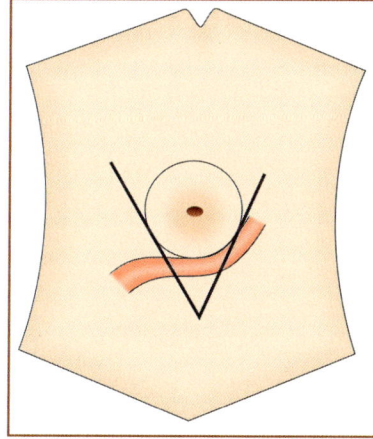

Fig. 24.108A: Enterogenous cyst—excision along with bowel is the treatment

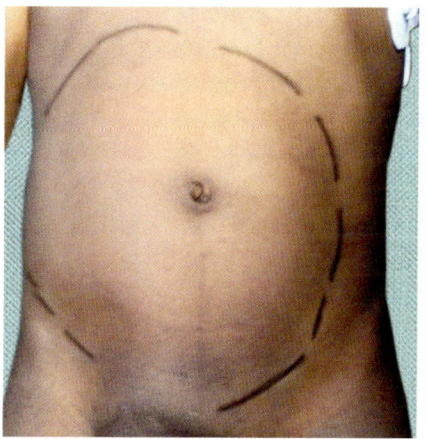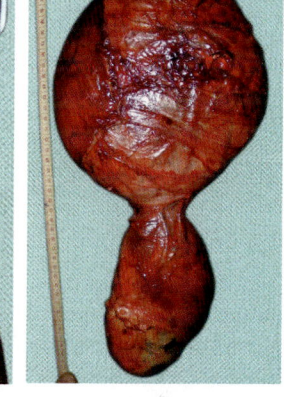

Fig. 24.108B: Retroperitoneal cyst confused for mesenteric cyst. Carefully watch the specimen. It was extending into the scrotum (*Courtesy:* Dr Chethan K, Prof of Surgery, KMC, Manipal)

3. **Stomach mass:** Any large stomach mass can extend from epigastrium to umbilical region. Gastrointestinal stromal tumours and carcinoma stomach are the differential diagnosis. In cases of carcinoma pyloric antrum, a peristaltic wave (contractions) of the stomach can be confused for a mass.

4. **Pancreatic mass:** Just like stomach, a large pancreatic mass can be felt in the umbilical region specially cystadenoma pancreas. Typically mass does not move with respiration, has treetop mobility. These have been described earlier.

5. **Mesenteric masses** (Figs 24.105 to 24.108)

   a. **Mesenteric cyst:** Line of mesentery extends form left of 2nd lumbar vertebra to the right sacroiliac joint. Mesenteric cyst is the most common cystic mass in the children or young adults. Typically, it s a tensely cystic mass, **may feel firm in the umbilical region and moves at right angles to the direction of the mesentery.** Swelling is dull, surrounded by resonance and traversed by band of resonance. These three features have been described as **Tillaux's triad.** Acute abdominal pain is due to torsion of the cyst or due to haemorrhage. Many patients present only with abdominal distension. Diagnosis is easily made by ultrasound examination. Chylolymphatic cysts are

common. They can be treated by simple enucleation. Enterogenous cysts are removed with the intestines because they arise from the intestines.

b. **Lymph nodal mass** (Fig. 24.109)

   • Large enlargement of para-aortic lymph nodes will form a nodular mass in the epigastrium and umbilical region. Examine the testis first and rule out testicular tumour in young patients. It is usually seminoma testis. Consider lymphoma next and examine other group of lymph nodes, liver and spleen. Look for any pigmented lesions—malignant melanoma, operated or not operated. If ascites and bowel gurgling is present, think of tuberculosis also.

   • Advanced gastrointestinal tract malignancies can give rise to large para-aortic lymph nodes . Primaries can be from stomach, pancreas and colon. These nodes are hard and fixed.

   • Tuberculosis of mesenteric lymph nodes also can produce lump abdomen in the umbilical region. However, the mass can be a complex mass with lymph nodes, matted bowel loops (gurgle), cold abscess (within leaves of mesentery). Such abscesses have been described as pseudo-mesenteric cyst.

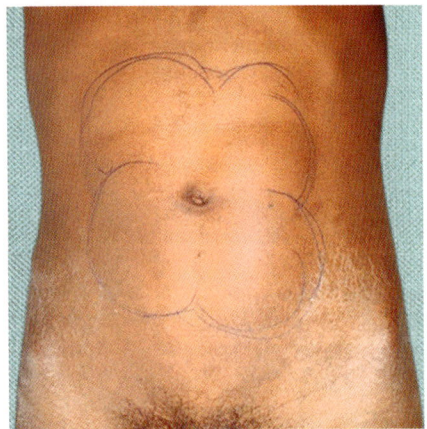

Fig. 24.109 : Para-aortic lymph node mass due to seminoma

6. **Retroperitoneal mass** (Fig. 24.110): Typically retroperitoneal masses attain huge sizes, does not move with respiration and does not fall forwards in the knee-elbow position. Retroperitoneal cyst and retroperitoneal sarcoma are the two differential diagnoses. Cysts are lymphatic cysts, patients do not have loss of weight and general condition of the patient is good. Liposarcoma is the most common sarcoma in the retroperitoneum which feels hard, irregular and weight loss is a feature. Both are treated by excision.

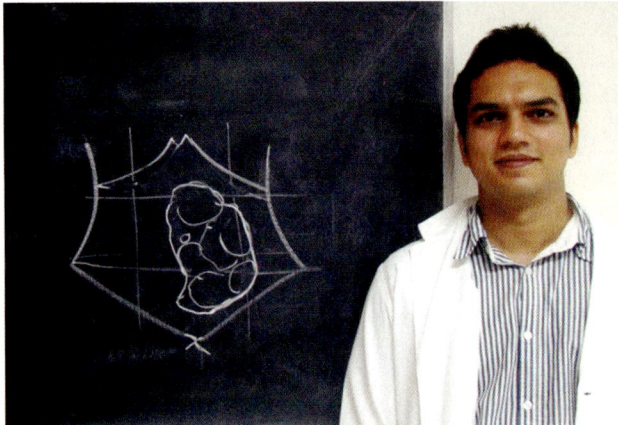

Fig. 24.110: Retroperitoneal tumour (*Courtesy*: Dr Zeeshan Hameed, postgraduate student 2011, KMC, Manipal)

MASS IN THE LEFT LUMBAR REGION

1. **Renal masses** (consider renal masses first): When you find a mass in the lumbar region, as already been discussed under mass in the right lumbar region, hydronephrosis, renal cell carcinoma, polycystic disease of the kidney are the important causes. The most confusing picture is when spleen is enlarged. This has been already discussed under splenic masses.

2. **Carcinoma descending colon**: In the right lumbar region, not only carcinoma but tuberculosis is an important differential diagnosis of the mass arising from intestines. It is very rare for tuberculosis to affect descending colon. Hence, if there is a mass in the left lumbar region which is not kidney—not ballotable, one can consider carcinoma descending colon

as a diagnosis. Again descending colon is not the common site—rather rectosigmoid junction is a common site on the left colonic malignancy. Middle aged patients who have change in the bowel habits, constipation, bleeding per rectum are the victims. The mass is hard and irregular—sometimes indentable because of faecal matter in the proximal colon. Colonoscopy to confirm the diagnosis followed by left hemicolectomy is the treatment of choice.

3. **Splenomegaly**: It is always a mass in the left hypochondrium extending into lumbar region. Details can be got under mass in the left hypochondrium.

4. **Retroperitoneal mass**: Again by the time retroperitoneal mass presents, it usually occupies not only lumbar region but also umbilical region, hypochondriums, etc.

MASS IN THE RIGHT ILIAC FOSSA

This is a common long case for students because of many interesting masses. Once a challenging problem for surgeons when only clinical diagnosis was important, many of these masses are now diagnosed with ease with investigations such as ultrasound and CT scan. However, students are requested to use their clinical sense (thinking) rather than look at the diagnosis by investigations and give the diagnosis. Please draw simple diagrams which help you many times. The masses can be classified as parietal swellings and intra-abdominal swellings.

Parietal Swellings

a. Parietal wall abscess—chronic may be due to tuberculosis of spine
b. Desmoid tumour
c. Endometriosis
d. Lipoma
e. Neurofibroma
f. Hernias which can be called parieto-intra-abdominal masses.

Intra-abdominal Swellings

a. Arising from normal structures
b. Arising from abnormal structures

From Normal Structures

I. **Intestines**
  1. Appendicular mass
  2. Appendicular abscess
  3. Ileocaecal tuberculosis
  4. Carcinoma caecum
  5. Amoeboma
  6. Intussusception
  7. Actinomycosis

II. **Lymph nodes**
  1. Acute lymphadenitis
  2. Lymphoma
  3. Secondaries

III. Retroperitoneal structures
1. Sarcoma
2. Aneurysm
3. Iliopsoas abscess
4. Chondrosarcoma

IV. In females
1. Ovarian cyst
2. Fibroid
3. Tubo-ovarian mass

From Abnormal Structures

1. *Undescended testis*: Seminoma.
2. *Unascended kidney*: Hydronephrosis, renal cell carcinoma, etc.

DIFFERENTIAL DIAGNOSIS OF MASS IN THE RIGHT ILIAC FOSSA

Parietal swelling: Parietal swellings are extra-abdominal. On head or leg raising test, they become more prominent. These are a few swellings.

a. **Parietal wall abscess:** It is a pyogenic abscess which can occur in a haematoma, or a pyaemic abscess which can occur as a part of pyaemia as in diabetic patients. Such abscesses are very tender, with warm surface and are associated with fever, chills and rigors. Treated by incision and drainage with antibiotic treatment.

b. **Cold abscess:** A tubercular abscess arising from a costo-chondral junction may track down, either lateral or medial to the linea semilunaris. If it extends lateral to the rectus, it spreads down between the internal oblique and transverse abdominis muscles, but if it extends medial to the linea semilunaris, it may spread into the rectus sheath and may extend downward behind the rectus muscle. **Cold abscess arising primarily from muscles is extremely rare because muscles have high lactic acid content. They lack of reticulo-endothelial tissue in muscle, lack of lymphatic tissue and the abundant blood supply.**

c. **Desmoid tumour:** It is an unencapsulated fibroma occurring in the abdominal wall and occurs in multiparous females. Repeated stretching of abdominal layers (due to pregnancy) is supposed to initiate formation of tumour. It can also occur following abdominal wall injury including laparotomy. It is a firm to hard swelling. It has no capsule. Hence, it should be treated with wide excision. It does not undergo sarcomatous change. After wide excision, the abdominal wall has to be reconstructed by using mesh.

d. **Recurrent tumours:** Abdominal wall recurrence due to the tumour seeding directly, at the drain site or later due to metastasis have been described in Fig. 24.111.

INTRA-ABDOMINAL SWELLING

A. Arising from structures normally present in the right iliac fossa

1. **Appendicular mass:** It is a tender, soft to firm mass which develops 48–72 hours following acute appendicitis. It is

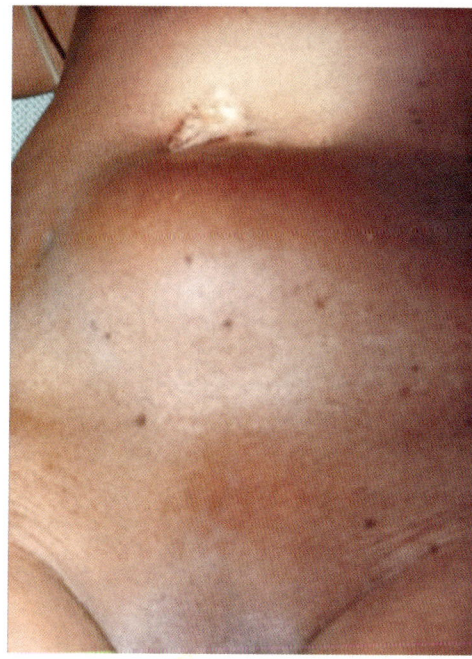

Fig. 24.111: Abdominal wall recurrence following hemicolectomy for carcinoma colon

nature's attempt to limit the spread of infection by forming a mass consisting of omentum, terminal ileum, caecum with pericaecal fat and inflammatory oedema. It is managed conservatively by **Ochsner-Sherren's regime** in the form of nil per oral, antibiotics, maintaining the basic charts such as temperature, pulse rate and respiratory rate and diameter of the mass (today it is done best with ultrasound), intravenous fluids and relief of pain. An attempt to remove the appendix may result in faecal fistula. During follow up an option can be given to the patient about elective appendicectomy after 6–8 weeks or observe. In case of recurrence of symptoms, consider for apendicectomy. If the mass is tender and associated with high grade fever with chills and rigors and extremely tender, it is appendicular abscess which needs to be drained.

2. *Ileocaecal tuberculosis:* Hyperplastic variety of tuberculosis of intestines results in a a chronic cicatrising granulomatous reaction involving terminal ileum, caecum and part of ascending colon resulting in a mass in right iliac fossa. It is a chronic, nontender, firm, nodular mass, with some degree of mobility, situated in the lumbar region, slightly on the higher side. Features of tuberculosis may be present. It is treated by limited resection followed by ileocolic anastomosis (Fig. 24.112).

Clinical Wisdom

Abdominal mass from tuberculosis
1. The matted bowel loops
2. Granular omentum
3. Mesenteric lymph nodal mass
4. Ascites
5. Cold abscess

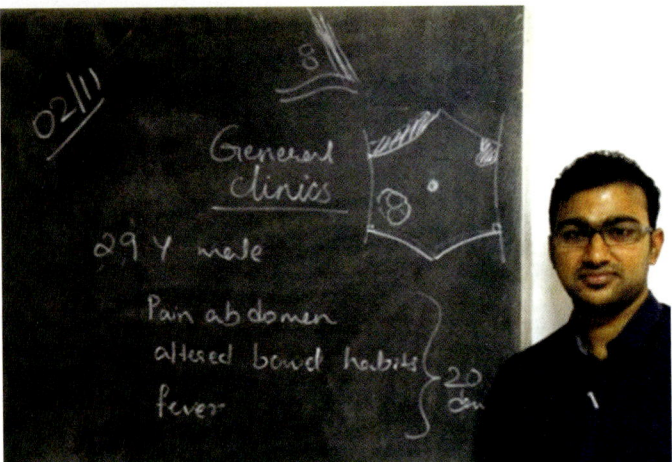

Fig. 24.112: Ileocaecal tuberculosis—caecum is pulled up and more medial (*Courtesy*: Dr Mohan Amresh, postgraduate student, KMC, Manipal)

3. ***Carcinoma caecum:*** It is more common in females, around 40–50 years of age. The patient presents with altered bowel habits, bleeding per rectum, severe anaemia, and weight loss. In fact many of these patients are evaluated and treated by physicians for anaemia. Examination reveals pallor, and a hard, irregular mass in right iliac fossa with fixity or restricted mobility. Psoas spasm indicates infiltration into psoas muscle.

- Diagnosis is by colonoscopy. Barium studies is mostly not done nowadays. However, if done it may show apple core deformity suggesting carcinoma. If colonoscopy cannot be done, barium study may be done. CT scan is done to find out the local infiltration.

- It is treated by right radical hemicolectomy (Figs 24.113 to 24.118) which includes removal of terminal 5 cm of the ileum, caecum, ascending colon and right one-third of transverse colon with regional lymph nodes.

- Study Table 24.5 to differentiate 3 common abdominal masses

- Study Clinical Case Capsule given in the next page.

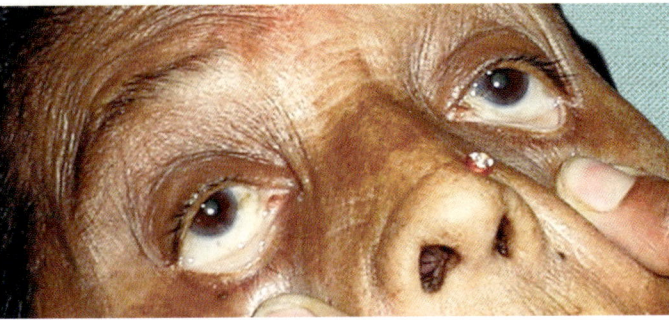

Fig. 24.114: Gross pallor in 60-year-old lady

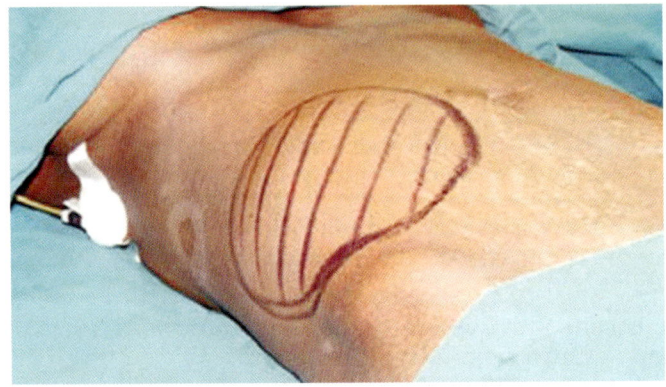

Fig. 24.115: Surface marking of the mass abdomen

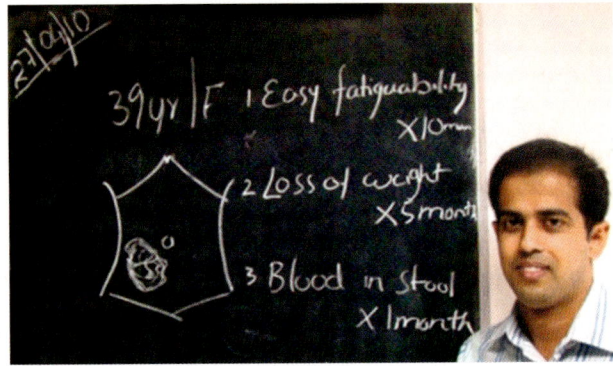

Fig. 24.116: Blackboard sketch (*Courtesy:* Dr Sunilkrishna, postgraduate student, year 2010, KMC, Manipal)

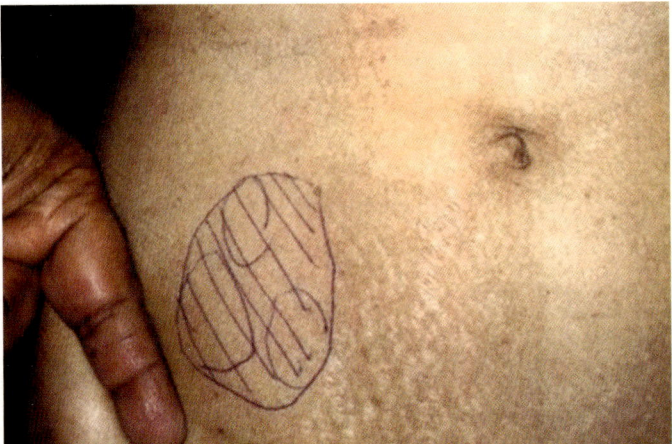

Fig. 24.113: Clear space between lower border of the mass and iliac bone and inguinal crease. It rules out ovarian tumour

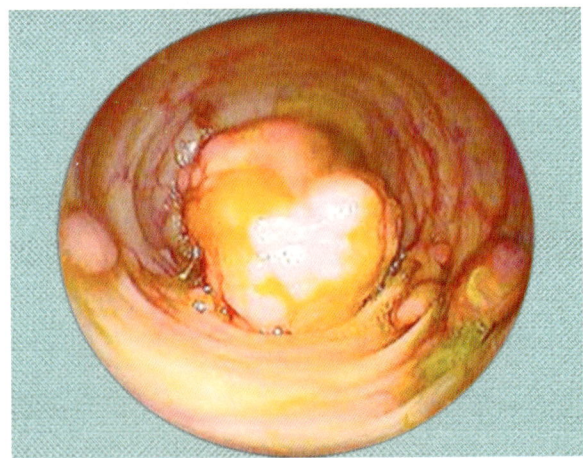

Fig . 24.117: Colonoscopy showing multiple polyps and growth

Table 24.5: Differntiating features of three bowel masses

Features	Carcinoma	Tubeculosis	GIST
Age	Above 50 years	30–40 years	20–40 years
Symptoms	Blood and mucus, anaemia	Mass, fever	Blood
General condition	Not good, loss of weight present	Not good, loss of weight	Good
Mass	Irregular, hard, restricted mobility	Irregular, firm to hard, mobile	Nodular or bosselated, mobile
Colonoscopy	Ulcerative growth and biopsy	Ulcers and biopsy	May be missed, ulcer if seen biopsy to be taken
CT scan	Confirms location and infiltration	Confirms location	Confirms the origin—extra luminal
Treatment	Right radical hemicolectomy	Limited colectomy in cases of obstruction with ATT	Excision, resection of involved bowel, limited colectomy

Table 24.6: Differentiation of ileocaecal tuberculosis from carcinoma caecum

Features	Ileocaecal tuberculosis	Carcinoma caecum
Age	Young	>50 years
Sex	Male = Female	Female > Male
Clinical presentation	Low grade evening rise in temperature Diarrhoea—watery, foul smelling, weight loss Pulmonary symptoms +/–	Loss of weight and appetite—cachexic Diarrhoea—mucus, occult blood Features of anaemia—weakness
Family history	H/o tuberculosis	Breast, ovary, colon malignancy
Pallor	+/–	++
Details about the mass: Location	High up—may be lumbar region	Right iliac fossa
Consistency	Firm, irregular	Hard, nodular
Mobility	Mobile	Restricted mobility or fixed
Haemoglobin	Normal	Low
Stool	Blood may be present	Occult blood
Chest X-ray	May show pulmonary tuberculosis	**Cannon ball secondaries**
Ultrasound abdomen	Mass arising from pulled up caecum	Colonic mass, ascites, para-aortic nodes
Colonoscopy and biopsy	Multiple ulcers	Proliferative growth, ulcer with everted edge
Biopsy	Casseating granuloma Giant cells of Langerhans	Adenocarcinoma
Barium enema	Contracted, pulled up caecum	Apple core deformity
CEA (Carcino-embryonic antigen)	Negative	May be elevated—prognostic value
Treatment	1. ATT for 6–9 months if no obstruction 2. Limited colectomy and postop anti-tubercular treatment for 6–9 months	Metastatic work up—CT followed by Right radical hemicolectomy followed by ileocolic (transverse colon) anastomosis

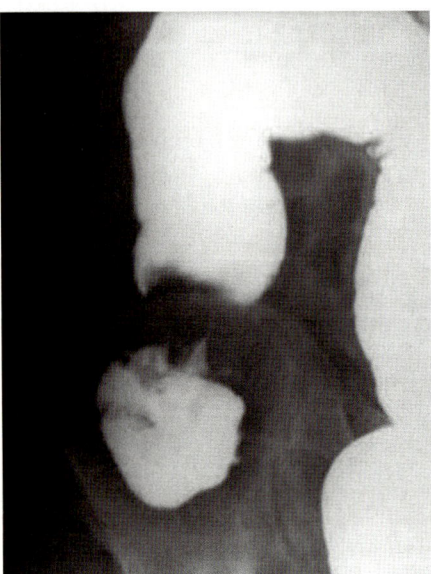

Fig. 24.118: Barium enema showing apple core deformity (different case)

Clinical Case Capsule

A 65-year-old lady was admitted and evaluated by physician for the complaints of fatigue and weakness. All tests showed anaemia. Ultrasound abdomen was normal. She also said occasional blood in stools. Upper gastrointestinal scopy was normal. Proctoscopy showed haemorrhoids. She was treated with iron supplements. After 2 months patient presented with severe abdominal pain with gurgling contracting mass in the right iliac fossa. Ultrasound revealed intussusception. At laparotomy, there was ileocolic intussusception due to carcinoma caecum (Fig. 24.120).

- Right-sided colonic tumours can present with anaemia, intussusception and acute appendicitis. A few cases who undergo only appendicectomy will come back with discharging faecal matter in the right iliac fossa.

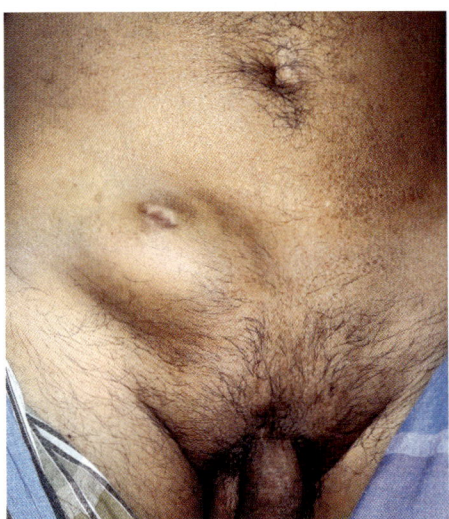

Fig. 24.119: Advanced carcinoma caecum with perforation, with an abscess in the abdominal wall (*Courtesy*: Dr Prem Kumar, Dr Vimal Kumar, Dr Rajesh Kumar, Dr Sunay Bhatt, Department of Surgery, PSG Medical College, Coimbatore, Tamil Nadu, CME 2017)

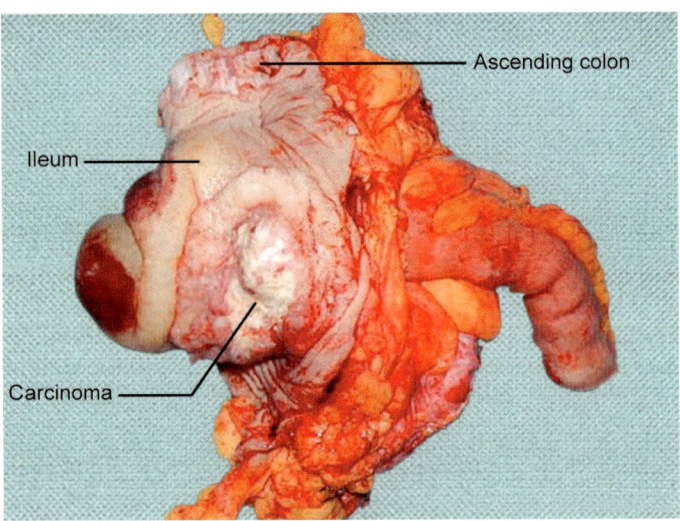

Fig. 24.120: Carcinoma caecum presenting as intussusception

4. **Intussusception**: Invagination of one segment of intestine within another segment is called intussusception.

- *Acute intussusception* can give rise to a mass in the right iliac fossa/umbilical region which is tender and soft to firm. Weaning of diet results in change in bacterial flora of the gut and swollen Payer's patches has been considered as the chief factor. This occurs in children and is described as idiopathic intussusception. The mass is not in the right iliac fossa but it is higher in the umbilical region. In fact right iliac fossa is empty—**Signe de dance**. Contracting mass with concavity towards umbilicus is a feature. Every attempt should be made to reduce the intussusception. Reduction is done only at surgery.

- *Chronic intussusception* is always due to some pathology related to or within the bowel. The common causes are **submucous lipomas, polyps, Meckel's diverticulum, carcinoma caecum, carcinoid tumours,** etc. All these will act like a triggering factor for the initiation of the intussusception. The mass is usually nontender, firm, mobile and contractions of the bowel may be felt while palpating the mass. Gurgle is also a feature. The mass may disappear spontaneously also. It is treated by resection of the bowel and anastomosis (Fig. 24.120). Also see Fig. 24.121, patient with Peutz-Jeghers syndrome presented with acute intussusception.

Clinical Wisdom

Microcytic hypochromic anaemia evaluation: Rule out carcinoma stomach —do upper GI scopy. If it is normal, rule out carcinoma caecum.

5. **Amoeboma**: It can be acute or chronic. It follows an attack of amoebic typhilitis (inflammation of the caecum). An **amoeboma,** also known as an amoebic granuloma, is a rare complication of *Entamoeba histolytica* infection where, in response to the infecting *amoeba* there is formation of annular colonic granulation, which results in a large ulcerative

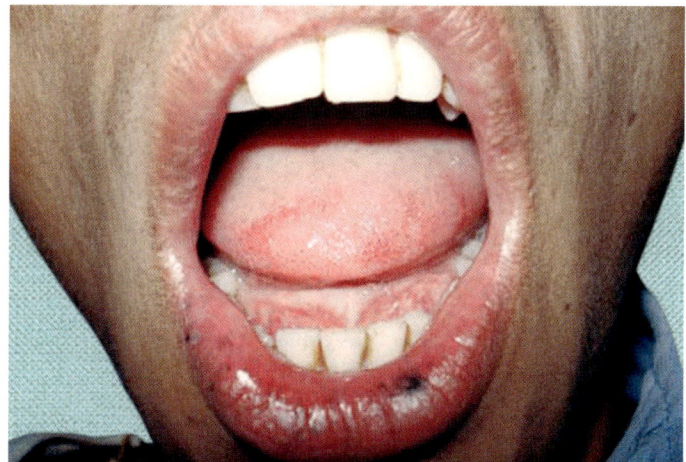

Fig. 24.121: 35-year-old man with chronic intussusception. He had pigmentation of lips. Case of Peutz-Jeghers syndrome

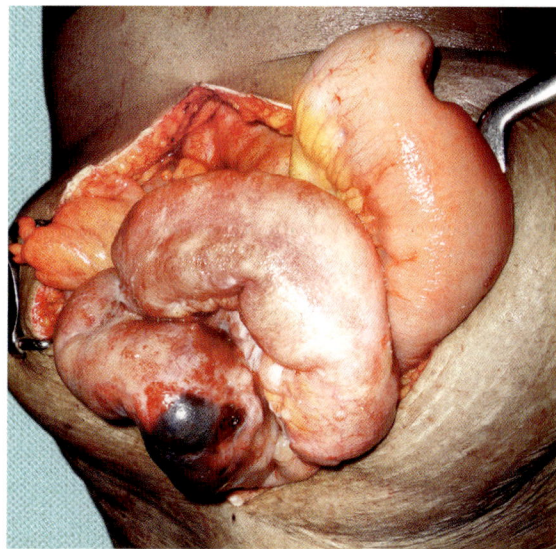

Fig. 24.122: Non-Hodgkin's lymphoma affecting terminal ileum at surgery

local lesion of the bowel. **Amoeboma is tender and firm.** Complications of amoeboma include perforation, obstruction and bleeding. It is not common to find amoebomas nowadays because of effective treatment of amoebiasis with metronidazole, tinidazole, etc.

6. **Actinomycosis:** This is a rare mass in the right iliac fossa which usually develops 2–3 months after appendicectomy. Actinomycosis is an *infectious bacterial* disease caused by *Actinomyces* species such as *Actinomyces israelii*. A woody hard, indurated tender mass with multiple sinuses is characteristic of this condition. Sinuses discharge sulphur granules which can trickle down. Unlike tuberculosis, narrowing of lumen of the gut and lymph node enlargement does not occur. Treatment is difficult.

7. **Lymphoma involving ileocaecal region and greater omentum**

   Lymphoma of the abdomen: This should not be the primary diagnosis. This is diagnosis by exclusion.

   Hodgkin's disease: Here hepatosplenomegaly and paraaortic node enlargement are common. It has been already discussed.

   Non-Hodgkin's lymphoma: The gastrointestinal tract is the most common extranodal site involved with lymphoma accounting for 5–20% of all cases. Diffuse large B-cell lymphoma can be dangerous, infiltrating the peritoneum and omentum and presenting with ascites and pleural effusion. Such patients deteriorate fast unless treated fast. Multiple intra-abdominal organ infiltration or disseminated peritoneal lymphoma is called peritoneal "lymphomatosis". There are two types of lymphoma: Diffuse, large B-cell lymphoma (most common) and follicular lymphoma. Presentation can be with peripheral lymphadenopathy or with symptoms of B-cell lymphoma. Abdominal pain may be vague with occasional radiation to the back. Diagnosis is by CT scan and CT guided biopsy or laparoscopy and biopsy. Treatment is by radiotherapy and chemotherapy (Fig. 24.122).

8. **Lymph node mass**
   - **Acute mesenteric lymphadenitis** is common in children. It produces tender, nodular and firm mass in right iliac fossa. The child usually has fever. Acute lymphadenitis can also involve **external iliac nodes** as in filariasis. It is non-specific in aetiology, may be due to viral. It is confused for acute appendicitis. Ultrasound and blood tests can help. When in doubt, specially when acute appendicitis cannot be ruled out, exploratory laparotomy, appendicectomy and lymph node biopsy are done.
   - **Lymphoma involving external iliac nodes** can be mass in the right and left iliac fossa. Mass is nodular, firm, deep seated and retroperitoneal. Transmitted pulsations from iliac artery may be present. Other group of lymph nodes, liver, spleen, if palpable will clinch the diagnosis.
   - **Secondaries in lymph nodes (external iliac) from carcinoma ovary, cervix, etc.** Nodes are hard and fixity is a feature. Mass is not only from lymph node but a complex mass from ovary, lymph nodes, peritoneal nodules, etc.

9. **Retroperitoneal sarcoma** (Fig. 24.123): This is common in young patients, presents as huge, irregular/ nodular, fixed lump involving lumbar, umbilical and right iliac fossa. Recent increase in size draws the attention of the patient. It is fixed

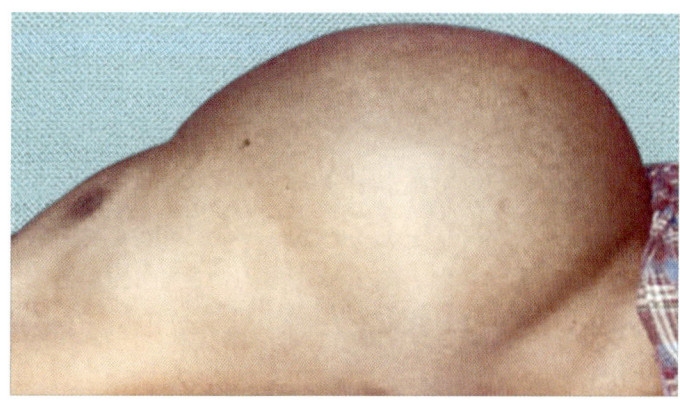

Fig. 24.123: Retroperitoneal liposarcoma

to posterior abdominal wall. It compresses the retro-peritoneal structures such as inferior vena cava resulting in bilateral pedal oedema, and ureters causing hydronephrosis.

Liposarcoma is the commonest and may arise from pre-existing lipoma. R-0 resection should be the aim. Fibrosarcoma, haemangiosarcoma, leiomyosarcoma are other sarcomas. They are treated by wide excision followed by radiotherapy. Chemotherapy is also helpful, when it is not possible to remove the entire mass. Debulking also can be done even if it is an advanced case.

Clinical Wisdom

- Compression on inferior vena cava results in bilateral pedal oedema
- Compresses on common iliac vein results in unilateral limb oedema.

10. **Aneurysm**: Iliac artery aneurysm is rare and occurs in old-aged patients. It produces a soft, pulsatile swelling in the right iliac fossa. Bruit or thrill is usually present. They occur due to atherosclerosis. Evidence of atherosclerosis in the form of locomotor brachialis, hypertension, obesity may be present. Ultrasound, CT angiogram are the investigations. Repair of aneurysm is the treatment of choice by using polytetrafluoroethylene (PTFE) graft.

11. **Iliopsoas abscess** (Figs 24.124 and 24.125): It is the result of tuberculosis of thoracolumbar spine. It should be suspected when a young patient complains of pain in the back referred to abdominal wall. Spine movements are limited. On examination, tenderness over the spine is the clue to the diagnosis. Gibbus can be present. Initially, it forms paravertebral abscess and later it **gravitates down beneath the medial arcuate ligament and forms psoas abscess. Psoas abscess burrows into the thigh under inguinal ligament and forms iliopsoas abscess.** Fluctuation is present on both sides of the inguinal ligament. It is described as **cross-fluctuation test**. Diagnosis is by plain X-rays of the involved bones, CT scan and other relevant investigations. Treatment in early cases is antituberculosis treatment for 12 months. Decompression, drainage of cold abscess, fusion of spines are other types of treatment.

12. **Chondrosarcoma of the iliac crest**: It is a hard, fixed tumour which cannot be separated from the bone. **Iliac crest is one of the sites of chondrosarcoma.** It presents as a slow growing swelling. Patients are young may complain of dull aching pain. If the tumour is near a neurovascular bundle, as in iliac bone chondrosarcoma, the patient may present with nerve dysfunction of the lumbosacral plexus or the sciatic or femoral nerves. If a chondrosarcoma is close to a joint, it may limit the joint's range of movement. It is resistant to *chemotherapy* and *radiotherapy*.

SPECIFIC MASSES IN FEMALES

13. **Ovarian cyst**: It is usually unilateral. To start with, the cyst develops in the pelvis and gives rise to discomfort in the lower abdomen. As the cyst grows, it comes out of the pelvis

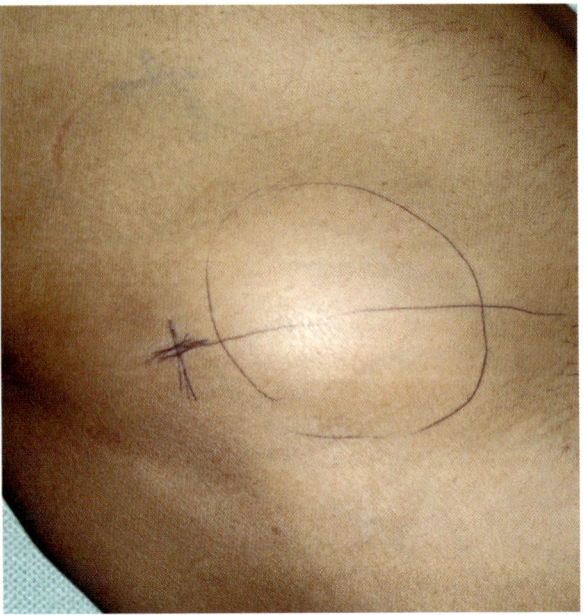

Fig. 24.124: Iliopsoas abscess due to tuberculous spine resulting in swelling above and below the inguinal ligament. Cross fluctuation is positive and tenderness was present in the lower thoracic spine

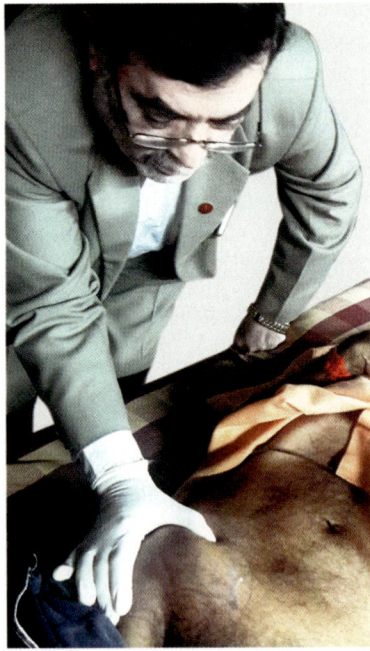

Fig. 24.125: Checking for the extent of the swelling—both above and below the inguinal ligament

and forms a mass in right iliac fossa. It has smooth surface, round borders, is cystic but feels firm, freely mobile and can be pushed back into the pelvis. Sometimes, the cyst can attain huge size. Typically lower border is not felt. Even if lower border is felt, a large mass can still be ovary, if it has completely come out of pelvis. Such freely mobile ovarian cysts have a long pedicle. Per vaginal examination gives the clue to the diagnosis. Following examination findings will help you to make a clinical diagnosis of ovarian cyst (Figs 24.126A, B and 24.127).

- Also careful palpation reveals the wall of the cyst. Try pushing the ovarian cyst upwards. Obviously the ovarian pedicle is stretched and patient experiences the pain.
- Large ovarian cysts are confused for ascites.

    • **Ruler test** will help in such cases. **A flat ruler is firmly applied over the lower abdomen just above anterior iliac spine and firmly pressed backwards. In cases of ovarian cyst aortic pulsations are felt,** not in cases of ascites.

- Large Krukenberg's tumours from carcinoma colon, carcinoma stomach, carcinoma breast can present as large abdominal masses.

14. **Fibroid of the uterus:** It presents as a firm to hard nodular mass in the suprapubic region and in the right and left iliac fossa. Typically lower border is not felt. Pain in the fibroid is due to red degeneration or inflammation. It is not uncommon to find a large fibroid with secondary inflammation resulting in bowel complaints such as colicky abdominal pain and even intestinal obstruction.

15. **Tubo-ovarian mass:** Women between the age of 20 and 40 are affected. The patient presents with lower abdominal pain, discomfort and fever. On examination, mass is felt in the right and left iliac fossa (often bilateral) usually tender, soft to firm. It is felt more in the hypogastrium with extension into the iliac fossa. Pelvic infection is usually present. Masses can be felt on the lateral wall of both fornices during vaginal examination.

B. Mass arising from structures which are not normally present

1. **Unascended kidney:** It can be either in the pelvis-pelvic kidney or in the iliac fossa. Such kidney is usually not very well-developed. It presents as a lobular mass. The mass is usually hydronephrosis due to the angulation of the ureters.

2. **Normal mobile kidney:** It can be felt in lumbar region, iliac fossa and can be pushed back into the loin.

3. **Undescended testis** (Fig. 24.128): It is palpable in right iliac fossa only when it is involved by seminoma—the most dangerous complication of undescended testis. Incidence of malignancy in intra-abdominal testis is 80%. The tumour is seminoma. It is hard, irregular, fixed mass. Absent testis in the scrotum clinches the diagnosis. Patient may have palpable para-aortic nodes, **supraclavicular nodes.** (Details about testicular tumours discussed under examination of testis and scrotum.)

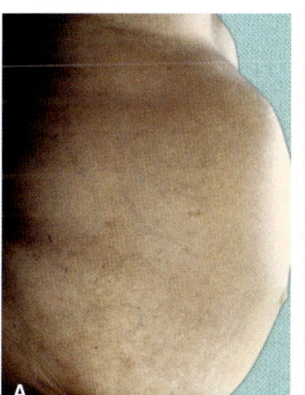
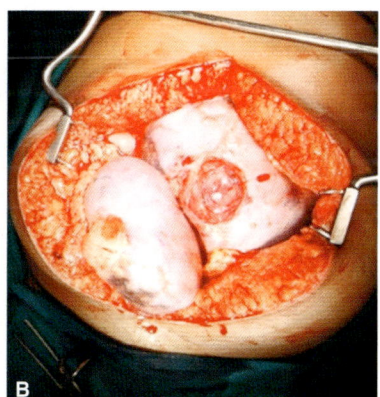

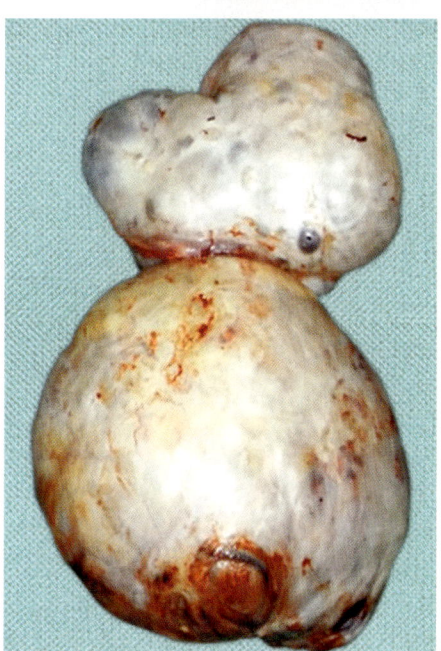

Figs 24.126A, B and 24.127: Showing distension of abdomen, large Krukenberg tumour at surgery and removal of the ovarian masses (specimen)

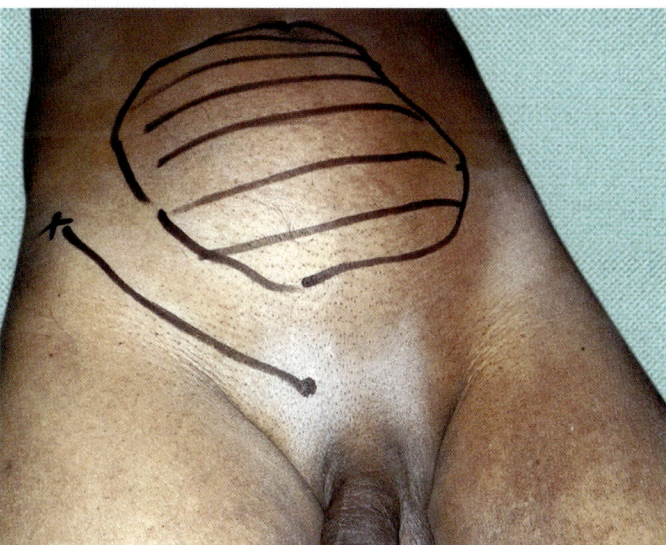

Fig. 24.128: Large testicular tumour arising in undescended testis

MASS IN THE HYPOGASTRIUM

When a mass is felt in the hypogastrium, first thing to consider is a mass arising from pelvic organs or masses arising from other regions and extending to hypogastrium. **Before examination, first ask the patient to void urine. Otherwise distended urinary bladder can be confused for a pathologic mass.** Also remember in elderly patients, even after voiding, urinary bladder may be significantly palpable and patient may not have symptoms such as pain. This is due to chronic retention of urine due to benign enlargement of prostate.

1. **Parietal swellings**

   a. **Desmoid tumour:** Desmoid tumours and endometriosis are the other 2 swellings to be considered in female patients. Desmoid tumours usually occurs in the abdominal wall of women of childbearing age during or after pregnancy. Clinically, the lesions present as deep-seated, firm, nonencapsulated, slow-growing, locally invasive and painless masses, become more prominent on abdominal muscle contraction. Mass is in the abdominal wall and is firm to hard in consistency. Desmoids are uncapsulated fibroma having a tendency to recur even after a wide excision. Stretching of the muscles and aponeurosis influenced by female hormones are responsible for the growth of the tumour. It is treated by wide excision (Figs 24.129 and 24.130).

   b. **Endometriosis** (Figs 24.131 and 24.132)**:** It occurs due mechanical implantation of endometrial cells during surgery (Clinical Box 24.8). Painful, palpable swelling, more symptomatic at the time of menstruation are characteristic features. Perimenstrual cyclical bleeding can occur. Oral contraceptive pills may control the symptoms. Otherwise, excision of the nodule has to be done.

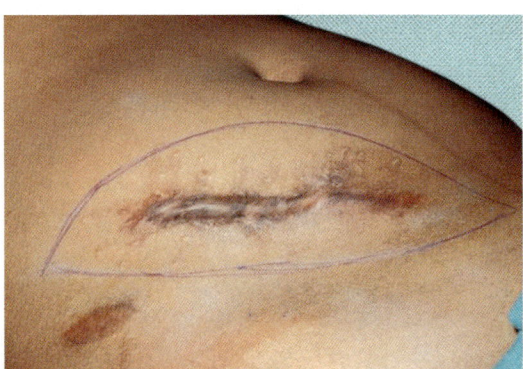

Fig. 24.129: Ugly bad scar following open appendicectomy for perforated appendicitis. Patient presented with 3 × 4 cm growing lump. It was firm in consistency with restricted mobility when oblique muscles were contracted (straining test)

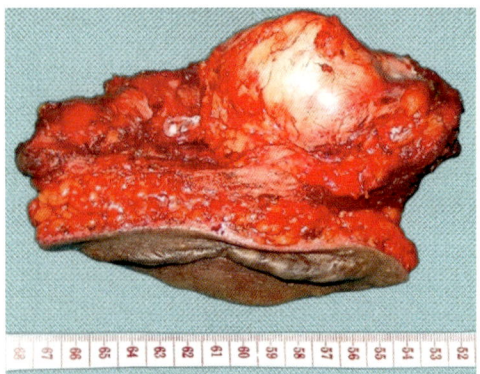

Fig. 24.130: Excised specimen along with normal tissue—wide excision

   c. **Urachal cyst:** The ventral urogenital sinus which forms the urinary bladder is continued cranially as urachus which extends into the umbilical cord—allantoic stalk. If this portion persists, patent urachus forms which connect umbilicus with urinary bladder. If it is fibrosed, as it occurs normally, it is called median umbilical ligament. A patent

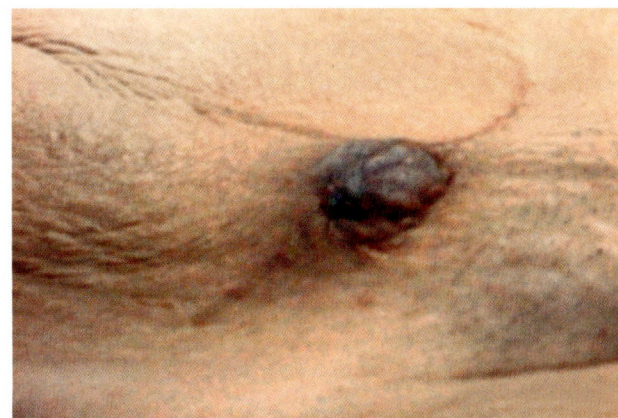

Fig. 24.131: Endometriosis in a scar of caesarean section

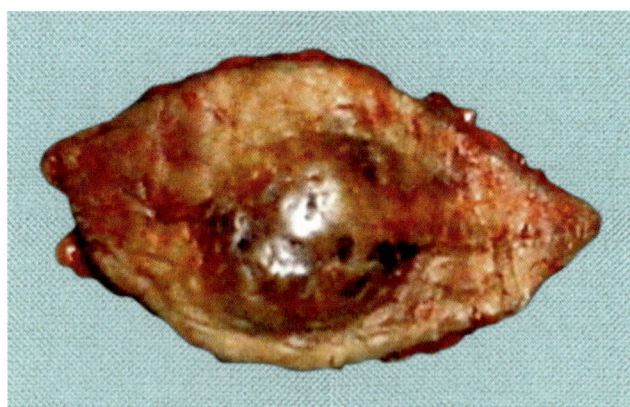

Fig. 24.132: Excised specimen

urachus may manifest as urinary discharge from umbilicus. It manifests usually in childhood and early adult life. **In most cases, there will be some kind of obstruction to the normal passage of urine.** Entire urachus is excised after correcting distal obstruction. Closure of cranial end (umbilical) and caudal end (bladder) and persistence of the central portion of the urachus results in urachal cyst. It is a cystic swelling deep to the abdominal muscles.

   d. Other swellings are neurofibromas, lipomas—they are the part of generalized diseases.

2. *Intra-abdominal swellings:* These can occur from the urinary bladder, uterus and its appendages, small intestines and pelvis.

Urinary bladder

a. Chronic retention of urine occurs in elderly patients. Often it is due to benign prostatic hypertrophy (BPH). Typically, it forms a globular swelling in the midline above the pubis. Typically, lower border cannot be palpated. It is a tensely cystic mass, easily felt. Retroperitoneal tumours can compress on the urinary bladder and give rise to retention of urine (Fig. 24.133). On percussion it is dull. Normal resonant note in the hypogastrium is due to small intestinal coils. They will be displaced by enlarged bladder. Palpable urinary bladder can occur in many conditions including bladder neck contractures, stricture urethra, phimosis, etc. This is one mass which appears and disappears. Examples of such masses are given in Clinical Box 24.9.

Note: First 3 are physiological and last 3 are pathological.

b. **Carcinoma urinary bladder** *may be palpable as hard mass.* The patient is elderly male, often a smoker, between 60 and 70 years of age who complains of haematuria.

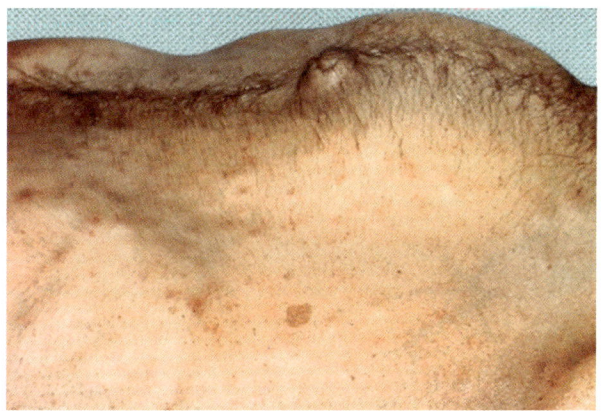

Fig. 24.133: Neurofibrosarcoma in a von Recklinghausen's disease causing retention of urine

---

Clinical Box 24.9

Appearing and disappearing masses
- Normal pregnancy
- Urinary bladder
- Loaded colon
- Intussusception
- Hydronephrosis—Dietl's crisis
- Ruptured pseudocyst

When the mass is palpable, it is fairly advanced. Patients do complain of suprapubic pain, strangury (painful micturition with bleeding), loin pain due to hydronephrosis, perineal pain due to infiltration of nerves. Cystoscopy to take a biopsy and CT scan to know the infiltration of the muscle layers are the main investigations. Transurethral resection of the tumour for early cases (T-1 lesions) and radical cystectomy for T-2 lesions involving muscle layers are done followed by chemotherapy and radiotherapy.

c. **Uterine masses** (Fig. 24.134): Two important masses have to be considered. One physiological, that is pregnancy. Amenorrhoea, child bearing age group, smooth enlargement of the uterus are the features. Second mass is pathological mass, that is fibroids. They can attain large sizes also. Typically the surface is nodular. Menorrhagia may be the feature. Sometimes it is difficult to appreciate the lower border. So, In a female if a large midline mass is palpable, differential diagnosis includes not only bladder mass and retroperitoneal mass but also uterine masses. Ovarian masses are typically on one side of the midline but a large ovarian cyst can present as midline masses with extension to one of the sides.

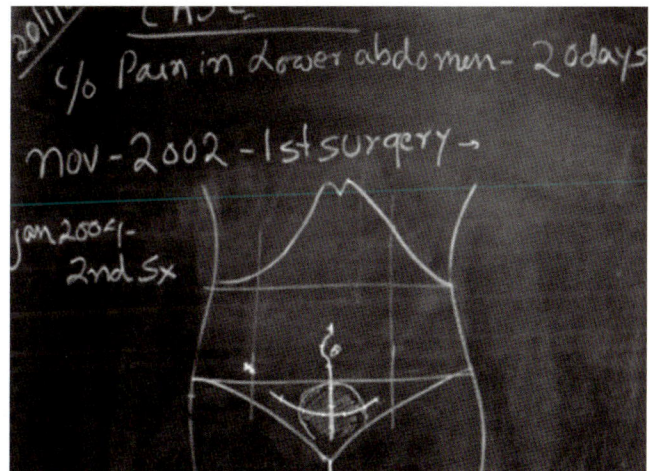

Fig. 24.134: Uterine fibroid. Blackboard sketch. Observe—lower border cannot be made out

3. *Ovarian mass:* Mostly it is a benign cyst but can be malignant. Malignant ovarian cysts often present with ascites which is detectable by shifting dullness. The real problem is to differentiate a large ovarian cyst from ascites. Ovarian cyst is dull in the center and resonant in the periphery because coils of bowel are displaced. In cases of ascites, periphery is dull because of fluid and resonance is in the centre because of floating intestines.

Ruler test (this has been discussed in page 405)

4. *Other causes:* For completion sake, in females, mass from the ruptured tubal gestation when the leakage is slow, hydrosalpinx and broad ligament cysts have to kept in mind for differential diagnosis.

MASS IN THE LEFT ILIAC FOSSA

Parietal Swelling

a. Parietal wall abscess
b. Desmoid tumour

Intra-abdominal

a. Arising from normal structures
b. Arising from abnormal structures

From Normal Structures

I. *Sigmoid colon*

a. **Carcinoma sigmoid colon:** Increasing constipation requiring increasing doses of purgatives is the typical symptom. Symptoms are of short duration of 1 or 2 months. Typically the patient is male in the middle age group. Occasional bleeding per rectum may be present. Rectosigmoid lesions present with features of intestinal obstruction in the form of colicky abdominal pain, distension and failure to pass stools and gas (obstipation). Clinical examination reveals a lump in the left iliac fossa. Hard irregular lump (growth with or without lymph nodes) is definitely carcinoma. Often what is felt is loaded colon. In such cases, indentation can be found.

b. **Amoeboma:** It is an inflammatory mass of the colon. Caecum and sigmoid are the common sites. It can present as a mass or even as acute abdomen due to perforated circumferential mass in the sigmoid colon. It is often confused for carcinoma sigmoid colon. Although rare, amoeboma must be considered in differential diagnosis of cancer of any colonic mass.

c. It is common to find a thickened sigmoid with a gurgle in Indian patients. It is due to thickening of the sigmoid due to amoebiasis.

d. **Diverticulitis with mass** (Figs 24.135 and 24.136): Elderly patients are affected. Diverticuli can present with acute abdominal pain, high grade fever and abdominal distension due to perforation. The mass is inflammatory and very tender, with vague borders almost similar to left-sided appendicitis. History of flatulence, distension of the abdomen and bleeding per rectum are common. The mass is due to perforation of the diverticulum which gets sealed off soon. Diverticulitis is one of the examples for a cause for internal fistula (colovesical, colovaginal). Diagnosis is by CT scan. It should be managed conservatively with antibiotics, low residue diet and rest. Abscess should be aspirated with ultrasound guidance. First attack of diverticulitis can be managed conservatively and patient can be advised for follow up. Second attack will be an indication for surgery. Sigmoid colectomy is the treatment of choice. Some patients may be very sick. In such situations, drainage of pus followed by diversion colostomy is done. Once patient's condition is better, elective resection and anastomosis of the colon is done.

II. *Lymph nodes*

1. *Acute lymphadenitis:* Nodes are firm and tender. Fever with chills and rigors will give a clue to the diagnosis. Some infective focus in the limbs or skin of the gluteal region may be present. This is one place where careful history will help. Read the Clinical Case Capsule below.

■ Clinical Case Capsule

A 6-year-old child was admitted for fever, severe pain in the left iliac fossa and vomiting of 2 days duration. Clinical examination revealed tender nodular mass. Residents were thinking about the diagnosis and what to do next? Senior consultant asked child's mother—What precipitated these complaints. Mother replied that child had an injury to the leg and injections were given in the gluteal region. Diagnosis was acute infective lymphadenitis involving iliac group of lymph nodes.

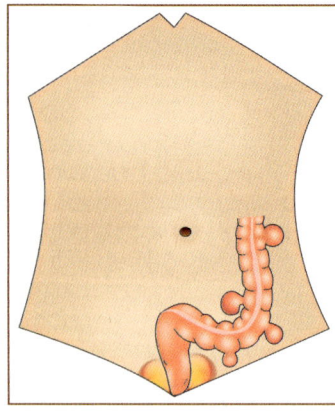

Fig. 24.135: Diagrammatic representation of sigmoid diverticuli

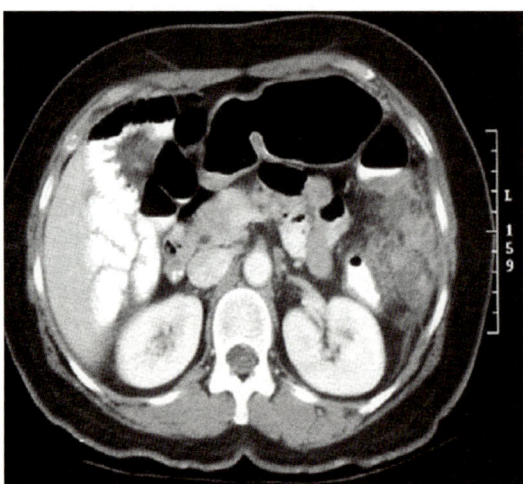

Fig. 24.136: Pericolic abscess secondary to diverticuli

2. *Lymphoma:* The lymph node mass is nodular, fixed, with or without enlargement of other group of lymph nodes and hepatosplenomegaly.

3. *Secondaries:* Iliac node enlargement is due to rectal carcinoma, ovarian carcinoma. Nodes are hard and nodular and often fixed.

III. *Retroperitoneal structures (already discussed)*

1. Sarcoma
2. Aneurysm
3. Iliopsoas abscess
4. Chondrosarcoma

IV. *In females*

1. Ovarian cyst (Figs 24.137 and 24.138)
2. Fibroid
3. Tubo-ovarian mass

From abnormal structures (already discussed)

1. *Undescended testis:* Seminoma
2. Unascended kidney

Authors' column: Thus, we have completed examination of all regions in the abdomen and differential diagnosis. However, certain interesting and specific masses have been discussed now because these are important. I hope you will like it.

THE CYSTIC MASS IN THE ABDOMEN

Intra-abdominal cystic swellings are interesting swellings. They occur in young children, adults, middle-aged persons. There are many cases of cystic swellings which have given a surprise at laparotomy (notoriously so in females). In children, cysts have confused many competent paediatricians. Being intra-abdominal cysts, it is not possible to elicit fluctuation and very often, they are firm due to increased tension. The details of important cystic swellings are given below.

▌ Clinical Case Capsule

A 2-year-child was shown to a paediatrician who diagnosed the case as ascites. Ultrasound also said it was ascites. Fluid was present in almost all regions. Ascitic tap was done, it was inconclusive. Paediatrician started the child on anti-tuberculous treatment (ATT) because he had seen many cases and tuberculosis is a common disease in India. After 3 months of ATT, the child was examined again, abdominal girth had increased with no relief. Paediatric surgeon who gave opinion said he could feel the wall of the cyst. This is not ascites but a large cyst occupying 9 quadrants. The child underwent surgery. A large cyst arising from greater omentum and occupying all 9 regions was removed. Histopathology was lymphatic cyst arising from omentum.

1. **Pseudocyst of pancreas** (Figs 24.137 and 24.138): Tensely cystic upper abdominal mass may feel firm and tender, and does not move with respiration. Getting above the swelling is possible. Transmitted pulsations of the aorta can be felt over the mass which disappears on knee-elbow position. History of acute pancreatitis or blunt injury abdomen gives the clue to the diagnosis.

2. **Hydatid cyst of liver** (Fig. 24.139): This swelling is of long duration, is symptomless or with dull pain in the upper abdomen. The cyst is spherical with smooth surface, rounded borders and feels firm. Since it is a mass arising from liver, it moves with respiration and getting above the swelling is not possible. Classical hydatid thrill, mentioned in the books, is rarely appreciated. Simple cyst of the liver can also present as a cystic mass (Fig. 24.139).

3. **Mesenteric cysts (for more details see page 397):** These are congenital cysts, enterogenous or chylolymphatic, manifest in young children or during adolescence. Typically, the cyst is located in the umbilical region which moves at right angles to the direction of mesentery.

   Types of mesenteric cyst (Clinical Box 24.10 and Fig. 24.140)
   a. *Chylolymphatic cyst* is a lymphatic cyst arising from mesentery of ileum. It is a thin-walled cyst with clear fluid or chyle. It has a separate blood supply. Hence, enucleation is the treatment without sacrificing the bowel.
   b. *Enterogenous cyst* is a duplication cyst from the intestine or due to diverticulum of the mesenteric border of the intestine. It is thick walled and contains mucus. This cyst is treated by excision of cyst with bowel segment because both share the same blood supply.

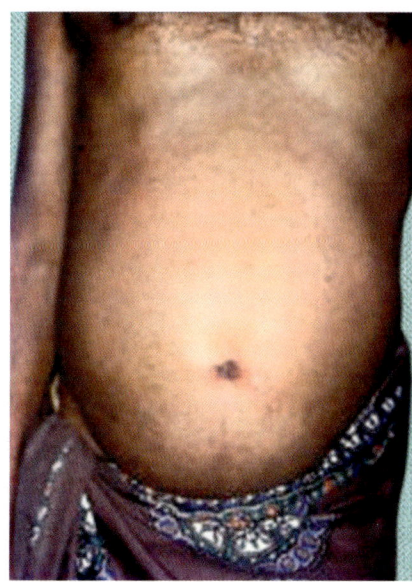

Fig. 24.137: Pseudocyst of pancreas—distension was more in the umbilical region

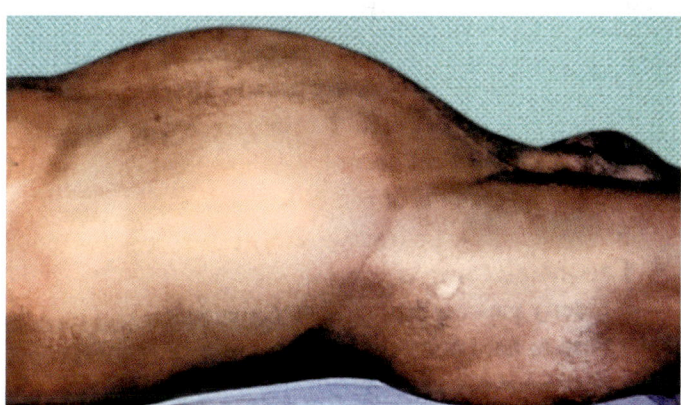

Fig. 24.138: Pseudocyst of pancreas. Distension was in the epigastrium and in the umbilical region

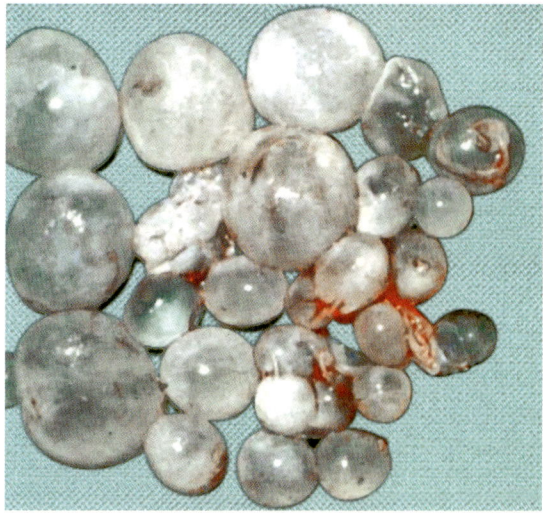

Fig. 24.139: Hydatid cyst

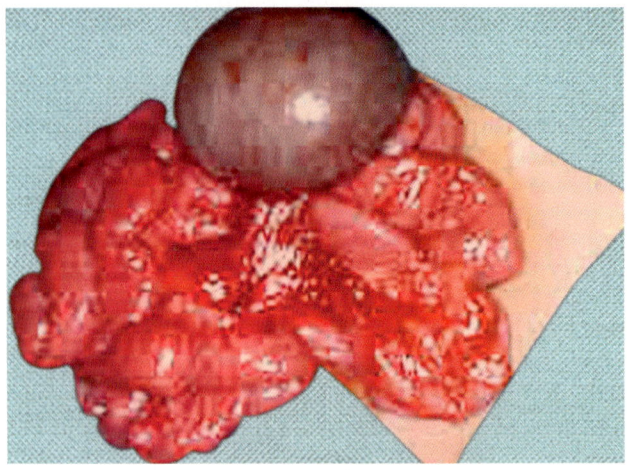

Fig. 24.140: Enterogenous cyst at surgery

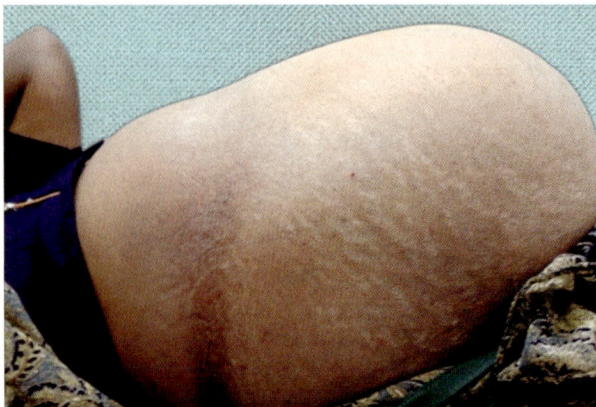

Fig. 24.141: Large right ovarian cyst filling all quadrants of the abdomen

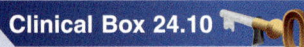

Clinical Box 24.10

Mesenteric cyst—types
- Chylolymphatic cyst
- Enterogenous cyst
- Urogenital remnant
- Teratomatous dermoid cyst

4. *Hydronephrosis:* Large hydronephrosis can attain a huge size without producing any symptoms. Bulk of the swelling is confined to one side of abdomen, with prominent bulge in the loin. It is difficult to elicit fluctuation in a tensely cystic intra-abdominal mass. Bimanual palpation and ballotability give the clue to the diagnosis. One of the large cysts of polycystic kidney can present as a large renal cyst.

5. *Ovarian cyst* (Figs 24.141 and 24.142): It is a freely mobile, firm or soft mass in any quadrant of the abdomen. Such ovarian cysts, once they come out of pelvis will have free mobility. On pushing **the mass upwards there will be traction** on the pedicle, which may result in pain (Fig. 24.28). In any female patient who presents with lower abdominal mass, ovarian mass has to be considered first, and only then consider other possibilities.

6. *Retroperitoneal lymphatic cyst:* Retroperitoneal cyst is one of the commonest of lymphatic cysts, which grows slowly to attain large size. Typically, it is painless, seen in young patients and is tensely cystic. The bowel loop may be felt over the mass (retroperitoneal mass), or bowel loops may be pushed to the side.

7. *Encysted ascites:* This consists of ascitic fluid loculated by many loops of intestine along with omentum. Loss of weight, fever, anorexia, emaciation are the other features.

8. *Rare cystic swellings in the abdomen* (Figs 24.143 and 24.144):
   - *Large serous cyst from the liver and omental cyst can give rise to abdominal distension. Omental cyst is usually a lymphatic cyst which occurs in children and can attain a huge size. Sudden enlargement indicates haemorrhage. Excision is easy.*

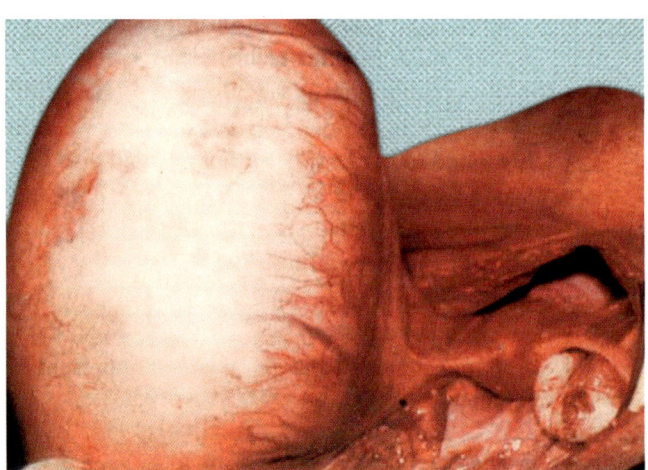

Fig. 24.142: Ovarian cyst

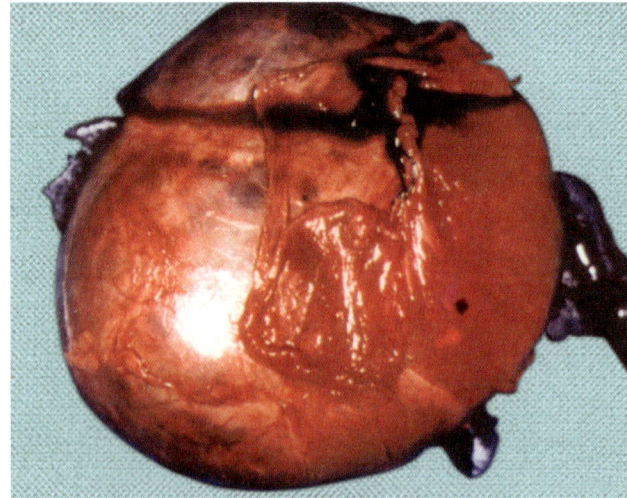

Fig. 24.143: Large lymphatic cyst arising from omentum

LARGE MASSES IN THE ABDOMEN

It is difficult to define large masses but generally, when a mass occupies almost 5–6 regions or quadrants, it is considered as

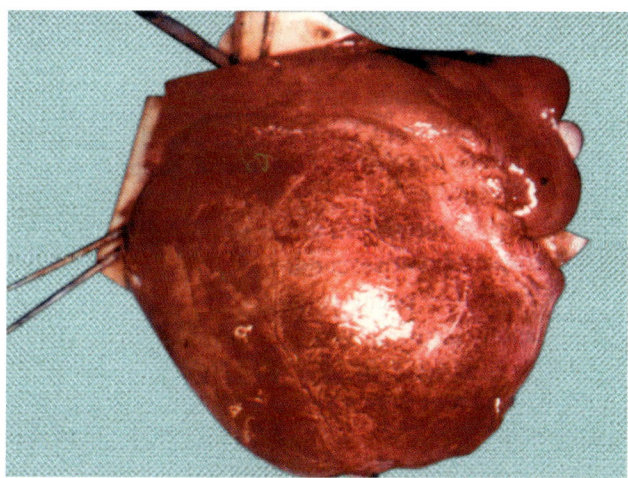

Fig. 24.144: Intra-abdominal cyst: Serous cyst in the liver

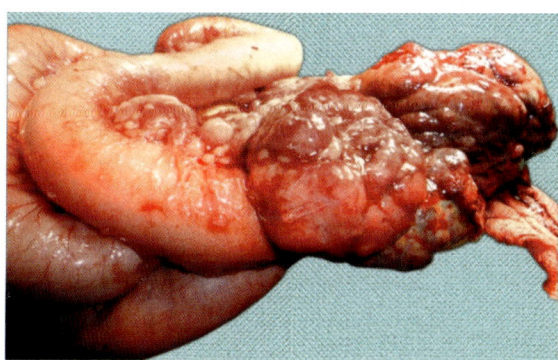

Fig. 24.145: Large intra-abdominal mass due to advanced carcinoma right colon

large mass. Following differential diagnosis should be considered in such cases

1. **Disseminated malignancy**: Majority of them arise from gastrointestinal tract. Either the presentation is late or multiple masses are due to recurrence.

2. **Large hepatomegaly**: This can occur in advanced hepatoma. More often seen when the liver is involved with multiple metastasis—secondaries in the liver. Other causes of massive enlargement are—large polycystic liver, portal hypertension, etc.

3. **Large GIST**: Stomach is the most common site of the GIST. It can attain huge size. However, it is mobile and firm.

4. **Retroperitoneal sarcoma**: These tumours are usually liposarcomas.

5. **Cystic swellings** (already discussed).

6. Large hydronephrosis which can be confused for ovarian cyst specially when it occupies 3–5 regions of the abdomen. (Refer to Clinical Case Capsule.)

THREE INTERESTING CLINICAL CASE CAPSULES

1. Clinical Case Capsule (Figs 24.28 and 24.29)

CME, Government Medical College, Mysore-2016

A 45-year-old lady presented with mass abdomen predominantly on the left side of the abdomen. Lower border was easily palpable. Following is the discussion by three senior faculty:

Faculty 1: Ovarian cyst can grow big size and occupy abdomen where it comes out from pelvis. Lower border can be felt easily. It is freely mobile. On percussion, dull note was heard all over the mass. Hence, it is a ovarian mass.

Faculty 2: Large swelling in the loin—renal pathology should be considered. Hydronephrosis feels firm (tensely cystic swelling. Even though there was no ballotability, it had a doubtful movement with respiration and some tympanitic note could be elicited.

Faculty 3: Retroperitoneal cyst because it has smooth surface, round borders and a tympanitic note could be elicited in a few areas. He also offered cystadenoma pancreas as another diagnosis

Final diagnosis

- A senior clinical professor said, it is hydronephrosis in unascended kidney. In fact, it was the correct proved later by CT/ultrasound. He said loin swelling started first.

- Slight movement with respiration, direction of enlargement suggests kidney mass. Since it did not have classical kidney features, it was unascended kidney. Hence, the final diagnosis was hydronephrosis.

A word of caution: Postgraduates are requested to give common diagnosis. for example, in this case ovarian cyst, hydronephrosis and retroperitoneal cyst.

2. Clinical Case Capsule (Figs 24.146 and 24.147)

A 30-year-old male, otherwise healthy, presented with intermittent episodes of melena and generalized weakness. He was pale. There was a mass palpable more laterally in the epigastrium. It was moving with respiration. It was looking like spleen but without any notch in the anterior border. Percussion note was resonant. The picture was confusing. The candidate wanted to give a diagnosis of portal hypertension with palpable spleen but clinical signs are not fitting in. Now look at the blackboard sketch and marking in the abdomen of patient. It was a more medially situated swelling. It was fitting in for a diagnosis of GIST of the stomach. It was proved after CECT scan and laparotomy.

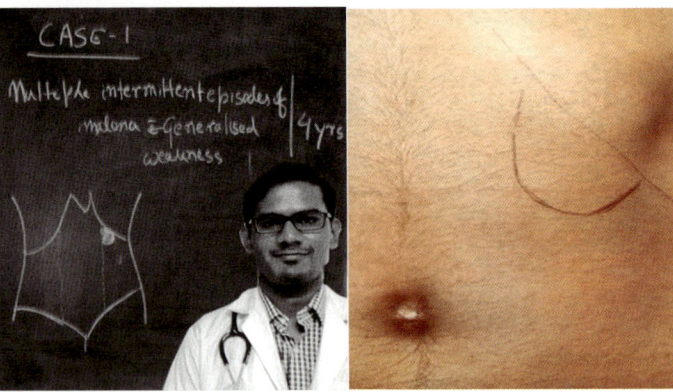

Fig. 24.146: Black board sketch of the mass abdomen.
Fig. 24.147: Mass is marked (*Courtesy:* Dr Nagesh Biradar, Asst Professor, Dept of Surgery, KMC, Manipal)

3. Clinical Case Capsule (Figs 148 and 24.149)

INTERESTING CASE OF MASS ABDOMEN

A 20-year-old lady with no previous medical history was admitted to the hospital with dull aching pain and mass in the abdomen of 20 days duration. She had one episode of vomiting containing food particles. She also had weight loss of 4 kg in the past 2 months. On examination, vitals were stable. On inspection, a visible swelling was noticed in the left upper quadrant of the abdomen. On palpation, a mass of size 20 × 15 cm was felt in left upper quadrant occupying left hypochondrium, epigastrium, umbilical region and left lumbar region. The mass moved with respiration, was firm and upper border could not be felt since fingers could not be inserted below left costal margin. No notch was felt, no pulsations were felt over the mass, the mass was not ballotable and not bimanually palpable. The mass was dull on percussion. Rest of the examination including systemic examination were normal.

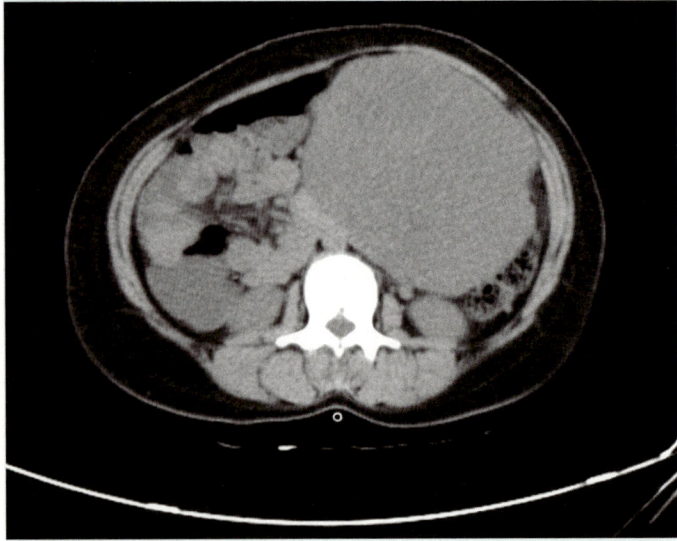

Fig. 24.148: CECT showing a large hypodense mass

Clinical discussion: What is the diagnosis?

Professor 1: Mostly it is **cystadenoma pancreas** because it is a large swelling in a young female. Tensely cystic intra-abdominal swelling, feel firm in consistency, lies close to spleen and hence moves with respiration. Mass is very large and hence upper border cannot be palpated.

Professor 2: It is **splenic mass,** may be some congenital masses such as splenic haemangioma, dermoid cyst etc, reasons being the location, free movement with respiration, finger insinuation was not possible and dull on percussion everywhere.

Professor 3: It is a **retroperitoneal mass, may be a sarcoma.** It is so large that stomach and intestines have been displaced and hence dull on percussion. It moves with respiration because it is close to spleen and diaphragm. She also has weight loss.

CT- scan report

A well-defined, heterogeneously enhancing, soft tissue hypodense mass lesion occupying the left retroperitoneum region which is very close and compressing on stomach anteriorly, spleen laterally, kidney posteriorly and looks like originating from pancreas. Possibility of solid pseudopapillary tumour of the pancreas.

Exploratory laparotomy: Retroperitoneal mass excision + splenectomy.

Histopathology diagnosis: Reactive nodular fibrous pseudotumour arising from retroperitoneum. Spleen and lymph node are free.

Lessons learnt from this mass abdomen

1. Try to give 2 or 3 differential diagnosis: In this case pancreas, spleen and retroperitoneum were considered.

2. Also explain the symptoms and signs after correlating your physical findings. Patient had vomiting and loss of weight. She was probably not able to eat properly due to extrinsic compression on the stomach. Patient never had backache.

3. Do not give histological diagnosis in your university examination as given here. Think of common conditions arising from the organ with relevance to the age of the patient and symptoms. Remember, abdomen is called a Pandora's box.

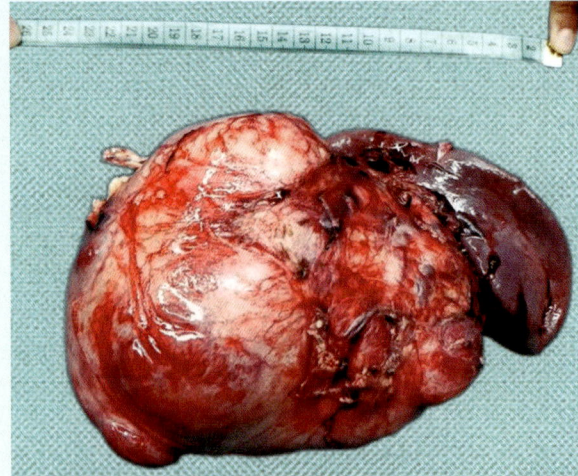

Fig. 24.149: Retroperitoneal mass excised along with spleen (*Courtesy:* Dr Richa Todi, Dr Keerthan Upadhya, Dr Sunilkrishna KMC, Manipal)

25

Examination of Anorectal Case

INTRODUCTION

Usually, these are the cases not kept in the clinical examination but definitely these cases are encountered in the outpatient department. These cases have some common complaints which can be grouped as rectal complaints. They are bleeding per rectum, discharge per rectum, discharge around the anal opening, itching around the anal canal, altered bowel habits and sometimes a mass coming out of the rectum (prolapse rectum or prolapse piles). Also rectal and anal canal diseases are very common problems. Hence, students should have clear picture about all these conditions.

Before examining the anorectum, some important anatomical considerations of the anal canal have to be studied. Anal canal is about 4 cm long. It is divided by the dentate line into surgical and anatomical anal canal.

COMPARISON OF ANAL CANAL ABOVE AND BELOW THE DENTATE LINE

Note: Understanding these differences will help the students and surgeons to do the complete

Above the dentate line	Below the dentate line
• Surgical anal canal	Anatomical anal canal
• Postallantoic gut	Proctodeum
• Cuboidal epithelium	Stratified squamous epithelium
• Pink	Pale or skin colour
• Parasympathetic nerve supply—no pain	Spinal nerves—painful
• Portal system	Systemic system
• Para-aortic nodes	Superficial and deep inguinal lymph nodes

examination and also help in better knowledge about the diseases. *Example*: If any suspicious lesion such as malignant melanoma is detected in the lower anal canal (Fig. 25.1), inguinal nodes have to be examined. Haemorrhoids occur above the dentate line (parasympathetic nerves) hence are painless but fissure occurs in the lower anal canal (spinal nerves) hence are very painful. **(Please study the two Clinical Case Capsules given in the next page)**.

COMPLAINTS: HISTORY OF PRESENT ILLNESS

- *Bleeding*: This is one of the common complaints. When did it occur? How many times? Was it bright red in colour? Did you notice the blood after

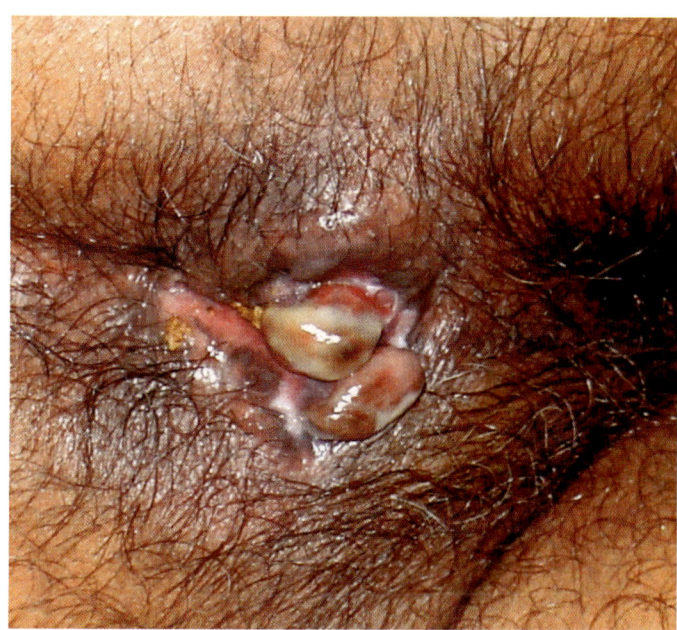

Fig. 25.1: Separation of buttocks revealed purplish black swellings. A case of malignant melanoma

Clinical Case Capsules

1. A 38-year-old female was getting treatment for itching and burning in and around anal canal for 2 months with ointments and sitz bath. After 2 months, she developed inguinal lymph nodes. Initially, they were treated as infective and antibiotics were given. There was no response. Swelling was increasing. Postgraduate who examined the case considered possible causes of enlargement of lymph nodes such as infective, tuberculosis and lymphoma. He could not correlate the anal complaints. He examined the anal canal and saw a few swellings which he diagnosed as purplish-black prolapsed piles. **Biopsy of the inguinal lymph nodes confirmed malignant melanoma of the anal canal.** In cases of persisting inguinal lymph-adenopathy, keep in mind lesions of the anal canal also in addition to lesions in the limb, abdominal wall, and scrotal skin (Fig. 25.1).

2. A 28-year-old boy with recurrent abdominal pain was diagnosed to have a mass in the umbilical region. Careful examination revealed a tympanic mass and it was contracting. Was it intestinal obstruction? What can the mass be? Tuberculosis or malignancy. While doing general physical examination, there were a few pigmented spots in the lips. Postgraduate student who examined this case did not give importance to this finding. He was asked whether he had done rectal examination. He said, yes and it was normal. He had done the rectal examination but had not inspected the anal region carefully after spreading the buttocks apart. There was also pigmentation of the anal skin. This was a case of Peutz-Jeghers syndrome and the contracting bowel mass was due to intussusception. (*Courtesy:* Prof. Sreevatsa, MS Ramaiah Medical Collage, Bangalore).

passing stools or was it mixed with stools? What about quantity? Was it a few drops, a few ml or was it massive? Was the bleeding associated with pain? Fresh bleeding without pain after defaecation—what is described **as splash in the pan is due to haemorrhoids** (Clinical Box 25.1). Fresh blood—a drop of blood, associated with pain at the end of defaecation is usually due to fissure-in-ano. Fresh bleeding in a child is due to juvenile polyps. Blood mixed with stools is an indication of bleeding coming from the colon as typically happens in carcinoma colon. Blood and mucus mixed with stools indicates carcinoma colon. **Bloody slime** refers to mucus with streaks of blood. Frequent stools with blood and mucus for months indicate inflammatory bowel diseases such as

---

Clinical Box 25.1

- Splash in the pan—haemorrhoids
- Drops of blood—fissure-in-ano
- Blood and mucus—long duration—ulcerative colitis
- Fresh bleeding in elderly—diverticular disease
- Blood mixed with stools—carcinoma colon
- Fresh bleeding in a child—Juvenile polyp

---

ulcerative colitis. Often these patients are young, emaciated, anaemic and look unwell. Diverticular disease of the colon can also give rise to fresh bleeding separate from stools—sometimes in small quantity and sometimes with **massive bleeding**.

- *Altered bowel habits*: Do you have diarrhoea or constipation? Anorectal lesions which are proliferative will give rise to mucus diarrhoea with bleeding. Typical example is growth in the ampulla of rectum. There is a partial obstruction with bleeding and mucus. Overnight accumulation of large quantity of mucus results in distension of the ampulla of rectum which causes an urgency to pass stools in the morning—what has been called **early morning spurious diarrhoea.** This can also be associated with tenesmus—painful straining of stools without good result. Stricture at rectosigmoid junction gives rise to increasing constipation. Stools are hard and less in quantity. Patient says he has to strain a lot.

- *Discharge per rectum*: Purulent discharge around the anus indicates fistula-in-ano. Usually, there is no pain. Patients complain of pain, if the fistula gets blocked partially, gets infected and an abscess is developed. Passage of large quantity of mucus indicates Crohn's disease, severe colitis (amoebic, bacillary) or colloid carcinoma rectum.

- *Pain*: All problems which occur below the dentate line or Hilton's line are painful—classical example being fissure-in-ano (anatomical anal canal—last 2 cm) and painless when they occur above the dentate line, example being haemorrhoids (surgical anal canal). What is the nature of the pain? Is it severe or throbbing? Severe pain which starts with act of defaecation and persists even after defaecation for about half an hour suggests fissure-in-ano. In fact, many patients describe it as burning in nature. Throbbing pain indicates anorectal abscess. Another severe painful condition is ischiorectal abscess typically common in diabetic patients. Often the patient is ill with high grade fever and unable to sit. Following are a few dictums that must be remembered.

A. *Carcinoma rectum is painless*: Pain indicates infiltration into surrounding structures. Severe backache and pain radiating down the legs indicate carcinoma rectum infiltrating the sacral plexus of nerves.

B. *Haemorrhoids are painless*: Pain indicates thrombosed piles.

C. Fistula-in-ano is painless: Pain indicates it is blocked and abscess is present.

- **Prolapse:** It is common for patients with haemorrhoids to tell you that when they strain at stools, something comes out. It is usually prolapsed piles. Often it goes inside spontaneously. Ask the patient whether it goes inside spontaneously or does he have to do it manually. Sometimes the patient can present with severe pain in and around anus and a prolapsed pile which is irreducible. It is a surgical emergency. Prolapsed rectum should not be confused for prolapsed piles. This can be made out on inspection. If a child is brought with prolapsing reddish pile mass like lesion, it is a **pedunculated polyp.**

- **Pruritus ani:** Do you have itching around anal opening? Most important cause of itching in and around anus is mucus discharge. Fistula-in-ano, colloid carcinoma rectum, and Crohn's disease are a few causes. **In females, vaginal infections such as moniliasis and** *Trichomonas vaginalis* **have to be ruled out.** In children, threadworm infections are common. Poor hygiene, lack of cleanliness, excessive sweating and wearing tight and rough underclothing are common causes. Psychoneurosis allergy, and diabetes are the other causes.

Clinical Wisdom

Sexually transmitted diseases such as herpes, anal warts and HIV infection must be excluded in all cases of pruritus ani.

INSPECTION OF THE ANAL REGION

- Explain to the patient what you are doing.
- A nurse should always be present.
- Good illumination is a must.
- In the left lateral position, anal region is inspected by separating the gluteal folds.
- Always use double gloves.

Conditions which can be diagnosed by inspection alone (refer to page 416):

- **Anal tag of skin:** They do not reflect any particular pathology.
- **Sentinel pile:** It is not a pile but a hypertrophied skin present in the midline posteriorly at the distal most end of the anal fissure. (Sentinel pile is a misnomer.)
- **Anal fissure:** A longitudinal ulcer may be visible when the gluteal folds are separated. It is fissure-in-ano—typically located in the midline posteriorly.

- **Piles can be seen only when they are prolapsed outside:** They may be blackish, if patients come late due to strangulation of the pile masses or if external piles can be seen (Fig. 25.2).

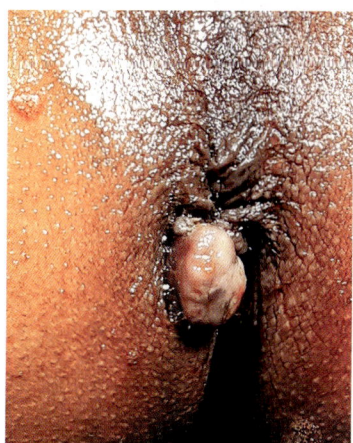

Fig. 25.2: External piles are visible on inspection

- **Fistula-in-ano:** The external opening of the fistula is noted anteriorly or posteriorly. Note whether there is a single opening or there are multiple openings. Note any discharge from the opening. Refer **Goodsall's rule for the direction of the fistula** (page 421).

- **Anal carcinoma:** Anal carcinoma is uncommon. It is an **epithelioma** and can present as a proliferative growth.

- **Malignant melanoma** of the anal canal presents as a pigmented ulcerative lesion or a pigmented swelling which can be confused for a prolapsed pile mass (many patients present late with inguinal nodes).

- **Condylomas** are papilliferous lesions—these are of 2 types. Pedunculated condylomas are due to viral aetiology. These can spread over a large area in the perineum. These are self-limiting. These are called **condyloma acuminata. In secondary syphilis,** condylomas are flat, raised, white, hypertrophic epithelium and classically located at the mucocutaneous junction of the anus. These are called **condyloma lata.**

- Rarely **intussusception** can be seen outside, especially in paediatrics age group.

- Pigmentation of the perianal region is characteristic of **Peutz-Jeghers syndrome.**

- Prolapse rectum can be diagnosed.

- Diagrammatic representation of various lesions has been given in Fig. 25.3.

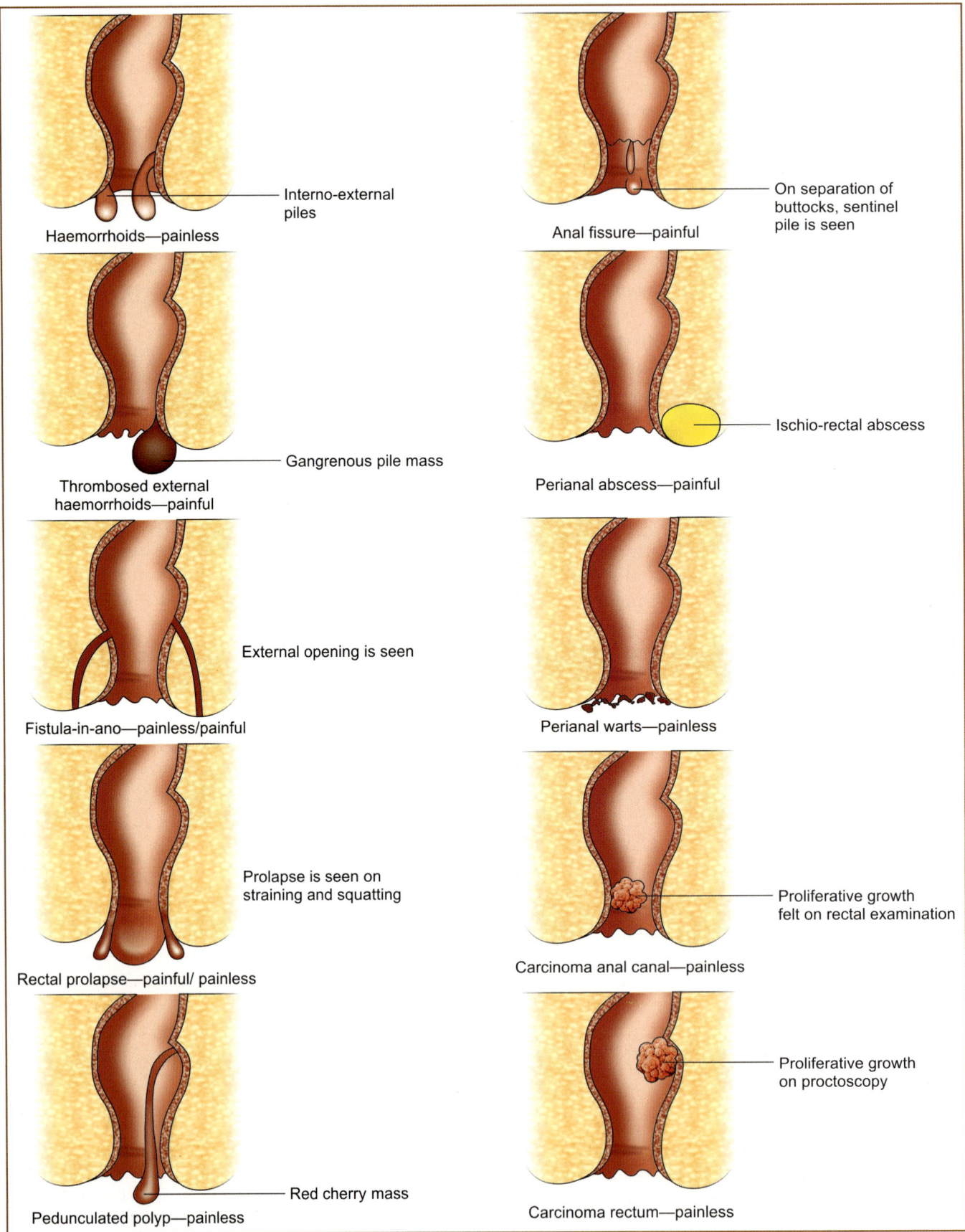

Interno-external piles

Haemorrhoids—painless

Gangrenous pile mass

Thrombosed external haemorrhoids—painful

External opening is seen

Fistula-in-ano—painless/painful

Prolapse is seen on straining and squatting

Rectal prolapse—painful/ painless

Red cherry mass

Pedunculated polyp—painless

On separation of buttocks, sentinel pile is seen

Anal fissure—painful

Ischio-rectal abscess

Perianal abscess—painful

Perianal warts—painless

Proliferative growth felt on rectal examination

Carcinoma anal canal—painless

Proliferative growth on proctoscopy

Carcinoma rectum—painless

Fig. 25.3: Common diseases of anorectum. These are the common anal/perianal conditions which can be diagnosed by inspection. A few can also be diagnosed by palpation and by per rectal examination/proctoscopic examination

RECTAL EXAMINATION

Various positions for rectal examination:

1. *Left lateral position*: Most common.

2. *Right lateral*: Inconvenient position as majority of the surgeons are right handed. However, pelvirectal growths fall towards anal side and hence can be palpated sometimes.

3. *Knee elbow position*: This method can be followed to palpate prostate and seminal vesicles.

4. *Dorsal position*: Often patients are sick and one has to do the rectal examination—it may be a case of impacted faeces or bleeding per rectum. In such cases, patient lies down supine. Flex the hip. Right hand and forearm are passed under the patient's thigh and rectal examination is carried out. At the same time, the left hand can be used to palpate the suprapubic region or lower abdomen for any pelvic mass.

- **Explain to the patient what you plan to do** (Fig. 25.4). Provide him with privacy. The most popular and commonly used position is **left lateral position—called Sims position.** Both hips and knees are well flexed. Buttocks should project over the edge of the table. Inspect the anal opening first. Lubricate the finger with lignocaine jelly. Spread the jelly all around the anal opening. Gently apply pressure on the external sphincter (anal opening) and slowly introduce the finger. Polyps, papillomas, carcinomatous growths, strictures, and thrombosed piles can be felt. Poor sphincter tone as in prolapse rectum, and spinal cord paralysis cannot be missed.

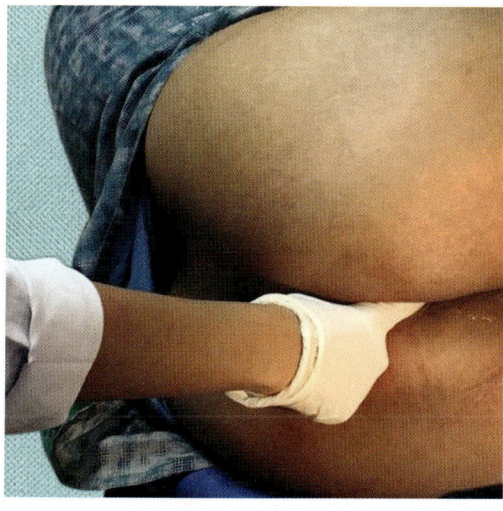

Fig. 25.4: Digital rectal examination

- *Severe pain while doing a rectal examination indicates acute fissure-in-ano. Better avoid proctoscopic examination in such cases.*

- It is possible to insert examining finger between anal margin and intussusception but not in a case of prolapse rectum.

- Gloved finger when withdrawn, if stained with blood is an indication of bleeding per rectum. Causes are given later in this chapter.

Findings at Rectal Examination

They can be classified as those within the lumen, at the wall and outside the wall.

1. *In the lumen*: In vast majority of cases, one will feel normal stools, which are typically brownish yellow in colour and soft.

   - **Impacted stools** suggest some fault at the normal physiology. Either peristalsis is weak as in Hirschsprung disease or due to paralysis (patients with paraplegia or quadriplegia) or due to drugs which are used to treat psychiatric illness. Hot climatic conditions, elderly patients, less water intake and postponement of defaecation also contribute to constipation and hard stools. Sometimes they may be confused for mechanical obstruction and almost get operated. Absence of colicky and severe pain and haemodynamic instability will negate a mechanical obstruction (*refer* to Clinical Box 25.2).

   - **Rectum is empty and ballooned** out in intestinal obstruction.

   - Surprising findings can be a **foreign body** in the rectum. This could have been inserted by the patient himself (again they are psychiatric patients) or occasionally fish bone and even chicken bone also.

2. *Examination of the wall of the rectum*: Once finger is introduced inside the rectum gently, rotate it all around. Within 2 cm of the anal canal inter-

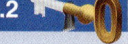

Clinical Box 25.2

Impacted stools
- Peristalsis is weak
- Paralysis—hemiplegia/paraplegia
- **P**sychiatric illness
- **P**oor hydration
- **P**ostponement of defaecation
- Observe 5 **P**s

sphincteric groove can be felt between internal and external sphincters. One can ask the patient to voluntarily tighten the sphincter. The tone of the sphincter, groove can be easily appreciated. An ulcer, growth, polyps can be detected.

- *Ulcer*: First note any ulcer in the anal canal or rectum. Painful tear or ulcer is **due to fissure.** The most important one being **carcinoma** rectum or anal canal. Typically, an irregular indurated ulcer can be felt in cases of carcinoma rectum. It bleeds on touch. Other causes are **sexually transmitted diseases. Solitary rectal ulcer** is not uncommon. It presents as bleeding per rectum. Blood is fresh red. Ulcer mimics malignancy. Biopsy will confirm the diagnosis.

- *Growth*: Majority of cases of carcinoma rectum can be easily felt by digital rectal examination. Typically, they are ulcerative or ulceroproliferative lesions cauliflower-like lesions. They **are friable and bleed on touch.** Feel the growth all around. Try moving the lesions. They move with mucosa. Hard, indurated, fixed lesions in the rectum are not uncommon. Patients come to the hospital late thinking that bleeding is due to haemorrhoids.

  Fixity anteriorly to prostate, seminal vesicles in males and posterior vaginal wall in females and posteriorly to sacrum, reflect advanced nature of the disease.

- *Adenomatous polyps*: These are benign lesions that can be felt. They are premalignant. They can be sessile or pedunculated. Larger the adenoma, higher are the chances of malignancy. A polyp which is irregular and hard should be considered malignant and investigated further. When more than hundred polyps are found, it is a case of familial polyposis coli.

- *Juvenile polyp*: This can be felt in children.

3. *Examination of the outer (surrounding) part of rectum*

- *Posteriorly*: This surface is easily felt and first one to be felt also. Sacrum and coccyx are the bones felt here. Try moving a growth, if felt, over the bone. Fixity to these bones by carcinoma makes it fairly advanced growth and necessitates neo-adjuvant chemoradiation followed by surgery. Many such patients have backache and radiating pain down the legs. Coccydynia is a condition wherein there is persistent dull aching pain over the coccyx region and it is worse on sitting posture. Sacrococcygeal teratoma and post-anal dermoid are the other swellings palpable in this location.

- *Laterally*: Laterally, one will feel side wall of the pelvis. Again fixation to side wall of the pelvis should be checked for carcinoma rectum. Ovarian tumours or cysts can be felt in the side wall of the pelvis (better felt per vaginal). In pelvic appendicitis, tenderness is present in the right lateral wall of the rectum during rectal examination. It has been called **differential tenderness**.

- *Anteriorly*: Normally, cervix can be palpable anteriorly. In males, urinary bladder, prostate, and seminal vesicles are the structures. Fixation of growth to these structures indicates advanced disease. **In tuberculosis, seminal vesicles can be palpable and they are thickened and irregular.** Advanced cases of carcinoma rectum infiltrating posterior vaginal wall can be felt and appreciated by rectal examination. Tender boggy swelling anteriorly may be due to pelvic abscess.

Proctoscopy—Diagnostic and Therapeutic

Do a *per* rectal examination and rule out painful condition (*fissure-in-ano*). Introduce the proctoscope with the obturator to full length. Withdraw the obturator slowly, use good illumination and note down the findings (Fig. 25.5).

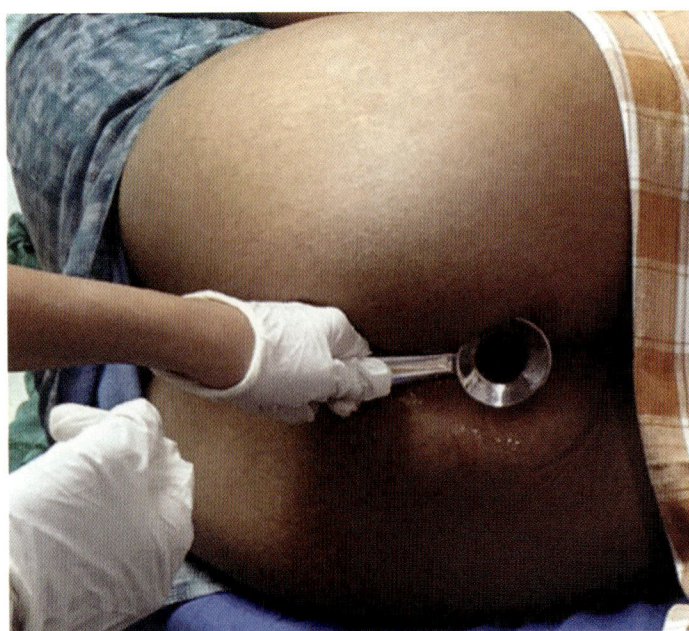

Fig. 25.5: Proctoscopy examination

- **Piles** are seen bulging into the lumen as **obturator is withdrawn. They are red cherry-like masses. With proctoscope in place,** pile masses can be injected with sclerosants (therapeutic use).

- **Growth** in the rectum can be visualised and a biopsy is usually taken. It easily bleeds as biopsy is taken.

- **Multiple, small, superficial pinpoint ulcers** in the rectum are due to ulcerative colitis. Biopsy is done.

- **Solitary ulcer** in the rectum can mimic malignancy. However, characteristic induration is missing.

- **Pelvic abscess** is diagnosed as boggy swelling in the anterior wall of the rectum. It can be drained through rectum.

Sigmoidoscopy (Figs 25.6 and 25.7)

- An enema is given before procedure.

- Flexible sigmoidoscope is 60 cm long. After doing a proctoscopy, the sigmoidoscope is introduced slowly under vision. Air insufflation helps in distension of the lumen so that the scope can be negotiated through curves of the rectum and sigmoid.

- **At no time should the scope be forced into the lumen.** By repeated advancement and withdrawal, the difficult bends, such as rectosigmoid junction, can be negotiated.

- Growth, ulcers, bleeding diverticulae, polyps, colitis can be diagnosed and biopsy can be taken. It may deflate and derotate sigmoid volvulus. Coagulation of bleeders and endoscopic polypectomy are the other uses of sigmoidoscopy.

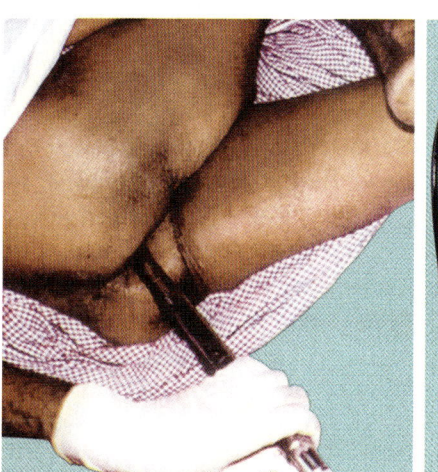 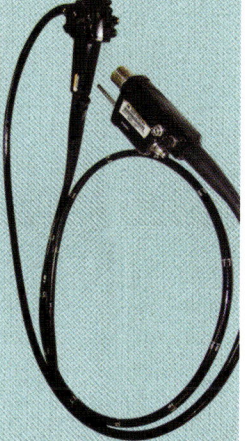

Fig. 25.6: Rigid sigmoidoscopy (almost abandoned now).
Fig. 25.7: Flexible sigmoidoscopy

- Suspect perforation **if a 'giving way' feeling is experienced by** the surgeon, if the patient experiences severe pain or intraperitoneal contents are seen. If perforation is suspected, X-ray abdomen, followed by treatment as per guidelines for colonic perforation should be initiated, urgently.

> **Clinical Wisdom**
>
> Digital rectal examination, proctoscopy and sigmoidoscopy are termed extended clinical examination.

DIFFERENTIAL DIAGNOSIS

1. *Haemorrhoids*: Most common anal canal lesions are haemorrhoids or piles. Painless fresh bleeding per rectum is the common presentation. Typically, a patient is male, young or old who complains of bleeding after the stools—what is described as **splash in the pan.** Bleeding is small in quantity and fresh red. As the condition advances, the pile masses slowly prolapse outside and go inside spontaneously. When they prolapse outside and cannot be replaced in, it is called as thrombosed piles. It produces severe pain. **Haemorrhoids cannot be diagnosed by digital examination unless thrombosed.** They are diagnosed during slow withdrawal of the obturator of the proctoscope. Slowly the pink red masses of piles, prolapse into the lumen of the rectum.

Grades of haemorrhoids

I. *Never prolapse*: Bleeding per rectum (Fig. 25.8)

II. *Prolapse on defaecation*: Something coming down and going back spontaneously (Fig. 25.9)

III. *Prolapse on defaecation*: Something coming down, but requires manual reduction. There is also bleeding, mucus discharge and pruritus.

IV. *Permanently prolapsed*: Acute pain, throbbing discomfort (Figs 25.10 and 25.11).

Treatment of Haemorrhoids

- Grade 1 haemorrhoids are conservative provided the bleeding is rare. Avoid constipation, add bulk purgatives and avoid spicy food. Grade 2 piles can be treated with Barron's band application or surgery. Grade 2 and 3 can be managed with excision—also called open haemorrhoidectomy. Recent surgery includes Stapler haemorrhoidopexy. Grade 4 haemorrhoids or thrombosed haemorrhoids are surgical emergencies. Treatment includes admission, rest, elevation of foot end of the bed, sitz bath, application of local anaesthetic agents such as lignocaine to the anal and perianal region and antibiotics. Generally, it takes 3 to 4 days for inflammation to settle down. Haemorrhoidectomy can be considered after this or it can be delayed by one or two weeks.

- Use of harmonic scalpel reduces significant blood loss in large long-standing grades 3 and 4 haemorrhoids.

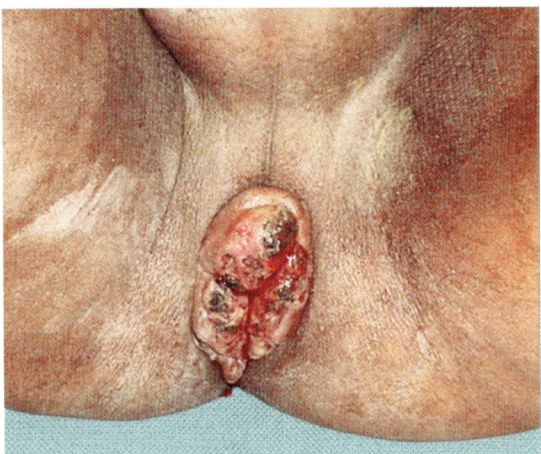

Fig. 25.8: Haemorrhoids at 3, 7, 11 o'clock position

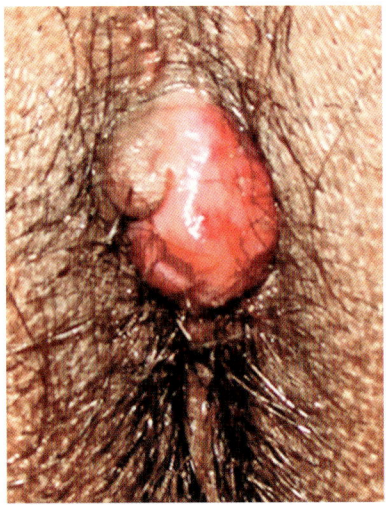

Fig. 25.9: Grade 3 piles which can be reduced

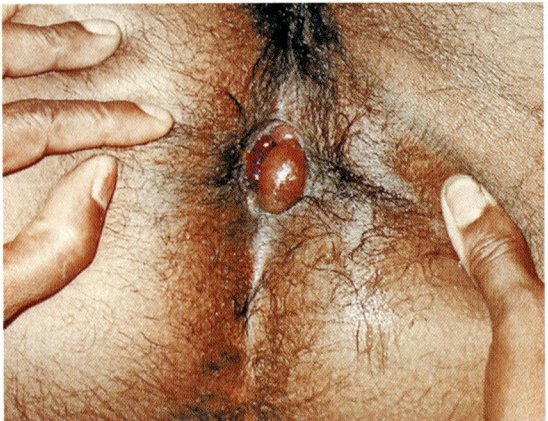

Fig. 25.10: Thrombosed external pile mass

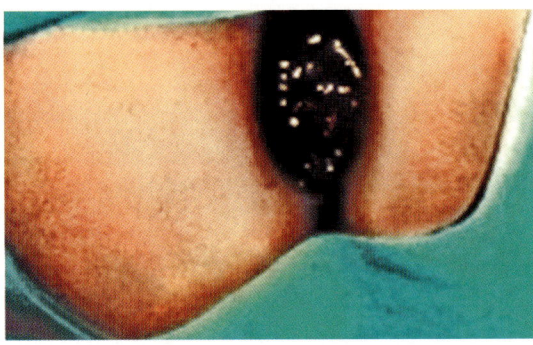

Fig. 25.11: Strangulated pile masses (grade 4 piles)

Clinical Wisdom

In all cases of recently diagnosed piles, do sigmoidoscopy to rule out a carcinoma rectum/sigmoid colon.

2. ***Fissure-in-ano***: Chronic fissure-in-ano is diagnosed by severe pain during defaecation, drop of blood at the end of defaecation and a tear at the lower anal canal. Posterior fissure is more common in men. In women, anterior fissure can also be seen (following delivery). Pain is severe, burning in nature, starts with the act of defaecation and lasts even after defaecation for a few minutes. Pain, constipation and internal muscle spasm form chain-like events thus resulting in chronicity of the condition. Diagnosis is clear while separating the buttocks—a canoe-shaped ulcer-crack is visible in the posterior part of anal canal. Hypertrophied skin—described in chronic conditions as **sentinel pile** is also seen. Rectal examination is painful and internal sphincter tone is very tight. It is treated with sitz bath, application of local anaesthetic agents such as lignocaine to the anal and perianal region and stool softening agents. In refractory cases, lateral sphincterotomy is the best surgery wherein a longitudinal cut

is given to internal sphincter around 8 o'clock position. It decreases spasm of internal sphincter and allows the fissure to heal. Refer to Table 25.1 to know the differences between acute and chronic fissure-in-ano.

3. ***Fistula-in-ano***: As soon as patient is positioned in lateral position, the diagnosis is made by visualisation of external opening. It can be single/multiple, with pouting granulation tissue, may discharge blood. Persistent seropurulent discharge keeps the part always wet. Previous history of anal gland infection, with recurrent abscess is the usual feature. Digital rectal examination reveals internal opening that is felt as a 'button hole' defect inside the rectum. Colloid carcinoma rectum can present with features of fistula—hence rule out carcinoma rectum. ***When tuberculosis is the aetiology, fistulae are not indurated and there is watery discharge not pus*** (Clinical Box 25.3) ***and this can be multiple*** (Fig. 25.12).

Clinical Box 25.3

Special types of fistula-in-ano
- **F**istula carcinoma
- **I**leitis—Crohn's
- **S**chistosomiasis
- **T**uberculosis
- **U**lcerative colitis
- **L**ymphogranuloma venereum
- **A**nal fissure abscess

Students can remember as FISTULA

Table 25.1: Differences between acute fissure in ano and chronic fissure in ano

Acute	*Chronic*
• Sudden onset—example after vaginal delivery or following hard stools	• A few months duration of symptoms
• Acute pain in the anal canal, severe burning after defaecation with bleeding	• Chronic pain in the anal canal, burning after defaecation with bleeding—few exacerbations
• No itching around anal opening	• Itching is usually present due to ulcer or hypertrophied skin— sentinel pile
• Severe sphincter spasm, small crack in the lower anal canal	• Sphincter spasm, chronic canoe-shaped ulcer in the lower anal canal
• No sentinel pile—tag of skin	• Sentinel pile—tag of skin is present
• PR: Very painful	• PR: Painful
• Proctoscopy—better to not try insertion	• Proctoscope—can be done with proper lignocaine application to the anal canal
• Usually responds to conservative treatment—local application of glyceryl trinitrate (GTN) 0.2% 3–4 times a day or diltiazem 2% twice a day	• Responds to conservative treatment but effect is temporary. Surgery is the treatment of choice
• Emergency sphincterotomy may be required in a few patients	• Lateral sphincterotomy or other procedures may be required

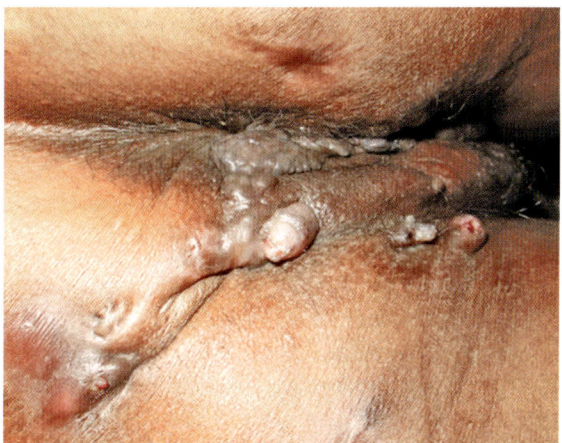

Fig. 25.12: Multiple fistulae due to tuberculosis

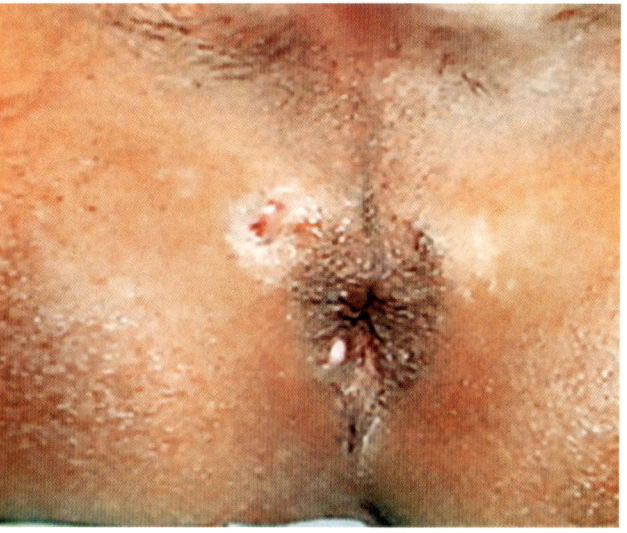

Fig. 25.13: Low fistula-in-ano

Various causes of special types of fistula can be remembered as **FISTULA** as given in Clinical Box 25.3. Fistulae are classified under **standard classification or Park's classification.** Subcutaneous, submucous, low anal (Fig. 25.13), high anal and pelvirectal are fistulae under standard classification and Intersphincteric, transsphincteric and supralevator under Park's classification. Refer **Goodsall's rule** to study the types of fistula and their significance. MRI (Fig. 25.15) is the best investigation specially in cases of high, supralevator and intersphincteric fistulae. Low fistulae can be treated with fistulectomy (Fig. 25.16) and high fistulae with fistulotomy. Rarely, diversion colostomy may be necessary to treat multiple high fistulae. Repeated and recurrent fistulae, as in Crohn's disease, are difficult problems to treat. Seton placement and tightening is a good, less traumatic alternative treatment.

Goodsall's rule: A fistula, with an external opening in the anterior half of anus within 3.75 cm tends to be direct type and in the posterior half, it is indirect type, curved or sometimes horseshoe type. It may communicate with the opposite side (Fig. 25.14).

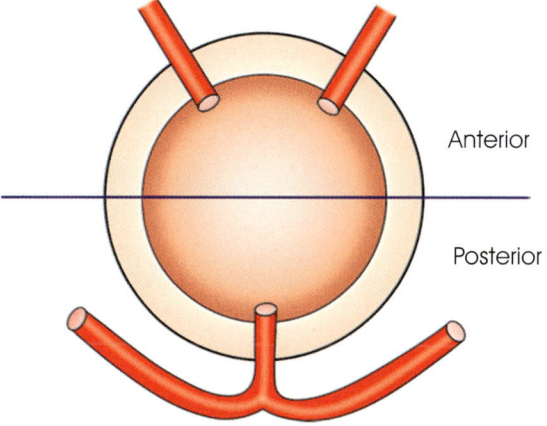

Anterior

Posterior

Fig. 25.14: Goodsall's rule

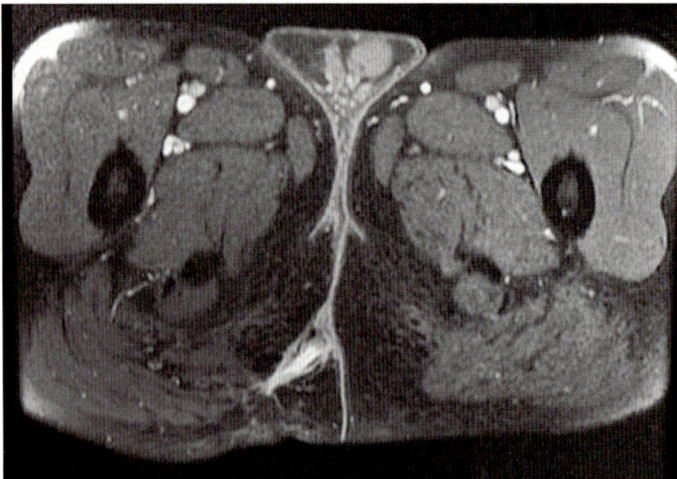

Fig. 25.15: MRI showing low fistula in ano. (*Courtesy:* Dr Rajgopal, Head, Dept of Radiology, KMC, Manipal)

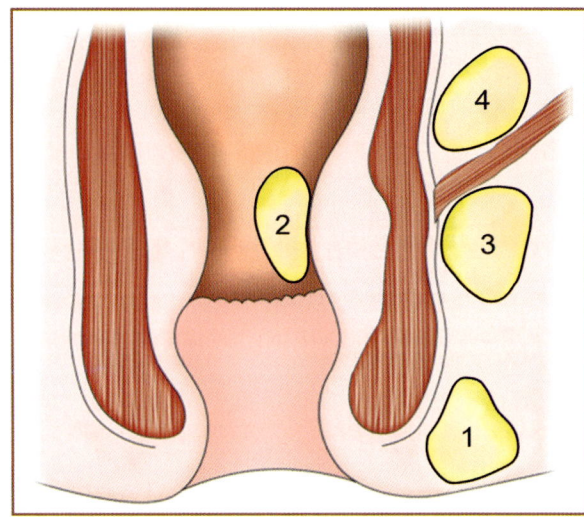

Fig. 25.17: Four types of anorectal abscess

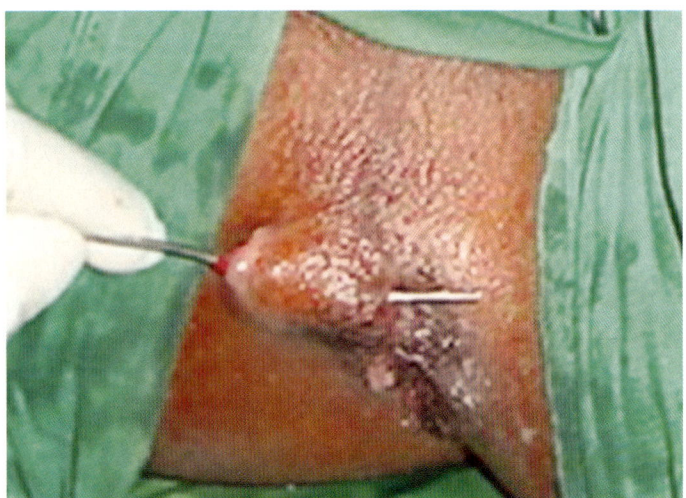

Fig. 25.16: Fistulectomy is being done

5. *Prolapse rectum:* Two types:
   A. **Partial prolapse** (Fig. 25.18): Protrusion of the mucous membrane or the entire rectum outside the anal verge. This condition is common in children and elderly patients. Prolapse can be partial or complete. When protrusion is between 1.25 and 3.75 cm, it is partial prolapse and it is mainly a mucosal prolapse. Any form of strain including **whooping cough or excessive straining** or due to **habitual constipation can give rise to partial prolapse of rectum.** It can follow an attack of diarrhoea resulting in **loss of fat** in the ischiorectal fossae, which support the rectum.
   B. **Complete/total prolapse** is also called procidentia (Fig. 25.19). Factors have been summarised below.
      • *Pelvic floor:* Weakness of pelvic floor can be due to birth injuries or collagen maturation.
      • *Large lateral ligaments:* These ligaments are condensation of pelvic fascia on each side of the rectum.
      • *Deep rectovesical pouch* is often found in prolapse rectum.

4. *Anorectal abscess:* This is more common in men especially diabetic. Blood-borne infection is common in diabetic patients. It mostly originates from the anal gland opening at the base of the anal crypts. Typically, patients present with high grade fever with chills and rigors. On examination, a tender, indurated swelling is found in the perianal region or in the ischiorectal fossa. Culture usually shows *E. coli* in about 70–80% of cases. *Staphylococcus aureus, Streptococcus, and Bacteroides* are the other organisms. Four types have been identified (Fig. 25.17). They are perianal abscess (1), ischiorectal abscess (3) (these two are common), submucous abscess (2) and pelvic abscess (4). Fever, throbbing pain and indurated tender swelling in the perianal region or ischiorectal fossa clinch the diagnosis. Rectal examination may reveal tender boggy swelling under anal mucosa as in perianal abscess. Ischiorectal abscess is surgical emergency. It should be treated by drainage as soon as possible. Control of diabetes is an important step in the management of ischiorectal abscess. Diabetic ketoacidosis, and septicaemia can follow in uncontrolled abscess.

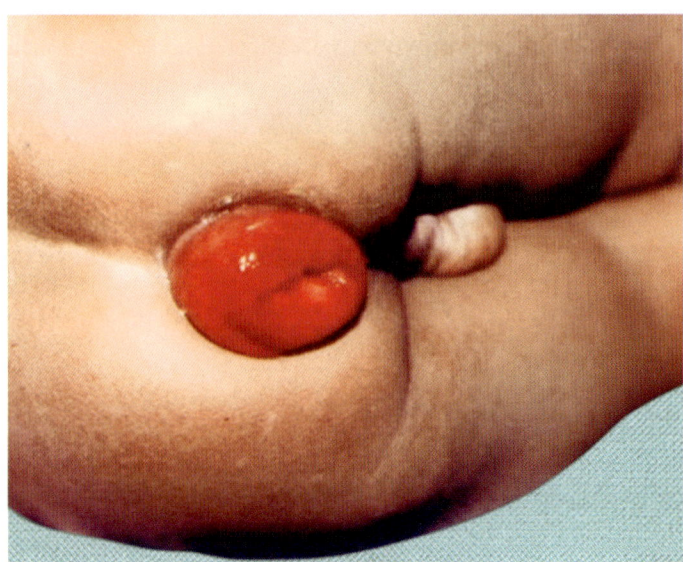

Fig. 25.18: Partial prolapse in a child

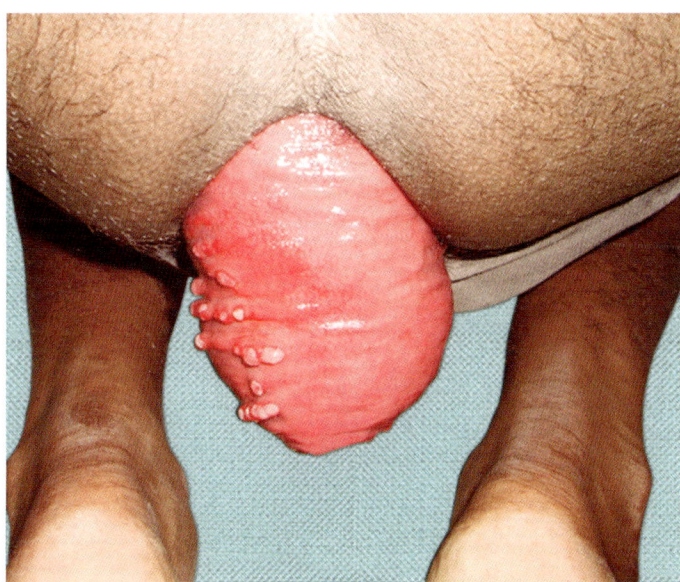

Fig. 25.19: Procidentia: Total prolapse of rectum

- *Fat supports the rectum.* Hence, any chronic illness and loss of fat may contribute to prolapse rectum. Excessive straining causes weakness of the supports of the rectum.
- Many people believe that prolapse of the rectum starts as an *intussusception* in the first stage, in anterior wall of rectum, where supporting tissues are weakest (refer to Clinical Box 25.4).

Clinical features and Management

- *This is common in elderly women who are multipara. It is probably due to repeated birth injuries* to the perineum causing damage to the nerve fibres. As age advances, muscles become weak. This, together with fatty degeneration of the muscle, results in prolapse rectum.
- Diagnosis is largely on clinical grounds. Manometric studies can also be done.
- Total prolapse in adults should be treated by laparoscopic or open mesh pexy by placing the mesh in the sacral hollow, reducing the deep rectovesical or uterine pouch and suturing the mesh to the sacrum posteriorly and to the side of the rectum.

Clinical Wisdom

In fact, the surgeon should see the prolapse of the rectum outside the anal canal when patient strains to make a clinical diagnosis.

Clinical Box 25.4

Prolapse rectum—causative factors

- **P**elvic floor weakness
- **E**xcessive straining
- **L**oose/lax lateral ligaments
- **V**esical pouch (rectovesical pouch) deep
- **I**mmature/defective collagen
- **C**hronic illness

You can remember as 'PELVIC'

6. *Pilonidal sinus* (Figs 25.20 and 25.21): Strictly speaking it has nothing to do with rectum and anal canal. Typically seen in the skin of gluteal cleft, diagnosis is often made by inspection alone. It is an acquired condition, commonly found in hairy males. **It is an acquired sinus due to following reasons:** It appears between the age of 20 and 30 years. Hairy men are more affected. The **hair follicle is never demonstrated in the wall of the pilonidal sinus** but hair is usually the content. Hair accumulates due to vibration and friction causing shedding of the hair. Thus, it accumulates in the gluteal cleft and enters the opening of the sweat glands. Pilonidal means **nest of hairs** in Greek. Also called **Jeep-bottom** because it was very common in jeep drivers. Obesity, male sex, dark skin are precipitating factors. External opening of the sinus is seen just above the anal verge in the midline over the coccyx. Other sites of pilonidal sinus are umbilicus and interdigital space in barbers. History of discharge of pus, history of recurrent abscesses which rupture discharging pus can be the presenting features. Pilonidal sinus is known for recurrences even after wide excision. It is better to define all tracks before surgery and excise all the stained tissues. Wound can be left open to heal by granulation tissue, secondary suturing can be done or a flap cover can be done.

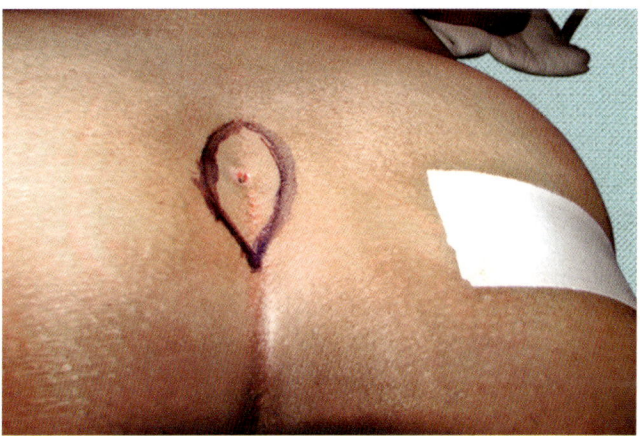

Fig. 25.20: Pilonidal sinus opening is marked before surgery

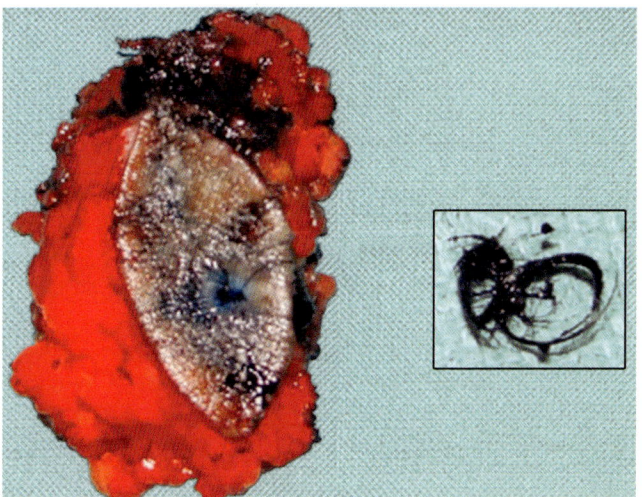

Fig. 25.21: Specimen of wide excision showing the skin, subcutaneous tissues, sinus tract and tuft of hair within the cavity of the pilonidal sinus

7. Carcinoma rectum (Figs 25.22 to 25.24): Typically, patients are middle-aged around 40–50 years who present with bleeding per rectum or passage of blood and mucus per rectum. Early morning spurious diarrhoea indicates growth in the ampulla of the rectum. Increasing constipation indicates growth in the rectosigmoid junction. Backache indicates sacral infiltration. Per rectal examination can detect almost all cases of carcinoma rectum. Typically, it is hard, indurated and friable—bleeds on touch. Infiltration to the structures around should be carefully looked into. Proctoscopy is an outpatient procedure to take a biopsy and diagnosis. If difficulty arises, sigmoidoscopy or even colonoscopy can be done. Ultrasound is done to rule out liver and lymph nodal metastasis. MRI is the best investigation to see for local infiltration such as bladder base, sacrum, posterior vaginal wall and side wall of the pelvis. When sphincter can be saved, surgery of choice is low anterior resection or high anterior resection. When sphincter cannot be saved, abdominoperineal resection (APR) with a permanent colostomy is the only operation to achieve cure. Adjuvant radiotherapy and chemotherapy are also given. Prognosis is very good for early lesions.

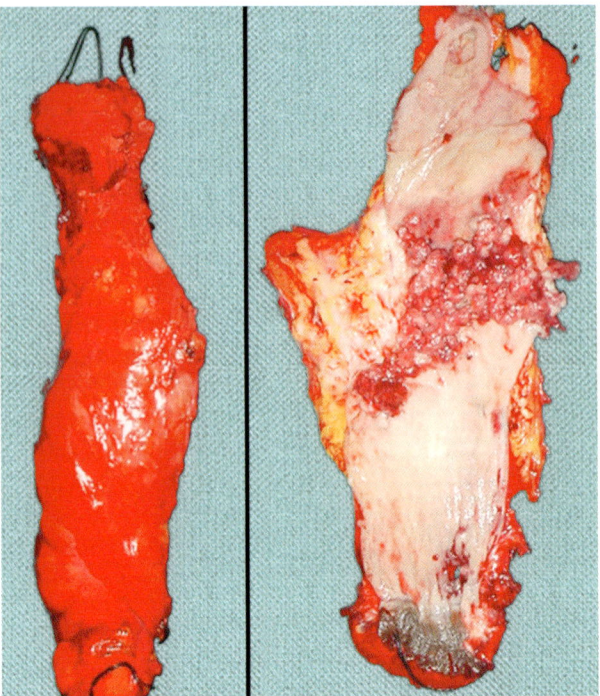

Fig. 25.23: Specimen of APR for carcinoma rectum   **Fig. 25.24:** Cut open specimen showing the growth

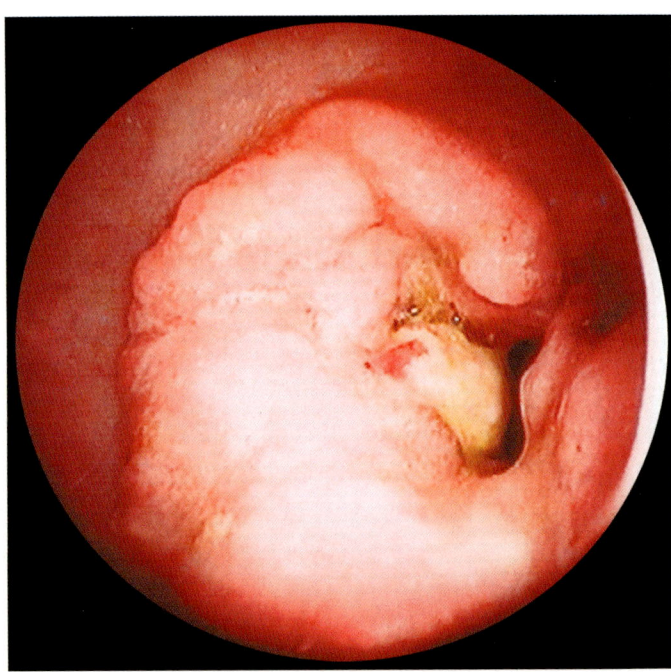

Fig. 25.22: Sigmoidoscopic view of carcinoma rectum—proliferative growth and narrowing of the lumen

8. Solitary rectal ulcer (Fig. 25.25): Commonly occurs in the anterior wall of lower rectum, an area of mucosal change. Mucosa is erythematous, heaped up and bleeds on touch. It is a single, depressed ulcer. The cause, even though not clear is probably due to trauma by anal digitation. Today, it is believed that it is due to **internal intussusception** or **anterior wall prolapse.** Clinical features are passage of blood and mucus in stools. Mucosal prolapse may also be a feature. A biopsy must be done to rule out carcinoma rectum. Treatment is conservative: Avoidance of constipation and straining may treat the prolapse.

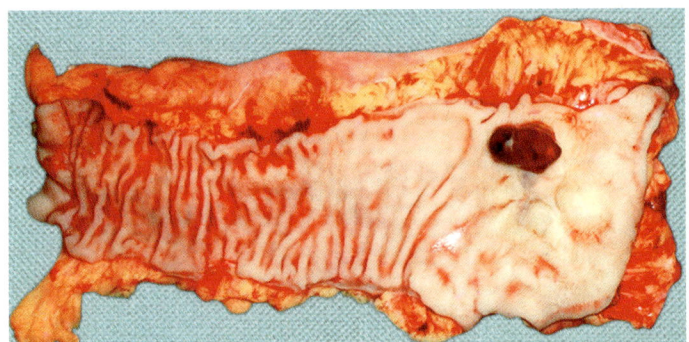

Fig. 25.25: Solitary rectal ulcer syndrome

9. Proctalgia fugax (fugax means fleetings): This condition is characterised by attacks of severe cramp-like pain arising in the rectum. Anxiety status, straining of stools and ejaculation are a few precipitating factors. The pain may be unbearable and may recur at irregular intervals. It is possibly due to segmental cramp in the pubococcygeus muscle. The pain usually lasts for a few minutes and subsides (fleeting perianal pain). Symptomatic treatment in the form of analgesics are given.

10. Pruritus ani: This is intractable itching around the anus. Mucous discharge is an intense pruritic agen. In all cases of pruritus, sexually transmitted diseases, such as herpes, anal warts and HIV infection must be excluded (Clinical Box 25.5). Treatment is in the form of hygienic measures, prednisolone topical cream 1% with antifungal agent (miconazole nitrate 2%) and moisturising cream/lotion and antihistamine-promethazine hydrochloride 10–25 mg at night-time.

1. **Perianal and anal discharge:** Anal fissure, fistula-in-ano, prolapsed piles, polyps, and genital warts are a few conditions which render the anus moist.
2. **Poor hygiene,** lack of cleanliness, excessive sweating and wearing tight and rough underclothing are common causes.
3. **Parasitic causes**—threadworms
4. **Psychoneurosis**
5. **Allergy, diabetes** are the other causes

11. ***Sacrococcygeal teratoma:*** It is a congenital condition affecting the sacrococcygeal region. In this region, totipotent cells persist for a longer period compared to the rest of the area. Hence, it is the site of teratomas. 20% of the cases are stillborn babies. It is common in a female child. It presents as a swelling in the sacrococcygeal region pushing the rectum anteriorly. The surface of the swelling ulcerates. Many cystic areas are present in the swelling. The swelling is fixed to the sacrum and coccyx from which it is impossible to separate/isolate. **Complications are** ulceration, secondary infection, haemorrhage, terato-carcinomatous change occurring by one year of age. Treatment is by excision of the teratoma with a part of sacrum and coccyx.

12. ***Malignant tumours of anal canal:*** They are not uncommon tumours which present with bleeding per rectum, burning and itching in the anal region. The diagnosis is obvious in many cases once buttocks are separated or by digital examination. Tissue diagnosis is a must before radical treatment. Various types of tumour are:
    a. *Squamous cell carcinoma*: Papillomas are the chief predisposing factors. Local excision or APR (abdomino-perineal resection with external radiotherapy is the appropriate treatment. For sphincter preservation, chemoradiation can be used (Fig. 25.26).

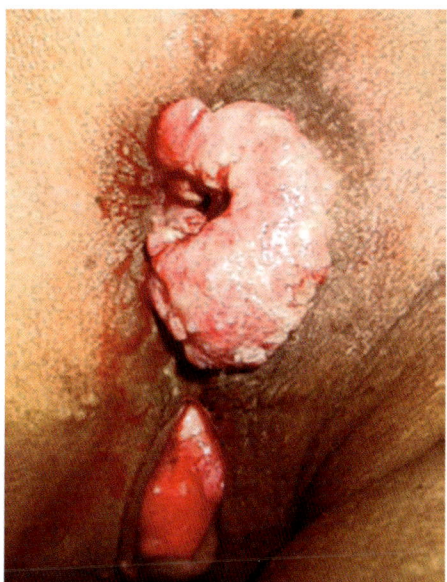

Fig. 25.26: Squamous cell carcinoma of anal canal

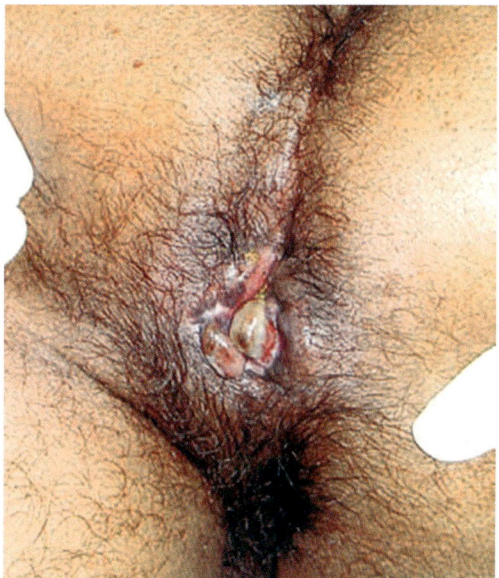

Fig. 25.27: Malignant melanoma of anal canal

b. *Basaloid carcinoma*: It is a highly malignant, non-keratinising, squamous cell carcinoma. Treatment is similar to squamous cell carcinoma.
c. *Melanoma*: Beware of a patient who comes with bilateral groin nodes which are bulky. Lesion in the anal canal is bluish/blackish ulcer in the anal canal. APR is potentially curative in early cases of melanoma. If metastasis is present, the prognosis is poor. **So, only local excision is done to provide palliation but colostomy is avoided** (Fig. 25.27).
d. *Adenocarcinoma* is rare. It can occur from the anal glands in pre-existing anal fistula. APR with 5-FU and radiation therapy are indicated.

13. ***Stricture of anal canal and rectum:*** There are many causes of stricture of anal canal. They are classified as given here.
    a. *Postoperative*: Haemorrhoidectomy, pull-through operations, repeated diathermy, fulguration of polyps.
    b. *Irradiation*: It occurs one to two years after irradiation.
    c. *Senile strictures*
    d. *Lymphogranuloma inguinale*: It is a sexually transmitted disease affecting both male and female patients. Initially **pararectal lymph nodes** are enlarged followed by development of multiple rectal strictures. More common in women.
    e. *Inflammatory bowel diseases*: Both ulcerative colitis and Crohn's disease result in rectal strictures (5–10%).
    f. *Rare*: Congenital, amoeboma, carcinoid, endometriosis, tuberculosis, and CMV colitis are other causes.

Clinical features: Increasing constipation is the characteristic feature of stricture of the rectum. It may be associated with hard stools, bleeding and pain in some cases. Per abdominal examination may reveal loaded colon with scybalous masses. Rectal examination can detect a stricture.

Treatment: Conservative treatment includes bulk purgatives and a vegetable diet. Regular dilatation may be necessary for the strictures situated low in the rectum and anal canal. Intractable strictures need to be resected. Always remember to treat the primary disease.

26

Examination of Urinary Tract and Renal Mass

INTRODUCTION

Entire urinary tract extends from kidney to external urethral meatus. The symptoms of upper urinary tract are different from lower urinary tract. It is important to realise that no patient will come and say that they have a renal mass. Renal masses being retroperitoneal, can be totally asymptomatic and may be detected only by ultrasound done for some other indication. They can present with backache and may consult an orthopaedician or may present with fever and consult a physician. Renal cell carcinoma is notorious to present with **fever, fatigue (suggests anaemia), fracture and fall**, thus delaying the diagnosis.

PATIENT DATA

1. *Age and sex*: Congenital hydronephrosis due to pelviureteric junction abnormalities can present in children and young adults. Wilms' tumour (nephroblastoma) commonly occurs in children under 4 years of age. Female children are affected more often than male children. Polycystic kidney though congenital, manifests between 30 and 50 years of age. Other common problem in the renal system is stone disease which affects young to middle-aged patients. Acute pyelonephritis is more common in women—at puberty, just after marriage and in pregnancy. Renal cell carcinoma occurs more in men than in women in the age group between 40 and 60 years of age.

2. *Occupation and habits*: Bladder cancer has been found to be more common in people who work in aniline dye industries (products such as benzidine and 3-naphthylamine are carcinogenic), rubber and printing, leather, and textile industries. Smoking increases the incidence of carcinoma bladder.

3. *Residence*: Calculus disease is more common in hot dry climates. In India, "stone belt" includes parts of Maharashtra, Gujarat, Punjab, Haryana, Delhi and Rajasthan. It is also more common in the Middle East, North Africa and Mediterranean regions.

HISTORY OF PRESENT ILLNESS (COMPLAINTS)

1. *Pain*: Ask questions such as when the pain started, how is it now/severe or dull aching, the nature of the pain, how is the progression, etc. Dull aching pain in the loin is due to stretching of the renal capsule (dragging pain) (Fig. 26.1). This is due to enlargement of the kidney as typically happens in

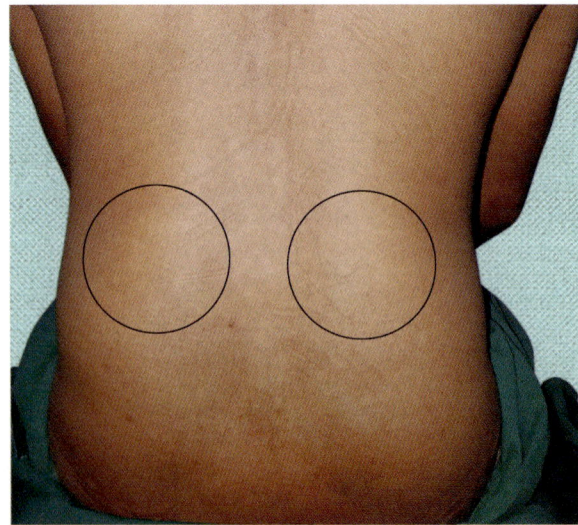

Fig. 26.1: Two renal angles (loin)—generally patient complains of pain in those areas

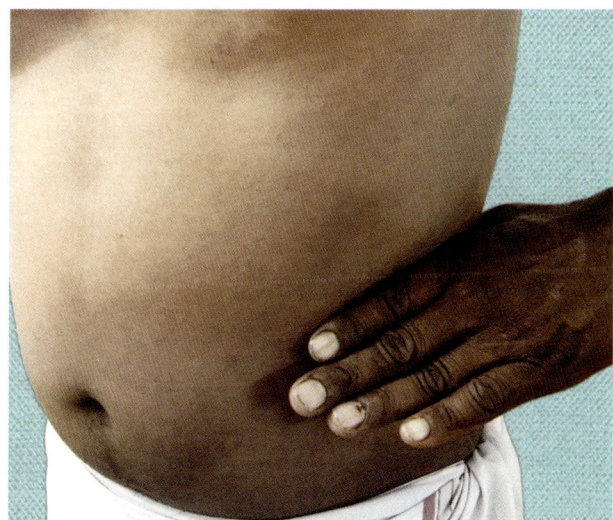

Fig. 26.2: Typical site of renal pain—costovertebral pain

renal cell carcinoma, hydronephrosis and polycystic kidneys. It is also described as pricking type of pain. It is also felt **posteriorly in the renal angle formed by the sacrospinalis and 12th rib.** (Murphy's kidney punch test demonstrates tenderness at renal angle.) The same pain may sometimes be felt anteriorly in the costal margin. Hence, it is described as **costovertebral pain** (Fig. 26.2). **Renal pain should not be described as colic as it is never a severe pain and never completely disappears like a colic.** When the stone is impacted in the pelviureteric junction or anywhere in the ureter, it results **in severe colicky pain originating at the loin** and **radiating to the groin,** testicles, vulva and medial side of the thigh. This may be associated with strangury (painful micturition with bleeding). The referred pain is due to **irritation of the genito-femoral nerve.** This typically happens when the stone is acutely obstructing the ureter. This is referred pain due to common innervations of the upper ureter and the testis (T11–T12) and lower ureter and inner side of the thigh (L1 through genitofemoral nerve). Common sites of ureteric stone getting impacted are given in Clinical Box 26.1.

Dietl's crisis: It is called intermittent hydronephrosis. This is common in calculus hydronephrosis. Following an attack of colic, ureteric obstruction occurs which results in enlargement of the pelvis of the kidney resulting in a palpable mass in the loin. After a few hours, the mass disappears after a large amount of urine is passed consequent to reflex polyuria or slipping of the ureteric stone.

2. *Pain* at the end of micturition referred to the tip of penis in young boys suggests urinary bladder stone. Pain is aggravated by jumping and jolting as in school going children. Pain is decreased on lying down because stone falls away from the trigone of the bladder. Typically, oxalate stones produce pain. Painful ineffective micturition with bleeding is described as strangury. **Loin pain in carcinoma bladder indicates** ureteric obstruction with hydronephrosis. **Suprapubic pain,** groin pain and perineal pain are due to infiltration of nerves. This indicates advanced nature of the carcinoma bladder. Difficulty in passing urine, painful micturition and sometimes with haematuria are due to involvement of prostatic urethra by carcinoma prostate.

3. *Nausea and vomiting* is due to intense sympathetic stimulation caused by stretching of renal capsule **mediated by coeliac plexus.**

4. *Haematuria:* Did you pass blood in the urine? Is it clots or liquid? Is it small quantity or large quantity? Stone disease, renal cell carcinoma and carcinoma urinary bladder are the three important diagnoses to be kept in mind in the surgery ward. In 90% of cases of carcinoma urinary bladder, initial symptom is painless, intermittent haematuria. Later painful, blood-stained micturition can occur. Strangury is also a feature. Haematuria is rare in BPH. It is due to congestion of prostatic venous plexuses resulting in hyperaemia and haematuria.

Clinical Box 26.1

Various sites of impaction of the stone
1. Pelviureteric junction
2. Crossing of the iliac artery
3. Crossing of the vas deferens or broad ligament
4. Site of entry into the bladder wall
5. Ureteric orifice

Clinical Box 26.2

Common causes of haematuria

Renal conditions	Urinary bladder conditions
1. Renal stone, ureteric stone	1. Papilloma of the bladder
2. Carcinoma kidney	2. Carcinoma bladder
3. Papilloma of kidney	3. Cystitis
4. Polycystic disease of kidney	4. Bladder stone
5. Renal tuberculosis	5. Bilharziasis of the urinary bladder

5. *Frequency, urgency and hesitancy form the triad of BPH.* **Frequency is the earliest symptom of bladder stone**. It is due to cystitis.

To start with, frequency is present during the day-time followed by day and night (5–10 times during the night). It is due to ineffective emptying of the bladder. It results in residual urine in the bladder precipitating cystitis.

Urgency: As the prostate enlarges, there is **vesical introversion of sensitive mucous membrane of prostatic urethra within the bladder.** This causes the internal sphincter to stretch and prevents contraction. This results in a few drops of urine trickling down the posterior urethra resulting in an urgent desire to pass urine (urgency).

Hesitancy: The patient hesitates to pass urine because it is so ineffective due to obstruction caused by BPH.

6. *Frequency* is the earliest symptom of tuberculosis. It is due to renal tubular inflammation and later due to tubercular cystitis.

7. *Retention of urine*: Patients with BPH can present with acute and chronic retention of urine. Acute retention of urine occurs due to postponement of micturition, following alcohol or drugs like mydriatics. Many of the patients present with chronic retention of urine, with painless enlarge-ment of the urinary bladder. Acute retention of urine can also be a feature of carcinoma bladder and occurs in about 10% of patients.

8. *Backache, multiple bony pains*: Confused for rheumatism, is due to multiple metastasis from carcinoma prostate. It typically occurs in patients above the age group of 60 years.

Clinical Wisdom

Elderly man with bilateral sciatica with metastasis in the thoraco-lumbar vertebrae may be having carcinoma prostate with bone metastasis.

Clinical Wisdom

Men are somewhat protected from ascending infection because of long urethra and antibacterial properties of prostatic secretions.

---

9. *Frequency dysuria and fever*: This indicates urinary tract infection/cystitis. It may be a presenting feature in bladder stone, stricture urethra or BPH also. Urinary tract infection is more common in women because of short and straight urethra. Evening rise in temperature, loss of weight and appetite indicate tuberculosis. In acute gonococcal urethritis, discharge is purulent, profuse and painful. In chronic cases, it is white-coloured and is called **Gleet**. Typically, it is discharged in the morning.

10. *History of straining* indicates urethral stricture. In young patients, it can be due to gonococcal urethritis and history of exposure to sexually transmitted diseases. History of surgery—specially instrumentation of urethra is also one of the common causes of stricture urethra. *Examples,* following transurethral resection of the prostate (TURP) or traumatic rupture urethra.

11. *Thirst, vomiting, abdominal distension* due to paralytic ileus, anuria, uraemic smell and coated tongue are the features of renal failure. This can be the first manifestation of polycystic kidney. Abdominal distension may be the only symptom in children and in polycystic disease. The abdominal distension is due to hugely enlarged kidney, which feels nodular on palpation. Rarely, Wilms' tumour is bilateral.

12. *Incontinence*: Leakage of urine due to defective sphincter control results in incontinence. Enquire whether the patient had undergone any surgical procedure. Following prostatectomy, or any history of trauma, repairs done for urethral injuries or road traffic accidents can result in automatic bladder (Clinical Box 26.3).

Clinical Box 26.3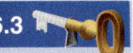

Types of incontinence
- *True incontinence*: Here, bladder remains empty and patient passes urine without any warning.
- *False incontinence*: Classically, it happens in BPH cases. Here it is due to overdistended bladder. Hence, it is called **overflow incontinence**.
- *Automatic bladder*: Typically happens in cases of spinal injury wherein spinal cord is involved. Periodic contractions of bladder occur without patient knowing about it and **he has no control over the problem.**
- *Stress incontinence*: This happens more in elderly patients. Coughing, sneezing or straining result in passage of a few drops of urine. Typically seen in female patients.

Past History

History of pulmonary tuberculosis must be enquired in the form of cough, haemoptysis, and rise in temperature. **Genitourinary tuberculosis is always secondary to pulmonary tuberculosis.** Any exposure to venereal diseases.

General Physical Examination

- Dry coated tongue, drowsiness and delirium are the features of renal failure.

- Pallor is an important feature of chronic renal failure (due to defective erythropoietin synthesis) and renal cell carcinoma.

- Cheyne-Stokes respiration can be seen in uraemia.

- Blood pressure is elevated in cases of polycystic kidney, renal cell carcinoma and renal ischaemia.

REGIONAL EXAMINATION OR LOCAL EXAMINATION

Inspection

1. *In recumbent position*: In vast majority of the cases, inspection is normal unless there is a large renal mass such as hydronephrosis or Wilms' tumour in children. If you see a mass, describe it otherwise use the word—fullness. (Fullness has no dimensions.)

2. *Any suprapubic swelling should be considered as distended urinary bladder unless proved otherwise.* Chronic retention of urine is painless.

3. *Look at the scrotum.* If it is empty, think of undescended testis.

4. *Any sinuses in the scrotum, think of tuberculous epididymo-orchitis.* Gumma of the testis (tertiary stage of syphilis) is not seen nowadays. Since it affects testis, sinuses are anterior. Tuberculosis affects epididymis, the sinuses are posterior (Fig. 26.3). This can be reversed, if it is a case of situs inversus, where testes will be posteriorly situated.

5. Swelling of the scrotum can be a hydrocoele or hernia (*refer* to Examination of Hernia and Hydrocoele, Chapters 27 and 28).

Clinical Wisdom

Remember, ruptured retrocaecal appendicitis can present as backache. Often these patients get admitted in orthopaedics department or urology department.

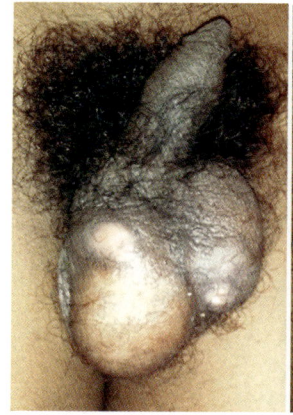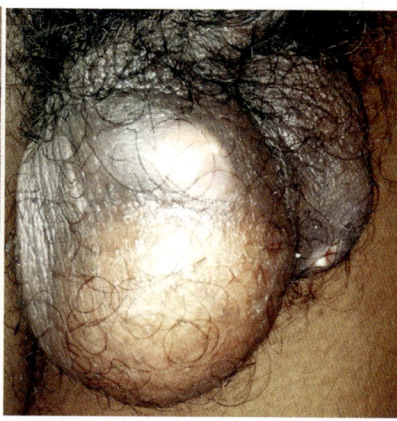

Fig. 26.3: Tuberculous epididymo-orchitis in a 24-year-old boy. Multiple sinuses in the scrotum. Craggy epididymis and beaded vas are typical features (*Courtesy:* Dr Kabalimurthy, Dr Ramesh, Dr Junior Sundaresh, Shri Raja Muttayya Medical College, Chidambaram, Tamil Nadu)

6. *In the sitting position*: Inspect the back—below the 12th rib and lateral to erector spinae muscles (renal angle). Kidney being a posterior structure, enlargement is often visible posteriorly. Any redness or wrinkled skin in the renal angle suggests infections such as **perinephric abscess.**

Palpation

- After feeling the mass, make a note of the location, size, shape, surface, borders, consistency, mobility and plane of the swelling. Typically, the kidney is reniform when it is uniformly enlarged. The shape will be lost when the lesion affects one of the poles as in renal cell carcinoma. Upper border of the renal swelling is difficult to appreciate because it is covered by lower ribs but still it may be possible to insinuate the fingers. Restricted mobility is typical of renal cell carcinoma.

- Renal masses move with respiration because fascia of Gerota blends with the diaphragm above.

- Two other important signs have to be elicited for a renal mass. They are bimanual palpation and ballotability. Kidney is best palpated by using the bimanual method because it is covered by lower ribs.

1. *Bimanual palpation* (Fig. 26.4): Grossly enlarged swellings in the lateral abdomen may be bimanually palpable such as liver, spleen and kidney. The patient is asked to lie down and a pillow is kept under the knees. The left hand is kept flat, with palm facing upwards, behind the loin and right hand is kept anteriorly below the costal margin with palm facing opposite

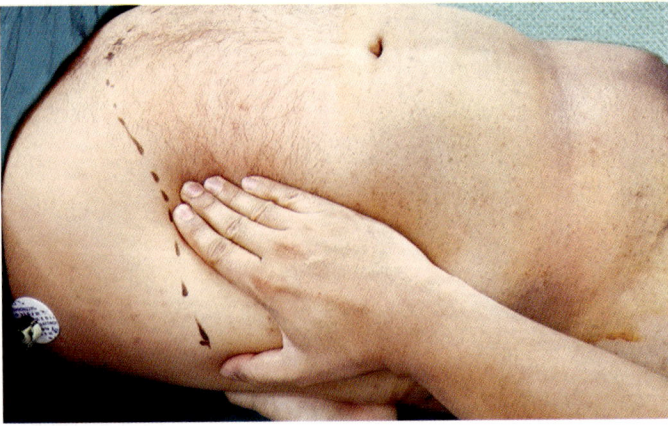

Fig. 26.4: Bimanual palpation of left renal mass (*Courtesy: Dr Zeeshan Hameed, Assistant Professor, Department of Urology, KMC, Manipal*)

direction. The patient is asked to breathe comfortably. Thus when muscles are relaxed, one cannot only feel the kidney anteriorly and posteriorly but also appreciate movement with respiration. At the same time, note down the features of the mass such as size, shape, surface, borders, consistency and mobility.

2. *Ballotability:* 'Ballot' means to toss about. To ballot, the swelling should be bimanually palpable and there should be a gap or space between the hands which are kept anterior and posterior to the mass. Kidney swellings being retroperitoneal and peripheral are suited for ballotability. Typically, renal swellings are **ballotable.** This test is done when the patient is in supine position, by keeping one hand anteriorly in the lumbar region over the swelling and the other hand posteriorly in the renal angle. A gentle push is given from behind and the swelling touches the hand which is placed anteriorly and it goes back. **Ballotability** is **because of perirenal pad of fat and due to** the presence of renal pedicle. (More details have been described in Chapter 24.)

Clinical Wisdom

All ballotable swellings are usually bimanually palpable but all bimanually palpable swellings need not be ballotable.

Percussion

Resonant note is elicited both anteriorly and posteriorly due to colon. It can be obliterated when the colon or small intestines are pushed by the large renal mass (polycystic kidney, hydronephrosis, renal cell carcinoma).

Auscultation

Systolic bruit can be heard in cases of renal artery stenosis or aneurysm of renal artery.

EXAMINATION OF THE URINARY BLADDER

- Any lower abdominal midline swelling has to be diagnosed as urinary bladder unless proven otherwise. In the Fig. 26.5, a retroperitoneal mass has been shown in the hypogastrium mimicking urinary bladder. However clinical features of urinary bladder mass are different and have been given in Clinical Box 26.4. Normal urinary bladder is not palpable. It is said that minimum of 150 ml of urine should be collected before it is palpable.

- Therefore, it is a dictum, especially in women to empty the bladder or catheterise the bladder before doing a pelvic examination.

- *Bimanual palpation of the urinary bladder:* The urinary bladder is felt with 1–2 fingers of one hand placed in the rectum/vagina and pushing anteriorly and the other hand placed on the abdomen in the

---

Clinical Box 26.4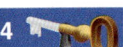

Typical signs of urinary bladder mass
1. Typical location—in the hypogastrium
2. Smooth oval swelling
3. Elastic, tensely cystic swelling—pressure produces urge to pass urine
4. Dull to percuss
5. Lower border cannot be made out

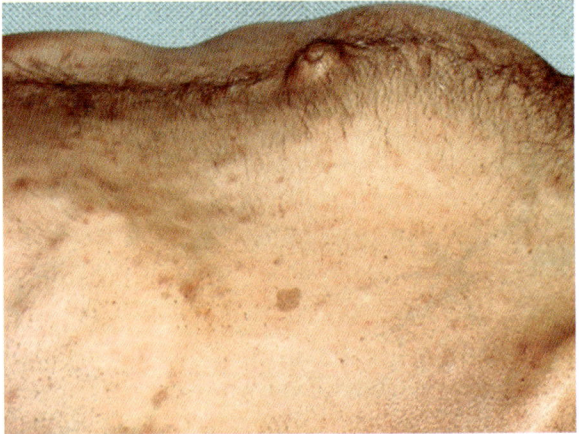

Fig. 26.5: A large suprapubic mass with all features of urinary bladder. It was hard on palpation and dull on percussion. Postgraduate gave a diagnosis of carcinoma urinary bladder. It is such a large mass with no complaints of any urinary disturbances including haematuria. You should think of something outside. This patient had multiple café au lait spots. It was a case of retroperitoneal neurofibrosarcoma arising from one of the pelvic nerves

suprapubic region pressing posteriorly and towards the pelvis. The extent of vesical neoplasm can be made out as an indurated mass.

A few masses arising from the bladder
1. Distended bladder—most common cause being benign prostatic hypertrophy.
2. Carcinoma of the bladder—hypogastric mass which is hard and irregular.
3. A large diverticulum of the urinary bladder (more of an exclusion diagnosis).

Clinical Wisdom

Tuberculosis of the urinary bladder will not produce a palpable mass because the urinary bladder will be contracted and become small (thimble bladder).

RECTAL EXAMINATION

Prostate can be palpated only through the rectum. The left lateral position is most commonly used and also comfortable for the patient. Knee elbow position also may be used.

1. Carcinoma prostate: It presents as a hard nodule on the anterior wall of the rectum with obliteration of median sulcus. The rectal mucosa cannot be moved over the prostate but it is not ulcerated. (Fascia of Denonvilliers prevents the spread of carcinoma prostate into the rectum.)

2. BPH: Enlarged lateral lobes can be easily felt. Normal consistency of the prostate is like a rubber. Rectal mucosa is free in an enlarged prostate gland. In case of carcinoma of prostate, the mucosa of the rectum cannot be moved, if it has infiltrated into the rectum.

Prostatic massage: Contraindications for **prostatic massage** are malignancies, acute prostatitis and in acute urethritis.

3. Seminal vesicles: These are better felt in knee elbow position.

- Tender and soft palpable seminal vesicle is felt in gonococcal urethritis.
- In tuberculosis, seminal vesicles are indurated and irregular.

Grading of prostate is done as follows

I. The prostatic lobes protrude minimally into the rectal lumen by 1–2 cm, the median sulcus is palpable.

II. Prostatic lobes protrude >2 cm but <3 cm into the rectal lumen and the median sulcus is obliterated.

III. 3–4 cm protrusion.

IV. >4 cm protrusion of lobes, most of the rectal lumen is filled by the projecting prostatic lobes.

DIFFERENTIAL DIAGNOSIS OF RENAL MASS

I. NONTENDER MASS

Three common masses arising from the kidney are hydronephrosis, renal cell carcinoma and polycystic disease. Solitary renal cyst and hydatid cyst of the kidney are other cystic swellings. Last two cysts have been mentioned here only for completion sake. With imaging done frequently today, asymptomatic renal cysts have been diagnosed more often.

a. **Hydronephrosis:** The common variety of hydronephrosis in young patients is due to pelviureteric junction dyskinesia. Enlargement is huge and bilateral. Since it is painless, patients often present late to the hospital. A large renal mass with smooth surface, round borders, tensely cystic and a firm feel clinches the diagnosis.

- Hydronephrosis can be unilateral or bilateral. Bilateral hydronephrosis occurs when the obstruction is at or below the internal meatus of the urinary bladder. Common causes are BPH, bilateral ureteric infiltration from malignancies such as carcinoma rectum in males and carcinoma cervix in females. Do not forget phimosis and urethral stricture as causes for bilateral hydronephrosis. Please refer to the Fig. 24.103. The most common cause of unilateral hydronephrosis is ureteric stone. Other causes are strictures, lymph nodal mass (para-aortic lymph nodes), compressing the ureter as in lymphoma, aberrant vessels and PUJ dyskinesia (can be unilateral also).
- Diagnosis is by ultrasound and CT scan examination which also help in identifying the cause of hydronephrosis. In all cases, when the cause is identified, treatment of the cause will cure hydronephrosis. Classical examples are basketing of ureteric stone, transurethral resection of the prostate for BPH, circumcision for phimosis, dilatation of urethral stricture, etc. Congenital hydronephrosis is treated by Anderson-Hynes pyeloplasty. Principles of this surgery include excision of redundant pelvis, disconnection of PUJ which is not functioning and construction of new ureteropelvic anastomosis is done in such a way that urine should drain by gravity. For other details, please refer *Manipal Manual of Surgery.*

b. **Renal cell carcinoma**: A middle-aged person presenting with intermittent haematuria, dragging pain in the loin and renal mass is typical presentation. Anaemia disproportionate to haematuria is a feature. It is due to decreased production of erythropoietin. Fever can be the only presenting feature and patients are often investigated for pyrexia of unknown origin and treated by physicians. Pulsatile secondaries can be the presenting feature. Kidney is enlarged, hard and irregular. Loss of appetite and weight loss are the other features. Diagnosis is clinical and with imaging. Renal cell carcinoma is known to spread by blood. Tumour often grows

Pain, **P**yrexia, **P**allor, **P**edal oedema (nephrotic syndrome), **P**ressure (hypertension), **P**olycythaemia, **P**alpable mass, **P**ulsatile secondaries, **P**athological fracture and **P**araneoplastic syndromes are the presenting features **(observe 10 Ps)**.

- **P**ain ⎤
- **P**yrexia ⎟ Common
- **P**allor ⎟ symptoms
- **P**alpable mass ⎦

into the lumen of inferior vena cava and thus cannonball secondaries and bone metastasis easily occur. Tissue diagnosis is not required. Radical nephrectomy for renal cell carcinoma and extended nephrectomy for transitional cell carcinoma arising from urothelium is the treatment of choice (Figs 26.6 and 26.7). Refer to the clinical discussion.

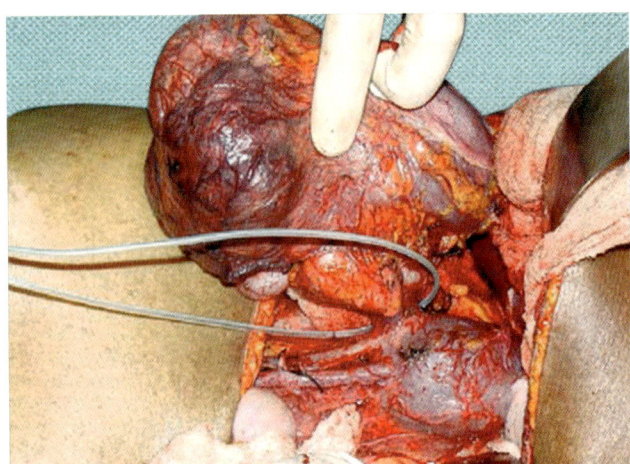

Fig. 26.6: Renal cell carcinoma with tumour thrombus in inferior vena cava (*Courtesy*: Professor Joseph Thomas, Professor of Urology, KMC, Manipal)

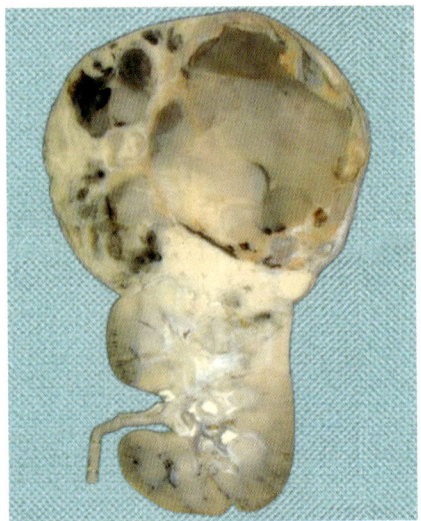

Fig. 26.7: Specimen of nephrectomy showing upper polar lesion—common site. Reniform shape is lost

c. *Polycystic kidney*: It is usually seen in a middle-aged patient who presents with haematuria or headache due to hypertension. On examination, both kidneys are grossly enlarged. Typically, they are bosselated and firm. Look for evidence of renal failure—thirst, coated tongue and oliguria. In such cases, urgent dialysis followed by renal transplantation is the treatment of choice. A few cases are asymptomatic—detected by ultrasound. They require follow up. Hypertension needs to be treated.

Clinical Wisdom

Haematuria, hypertension, bilateral huge kidney means it is polycystic kidneys.

CLINICAL DISCUSSION

1. **Why it is carcinoma kidney?**
   - Renal enlargement classically in the upper pole, hence upper border cannot be felt
   - Hard in consistency
   - Restricted mobility
   - Anaemia, weight loss
   - Haematuria in elderly patients.
2. **Why it is hydronephrosis?**
   - Young patient
   - May be bilateral
   - Smooth surface, round border
   - Tensely cystic and hence feels firm
   - General condition is good.
3. **Why not polycystic kidney?**
   - Usually bilateral
   - Both kidneys are grossly enlarged
   - Surface is nodular/bosselated
   - Firm in consistency
   - Hypertension is usually present.
4. **What other masses can arise from kidney?**
   Pyonephrosis and perinephric abscess—both are acute cases.

*Common three renal masses have been compared in Table 26.1.

d. *Horseshoe kidney*: When it is not enlarged, difficult to diagnose a horseshoe kidney. During development, two mesonephric buds appear on the side of the future vertebral column and grows into metanephros. Mesonephric buds form ureter and metanephros kidneys. **If fusion occurs at lower pole**, it results in a classical **horseshoe kidney. Inferior mesenteric artery crosses the isthmus at the level of L3–L4. Hence, horseshoe kidney cannot ascend.** It is felt lower down in the abdomen. It can be asymptomatic for many years. A palpable mass below and to the right and to the left of umbilicus or umbilical region can be a horseshoe kidney. **Recurrent urinary tract infection (UTI) is common because the ureters are angulated over the kidney isthmus. They are more prone for hydronephrosis due to the angulation of ureters.**

- *Rovsing sign*: Hyperextension of the spine results in abdominal pain, nausea or vomiting due to stretching of

Table 26.1: Renal mass in surgical ward

	Hypernephroma	*Hydronephrosis*	*Polycystic kidney*
1. Chief symptoms	Haematuria, pain in the loin, renal mass	Asymptomatic, distension, abdominal pain	Mass abdomen, hypertension, haematuria
2. Age of the patient	Over 50 years	20–30 years	30–40 years
3. Sex	Common in males	Common in females	Common in females
4. Anaemia	Present	Absent	May be present
5. Features of renal failure	Absent	Can be present in bilateral cases (rare)	May be present
6. Renal mass	Unilateral, nodular, hard, may be fixed, nontender	Can be bilateral, smooth, cystic, feels firm	Bilateral, bosselated, nodular, not fixed, nontender
7. Features of kidney mass	May not have free mobility due to fixity	Not fixed, nontender	Present
8. IVU	Irregular calyces	Gross dilatation of pelvicalyceal system	Spider-leg deformity of calyces
9. CT scan	Enhancing mass	Dilated pelvicalyceal system with uniform filling of contrast	Multiple hypodense areas without enhancement
10. Treatment	Radical nephrectomy	Pyeloplasty	Symptomatic—renal transplantation

the capsule. Diagnosis is by ultrasonography (USG), to locate the kidney and CT scan.

- Treatment is indicated only when there are complications. Removal of the stone or repair and reconstruction of the hydronephrosis are done in the usual manner.

II. TENDER RENAL MASS

a. *Pyonephrosis:* In this condition, the entire kidney is converted into a sac containing pus or purulent urine—almost always the renal parenchyma is destroyed totally. **Renal calculous disease** is the most common cause of pyonephrosis. Other causes are **acute pyelonephritis** in children and in females. Inadequately treated cases may develop into pyonephrosis, especially when pyelonephritis is associated with urinary tract obstruction. **Infection** of a hydronephrosis is another cause. Anaemia and fever, renal swelling, large tender swelling in the back with high grade fever with chills and rigors suggest an imminent danger of septicaemia and calls for an immediate drainage of pus.

b. *Perinephric abscess:* It refers to the collection of pus in the perirenal area. Infection in a perirenal haematoma, ruptured pyonephrosis, tubercular perinephric abscess and pus from retrocaecal appendicitis can extend into the loin in the perinephric area and may present as an abscess. High swinging temperature, rigidity, tenderness, fullness in the loin and oedema in the loin are the clinical features. Total counts are raised above 20,000 cells/mm³. X-ray spine: Scoliosis with concavity towards abscess is characteristic. Ultrasound and CT scan are the diagnostic imaging tests done today. **Pigtail insertion of the catheter under antibiotic cover with ultrasound guidance is the first choice of treatment.** Recurrent and multiloculated abscesses are managed by

incision and drainage. Treatment of the underlying disease is an important part of the surgery.

III. RENAL MASS IN A CHILD

Wilms' tumour (nephroblastoma) (Fig. 26.8): This is a malignant tumour of the kidney occurring in **children**. The tumour is composed of epithelial and mesothelial elements. Thus, it may contain bone, cartilage, muscle, etc. Hence, it is called **nephroblastoma (immature embryonic tissue)**. The tumour arises in one of the poles, distorting the reniform shape of the kidney. Microscopic features include connective tissue elements, cartilage, spindle cells, smooth striated muscle cells and

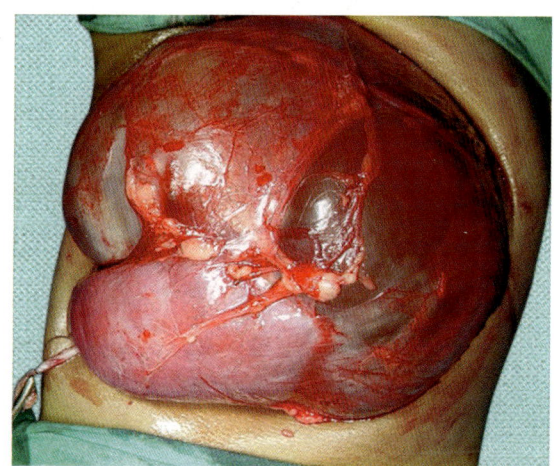

Fig. 26.8: Wilms' tumour (*Courtesy:* Dr Vijay Kumar, HOD, Dr Sandeep, Dr Santosh Prabhu, Department of Pediatric Surgery, KMC, Manipal)

epithelial elements. Common in **female children**, around 2–4 years. Upper limit of age is 7 years. Rarely it may occur in adolescents. The child is brought with **abdominal distension**, due to hugely enlarged kidney which on palpation feels nodular. Rarely, Wilms' tumour can be bilateral. **Haematuria** is a bad prognostic symptom. It is an indication of rupture of tumour into the pelvis of kidney. **Low grade fever** can occur in rapidly growing tumour due to tumour necrosis, which releases pyrogens. Rapid deterioration of health is characteristic.

OTHER DISEASES OF KIDNEY

1. *Renal stone* (Figs 26.9 to 26.12): Typically, the patient is between 20 and 40 years of age group who complaints of pain in the back and in the hypochondriac region. The pain can be very severe which becomes worse on movements, jolting, walking up the staircase and partially relieved on taking rest. Haematuria may be the presenting feature. Many cases are asymptomatic. The stones are detected by routine ultrasound examination or during a plain X-ray abdomen. Pyuria may also be found. A few can present with secondary infection with pyonephrosis or anuria due to damage to the kidneys (rare nowadays). As a rule, kidney is not palpable unless there is hydronephrosis. Plain X-ray KUB (kidney, ureter, bladder region) demonstrates the stones in more than 90% cases. They are calcium-rich stones except phosphate stones. Today vast majority of the stones are detected by ultrasound examination. Renal function is assessed. Asymptomatic small stones are left alone. Otherwise they are treated by percutaneous

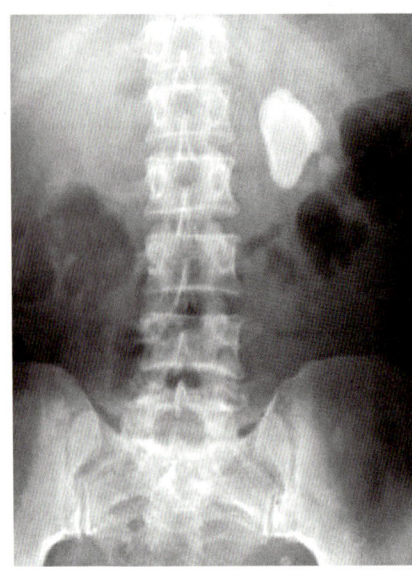

Fig. 26.11: Plain X-ray KUB showing stone in the left kidney

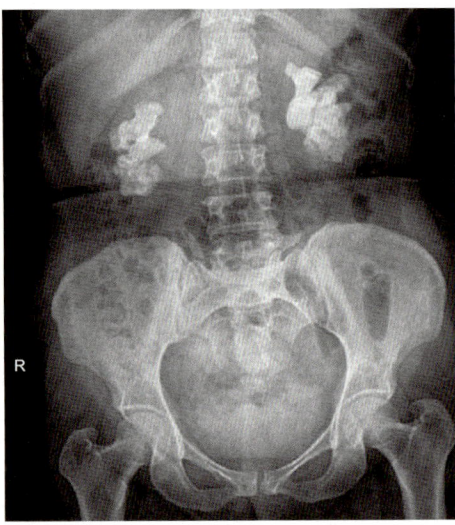

Fig. 26.12: Plain X-ray showing bilateral staghorn calculi (*Courtesy:* Dr Arun Chawla, HOD, Urology, KMC, Manipal)

nephrolithotomy or extracorporeal shock wave lithotripsy.

2. *Renal tuberculosis:* More details are given in *Manipal Manual of Surgery,* 4th edition. It is common in males, in the 20–40 age group. Infection is always **haematogenous**. Often one may not find any active lesion in the lung or in the lymph nodes. It is usually unilateral. Frequency is the earliest symptom of tuberculosis and is present in the day and night. It is due to renal tubular inflammation and later due to tubercular cystitis. **Abacterial acid pyuria** refers to opalescent, pale or yellow urine which is acidic on reaction and no organisms/bacteria are grown on repeated culture. *Sterile pyuria is seen in tuberculosis, stones and in carcinoma in situ.*

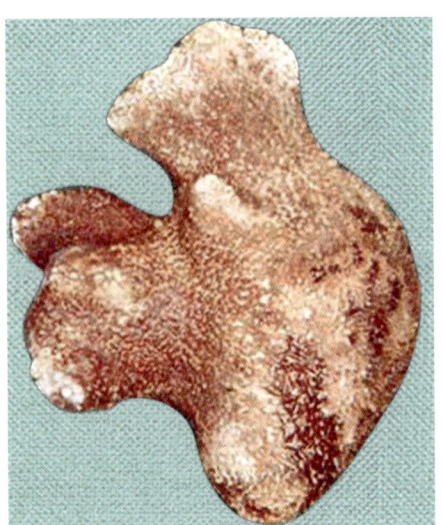
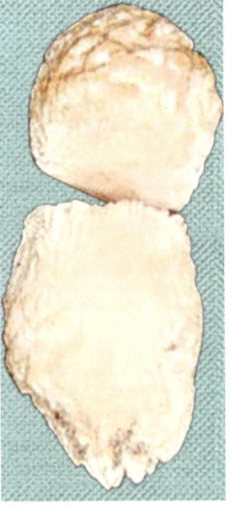

Fig. 26.9: Staghorn calculi   **Fig. 26.10:** Phosphate calculi

(*Courtesy:* Dr Natrajan, Associate Professor, Department of Urology, KMC, Manipal)

Various manifestations of renal tuberculosis
1. Ulcerative form
2. Ulcerocavernous form
3. Pseudocalculi
4. Hydronephrosis
5. Tuberculous perinephric abscess
6. Tuberculous pyonephrosis
7. Contracted kidney
8. Multiple tubercles—miliary tuberculosis
9. Entire kidney is a mass of caseous material (Fig. 26.13)

Haematuria is not uncommon. Usually, it is a small quantity due to ulcerocavernous variety. Evening rise of temperature, loss of appetite and loss of weight may be seen. As a rule, kidney is not palpable. Opposite kidney (normal side) may be palpable due to compensatory hypertrophy. Chest X-ray should be taken to look for any tubercular lesions such as cavity. If lymph nodes are palpable, biopsy should be done. Early morning sample of urine for 3 days—has to be examined which gives the highest concentration of AFB. Plain X-ray KUB may show calcified kidney. Cystoscopy clinches the diagnosis. Initially small ulcers are seen around ureteric orifice. They join together resulting in a big ulcer. Due to extensive periureteric fibrosis, the ureter becomes thickened, shortened and straight. The ureteric openings are lifted upwards and they are gaping which means it does not contract/does not close when bladder contracts. Such contracted, elevated, permanently opened, lower end of ureter is called **golf hole ureter**. As a result of this, with each act of contraction of bladder, there is reflux of urine into the kidney causing damage. When the disease involves the urinary bladder, it results in fibrosis. It becomes small and contracted with ineffective function. Storage capacity is lost resulting in intractable frequency, with a few drops of urine. There is bleeding. Micturition is painful and is called strangury. There is also severe pain in the suprapubic region which is referred to the tip of the penis. Such a small, contracted, nonfunctioning urinary bladder is called **thimble bladder** (Figs 26.14 and 26.15).

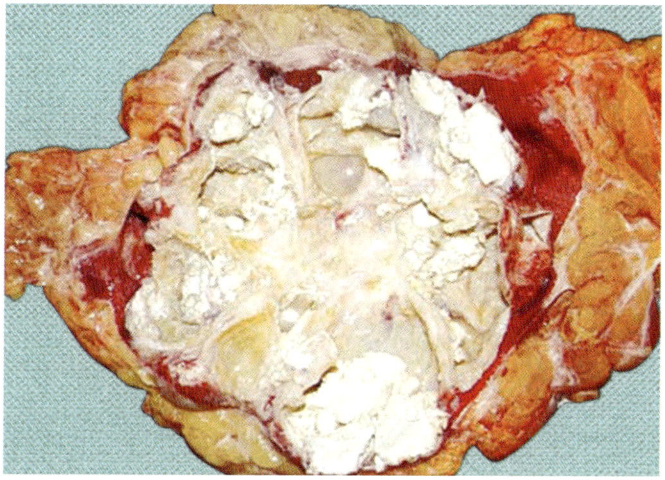

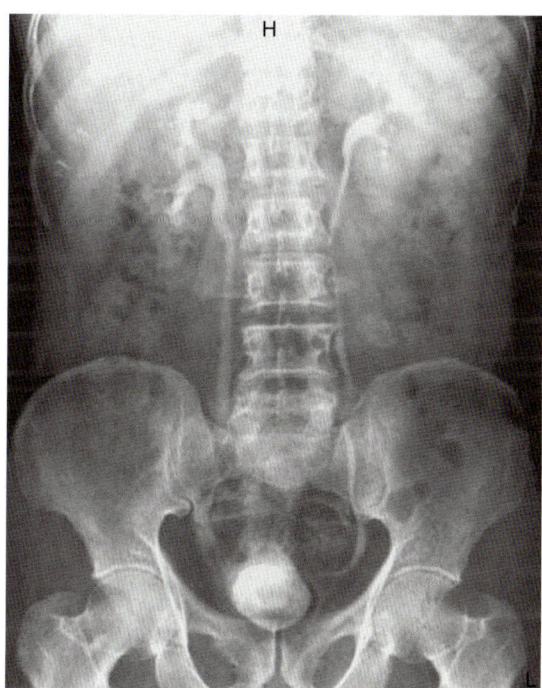

Fig. 26.14: Left kidney is normal. Right kidney shows hydro-ureteronephrosis. The urinary bladder is contracted—thimble bladder

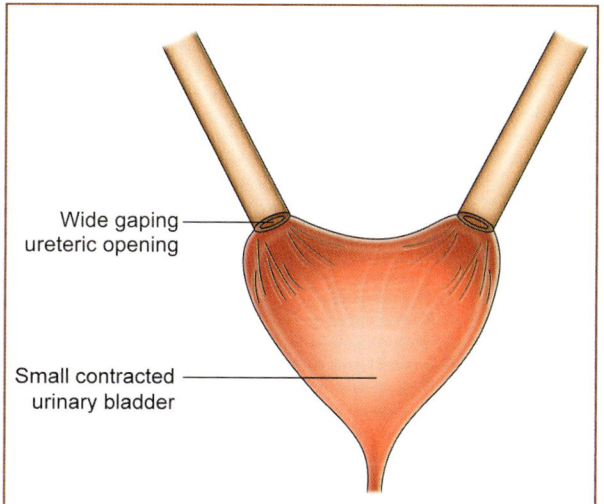

Fig. 26.13: Renal tuberculosis—entire kidney is a mass of caseous material (*Courtesy:* Dr Padmaraj Hedge, Dr Natarajan, Professor, Department of Urology, KMC, Manipal)

Fig. 26.15: Thimble bladder with golf hole ureter (TB)—diagrammatic representation

DISEASES OF URETER AND BLADDER

1. *Ureteric colic*: It is the most severe form of abdominal pain. Stones come down from pelvis of the kidney and may get impacted at any site of anatomical narrowing of ureter, namely:

a. Pelviureteric junction

b. Crossing of the iliac artery

c. Crossing of the vas deferens or broad ligament

d. Site of entry into the bladder wall

e. Urethral orifice.

This may lead to hydroureteronephrosis, renal parenchymal atrophy, infection and pyonephrosis. Typically, pain is felt in the loin and radiates to groin. Pain is severe, colicky, intolerable and lasts for a few hours. When stone descends into the lower ureter, pain radiates to the testicles, labia majora and to the upper portion of thigh due to **irritation of genito-femoral nerve.** Colic lasts for about 4–6 hours and is relieved by antispasmodics, narcotics and NSAIDs. They can have an attack of haematuria or pyuria. Guarding and rigidity of the abdominal wall, if present on the right side, is confused with acute appendicitis. Many stones may pass into the bladder with conservative treatment. A few other stones require cystoscopic basketing or rarely ureterolithotomy.

2. *Ectopia vesicae*: A rare congenital anomaly seen more in males (4 times more common than female children). This occurs due to failure of development of lower abdominal wall and anterior wall of the urinary bladder. As a result, the posterior bladder wall is seen protruding out below the umbilicus. **Hence, it is exstrophy of the bladder. Two types have been identified.** *Complete:* Pubic symphysis is not formed, complete epispadias in male or bifid clitoris in female. *Incomplete:* Pubic symphysis, penis and clitoris are normal. On examination, **posterior bladder wall is seen in the lower abdomen** as a pink to red mucosa, partially inflamed (Fig. 26.16). Umbilicus is usually absent. **Penis is rudimentary** and epispadias may be present. **Testis descends normally into a well-developed scrotum.**

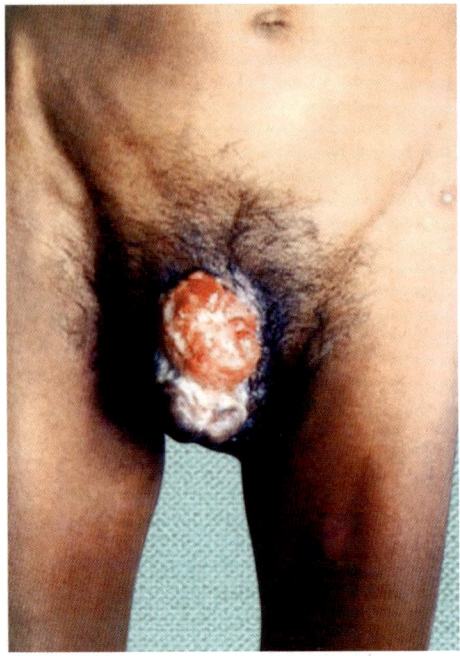

Fig. 26.16: Carcinoma bladder in a case of ectopia vesicae (*Courtesy*: Dr PS Aralikatti, Associate Professor, BIMS, Belgaum, Karnataka)

Pubic symphysis is widely separated. It has the advantage in female patients in that it facilitates the delivery. In **female children—umbilicus is absent**, external genitalia are poorly developed, and clitoris is bifid. There is constant dribbling of urine outside and hence they smell of urine. They will have recurrent urinary tract infections (UTI). Complications such as renal failure due to recurrent UTI, adenocarcinoma of bladder at an early age and ammoniacal dermatitis of the skin can occur. Treatment is difficult. Reconstruction of the anterior wall of the bladder along with reconstruction of the bladder sphincter is done in incomplete cases. A total cystectomy followed by urinary diversion by implanting the ureters in the sigmoid colon (ureterosigmoidostomy) is done in the complete variety. If the patient has urinary incontinence, reconstruction of anterior abdominal wall is also done.

3. *Vesical calculus*: Stones are 8 times more common in males than in females and in young patients. However, no age is exempted from the disease. Primary stones develop in sterile urine. **Secondary stone** develops in the presence of infection (Fig. 26.17) and stasis due to obstruction to the urinary flow. Following are a few types of stones:

a. *Oxalate stone*: Moderate size, uneven surface, mulberry stone is dark brown or black because of incorporation of blood pigment in it.

Clinical Box 26.7

Ectopia vesicae

1. **P**osterior bladder wall is protruding out.
2. **P**ubic symphysis is widely separated.
3. **P**enis is rudimentary.
4. **P**oor stream of urine hence constant dribbling.
5. **P**rogression to adenocarcinoma bladder.

Observe **5 Ps**

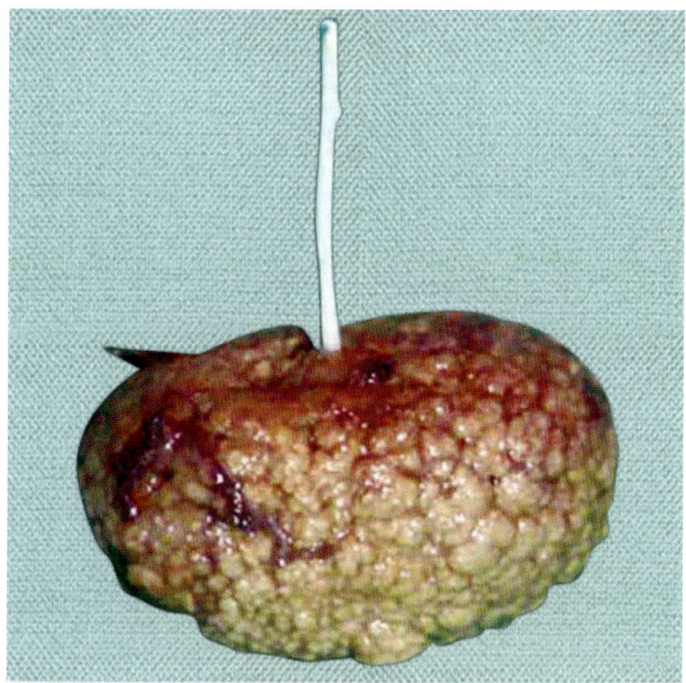

Fig. 26.17: Migrated copper T into the urinary bladder resulting in a stone (*Courtesy:* Dr Rajiv Shetty, Ex-Dean, ESI Medical College, Bangalore)

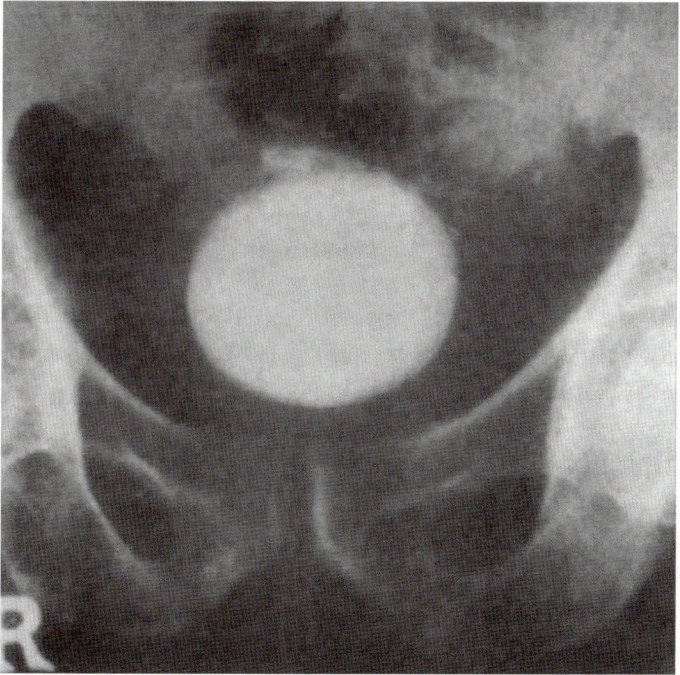

Fig. 26.18: Plain X-ray showing urinary bladder stone which is round. Usually triple phosphate stone

b. *Uric acid stone*: Round to oval, smooth, pale yellow, not opaque to X-rays. They are primary stones (Fig. 26.18).

c. *Cystine*: Radio-opaque due to high sulphur content.

d. *Triple phosphate*: These stones consist of ammonium, magnesium and calcium phosphates. **They occur in urine infected with urea-splitting organisms**. The stones are dirty white in colour. **Frequency of micturition is the earliest symptom of bladder stone. It is due to cystitis. Pain** at the end of micturition referred to tip of the penis in young boys suggests bladder stone. In school going children, pain is aggravated by jumping and jolting. Pain is decreased on lying down because stone falls away from the trigone of the bladder. Typically, oxalate stones produce pain. Painful ineffective micturition is described as strangury. **Haematuria** is due to stone causing abrasions in the bladder mucosa. **Acute retention of urine can occur** due to the calculus obstructing the internal meatus. **This is treated by litholapaxy.** By introducing a cystoscopic lithotrite, stone is grasped firmly and broken. Small fragments of stone are evacuated by using evacuator.

4. *Carcinoma bladder*: Cigarette **smoking is an important factor for carcinoma bladder.** Incidence is more in **aniline dye workers**. Products such as **benzidine and 3-naphthylamine** are carcinogenic. Other professions which are vulnerable are leather industry, paint industry and rubber industry. **Bilharziasis or schistosomiasis** increases the chances of bladder cancer (squamous cell carcinoma). In 90% of cases, initial symptom is **painless, intermittent haematuria. Severe cystitis** like symptoms occur in carcinomatous ulcer. Later painful, **blood-stained micturition** can occur. **Strangury:** Painful micturition with bleeding and incomplete emptying of bladder. **Loin pain** is due to ureteric obstruction with hydronephrosis. **Suprapubic pain,** groin pain, and perineal pain are due to infiltration of nerves. This indicates advanced nature of the growth. IVU if done may show filling defect in the urinary bladder (Fig. 26.19). Cystoscopy to confirm the diagnosis and take a biopsy followed by CT scan (Fig. 26.20) to know the infiltration of the bladder wall and surrounding tissues are the investigations of choice. Partial or radical cystectomy should be done depending upon the staging.

5. *Acute cystitis*: Acute uncomplicated bacterial cystitis predominantly affects women. The ascending faecal–perineal–urethral route is the primary source of infection. Men are somewhat protected from ascending infection because of long urethra and antibacterial properties of prostatic secretions. 80% of bladder infections in women are caused by *E. coli*

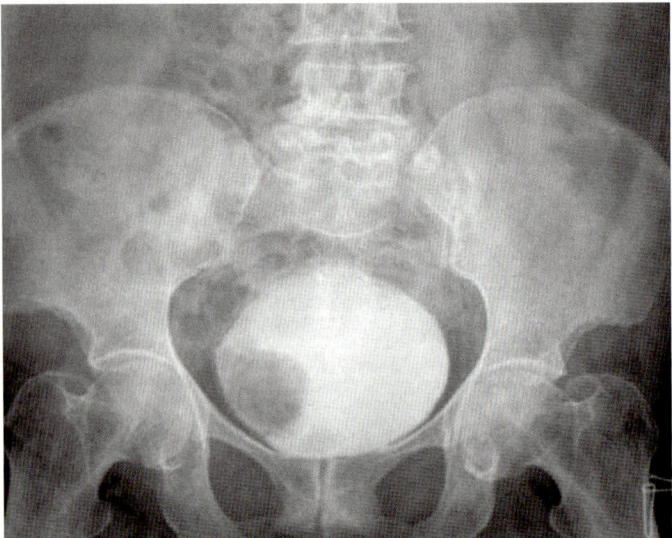

Fig. 26.19: IVU showing irregular filling defect in the urinary bladder

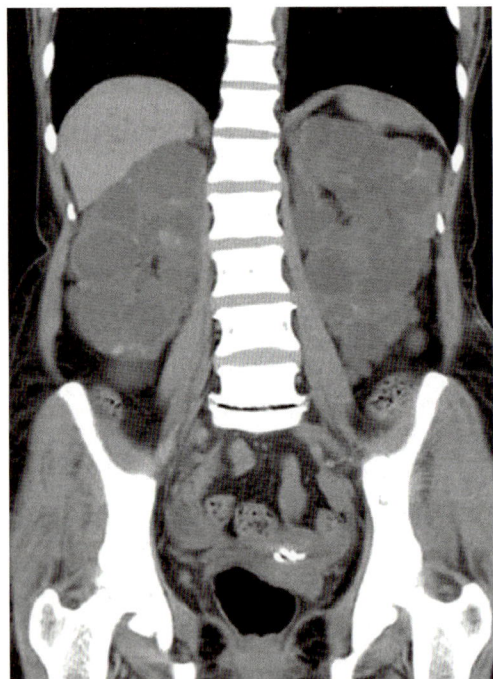

Fig. 26.20: CECT abdomen and pelvis showing a large tumour in the right lateral wall of bladder with right hydroureteronephrosis

followed by other gram-negative organisms such as *Klebsiella* and *Proteus* species. Irritative voiding symptoms (frequency, urgency, dysuria) are the hallmarks of cystitis. Low backache and suprapubic pain are other complaints. Fever and other constitutional symptoms are usually present. Physical examination is frequently unremarkable except for suprapubic tenderness. **Urinary microscopy** is the mainstay of diagnosis. Diagnosis is strongly considered positive, if microscopy shows **>5 WBCs/**

high power field in females and 2–3 WBCs/high power field in males. **Urine culture** not only confirms the diagnosis but also identifies the causative organisms. Antibiotic therapy based on the culture and sensitivity report given for a period of 7–10 days, is curative. Symptomatic treatment in the form of antipyretics, urinary analgesics and antispasmodics may help.

6. *Diverticula of the bladder:* True diverticulum—congenital (situated midline anterosuperiorly) is rare and usually symptomless. They represent the **unobliterated vesical end of the urachus.** They may require excision if chronic infection persists. Acquired diverticula are more common. They are pulsion diverticula and occur due to bladder outflow obstruction. They are found more commonly in males (95%) and seen after the age of 50 (Fig. 26.21).

   a. Symptoms of recurrent urinary infection: Suprapubic pain, frequency of micturition, fever with chills, etc.

   b. Symptoms of lower urinary obstruction: frequency, urgency, hesitancy, etc.

   c. Symptoms of pyelonephritis: Backache, fever, renal angle tenderness, etc.
    Complications include recurrent urinary infections, bladder stones, hydronephrosis and hydroureter due to peridiverticular inflammation, fibrosis and neoplasm (squamous metaplasia

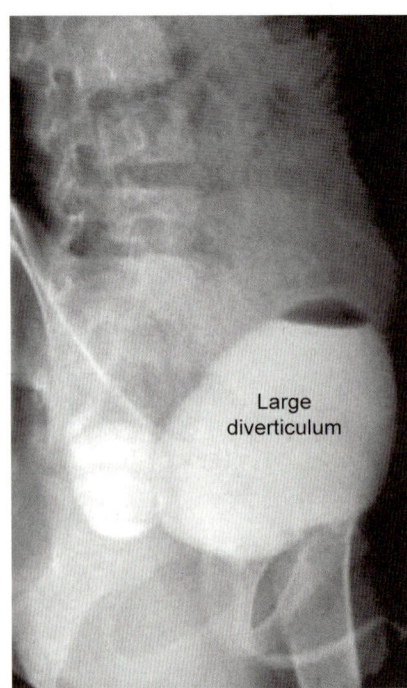

Large diverticulum

Fig. 26.21: Bladder diverticulum arising from the posterior wall. Ureter is seen entering the diverticulum

and leukoplakia). Ultrasonogram will detect the diverticulum. Treated by excision in symptomatic cases.

7. *Urinary fistulae*: Urinary fistulae are not an uncommon problem encountered by surgeons. They are broadly classified into congenital and acquired. A few of them are congenital in origin such as ectopia vesicae, patent urachus and in association with imperforate anus. More important ones are acquired fistulae. Traumatic fistulae are common. Other important fistula is vesicovaginal fistula. It is discussed here. Protracted or neglected labour, gynaecological operations such as total hysterectomy and anterior colporrhaphy, radiation causing avascular necrosis of the bladder, carcinoma cervix infiltrating into the bladder can also cause fistulae.

- Also *refer* to Clinical Box 26.8.

Clinical features: Typically after the surgery, leakage of urine from vagina happen after 7 days. Excoriation of the vulva is typical. Diagnosis is by digital vaginal examination which may reveal thickening on the anterior wall of vagina. Vaginal speculum examination demonstrates dribbling of urine into vagina. Swab test: Methylene blue is injected into the urethra and if vaginal swab is coloured blue, it is vesicovaginal fistula.

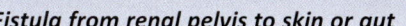

Clinical Box 26.8

Fistula from renal pelvis to skin or gut
- Tuberculosis causes caseation and may result in fistula in the loin
- Large staghorn calculi
- Pyonephrosis
- Crohn's disease of the renal pelvis

Treatment: Low fistula: Transvaginal repair and high fistula: Suprapubic approach and repair.

8. *Interstitial cystitis*: It is also called **Hunner's ulcer**. Initial symptoms are increased frequency and pain. It is relieved by micturition and aggravated by overdistension of bladder. The characteristic linear bleeding ulcer is caused by splitting of mucosa when the bladder is distended under anaesthesia. It is common in Western female patients. Many of them are psychiatric patients. There is severe fibrosis of the urinary bladder due to pancystitis, resulting in a small thimble bladder. (In India, tuberculosis must be considered.) Frequency of micturition and pain due to decreased bladder capacity are the features. It causes sterile pyuria. Cystoscopy and biopsy will confirm the diagnosis. Treatment is difficult—hydrostatic dilatation, instillation of dimethyl sulphoxide or surgical procedures such as ileocystoplasty have been tried.

9. *Schistosoma haematobium*: It is the commonest cause of calcification in the bladder wall. It is called urinary bilharziasis. The disease is caused by embryos (cercariae) of Schistosoma, which enter the body through penetration of the skin and reach the bladder *via* the portal vein in a retrograde manner. In the bladder, ova are released which are excreted back into the fresh water *via* the urine. Fresh water snail is the intermediate host. Multiple pseudotubercles, nodules, granulomas and fibrosis are the **prominent pathological** features. Diagnosis is suspected by painless terminal haematuria, which lasts for 5 days (swimmer's itch), fever and eosinophilia. Cystoscopy and biopsy confirms the diagnosis. It is treated by long-term praziquantel and surgery may be required (ileocystoplasty). ***Urinary bilharziasis is a premalignant condition.***

27

Examination of Hernia

INTRODUCTION

Hernia is a common condition affecting patients, especially inguinal hernia in males and incisional hernia in females. Even though several types of surgery have been described for hernias, mesh hernioplasty remains the gold standard treatment. Majority of the hernias require surgical treatment except small asymptomatic direct hernias in elderly. Today, laparoscopic hernia repair is becoming very popular. Obstructed hernia is an emergency and late cases carry significant mortality. As far as students are concerned, hernia is the most common case in the examination. Hence, detailed clinical examination of hernia, its complications, various types of hernias and their treatment have been described in this chapter.

Hernia means **to bud, protrude or rupture** (Latin).

Definition

Abnormal protrusion of a viscus or a part of it through a weak point in the body (opening) is known as a hernia. Inguinal hernia occurs either through the deep inguinal ring (indirect hernia), or through the posterior wall of the inguinal canal (direct hernia).

INDIRECT HERNIA

It is a herniation of abdominal contents through the deep ring into the inguinal canal. **Indirect hernia occurs due to persistent processus vaginalis sac.** It is the most common type of hernia in the body. The preformed sac passes through the deep ring, traverses the inguinal canal and may extend into the scrotum through the external ring. As it comes into the inguinal canal, it is invested by the following coverings from inside out:

- Internal spermatic fascia from fascia transversalis.
- Cremasteric fascia derived from internal oblique.
- External spermatic fascia derived from external oblique aponeurosis.

Types of Indirect Hernia (Figs 27.1 and 27.2)

1. *Complete hernia (scrotal):* When the sac is patent up to the bottom of the scrotum, it is a **complete scrotal hernia.**

2. *Funicular:* When the processus vaginalis sac is patent up to the root of scrotum, it is an **incomplete indirect hernia.**

3. *Bubonocoele:* Processus vaginalis sac is confined to the inguinal region or the inguinal canal only. Such hernias are seen in young patients.

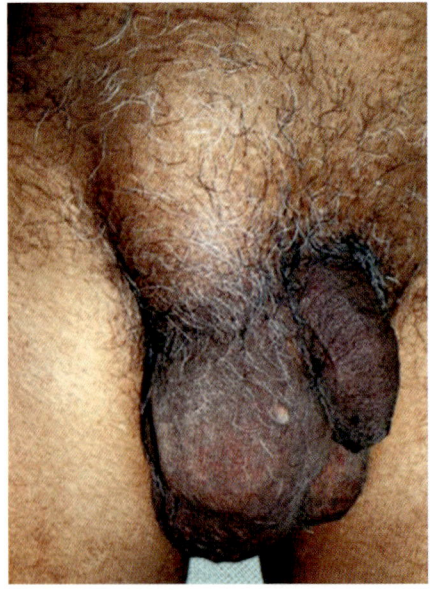

Fig. 27.1: Indirect hernia extending into scrotum

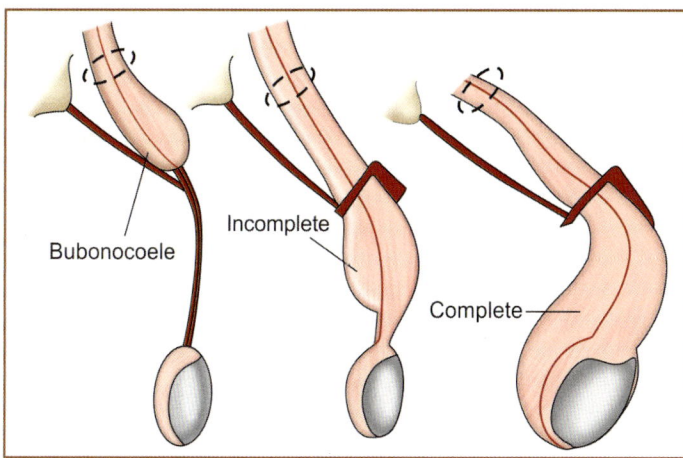

Fig. 27.2: Three types of indirect hernia

DIRECT HERNIA

It is a herniation occurring through the posterior wall of inguinal canal either due to weakness of posterior wall or due to congenital absence of a few muscles and fascial fibres (congenital). Since posterior wall is formed by transversalis fascia and the sac is posterior to it, direct hernia is usually confined to a medial bulge in the inguinal region and rarely descends into the scrotum.

CLINICAL EXAMINATION OF INGUINAL HERNIA

Patient Data

- Majority of groin hernias are seen in men. Direct hernias are common in the elderly and the indirect hernias are common in the young. It can also be seen in infants.
- Femoral hernias are common in females (middle age).

History of Present Illness

- What is your complaint? Why have you come to hospital? How long have you had this problem? Swelling and pain are 2 common complaints for which a patient comes to the hospital. To begin with, the swelling in the inguinal region is small but gradually progressing over a few months or years, it increases to attain the present size. The patient says the swelling disappears on lying down, and increases on straining, walking, etc. Some of them present late to the hospital and say that earlier they could push the swelling inside but now they cannot. This is called irreducibility, and it occurs due to adhesions. Sudden appearance of hernia may be attributed to violent coughing or straining

resulting in rupture of few fibres and causing hernia.

- **History of dragging pain** indicates omentocoele. Since the omentum is attached to the stomach above, and is supplied by T10, sympathetic nerve, the pain is referred to the umbilical region (the umbilicus is supplied by T10 intercostal nerve).
- Sudden, severe pain in the hernia, vomiting and irreducibility indicate **'obstructed hernia'.**
- **Chronic smoking:** Obtain details about pack years of smoking and cough. Chronic bronchitis, and obstructive (*refer* to page 109) pulmonary disease are important factors responsible for development of hernia. **History of chronic cough, constipation, and difficulty in passing urine** should be elicited. If present, it may suggest the cause of hernia. For example, straining on urination in an elderly patient is due to benign prostatic hypertrophy. Straining in younger patients is due to stricture urethra, caused by gonococcal urethritis. This can be suspected, if there is a history of exposure to multiple sexual partners, and thus venereal diseases. Its incidence has reduced considerably. Chronic cough due to cigarette smoking or due to chronic bronchitis can precipitate hernia.
- Instrumentation and trauma are other causes of stricture. Thus in appropriate cases, you have to ask a leading question—Did you fall or have any injury to perineum?
- History of constipation in the elderly may be due to carcinoma of left colon (rectosigmoid stricture). Such patients can also develop hernia.
- If the patient says that the swelling becomes bigger at the commencement of micturition, it suggests that the hernial sac contents include urinary bladder. Usually, it is of sliding variety. (Details later.)

Past History

- **History of appendicectomy: Did you undergo any surgery?** Division of ilioinguinal nerve during appendicectomy may cause denervation of fibres of the right transversus abdominis, which forms a U-shaped ring in the inguinal canal. It results in weakness of the abdominal wall.
- **History of surgery for hernia in the past.** Get details about postoperative cough, wound infection, discharge, etc.
- Look at the scar. Ragged edges indicate infection, a cause for recurrent hernia.

Personal History: History of Smoking

Inspection

It should be done in the **standing position. Both sides should be checked.**

- Direct hernia pops out as soon as the patient stands and is often bilateral. Indirect hernia takes some time to appear and becomes more prominent when the patient is asked to cough.

- Ask the patient to cough—look for **expansile impulse to confirm presence of hernia.** Expansile impulse on cough is diagnostic of hernia.

Clinical Box 27.1

Expansile impulse on cough
- Hernia
- Meningocoele
- Dermoid cyst with intracranial communication
- Laryngocoele
- Lymphatic cyst in children
- Empyema necessitans

- Once the swelling is obvious, describe it. For example: There is a swelling in the inguinal region extending up to the root of the scrotum measuring about 6 × 3 cm, pyriform in shape. **Its surface is smooth, borders are round, skin over the swelling is normal.** If peristalsis is present, it indicates presence of enterocoele.

- Presence of scar indicates a recurrent hernia. Ragged scar indicates infection.

- Look at the scrotum and testis. Empty scrotum indicates undescended testis.

- Look at the penis for any abnormalities. Mention circumcision has been done or not.

Palpation

1. Inspectory findings should be confirmed. Measure with a tape and confirm the extent. Start palpating the hernia and its contents gently. Swelling is soft and gurgles, if it is an enterocoele. It may be firm or granular, if it is an omentocoele.

2. *Ask the patient to cough*—expansile impulse may be felt at the root of scrotum (Figs 27.3 and 27.4).

3. *Getting above the swelling* (Fig. 27.5): This should be done in the standing position. At the root of scrotum, the spermatic cord is palpated between the

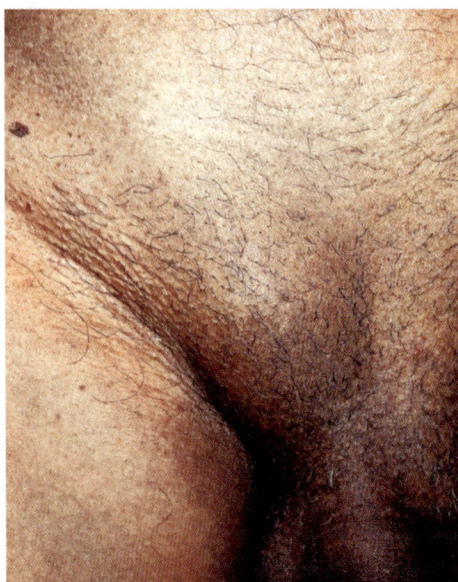

Fig. 27.3: Inspection in the standing position—small bulge is seen just above inguinal ligament on the medial side

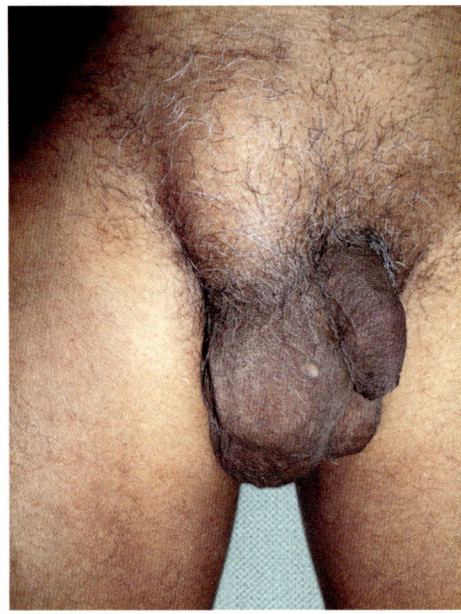

Fig. 27.4: On asking the patient to cough, an expansile impulse is seen and swelling is increased in size

finger and the thumb. In cases of complete indirect hernia, spermatic cord cannot be felt as a naked structure because it is covered anterolaterally by the sac. This is called **getting above the swelling not possible** (negative). *Getting above the swelling is a test to differentiate scrotal* swellings from inguino-scrotal swellings. (Clinical Box 27.2)

Clinical Wisdom

Getting above the swelling has no relevance in bubonocoele and in femoral hernia.

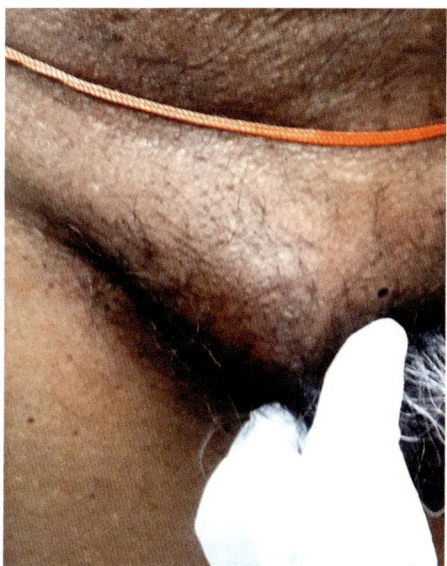

Fig. 27.5: The swelling is palpated at the root of the scrotum. Getting above the swelling is not possible. A case of incomplete hernia

Common inguinoscrotal swellings
- Complete and incomplete hernia
- Infantile hydrocoele
- Hydrocoele en bisac
- Diffuse lipoma of the cord

4. *Reducibility* (Fig. 27.6): Ask the patient to lie down.

If the swelling becomes smaller or disappears, it is a hernia. (Hydrocoele is not reducible.) **Omentocoele:** Initially, reduction is easy but later, becomes difficult (due to adhesions). If it is difficult to reduce, ask the patient to reduce it. Otherwise, flex and medially rotate the hip and try to reduce it, a method called

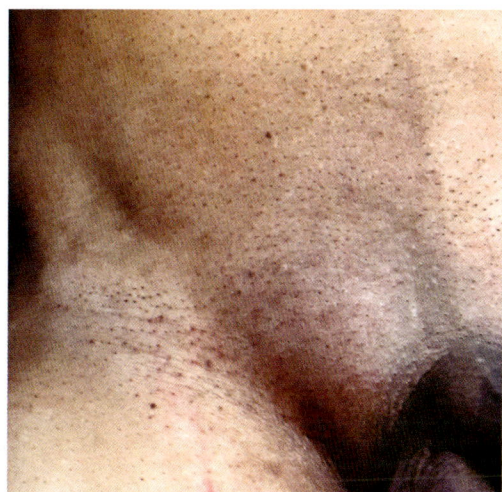

Fig. 27.6: On asking the patient to lie down, the swelling almost disappeared—sign of reducibility

taxis. If in spite of this the swelling is not reduced, it is called an irreducible hernia. **In long-standing hernias, and large hernias which are irreducible, suspect sliding hernia.**

5. *Deep ring occlusion test—internal ring occlusion test* (Fig. 27.7 and Clinical Box 27.3): Reduce the swelling first. Run the fingers along the groin crease. First bony point felt laterally is the anterior superior iliac spine. Mark this point. The most medial bone which is felt is the pubic tubercle. Just medial to it in the midline is pubic symphysis. Locate the deep ring above the midpoint between anterior superior iliac spine and symphysis pubis. Occlude the deep ring with the thumb and ask the patient to cough. If an impulse and a swelling are seen, it is a direct hernia because it occurs in the Hesselbach's triangle (medial to deep ring). If the swelling is not seen, it is an indirect hernia. Deep ring occlusion test can be done with the patient in both standing and supine positions.

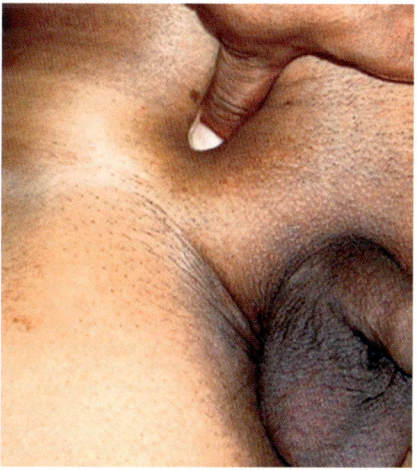

Fig. 27.7: Deep ring occlusion test. Swelling is not seen on coughing. A case of indirect hernia

Clinical Wisdom
- When you try to reduce the swelling, it may be displaced into inguinal region—may happen in infantile hydrocoele.
- To avoid confusion, avoid using the terms positive and negative. Use the words—swelling is 'seen' or 'not seen' in deep ring occlusion test.

Problems with deep ring occlusion test (fallacies)
a. If deep ring occlusion is not done properly, results may vary
b. If deep ring is wide, results may vary
c. If patient is very obese, occlusion may not be proper
d. Pantaloon hernia (Romberg hernia, saddle bag hernia, dual hernia). It is a direct hernia having indirect component, results may vary

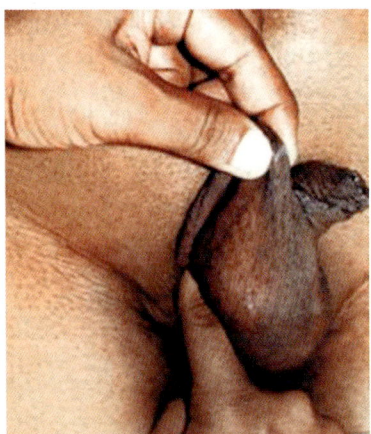

Fig. 27.8: External ring invagination test—finger goes directly backward. A case of direct hernia

6. *External ring invagination test* (Fig. 27.8): At the root of the scrotum, skin is gathered and lifted up with the index finger and thumb. Little finger is then invaginated into the external ring. As the external ring is stretched in case of indirect hernia, the finger goes obliquely and laterally. In a direct hernia, the finger goes backwards and the superior ramus of the pubic bone can be felt as a bare bone. On asking the patient to cough, the impulse is felt at the pulp of the finger in direct hernia, and at the tip in indirect hernia.

The strength of two pillars of external oblique aponeurosis and sphincteric action of conjoined tendon can also be assessed.

CLINICAL DISCUSSION
ABOUT EXTERNAL RING INVAGINATION TEST

- The test has no relevance in females. It cannot be done in female patients because the labial skin is thick and not lax. Hence, it is not a relevant test.
- When hernia descends into scrotum, external ring is stretched wide. In such cases, it is easy to do and it does not cause discomfort to the patient.
- In bubonocoele, the external ring is not stretched. In such patients, it may cause discomfort or pain to the patient.
- When I asked a senior professor about the relevance of this test, he said that in very early cases of indirect hernias, impulse can be detected near the deep ring in this test (**very subjective**).
- That was the answer. Today, this is easily detected by ultrasound examination.
- I do not do this test.

---

7. *Zieman's method* (Figs 27.9A and B): Three-finger method. Keep index finger at deep ring, middle finger on the posterior wall above and lateral to the external ring and ring finger at femoral ring. Now ask the patient to cough. Depending upon the type of hernia, impulse is felt.

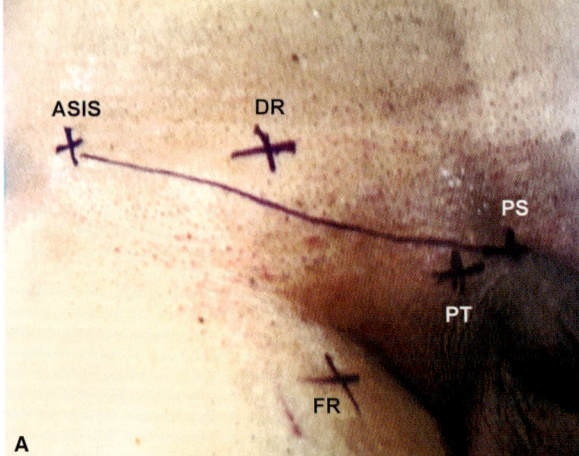

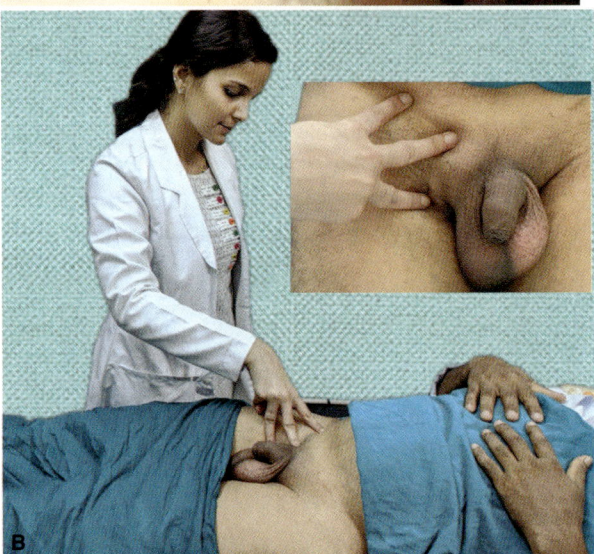

Figs 27.9A and 9B: Zieman's method: Anterior superior iliac spine (ASIS), deep ring (DR), pubic symphysis (PS), pubic tubercle (PT) and femoral ring (FR) have been marked for doing Zieman's test

- Impulse near the deep ring—indirect hernia
- Impulse near the superficial ring—direct hernia
- Impulse near the femoral ring—femoral hernia

8. *Leg raising test or head raising test* (Fig. 27.10): The patient is asked to raise the legs without bending

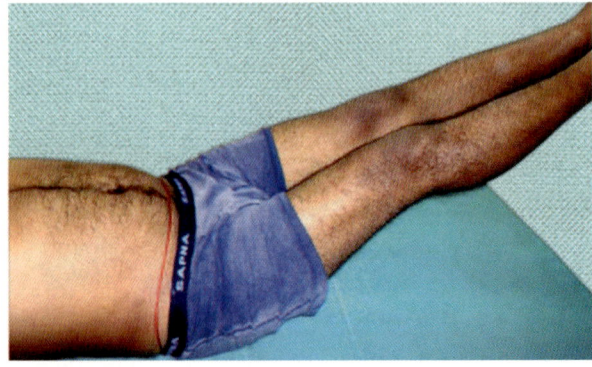

Fig. 27.10: Leg raising test: Muscle tone is good

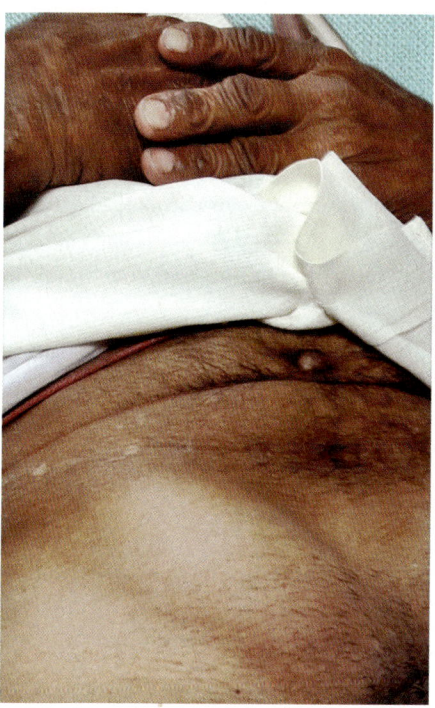

Fig. 27.11: Head raising test: Malgaigne's bulgings

the knee, or to raise the head with arms folded over the chest. Bulges, if seen above the inguinal ligament laterally are called Malgaigne's bulgings (Fig. 27.11). These indicate weakness of the oblique muscles of the abdominal wall. This test was used to detect poor muscle tone, a guide for the surgeon performing hernioplasty using a mesh. However, today all hernia repairs are done using a mesh.

9. *Per abdomen*: Rule out any mass (colonic), ascites, or ovarian tumours.

10. *Examination of external genitalia*: Look for phimosis/stricture urethra. Young patients experiencing urinary complaints with hernia may suffer from stricture urethra. Lift the scrotum and feel for any strictures in the bulbar urethra in the midline through scrotal skin. Strictures are felt to have consistency like button hole. Retract skin of prepuce and rule out phimosis.

11. *Per rectal examination* should be done in elderly patients to rule out prostatic enlargement.

12. *Examination of respiratory system* is done to rule out chronic bronchitis, tuberculosis, etc. Look for crepitations and rhonchi.

Clinical Wisdom

Examine the opposite side, examine the umbilicus and epigastrium—all possible sites of hernia.

Clinical Examination of a Hernia in a Child

- Swelling may not be visible at first as it may be covered by thick pad of fat. Examine when a child strains (cry), or after child's play (jumping, etc.). Examine the root of scrotum—may find hernial sac (thickening).

- **Gornall's test:** By gentle compression on child's abdomen (hold the child on its back), hernia may become apparent.

Diagnosis: When giving a diagnosis, give a complete diagnosis. Mention the side, type, contents and presence or absence of complications. Two examples are given below.

- Right sided, indirect, incomplete, reducible, hernia with enterocoele as content.

- Bilateral direct, reducible, hernia with possibly an enterocoele.

CLINICAL DISCUSSION

1. What hernias are common in young patients?
Bubonocoele.

2. What causes dragging pain?
Omentum.

3. What are the other causes of groin pain?
Muscular strain in sports men

4. Direct hernia comes out of what structure?
Hesselbach's triangle.

5. What are the boundaries of Hesselbach triangle?
Medially by lateral border of rectus abdominis, laterally by inferior epigastric vessels and inferiorly by inguinal ligament.

6. What causes indirect hernia?
Persistent processus vaginalis sac.

7. What is pantaloon hernia?
It is double or **Romberg or saddle bag hernia.** It is concurrent direct and indirect hernias—hernias are on both sides of inferior epigastric vessels. In majority, direct component is bigger than indirect component.

8. Why should you look for pantaloon hernia?
Missing one sac at surgery may result in recurrence of hernia.

9. How does smoking cause hernia?
Chronic cough results in chronic bronchitis. Other reason is **smoking decreases elastin** content in the abdominal muscles thereby decrease strength.

10. Why direct hernia does not descend into scrotum?
Transversalis fascia which forms posterior wall is anterior to the sac. It prevents the descent of the sac. However, if a few fibres of transversalis fascia are absent congenitally or ruptured, it can descend into scrotum.

11. What are the parts supplied by ilioinguinal nerve?

Supplies the skin of the upper and medial parts of the thigh, scrotum and vulva.

12. What is European classification?

The European Hernia Society classification:

- It considers following aspects. Primary (P), Recurrent (R)
- Lateral (L), Medial (M), Femoral (F)
- Defect size assumed to be 1.5 cm

   Thus, primary direct hernia with 3 cm defect size is written as PM2.

13. What are the differences between indirect and direct hernias?

Refer to Table 27.1

14. What are the differences between inguinoscrotal hernia and vaginal hydrocoele?

Refer to Table 27.2

15. What are the investigations for hernia?

Hernia is a clinical diagnosis. Other than investigations for fitness for surgery, no other investigations are required. However, in large hernias, sliding hernias, recurrent hernias, perineal hernias and obturator hernia, CT scan can give all the details of the structures and anatomy of the hernia. Thus, surgeon will be able to protect a few important structures such as urinary bladder, ureters, etc.

16. When do you do MRI in cases of hernia?

Groin pain in sportsmen may be confused for hernia pain. MRI can clearly define any muscular aetiology (a few ruptured fibres—Gilmore groin).

17. What is the treatment of inguinal hernia?

Lichtenstein's inguinal hernioplasty. High ligation of the sac is done first followed by excision of sac as close to the deep ring as possible. A 15 × 10 cm prolene mesh which is trimmed at all 4 corners, is placed over the transversalis fascia and sutured above to the conjoint tendon, inferiorly to the inguinal ligament (continuous sutures), medially in the midline across the pubic symphysis. Laterally, the mesh is split in the inferior one-third width area so as to allow a passage for the spermatic cord (*refer to* Flowchart 27.1 given in the next page).

18. What is Lytle's repair ?

When the deep ring is stretched wide, it is better to narrow the deep ring by a few sutures on the internal oblique fibres. This repair is called **Lytle's repair.** (You can remember as a **small little repair** done at deep ring is called **Lytle's repair.**)

19. What are the important causes for recurrence?

Low ligation of the sac, suturing with tension, small size mesh (mesh contracts), haematoma, infection, straining/coughing in the pre- and postoperative period and poor muscle tone are important factors.

20. What is modified Bassini herniorrhaphy?

In this operation, conjoint tendon is sutured to the inguinal ligament by using non-absorbable interrupted sutures. Suture material used is prolene 2–0. It is a simple operation. However, compared to meshplasty, the approximation of the conjoined tendon to inguinal ligament will produce some degree of tension, the reason for increased incidence of recurrence.

21. The patient says swelling descends into scrotum. What does that mean? Is it incomplete or complete hernia?

It is indirect hernia because processus vaginalis sac traverses through inguinal canal and descends into scrotum.

22. Why not direct hernia?

Direct hernia rarely descends into scrotum.

23. Rarely direct hernia also descends into scrotum. What may be the reason?

- May be a few fibres of transversalis fascia are weak or missing.
- It may be sliding hernia also.

24. What is the relationship of indirect hernia sac to the cord structures?

It is anterolateral.

25. What is the shape of deep ring?

It is inverted U-shaped.

26. What is the common mistake done by students while doing deep ring occlusion test?

Not identifying the exact location of deep ring.

27. Where is the deep ring located?

1.25 cm above midinguinal point.

28. What are the identification points at surgery to find out deep ring?

Inferior epigastric artery and extraperitoneal pad of fat.

29. What is taxis?

In case of irreducible hernia—an attempt is made to reduce by flexion of hip and medial rotation (relaxes the muscles)

30. What are the problems of forceful taxis?

Hernia may be reduced but obstruction is not relieved. If there is gangrene, it easily spreads within peritoneal cavity.

31. What is the shape of femoral hernia as it spreads across saphenous opening into loose areolar tissue?

It is retort shaped, white bulbous portion towards inguinal ligament.

32. Where is the saphenous opening located?

4 cm below and lateral to pubic tubercle as a defect in the fascia lata. Saphenous opening is called fossa ovalis.

33. What test do you do to check for tone of the muscles?

Head raising test or leg raising test.

34. Where do you look for Malgaigne's bulging?

Above the inguinal ligament on the lateral part of lower abdomen.

35. What is the significance of these findings?

Patient requires hernioplasty not herniorrhaphy.

Table 27.1: Differences between direct and indirect hernias

	Direct hernia	Indirect hernia
1. Age	Common in elderly	Can occur in any age group
2. Aetiology	Weakness of posterior wall of inguinal canal	Preformed (PV) sac
3. Precipitating factors	Chronic bronchitis, enlarged prostate	—
4. On standing	Pops out	Does not pop out
5. Side	Usually bilateral	Unilateral (30% bilateral)
6. Deep ring occlusion test	Swelling is seen	Swelling is not seen
7. Malgaigne's bulgings	May be present	Absent
8. Obstruction and strangulation	Not common because neck is wide	Common, neck is narrow
9. Relationship of sac to the cord	Sac is posterior to the cord	Sac is anterolateral to the cord
10. Direction of the sac	It comes out of Hesselbach's triangle	Comes through the deep ring

Table 27.2: Clinical differences between hernia and hydrocoele

	Indirect complete hernia	Vaginal hydrocoele
1. Standing position	Swelling of scrotum and inguinal region	Swelling confined only to scrotum
2. Impulse on coughing	Present	Absent
3. Getting above swelling	Not possible	Possible
4. Reducibility	Usually present unless complicated	Not reducible
5. Consistency	Soft and elastic	Soft, fluctuant
6. Transillumination	Absent	Present

Flowchart 27.1: Management of inguinal hernia

Herniotomy in children	Herniorrhaphy • Modified Bassini • Shouldice • Desarda repair	Hernioplasty • Lichtenstein • Stoppa • Gilbert	Laparoscopic repair • TEP • TAPP

SUMMARY OF VARIOUS TYPES OF SURGERY FOR INGUINAL HERNIA (Refer textbooks for more details)

1. **Herniotomy:** It means excision of the hernia sac. No repair is required. This is done in children within 16 years of age group. Reason for development of hernia is patent processus vaginalis (PV) sac. Hence, simple excision of the sac is the treatment of choice.

2. **Herniorrhaphy**

   A. **Modified Bassini's repair:** In this surgery, approximation of posterior wall of inguinal canal is done by suturing conjoint tendon to inguinal ligament by using nonabsorbable sutures.

   B. **Shouldice:** This repair involves division of all layers of the posterior wall of the inguinal canal upto peritoneum followed by layered reconstruction involving three to four suture lines by overlap (double breasting) technique.

   C. **Desarda technique:** In this operation, a strip of external oblique aponeurosis is prepared and isolated but still connected medially and laterally to external oblique muscle and sutured to conjoint tendon and inguinal ligament below.

3. **Hernioplasty:** Basic principle is strengthening of posterior wall of inguinal canal
   A. **Lichtenstein:** It has been already discussed.
   B. **Stoppa:** It is called as Giant prosthetic reinforcement of the visceral sac (GPRVS). A broad prosthetic mesh is placed over the preperitoneal space, thus covering myopectineal orifice of Fruchauds.

   C. **Gilbert:** Depending upon the size of the defect and type of hernia, herniorrhaphy and hernioplasty are done. When the defect is large as in few cases of direct hernias, a purse string closure of the defect followed by hernioplasty is done. In few other cases of indirect hernias, a cone-shaped plug of polypropylene mesh that when inserted into the internal inguinal ring, it would deploy like an upside-down umbrella and occlude the hernia. This plug is sewn to the surrounding tissues, held in place by an additional overlying mesh patch.

4. **Laparoscopic hernia repair**

   A. **TEP:** Totally extraperitoneal repair: A 15 × 15 cm mesh is placed in the extraperitoneal space which is created between the rectus abdominis muscle and posterior rectus sheath after excision of the sac. The main advantage is that both sides can be done with same ports and peritoneum is not opened.

   B. **TAPP:** Trans Abdominal Pre Peritoneal repair—here the size of the mesh and placement are similar to TEP but abdomen is entered through peritoneum. The peritoneum is incised, access to the inguinal canal is gained through it and repair is done.

DIFFERENTIAL DIAGNOSIS OF A GROIN SWELLING

Groin refers to the junction of lower abdomen with the thigh—above and below inguinal ligament. Hence, swellings in the inguinal region and upper thigh close to the inguinal ligament are included under groin swellings.

1. **Inguinal hernia** (Fig. 27.12): Sac is above inguinal ligament in bubonocoele, and above and medial in indirect hernia descending into scrotum.

2. **Femoral hernia**: The main sac is below and lateral to pubic tubercle (Fig. 27.13).

3. **Vaginal hydrocoele**: Fluctuation and transillumination tests are usually positive and getting above swelling is possible in vaginal hydrocele. However, in infantile hydrocoele and hydrocoele *en bisac*, getting above swelling is not possible, and they also will have inguinal component (Fig. 27.14).

4. **Retractile testis**: It can present as a firm swelling in the inguinal region. Scrotum is empty (Fig. 27.15). However, it is well developed.

5. **Saphena varix**: The patient can present with a swelling in the thigh. Swelling is usually about 2.5 cm below the pubic tubercle. A swelling that disappears on elevation of the leg is characteristic of a swelling of venous origin (Fig. 27.16).

6. **Funiculitis**: A funiculitis can occur with or without acute epididymo-orchitis. Severe pain in the inguinal region, tender swelling, high grade fever with chills and rigors are characteristic. Spermatic cord is thickened and swelling is not reducible (Fig. 27.17).

7. **Inguinal lymphadenitis**: Pain and presence of nodular swelling below inguinal ligament is a feature. It is not reducible and some source of infection in the lower limb is usually present (Fig. 27.18).

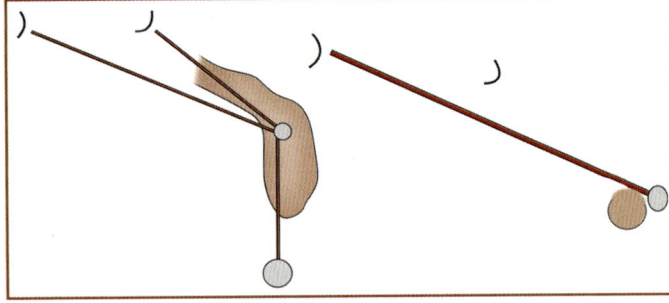

Fig. 27.12: Inguinal hernia   **Fig. 27.13:** Femoral hernia

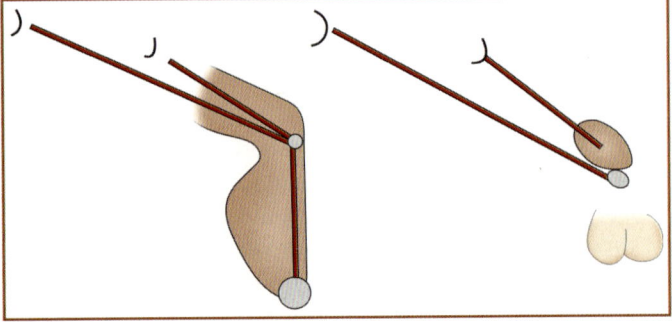

Fig. 27.14: Infantile hydrocoele   **Fig. 27.15:** Retractile testis

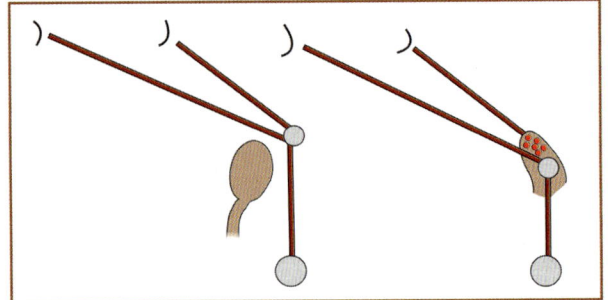

Fig. 27.16: Saphena varix   **Fig. 27.17** Funiculitis

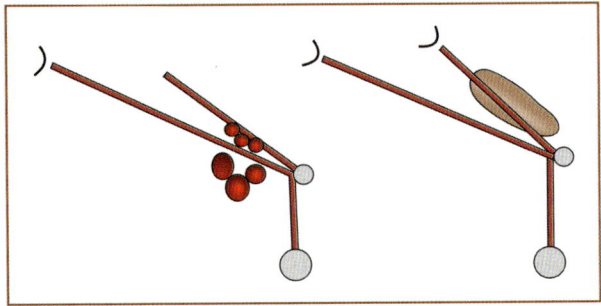

Fig. 27.18: Inguinal lymphadenitis   **Fig. 27.19:** Lipoma of the cord

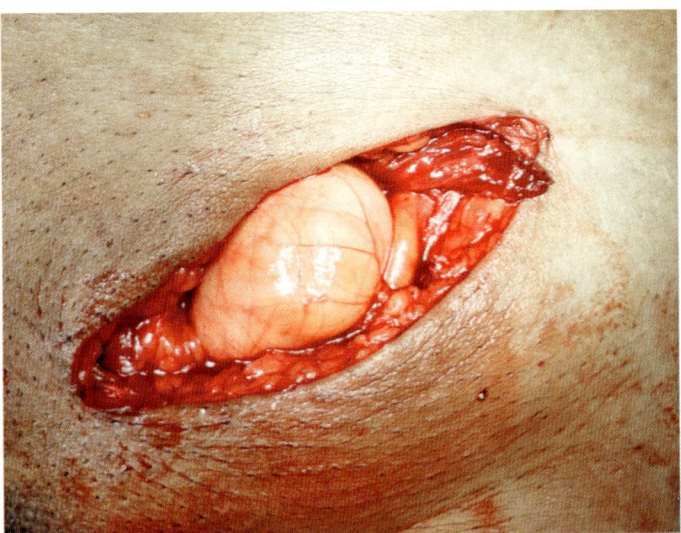

Fig. 27.20: Lipoma of the cord—left inguinal region

8. **Lipoma of the cord**: It presents as a soft, lobulated but irreducible swelling in the inguinal region (Figs 27.19 and 27.20).

MORE DETAILS ABOUT INGUINAL HERNIA

Basically, there are two types of hernia: Indirect and direct. Indirect hernia comes through deep inguinal ring into inguinal canal and then descends into scrotum. Direct hernia occurs as a protrusion or a bulge through transversalis fascia, on the medial side and rarely descends into scrotum.

ANATOMICAL CLASSIFICATION

1. *Indirect hernia*: Common in young and middle age group. More common in men. Persistent processus vaginalis is the chief cause for this hernia. Other factors which cause hernia are chronic cough, chronic bronchitis, chronic asthma, etc. The test which distinguishes indirect hernia from direct is the deep ring occlusion test, in which swelling does not reappear after reduction. The following types of hernia are described based on anatomy:

A. Depending upon the descent

- *Bubonocoele*: Hernia confined to inguinal canal. It is common in young children and adolescent age group.

- *Incomplete*: Hernia reaches the root of the scrotum.

- *Complete*: Hernia descends into the bottom of the scrotum.

B. Depending upon the contents

- *Enterocoele*: Elastic, tympanitic, reduces with gurgle.

- *Omentocoele*: Doughy, granular, dull, reduces with ease in the beginning but difficult at the end (due to adhesions).

C. Depending upon the duration

- *Congenital*: The whole processus vaginalis sac is patent and hence it is usually a complete hernia. It can be seen in infants but often seen in adults also. Congenital funicular hernia refers to the hernia that stops at the root of the scrotum.

- *Acquired*: It takes a few years for the hernia to protrude into preformed sac. It takes a long time to develop into complete hernia.

2. *Direct hernia*: This is more common after 40 years of age. Chronic cough, carrying heavy load on back and benign prostatic hypertrophy are a few common causes. It is spherical in shape and rarely descends into scrotum. Because of its wide neck (defect in the transversalis fascia), it is not prone to strangulation. Usually bilateral, it just pops out as soon as the patient stands. The following types have been identified.

A. Depending upon the descent

- *Incomplete*: Hernia in the medial part of inguinal canal.

- *Complete*: Hernia descends into scrotum (rare).

B. Depending upon the contents

- *Enterocoele:* Elastic, tympanitic, reduces with gurgle.

- *Omentocoele:* Doughy, granular, dull, reduces with ease in the beginning but difficult at the end (due to adhesions).

- *Cystocoele:* It is a direct hernia with urinary bladder being the content. Very often it is also a sliding hernia (details are given later). Usually, they are partially reducible. An attempt to reduce this may result in desire for micturition.

CLINICAL CLASSIFICATION

These are complications of hernia

1. *Irreducible hernia*: When hernia cannot be reduced completely, it is called irreducible hernia. Irreducibility is usually due to presence of adhesions between omentum and sac, omentum and intestines or adhesions between any contents. Sliding hernias are usually irreducible. It is nontender and blood supply of contents is not affected. When the hernia is irreducible, one need not perform invagination test and deep ring occlusion test. The best technique to reduce this hernia is known to the patient.

2. *Obstructed hernia*: It is a surgical emergency. Typically, a patient with hernia of a few months or years presents with severe abdominal pain and vomiting. Pain is colicky due to obstruction of the lumen of the intestines resulting in hyperperistalsis. Vomiting is frequently projectile, and contains food contents. Faeculent vomiting suggests terminal ileal obstruction. Hernia is tense, may be tender. There will not be impulse upon coughing. It is irreducible. It is treated by emergency hernioplasty.

3. *Strangulated hernia* (Clinical Box 27.4)**:** It is a combination of irreducibility + obstruction + impairment of blood supply resulting in gangrene of the bowel. It is a serious emergency. During surgery,

---

Clinical Box 27.4 🔑

Strangulated hernia—clinical diagnosis
- Tense
- Tender
- Irreducible
- Impulse on cough is absent
- Recent increase in size is present

constriction at the deep ring should not be released first because contents from the hernia sac which are toxic can easily enter the peritoneal cavity and may result in septic shock. Once the sac is opened, the contents are sucked out, and the constricting ring is divided. The gangrenous bowel is then resected and end-to-end anastomosis performed. Mesh placement is not recommended. Tissue repair, such as Bassini, can be done.

4. Incarcerated hernia: It is an obstructed hernia, but obstruction is not due to the deep ring or any other constriction, but it is due to solid faecal matter present in the colon. This can happen in large, giant hernias of long-standing or sliding hernias. It can also happen in umbilical hernias wherein transverse colon is the content. Indentation, if present during palpation of the contents, may suggest an incarcerated hernia. Treatment is hernioplasty.

5. Inflamed hernia: It is a misnomer. Hernial sac is inert and it does not get inflamed but contents can get inflamed, e.g. appendicitis, Meckel's diverticulitis. It is difficult clinically because it mimics strangulated hernia. However, features of intestinal obstruction are absent. Skin will be reddish and erythematous. Ultrasound/CT scan is an ideal investigation in such cases. Treatment is to treat the primary disease. If a conservative approach is followed, strangulation has to be ruled out.

A few uncommon Types of Hernia

1. Sliding inguinal hernia (Figs 27.21 to 27.23)/**hernia-en-glissade:** Incidence: 1–2%. It is always an acquired hernia. It occurs as a result of the slipping of posterior peritoneum along with the retroperitoneal viscus under the cellular tissue. As a result of which, the caecum on the right side and the sigmoid colon on the left side, form the posterior wall of the sac. Weakness of the abdominal wall at the deep ring lateral to inferior epigastric vessels is also a contributing factor. **If the caecum and appendix are the contents of the hernia sac, it is not a sliding hernia.** Omentum, small bowel and urinary bladder can also be the contents of the hernia sac (Figs 27.21 and 27.23). It generally occurs in males. It can be suspected when there is a large hernia descending down into the scrotum. Left-sided is more common than right-sided hernia. It almost always occurs in long-standing cases of inguinal hernia. **They are not completely reducible.** It can be direct hernia or an

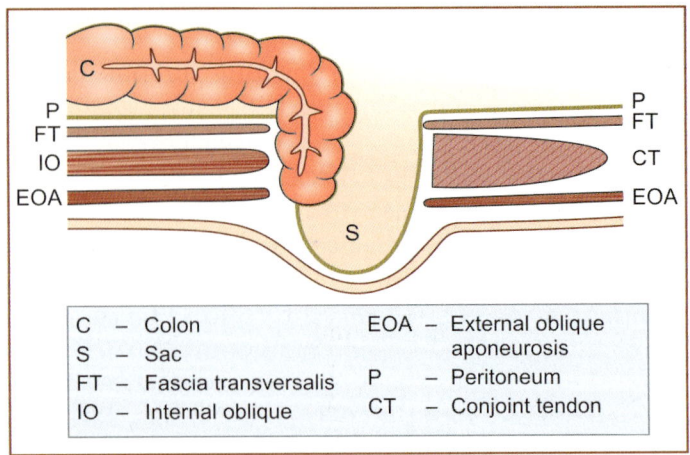

C – Colon	EOA – External oblique aponeurosis
S – Sac	P – Peritoneum
FT – Fascia transversalis	CT – Conjoint tendon
IO – Internal oblique	

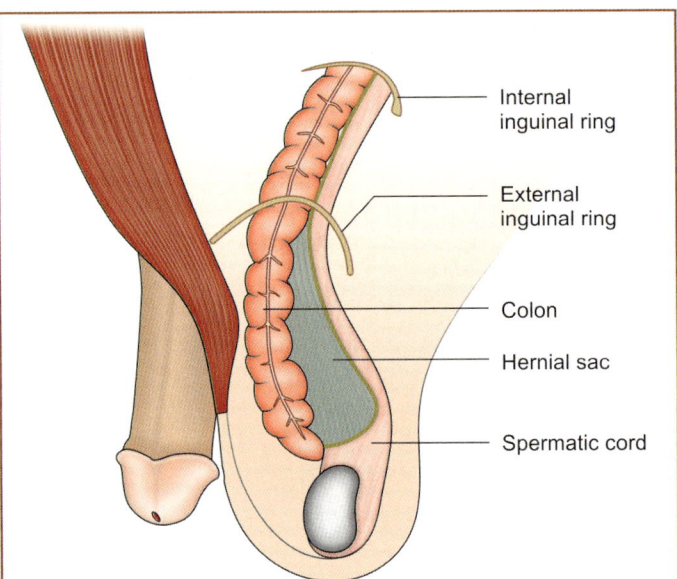

Figs 27.21 and 27.22: Diagrammatic representation of sliding hernia—coronal and sagittal view (*Courtesy:* Dr Chitra Y Bhat, Assistant Professor, Department of Surgery, KMC, Manipal)

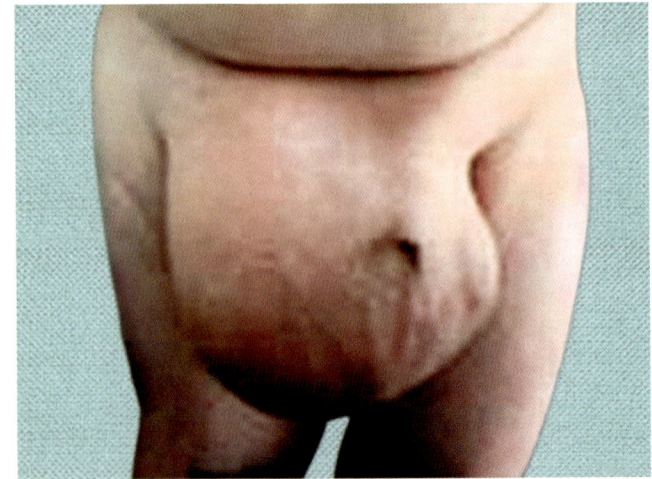

Fig. 27.23: Sliding hernia (*Courtesy:* Vladimir M Lobankov, Gomel State Medical University, Belarus)

indirect hernia. These hernias can easily strangulate and since its wall contents include the large intestine, the mortality and morbidity increases. **Truss is absolutely contraindicated.** Once the hernial sac is opened, the sac should not be twisted. A purse-string suture is applied within to avoid injury to caecum/sigmoid colon. The sac is removed and the hernia is repaired. In elderly patients, orchidectomy is advised as a permanent cure for hernia (Clinical Box 27.5).

2. *Giant hernia* (Fig. 27.24): A giant inguinoscrotal hernia is defined as a hernia that extends below the midpoint of the inner thigh in the standing position. Most patients would have had this hernia for several years. Often colon, small intestines and bladder are the contents. A few of these are also sliding inguinal hernias. Hence, it is more prone for complications like incarceration, intestinal obstruction and scrotal ulceration. The last complication is due to pressure necrosis or due to friction while walking or moving. Differential diagnosis includes scrotal elephantiasis. Surgery is the treatment of choice. A few precautions must be taken during surgery. These are: Preoperative

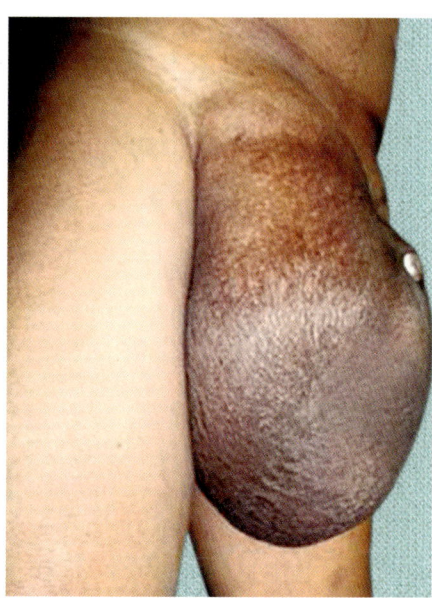

Fig. 27.24: Giant hernia

chest physiotherapy to decrease abdominal compartment syndrome. Catheterise all the patients to decrease the incidence of urinary bladder injury. Bowel wash before surgery because colonic resection is often required in these cases. If necessary, omentectomy and rarely colectomy may be required. If bowel is not resected, mesh can be placed safely. In cases of emergency and in patients with comorbid factors including cardiac problems, take consent for orchidectomy—divide the cord at the level of deep ring and close the deep ring. That will be best option.

3. *Dual hernia*: It has two sacs, one direct and another indirect, connected by an isthmus which is behind the inferior epigastric artery. It is also known as saddle bag hernia, **pantaloon hernia**, dual hernia or Romberg hernia. **Significance:** Deep ring occlusion test: The inference of the test may not be correct. It is the cause of recurrence, if one sac is not treated properly.

4. *Maydl's hernia (hernia-en-W)*: It is a **W** hernia wherein the intra-abdominal bowel loop segment becomes gangrenous very early but in the scrotum there are no signs of gangrene. The patient presents with obstructed hernia and upon operating, the inguinoscrotal segment has no gangrene. The intra-abdominal segment must be examined and the gangrenous portion should be excised. It can also be called retrograde strangulation. Clinically, there is tenderness above the inguinal ligament. High degree of suspicion is required to diagnose such cases. CT scan will help to know the viability of the intestines. Laparotomy and resection of the bowel are required.

5. *Richter's hernia*: When only part of circumference of bowel becomes strangulated, it is called Richter's hernia. It may spontaneously reduce. Thus, gangrene may be overlooked while operating. Even though the patient has features of intestinal obstruction, there will be diarrhoea and often blood in stools. Femoral hernia and obturator hernia are a few examples of Richter's hernia.

6. *Sportsman's hernia*: This is common in men who play rugby or football wherein the inguinal region may be hit by the ball. Pain is in the groin and radiates to scrotum and upper thigh. On examination, there may be tenderness in the inguinal region. Orthopaedic disorders must be ruled out first by MRI or CT scan. These are soft tissue injury in the groin, pubic bone diastasis, adductor spasm, etc. If hernia is due to

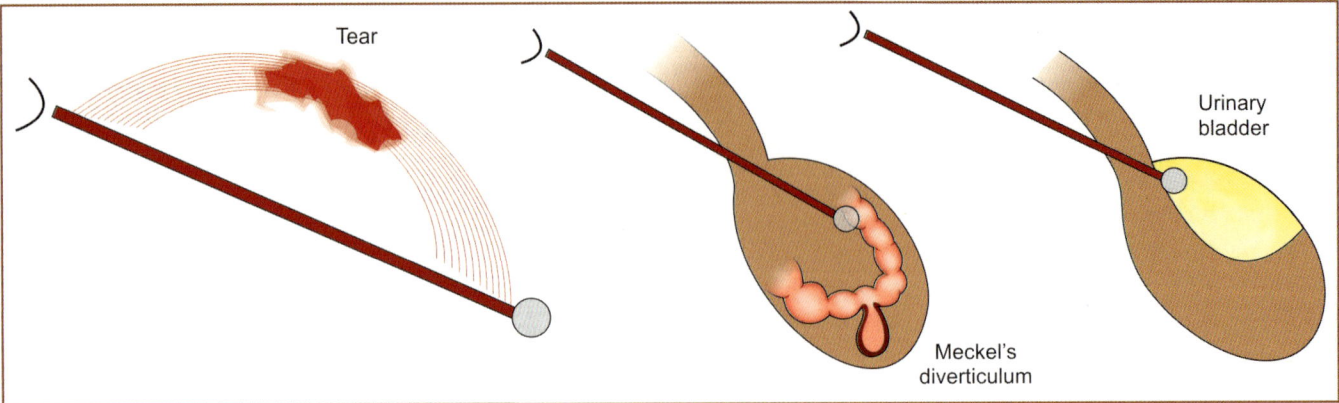

Fig. 27.25: Gilmore's groin   **Fig. 27.26:** Littre's hernia   **Fig. 27.27:** Prevesical hernia

tearing of muscles **(Gilmore's groin)**—it should be repaired in the usual manner (Fig. 27.25).

7. *Littre's hernia*: It refers to a hernia containing Meckel's diverticulum. When the diverticulum gets infected, such hernias are called inflamed hernias. The cause of infection may be precipitated by partial obstruction to the diverticulum by constricting agents. Treatment is by hernioplasty. It is better to resect Meckel's diverticulum so as to avoid confusion the next time the patient has abdominal pain (Fig. 27.26).

8. *Prevesical hernia*: It is also called **funicular direct hernia**. It is a hernia containing portion of the bladder with prevesical fat through the defect in the conjoined tendon on the medial side. History of the swelling becoming less prominent after micturition may be present. Due to its narrow neck, it is prone for strangulation (Fig. 27.27).

FEMORAL HERNIA

Herniation of intra-abdominal contents through the femoral canal is described as femoral hernia. Women are more often affected, as compared to men with the ratio being 2:1, which is doubled in parous women. However, it should be remembered that **in women, inguinal hernia is the most common type of hernia, followed by incisional hernia.** Femoral hernia is the third most common type of hernia. Commonly the hernia is unilateral, the right side being affected more often than the left side. It is bilateral in about 15–20% of the patients. Typically, the swelling is below and lateral to the pubic tubercle (inguinal hernia is above and medial to pubic tubercle) (Fig. 27.28). Very often the patient presents with intestinal obstruction and a

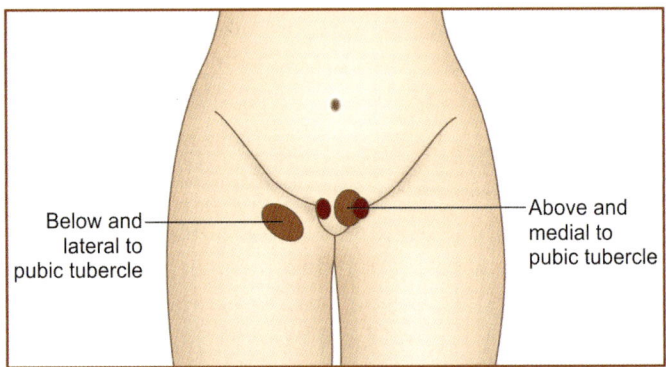

Fig. 27.28: Femoral hernia (R) and indirect hernia (L)

small obstructed femoral hernia in females may be missed. This highlights the importance of examination of hernial sites in cases of intestinal obstruction. Uncomplicated cases can be operated by low incision in the upper thigh directly over the sac, reduce the sac and suture the inguinal ligament anteriorly to Cooper's ligament posteriorly. When in doubt or when there is gangrene, it is better to adopt a high approach—inguinal incision, open transversalis fascia, reduce the sac and even resect the gangrene. Repair is similar to what has been described already.

CLINICAL DISCUSSION

1. Why is femoral hernia retort-shaped?

Hernia comes out of tight femoral canal and then suddenly comes out of saphenous opening and expands. However, further expansion is limited by attachment of Scarpa's fascia to the deep fascia of the thigh just below the saphenous opening.

2. Is femoral hernia congenital?

No. It is never congenital but is always acquired.

3. What is the lateral structure in femoral hernia?

Femoral vein.

4. What is Gaur sign?

Dilatation of superficial epigastric/circumflex iliac veins due to compression.

5. What artery is in danger during surgery of femoral hernia?

Abnormal obturator artery is sometimes found on the medial side of the femoral hernia sac near the lacunar ligament.

6. What is Narath hernia?

It is femoral hernia with congenital dislocation of the hip.

What is Cloquet hernia?

The hernia passes between the pectineus muscle and its fascia, behind the femoral vessels.

DIFFERENTIAL DIAGNOSIS OF FEMORAL HERNIA

1. *Inguinal hernia*: An inguinal hernia occurs above and medial to pubic tubercle. The femoral hernia occurs below and lateral to pubic tubercle (Fig. 27.28).

2. *Saphena varix*: It is the dilated, saccular, upper end of long saphenous vein with varicosity. It disappears on lying down because of gravity. Thrill may be felt on coughing (Fig. 27.29).

3. *Lipoma*: Soft and lobular, slips under palpating fingers (Fig. 27.30).

4. *Femoral artery aneurysm* is rare. It presents as a pulsatile swelling in the groin with a continuous murmur. Peripheral pulses are often weak (Fig. 27.31).

5. *Enlarged femoral lymph nodes* are firm and round. They can be enlarged in lower limb infections, abrasions, wounds in the perineum and also in carcinoma penis (Fig. 27.32).

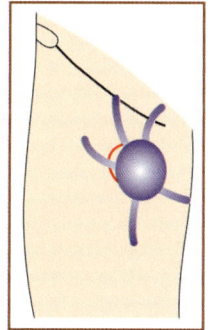

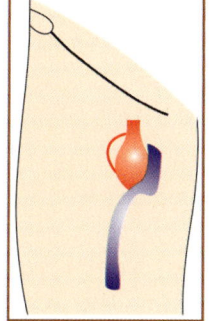

Fig. 27.29: Saphena varix

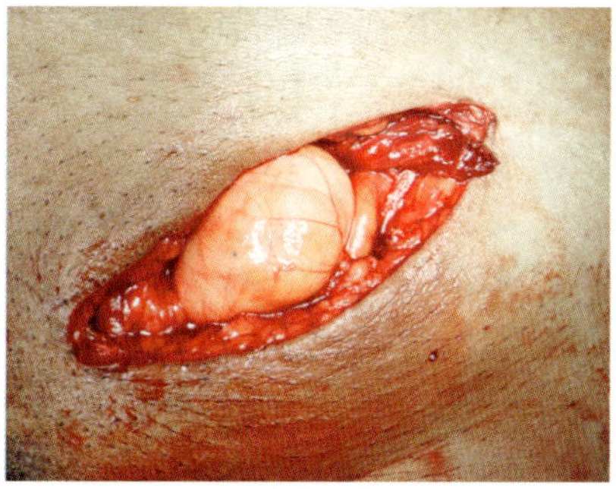

Fig. 27.30: Lipoma of the cord

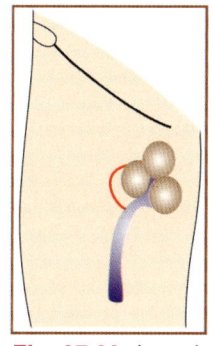

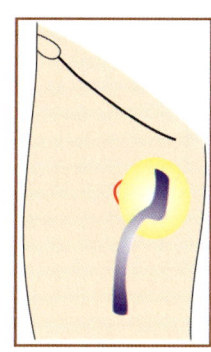

Fig. 27.31: Femoral artery aneurysm

Fig. 27.32: Lymph-adenitis

Fig. 27.33: Psoas bursa

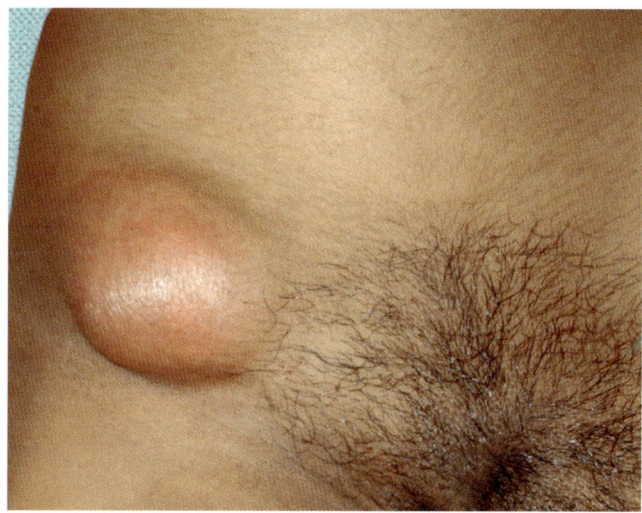

Fig. 27.34: Iliopsoas abscess (*Courtesy:* Dr Durganna, Head of the Department, Bangalore Medical College, Bangalore, 2016)

6. *Psoas bursa*: Osteoarthritis of the hip can produce distension of psoas bursa (Fig. 27.33), which disappears on flexing the hip. Tuberculosis of spine can present as iliopsoas abscess.

7. *Psoas abscess*: It is an iliopsoas abscess due to tuberculosis of spine. There are two swellings, one above and one below the inguinal ligament. Cross-fluctuation can be elicited between these two swellings. The tenderness over the spine and X-ray of the spine help in arriving at a diagnosis (Fig. 27.34). Typically, swelling is lateral to femoral vessels.

CASE OF UMBILICAL HERNIA OF ADULTS

- It is not a true umbilical hernia but it is a paraumbilical hernia in which the hernia occurs either above, below or to the side of the umbilicus, through the linea alba.

- The contents are the greater omentum, transverse colon or small bowel. Due to adhesions, it is often irreducible. Females in the 5th decade are commonly affected. Male:female ratio is 1:5. **Obesity** with flabby abdominal muscle predisposes to paraumbilical hernia. Repeated **pregnancies** also weaken the abdominal wall.

- Ascites may precipitate hernia specially in cirrhotic patients. The patient presents with a swelling in the umbilical region, which increases on straining or coughing. **Dragging pain** is usually due to the presence of omentum.

Clinical Examination

Inspection

- Describe the hernia as a swelling, with all other features (location, extent, size, shape, surface, borders, and skin over the swelling). Ask the patient

Table 27.4: Comparison between umbilical hernia in infants and adults

Features	Infants	Adults
Age in years	0–3	50–60
Sex	Common in male child	Common in females
Causes	Neonatal sepsis	Obesity, weak muscles, pregnancy
Defect	A small defect in the umbilical scar	Above or below the umbilicus
Symptoms	Symptomless	Symptoms are present
Strangulation	Rare	Very common
Treatment	Conservative (strapping), surgery (rare)	Mayo's repair

to cough—expansile impulse on cough is diagnostic of hernia. Look for any incisions in the lower abdomen specially vertical midline. (Often patients are referred with a diagnosis of umbilical hernia but on careful examination they are incisional hernias from the umbilical end of the incision.)

Palpation

- On palpation, details of the swelling are examined and documented. Typically, it is soft, reducible often with a gurgle. Omentum is felt as a granular mass.

- *Assessment of the defect*: Once the swelling is reduced, feel the defect all around and make a note—2-finger or 3-finger defect which amounts to about 2 to 4 cm size.

- *Defect occlusion test*: Now occlude the defect with fingers and ask the patient to cough—swelling is not seen.

- *Head raising test*: Swelling is more prominent. This happens because sac and the contents are almost in the abdominal wall.

Percussion

Not very important. Resonance can be due to presence of bowel within the sac.

Auscultation: Bowel sound may be heard.

Examination for other hernial sites: Abdominal wall incision, groin.

Diagnosis: Umbilical hernia. Mention, if any complications are present.

Treatment

Reduction of weight, **anatomical repair:** Small defects can be closed with nonabsorbable sutures such as nylon or prolene. **Most favoured** surgery for umbilical

hernia is **mesh repair**. It is a tensionless repair. It can also be done by **laparoscopic method** which is popular today.

*Refer Table 27.4 for comparison of umbilical hernia in infants and adults.

CLINICAL DISCUSSION

1. **What is IPOM?**
   Intraperitoneal onlay mesh repair.
2. **What are the complications of umbilical hernia?**
   Irreducibility, obstruction and incarceration.
3. **What are the factors causing irreducibility?**
   Adhesions between the contents of the sac, faecal matter (incarceration).
4. **Why do they get intertrigo?**
   As the sac enlarges, due to its weight and gravity, it sags down resulting in friction of the skin and this causes intertrigo.
5. **Any other complications?**
   Fistula due to thinning of the sac and opening in the skin.

INCISIONAL HERNIA

Herniation occurring through a weak point in the incision is called incisional hernia. Most of them occur in the anterior abdominal wall. It is commonly called ventral hernia. When it occurs after surgery in the loin, it is called lumbar hernia.

History of Present Illness (Figs 27.35 and 27.36)

- Often patient complains of some discharge (pink thin blood—serosanguinous) on the 4th post-operative day through the main suture line—it is a signal of development of wound dehiscence, partial or total. Such cases later develop an incisional hernia.

- Other patients report pus development after infection. History of infection during the first surgery may suggest the infection as a cause of hernia.

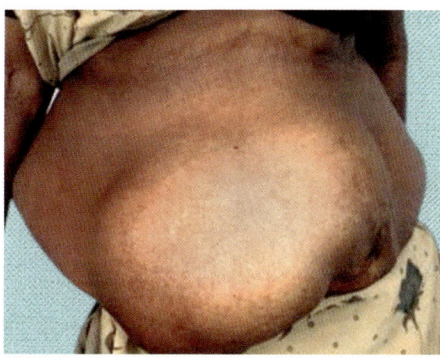

Fig. 27.35: Large incisional hernia. Recently, signs of irreducibility appeared (*Courtesy:* Dr CG Narasimhan, Consultant Surgeon, Mysore, Karnataka)

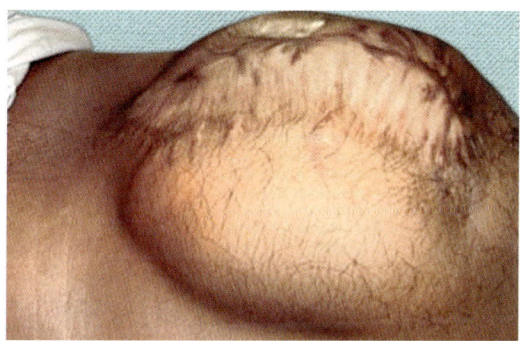

Fig. 27.36: Incisional hernia following three laparotomies done for intestinal obstruction—resection, anastomosis, leak and again laparotomy

- The patient may complain of cough in the post-operative period.
- Many patients have had multiple surgeries including caesarean sections or hysterectomy.

Clinical Examination

- There is a bulge/swelling in relation to the scar. The scar is thin and evidence of secondary healing in the form of irregular scar may be present.
- Expansile impulse on cough and reducibility may be present.
- After reduction of the contents, a defect can be palpated through the scar. The defect depends upon number of stitches that had given way.

Triad of Incisional Hernia Diagnosis

1. Incision (operated/traumatic)
2. Expansile impulse on cough
3. Reducibility—partial or total

Treatment

It is not easy to obtain good results in cases of incisional hernia if one takes it lightly especially when multiple surgeries and multiple recurrences have occurred. Basic principle is to repair the anterior abdominal wall defect with mesh. When the defect is small (less than 2 cm), simple closure can be done with non-absorbable sutures. Any hernia larger than that will require a mesh to close the defect. The best approached will be preperitoneal in open repair. Often rectus muscle is widely separated due to multiple operations. It may not be possible to keep the mesh in the preperitoneal space and it may become subcutaneous. It is still worth trying and the results are good, provided there is no infection. Laparoscopic repair—IPOM can still be attempted, if sac is small and reducible.

EPIGASTRIC HERNIA (Fig. 27.37)

It is also called **fatty** hernia of the linea alba. Hernia occurs in the epigastrium through the linea alba which extends between the xiphoid process and umbilicus. Sudden straining or heavy exercise results in the tearing of a few fibres of linea alba and is responsible for precipitating an epigastric hernia. Initially, there is a small protrusion of extraperitoneal pad of fat. Rarely, if it enlarges, it is due to the dragging of the peritoneal sac. The opening is very narrow. Hence, the hollow viscus cannot enter the sac. Diastasis of rectus muscles which results in a wide linea alba can also precipitate an epigastric hernia. It is common in muscular men and manual labourers (Clinical Box 27.6). Typically, the swelling is situated in the upper abdomen midway between xiphoid process and

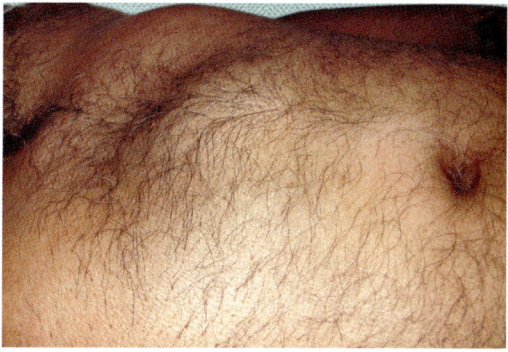

Fig. 27.37: Epigastric hernia (*Courtesy:* Dr Yashdip Sharma, Assistant Professor, KMC, Manipal)

Clinical Box 27.6

Peculiarities of epigastric hernia
- Common in muscular men
- Hernial sac is uncommon
- Hollow viscus in the sac is rare
- Impulse on cough is rare
- Reducibility is rare
- Tenderness is an important feature

umbilicus. Often, it contains only an extraperitoneal protrusion of fat. An expansile impulse on cough is rare. Dull aching pain is due to the fatty contents which are partially strangulated. However, tenderness is an important feature of epigastric hernia. Many cases are associated with peptic ulcer disease. On head-raising, it becomes more prominent. A small incision is made over the swelling and the fatty tissue is isolated. It is ligated and excised.

SPIGELIAN HERNIA

- It is an interstitial hernia which occurs through the Spigelian fascia. This is a thin strip of fascia which runs parallel to the outer border of rectus sheath from the tip of the 9th costal cartilage to the pubic tubercle (Figs 27.38 to 27.41).

- Since it is very wide in the region of umbilicus/ arcuate line, Spigelian hernias occur commonly at this level.

- Spigelian fascia contributes a few fibres to form rectus sheath.

Spigelian Belt

- It is a 6 cm horizontal transverse zone located within umbilicus and two anterior superior iliac spine.

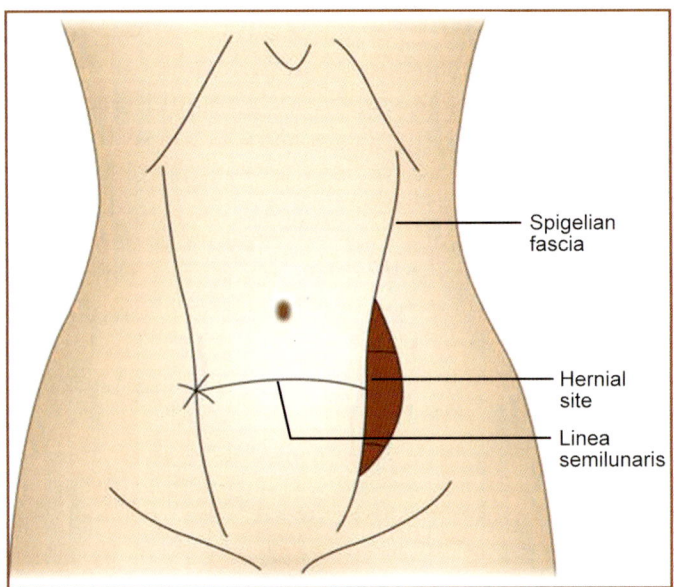

Fig. 27.38: Spigelian fascia and the site of hernia

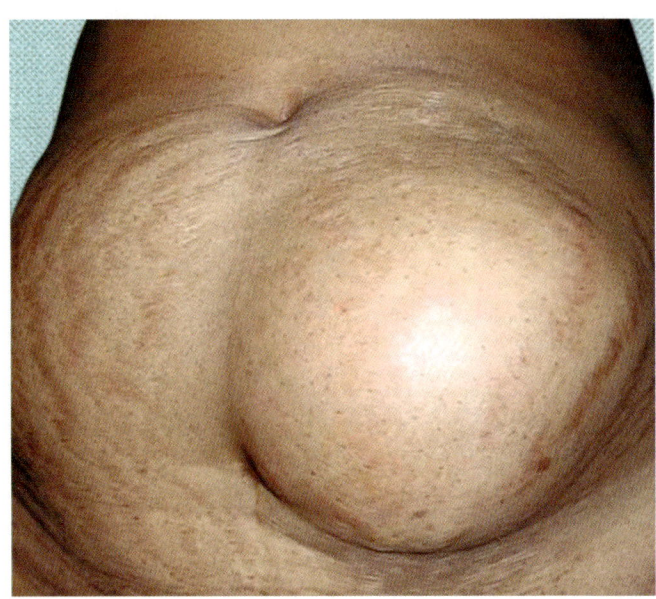

Fig. 27.39: Obstructed Spigelian hernia in a 70-year-old lady—first presentation to the hospital

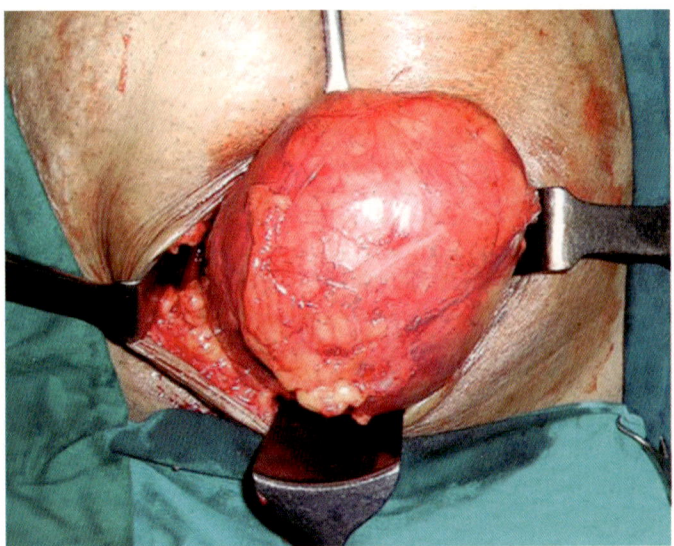

Fig. 27.40: Delivery of the sac

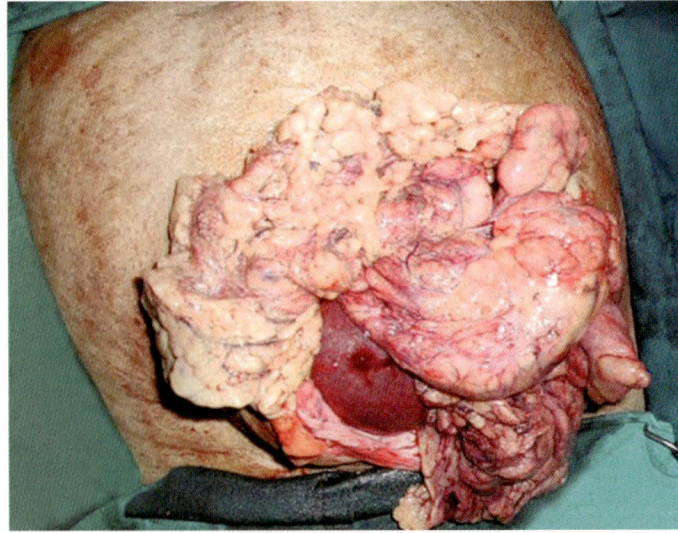

Fig. 27.41: Contents of the sac

- A Spigelian hernia starts as a direct protrusion behind rectus abdominis.
- It is intramural; sac penetrates across transverse muscles and lies behind external oblique muscles.

Precipitating Factors

Repeated pregnancies, advancing age, obesity, muscular degeneration, sudden strain due to coughing, weight lifting, etc. give rise to Spigelian hernias.

Clinical Features

- It is seen in both sexes equally around 50 years of age.
- A round, soft, reducible swelling situated just below and lateral to the umbilicus. It is located typically at the junction of the arcuate line and lateral border of rectus abdominis. Sometimes, it is tender.
- **The swelling gives rise to an expansile impulse on cough.**
- As the hernia enlarges, it insinuates between external and internal oblique muscle. Hence, it is an example for interparietal hernia.

Investigations

1. An ultrasound examination can define the defect in the semilunar line.
2. X-ray abdomen, lateral view, shows coils of bowel outside the peritoneal cavity.

Differential Diagnosis

- **Haematoma** within the rectus sheath. However, it will not give rise to impulse on cough. It occurs suddenly and it will be a tender swelling.
- **Pyogenic or pyaemic abscess** can occur in the abdominal wall, more so in diabetic patients. Tenderness and high temperature clinches the diagnosis.

Complication

Strangulation is common due to the rigid fascial rings surrounding the hernial sac. Richter's hernia also can occur here.

Treatment

- An incision of about 5 to 6 cm is made over the swelling and abdominal wall muscles are split or cut. The sac is excised after reducing the contents and the defect is repaired.
- Recurrence occurs in about 5% of the patients.

LUMBAR HERNIA

Two types of lumbar hernia are well-recognised. They are as follows:

1. *Primary* which occurs through an anatomical defect (Fig. 27.43):
   - **Through the inferior lumbar triangle of Petit.** Its boundaries are (Fig. 27.42):
     - *Inferiorly:* Iliac crest
     - *Laterally:* External oblique
     - *Medially:* Latissimus dorsi
   - **Through the superior lumbar triangle of Grynfeltt.** Its boundaries are:
     - *Above:* 12th rib
     - *Medially:* Sacrospinalis
     - *Laterally:* Internal oblique

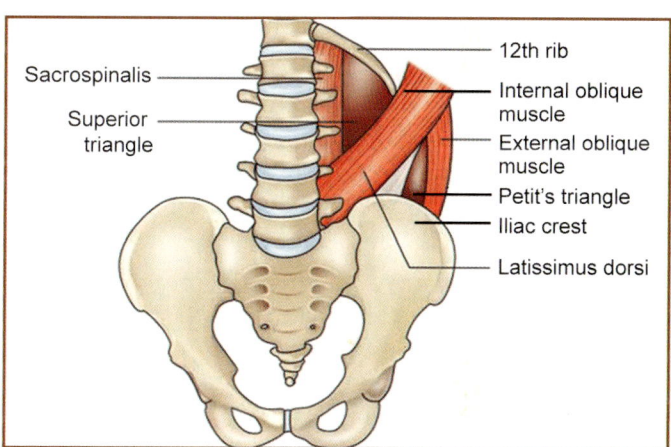

Fig. 27.42: Petit's triangle

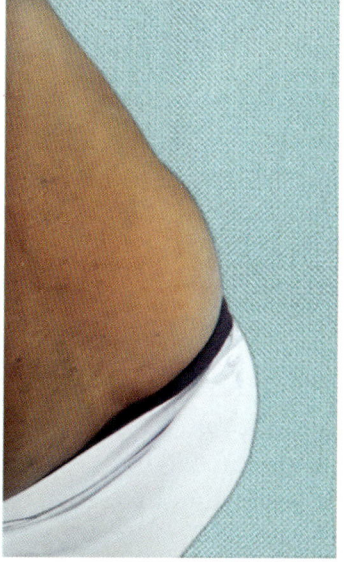

Fig. 27.43: Primary lumbar hernia (*Courtesy*: Dr Chethan K, Dr Nagesh Biradar, Dept of Surgery, KMC, Manipal)

2. *Secondary* to a renal (Fig. 27.44) operation done through a loin incision. It is an example of a *lumbar incisional hernia,* which occurs due to either infection or weakness of loin muscles. The operation done for tuberculosis of spine through a loin incision, very often gives rise to a secondary lumbar hernia (it is an incisional hernia). It is treated depending upon the size of the defect. Small defects can be closed with simple sutures. Large defects need to be closed with or without mesh.

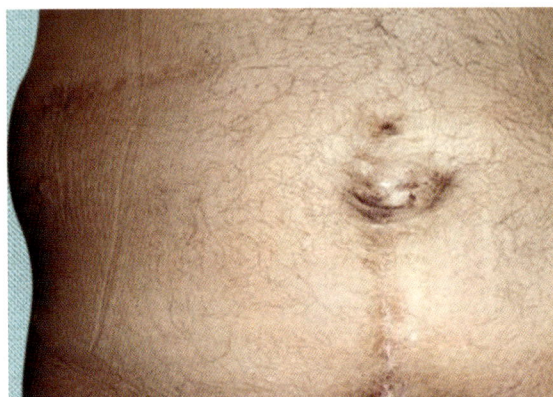

Fig. 27.44: Lumbar hernia (*Courtesy:* Prof SS Prasad, Dr Rajendra, Dr Vijendra, Department of Surgery, KMC, Manipal)

Clinical Features

Swelling with expansile impulse on coughing, reducibility on lying down and the location are the important features.

Differential Diagnosis

1. *Lipoma* is common in the lumbar region (loin). It is soft, lobular, and slips under the palpating fingers.
2. *Cold abscess* secondary to tuberculosis of the spine gives rise to a nontender swelling in the para-vertebral space. Tenderness is present over the spine which gives a clue to the diagnosis. Patients may have deformity of the spine in the form of gibbus.

OBTURATOR HERNIA

- This hernia occurs through the obturator canal which is bounded above by the superior ramus of pubis and below by the sharp edge of the obturator membrane.
- As the hernia is covered by the pectineus muscle, it is often overlooked.

 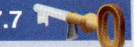
Precipitating Factors

- In females, the **obturator foramen** is wider in the transverse direction (it is triangular in shape in females and oval in males).
- Repeated pregnancies
- Loss of body weight
- Chronic lung diseases

Clinical Features

- The **most common presentation** is acute intestinal obstruction **with strangulation** (80%). Recurrent attacks of intestinal obstruction which get resolved spontaneously is also common (Clinical Box 27.7).
- This hernia causes more pain than any other type of hernia. Pain often radiates along the obturator nerve and may even be referred to the knee *via* its geniculate branch called *Howship-Romberg sign.* The leg is usually kept in the *semiflexed position* and movement of the limb gives rise to pain. If the limb is flexed, abducted and rotated outwards, the hernia becomes prominent. Patients are usually over 60 years of age and women are more frequently affected than men.
- Due to strangulation and blood in the hernial sac, bruising is seen below the medial edge of the inguinal ligament.
- A few patients (20%) complain of palpable *hernial mass* in the groin.
- Per vaginal examination can reveal a tender lump on the lateral side of the vault.

Treatment

The constricting agent in case of obstruction is the **obturator fascia,** which needs to be divided. Nerves and vessels are posterolateral to the hernial sac. Since majority of the cases present with intestinal obstruction and strangulation, a lower laparotomy is done. A grooved director is used to divide the obturator fascia.

28

Examination of Scrotum and Testis

INTRODUCTION

Diseases involving scrotum and testis are interesting and specific to these parts. Examples are: Scrotum is the site of multiple sebaceous cysts and carcinoma. Fluid collection inside tunica vaginalis, the sac that covers the testis inside the scrotum, is called **hydrocoele.** Important diseases of testis are testicular tumours and torsion. Tuberculosis affects epididymis and spermatic cord more often than testis. Syphilis affects testis more than epididymis. Thus, when you start examining these organs, keep in mind these diseases and start asking questions.

HISTORY OF PRESENT ILLNESS

What is your complaint? Why have you come to the hospital? How old are you? How long have you had this problem? What is your problem, is it swelling, ulcers or pain? Is there any history of trauma? Swelling and pain are two common complaints for which a patient comes to the hospital.

Age at presentation: Hydrocoele is more likely in younger patients. Testicular tumours notoriously occur in young age—teratoma around twenties and seminoma around thirties.

Swelling and pain: The most common complaint is painless swelling of the scrotum of a few years duration. It is hydrocoele (accumulation of fluid in the tunica vaginalis sac) (Fig. 28.1). Pain is not a feature of hydrocoele. However, **trauma may result in haematocoele** and can give rise to pain. **Infected hydrocoele or pyocoele causes pain.** It is not common because tunica vaginalis sac is relatively avascular and protects the contents of hydrocele sac

from getting infected. Pain and fever with swelling of the scrotum indicates acute epididymo-orchitis. In coastal parts of India such as Karnataka and Andhra Pradesh, filariasis is still a common problem.

Malignant tumours of the testis present with painless enlargement of the testis. Since pain is absent, it is not uncommon to find patients who present with supraclavicular swellings (lymph nodes), abdominal distension (para-aortic nodes) and testicular swelling (tumour).

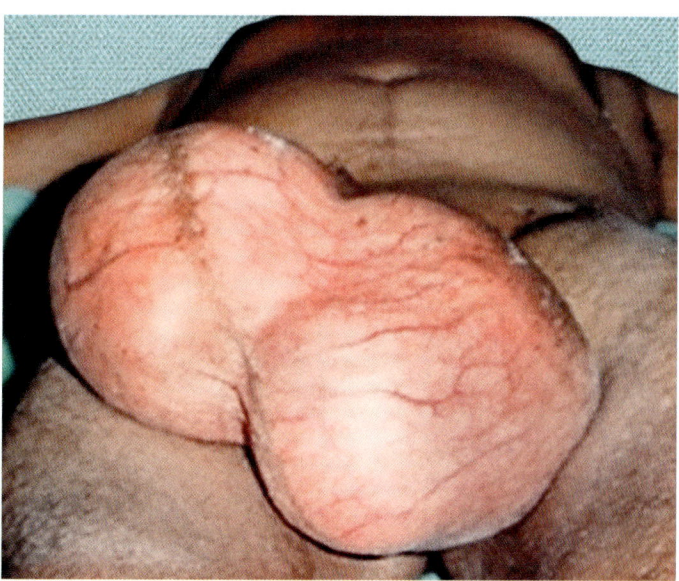

Fig. 28.1: Bilateral hydrocoele—swelling of the scrotum 10 years duration

- Painless multiple swellings of the scrotum (Fig. 28.2) are sebaceous cysts. Patients may not come to hospital early. Infected cysts result in severe pain—infected sebaceous cyst, almost presents like an abscess. Ruptured cyst presents with foul

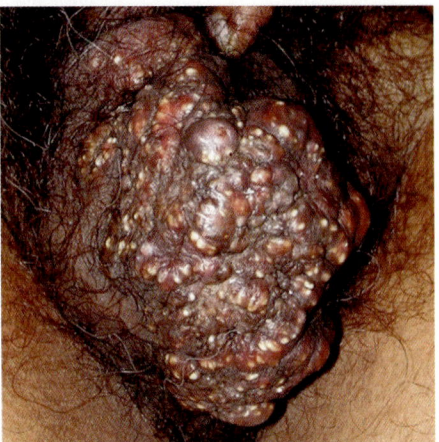

Fig. 28.2: Calcified multiple sebaceous cysts (dystrophic calcification) (*Courtesy:* Prof Abdul Majeed, Yenepoya Medical College, Mangaluru)

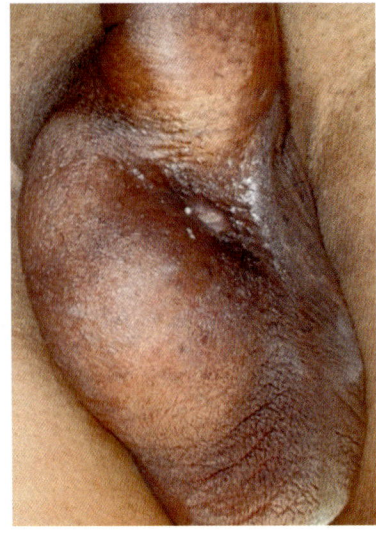

Fig. 28.4: Tuberculous sinus

smelling discharge. Torsion of the testis is a surgical emergency. Patients are young boys who present with severe pain in the testis. There is no history of fever. Factors which precipitate torsion are vigorous exercises, lifting of weight, coitus, etc. Sometimes it can occur during sleep, sometimes several hours after physical activity. Torsion of the appendix of testis and epididymis also cause severe pain in the testis.

Fever: Funiculitis/ acute epididymo-orchitis caused by filariasis results in pain in the inguinal region, scrotum with high grade fever, chills and rigors. Net result is fluid collection in the tunica vaginalis sac called **chylocoele. Such recurrent attacks of funiculitis result in**

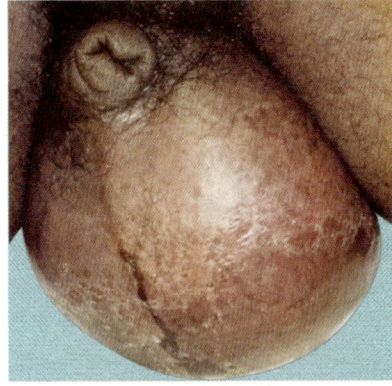

Fig. 28.3: Grossly thickened scrotal skin—filarial hydrocoele

chylocoele and thickened skin due to lymphoedema (Fig. 28.3). Swelling of the epididymis, evening rise in temperature may indicate tubercular aetiology. Tuberculosis cause chronic epididymo-orchitis.

Discharge: White cheesy discharge means a sinus typical of tuberculous epididymo-orchitis (Fig. 28.4). Sebaceous cyst also can present with discharge which is white and with foul odour.

Ulcers: Rarely scrotum is one of the sites of epithelioma (squamous cell carcinoma). It happens when there is chronic irritation due to tar, oil or soot.

It has been called **chimney sweep's cancer or soot wart**. It is less common nowadays due to awareness and wearing tight fitting clothes thus avoiding accumulation of soot between the scrotal skin folds.

CLINICAL DISCUSSION

1. **What are the common painless swellings in scrotum and testis?**
   a. Hydrocoele
   b. Varicocoele
   c. Spermatocoele
   d. Epididymal cyst
   e. Chronic tuberculous epididymo-orchitis
   f. Testicular tumours—it is a feeling of heaviness. If there is bleeding within the testis, it can be painful.

2. **What are the common painful swellings in scrotum and testis?**
   a. Acute epididymo-orchitis—filarial or nonfilarial
   b. Haematocoele—traumatic
   c. Torsion of the testis
   d. Infected sebaceous cyst

Past History

Relevant past history includes tuberculosis, recurrent fever with chills and rigors or any previous surgery—such as surgery for undescended testis.

REGIONAL EXAMINATION

Inspection

Inspect the scrotum on both sides, look at median raphe, look for any visible swelling, any discharge, opening or scars? Also look for any obvious penile lesions.

- When the swelling is obvious like a case of hydrocoele, you can start describing the swelling in the usual way: Location, size, shape, surface, borders, skin over the swelling, dilated veins, pulsations, etc. Typically vaginal hydrocoele is confined to scrotum, smooth surface with round borders (Fig. 28.5), skin is stretched. Carefully look at the extent of the swelling. Does the swelling extend into the inguinal region? If so, it may be hernia or infantile hydrocoele. Thin veins are seen in a tense hydrocoele. Spermatocoele and epididymal cysts are usually not visible.

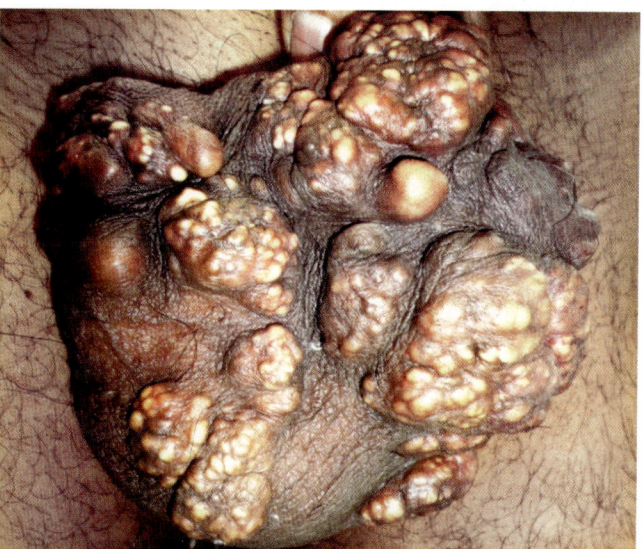

Fig. 28.6: Multiple sebaceous cysts

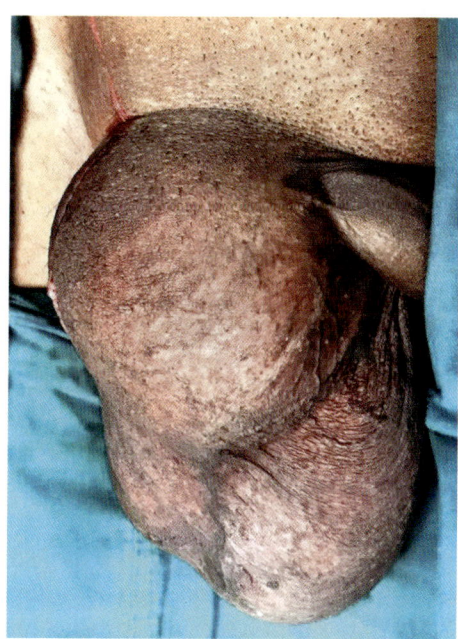

Fig. 28.5: Vaginal hydrocoele

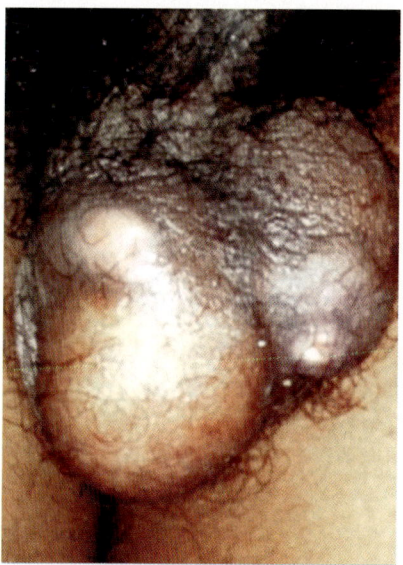

Fig. 28.7: Tuberculous epididymo-orchitis—both sides

- Ask the patient to cough and rule out expansile impulse on coughing. If present, it is an inguino-scrotal hernia.

1. Skin of the scrotum

- Normal scrotal skin is wrinkled with **rugosity.** Rugosity is lost when it is stretched as in hydrocoele.
- **Multiple sebaceous cysts** of scrotum are not uncommon (Fig. 28.6).
- If any discharge is seen, explain it. Tuberculous epididymo-orchitis results in a sinus posteriorly. Cheesy white-coloured discharge is classical (Fig. 28.7).
- Gumma (not seen nowadays), caused by syphilis, affects testis and results in a sinus anteriorly.
- **Extensive necrosis** of the scrotal skin (gangrene) is a feature of Fournier's gangrene. The present

terminology is necrotising fasciitis of the scrotum and perineum (Figs 28.8 and 28.9).

- If any ulcer is present, describe the ulcer in the usual manner.
- **Gross thickening** of scrotal skin and subcutaneous tissues is seen in elephantiasis of the scrotum. It can be seen in filariasis and also following radiation given to groin nodes (lymphoedema scrotum). **Lymph scrotum** is the name given to cases wherein cutaneous vesicles appear and continuous leakage of lymph occurs and soaking the undergarments. This is called **lymphorrhagia.** When skin and subcutaneous tissues of the penis are thickened, it is called **Ram's horn penis** (Fig. 28.10).

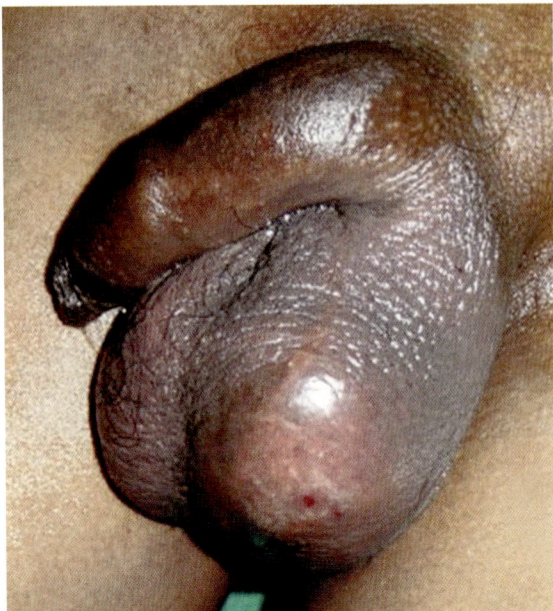

Fig. 28.8: Initial stage of Fournier's gangrene with scrotal abscess—you can see redness and few areas of suppuration

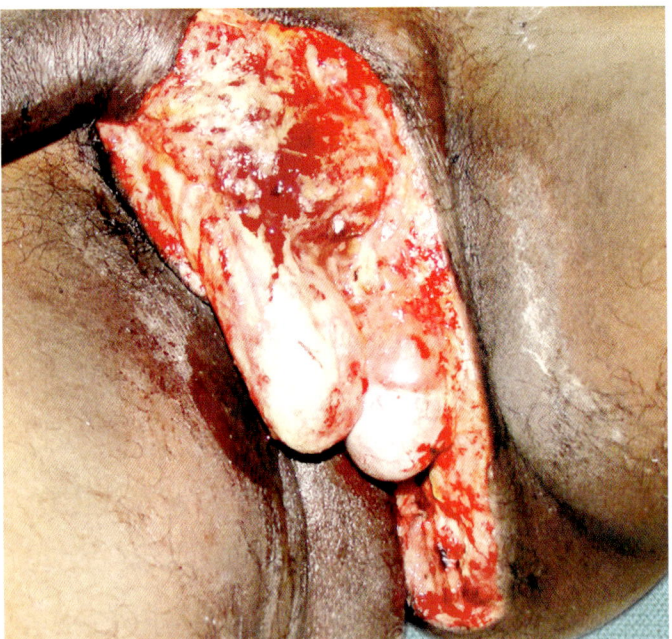

Fig. 28.9: Fournier's gangrene—after debridement of scrotal skin and dead tissues

2. Oedema of the scrotum

- Gross swelling of scrotum is seen in **ascites** secondary to liver diseases (cirrhosis), nephrotic syndrome and cardiac failure.

- It is also important to know that **retroperitoneal inflammation** such as retrocaecal abscess following appendicitis can track down into scrotum and can involve the scrotal layers and can result in necrosis and sepsis.

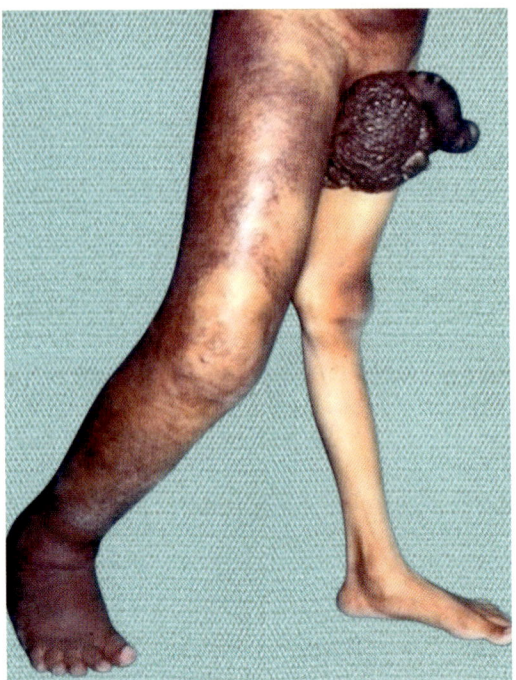

Fig. 28.10: Ram's horn penis

Palpation

General rules of palpation will apply here also. Check local rise in temperature and tenderness. Describe the swelling in the usual manner such as location, extent, size and shape, surface, skin over the swelling and surrounding area. During palpation, ask the patient to cough and rule out an inguinoscrotal hernia. If any ulcer is seen, describe it in the usual manner. Local rise in temperature and tenderness indicate inflammatory conditions such as cellulitis of the scrotum, infected sebaceous cyst or pyocoele. The commonest scrotal swelling is vaginal hydrocoele. Three important tests that must be done here are:

1. *Getting above the swelling:* It is possible to feel the cord above the swelling at the root of the scrotum. That means it is a scrotal swelling. The cord is palpated between index finger posteriorly and thumb anteriorly.

2. *Hydrocoele is soft and fluctuant.* The ring and little fingers of the both hands are used to stabilise the swelling by pushing them under the swelling as shown in Fig. 28.11. The thumb and index fingers are used to demonstrate fluctuation.

3. *Transillumination.* Hydrocoele is brilliantly transilluminant because it contains clear serous fluid. Hydrocoele is held tense and a light source (pen torch) is applied laterally over the swelling. One

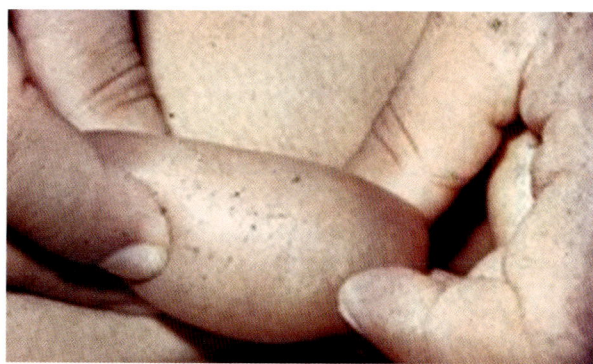

Fig. 28.11: Demonstration of fluctuation

can easily see the red glow of the light. It is better appreciated by an X-ray film which is rolled into a tube and used on the other side. One can see the transillumination (Figs 28.12 and 28.13).

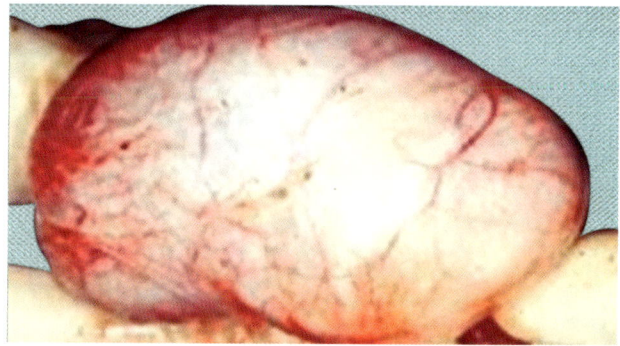

Fig. 28.12: Thin sac with clear fluid reason why it is transilluminant

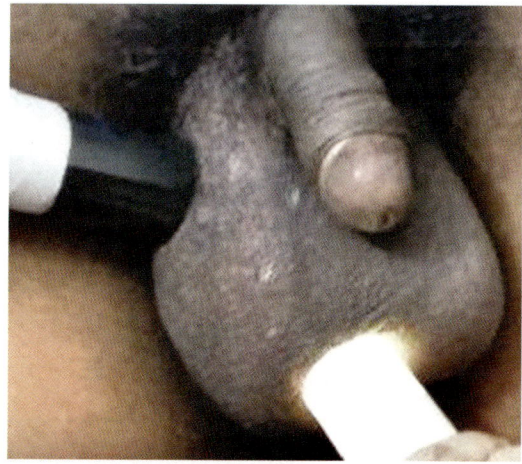

Fig. 28.13: Light is directed towards the swelling avoiding testis

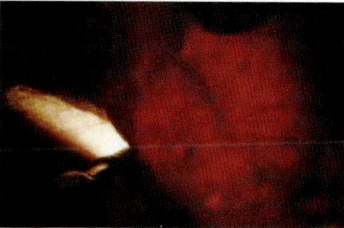

Fig. 28.14: Transillumination should be tested in dark room. You can see the transillumination in this case

- **Precautions that must be taken before transillumination:** This is better done in a dark room. Light should not be applied from the posterior aspect of scrotum because testis will block the illumination.

- Once you do these 3 tests, check reducibility and impulse on coughing. Both will be negative in a case of hydrocoele. These are the points that differentiate hydrocoele from hernia.

CLINICAL DISCUSSION

1. **In which type of hydrocoele, is transillumination negative?**

   When you suspect hydrocoele and if transillumination is negative, it can be haematocoele, chylocoele or pyocoele. Rarely long-standing hydrocoele may not be transilluminant because the wall is thick.

2. **In which type of hydrocoele, getting above the swelling may not be possible?**

   Infantile hydrocoele (*page 466*)

3. **Infantile hydrocoele is seen only in infants. Is it true?**

   It is a misnomer. It is not only seen in infants but also in adults. In this condition, the processus vaginalis sac is patent up to the deep ring (from the scrotum).

4. **What is hydrocoele en-bisac and what is its relevance to reducibility?**

   Hydrocoele en-bisac: It is also called bilocular hydrocoele. In this condition, the scrotal sac communicates with another sac underneath the anterior abdominal wall musculature. Diagnosis is made by eliciting **cross-fluctuation** test. When you try to reduce the swelling, some amount of fluid may enter into the second compartment and one may feel reducibility is present and a diagnosis of hernia is made. If you wait for a few minutes, you will see that the fluid accumulates again.

5. **What happens to reducibility in congenital hydrocoele?**

   As a rule, when the legs of a child are elevated, fluid will gravitate slowly into peritoneal cavity and the scrotum will be empty. However, when an examiner tries to reduce the swelling it may not be possible because of **inverted ink bottle effect.**

6. **What is blue dot sign?**

   In cases of torsion of the appendix of the epididymis or testis, blue dot may be visible in the scrotal skin—a tender nodule with **blue** discoloration on the upper pole of the testis.

Palpation of the Testis/Epididymis/Spermatic Cord/Vas Deferens

- Testis is palpated using both hands. Note down whether it is normal in position or shape, enlarged or atrophic, smooth or irregular, firm or hard, testicular sensations are present or absent.

- Normal testis is vertically oval in position and left testis hangs slightly lower level than the right testis. If the testis is horizontal, it is a congenital anomaly, with undue mobility which predisposes to torsion. It has been described as **bell clapper deformity**.

- In a classical case of vaginal hydrocoele, testis cannot be palpated.

- **If testis is enlarged, it is pathological**. In such cases, testicular tumour should be considered first. Other pathology is gumma which is hardly seen nowadays. Testicular sensations are lost in malignancy and gumma (tertiary stage of syphilis). Gentle pressure on the testis results in a sickening feeling. This has been described as normal testicular sensation.

- Tenderness is a feature of haematocoele or epididymo-orchitis.

- Testis is enlarged, can be firm or hard. Surface is smooth in seminoma and lobular or irregular in teratocarcinoma.

- In cases of anteverted testis, epididymis is felt anteriorly and the body of the epididymis is felt posteriorly. In cases of inverted testis, globus major of the epididymis lies inferiorly.

- Normal epididymis is felt posteriorly as a firm nodular structure. It is firmly attached to the testis and hence cannot be moved separately. Globus major is the large portion of the epididymis which gets affected in cases of blood spread infections. On the other hand, tail or globus minor gets affected in cases of tuberculosis of genitourinary tract, an infection spreads retrogradely from the urinary bladder. In initial stages of urinary tuberculosis, epididymis is enlarged and firm. **Then it gets thickened and craggy (rough or irregular)**. Within 1 or 2 months, softening occurs due to cold abscess formation (Fig. 28.15). Rupture of this results in a sinus formation in the posterior part of the scrotum. Spermatic cord is tender and thickened in epididymo-orchitis. Spermatic cord is thickened but nontender in testicular tumours due to cremasteric hypertrophy.

- **Sign of vas:** Vas is never thickened or involved in testicular tumours. It has been described as **sign of vas is negative.**

- If you suspect testicular tumour, after completion of examination of genitalia, para-aortic group of lymph nodes should be examined. They are felt in epigastrium or umbilical region as a nodular, firm, retroperitoneal mass (does not move with respiration).

- Cysts of epididymis (Fig. 28.16) is felt at the upper pole of the testis as a soft fluctuant swelling. Transillumination is brilliantly positive. It has been called 'Chinese lantern appearance' or tesselated appearance.

- Cysts of spermatic cord appear as a fluctuant but not transilluminant swelling.

- **Examination of left supraclavicular lymph nodes:** Seminoma testis spreads mainly by lymphatics. Initial draining nodes are para-aortic lymph nodes (Fig. 28.17) followed by mediastinal and then supraclavicular lymph nodes.

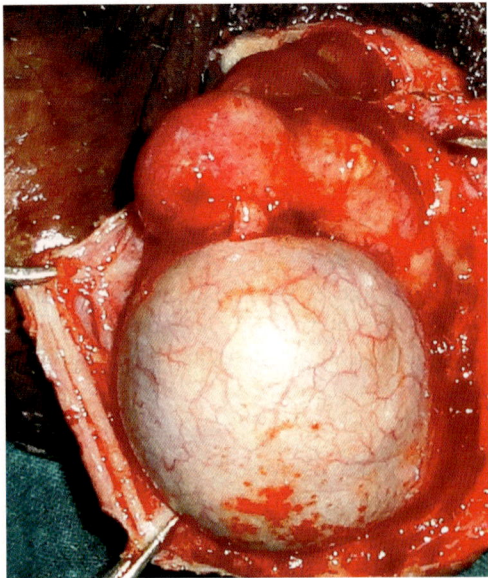

Fig. 28.15: Tubercular epididymo-orchitis resulting in cold abscess in the epididymis at surgery. Testis is normal. Findings at surgery

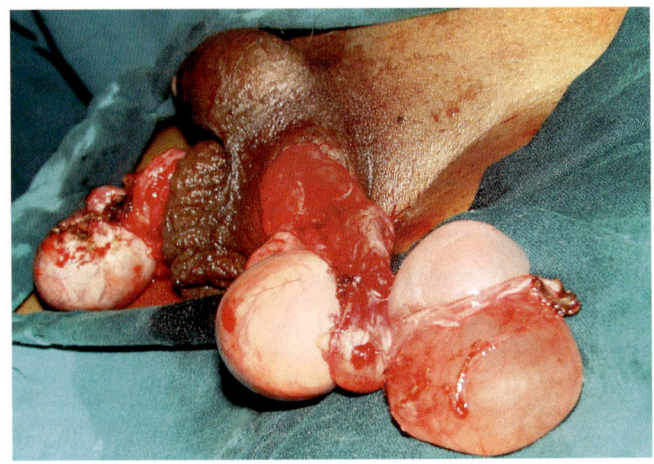

Fig. 28.16: Bilateral cysts of the epididymis

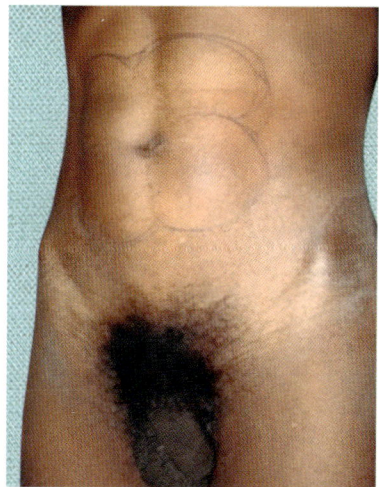

Fig. 28.17: Left testicular tumour with para-aortic lymph nodes. The patient presented with abdominal distension and epigastric pain. He had minimal discomfort in the scrotum

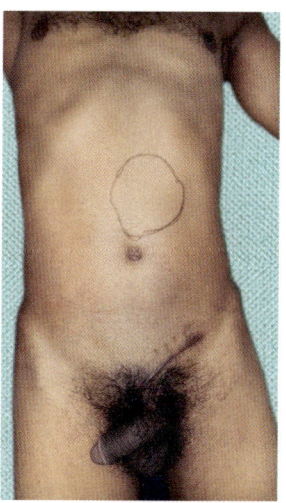

Fig. 28.18: Patient presented with upper abdominal distension and backache. On examination there was an inguinal scar. Testis was absent in the scrotum. **Fig. 28.19:** Palpation of the epigastrium revealed para-aortic lymph nodes mass (as in case of Fig. 28.18) (*Courtesy:* Dr P Sampath Kumar, Prof of Surgery, KMC, Manipal)

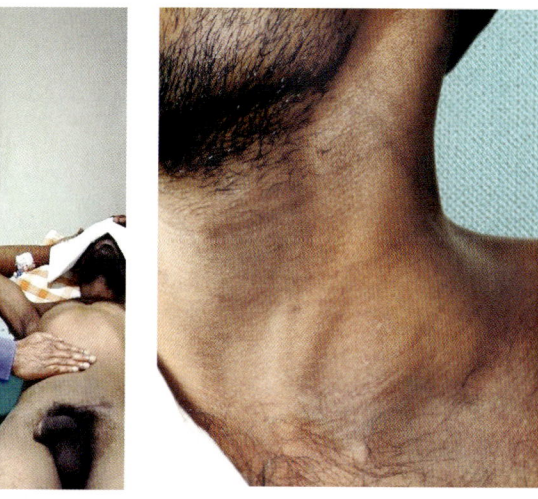

Fig. 28.20: Seminoma with supra-clavicular lymph nodes. Ultrasound revealed a testicular mass

CLINICAL DISCUSSION

1. **If you find a testicular tumour, what else you will examine?**
   - Para-aortic lymph nodes and supraclavicular lymph nodes. They can get enlarged in seminoma testis.
   - Gynaecomastia can occur due to secretion of human chorionic gonadotrophins.

2. **What happens to epididymis in testicular tumour?**

   Initially it is normal. Later it is flattened behind the testis. Slowly it gets incorporated within the growth. In such cases, it is not palpable.

3. **What is the diagnostic sign of epididymal cyst?**

   Brilliant transillumination: The appearance is like a Chinese lantern.

4. **Is spermatocele transilluminant?**

   Mostly not because it contains opalescent, barley water-like fluid that contains *spermatozoa.*

5. **Why should a chest X-ray be done?**

   To look for evidence of tuberculosis in cases of genito-urinary tuberculosis and cannonball secondaries in the lung from testicular tumours.

6. **What are the signs of tuberculous epididymo-orchitis?**

   Craggy epididymis, beaded vas and secondary hydrocoele.

DIFFERENTIAL DIAGNOSIS

1. *Primary hydrocoele:* This is the most common swelling of the scrotum. Majority of these are primary hydrocoele. It is also called congenital hydrocoele. They occur due to collection of fluid in the tunica vaginalis sac due to partially or totally patent processus vaginalis sac. The history is usually of a painless swelling growing slowly, over a few months to years. Swelling is soft, fluctuant and transilluminant. It is not reducible and there is no impulse on cough. Typically getting above the swelling is possible. Testis is not palpable separately and there is no other pathology in the testis or in the epididymis. Diagnosis is based on clinical grounds and treated by partial excision and eversion of the sac. Different types of primary hydrocoele are given below.

A. **Primary vaginal hydrocoele** (Figs 28.21 and 28.22): It occurs when hydrocoele sac is patent only in the scrotum (details given above).

B. **Infantile hydrocoele** (Fig. 28.23): The sac from the scrotum is patent up to the deep inguinal ring.

C. **True congenital hydrocoele** (Fig. 28.24): In this condition, the scrotal sac communicates with the peritoneal cavity. It is seen in infants. It can also be due to tuberculous peritonitis. The scrotal swelling appears when the child assumes an erect posture for a long time and it may not reduce due to **inverted ink bottle** effect. Hence, congenital hydrocoele is not reducible. It regresses in size, if the child assumes supine position while sleeping. Treatment is by herniotomy.

D. **Encysted hydrocoele of the cord** (Figs 28.25 to 28.27): In this condition, the sac is obliterated above (inguinal canal) and below (scrotum) but patent at the root of the scrotum around spermatic cord. It presents as a soft, cystic, fluctuant, and transilluminant swelling separate from testis, well above the testis. Diagnosis is established by **traction test:** The swelling has got free mobility but when traction is applied to testis gently, the swelling becomes fixed and it moves down when testis is pulled down. This variety of hydrocoele is treated by excision of the sac.

E. **Hydrocoele en-bisac** (bilocular hydrocoele) (Fig. 28.28): In this condition, the scrotal sac communicates with another

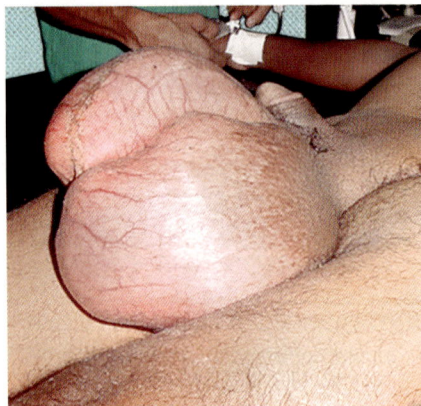

Fig. 28.21: Bilateral primary vaginal hydrocoele

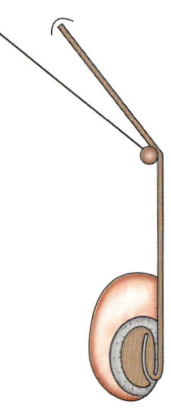

Fig. 28.22: Primary vaginal hydrocoele

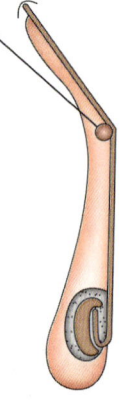

Fig. 28.23: Infantile hydrocoele

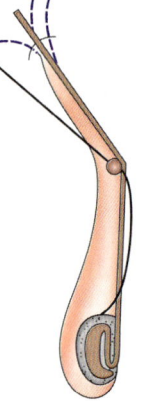

Fig. 28.24: True congenital hydrocoele

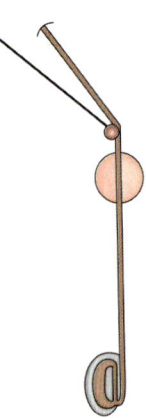

Fig. 28.25: Encysted hydrocoele

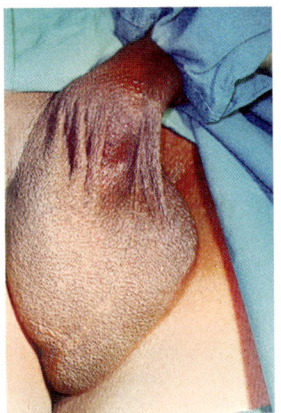

Fig. 28.26: Encysted hydrocoele

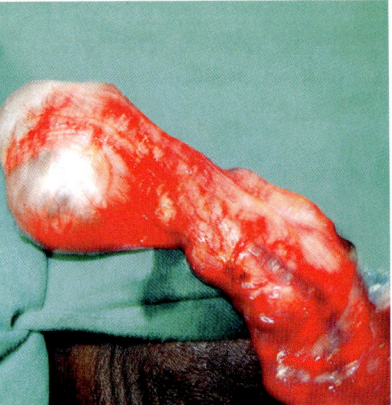

Fig. 28.27: At surgery

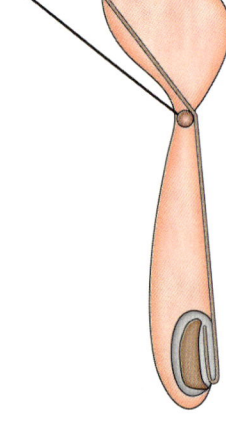

Fig. 28.28: Hydrocoele en-bissac

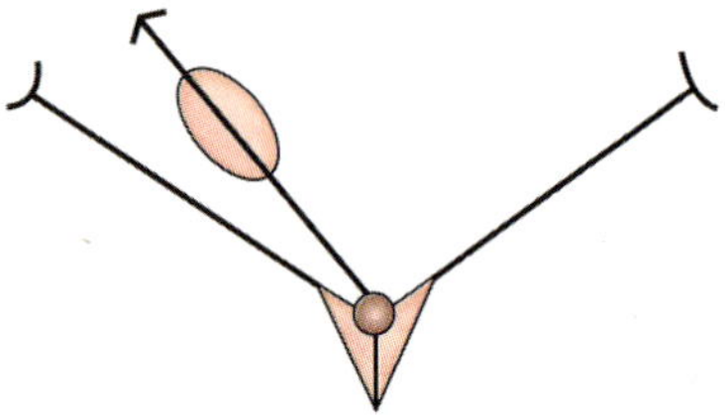

Fig. 28.29: Hydrocoele of canal of Nuck

sac underneath the anterior abdominal wall musculature. Diagnosis is made by eliciting **cross-fluctuation** test. This variety of hydrocoele can be confused for inguinal hernia because when you try to reduce the swelling, fluid may gravitate or shift to the second cavity thus giving a false impression of reducibility. Also there is no impulse on coughing. In females, hydrocoele can occur in the **canal of Nuck** (Fig. 28.29).

2. Secondary hydrocoele: It results due to disease of the epididymis or disease of the testis. A few causes have been listed below.

A. Acute bacterial–non-filarial epididymo-orchitis: This occurs due to retrograde infection from urethra, prostate or seminal vesicles. Bacteria that cause sexually transmitted diseases, such as gonorrhoea, chlamydia and syphilis can cause orchitis. It is typically seen in young patients between the ages of 19 and 35 years. People may be at risk, if they have many sexual partners. Gonococcal infections were common earlier. Today, instrumentation or postsurgical or postcatheterisation of the bladder are the common causes. Infective organisms are E. coli, Klebsiella, Streptococci or Staphylococcus, Proteus or Pseudomonas, etc. Scrotal skin will

be oedematous and red. Fluid accumulates in acute phase and generally subsides after treatment.

B. Acute/subacute filarial epididymo-orchitis: The disease is caused by microfilaria of Wuchereria bancrofti. Typically, young patients are affected (Fig. 28.30). Severe pain in the scrotum, fever with chills and rigors are characteristic. Globus major is affected. Epididymis is swollen, tender and firm. Testis is affected later. Unlike tuberculous epididymo-orchitis, cold abscess and sinus formation will not occur.

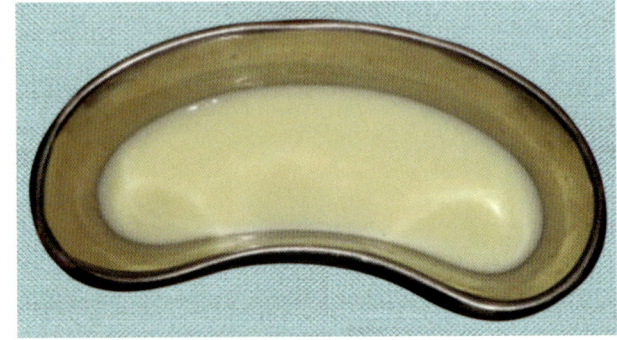

Fig. 28.30: Chylous fluid drained from hydrocoele sac

C. **Chronic tuberculous epididymo-orchitis:** Retrograde infection from the seminal vesicles is more common. In such cases, globus minor is affected first. In blood-borne infections—globus major is affected. Epididymis becomes hard and irregular (rough surface). It has been called craggy. Vas deferens feels like beads, called **beaded vas.** Secondary hydrocoele occurs in 30% of the cases. Eventually it forms **cold abscess** which ruptures and results in sinus posteriorly, in the scrotum. Tuberculosis never involves the testis proper.

D. **Gumma:** It is due to hypersensitivity reaction to tertiary syphilis. It manifests as subcutaneous swellings, bony swellings and swellings in the midline, etc. Gummas have a firm, necrotic centre surrounded by inflamed tissue. Central softening occurs due to *coagulative necrosis,* eventually leads to sinus formation. Typically, syphilis affects testis and the sinus will be anterior unless in cases of anteverted testis.

   • In secondary syphilis, testis is converted into hard, freely mobile lump. It has been described as **billiard ball testis**.

3. *Testicular tumours:* Seminoma and teratoma are the two common testicular tumours. Other uncommon tumours are lymphoma, interstitial tumours and others. They occur in young patients—teratoma between 20 and 30 years and seminoma between 30 and 40 years. All tumours of the testis should be considered malignant unless proved otherwise. Painless swelling of the scrotum is the common presentation. History may be of 1 or 2 months. Rarely hurricane variety can present with acute pain in the testis and rapid deterioration of health. Pain may mimic acute epididymoorchitis. History of undescended testis or late orchidopexy for undescended testis may be present. History of abdominal distension is due to para-aortic lymph nodes. Left supraclavicular swelling is due to lymph node enlargement. Clinical examination reveals a scrotal swelling with smooth surface in seminoma and irregular or nodular in teratoma. Consistency is firm or even hard sometimes. Testicular sensation is lost. Be gentle in eliciting this because of fear of tumour embolisation. **Secondary hydrocoele may be present.** Transillumination may be negative due to collection of blood- stained fluid. Look for gynaecomastia (Klinefelter syndrome). Ultrasound of the scrotum and abdomen is done. CT scan is more objective. CT scan (Fig. 28.31) of the chest is more reliable to detect small lesions that are not picked by chest X-ray (cannon-ball appearance). **High orchidectomy (inguinal—Fig. 28.32) or radical inguinal**

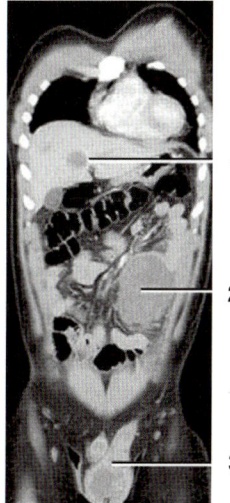
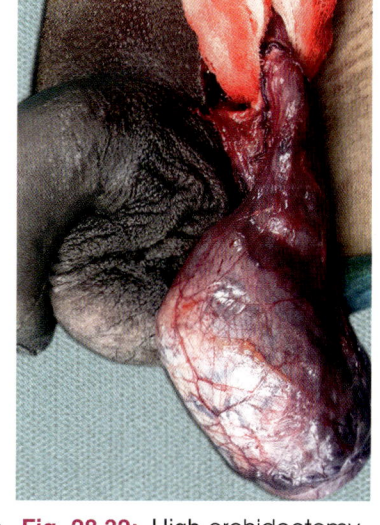

Fig. 28.31: 1. Secondaries in the liver, 2. Para-aortic lymph nodes; and 3. Testicular swelling

Fig. 28.32: High orchidectomy (*Courtesy:* Dr Zeeshan Hameed, Associate Professor, KMC, Manipal)

orchidectomy is the treatment of choice for all malignant tumours of the testis. Radiotherapy, chemotherapy and retroperitoneal lymph node dissection are the other treatment options depending upon the histological type of the tumour. Comparison of seminoma and teratoma is given in Table 28.1.

4. *Cystic swellings of the spermatic cord and epididymis:* Epididymal cyst and spermatocoele are the 2 common cystic swellings. Both produce fluctuation but epididymal cyst is brilliantly transilluminant and spermatocele is not. Two swellings have been compared in Table 28.2. Spermatocele is a *retention cyst* of a *tubule* of the *rete testis* or the head of the *epididymis*.

5. *Torsion of the testis:* **Inversion of testis** is the commonest cause where testis lies horizontally or upside down. **High investment** of tunica vaginalis—the bell clapper deformity is another important cause for torsion testis. In cases where the body of testis is separated from the epididymis, **sudden contraction** of spirally attached cremasteric muscle leads to rotation of testis around the vertical axis during straining at stools, lifting heavy weight, coitus. **A long redundant spermatic cord**

Table 28.1: Comparison of seminoma with teratoma

	Seminoma	Teratoma
1. Cell of origin	Seminiferous tubules in the mediastinum of the testis	Totipotential cells in the rete testis
2. Incidence	35–40%	30%
3. Age group	30–40 years	20–30 years
4. Shape of testis	Retained	Not retained
5. Surface	Smooth	Irregular
6. Cut surface	Smooth	Variegated—nodules, cysts
7. Consistency	Firm	Firm or soft (cystic)
8. Spread	Mainly lymphatic	Predominantly blood
9. Tumour markers	—	HCG—malignant teratoma
10. Radiation response	Excellent—melts like snow	Less sensitive

Table 28.2: Comparison of epididymal cyst with spermatocoele

	Epididymal cyst	Spermatocoele
1. Aetiology	Cystic degeneration of the appendages of epididymis—congenital	Obstruction to the sperm conducting mechanism; acquired—retention cyst
2. Site	Behind and above the testis in the region of epididymal head	Behind the body of the testis
3. Loculi	Multilocular	Unilocular
4. Contents	Crystal clear, watery	Barley water-like
5. Transillumination	Brilliant (Chinese lantern pattern)	Poor transillumination—very often negative
6. Aspiration	Results in recurrence as the cyst is multilocular	May cure as the cyst is unilocular
7. Excision	Excision may be necessary, if the cyst is large	May be excised, if aspiration is not successful

allows twisting of the testis on its own axis. **Two types of testicular torsion:** *Extravaginal torsion*: It is diagnosed in newborns and is caused by non-adherence of tunica vaginalis to the dartos layer. As a result, spermatic cord and tunica vaginalis are rotated as a unit. *Intravaginal torsion*: It is usually diagnosed in boys of 12–18 years of age, but it can occur at any age. **Typically occur in the age group of** 10–25 years who present with sudden agonising pain in the groin and lower abdomen. Vomiting is a feature. **Scrotum is empty** and oedematous on the side of lesion. Following few signs have been described.

- **Tender lump at the external abdominal ring may be palpable.** It is the testis which is positioned high (**Deming's sign**).
- **Prehn's sign:** Elevation of scrotum increases pain in torsion of completely descended testis (decreases pain in epididymo-orchitis).
- **Angell sign** refers to horizontal position of the normal testis.

Doppler is superior to all clinical tests and can clearly distinguish normal testis from ischaemic or gangrene testis.

Low orchidectomy in cases of gangrene and fixing the normal testis is the treatment of choice (Fig. 28.33).

7. *Scrotal oedema*: Scrotal oedema can result in all acute cases such as epididymo-orchitis, torsion testis, torsion of appendix of the testis, etc. Acute idiopathic scrotal oedema is a self-limiting condition in children which can present as severe pain and erythema of the scrotal skin. Doppler shows hypervascularity of the scrotal skin and it helps to rule out other painful conditions such as torsion testis.

8. *Fournier's gangrene* (Figs 28.34 and 28.35): Even though Fournier's gangrene is called idiopathic gangrene, certain factors precipitate the scrotal gangrene such as low socioeconomic group patients, unhygienic conditions, minor trauma including scratching, cut or bruise in the scrotal skin, perianal abscesses, and urogenital instrumentation. Extensive gangrene of the scrotum and perineum including abdominal wall can occur and hence it is included under **necrotising fasciitis**. **Causative organisms are:** Microaerophilic haemolytic Streptococci, Staphylococci, *E. coli*, anaerobes: *Clostridium welchii*.

It is common in young apparently healthy individuals. There is sudden appearance of scrotal inflammation—red, swollen, very painful. Patient is toxic with fever, prostration. Within one/two

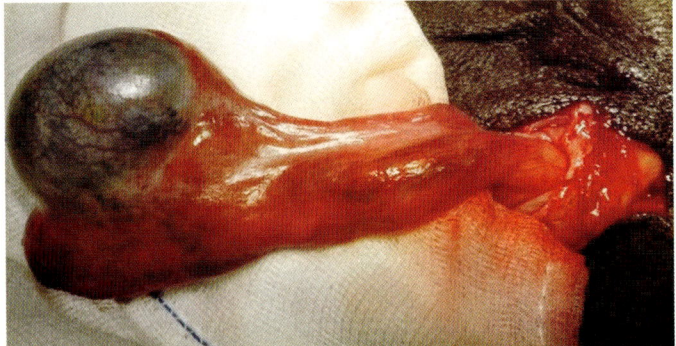

Fig. 28.33: Torsion of the testis and gangrene

6. *Elephantiasis of the scrotum*: This is the result of filariasis. Lymphatics of the scrotum are dilated. Later they are fibrosed and thus gets obliterated. As a result of this, vesicles appear in the scrotal skin which discharge lymph on rupture. This has been called lymphorrhagia. Over a period of time, skin of the scrotum is thickened, firm, and rugosity of the scrotum is obliterated. Filariasis is an important cause for lymphoedema of the scrotum, other cause being radiotherapy given to the groin lymph nodes in carcinoma penis and in any other such conditions.

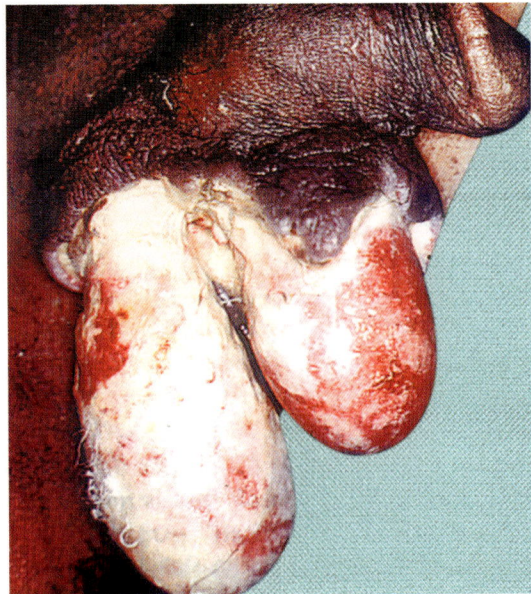

Fig. 28.34: Fournier's gangrene (*Courtesy:* Prof Santhosh Pai, MMMC, Manipal)

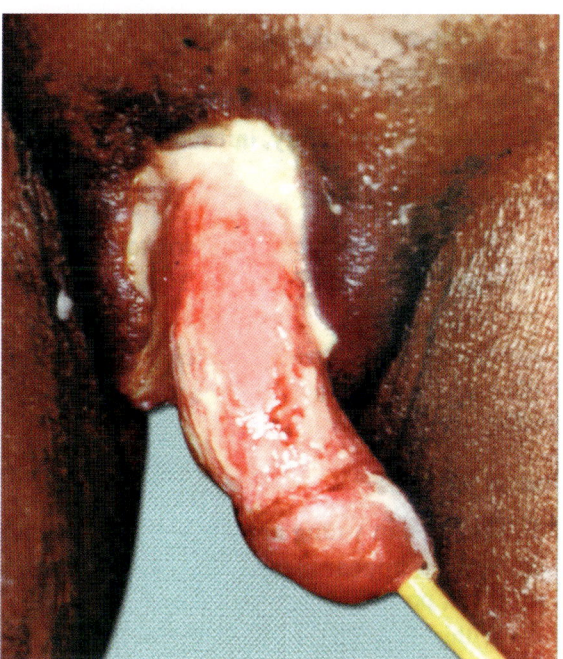

Fig. 28.35: Perineal phlegmon (*Courtesy:* Dr Ramachandra L, Consultant Surgeon and Head, Dept of Surgery, KMC, Manipal)

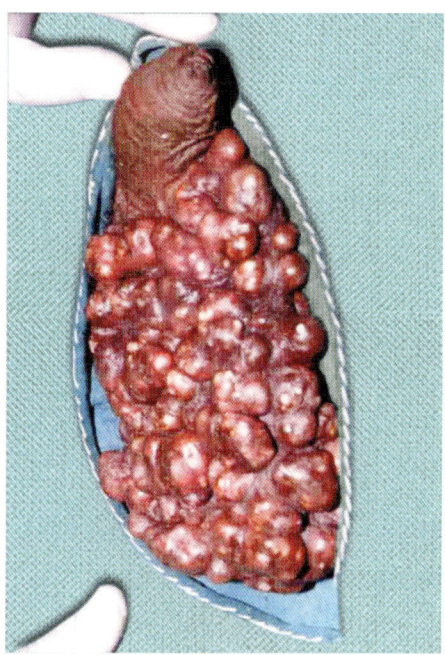

Fig. 28.36: Strawberry scrotum (*Courtesy:* Dr Umesh Bhat, General Surgeon, Kundapur, Karnataka)

days, extensive gangrene of the scrotal skin occurs resulting in sloughing of the scrotal skin exposing the testicles. In a few cases, the gangrene can involve skin of the penis, anterior abdominal wall, medial side of thigh, perianal region. In such situations, it is described as **perineal phlegmon.** Luckily, the testis does not get involved in Fournier's gangrene because of thick tunica albuginea.

Treatment: Broad spectrum antibiotics are given once pus is sent for culture and sensitivity, e.g. metronidazole for anaerobes, gentamicin for gram-negative organisms, cephalosporins may have to be added if required. Gangrenous portion of the scrotum has to be excised, as soon as possible which brings a dramatic reversal of general condition of the patient from toxic to near normal. If the testicles are exposed, they can be implanted in the thigh and once the inflammation subsides, skin grafting is done to cover testicles.

9. *Multiple sebaceous cysts*: Scrotum is one of the common sites of multiple sebaceous cysts. Scalp and back are the other 2 common sites. They are common in young patients. Sebaceous duct obstruction or influence of testosterone hormones may be responsible for sebaceous cysts. They can be asymptomatic in the beginning. When scrotal skin shows nodularity, it has been called as strawberry scrotum (Fig. 28.36). Typically, they are multiple and dome-shaped or hemispherical swellings. A few of them may be seen discharging cheesy-like material (that is

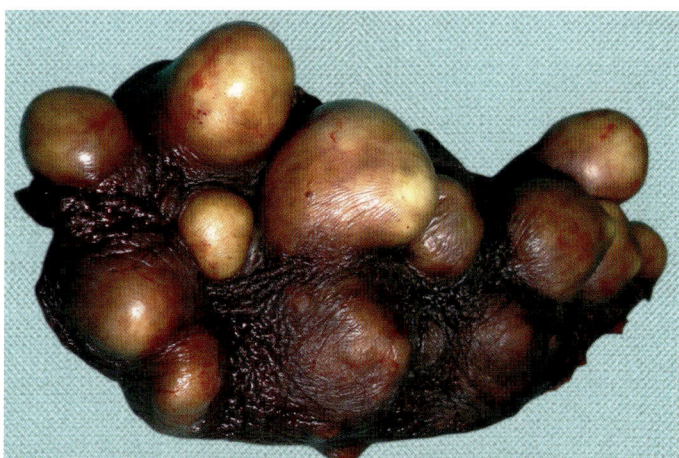

Fig. 28.37: Multiple sebaceous cysts of the scrotum excised with the skin

keratin not sebum). Diagnosis is by clinical examination. No investigations are required. Excision includes scrotal skin also (Fig. 28.37). Otherwise recurrence is possible. Direct suturing of the skin is possible in many cases because scrotal skin is lax. Otherwise flap reconstruction may have to be done by using pedicled inguinal flap.

29

Examination of Penis

INTRODUCTION

Diseases involving penis are interesting and specific to these parts. *Examples are*: Phimosis (inability to retract prepucial skin), paraphimosis (retracted skin cannot be returned back over the glans), hypospadias, epispadias (anomalous urethral openings), carcinoma penis (Fig. 29.1), etc. Being a sexual organ, it is vulnerable for variety of sexually transmitted diseases such as syphilis, gonorrhoea, chancroid, warts due to HPV (human papillomavirus) infections. Thus when you start examining penis, keep in mind these diseases and start asking questions.

COMPLAINTS/HISTORY OF PRESENT ILLNESS

1. *Ulcer over the penis*: The usual questions are what is the duration of the ulcer? How did the ulcer occur?

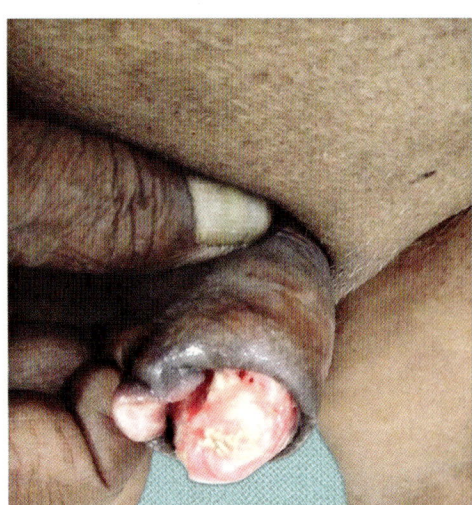

Fig. 29.1: Carcinoma penis—proliferative lesion started in the subpreputial region

When did it occur? How is the progress and how is the discharge? Have you taken any treatment? Is it becoming small? Is it increasing? Is there foul odour? In adults, ulcers are mostly due to sexually transmitted diseases (STDs). History of exposure to venereal diseases should be enquired. Sexual relationship with multiple partners, and high-risk sexual exposures are the causes. **Syphilis** is rare nowadays but can still occur. Typical syphilitic chancre occurs within 4 weeks after exposure to the disease. **Chancroid** occurs after 4 days. Painless vesicle or indurated papule over the penis within 1 to 4 weeks is usually due to **granuloma inguinale**. *Painless ulcer without history of exposure to venereal diseases may be due to carcinoma of penis.*

2. *Discharge*: **Attention should be given to find out where exactly the discharge is coming from—is it from the prepuceal sac, glans penis or from the urethra?** Purulent discharge suggests highly infective contagious diseases such as chancroid and **balanoposthitis**. (Inflammation of glans—balanitis and prepuce—posthitis.)

Blood-stained discharge suggests ulcers specially carcinomatous ulcers. Urethral discharge suggests gonococcal or nongonococcal urethritis. Foul characteristic odour of carcinoma penis cannot be missed.

3. *Pain*: Pain is due to ulcerations and it is a dull ache or pricking type of pain. Secondary infection is common. Urethritis and prostatic abscess will give rise to pain while passing urine. Genital warts, genital herpes or STDs can cause pain independent of micturition. Pain radiating to the tip of penis is usually due to bladder stone and it occurs after micturition. Pain during intercourse can be due to Peyronie's disease.

Recurrent pain in the prepuceal region and recent inability to retract the skin of the prepuce suggest development of diabetes.

4. *Inability to retract the prepuce*: It may be congenital. Some patients will complain of recent inability to retract the prepuceal skin. If it is associated with diabetes and pain, it is due to recurrent balanoposthitis. But recent phimosis can also be due to subpreputial carcinoma penis (Fig. 29.2).

5. *Poor stream while passing urine*: This is due to narrowing of the external meatus. In children, it is due to pinhole meatus. A tight phimosis also results in poor stream of urine with ballooning of the prepuce while passing urine.

6. *Bifid stream of urine*: Some patients point out and say that urine flows out of two places while passing urine, one through external urinary meatus and the other through some part of the penis. This is due to a fistula which has developed between distal urethra and the growth. This happens in advanced cases of carcinoma penis. Sometimes mother may complain that her son is passing urine with good stream but wetting of clothes is present. It is due to hypospadias (page 473).

7. *Swellings in the groin*: Did you notice any swelling in the groin? It is due to enlarged lymph nodes (Figs 29.3 and 29.4).

8. History of sexual contact with multiple partners should be enquired.

Inspection

• First comment on circumcision status. Mention whether the patient has undergone circumcision or not. Otherwise ask him to retract the prepuce and show the lesion or ulcer.

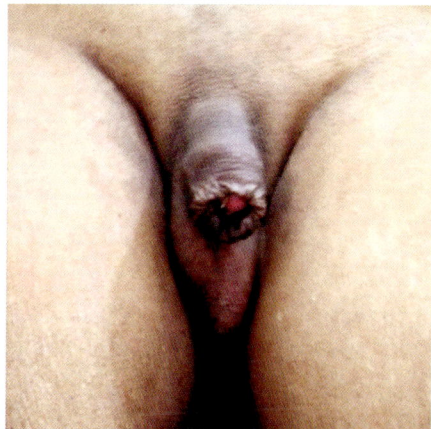

Fig. 29.2: This patient had phimosis. He developed phimosis due to subpreputial growth

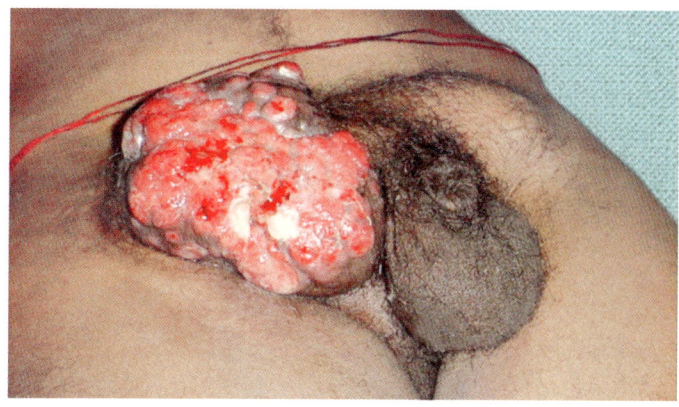

Fig. 29.3: This patient presented with fungating inguinal lymph nodes. Observe the penis—he has undergone partial amputation of the penis 2 years back. There is a swelling in the left side also due to inguinal lymph nodes.

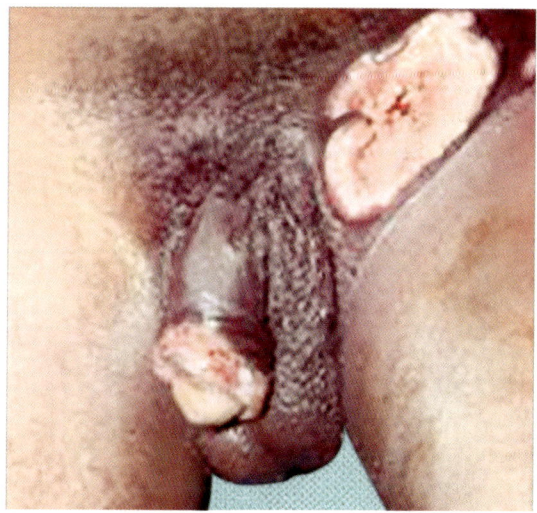

Fig. 29.4: Carcinoma penis—difficult to find external urinary meatus—ask the patient where he passes urine—he will show you the urinary meatus

• Look at the external urinary meatus. Specially in children, pinhole meatus due to meatal narrowing is not uncommon.

• A red, raw lesion on the glans or inside the prepuce—**erythroplasia of Queyrat** or Paget's disease of penis—is a precancerous condition.

• Persistent nonspecific patches in the glans or in the preputial skin are called leukoplakic patches. In the penis, leukoplakic patches are not white.

• If any ulcer is visible, describe it. Classically malignant ulcers have everted edge, unhealthy floor, oedematous surrounding area. Foul odour is characteristic. Syphilitic chancre or hunterian chancre (hard chancre) is a well-defined ulcer with punched out edge and it is single. If you see multiple ulcers, it is usually chancroid (soft sore).

- Exophytic lesions can be due to verrucous carcinoma. Warty lesions occur in **Buschke-Löwenstein** tumours (giant condylomata). Venereal warts are commonly located around coronal sulcus.

- When urethral opening is in the undersurface (ventral) of penis, it is hypospadias and if it is on the dorsal aspect, it is epispadias. Hypospadias is more common than epispadias.

Palpation

- If growth is visible, start palpating and describe it in the usual manner. Induration and fixity are the two important points to be noted under palpation. Typical lesion is ulceroproliferative growth with everted edges and induration of the base and edge. Growth is friable and bleeds easily on touch (Fig. 29.5)

- **The induration is much more extensive** than the lesion. Hence, entire shaft has to be examined for evidence of induration. Deep part of the shaft or body of the penis is felt through the scrotum in the midline.

- **Urethra is rarely involved** (Fig. 29.6) in carcinoma of penis because it is protected by the tough Buck's fascia, which is a part of pelvic fascia.

- In large fungating lesions, it may be difficult to identify the external urinary meatus. In such situations, the patient will point out at the external urinary meatus.

Examination of Lymph Nodes

Horizontal group of deep inguinal nodes are enlarged due to metastasis. Metastatic nodes are usually hard and nontender. If the enlargement is due to infection, they are tender and soft or firm.

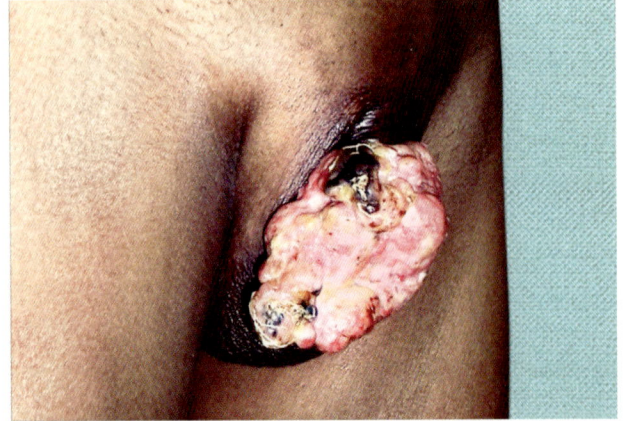

Fig. 29.5: Carcinoma penis—proliferative lesion (exophytic) with destruction of penis. (Advances lesion.)

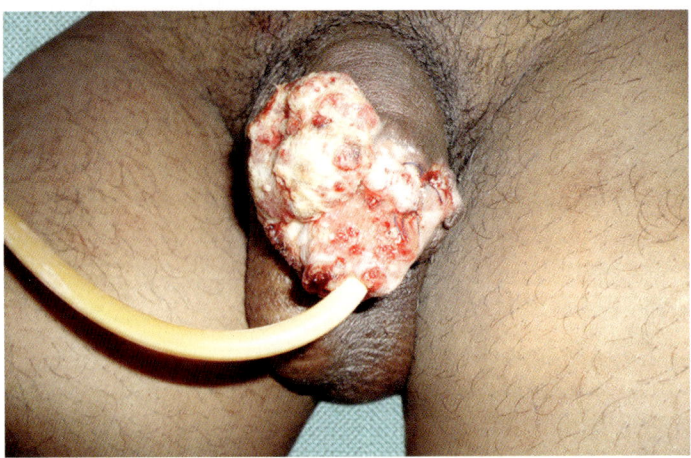

Fig. 29.6: Carcinoma penis—proliferative lesion with bifid stream hence, patient was catheterised

CLINICAL DISCUSSION

1. **What is the most common site of carcinoma penis?**
   Glans penis
2. **How does phimosis predispose to carcinoma penis?**
   Smegma collects underneath the preputial skin and that results in chronic irritation causing carcinoma penis.
3. **What is Buck's fascia?**
   Buck's fascia (deep fascia of the penis) is a layer of *deep fascia* covering the three erectile bodies of the *penis*. It is continuous with the *external spermatic fascia* in the *scrotum* and the *suspensory ligament of the penis*. On its ventral aspect, it splits to envelop corpus spongiosum in a separate compartment from the tunica albuginea and corporal bodies.
4. **What are the other names for syphilitic chancre?**
   Hard sore or hunterian chancre.
5. **Is HIV a premalignant condition?**
   No.
6. **What is the speciality of blood supply of corpora cavernosa?**
   Corkscrew-shaped arteries or helicine arteries.
7. **Which artery supplies blood during erection?**
   Deep artery of penis.
8. **What is the medical treatment for genital warts?**
   Podophylline.
9. **In case of phimosis, how do you take biopsy?**
   Dorsal slit and do biopsy
10. **In proliferative lesions, what type of biopsy is done?**
    A wedge of tissue is taken from the edge of the lesion.
11. **Why biopsy from the edge of the lesion?**
    It is the most proliferative site
12. **What is the biopsy result expected?**
    Squamous cell carcinoma
13. **How will you assess lymph nodes?**
    Ultrasound can detect the enlarged lymph nodes, change in the shape, loss of fatty hilum, etc.
14. **What other investigations are done?**
    Ultrasound of the abdomen to rule out iliac and para-aortic lymph nodes.

DIFFERENTIAL DIAGNOSIS

PHIMOSIS

Inability to retract preputial skin is called phimosis.

Cause can be congenital: Most common type seen in young patients. Secondary to **chronic balanoposthitis**: Balanitis means inflammation of glans penis and posthitis means inflammation of the prepuce. Balanoposthitis is common in diabetic patients. **Chancre** also can cause phimosis. **Carcinoma** of the penis can present as a recent phimosis. The patient complains of inability to retract the prepuce. In children, ballooning of the prepuce (second bladder) can be seen, which is diagnostic of phimosis. It makes them more prone for balanoposthitis because of the inability to clean the glans. Carcinoma of the penis and paraphimosis are the complications. Treatment is by circumcision means removal of the prepuce.

PARAPHIMOSIS

In this condition, the retracted skin of the glans penis (prepuce) cannot be pulled forwards. As a result of this, the retracted skin acts like a tight constricting agent which compresses the corona resulting in venous congestion. As venous congestion increases, glans swells up resulting in paraphimosis. This can follow after a sexual intercourse. During catheterisation, if the retracted prepuce is not pulled forwards, it results in paraphimosis. **Severe pain in the glans penis, gross swelling of retracted prepucial skin and oedema of the distal glans penis are the clinical features.** Urgent reduction of paraphimosis with or without injection hyaluronidase into the constriction ring is done. In difficult cases, dorsal slit is given so that reduction can be done. Complications include ulcers of glans and gangrene of glans penis in later stages.

HYPOSPADIAS

In this condition, some portion of distal urethra is not developed, as a result of which external meatus is situated in the under surface of penis. Usually this is associated with chordee and hooded prepuce.

Types (Fig. 29.7)

1. Glandular variety: In this, the external meatus is situated a few mm away from normal site within the glans.

2. Coronal variety: It occurs due to failure of development of urethra which runs in the glans penis. As a result of this, urethra opens at the corona gland is—junction of glans and shaft of penis. Both these varieties do not give major problems functionally. It can be left alone without treatment.

3. Penile hypospadias: In this, the external opening is situated somewhere on the under surface of the penis.

4. Penoscrotal/perineal hypospadias: In this condition, the entire urethra is not developed. Penis is rudimentary.

- Urethral opening is seen in-between two halves of the scrotum and often it is split.
- Cases may be associated with undescended testes.
- In such cases, it is difficult to differentiate the sex of the child. Occurs in 1:350 males.

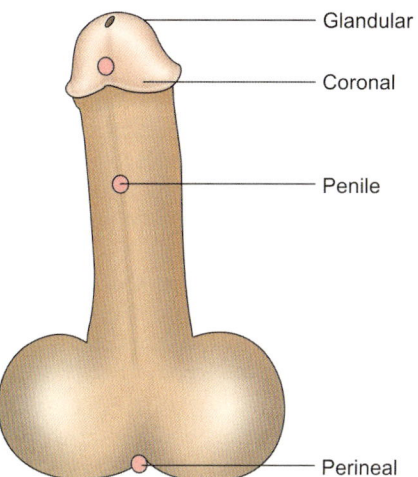

— Glandular
— Coronal
— Penile
— Perineal

Fig. 29.7: Various types of hypospadias

- *Micturition*: Stream is good, but it wets the clothes in 3rd and 4th varieties.
- *Chordee*: Many of the cases are associated with bending of penis. Sexual intercourse will be difficult.
- Hooded prepuce. In severe hypospadias, possibility of intersex problem is settled by **karyotyping**.

Treatment

One-stage urethroplasty: Chordee correction: Always confirm by inducing artificial erection. Urethral tube formation by tubularising urethra—inner preputial island tube urethroplasty.

Two-stage urethroplasty: When the child is 6–12 months old, chordee is corrected by straightening the penis. This is called orthoplasty. When the child is 5–6 years old, reconstruction of the urethra is done by using locally available skin either from the prepuce or from penile shaft. This is called urethroplasty. Hence, **circumcision should not be done in hypospadias.**

CONDYLOMA ACUMINATUM

It refers to an epidermal manifestation attributed to the human papillomavirus (HPV). They are also called anogenital warts. They are usually benign such as condyloma but malignancy is often detected by pathologist such as **low grade intraepithelial neoplasia, high-grade squamous intraepithelial neoplasia, especially in immunocompromised individuals**. Most patients with anal condylomata present with perianal growth, pruritus ani, discharge, bleeding, and sometimes with tenesmus. On examination, the classic cauliflower-like lesion or warty lesions are found. They tend to run in radial rows out from the anus. The warts may be single or multiple, or coalesce to form polypoid masses. Individual warts can be sessile or pedunculated, isolated, or clustered.

BUSCHKE-LÖWENSTEIN TUMOUR

They are called the Giant Condyloma of Buschke and Löwenstein (GCBL). They are slow-growing, locally destructive verrucous plaque that typically appears on the penis but may occur elsewhere in the anogenital region. It is a type of verrucous carcinoma occurring in the penis. *Buschke-Löwenstein tumour* (i.e. giant condyloma) is a fungating, locally invasive, low-grade cancer attributed to HPV.

CARCINOMA PENIS

It is common in Asian countries including India wherein routine circumcision is not done. **Circumcision done immediately after birth and in early infancy** is the protective factor against development of carcinoma penis. Phimosis results in collection of smegma under the prepuce and thus is considered as one factor for carcinoma penis. It is common in the 6th or 7th decade and common in poor socioeconomic patients.

- Genital warts, leukoplakia, **erythroplasia of Queyrat** and Bowen's disease are premalignant conditions. Glans penis is the commonest site (45%) followed by preputial skin (25%). **Most common type is squamous cell carcinoma.**

- Typically, the patient is an elderly round 60 years of age who presents with nonhealing ulcer. Foul smelling discharge is common and occasionally it is blood stained. Recent phimosis due to growth underneath the prepuce may be the complaint.

- On examination, often there is an ulceroproliferative growth with everted edges and induration of the base and edge. The induration is much more extensive than the lesion. Hence, entire shaft has to be examined for evidence of induration. **Urethra is rarely involved in carcinoma of penis** because it is protected by the tough Buck's fascia, which is a part of pelvic fascia. In large fungating lesions, it may be difficult to identify the external urinary meatus. In such situations, **the patient will point out at the external urinary meatus.**

- Spread is first by local spread involving the shaft of penis and entire glans and in late stages urethra. The skin of the penis and prepuce drain primarily to the superficial inguinal nodes on the medial side.

- The lymphatics of the glans may drain to the superficial inguinal nodes or drain directly to the deep inguinal nodes or even the external iliac group. The lymphatics of the corporal bodies may drain to the superficial, inguinal nodes or directly to the external iliac nodes. Because of these reasons, ilioinguinal block dissection is favoured than inguinal block dissection.

Differential Diagnosis of Ulcer Penis (refer to Table 29.1)

Lymphatic spread: Inguinal nodes are enlarged. 30% cases are due to infection. Nodes are firm and tender in infection. Hard nodes suggest metastases. Later, internal iliac and para-aortic nodes can also get enlarged. In advanced cases, the lymph nodes may show fungation, as in Fig. 29.2.

Wedge biopsy from the edge of the growth, proves the diagnosis of squamous cell carcinoma. MRI is helpful in lesions invading corpora cavernosa (soft tissue details). When the growth is confined to the prepuce, **circumcision** is the treatment of choice. Regular follow-up is required. Growth involving the glans and part of shaft: **Partial amputation** with at least 2 cm margin from the palpable indurated edge of the tumour. Major advantage of partial amputation is preservation of normal passage of urine. **Total penectomy with perineal urethrostomy**

Table 29.1: Differential diagnosis of ulcer penis

	Nature of the ulcer	Inguinal region	Other features/findings
1. Hunterian chancre (syphilitic chancre, hard chancre)	Single, round, painless ulcer—coronal sulcus, frenulum, glans are the sites; base is indurated	Multiple, shotty, painless inguinal lymph nodes	Incubation period—3 weeks; organism—*Treponema pallidum*
2. Chancroid (soft sore)	Multiple painful ulcers; oedematous edges, slough and discharge—plenty of bubo and sinuses	Multiple nodes—above and below inguinal region—bubo; suppuration	Incubation period 3–4 days; organism—Ducrey's bacilli
3. Lymphogranuloma venereum (LGV) (lymphogranuloma inguinale, tropical tubular bubo)	Painless vesicles or papules, fleeting duration, heals spontaneously	Multiple nodes above and below in the inguinal region form sign of groove, later give rise to bubo and sinuses	Incubation period 1–2 weeks; virus *Chlamydia trachomatis*; rubbery rectal stricture; can occur in females
4. Granuloma inguinale (granuloma venereum)	Painless vesicle, changes into an ulcer with exuberant granulation tissue; highly contagious ulcer; bleeds but painless	Inguinal region may be involved, but inguinal lymph nodes are not involved unless secondary infection supervenes	Incubation period—10–40 days; organism—*Donovania granulomatis* (bacilli)
5. Balanoposthitis ulcers	Multiple, painful ulcers, difficulty in retracting prepuce	Lymph node enlargement uncommon	Recurrent balanoposthitis common in diabetic patients
6. Herpes progenitalis	Vesicles and pustules on the prepuce or on the glans	Inguinal lymph nodes are not enlarged	Neuralgic pain and itching occur before the onset of ulcer
7. Carcinomatous ulcer	Painless, indurated ulcer with everted edges; bleeds on touch	Tender nodes, hard nodes, metastasis	Phimosis is one aetiological factor

is done if adequate shaft cannot be retained. **Complications of perineal urethrostomy include ammoniacal dermatitis** of scrotum and stricture of perineal urethra. To prevent ammoniacal dermatitis, the patient has to lift the scrotum to pass urine. **Stricture of perineal urethra** can be dilated by Hegar's dilators.

PEYRONIE'S DISEASE (PENILE FIBROMATOSIS)

Aetiology

- Past trauma has been considered as one of the factors.
- Venereal diseases also have been blamed.
- Association with Dupuytren's contracture, retroperitoneal fibrosis and plantar fasciitis.

Clinical Features

- Hard plaques of fibrosis can be palpated along the length of the penis in the sheath of corpora cavernosa (induration—penis—plastica).
- As a result of hard plaques, erection is not proper, and erected penis tends to bend towards the side of the plaque.

Treatment

Medical: Steroids, vitamin E, tamoxifen (not good results), colchicine therapy, intralesional verapamil.

Watch and observe some cases. It may recur after a few years.

Surgical: Straightening of the penis is recommended, if the deformity is distressing.

1. **Nesbitt's operation:** Straightening the penis by placing non-absorbable suture in corpora cavernosa opposite the plaque.
2. **Gelhard's operation:** Multiple incisions over fibrous plaques and temporal fascia bridging.

FRACTURE OF PENIS

- It is a misnomer.
- It is traumatic rupture of corpora cavernosa. It is considered a urologic emergency.
- Sudden blunt trauma or abrupt lateral bending of penis in an erect state can break the markedly thinned and stiff tunica albuginea (Fig. 29.8).

- One or both corpora may be involved and concomitant urethral (38%) injury can be, if both corpora are involved.
- *Causes:* Sexual activity, masturbation, gunshot wounds, industrial accidents, mechanical trauma.
- Diagnosed clinically.
- In equivocal cases—cavernosonography or MRI.
- Preoperative retrograde urethrography, if urethral injury is suspected.

Treatment

a. **Medical:** Fluids, antibiotics.

   If surgical therapy is delayed due to urethral injury, initial medical therapy consists of cold compresses, pressure dressings, anti-inflammatory medications and suprapubic cystostomy.

b. **Surgical:** Evacuate haematoma, identify site of injury, correct the defect in tunica albuginea and repair urethral injury. Urethral catheter is removed after 2 weeks.

Complications

Erectile dysfunction, abnormal curvature, painful erections, urethrocutaneous fistula, corpora-urethral fistula and painful nodules are a few complications

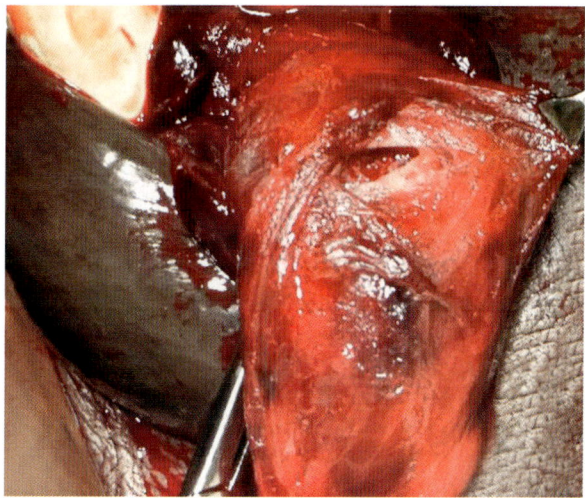

Fig. 29.8: Fracture penis (*Courtesy:* Dr TS Rao, Consultant Surgeon, Hitech Hospital, Udupi)

30

Viva Voce Examination

INTRODUCTION

One of the sessions in the undergraduate and postgraduate examinations is on X-rays and images. More and more images, such as ultrasound, CT scan, MRI and PET scan, etc., have been used. Hence, I have added a few of them here. Several CT images have been included in the book. This is only an exercise for you to perform better in the final examination.

I. Plain X-ray Abdomen showing Collection of Free Gas Under the Right Dome of the Diaphragm (Fig. 30.1)

Normally, fundic air bubble is present on the left side. Hence, importance is given to the gas on the right side.

1. What are the causes of free gas under the right dome of the diaphragm?

- Perforation of hollow viscus. Examples:
  - Duodenal ulcer, gastric ulcer
  - Perforation of enteric ulcer
  - Perforation of Meckel's diverticulum
  - Malignant ulcers—colonic, gastric
  - Perforation of the tuberculous ulcer—ileum
- Abdominal stab injury
- Laparotomy
- Tubal insufflation test done for tubal patency.

2. Is there any other finding in the X-ray?

- Ground glass appearance indicates significant fluid in the peritoneal cavity.

3. How do you manage a case of perforated duodenal ulcer?

- With antibiotic coverage, Ryle's tube aspiration and early resuscitation with intravenous fluids, exploratory laparotomy is done. The site of perforation is identified which is in the first part of the duodenum. The perforation is closed by using nonabsorbable sutures. Pedicled omentum can be used to reinforce the suture line. This is called Roscoe Graham operation. Tube drain is used to drain the peritoneal cavity.

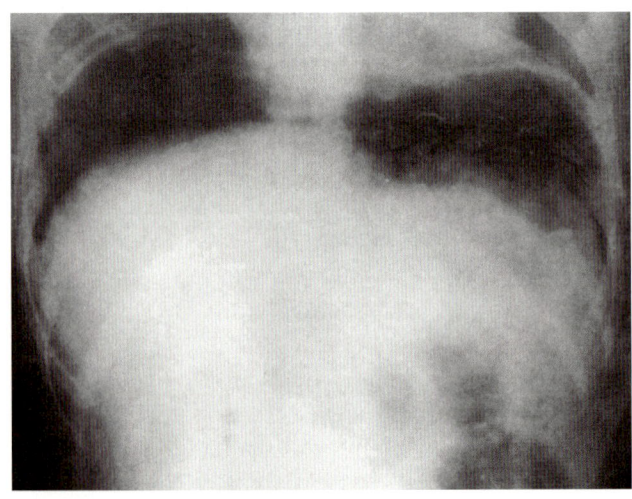

Fig. 30.1: Plain X-ray abdomen showing collection of free gas under the right dome of the diaphragm

4. Will you do elective surgery such as GJ and vagotomy or HSV at this stage?

- Since the general condition of the patient will be very poor at this acute stage because of hypovolaemic and septic shock, elective surgery is not done.
- Most of the ulcers which perforate today are NSAID induced with or without *Helicobacter pylori.*

5. What are the stages of duodenal ulcer perforation?

- Stage of chemical peritonitis
- Stage of illusion or delusion
- Stage of bacterial peritonitis

II. Plain X-ray Abdomen showing Multiple Gas and Fluid Levels (Fig. 30.2)

1. What is the diagnosis?

- Since jejunal loops are prominently seen and loops are centrally located, it is probably terminal ileal obstruction.

2. What are the common causes of terminal ileal obstruction?

1. Tuberculous stricture
2. Bands—congenital
3. Adhesions
4. 'Worm ball' in children
5. Obstructed hernia

3. How do you identify jejunum, ileum and colon in a plain X-ray?

- Jejunum—valvulae conniventes—regularly placed mucosal folds placed opposite to each other.

- Ileum—no character—**characterless loop of Wangensteen**.
- Colon—**haustrations**—large incomplete mucosal folds **not placed** opposite to each other.

4. How do you treat tuberculous strictures?

- Resection and end-to-end anastomosis

5. Can any other surgical procedure be done?

- Stricturoplasty (like pyloroplasty)

III. Plain X-ray Abdomen showing Radio-opaque Shadow in the Right Upper Abdomen (Fig. 30.3)

1. What is the diagnosis?

- Probably renal stone

2. Why is it not a gallstone?

- The location of the stone is at lower level when compared to gallstone.
- The shape of the stone suggests that it is a stone in the pelvis growing within calyces.

3. What do you call such a stone?

- Staghorn calculus

4. What type of X-ray is ideal to distinguish renal stone from gallbladder stone?

Lateral view

5. What will be the findings in case of renal stones in a lateral picture?

- Renal stones are found superimposed on vertebral bodies. On the other hand, gallstones are found anterior to it.

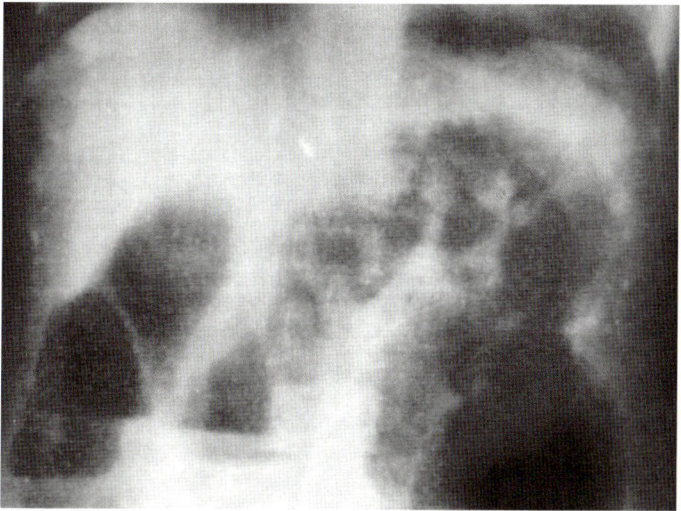

Fig. 30.2: Plain X-ray abdomen showing multiple gas and fluid levels

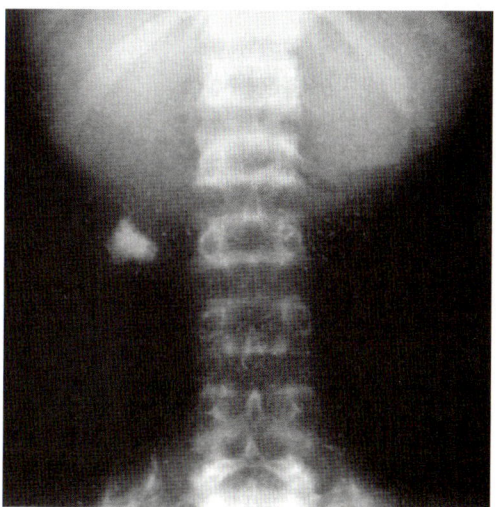

Fig. 30.3: Plain X-ray abdomen showing radio-opaque shadow in the right upper abdomen

IV. Plain X-ray Abdomen showing Radio-opaque Shadow in the Region of Gallbladder (Fig. 30.4)

1. What is the diagnosis?

- Probably gallstone

2. What percentage of gallstones are visible in a plain X-ray?

- Only 10%

3. What is the reason for that?

- The calcium content in gallstones is very less.

4. What are the causes of radio-opaque shadow in the abdomen?

- Gallstones
- Renal stones
- Pancreatic stones
- Renal tuberculosis
- 'Chip' fracture of the transverse process of the vertebrae
- Calcified lymph nodes—tuberculosis
- Faecoliths
- Phleboliths

5. What is the treatment of symptomatic gallstones?

- Laparoscopic cholecystectomy

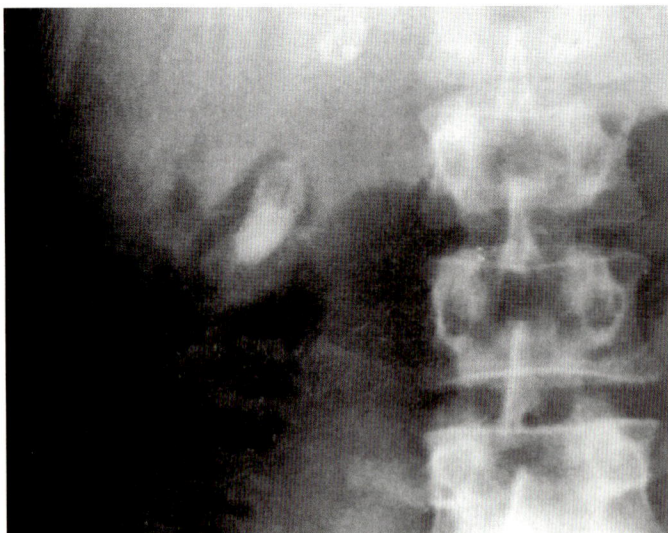

Fig. 30.4: Plain X-ray abdomen showing radio-opaque shadow in the region of gallbladder

V. X-ray Chest PA view showing Multiple Round Shadows in Both Lung Fields (Fig. 30.5)

1. What is the diagnosis?

- Bilateral chest secondaries

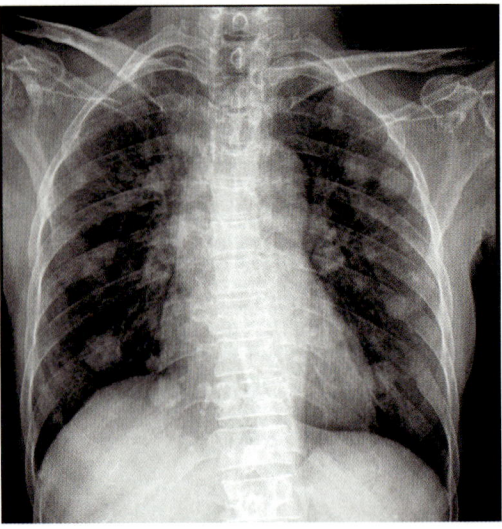

Fig. 30.5: X-ray chest PA view showing multiple round shadows in both lung fields

2. What are they called?

- Cannonball secondaries

3. Why are secondaries in the lung round?

- Lung is an elastic tissue, it has resilience. Hence, during the act of inspiration and expiration, equal amount of pressure is exerted on secondaries, which are growing. Hence, they tend to become round.

4. What are the common causes of chest secondaries?

- Carcinoma breast
- Carcinoma testis
- Malignant melanoma
- Colonic carcinoma
- Renal cell carcinoma
- Sarcoma

5. Is there any other differential diagnosis?

- *Miliary tuberculosis*: The shadows will be very small and numerous.

VI. X-ray Cervical Vertebrae with Upper Ribs showing Bilateral Cervical Ribs (Fig. 30.6)

1. What is a cervical rib?

- It is an extra rib arising from 7th cervical vertebra.

2. What are four types of cervical rib?

- Incomplete bony
- Complete bony with anterior expanded bony end
- Partly fibrous, partly bony

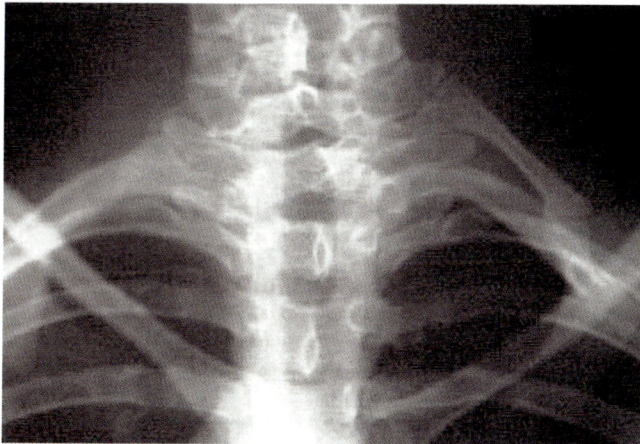

Fig. 30.6: X-ray cervical vertebrae with upper ribs showing bilateral cervical ribs

- Complete fibrous band

3. What variety gives rise to vascular symptoms?

- The fibrous band variety

4. What is your finding here?

- On the right side, it is complete variety and on the left side, it is incomplete.

5. If cervical rib is symptomatic, what is the treatment?

- Extraperiosteal excision of cervical rib which means removal of the rib along with the periosteum. Some surgeons also do cervical sympathectomy to decrease vasomotor tone of vessels.

VII. Barium Swallow showing Intrinsic, Irregular, and Persistent Filling Defect in the Lower Oesophagus (Fig. 30.7)

1. What is the diagnosis?

- Carcinoma lower one-third of oesophagus

2. What are the other findings?

- Proximal shouldering is very characteristic of malignancy.

3. How do you confirm the diagnosis?

- Oesophagoscopy and biopsy

4. If biopsy report is adenocarcinoma, what is the treatment?

- Operable—oesophagogastrectomy
- Inoperable—to relieve dysphagia, metallic stents can be introduced. Thus, surgery can be avoided.

5. What are the premalignant conditions?

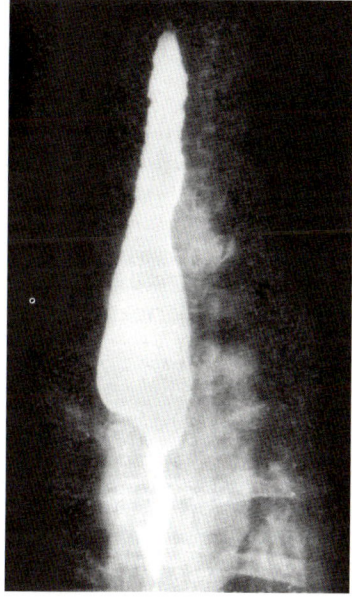

Fig. 30.7: Barium swallow showing intrinsic, irregular and persistent filling defect in the lower oesophagus

- Achalasia cardia
- Barrett's oesophagus
- Corrosive stricture
- Plummer-Vinson syndrome

VIII. Barium Swallow showing Extensive and Irregular Filling Defect involving Middle One-third of Oesophagus (Fig. 30.8)

1. What is the diagnosis?

- Carcinoma middle one-third of oesophagus

2. How do you confirm the diagnosis?

- Oesophagoscopy and biopsy

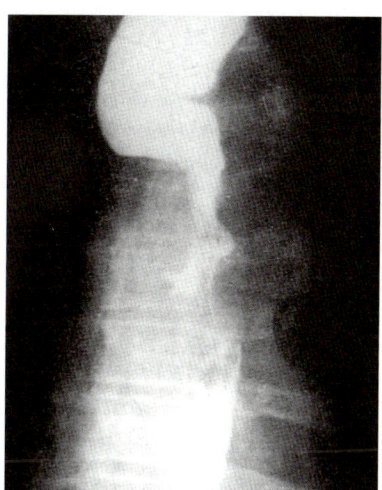

Fig. 30.8: Barium swallow showing extensive and irregular filling defect involving middle one-third of oesophagus

3. What will be the biopsy report?

- Squamous cell carcinoma

4. What other investigations are necessary in such case?

- Bronchoscopy, CT scan of the chest and endosonography are important investigations.

5. Looking at this advanced lesion, what is probably the best treatment for this patient?

- Chemoradiotherapy followed by dilatation of the oesophagus, since chances of fibrosis and narrowing of the lumen following radiotherapy are high.

IX. Barium Meal showing Intrinsic, Irregular, and Persistent Filling Defect involving Pyloric Antrum (Fig. 30.9)

1. What is the diagnosis?

- Carcinoma pyloric antrum

2. How do you confirm diagnosis?

- Gastroscopic biopsy (6 pieces)

3. What will be the biopsy report?

- Adenocarcinoma

4. What is the treatment, if it is operable?

- Subtotal gastrectomy

5. What structures are removed in the operation?

- Growth along with 60–70% of distal stomach, omentum, enlarged regional nodes such as prepyloric, suprapyloric, infrapyloric, left and right gastric nodes are removed, followed by gastrojejunal anastomosis.

X. Barium Meal X-ray showing Enormous Dilatation of the Stomach and Failure of Barium to Fill into the Distal Intestine (Fig. 30.10)

1. What is the diagnosis?

- Gastric outlet obstruction due to chronic cicatrised duodenal ulcer. (Pyloric stenosis is an old terminology.)

2. Why is it not due to carcinoma pyloric antrum?

- There is no filling defect in the pyloric antrum.

3. How do you treat this case?

- With a preoperative stomach wash, adequate intravenous fluids, total truncal vagotomy with GJ is the treatment of choice.

4. Why GJ and vagotomy?

- After vagotomy, motility of the stomach is lost and in pyloric stenosis, there is already obstruction at the pyloric antrum. Hence, gastrojejunostomy is the drainage procedure of choice.

5. Why not pyloroplasty or highly selective vagotomy?

- Pylorus is scarred and deformed. Hence, it is not safe to do pyloroplasty. HSV is contraindicated in the presence of pyloric obstruction.

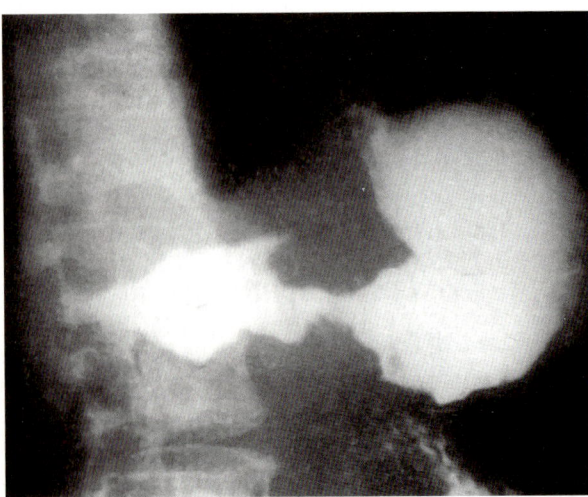

Fig. 30.9: Barium meal showing intrinsic, irregular and persistent filling defect involving pyloric antrum

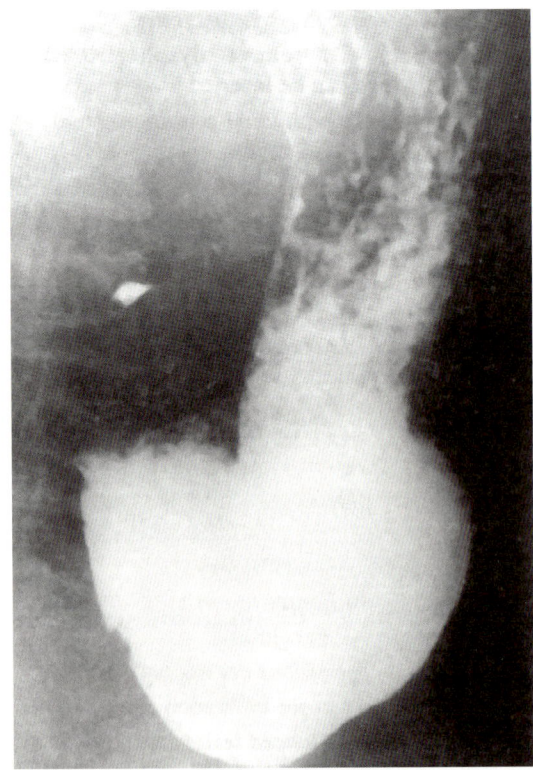

Fig. 30.10: Barium meal X-ray showing enormous dilatation of the stomach and failure of barium to fill into the distal intestine

XI. Barium Enema showing the Left Colon, Transverse Colon and a Part of Ascending Colon (Fig. 30.11)

1. What is the diagnosis?

- Ileocolic intussusception

2. Why do you say so?

- The 'claw' like ending or pincer ending is typical of intussusception.

3. What are the causes of intussusception in adults?

- Submucous lipoma, or polyps
- Meckel's diverticulum
- Growth in the caecum
- Leiomyoma of the ileum

4. In a child, what are the causes?

- Weaning of the diet or viral infection

5. What is the treatment of adult intussusception?

- Resection because there is a precipitating cause.

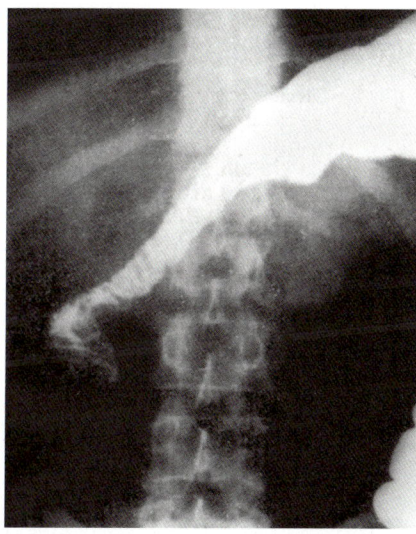

Fig. 30.11: Barium enema showing the left colon, transverse colon and a part of ascending colon with pincer ending

XII. Barium Enema showing Intrinsic, Irregular and Persistent Filling Defect in the Ascending Colon (Fig. 30.12)

1. What is the diagnosis?

- Carcinoma ascending colon

2. What is the confirmatory investigation?

- Colonoscopy and biopsy

3. What is the report, if it is carcinoma?

- Adenocarcinoma

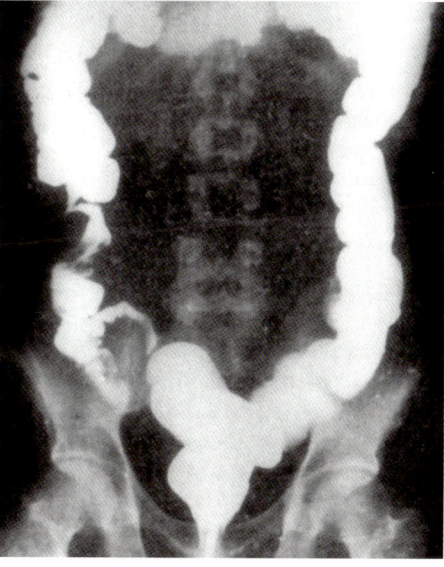

Fig. 30.12: Barium enema showing intrinsic, irregular and persistent filling defect in the ascending colon

4. What is the treatment?

- Right radical hemicolectomy, if it is operable. Structures removed in this operation include terminal ileum (6–8 cm), caecum including appendix, ascending colon and 1/3rd of right transverse colon. If it is inoperable, part of ileum is anastomosed to the transverse colon to prevent or relieve intestinal obstruction (side-to-side). One need not remove two feet of ileum.

5. What is the differential diagnosis?

- Ileocaecal tuberculosis: In this condition:

    a. Irregular filling defect is not seen.

    b. Caecum is usually pulled up and then ileocaecal angle becomes obtuse.

XIII. Barium Enema showing Loss of Haustrations in the Left Colon, Small and Multiple, Regular Filling Defects due to Pseudopolyposis (Fig. 30.13)

1. What is the diagnosis?

- Ulcerative colitis

2. What is pseudopolyposis?

- An attempt at healing in-between the ulcers produces granulation tissue which have the appearance of polyps. Hence, pseudopolyposis.

3. What are the dangerous complications of ulcerative colitis?

- Haemorrhage, toxic megacolon, perforation and malignancy.

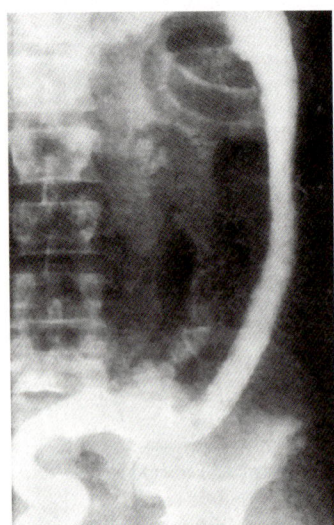

Fig. 30.13: Barium enema showing loss of haustrations in the left colon, small and multiple, and regular filling defects due to pseudopolyposis

4. What are the drugs used in the treatment of ulcerative colitis?

• Salazopyrines and corticosteroids

5. What are the surgical treatments?

• Total colectomy, creation of a pouch with anastomosis of the pouch to the anal canal.

XIV. X-ray Lateral View of the Skull showing a Large Swelling with Erosion in the Pericranium (Fig. 30.14)

1. What is the diagnosis?

• Secondary deposit in the skull

2. Why is it not a lipoma or neurofibroma?

• Erosion of the bone is seen in malignancy, not in benign tumours.

3. If this patient is a female aged 40 years, what are the causes?

• Follicular carcinoma thyroid
• Carcinoma of the breast
• Renal cell carcinoma

4. What is the treatment, if this is follicular carcinoma thyroid?

• Total thyroidectomy followed by radio-iodine ablation and external radiotherapy for isolated metastasis in bones.

5. How do you diagnose follicular carcinoma thyroid histologically?

• Angioinvasion and capsular invasion

XV. Endoscopic Retrograde Cholangiopancreatography (ERCP) showing the Biliary and Pancreatic Systems (Fig. 30.15)

1. What is the diagnosis?

• Chronic pancreatitis

2. Why do you say so?

• Extensive calcification involving head, body and tail of pancreas.

3. What is the simple investigation to diagnose chronic pancreatitis?

• Plain X-ray abdomen showing calcification.

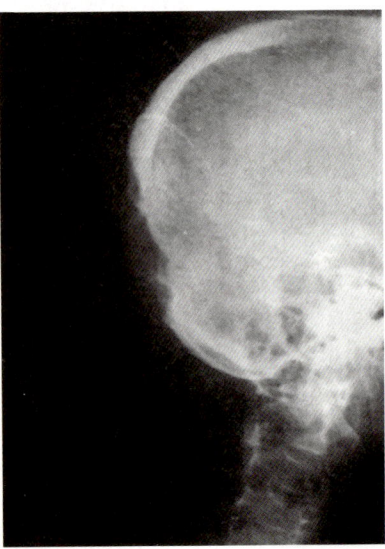

Fig. 30.14: X-ray lateral view of the skull showing a large swelling with erosion in the pericranium

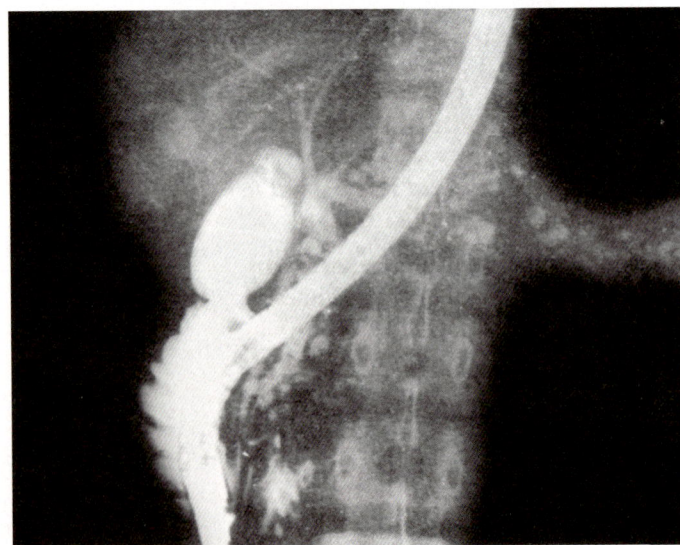

Fig. 30.15: Endoscopic retrograde cholangiopancreatography (ERCP) showing the biliary and pancreatic systems

4. Why is ERCP done in this patient?

- To know whether the pancreatic duct is dilated or not.

5. If pancreatic duct is dilated more than 6 to 8 mm in a patient with severe abdominal pain with chronic pancreatitis, what is the treatment?

- Longitudinal pancreaticojejunostomy—Puestow's operation. In this operation, pancreatic duct is laid open, strictures are divided and the duct is anastomosed to jejunum.

XVI. T-tube Cholangiography showing a Filling Defect in the Lower End of the Common Bile Duct (CBD) (Fig. 30.16)

1. What is the diagnosis?

- Postcholecystectomy—residual stone in the CBD

2. What is the surgery done for this patient?

- Cholecystectomy and choledocholithotomy

3. Why do you insert a T-tube after CBD exploration?

- In case of distal obstruction by a residual stone, the bile starts leaking from the suture line on the CBD and may result in biliary peritonitis. In such situations, T-tube helps in drainage of the bile.

4. What material is T-tube made of?

- Latex

5. How do you treat this patient in order to extract the stone?

- Endoscopic sphincterotomy and extraction of the stone.

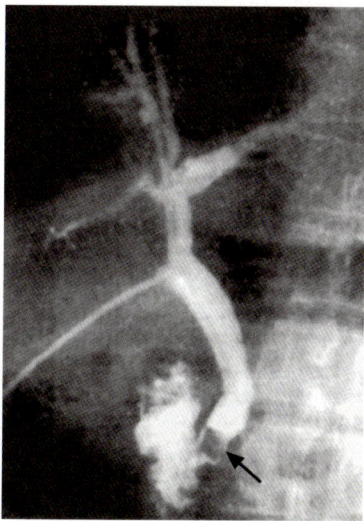

Fig. 30.16: T-tube cholangiography showing a filling defect in the lower end of the common bile duct (CBD)

XVII. Splenoportovenography (SPV) showing Extensive Collaterals in the Region of Spleen (Fig. 30.17)

1. What is the diagnosis?

- Portal hypertension

2. What is the type of portal hypertension?

- Hepatic type

3. Why do you say so?

- Splenic vein, portal vein and its branches within the liver are visualised.

4. What is the probable cause in this patient?

- Cirrhosis of the liver

5. What is the first line of specific treatment for bleeding oesophageal varices?

- Endoscopic banding/sclerotherapy
- Banding is costly and needs more expertise
- Sclerotherapy can be perivariceal or intravariceal—injection of 2% solution of sodium tetradecyl sulphate.
- Sclerotherapy is given at multiple sites and in multiple sittings.

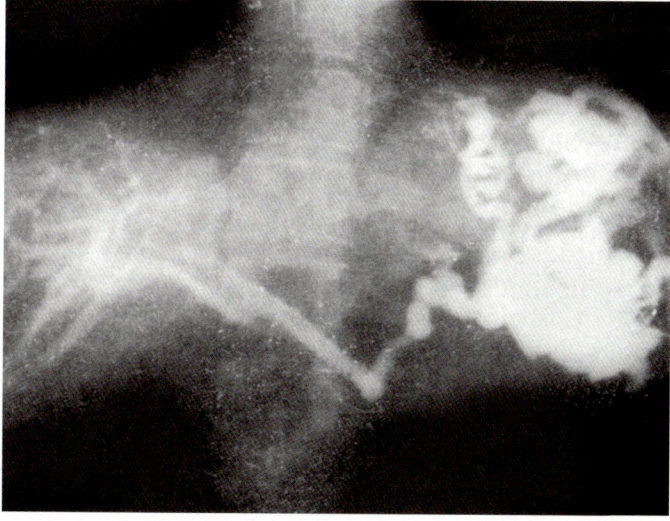

Fig. 30.17: Splenoportovenography (SPV) showing extensive collaterals in the region of spleen

XVIII. Retrograde Angiography showing Occlusion of Femoral Artery on the Left Side (Fig. 30.18)

1. What is the technique employed in this angiography?

- Seldinger's technique—percutaneous, transfemoral, retrograde.

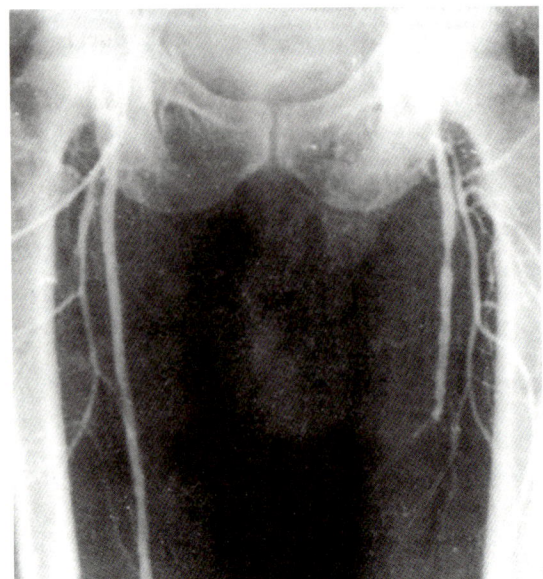

Fig. 30.18: Retrograde angiography showing occlusion of femoral artery on the left side

2. What is the probable cause in our country?

• Buerger's disease (thromboangiitis obliterans).

3. Why do you say so?

• Buerger's disease affects medium-sized vessels and narrowing of femoral artery is segmental in this radiograph.

4. What is the surgical treatment for Buerger's disease?

• Lumbar sympathectomy

5. How does lumbar sympathectomy help these patients?

• By reducing the sympathetic tone of the lower limb, arterioles and capillaries get dilated allowing cutaneous ulcers to heal.

XIX. Contrast-enhanced (CE) CT Abdomen showing Mass in the Right Iliac Fossa (Fig. 30.19)

1. What is this investigation?

• Contrast-enhanced CT scan

2. How to interpret the CT scan?

• Structures imaged appear as densely white or black.

3. What is the name used to the picture in terms of number of units?

• Hounsfield units

4. Why do you give contrast?

• This is to increase the density between various structures. Example: Aorta appears bright with contrast.

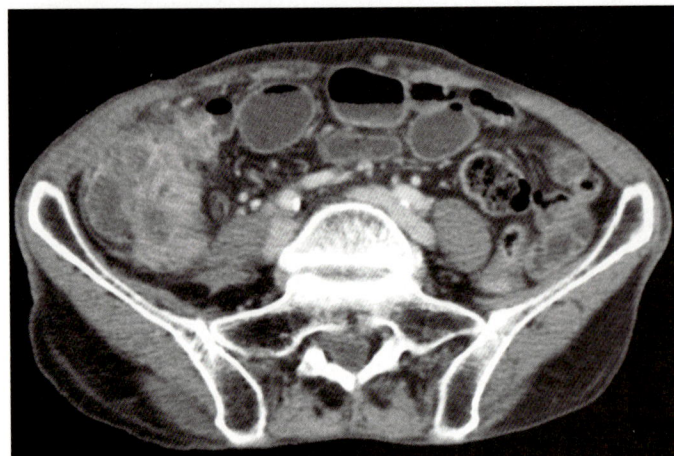

Fig. 30.19: A hypodense mass in the right iliac fossa involving caecum

5. What are the precautions?

• Pregnancy is a contraindication. Iodine containing contrast can give rise to nephropathy. Allergy to contrast can happen. Hence, dehydration should be corrected. Serum creatinine should be checked before contrast.

6. When do you use oral contrast?

• While studying abdominal viscera, e.g. if leak is suspected.

7. What is the finding here?

• It is showing a hypodense lesion in the right iliac fossa.

8. What is the diagnosis?

• Mostly carcinoma caecum

9. Why do you say so?

• Anatomically, it is a lesion occupying the right iliac fossa involving caecum.

10. How do you describe this?

• It is a hypodense mass with solid and cystic areas. Cystic areas represent tumour degeneration.

11. What else is seen in this picture?

• Fat planes between the mass and the abdominal wall is obliterated.

12. What is the importance of that?

• Probably, it is infiltrating the abdominal wall.

13. Why do you want to know this information?

• At surgery, the involved portion of the abdominal wall has to be removed.

14. How do you confirm the diagnosis?

- Colonoscopy and biopsy

15. What will be the report expected?

- In majority of the cases, it is adenocarcinoma.

16. What is the treatment, if it is operable?

- Right radical hemicolectomy

17. If it is inoperable, what is the treatment?

- Palliative ileotransverse anastomosis.

XX. Positron Emission Tomography (PET) Scan (Fig. 30.20)

1. Name this investigation.

- PET-CT scan

2. What is PET scan?

- Positron emission tomography

3. What is the most commonly used positron emitting radionuclide?

- Fluorodeoxyglucose (FDG)

4. What are the chief uses of PET scan?

- For myocardial perfusion and viability, detection of metastasis from cancer—carcinoma lung, colon, nasopharynx, etc.

5. What are the disadvantages?

- Very expensive and limited availability

6. What does this picture show?

- Hilar mass with a nodule anteriorly on the left side of pleura.

7. What may be the diagnosis?

- Carcinoma lung

8. How do you confirm the diagnosis?

- Bronchoscopy and biopsy

9. If the report is adenocarcinoma lung, what is the next step?

- To stage the disease by whole body bone scan, PET scan, and CT scan.

10. If confined to lung, what is the treatment?

- Lobectomy/pneumonectomy

XXI. MRI of the Thigh (Fig. 30.21)

1. Name this investigation.

- Magnetic resonance imaging.

2. What are the principles of MRI?

- Certain atomic nuclei, which possess unpaired protons or neutrons, possess an inherent spin. The nucleus is positively charged and, therefore, creates a small magnetic field around itself, when it spins. The human body contains in abundance such spinning nuclei in the atoms of hydrogen, which is found in water and lipids.

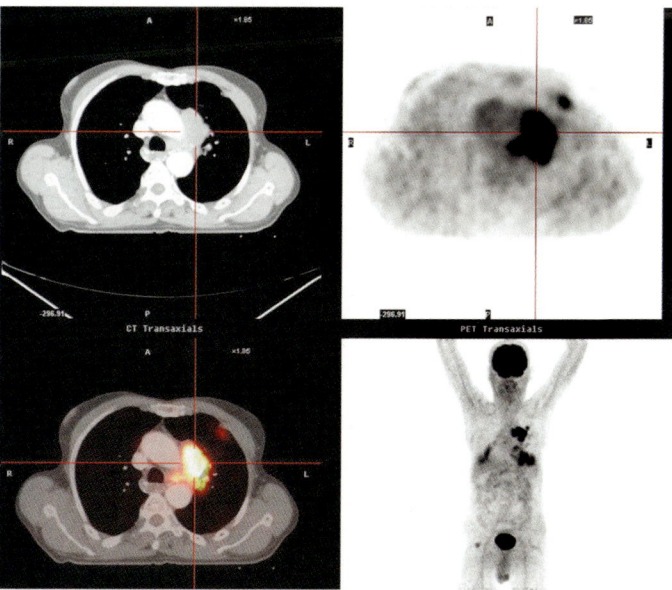

Fig. 30.20: CT and PET of lung: PET-CT of a patient who was diagnosed to have carcinoma lung on bronchoscopy. PET-CT shows a hilar mass with a nodule anteriorly on left side of pleura. It also shows pneumonic patch on lower zone of left lung which is FDG avid

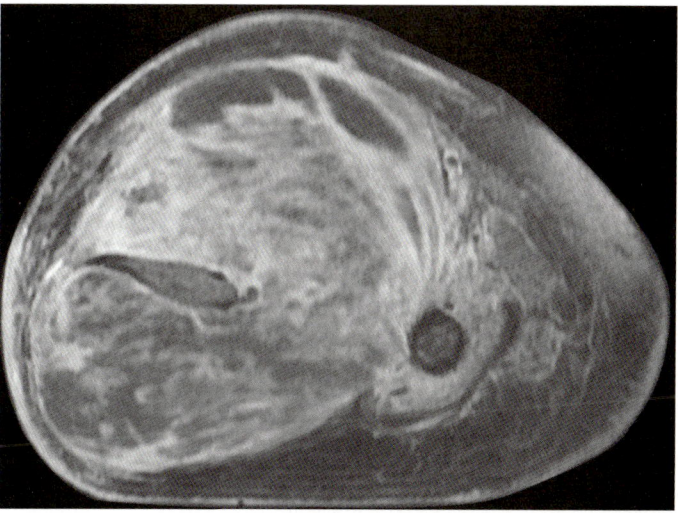

Fig. 30.21: MRI of the thigh

3. What are the chief advantages of MRI over CT scan?

- It is noninvasive and does not involve the use of ionising radiation. Hence, it is safe.

4. What are the disadvantages of MRI?

- The imaging time is long. Hence, movement of the patients may produce artefacts.
- Expensive
- Patients with pacemakers, metallic implant and critically ill patients cannot be scanned.
- Claustrophobia

5. What does this picture show?

- A hyperintense mass occupying the thigh region.

6. What is the diagnosis?

- Soft tissue sarcoma

7. How do you confirm the diagnosis?

- Tru-cut biopsy

8. Why not FNAC?

- FNAC cannot diagnose the type of sarcoma

9. What are common tumours in this location?

- Malignant fibrous histiocytoma (MFH) and lipo-sarcoma.

10. What is the treatment?

- Wide excision with 2–3 cm margin

Please note: X-rays discussed here are the common X-rays which are asked in the MBBS examination. However, modern investigations such as mammogram, ultrasound, CT scan and MRI also may be asked. You are requested to read the chapters on radiology and breast for more details about these investigations in 'Manipal Manual of Surgery'.

INSTRUMENTS

Artery Forceps (Haemostat)

- It is also called **Spencer Well's artery forceps**. It has a ratchet and two blades with uniform serrations.
- It is used to control bleeding, not only from arteries but also from veins and capillaries. Once the bleeding points are caught, they are coagulated or ligature is applied.
- The curved artery is commonly used (Fig. 30.22A).
- The smaller version of this is called mosquito forceps (Fig. 30.22B). This is extremely useful in repair of harelip, cleft palate or other plastic surgery operations.
- It is also available as straight artery forceps which is used to hold the stay sutures (Fig. 30.22C).

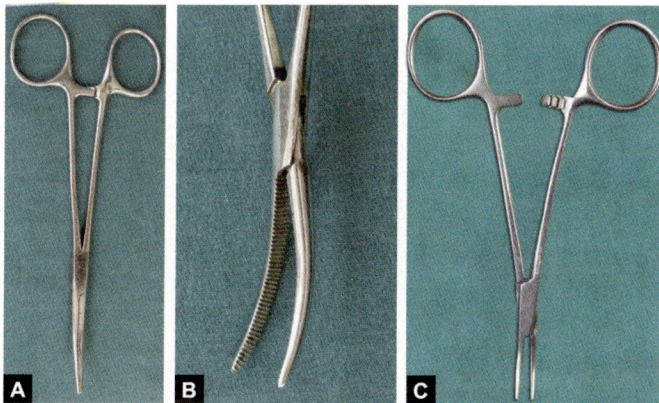

Figs 30.22A to C: (A) Mosquito forceps, (B) curved artery forceps, (C) straight artery forceps

Allis Tissue-holding Forceps (Fig. 30.23)

- It has a ratchet and triangular expansion at the tip, where serrations are present.
- It can be used to **hold tough structures** such as fascia, aponeurosis, etc.
- Even though it can cause trauma, because of its better grip, it can be used to hold the duodenum for duodenal closure during gastrectomy.

Kocher's Forceps (Fig. 30.24 and Clinical Box 30.1)

- This is similar to an artery forceps with serrations. It is available as curved and straight.
- There is a sharp tooth at the tip of the instrument. Hence, it has a better grip.
- Kocher's forceps can be used to **hold tough structures** such as **aponeurosis, fascia**, etc.

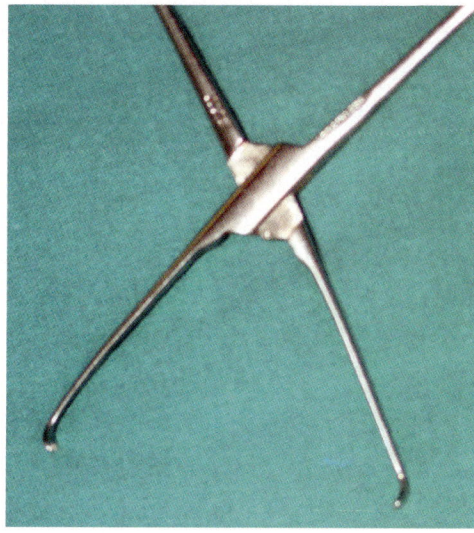

Fig. 30.23: Allis forceps

- During thyroidectomy, it can be used to hold the strap muscles for dividing them.
- Theodor Kocher, a German surgeon, got the Nobel prize for his contribution to thyroid surgery.

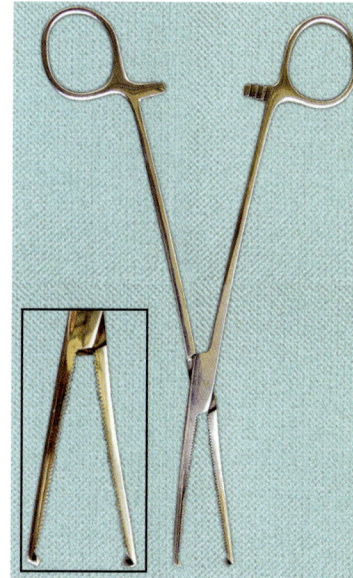

Fig. 30.24: Kocher's forceps

Clinical Box 30.1

Remember
- Kocher's forceps
- Kocher's test
- Kocher's thyroid dissector
- Kocher's vein
- Kocher's subcostal incision
- Kocher's gland-holding forceps

Sinus Forceps (Fig. 30.25)

- This is like an artery forceps which has no **ratchet**.

- Serrations are confined to the tip so as to hold the wall of an abscess cavity, for biopsy.

- In *Hilton's method* of drainage of an abscess, once the incision is made, the sinus forceps is thrust into the abscess cavity and by opening the blades in all directions, the loculi are broken. To facilitate free opening of the blades, sinus forceps has no ratchet.

Swab-holding Forceps (Fig. 30.26)

- This has a ratchet and two long blades.

- Operating end is rounded with serrations.

- It is used to hold the swab (gauze pieces) to prepare the parts with antiseptic agents at the time of surgery.

- This instrument can also be used as a blunt 'dissector' with the swab, while dissecting at a depth, e.g. lumbar sympathectomy, vagotomy.

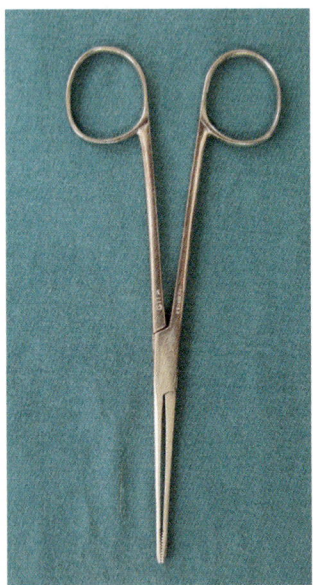

Fig. 30.25: Sinus forceps

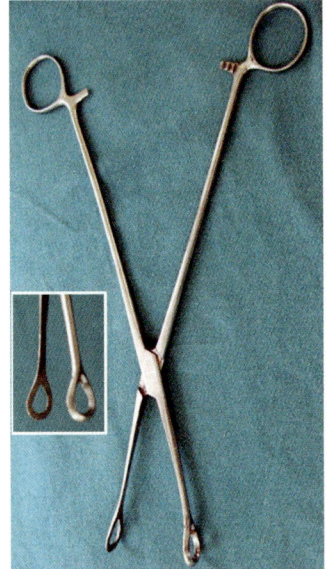

Fig. 30.26: Swab-holding forceps

Babcock's Forceps (Fig. 30.27)

- An instrument with a ratchet and a triangular expansion with fenestrations at the operating end. It does not have any teeth. Thus, it is used to hold intestines during anastomosis or resection.

- This instrument can also be used to hold many other structures such as thyroid gland, meso-appendix, uterine tubes, etc.

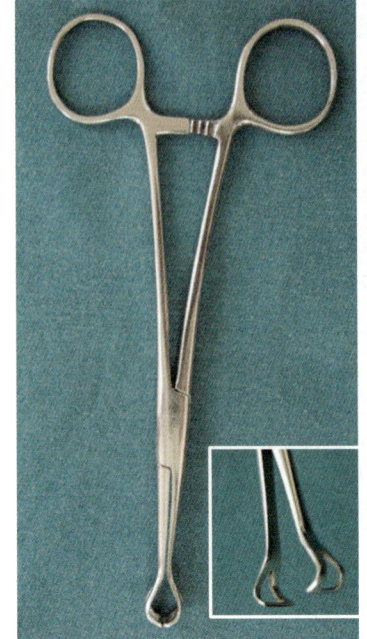

Fig. 30.27: Babcock's forceps

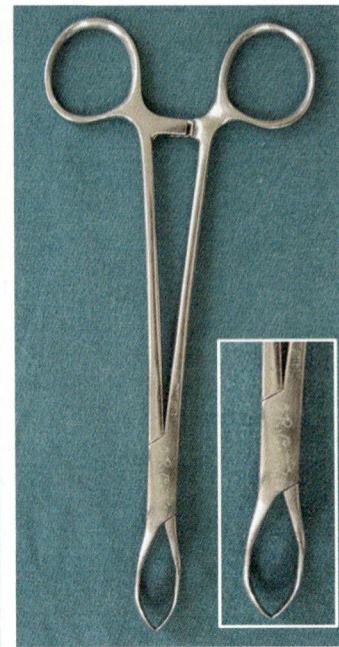

Fig. 30.28: Lane's forceps

Lane's Forceps (Fig. 30.28)

- This is similar to Babcock's forceps but the tip is more broad, expanded with a bigger opening.

- It is used to hold the appendix.

- However, it does not seem to have any additional advantage when compared to Babcock's forceps.

Dissecting Scissors

- This is also called **Mayo's scissors** (Clinical Box 30.2 and Fig. 30.29).

- It does not have ratchet and operating end is sharp.

- This is used to dissect tissue planes during surgical operations and to cut or divide important structures.

- It is popularly called **tissue scissors**.

Clinical Box 30.2

Remember
- Mayo's scissors
- Mayo's herniorrhaphy
- Mayo's posterior GJ
- Mayo's vein
- Mayo's needle (used for hernia repair)

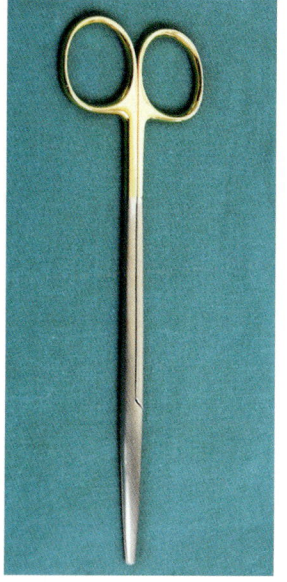

Fig. 30.29: Mayo's scissors

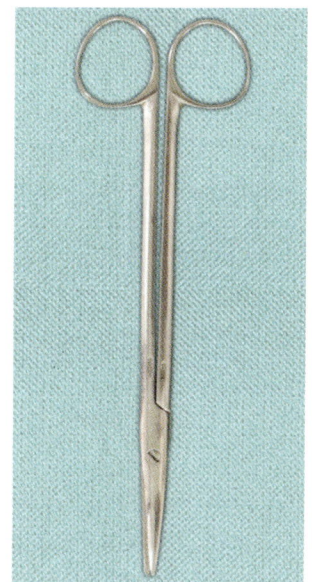

Fig. 30.30: Straight scissors

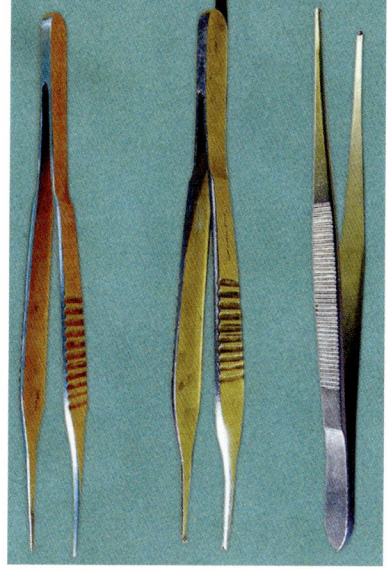

Fig. 30.31: Dissecting forceps

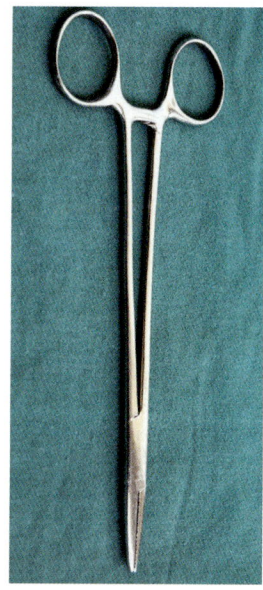

Fig. 30.32: Needle holder

Straight Scissors (Fig. 30.30)

It is used to cut the sutures or knots. Hence, called suture-cutting scissors.

Dissecting Forceps (Fig. 30.31)

- This is a toothed forceps. It is also available as non-toothed forceps.
- Dissecting forceps with dissecting scissors makes good 'tool' for a surgeon to develop a tissue plane in majority of surgeries.
- The forceps is very useful to 'pick' individual layers such as serosa, seromuscular layers, mucosa, etc. during anastomosis.

Needle Holder (Fig. 30.32)

- This is a long instrument with a ratchet at non-operating end.
- The operating end has two small blades with serrations.
- The instrument is used to **hold the curved needles** which are used to suture the parts.
- A firm grip is essential to apply proper sutures.

Scalpel with Blade (Fig. 30.33)

- This is popularly called **surgeon's knife.**
- This is used to incise the skin and subcutaneous tissue.
- Due to the sharp nature, it can be used to divide a major vascular pedicle once ligatures are applied.

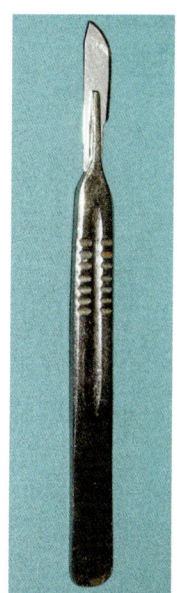

Fig. 30.33: Scalpel with blade

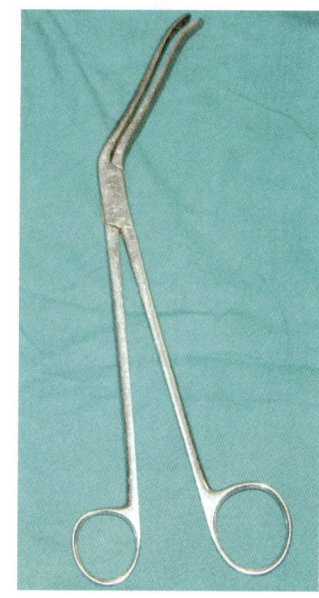

Fig. 30.34: Cheatles forceps

Cheatles Forceps (Fig. 30.34)

- It is a long instrument having a curved shaft.
- The **handle has no lock.**
- It is kept dipped in antiseptic solutions.
- This instrument is used to pick up sterilised articles such as sponges, gauze pieces or other instruments and to transfer to the instrument trolley.

Deaver Retractor (Fig. 30.35)

- This is popularly called **Deaver liver retractor.**
- It has a long blade and operating end is curved.

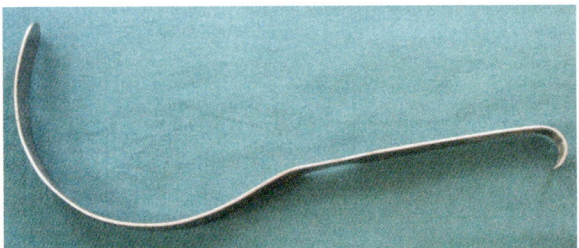

Fig. 30.35: Deaver retractor

- It can be used to retract the liver during vagotomy, cholecystectomy or gastrectomy, etc.
- Since it has long blades, it can be used to retract the kidney upwards, during lumbar sympathectomy or to retract the urinary bladder during surgery on the rectum.

Morris Retractor (Fig. 30.36)

- This is a long instrument with broad operating end.
- This is used **to retract the abdominal wall**, once the peritoneum is opened.
- However, if a self-retaining retractor is used to widen the laparotomy wound, the use of Morris retractor gets limited.

Czerny Retractor (Fig. 30.37)

- This is a double-hooked retractor on one side and a single blade on the other side.
- This is a **superficial retractor**, can be used to retract layers of the abdominal wall, muscles, etc. Thus, during appendicectomy, herniorrhaphy or thyroidectomy, this instrument is very useful.

Langenbeck Retractor (Fig. 30.38)

- This instrument has only **one blade.**
- The uses of this are similar to that of Czerny's retractor.

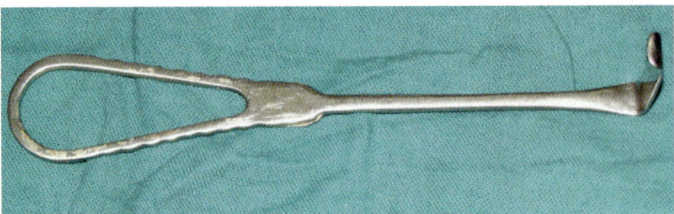

Fig. 30.38: Langenbeck retractor

Moynihan's Straight Occlusion Clamp (Fig. 30.39)

- This is a long instrument with a ratchet. The operating end has two long blades with serrations in the line of blades.
- This instrument is used to **occlude the intestinal lumen** to prevent spillage of intestinal contents during intestinal resection or intestinal anastomosis.
- This does not interfere with the vascularity of the intestine.

Payr's Crushing Clamp (Fig. 30.40)

- This is a heavy instrument with **double lever system**, because of which it has a better grip.
- The two short blades have uniform serrations.
- During gastrectomy, when portion of the stomach is excised, this instrument is applied on the stomach

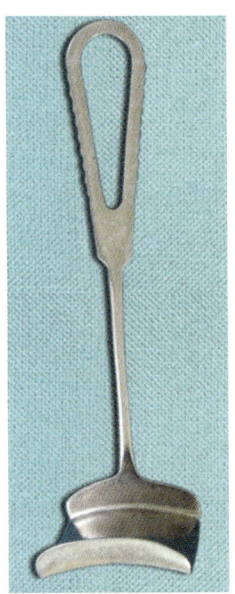 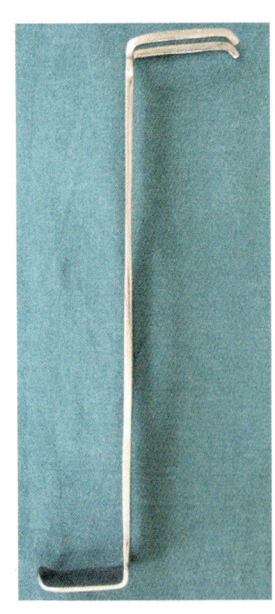 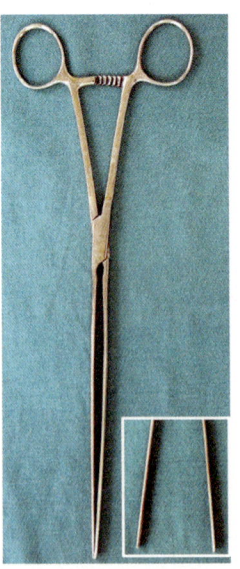 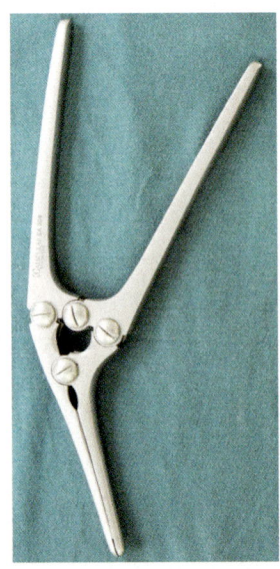

Fig. 30.36: Morris retractor   **Fig. 30.37:** Czerny retractor   **Fig. 30.39:** Moynihan's occlusion clamp   **Fig. 30.40:** Payr's crushing clamp

side so that the stomach with this instrument is excised.

Desjardin's Choledocholithotomy Forceps (Fig. 30.41)

- This is a long curved instrument with no **ratchet.**
- The operating end is expanded with fenestrations.
- The tip is blunt.
- It is used to **extract stones from common bile duct**. It can also be used to extract stones from the ureter.
- Since there is no ratchet, free opening is possible, and the stones do not get crushed.

Bake's Dilator (Fig. 30.42)

- This is a long malleable instrument available in various diameters.
- It has a handle, long body and the tip is blunt.
- Once common bile duct exploration is completed, this dilator is passed, to assess for any distal obstruction.
- The free passage of Bake's dilators of different sizes indicates that there is no distal obstruction (however, to be confirmed by cholangiogram).

Kocher's Thyroid Dissector (Fig. 30.43)

- This has a long handle and the operating end is small and blunt with an opening.
- A few longitudinal serrations are present at the tip.
- This was used to dissect the upper pole of thyroid gland.

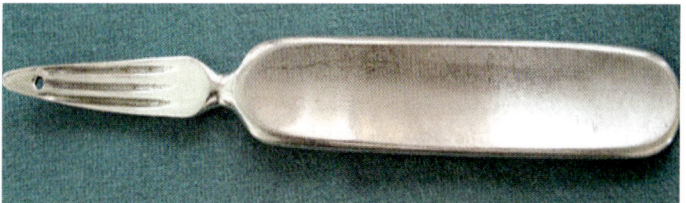

Fig. 30.43: Kocher's thyroid dissector

- This instrument can also be used to dissect the isthmus of the thyroid gland from the trachea.
- **Silk thread can be fed** into the opening so as to ligate the vascular pedicle or isthmus.
- With the availability of the right-angled forceps, this instrument is not in routine use nowadays.

Aneurysm Needle (Fig. 30.44)

- It is a long instrument with an *eye* at the operating end.
- It is called aneurysm needle because it was used to ligate the feeding artery in an aneurysm. However, today, this instrument is of limited use.
- During **venesection or cut down**, the silk suture can be threaded within the *eye*, passed round the vein and it is tied.

Trocar and Cannula (Fig. 30.45)

- This has two parts. The inner sharp part is the trocar and outer blunt part is cannula.
- It is used to drain hydrocoele fluid.

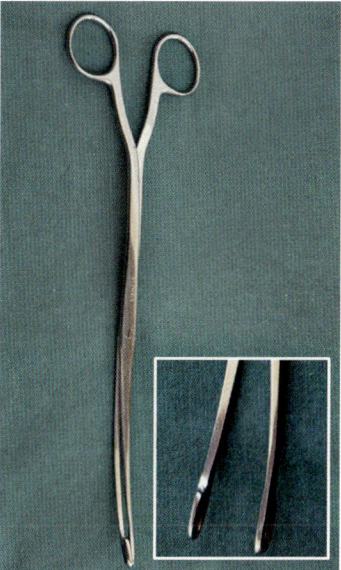

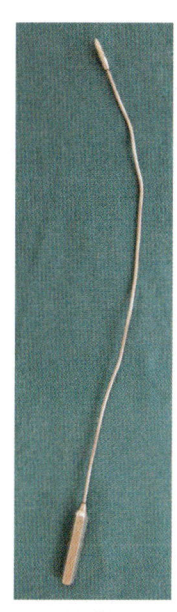

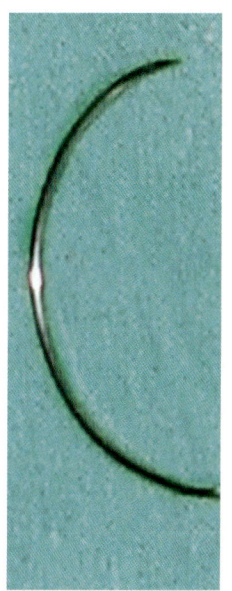

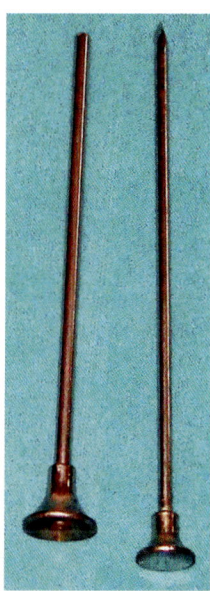

Fig. 30.41: Desjardin's forceps **Fig. 30.42:** Bake's dilator **Fig. 30.44:** Aneurysm needle **Fig. 30.45:** Trocar and cannula

- Once hydrocoele sac is delivered, it is punctured with trocar and cannula, the trocar removed and the fluid drained.

- Make sure that trocar and cannula should match, otherwise injury to the deeper structures (testis) can occur.

Humby's Knife (Fig. 30.46)

- This instrument has a handle and a long sheath.

- When in use, a disposable blade can be attached to it.

- The instrument is used to take skin graft. Hence, it is also called skin grafting knife.

- To facilitate the exact thickness of the skin to be removed, there is a screw at the operating end, with which, prior adjustment should be done.

Myer's Metal Stripper (Fig. 30.47)

- This is a long metallic chain or a stripper used in varicose vein surgery.

- It has a handle which is T-shaped and the 'advancing' end which enters the vein. This is blunt. Once this end comes out of the cut end of the vein, a medium-sized head is connected to it.

- With gentle force (traction) exerted on the handle, the varicose vein can be stripped.

- Hence, it is also called vein stripper.

Self-retaining Retractor (Fig. 30.48)

- It is a strong, heavy instrument, with two blades.

- This is used to spread the laparotomy wound. Hence, it is called self-retaining retractor.

Rib Spreader (Fig. 30.49)

- This is also a strong heavy instrument with two long blades.

- Once an incision is deepened through the intercostal spaces and the pleura is opened, the rib spreader is used and by rotating the latch handle, the ribs are spread apart.

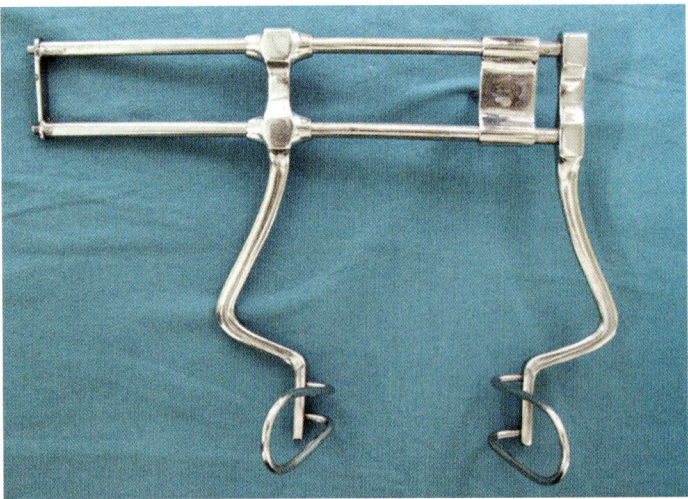

Fig. 30.48: Self-retaining retractor

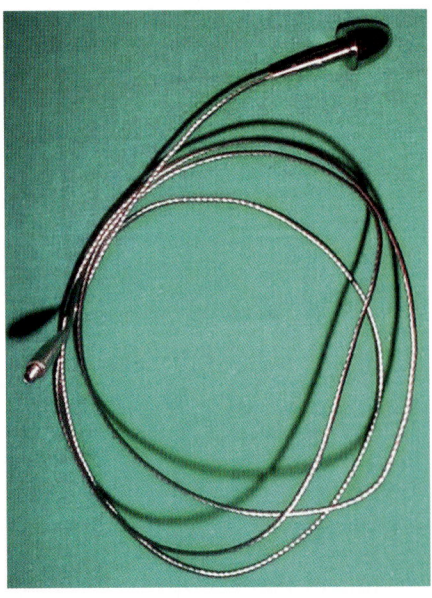

Fig. 30.46: Humby's knife   **Fig. 30.47:** Myer's metal stripper

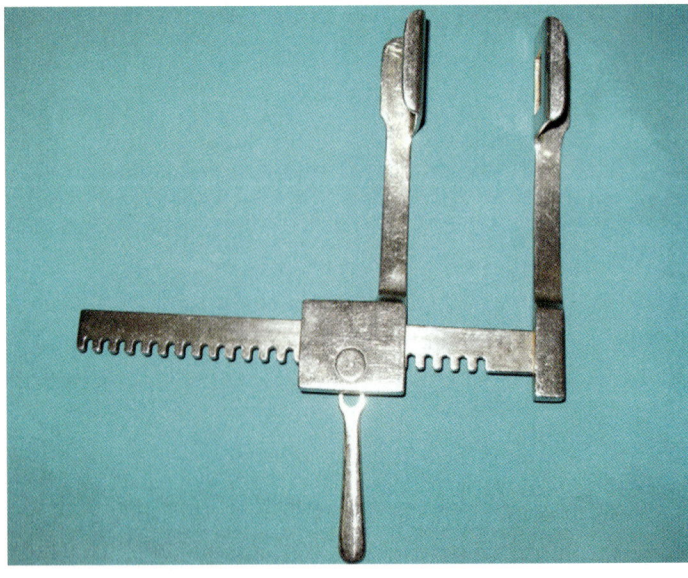

Fig. 30.49: Rib spreader

Proctoscope (Figs 30.50)

- This is an instrument used to visualise the rectum and the anal canal.
- It has an outer sheath with the handle (Fig. 30.50A).
- An inner blunt part is called obturator (Fig. 30.50B).

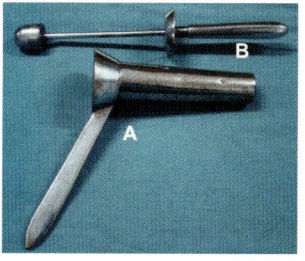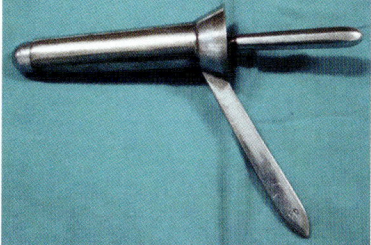

Fig. 30.50: Proctoscope

- Before introducing the proctoscope, one must make sure that obturator and the outer sheath must match. Lubricate the instrument well before introducing.
- In painful conditions, such as fissure in ano, proctoscopy is contraindicated.
- Once rectal examination is done, proctoscope is held firmly with the left hand (buttocks separated), the obturator is supported by the right hand. The instrument is slowly introduced inside. The obturator is removed and rectum is visualised using light source.
- Proctoscope is used to diagnose haemorrhoids, carcinoma rectum or rectal ulcers, etc. Biopsy can be taken with a biopsy forceps in nonhealing ulcers of the rectum. Haemorrhoids can be injected and pelvic abscess can be drained into the rectum with the help of a proctoscope.

Lister's Metal Dilator (Lister's Bougie)

- This is a long instrument curved at the tip. Its diameter is written near the handle. It is available in various diameters. The difference between the two numbers is 3. The maximum size of the Lister's dilator is 9/12 (Fig. 30.51).

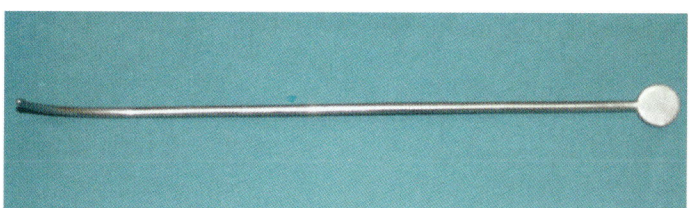

Fig. 30.51: Lister's dilator

- The tip is olive-pointed and the end of the handle is round. The minimum and maximum diameter of the instrument is written on the handle. The other type of bougie is Glutton's bougie with a plain tip and the end of the handle is trapezoid. The maximum size of Glutton's bougie is 24/28 and difference between the two numbers is 4.

Male Metallic Catheter (Fig. 30.52A)

- These catheters are used to drain urine in cases of retention of urine when rubber catheter fails.
- It is a long instrument which is curved because the male urethra is long and curved.
- It has two eyes at the distal end which are situated laterally and at different levels so that the instrument does not become weak at that spot.
- Once the urine is drained, the catheter can be left in place by passing a thread through the two rings present at the proximal end and fixing them to patient's thigh.
- Due to the fear of false passage, injury to the urethra and introducing infection, this catheter is not used nowadays. It is replaced by trocar suprapubic cystostomy.

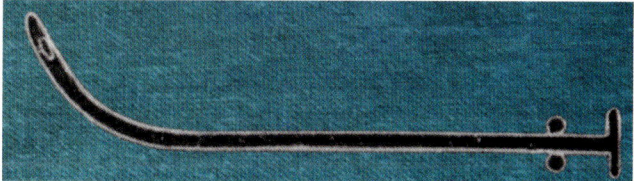

Fig. 30.52A: Male metallic catheter

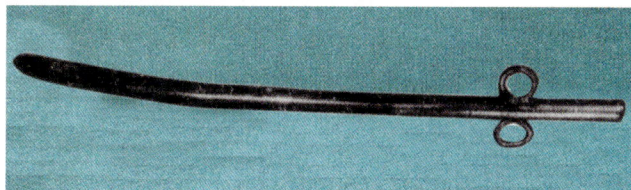

Fig. 30.52B: Female metallic catheter

Female Metallic Catheter (Fig. 30.52B)

- Used to drain urine in females.
- This is a short and straight instrument because the urethra is short and straight in females.
- It has multiple holes at the tip.
- Indications for usage of this catheter are very rare because acute retention of urine is rare in females and even if it occurs, a red rubber catheter can be passed.

- It is used to empty bladder before vaginal hysterectomy and other gynaecologic surgeries.
- Emptying the bladder is mandatory before any gynaecological examination of a patient.

Towel Clip (Fig. 30.53)

- This instrument has a ratchet and the operating end is sharp.
- This is available in different sizes.
- Once the part is cleaned and draped, the clips are used to hold the towels in place.

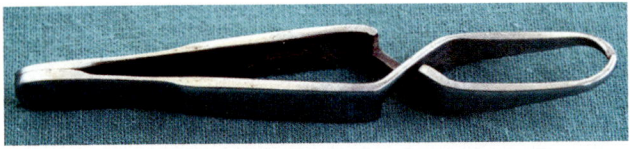

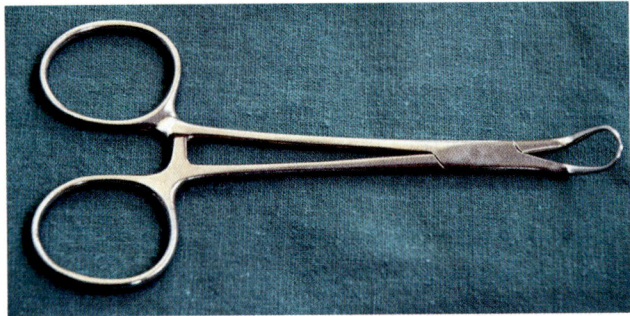

Fig. 30.53: Towel clip

Right-angled Forceps (Lahey's Forceps)

- This is a long instrument with right angle at the operating end (Fig. 30.54).

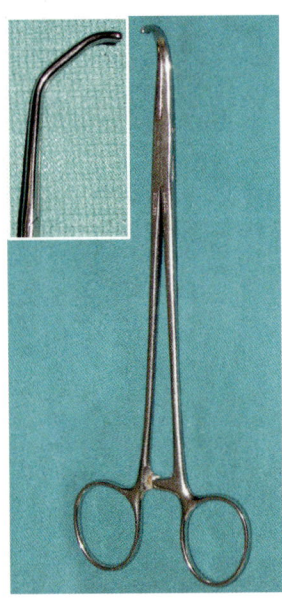

Fig. 30.54: Right-angled forceps

- This instrument is extremely useful in **ligating the major vascular pedicles**, e.g. superior thyroid pedicle—thyroidectomy.
- Cystic artery: Cholecystectomy.
- Lumbar veins: Lumbar sympathectomy.

Hudson's Brace and the Burr (Fig. 30.55)

- This is a heavy instrument with a brace and the burr (drill).
- This is used to create **openings into the cranium** so as to get an access to the structures within.
- Thus, once a 'burr' is made, drainage of blood, fluid or pus can be done.

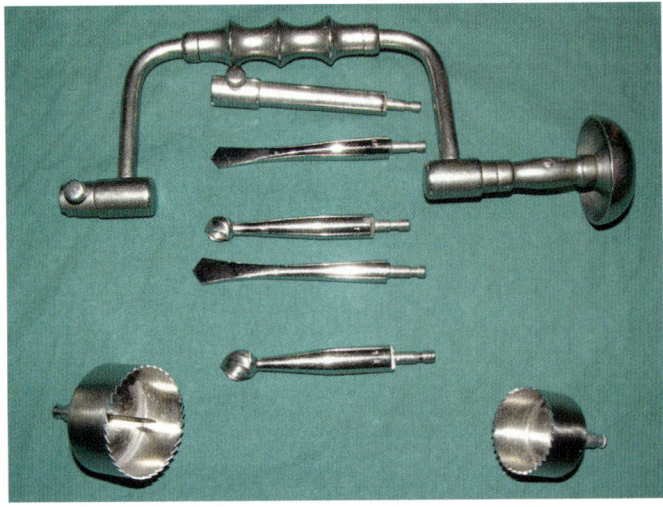

Fig. 30.55: Hudson's brace and the burr

Cricoid Hook (Fig. 30.56)

- This has a broad handle and a thin shaft with a hook at the operating end.
- This is used to stabilise the trachea by hooking the cricoid cartilage 'up'.
- This step is essential in children wherein veins are very superficial and can get injured easily when child moves the head and neck. By stabilising the trachea, it is easy to incise the trachea, without injuring the vessels.

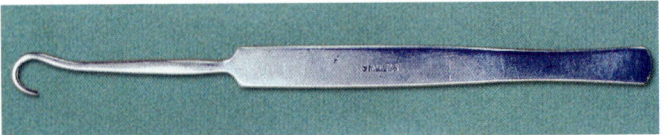

Fig. 30.56: Cricoid hook

Tracheal Dilator (Fig. 30.57)

- This is an instrument with **no ratchet at** the nonoperating end.
- The operating end is blunt and curved.
- The peculiarity of this instrument is that **when the handle is opened, operating end is closed** and **when the handle is closed, operating end is opened**.
- Tracheal dilator is used in the **post-tracheostomy period**, when the tube has to be changed due to blockage. In such situations, once the tube is removed, tracheal dilator is introduced, the opening in trachea is kept open, and the new tube is introduced. However, once the track is formed, tracheal dilator need not be used.

Fergusson's Amputation Saw (Fig. 30.58)

Amputation saw has teeth on its cutting edge to facilitate cutting through the bone and is of different sizes. They are manufactured with one- or two-sided cutting edge for limb amputations.

Uses: In lower limb, amputations commonly—above knee (AK) amputation and below knee (BK) amputation.

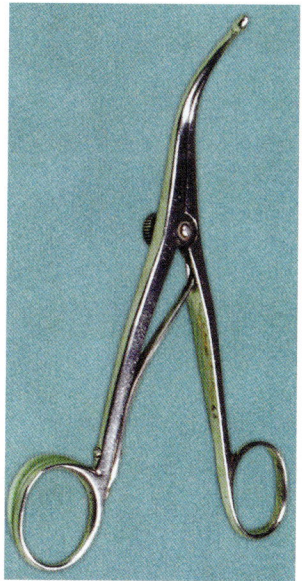
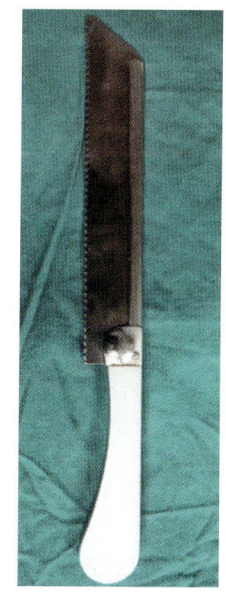

Fig. 30.57: Tracheal dilator   **Fig. 30.58:** Fergusson's amputation saw

Bone Nibbler (Fig. 30.59)

It is also called double action bone nibbler, identified by long handle and small jaws, top jaw is used for cutting and lower jaw is used to hold the tissue firmly.

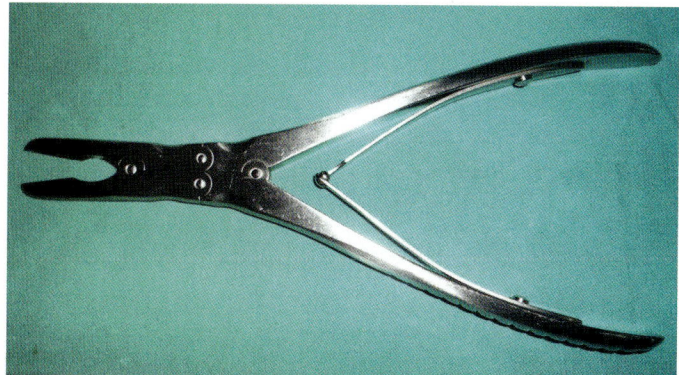

Fig. 30.59: Bone nibbler

Uses: To make cut end of the bone smooth after amputation, rib cutting and to enlarge burr hole.

Bone File/Raspatory (Fig. 30.60)

One side of the raspatory is used to hold as a handle, while its other side has sharp projections with both fine and coarse teeth on both sides with a flat blade.

Uses: Blunt separation of the periosteum and connective tissue from the surface of the bone, smoothening of sharp bony edges after amputation and before fixing fractures.

Volkmann Curette (Fig. 30.61)

The edges of the distal spoon-shaped part of this instrument are sharp which make it possible to remove the tissues.

Uses: Scoop the granulation tissue, to clean the base of the infected wound, and to remove the infected bone in the case of osteomyelitis.

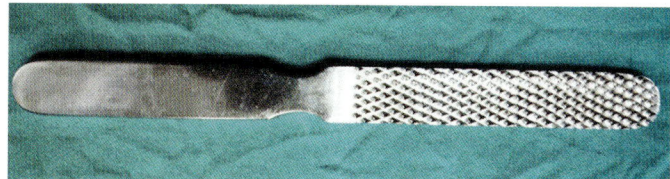

Fig. 30.60: Bone file

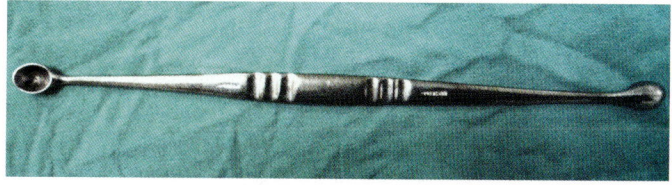

Fig. 30.61: Curette

DeBakey Forceps (Bayonet Style) (Fig. 30.62)

They are typically large—some examples are upwards of 12 inches (36 cm) long, and have a distinct coarsely ribbed grip panel, as opposed to the finer ribbing on most other tissue forceps, a type of atraumatic tissue forceps.

Uses: In vascular procedures to avoid tissue damage during manipulation. Less traumatic manipulation of tissue and used during suturing.

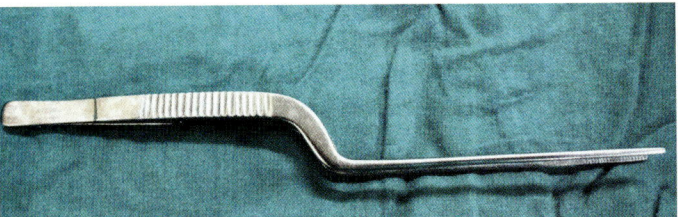

Fig. 30.62: DeBakey forceps

Beckman-Adson Laminectomy Retractor (Fig. 30.63)

It has hinged blades with 4 × 4 prongs, an adjustable swivel arms and a ratchet to hold tissue apart.

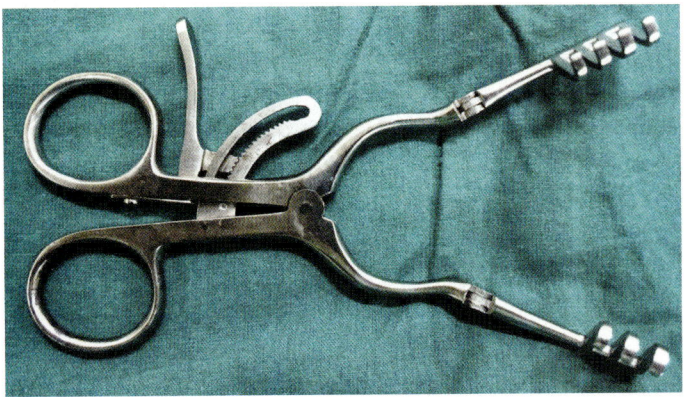

Fig. 30.63: Beckman-Adson laminectomy retractor

Uses: Retraction in procedures involving deep tissues like in laminectomy for spinal surgeries.

Ribbon-Malleable Retractor (Fig. 30.64)

A malleable or ribbon retractor (manual) may be bent to various shapes.

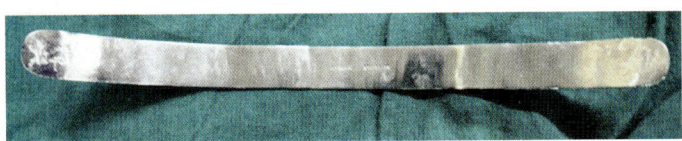

Fig. 30.64: Malleable retractor

Uses: It is used at the end of the case to keep the viscera away during the fascial closure and is also used to retract deep wounds.

The Harmonic Scalpel (Fig. 30.65)

The harmonic scalpel is a new device that has been introduced to surgery during the last decade. It is a device that uses high-frequency mechanical energy to cut and coagulate tissues at the same time.

It uses ultrasound technology to cut tissues while simultaneously sealing the edges of the cut.

Active tips of the harmonic scalpel employ a rigid active lower blade through which the vibrating energy is transmitted. The movable upper jaw is used to compress the vessel against the lower blade, thus allowing transfer of the vibrational energy.

The instrument is similar to an electrosurgery instrument and can be used in all open and laparoscopic surgeries, but superior in that it can cut through thicker tissue, creates less toxic surgical smoke and may offer greater precision especially during a laparoscopic surgery.

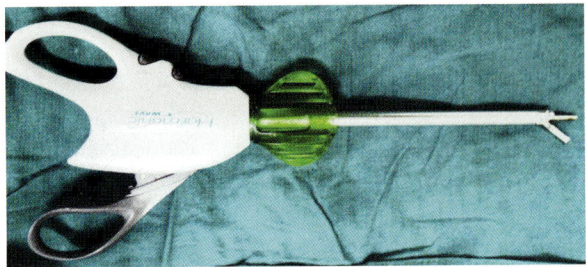

Fig. 30.65: Harmonic scalpel

Bipolar Cautery (Fig. 30.66)

When the electric current is passing between the two parts of the instrument, we call it the bipolar diathermy/cautery (e.g. bipolar forceps).

It makes possible to perform a more precise work and the size of the burned area is small and is more useful when haemostasis is required close to the nerves.

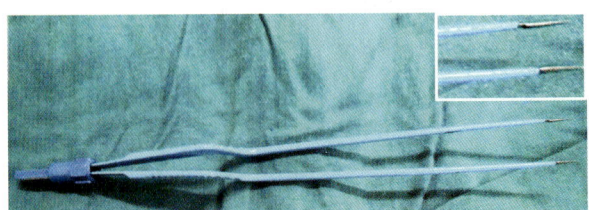

Fig. 30.66: Bipolar cautery

Uses: Thyroid surgery when close to RLN (recurrent laryngeal nerve) neurosurgery or spinal surgeries.

Allison's Lung Retractor (Fig. 30.67)

It is retractor with a special type of blade, made of wires, in the form of a net over one end and a handle at the other end.

Uses: For retraction of the lung in thoracotomy. It does not damage the lungs and the lungs can expand in between the wires.

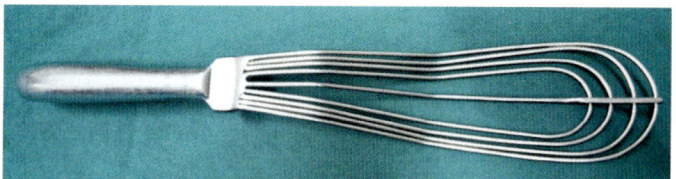

Fig. 30.67: Allison's lung retractor

Gigli Saw (Fig. 30.68)

Composed of a wire as a blade and two handles to hold the wire on either side.

Uses: It is commonly used bone cutting in amputation surgeries similar to amputation saw such as below knee and above knee amputations.

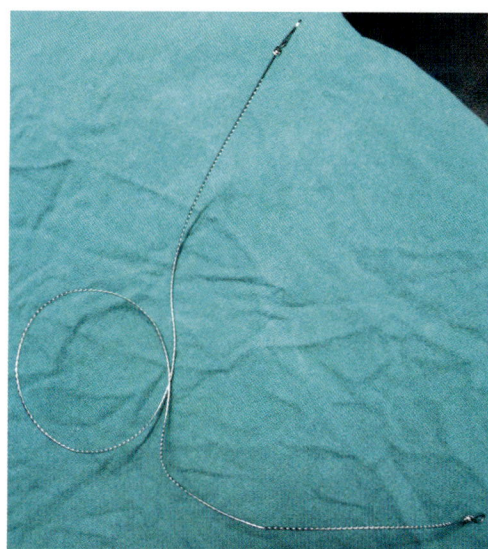

Fig. 30.68: Gigli saw

Joll's Thyroid Retractor (Fig. 30.69)

It is a self-retaining retractor, which is held by the two-towel clip-like forceps on both sides to hold the flaps and can be adjusted using a screw in between.

Uses: To retract skin flaps during thyroid surgery.

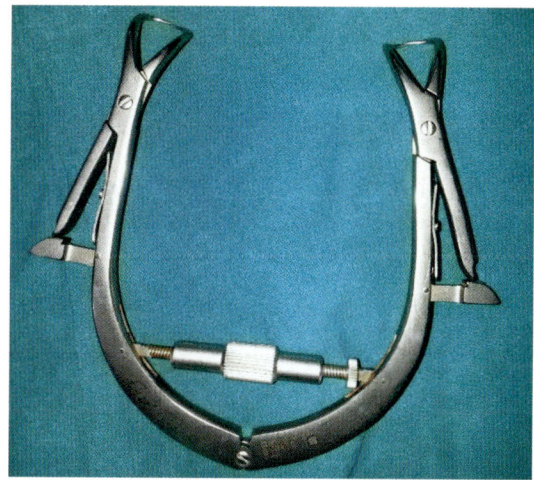

Fig. 30.69: Joll's retractor

Metal Tracheostomy Tube (Fig. 30.70)

- This has **two tubes**, the inner long and the outer short tube.
- This has no **cuff**.
- Once the tube is introduced, the tape is passed around the neck, passed through the opening and tied so as to keep the tube in place.
- If the tube is blocked, the inner tube can be removed, cleaned and reintroduced.
- Metal tracheostomy tubes are useful as permanent tracheostomy tube.

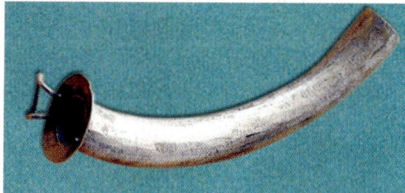

Fig. 30.70: Metal tracheostomy tube

Cuffed Tracheostomy Tube (Fig. 30.71)

- This is made of polyvinyl chloride. It is a **single tube**.

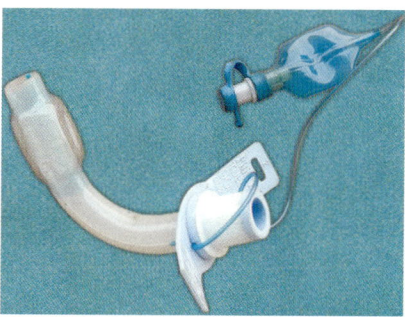

Fig. 30.71: Cuffed tracheostomy tube

- Once the tube is introduced within the trachea, the cuff is inflated by using 3–5 ml of air.
- The cuff prevents leakage of air and prevents **acid aspiration syndrome (Mendelson's syndrome)**.
- If this tube is blocked, it is an emergency. In such cases, the tube has to be cleaned and mucus plugs have to be removed. Otherwise, the tube is removed, the tracheal opening is kept open with the help of tracheal dilator and a new tube is introduced. Alternatively, endotracheal intubation may need to be done to ensure patency of the airway.

Corrugated Red Rubber Drain (Fig. 30.72)

- It is made of red rubber. It has corrugations on both sides. Whenever a major surgery is done, some amount of blood loss or anastomotic leakage is expected. This drain is used so that **fluid can escape freely outside**.
- Thus, it is used after thyroidectomy, gastrectomy, cholecystectomy, etc. The drain is removed after it stops draining. Usually, it takes about 3–5 days.
- After laparotomy for peritonitis, these drains are used to prevent residual abscess in the postoperative period.

Malecot's Catheter (Fig. 30.73)

This is made of red rubber. It has flower-shaped end and has a wide diameter. It is used to drain amoebic liver abscess. It is straightened with the help of an introducer and left in cavity and brought outside. It is a self-retaining catheter. This is used to drain urinary bladder after transvesical prostatectomy or can be used as feeding gastrostomy tube. It can also be used to drain empyema thoracis.

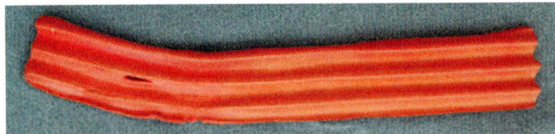

Fig. 30.72: Corrugated red rubber drain

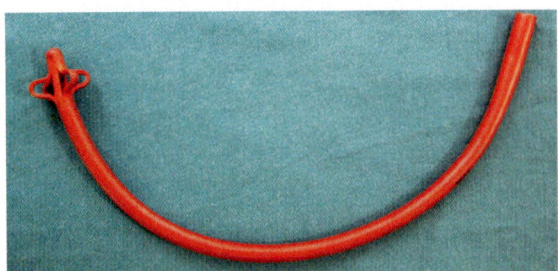

Fig. 30.73: Malecot's catheter

Mousseau-Barbin Tube (Fig. 30.74)

- This is also called MB tube. It is a funnel-shaped tube with Ryle's tube-like attachment. It is used in inoperable cases of carcinoma oesophagus to palliate dysphagia. It is stitched to the Ryle's tube which is brought out through the mouth and it is slowly drawn in by pulling the other end of Ryle's tube which is in the stomach, after doing a gastrostomy.
- Once the tube is below the level of growth, it is cut at a sufficient distance and is stitched to the stomach wall.
- With the availability of laser coagulation of the growth, and considering discomfort caused by the tube including its migration, the MB tube is not popular and not preferred.
- Self expanding metalic stents are popular nowadays.

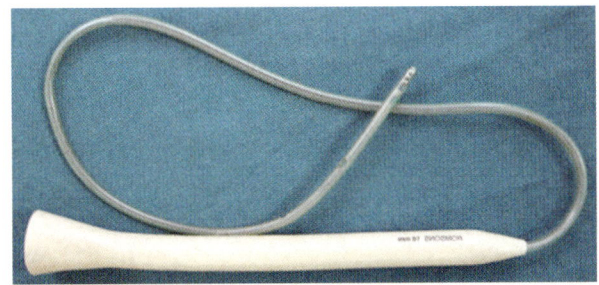

Fig. 30.74: Mousseau-Barbin tube

Foley's Self-retaining Urinary Catheter (Fig. 30.75)

- This is made of **latex with silicon coating**. At the tip, there is a bulb, capacity of which is written at the other end.
- Before inflating the bulb, one must make sure that **catheter is in the urinary bladder, not in the urethra**. This is assessed by free flow of urine.

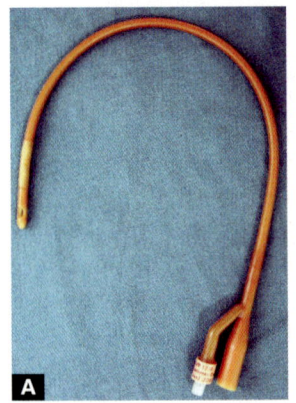 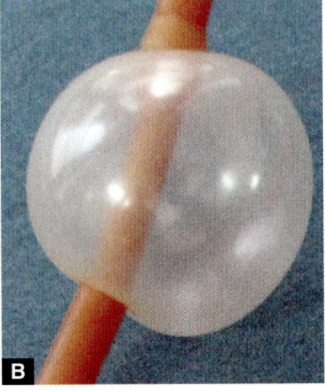

Fig. 30.75: (A) Foley catheter, (B) distended bulb

- After introducing the catheter, the bulb is inflated using saline. Thus, it becomes self-retaining. After the usage, it is removed by deflating the bulb. It can also be used to drain peritoneal cavity as in biliary peritonitis. Inflated bulb compresses the prostatic bed and controls bleeding after prostatectomy.

Red Rubber Catheter (Fig. 30.76)

This is used to drain urine temporarily. It causes urethritis, if it is left long in the urinary bladder. Once the urine is emptied, it is removed. It is not a self-retaining catheter. Not routinely used nowadays because of availability of Foley's catheter. It is more stiff than Foley catheter. Hence, **in cases of stricture urethra,** where **Foley's catheter cannot be passed, red rubber catheter may be used.**

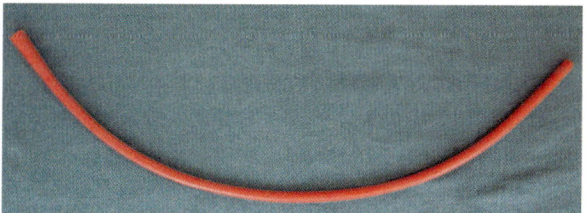

Fig. 30.76: Red rubber catheter

Nasogastric Tube/Ryle's Tube (Fig. 30.77)

- This is also called **nasogastric tube.** At the end of this tube, there are **lead shots.** After introducing within the stomach, its position is confirmed by pushing 5–10 ml of air and auscultating in the epigastrium or aspirating gastric juice. It is a long tube having 3 marks. When the tube is passed up to the 1st mark, it enters the stomach. Usually, it is passed

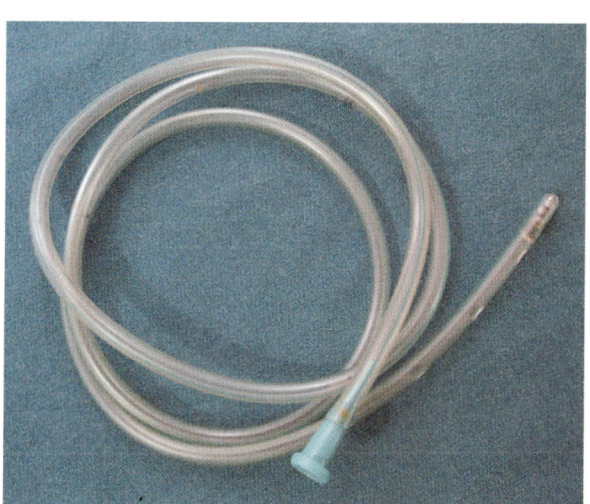

Fig. 30.77: Ryle's tube

up to 2nd mark. Life-saving use of **Ryle's tube** is in **acute gastric dilatation.**
- **In volvulus of the stomach, it is impossible to pass a Ryle's tube.**
- Ryle's tube is used to decompress the stomach as in intestinal obstruction or pyloric stenosis.
- It is used in the diagnosis of GI haemorrhage.
- It is also used to provide enteral nutrition to comatose patients or critically ill patients.

T-tube (Kehr) (Fig. 30.78)

- This is a flexible tube made of latex with a long vertical limb and a short horizontal limb.
- Whenever the **common bile duct (CBD) is incised,** it is sutured after inserting the T-tube. The short horizontal limb is placed vertically within the common bile duct after making 2–3 holes within. Some surgeons slit open the entire length of the short limb.
- The long limb is brought to the exterior from the most dependent part of the common bile duct and connected to a sterile container.
- Presence of the T-tube may prevent peritonitis due to biliary leakage in cases of residual stones blocking the lower end of the CBD.

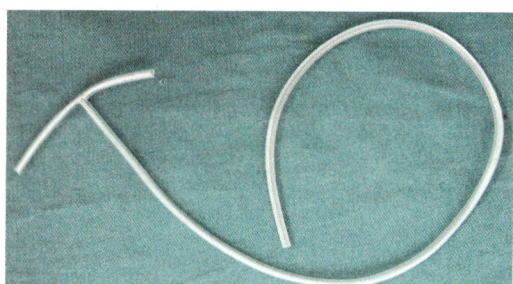

Fig. 30.78: T-tube (Kehr)

Removal of the Tube

About 7–10 days later, a T-tube cholangiography is done and the T-tube is removed with a gentle pull, provided following criteria are fulfilled.

- The dye flows freely into the duodenum.
- No filling defects in the CBD.
- After clamping the tube for 24 hours, there is no abdominal pain or fever.
- Patient is passing normal coloured stools.

Once the tube is withdrawn, some amount of biliary leak may persist for 2–3 days and it stops by itself provided there is no distal obstruction.

Sengstaken-Blakemore Double Balloon Triple Lumen Tube (Fig. 30.79)

- It is used in controlling bleeding **oesophageal varices.** It has 3 lumens and 2 balloons—a gastric balloon and an oesophageal balloon.

- **Gastric balloon is inflated** with about **200–250 ml** of air and oesophageal balloon is inflated with about **40–60 ml of air.** It is pulled upwards so as to snugly fit at the oesophagogastric junction and thus it acts by internal tamponade.

- Sengstaken tube should not be kept in place for more than 48 hours because it can cause pressure necrosis of oesophagus.

- It should be deflated for a few minutes after 24 hours.

- Sengstaken tube should be used by an experienced physician. Oesophageal secretions and saliva cannot be aspirated while using this tube, and if gastric balloon is deflated suddenly, it slides up and causes choking. The oesophageal balloon should be immediately deflated in such situations.

- **Modification of Sengstaken tube is called Minnesota tube or 4 lumen tube.** It has 4 lumens. The 1st to inflate oesophageal balloon, the 2nd to inflate gastric balloon, the 3rd to aspirate like a Ryle's tube, and the 4th lumen is used to aspirate oesophageal secretions. If there is any difficulty in breathing while using Sengstaken tube or Minnesota tube, bulb should be deflated or tube should be cut.

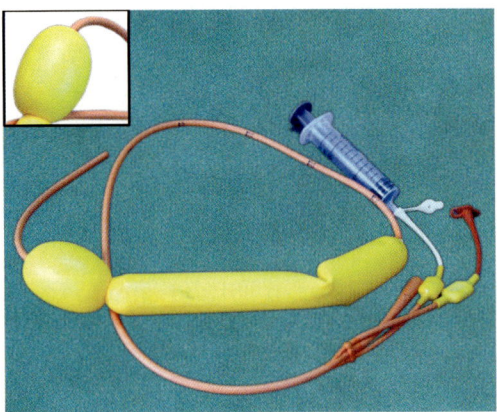

Fig. 30.79: Sengstaken-Blakemore double balloon triple lumen tube

Suturing Needles (Fig. 30.80)

Traumatic

- Round body needle is an eyed needle. They are used to suture soft tissues, muscles, tendons, vessels, intestines, etc.

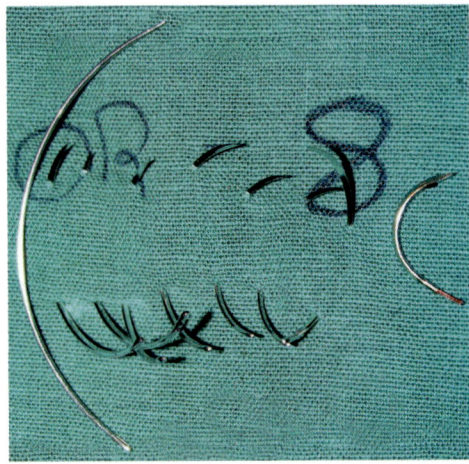

Fig. 30.80: Suturing needles

- Cutting needles are used to suture slim and some tough structures.
- Reverse cutting needles are used to suture muco-periosteum.

These needles have an eye. The eye is wider than body of the needle, so tissue trauma is more.

Atraumatic

These needles have no eye. **Suture** is attached to the needle by a process called **swaging**. Tissue trauma is less, and hence is used in suturing vessels or to repair a small tear in the bowl, etc.

SUTURE MATERIALS (Clinical Box 30.3)

ABSORBABLE

1. Plain Catgut (7-day Catgut)

- The word catgut is derived from kit-gut, which means the violin strings. It is the oldest suture material known.
- Catgut is derived from the submucosa of the sheep intestines.

Clinical Box 30.3

Colour	Suture material
• Yellow	Plain catgut
• Brown	Chromic catgut
• Violet	Vicryl
• Creamy yellow	Dexon
• Creamy	PDS
• Blue	Prolene
• Black	Silk
• White	Cotton

- The plain catgut lasts for **7–10 days**. Hence, its uses are minimal.
- It can be used to put 'fat stitches' (subcutaneous fat).
- It is biological, absorbable and monofilament.
- Sheep's submucosa has a rich content of elastic tissue.

2. Chromic Catgut (21-day Catgut)

- When plain catgut is mixed with chromic salts, chromic catgut is obtained.
- **The strength of the chromic catgut is about 15–25 days**.
- Chromic catgut is widely used in intestinal anastomosis, closure of urinary bladder, closure of common bile duct, gastrojejunostomy, etc.
- Catgut is biological, absorbable, monofilament suture material.
- Chromic catgut is packed along with round body needle.
- The number 2–0 refers to the thickness of the suture.
- Knotting property is good.
- The catgut is preserved in 70% alcohol and is kept soft due to 5% glycerine.

3. Vicryl (Polyglactin)

- This is a copolymer of glycolide and lactide.
- It is a synthetic and absorbable suture.
- Unlike catgut, this is absorbed by hydrolysis.
- **Since the strength and reliability is more than catgut, vicryl is being used more and more for small intestinal and colonic anastomosis. It has replaced catgut in suturing bile duct also.**
- Being synthetic, tissue reaction is less than that of chromic catgut.
- This has also replaced catgut while suturing common bile duct.
- Knotting property is good.
- Vicryl can be used in the presence of infection.

4. Dexon (Polyglycolic Acid)

- Synthetic absorbable
- Braided
- Used like Vicryl

5. PDS (Polydioxanone Suture)

- Like Vicryl

- Costly
- Creamy in colour

NONABSORBABLE

1. Prolene

- This is polypropylene and nonabsorbable.
- It is monofilament, artificial and uncoated. Does not harbour micro-organism. Hence, the chances of infection are less.
- Since it is nonabsorbable, prolene can be used for abdominal closure, repair of hernias, repair of incisional hernia, etc.
- It has high memory (recoiling tendency after removal from the pocket) and hence multiple knots are required.

2. Sutupack

- It is a monofilament or multifilament polyamide.
- Black in colour.
- It is braided, uncoated and nonabsorbable.
- Uses of sutupack are similar to prolene.
- Knotting property is not very good. Hence, it is mandatory to put 4–5 knots.

3. Mersilk

- This is nonabsorbable, braided silk, black in colour.
- It has been provided with a round body. This can be used in ligating bleeding points or anastomosis, etc.

4. Black Silk

- This is a nonabsorbable suture material.
- It is biological and derived from the **cocoon of the silkworm larva**.
- It is braided, coated with wax to reduce capillary action. Tissue reaction is much more with black silk because it is a foreign protein.
- In spite of this, it is widely used because of its easy availability and is cheap.
- Knotting property is excellent.

5. Cotton

- White in colour
- Multifilament—infection rate is high
- Nonabsorbable, cheap

SPECIMENS

I. Tuberculous (TB) Lymphadenitis (Fig. 30.81)

1. What is this specimen?

- Specimen of lymph nodes which are matted. Cut surface shows caseation. Hence, it is tuberculous lymphadenitis.

2. What is the microscopic picture?

- Central caseation surrounded by epithelioid cells, Langhans' type of giant cells.

3. What are the stages of TB lymphadenitis?

- Stage of lymphadenitis
- Stage of matting
- Stage of cold abscess
- Stage of collar stud abscess
- Stage of sinus formation

4. Why is matting seen in TB lymphadenitis?

- It is because of periadenitis

5. What is the treatment of cold abscess?

- Nondependent aspiration by using wide bore needle, to avoid sinus formation.

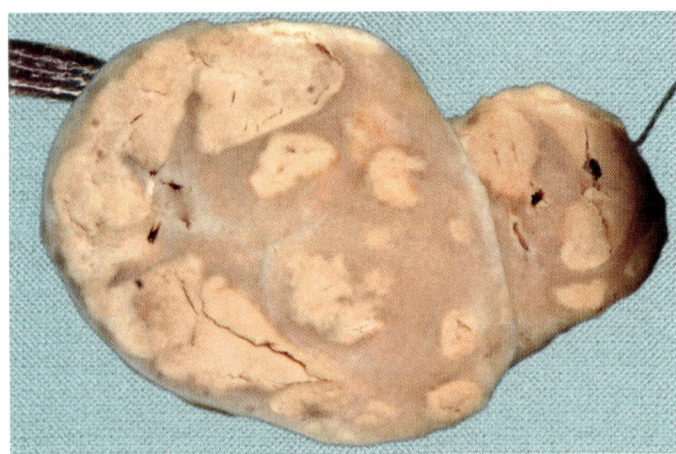

Fig. 30.81: Tuberculous (TB) lymphadenitis

II. Lymphoma (Fig. 30.82)

1. What is the diagnosis?

- Multiple lymph nodes which are discrete and not matted. Cut surface does not show caseation. It is homogenous. Hence, this is a specimen of Hodgkin's lymphoma.

2. How do you confirm the diagnosis?

- Lymph node biopsy.

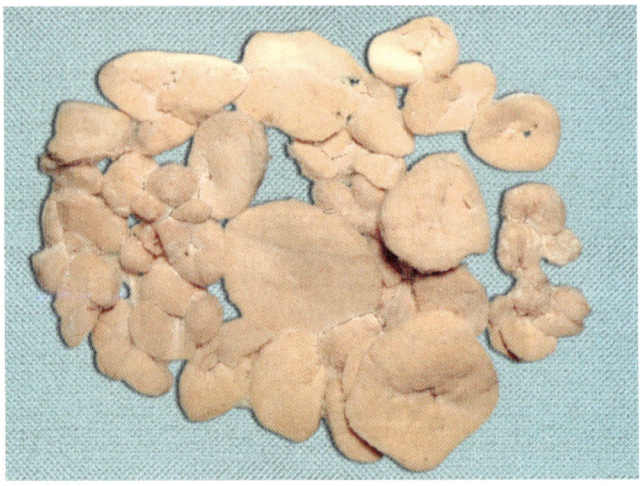

Fig. 30.82: Lymphoma

3. What is the microscopic picture?

- Cellular pleomorphism: Lymphocytes, histiocytes, eosinophils, monocytes with giant cells containing mirror image nuclei—Reed-Sternberg cell.

4. What are the common lymph nodes involved in Hodgkin's lymphoma?

- Cervical, axillary, para-aortic, iliac and inguinal lymph nodes.

5. Is Waldeyer's ring involvement seen in Hodgkin's lymphoma?

- No, it is usually seen in non-Hodgkin's lymphoma.

III. Specimen of Hemiglossectomy with Hemimandibulectomy (Fig. 30.83)

1. What is this specimen?

- Specimen showing growth arising from the tongue and infiltrating the mandible.

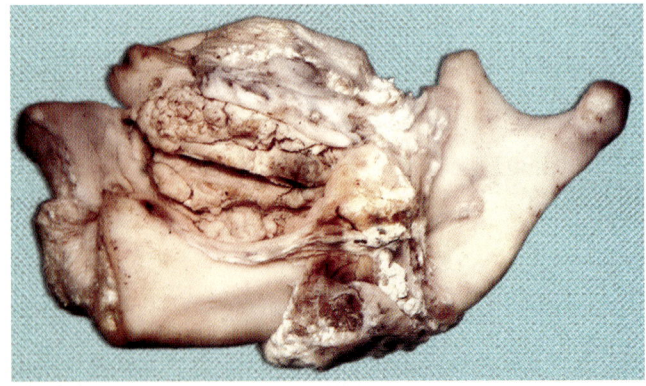

Fig. 30.83: Specimen of hemiglossectomy with hemimandibulectomy

2. What is the diagnosis?

- Advanced carcinoma tongue

3. Is radiotherapy indicated in this situation?

- No, because chances of radionecrosis of the mandible are high.

4. What type of X-ray is taken to look for involvement of the mandible?

- Orthopantomogram

5. What is Commando's operation?

- Hemiglossectomy with excision of the floor of the mouth, hemimandibulectomy, with radical block dissection of the neck done in a single stage, with *en bloc* removal.

IV. Chronic Gastric Ulcer (Fig. 30.84)

1. What is this specimen?

- Specimen of the stomach showing rugosity of the stomach. There is a deep ulcer crater along the lesser curvature.

2. What is the diagnosis?

- Benign gastric ulcer

3. Why is it a benign gastric ulcer?

- Since the rugae are of converging type, it is a benign gastric ulcer.

4. How do you rule out malignancy in a gastric ulcer?

- Endoscopic biopsy

5. What is the incidence of gastric ulcer turning into malignancy?

- 0.5 to 2%

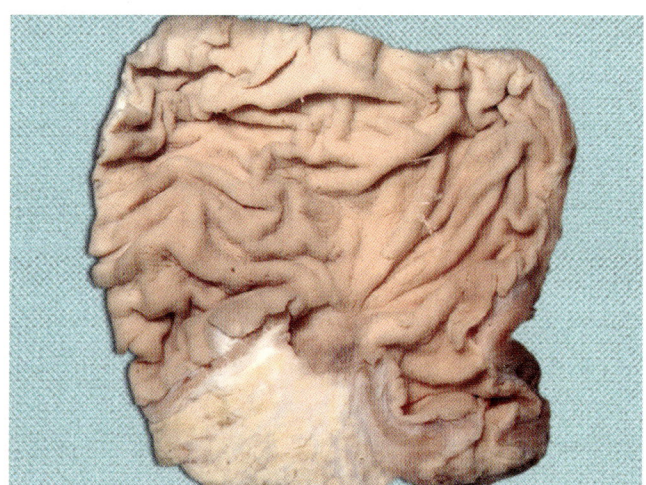

Fig. 30.84: Chronic gastric ulcer

V. Linitis Plastica (Fig. 30.85)

1. What is this specimen?

- Specimen of the stomach showing loss of normal rugosity. There is a nodular extensive infiltrating lesion along the entire length of the stomach.

2. What is the diagnosis?

- Linitis plastica—leather bottle stomach.

3. What is linitis plastica?

- It is an extensive fibrosis involving entire submucosa of the stomach initially and involves other layers also later.

4. What is the treatment for linitis plastica?

- Radical total gastrectomy

5. What is the prognosis?

- Very poor

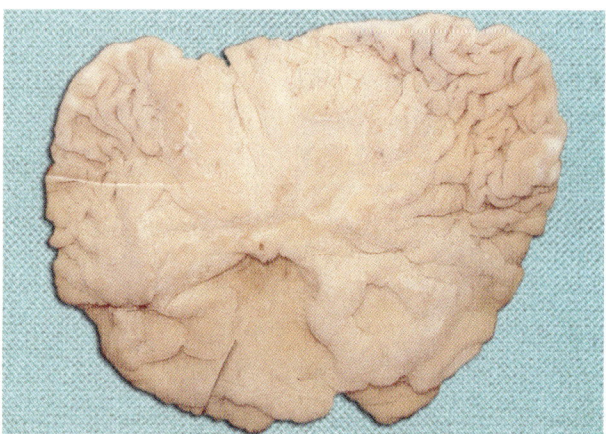

Fig. 30.85: Linitis plastica

VI. Intussusception (Fig. 30.86)

1. What is this specimen?

- Specimen of intestine showing one portion of bowel invaginated within the other.

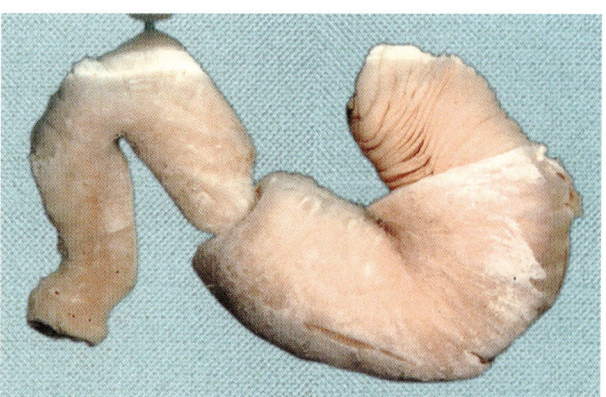

Fig. 30.86: Intussusception

2. What is the diagnosis?

- Intussusception

3. What is the common type of intussusception?

- Ileocolic

4. What are the parts of intussusception?

- Intussusceptum, intussuscipiens, neck and apex.

5. What is the treatment in children?

- Hydrostatic reduction or operative reduction.
- If there is gangrene—resection followed by end-to-end anastomosis.

VII. Carcinoma Rectum (Fig. 30.87)

1. What is this specimen?

- Specimen of rectum showing ulceroproliferative growth in the middle of the rectum. Specimen also shows entire rectum and anal canal.

2. What is the diagnosis?

- Carcinoma rectum

3. What is this surgery?

- Abdominoperineal resection (excision) (APR). In this operation, entire rectum, anal canal, part of the sigmoid colon, fat, fascia, lymphatics and regional nodes are removed *en bloc* followed by permanent colostomy in the left iliac fossa.

4. What are the indications for APR?

- Growth in the middle and lower rectum wherein sphincter cannot be saved.

5. What is the position of the patient during APR?

- Supine with lithotomy called Lloyd Davis position.

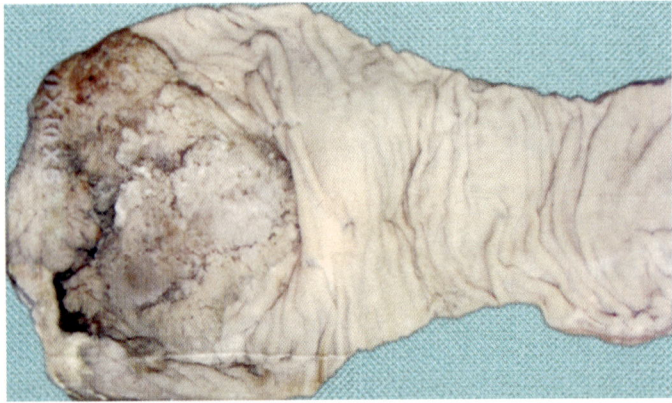

Fig. 30.87: Carcinoma rectum

VIII. Gangrenous Appendicitis (Fig. 30.88)

1. What is this specimen?

- It is an appendicectomy specimen showing blackish discolouration of the appendix.

2. What factors cause gangrene of the appendix?

- Gangrenous appendicitis occurs usually in elderly patients, where there is decreased vascularity due to atherosclerosis. It can also occur when the lumen is blocked due to faecolith, thereby causing ischaemia.

3. What is the one simple investigation which is useful in diagnosing appendicitis?

- Total WBC count. Above 10,000 cells/cu mm of blood with increased neutrophil count.

4. What are the complications of acute appendicitis?

- Appendicular mass (in untreated cases)
- Perforation with an abscess
- Perforation with generalised peritonitis
- Pylephlebitis, portal pyaemia
- Septicaemia, gram-negative shock

5. How do you treat an appendicular mass?

- Conservative line, Oschner-Sherren regime—aspiration, antibiotics, intravenous fluids, etc.

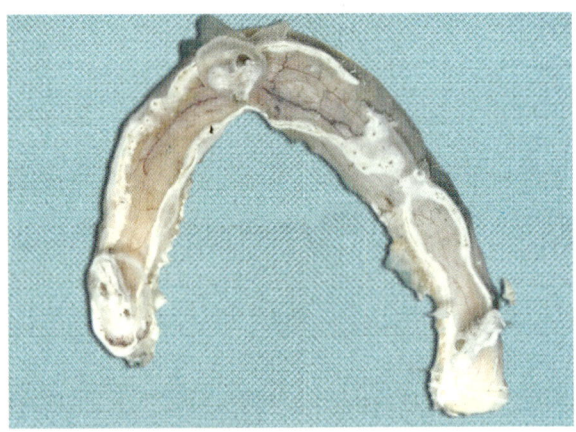

Fig. 30.88: Gangrenous appendicitis

IX. Carcinoma Ascending Colon (Fig. 30.89)

1. What is this specimen?

- Specimen of terminal ileum, caecum and right colon with removal of involved lymph nodes and fat fascia. Nowadays, only 4–6 cm of ileum is removed.

2. What is the surgery?

- Right radical hemicolectomy done for growth in the ascending colon.

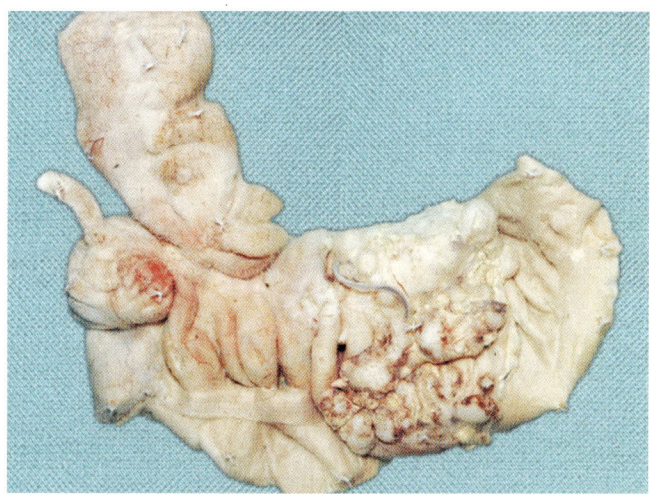

Fig. 30.89: Carcinoma ascending colon

3. How do you identify colon?

- *Taenia coli* and appendix are seen. The colon has a larger diameter compared to small intestine.

4. What are the investigations?

- Barium enema will show persistent filling defect. However, colonoscopy is the investigation because the growth can be visualised and biopsy can be taken.

5. What do you mean by limited resection?

- It is done for ileocaecal tuberculosis wherein diseased segment is removed.

X. Meckel's Diverticulum (Fig. 30.90)

1. What is the specimen?

- Resected specimen of intestine showing a diverticulum. Hence, it is a Meckel's diverticulum.

2. Why is it a Meckel's diverticulum?

- Because it is a single diverticulum arising from antimesenteric border of the intestine.

3. What are common symptoms?

- Bleeding per rectum, abdominal pain due to inflammation, intestinal obstruction and peritonitis due to perforation.

4. What is the cause and what are the types of bleeding?

- Ulcer in the ectopic gastric mucosa. Bleeding can be occult, in small quantities or rarely can be massive.

5. How do you diagnose Meckel's diverticulum?

- Radio-nuclear (^{99m}Tc pertechnetate) scan is helpful when there is active bleeding.

XI. Polycystic Kidney (Fig. 30.91)

1. What is this specimen?

- Specimen of kidney with multiple cystic lesions. Entire kidney is involved.

2. What is the diagnosis?

- Polycystic kidney

3. Why do you say it is polycystic kidney?

- Kidney is grossly enlarged
- Outer surface is bosselated
- Multiple cysts are present

4. What are clinical features of polycystic kidney?

- Women: 30–50 years
- Bilateral renal mass
- Hypertension
- Haematuria
- Renal failure

5. What is the treatment?

- If there is no renal failure, control hypertension.
- If there is renal failure—dialysis followed by renal transplantation.

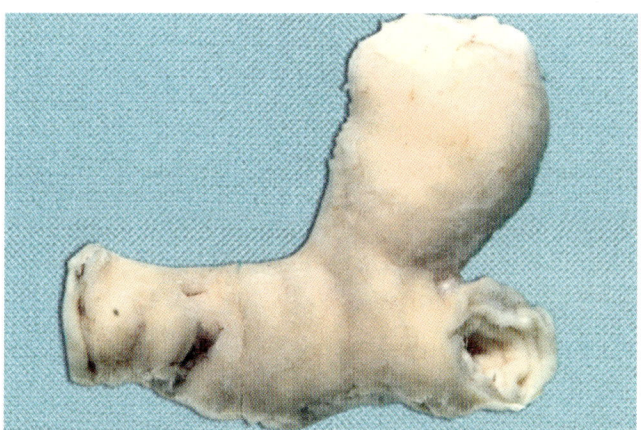

Fig. 30.90: Meckel's diverticulum

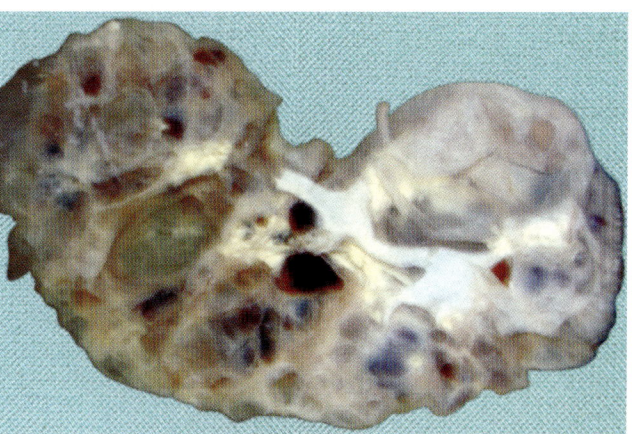

Fig. 30.91: Polycystic kidney

XII. Renal Cell Carcinoma (Fig. 30.92)

1. What is this specimen?

- Specimen of the kidney because it is reniform shaped, ureter and calyces are seen.

- In the upper pole, there is destruction of the calyces with solid mass. Cut surface is smooth.

2. What is the diagnosis?

- Renal cell carcinoma

3. What is the microscopic picture?

- Cuboidal or polyhedral clear cells with deeply stained rounded nuclei—clear cell carcinoma. Sometimes, dark cells can coexist. In some cases, walls of blood vessels are lined by tumour cells.

4. How does it spread?

- Lymphatic and blood spread

5. What are the primary malignant tumours which spread by blood?

- Renal cell carcinoma, follicular carcinoma thyroid, carcinoma prostate, carcinoma breast, bronchogenic carcinoma.

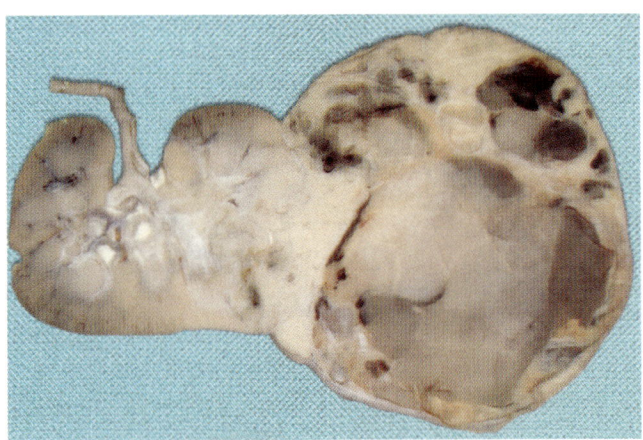

Fig. 30.92: Renal cell carcinoma

XIII. Hydronephrosis (Fig. 30.93)

1. What is this specimen?

- Specimen of the kidney with ureter showing dilatation of pelvicalyceal system. Calyces are club-shaped.

2. What is the diagnosis?

- Hydronephrosis—probably due to pelviureteric junction (PUJ) obstruction.

3. Why PUJ obstruction?

- Ureter is not dilated

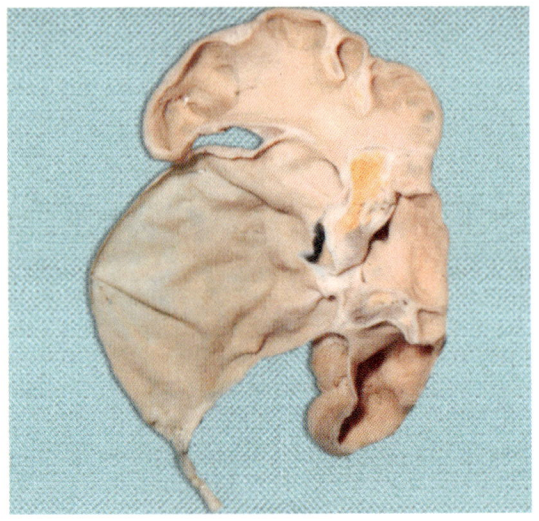

Fig. 30.93: Hydronephrosis

4. What are the common causes of obstruction at PUJ?

- Stone in the pelvis

- Aberrant vessels—a lower polar artery or vein arising from the main vessels in an aberrant position obstructs the upper ureter.

- PUJ dyskinesia—occurs due to incoordination between neuromuscular impulses and pelvis.

5. What is the treatment of PUJ dyskinesia?

- Anderson-Hynes pyeloplasty

XIV. Carcinoma Penis (Fig. 30.94)

1. What is this specimen?

- Specimen of penis, showing the glans. Prepuce is cut open showing the growth.

2. What is the diagnosis?

- Partial amputation done for carcinoma penis

3. What are the indications for partial amputation of the penis?

- Growth confined to the glans penis or to the prepuce

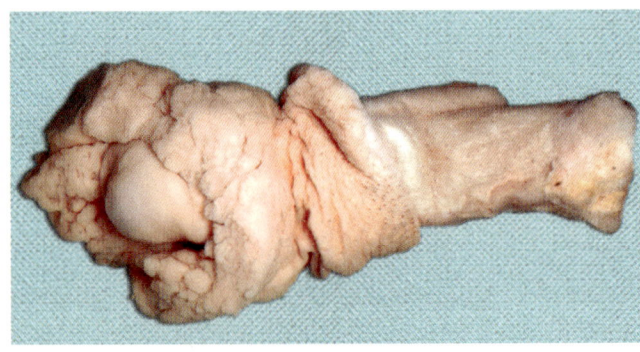

Fig. 30.94: Carcinoma penis

4. If shaft is involved, what is the treatment?

- Total amputation of penis followed by perineal urethrostomy.

5. What are the complications of perineal urethrostomy?

- Bleeding, dermatitis and stenosis. The stenosis should be dilated by using Hegar's dilators.

XV. Seminoma Testis (Fig. 30.95)

1. What is this specimen?

- Specimen of testis showing spermatic cord. Cut surface of the testis is smooth and homogenous with a tumour in the upper part.

2. What is the diagnosis?

- Seminoma

3. Why not a teratoma?

- In a teratoma, the cut surface is not homogenous.

4. How does seminoma spread?

- Mainly by lymphatics

5. What type of orchidectomy is done for testicular tumours and why?

- High orchidectomy, through an inguinal incision. If scrotum is incised, chances of alternate pathway of lymphatics opening up are high. Hence, inguinal exploration is the choice.

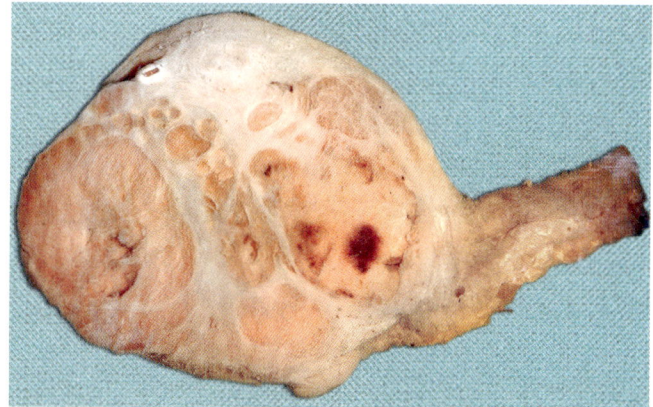

Fig. 30.95: Seminoma testis showing spermatic cord on the right side

XVI. Cholecystectomy for Gallstones (Fig. 30.96)

1. What is this specimen?

- Cholecystectomy specimen

2. What is the diagnosis?

- Multiple stones are present within lumen—diagnosis is probably chronic cholecystitis.

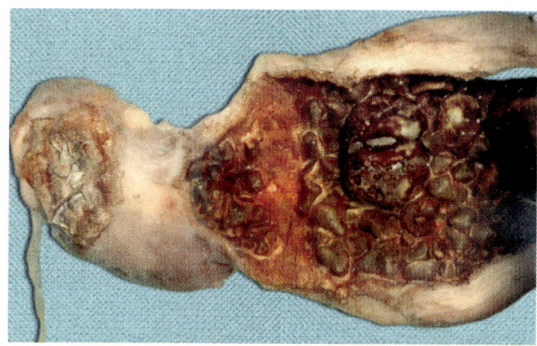

Fig. 30.96: Gallstones

3. Why do you say it is a gallbladder?

- It is pear-shaped with fundus, body and a narrow portion—cystic area.

4. What is Hartmann's pouch?

- It is the distal angulated portion of gallbladder wherein a stone commonly lodges.

5. What are the common symptoms of gallstones?

- Flatulent dyspepsia, gallstone colic, acute and chronic cholecystitis are common symptoms of gallstones. Mucocoele, empyema, perforation and gallstone pancreatitis are other complications.

XVII. Hydatid Cyst (Fig. 30.97)

1. What is this specimen?

- Specimen of laminated membranes—this layer is also called ectocyst. It is thick and elastic resembling onion skin appearance.

2. What is the diagnosis?

- Hydatid cyst—mostly liver

3. What are the other layers of hydatid cyst?

- Outermost layer is called adventitial layer which blends firmly with liver tissue. The middle layer is ectocyst, also called laminated membrane. Inner

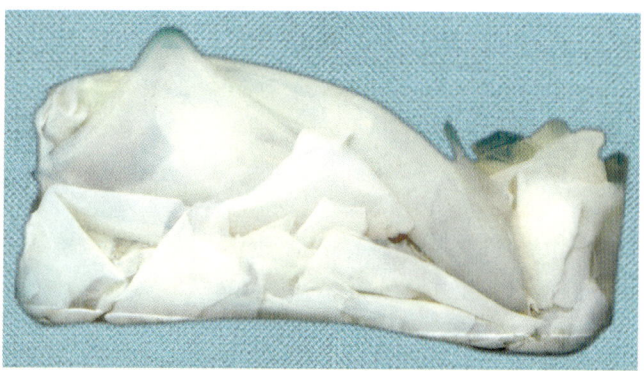

Fig. 30.97: Hydatid cyst

layer is germinal epithelium, also called endocyst within which brood capsules and daughter cysts are present.

4. What is the drug for hydatid disease?

- Albendazole 400 mg, a day for 15 days followed by no drug for 15 days. Then restart the cycle. Such treatment may have to continue for 6 months depending on the response rate.

5. What are the common complications of hydatid cyst of the liver?

- Infection, rupture, calcification, cholangitis with jaundice are a few complications.

XVIII. Radical Gastrectomy including Removal of the Colon (Fig. 30.98)

1. What is the specimen?

- Specimen of stomach with transverse colon

2. Why stomach and colon?

- It has lesser curvature and greater curvature—pylorus, body and proximal stomach. Colon is the immediate structure below the stomach

3. What does it show?

- Exophytic growth infiltrating the colon

4. What is the final diagnosis?

- Most probably it is carcinoma stomach infiltrating transverse colon.

5. What is the best investigation in such cases to identify local infiltration?

- CT scan

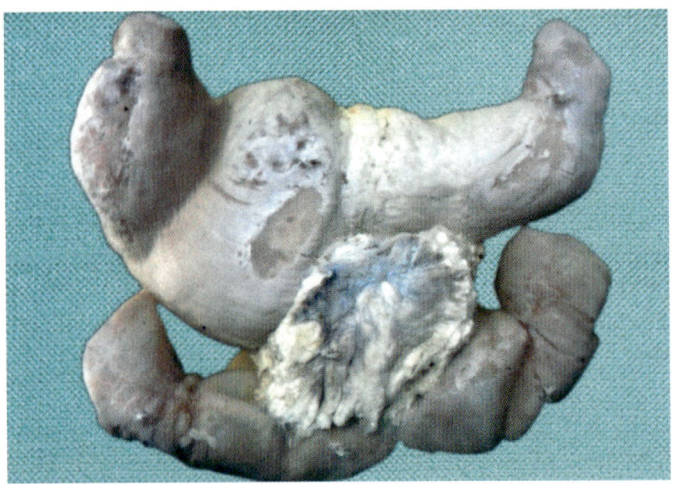

Fig. 30.98: Radical gastrectomy including removal of the colon

XIX. Lipoma (Fig. 30.99)

1. What is this specimen?

- Specimen of lipoma

2. Why do you say it is lipoma?

- It is lobular, yellow in colour

3. What is the commonest site and type of lipoma?

- Flank is the commonest site. Single and subcutaneous variety is the commonest type.

4. What are the common complications of lipoma?

- Liposarcoma and intussusception

5. Which type of lipoma give rise to intussusception?

- Submucosal type

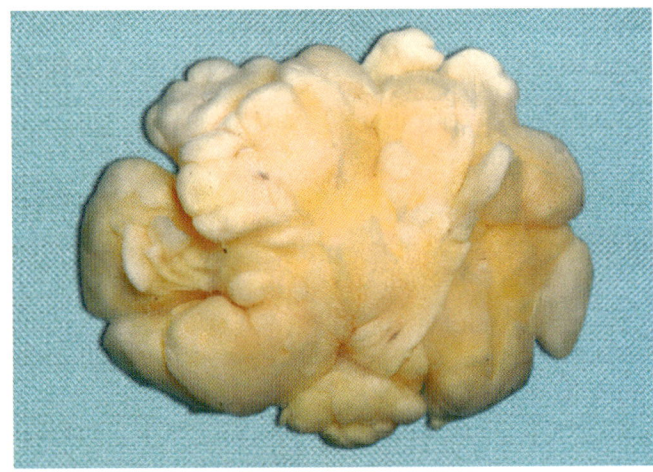

Fig. 30.99: Lipoma

XX. Malignant Melanoma (Fig. 30.100)

1. What is this specimen?

- Specimen of foot showing a large ulcerated growth in the sole of the foot.

2. What is the diagnosis and why do you say so?

- Malignant melanoma because the lesion is pigmented.

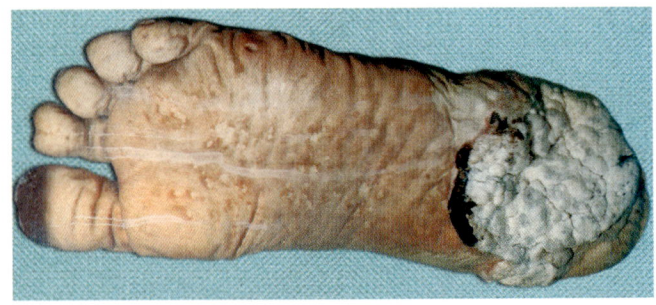

Fig. 30.100: Malignant melanoma

3. What is the commonest type of malignant melanoma?

- Superficial spreading is the first followed by nodular variety.

4. What are the staging systems available for this condition?

- Clark's level of invasion and Breslow's thickness are important staging systems in addition to TNM staging.

5. What are the ABCDE of melanoma?

- Asymmetry
- Border irregular
- Colour variegation
- Diameter >6 mm
- Elevation

XXI. Thyroidectomy Specimen (Fig. 30.101)

1. What is this specimen?

- Specimen of thyroid gland showing both lobes and isthmus.

2. What is the diagnosis and why do you say so?

- Probably it is a subtotal thyroidectomy specimen—surgery is done for multinodular goitre.

3. What is the commonest type of malignancy of the thyroid gland?

- Papillary carcinoma—63%. Second common type is follicular carcinoma thyroid.

4. What is the surgical treatment for well-differentiated carcinoma thyroid gland?

- Most centres follow total thyroidectomy. If the patient is in low-risk category, lobectomy can be done.

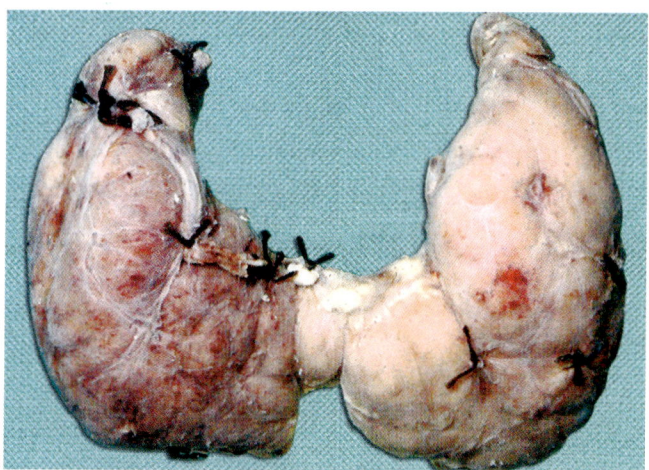

Fig. 30.101: Thyroidectomy specimen

5. What blood investigation is useful in the follow-up period of papillary carcinoma thyroid gland?

- Thyroglobulin

XXII. Wide Excision Specimen of Skin (Fig. 30.102)

1. What is this specimen?

- Specimen of skin which has been excised with normal skin. Hence, wide excision specimen.

2. What is the diagnosis and why do you say so?

- Probably it is a squamous cell carcinoma because edges are everted.

3. What are the common sites of squamous cell carcinoma skin?

- Areas with chronic irritation, e.g. Kangri cancer in the abdominal wall, chimney sweeper's cancer, etc.

4. What are the common precancerous lesions for squamous cell carcinoma?

- Leukoplakia, Bowen's disease, chronic irritation, scar tissues, etc.

5. What do you call squamous cell carcinoma arising in a scar tissue?

- Marjolin's ulcer

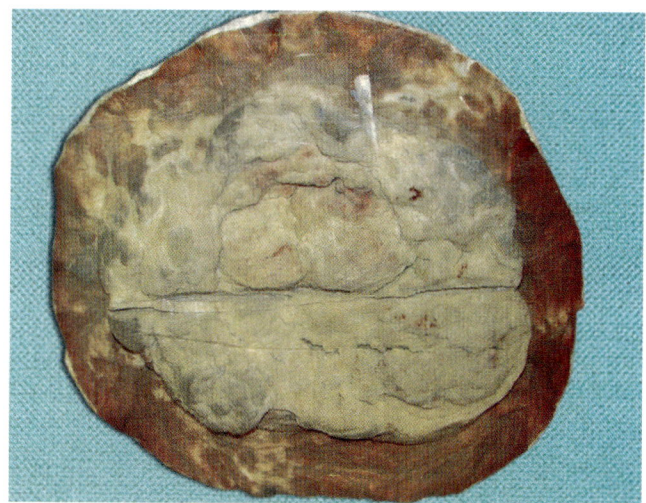

Fig. 30.102: Wide excision skin

XXIII. Whipple's Pancreaticoduodenectomy (Fig. 30.103)

1. What is this specimen?

- Specimen showing distal stomach, duodenum, proximal jejunum and pancreatic head.

2. What is the name of this operation?

- Whipple's pancreaticoduodenectomy

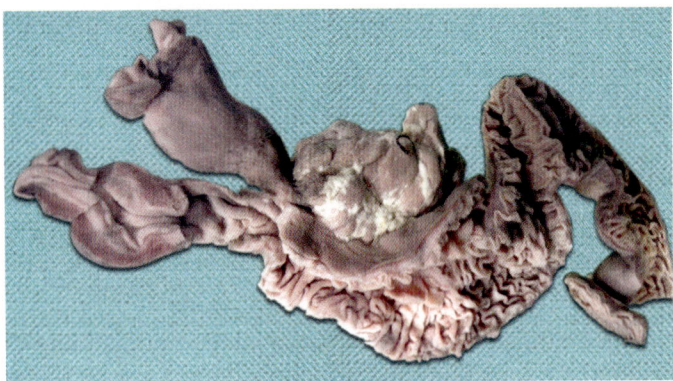

Fig. 30.103: Whipple's pancreaticoduodenectomy

3. Why is it done?

• Mostly due to periampullary carcinoma

4. How can you get histopathological diagnosis?

• Endoscopic biopsy

5. Is there any other indication for Whipple's surgery?

• Pancreatic head mass—doubt exists between chronic pancreatitis and carcinoma head pancreas. Provided experience of the surgeon is good.

XXIV. Right Hemicolectomy for Carcinoma Caecum (Fig. 30.104)

1. What is this specimen?

• Specimen showing distal ileum, caecum, part of the ascending colon and a few lymph nodes.

2. What is the name of this operation?

• Limited colectomy

3. Why is it done?

• Mostly due to ileocaecal tuberculosis

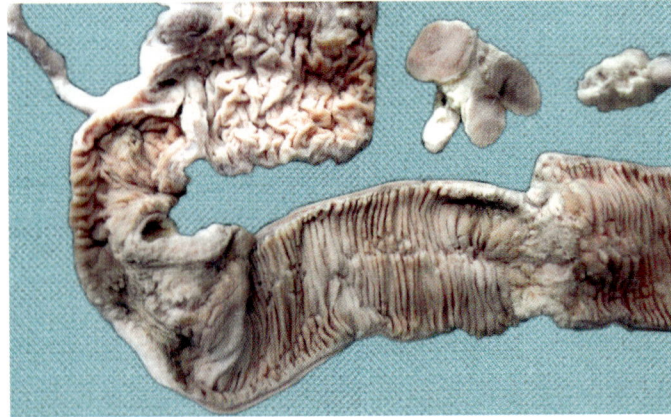

Fig. 30.104: Right hemicolectomy for carcinoma caecum

4. Why do you say so?

• Stricture is seen in the terminal ileum

5. What was the indication for surgery?

• Acute intestinal obstruction

XXV. Splenectomy Specimen (Fig. 30.105)

1. What is this specimen?

• Specimen showing spleen with laceration of the diaphragmatic surface.

2. Why laceration?

• Blunt injury is the most common cause of rupture spleen.

3. What will be clinical manifestation?

• Bleeding

4. What other surgery can be done for bleeding?

• Partial splenectomy or splenorrhaphy

5. What is the dangerous complication after splenectomy?

• Opportunistic post-splenectomy infections

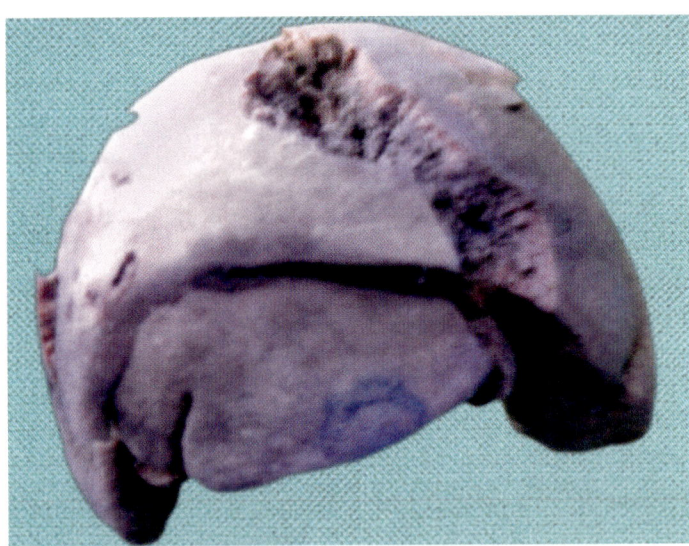

Fig. 30.105: Splenectomy specimen

Useful Tips

• Please look into the specimen carefully
• Please see both sides of the specimen
• Think which is the most likely organ involved
• Think what is the probable diagnosis.

OPERATIVE SURGERY

INTRODUCTION

Over a period of time, the number of operations an undergraduate is expected to know has become less and less. Today no MBBS doctor is supposed to do a surgical procedure because qualified surgeons are available even in a village. Hence, I have discussed a few surgical procedures in this chapter. These are common surgical procedures that an undergraduate student is expected to know. Every operation has been discussed along a certain basic pattern as given below and the keywords used are given in the keybox. *Students should study surgical anatomy before reading this chapter.*

Commonly Used Abbreviations (Clinical Box 30.4)

Clinical Box 30.4 🔑

Commonly used abbreviations

SA	Spinal anaesthesia
GA	General anaesthesia
LA	Local anaesthesia
OT	Operation theatre
NPO	Nil per oral
IV	Intravenous
RT	Ryle's tube

Steps of Operative Surgery

1. Indications
2. Contraindications
3. Position of the patient
4. Anaesthesia
5. Preparation of parts
6. Procedure
7. Closure
8. Postoperative management
9. Postoperative complications
10. Advice at discharge

Antiseptic Agents

- Povidone-iodine
- Spirit 70%
- Savlon

APPENDICECTOMY

Clinical Wisdom

Appendicectomy can be one of the easiest and sometimes one of the most complicated surgeries.

1. *Indications*

- Acute appendicitis—emergency appendicectomy
- Recurrent appendicitis—elective appendicectomy

2. *Contraindications*: Appendicular mass

3. *Position of the patient*: Supine

4. *Anaesthesia of the parts*: This surgery can be done either under GA or regional anaesthesia (spinal or epidural).

5. *Preparation*: Parts are cleaned with iodine and spirit, from the level of umbilicus above to the upper part of thigh below.

6. *Procedure*

Incision

A. **McBurney's grid-iron incision** is the most popular incision. It is at right angles to spinoumbilical line placed at McBurney's point. It is about 6–8 cm in length (Fig. 30.106).

B. **Lanz incision** is a curved transverse incision, placed at the McBurney's point. Cosmetically, it is a better incision (Fig. 30.107).

Table 30.1: Sterilisation

Agents for sterilisation	Common of items
1. Autoclaving	Linen, operative instruments, glass syringes
2. Dettol or phenol	Sharp instruments (scissors, needles, blades)
3. Glutaraldehyde	Endoscopy and laparoscopy equipment
4. Ethylene oxide, gamma radiation	Surgical catgut, syringes
5. Formaldehyde	Disinfect rooms like OT
6. Skin	70% spirit, povidone-iodine

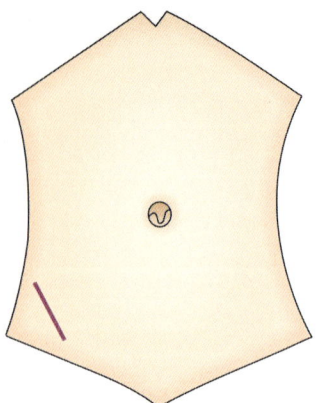

Fig. 30.106: Grid-iron incision

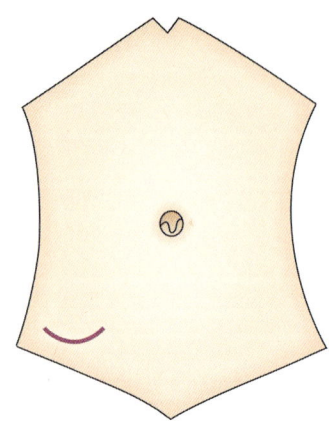

Fig. 30.107: Lanz incision

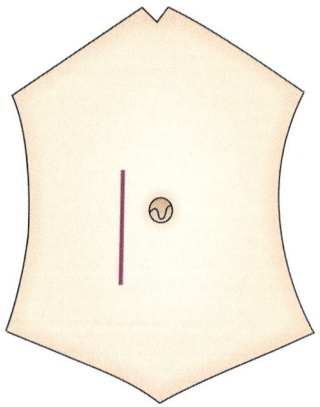

Fig. 30.108: Right paramedian incision

Today vast majority of appendicectomy is done via laparoscopic approach

Right paramedian incision is made when diagnosis is in doubt as a part of **exploratory laparotomy**. This is also preferred in females where there is a gynaecological pathology such as ovarian cyst which may be the cause of right iliac fossa pain (Fig. 30.108). *Today, all such cases are managed by lower midline incision.*

Layers opened
- Skin

- Two layers of subcutaneous tissue—superficial fatty (Campers), deep membranous (Scarpas). (C: comes first, S: later). There is no deep fascia in the abdomen.

- External oblique aponeurosis is seen running downwards and medially. It is incised in the direction of its fibres.

- Internal and transverse abdominal muscles are split (grid-iron—right angle to each other).

- Peritoneum is incised.

Features of acute appendicitis at operation
- Inflamed, turgid appendix
- Pus in the right iliac fossa
- Presence of omentum in the right iliac fossa
- Black or green appendix (gangrenous)
- Faecolith

Location of appendix
- Trace taenia coli. They will lead to the base of appendix (**all roads lead to Rome**).

- When you are tracing taenia coli, if you are not able to identify the appendix, it means most probably you are tracing taenia coli of the sigmoid colon.

Surgical procedure
- Appendix is gently held at mesoappendix by using Babcock's forceps and blood vessels in the mesoappendix are divided. These include appendicular artery, branch of ileocolic artery (accessory appendicular artery of Seshachalam, is a branch of posterior caecal artery). Once appendix is freed up to the base (caecum), a **purse-string suture** is applied all round appendix, taking bites from caecum, using 2–0 atraumatic silk (Fig. 30.109).

- Appendix is crushed at base and is held 1 cm above the crush. A tight silk ligature is applied at the crushed site and appendix is cut in between. Stump is cleaned with spirit, invaginated and purse-string is tightened. This is called burial of the stump. Perfect haemostasis is obtained (Fig. 30.110).

Clinical Wisdom
Look for Meckel's diverticulum, which may be the cause of right iliac fossa pain.

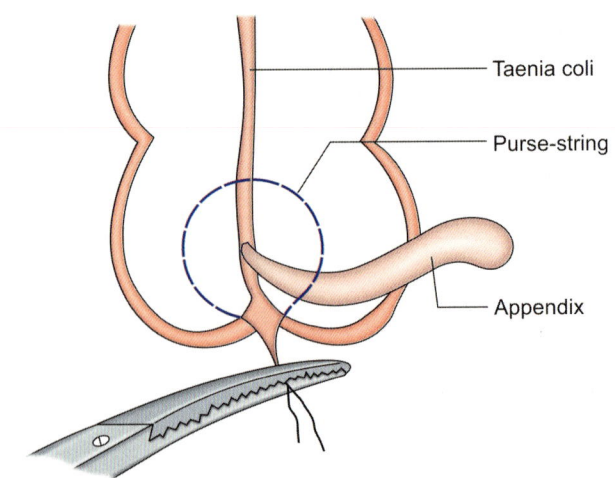

Taenia coli

Purse-string

Appendix

Fig. 30.109: Purse-string suture

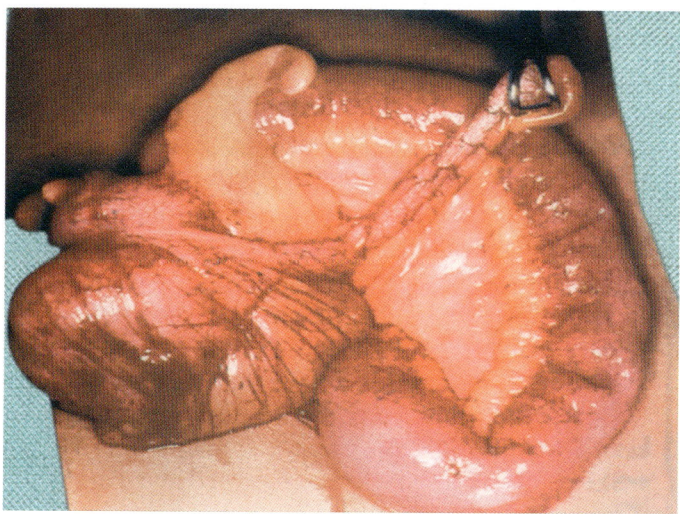

Fig. 30.110: Appendix at surgery

7. *Closure*

- Peritoneum—continuous 2–0 catgut/Vicryl
- Split muscles—sutured together by a few interrupted sutures using chromic catgut/Vicryl.
- External oblique is sutured with silk
- Subcutaneous fat is sutured with Vicryl
- Skin with interrupted silk: Instead of chromic catgut, 2–0 silk, 2–0 Vicryl is being used more often nowadays.
- Tube drain is not kept routinely unless there is gangrenous appendicitis or a lot of pus in the peritoneal cavity.

8. *Postoperative management*

- RT aspiration for one or two days
- IV fluids 100 ml/hr/day for one or two days
- Oral fluids are allowed once abdomen is soft and bowel sounds are heard.
- Appropriate antibiotics to cover gram-positive, gram-negative and anaerobic organisms.
- Suture removal by 7–10 days

9. *Complications after appendicectomy*

A. **Postoperative fever** can be due to various factors. Thrombophlebitis, urinary tract infection and IV fluids are common causes. In the absence of these, wound infection, intraperitoneal abscess secondary to gangrenous appendicitis, may have to be considered.

- Change of antibiotics according to culture and sensitivity reports of urine, pus and blood help in treating postoperative fever.

- Elderly patients may have a pre-existing pulmonary disease. Respiratory tract infection also has to be considered.

B. **Wound infection:** It is the most common complication after appendicectomy.

C. **Intra-abdominal abscess** needs drainage.

D. **Faecal fistula**—causes:

  a. Gangrene spreading into caecum

  b. Persistent infection

  c. Carcinoma caecum (elderly patients)

  d. Ileocaecal tuberculosis

  e. Crohn's disease (uncommon in India)

  f. Actinomycosis (rare)[1]

> **Clinical Wisdom**
>
> Most of the faecal fistulae will stop by themselves provided there is no distal obstruction.

E. Septicaemia, portal pyaemia, gram-negative shock in late cases of peritonitis due to perforated appendicitis are uncommon but dangerous complications.

- Mortality of appendicular perforation and peritonitis is around 2%.

10. *Advice at discharge*

- Not to strain for 15 days

MODIFIED BASSINI'S HERNIORRHAPHY AND LICHTENSTEIN REPAIR

- Herniorrhaphy means herniotomy and approximation of conjoined tendon to inguinal ligament to strengthen the posterior wall of the inguinal canal.
- Hernioplasty means herniotomy and strengthening the posterior wall of the inguinal canal
- In a large, long-standing hernias and in sliding hernias, especially in elderly patients, it is better to catheterise their bladder before surgery for two reasons. Firstly, to avoid injury to the urinary bladder and secondly, they invariably develop retention of urine in the postoperative period.

1. *Indication*: Indirect or direct hernia with good muscle tone.

---

[1]In viva, when a question is asked as to what is the common cause of faecal fistula following appendicectomy, the usual answer by students is actinomycosis. Remember it is the answer to be told last.

2. *Contraindication (relative)*: Severe cardiopulmonary insufficiency.

3. *Position of the patient*: Supine

4. *Anaesthesia*: Regional anaesthesia or G/A. **Local anaesthesia** can be preferred in **high-risk patients**.

5. *Preparation of the parts*: Like that for appendicectomy.

6. *Procedure*: Bassini's herniorrhaphy

Incision: 6–8 cm incision is made parallel to the inguinal ligament at the level of deep ring in the medial two-thirds of the inguinal ligament.

Layers opened

- Skin
- Two layers of superficial fascia
- External oblique is incised in the line of direction of fibres, till external ring is slit open.
- Thin cremasteric box is opened
- Identification of the sac—glistening white colour
  - Isolate the cord from the sac by blunt and sharp dissection. The cord is held separately by using cord holding forceps (Fig. 30.111).
  - The sac is mobilised up to the deep ring. Mobilisation is complete when inferior epigastric artery pulsations and extraperitoneal pad of fat are seen.
  - **The sac is opened and contents are examined.**
  - **The contents are reduced.**
  - **Twist the sac** so as to avoid injury to the contents of the sac (Fig. 30.112).
  - **Transfixation ligature** is applied as high as possible at the neck of sac and it is tightened.

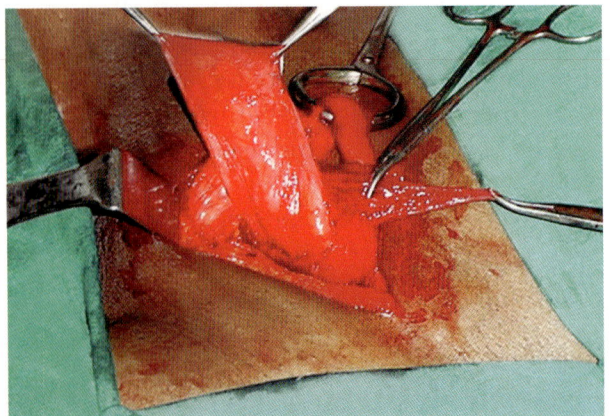

Fig. 30.111: Spermatic cord held with cord holding forceps

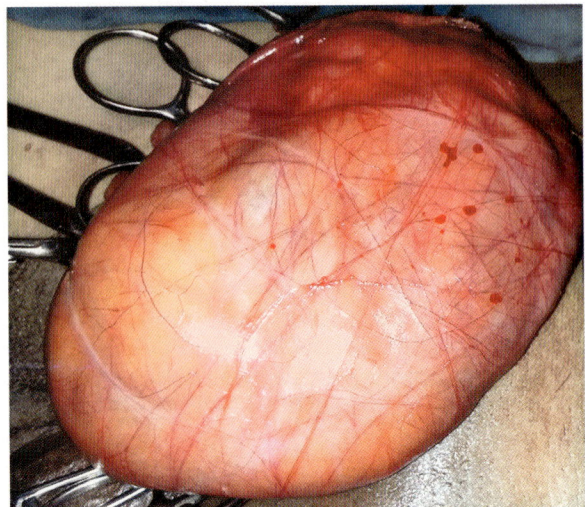

Fig. 30.112A: Large hernial sac is seen after opening inguinal canal

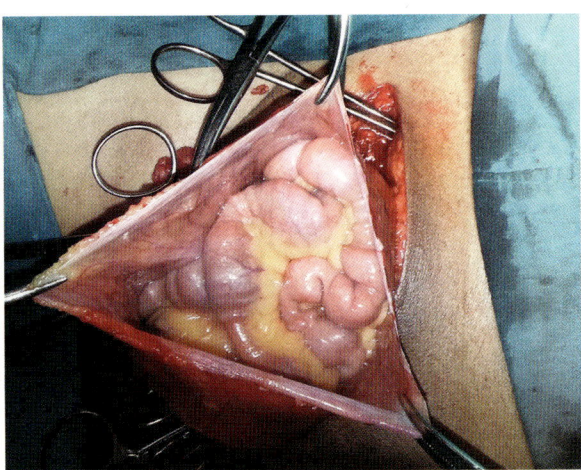

Fig. 30.112B: Sac is twisted, excised and opened. You can see the small intestines

  - **Excision of the sac:** After excision, see the excised sac and see whether omentum or intestine have been injured. Up to this stage, it is called **herniotomy**.

Repair

- Conjoined tendon above is approximated to the inguinal ligament below by using nonabsorbable suture such as nylon, silk or sutupack.
- Nonabsorbable suture is used so that its strength remains for a long time. This repair is called **Bassini's herniorrhaphy** (Clinical Box 30.5).

Clinical Wisdom

Do not twist the sac in direct hernias and in sliding hernias.

Precautions (Clinical Box 30.6)

1. Ilioinguinal nerve should not be caught in ligature.

2. Conjoined muscles should not be strangulated.

3. There should not be any tension in the suture lines.

7. *Closure*

- External oblique is sutured with chromic catgut or silk.

- Subcutaneous fat with absorbable catgut suture

- Skin with silk

8. *Postoperative management*

- NPO for 6–8 hours, oral fluids and soft diet later

- Analgesics

- Antibiotics—not always necessary

- Scrotal support, if the dissection is more (complete hernia).

- Suture removal after 7–10 days

9. *Postoperative complications*

1. **Immediate:** Haematoma due to injury to the pampiniform plexus of veins or improper haemostasis. It may need re-exploration.

2. **Wound infection** may result in discharging pus which is the cause of postoperative fever. Infection is the chief cause of recurrence.

3. **Severe periostitis pubis** (to avoid this nowadays, the repair is not done by taking bites through pubic bone). X-ray of the bone may have to be taken for diagnosis.

   It is managed by analgesics and in intractable cases, injection of corticosteroids locally may reduce the pain.

4. **Nerve entrapment** causing pain

10. *Advice at discharge*

- Not to strain or lift heavy weights (e.g. bucketful of water) or to carry load on the shoulders for 3 months.

- If there is any precipitating cause such as chronic cough or difficulty in passing urine, etc., they have to be treated first. Otherwise, hernia will recur once again.

   *Many surgeons have stopped doing Bassini's repair because of increase recurrence rates (6 to 8%). Lichtenstein repair is the most popular repair done today.

LICHTENSTEIN REPAIR

- Herniotomy is done first. Polypropylene mesh— 8 × 16 cm mesh is used tailored to patient's requirement.

- **Preparation of mesh:** Corners can be cut so as to give a round shape. A slit is given on the junction of one-third below and two-thirds below and two-thirds above laterally, to allow spermatic cord to pass thorough and to overlap two tails.

- It is sutured medially to overlap pubic tubercle and sutured over the tissue of symphysis pubis. Avoid taking suture bites through pubic bone.

- Laterally through the slit in the mesh, spermatic cord is brought out and mesh is sutured above to the conjoined tendon, inferiorly sutured to the inguinal ligament and laterally wrapping the spermatic cord.

SURGERY FOR HYDROCOELE

1. *Indication:* Vaginal hydrocoele. However, infantile and funicular hydrocoeles are also treated surgically in the same manner.

2. *Contraindication*: Secondary hydrocoele due to *testicular tumours*. They contain haemorrhagic fluid. **Biggest blunder** can be done here by incising the scrotum mistaking it to be a vaginal hydrocoele.

3. *Position of the patient*: Supine

Clinical Wisdom

Before incising scrotum, rule out testicular tumour. When in doubt, get ultrasound of testis.

---

4. *Anaesthesia*

- SA or GA
- It can also be done by using local infiltration anaesthesia.

5. *Preparation of the parts*: Savlon and spirit (iodine is better avoided because it can cause severe scrotal dermatitis and excoriation of skin, which can cause more discomfort to the patient than hydrocoele surgery).

6. *Procedure* (Clinical Box 30.7)

Incision: Hydrocoele is held tense by an assistant and 5–6 cm incision (depending upon size) is made over the most prominent part of the swelling parallel to the median raphe of the scrotum.

Layers opened
- Skin
- Dartos
- External spermatic fascia
- Cremasteric fascia
- Internal spermatic fascia

At this stage, hydrocoele sac is visible and is delivered outside the incision (Fig. 30.113).

Hydrocoele fluid is drained by using *trocar and cannula*. An opening is made in the tunica vaginalis sac and it is enlarged. All fluid is drained out. Testis and epididymis are inspected for any pathology, e.g. Craggy epididymis can be found in tuberculosis.

Clinical Box 30.7

Hydrocoele surgery
- Aspiration: Not advised
- Lord's plication: Small hydrocoele
- Jaboulay's: Large hydrocoele

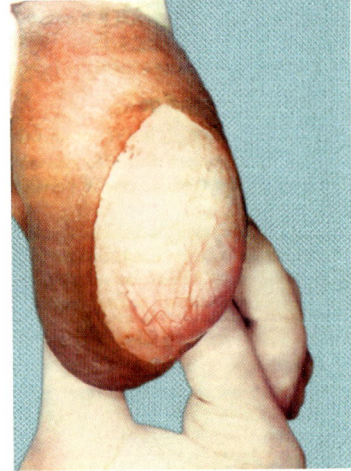

Fig. 30.113: Hydrocoele sac being delivered

Depending on the size of the hydrocoele and thickness of the wall of the sac, two types of surgery can be done.

a. **Small tunica vaginalis sac (TV sac):** The redundant tunica vaginalis is plicated by interrupted sutures. The sac gets crumpled up and surrounds the testis. This is called **Lord's plication** (Fig. 30.114).

b. **Sac is large and thick:** Partial excision and eversion of sac is ideal treatment. In this operation, after excision of the sac, cut edge of the sac is everted and sutured behind the testis. This is called **Jaboulay's operation. By eversion of the sac, the secreting surface of the testis becomes anterior and secretions are absorbed by subcutaneous lymphatics** (Figs 30.115A and B).

7. *Closure*

- A corrugated plastic drain is kept in the scrotum and brought out separately by making a stab

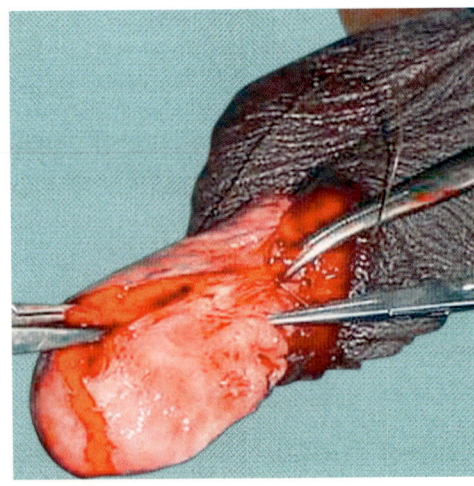

Fig. 30.114: The sac has been everted and edges of the sac sutured together

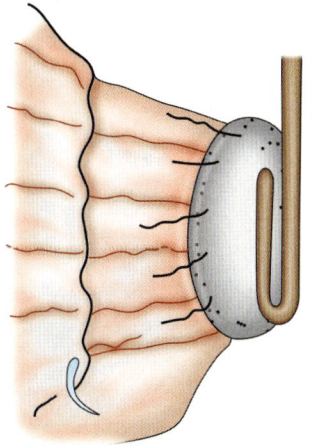

Fig. 30.115A: Lord's plication

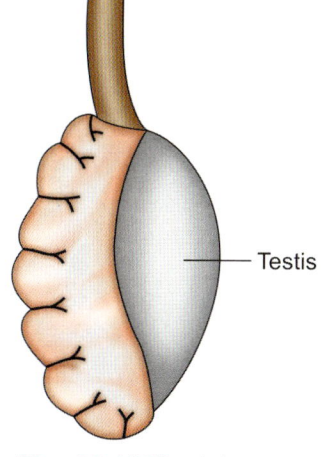

Testis

Fig. 30.115B: Jaboulay's operation

incision and is anchored to the scrotal skin by white thread.

- Subcutaneous layer by using absorbable suture such as chromic catgut or Vicryl sutures.

- Skin—interrupted thread (white)/catgut. Silk is avoided for skin closure over the scrotum as black colour of the silk is not seen clearly over dark pigmented skin of the scrotum, making stitch removal difficult. Absorbable sutures such as catgut or Vicryl can also be used.

- Scrotal support is given to reduce oedema.

8. Postoperative management

- NPO for 6 hours followed by soft diet

- Antibiotics and analgesics

- Suture removal after 7–8 days

9. Postoperative complications

- **Haematoma:** If it is large and increasing, wound should be reopened urgently and bleeders have to be ligated. It may be due to injury to the testicular artery, vein or pampiniform plexus of veins.

- **Wound infection** can result in pyocoele. Testis can undergo necrosis. Such cases are treated with orchidectomy.

- **Injury to the spermatic cord**

10. Advice at discharge: Rest for about a week

Clinical Wisdom

Even though surgery for hydrocoele is minor, it should not be taken lightly.

INCISION AND DRAINAGE (I and D)

1. Indication: Pyogenic abscess

2. Contraindication: Cold abscess

3. Position of the patient: Supine, prone or lateral depending upon site of abscess.

4. Anaesthesia

- GA is preferred because abscess is multiloculated and infiltration of lignocaine into the abscess cavity does not act because of the acidic pH of the pus.

- However, a superficial abscess which is pointing can be managed without GA.

5. Preparation of the parts: Iodine and spirit

6. Procedure

- **A stab incision** is made over the most prominent part of the swelling where skin is red, thinned out and is pointed.

- Pus that is drained is **sent for culture and sensitivity.**

- A sinus forceps or finger is introduced within the abscess cavity and all the loculi are broken. When fresh blood oozes out, it indicates the completion of the procedure.

- Cavity is irrigated with antiseptic agents such as iodine solution. It is followed by irrigation with normal saline.

- If cavity is large, it is packed with roller gauze soaked in iodine and it is removed after 24–48 hours. Packing helps in controlling the bleeding, and keeps the abscess cavity open. By 7–10 days, the cavity collapses, granulation tissue fills up the cavity and healing takes place.

7. Closure: An abscess should not be closed, as it contains pus, bacteria (*see* also breast abscess drainage).

8. Postoperative management

- Antibiotics

- Control of diabetes (if patient is diabetic)

- Regular dressings of the wound with antiseptic agents.

9. Postoperative complications

- During the process of breaking the loculi, vessels underneath may be injured causing haematoma which requires drainage. Otherwise no specific complications.

- Injury to vessels or nerves can occur, if basic principles of drainage of an abscess are not followed. When an abscess is located over a major vessel, as in axilla or neck, **do not make a stab incision**. An incision is made on the skin and subcutaneous tissue and sinus forceps is introduced. Later, it is treated like the treatment of an abscess. This method is followed to avoid injury to major vessels. It is also indicated in parotid abscess to avoid damage to facial nerve. This is called **Hilton's method of drainage**.

10. *Advice at discharge*: Control of diabetes (if present).

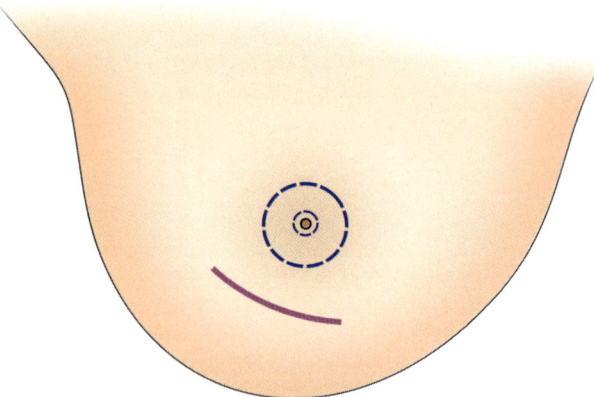

Fig. 30.116: Incision for breast abscess

INCISION AND DRAINAGE OF BREAST ABSCESS

1. *Indication*: Breast abscess (Clinical Box 30.8)

2. *Contraindication*: None

3. *Position of the patient*: Supine

4. *Anaesthesia*: GA

5. *Preparation*: Iodine and spirit

6. *Procedure* (Figs 30.116 and 30.117): A 5–6 cm long semicircular incision is made over the swelling where there is maximum tenderness. It is drained just like pyogenic abscess. Another stab incision is made in the dependent position and corrugated rubber drain/plastic is brought out through this incision.

7. *Closure*

- If infection is very severe, **do not close the incision**.
- Otherwise, main wound is sutured and corrugated red rubber drain is brought down at the dependent position. Once the drainage is minimal, the drain is removed.

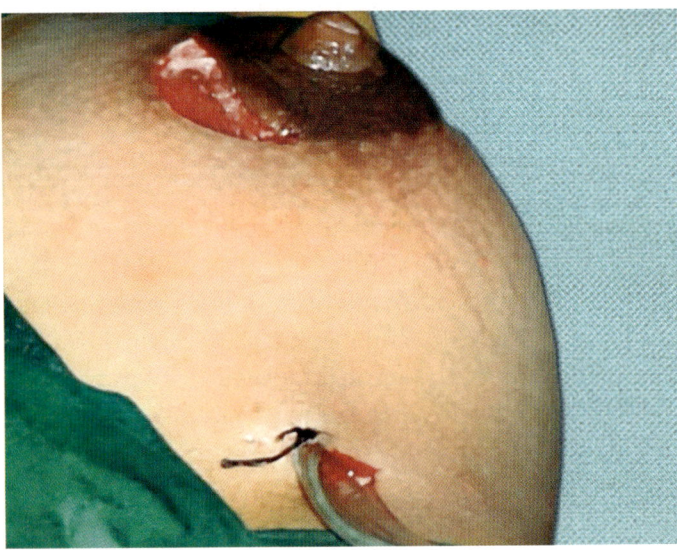

Fig. 30.117: Drainage and usage of corrugated rubber drain

8. **Postoperative management**
- NPO for about 6 hours.
- Antibiotic of choice is **cloxacillin** 500 mg 6th hourly because the common organism is *Staphylococcus aureus*.
- It may take 7–15 days for complete healing.
- One should not wait for fluctuation to develop in a breast abscess. If pain and tenderness does not subside by 48 hours, breast abscess is incised. Otherwise, breast tissue gets damaged.

9. *Postoperative complications*: Haematoma needs evacuation.

10. *Advice at discharge*: Lactating women should clean the nipple after every breastfeed and keep it clean.

Clinical Wisdom

Minor breast abscess need not be drained. One or two ultrasound guided aspirations may be curative in many cases.

Clinical Box 30.8 🗝️

Breast abscess drainage
- GA is preferred
- Do not wait for fluctuation
- Throbbing pain is an indication for surgery
- Small curved incision
- Keep in mind, mastitis carcinomatosa

Ultrasound-guided aspiration of breast abscess should be done first especially in unilocular breast abscess.

Clinical Wisdom

Do not use radial incision in breast surgery.

CIRCUMCISION

Circumcision refers to removal of the preputial skin.

1. *Indications*:

    a. Ritual: Religious

    b. Phimosis

2. *Contraindication*: Hypospadias

Clinical Wisdom

Preputial skin is required for repair of hypospadias.

3. *Position of the patient*: Supine

4. *Anaesthesia*

    a. In children—GA

    b. In adults—LA

5. *Preparation of the parts*: Savlon and spirit

Clinical Wisdom

Use plain lignocaine (without adrenaline) for LA during circumcision. Dose: 2% lignocaine 10–15 ml.

6. *Procedure*

In adults (Fig. 30.118)

- Skin of the tip of the penis is held in two places by using artery forceps, prepuce is separated from the glans and is slit up in mid-dorsal line to a point a little beyond the middle of the glans.

- Preputial layers are trimmed away in a line parallel to the corona. *On the ventral surface, frenular artery needs to be ligated by using figure of 8 stitch.* Two layers of prepuce are united by interrupted fine chromic catgut sutures/Vicryl. Dressings are applied.

In children (Fig. 30.119)

- Prepuce is held by two artery forceps and gentle traction is applied. A small artery clamp is applied distal to the glans and skin distal to the clamp is removed.

- Once clamp is removed, bleeding points are identified and ligated.

- Two layers of prepuce are approximated by using chromic catgut.

7. *Closure*: Two layers of prepuce by using chromic catgut/Vicryl.

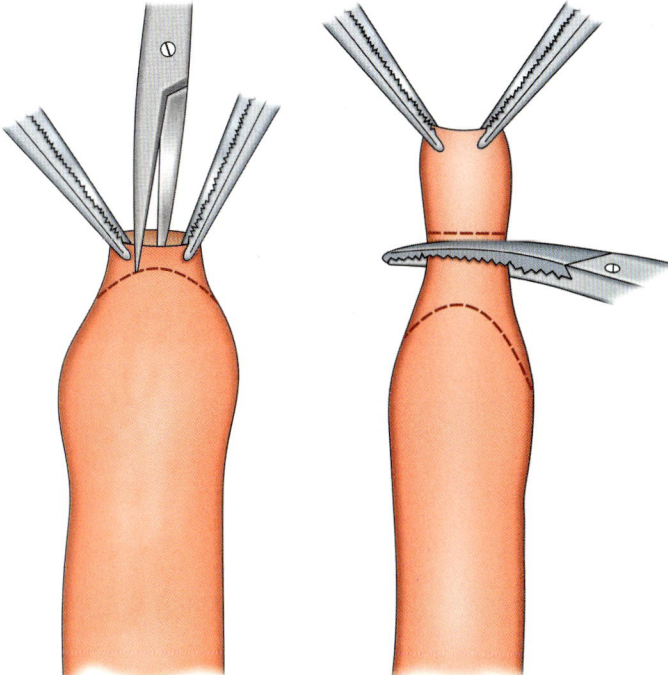

Fig. 30.118: Circumcision in adults

Fig. 30.119: Circumcision in children

8. *Postoperative management*

- Sedatives and analgesics

- Antibiotics

- Removal of sutures is very painful. Hence, **do not use nonabsorbable sutures**.

9. *Postoperative complications*

a. Injury to the glans penis can occur when there are extensive adhesions between prepuce and glans. It needs suturing.

b. **Haematoma:** Due to injury to the corpora cavernosa or due to the bleeding from cut edges.

c. **Tension at suture line,** if too much skin is removed. This may cause painful erection at a later date.

10. *Advice at discharge*: This surgery in adults is done on an outpatient basis. Patients are discharged within a few hours. Hence, patients are advised to report, if there is bleeding and also not to wet the area for 2–3 days.

VENESECTION OR CUT DOWN

1. *Indications*

- Shock: Hypovolaemic, haemorrhagic, burns, etc.

- When peripheral veins are not visible due to shock, burns or massive haemorrhage, an incision is made

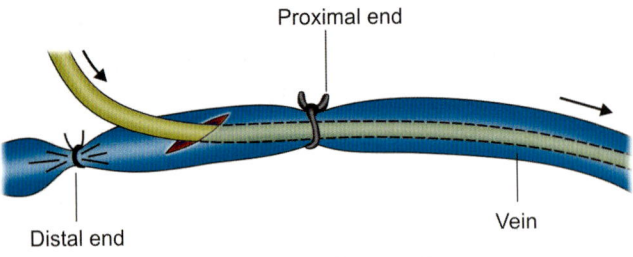

Fig. 30.120: Venesection

in the anatomical sites of the vein. The vein is identified, isolated and cannulated for transfusion of fluids. This procedure is called *venesection* or *cut down* (Fig. 30.120).

2. Contraindication: No

3. Position of the patient: Supine

4. Anaesthesia: Local infiltration by using 2% lignocaine 3–5 ml.

5. Preparation: Iodine and spirit

6. Procedure: Cephalic vein cut down is the most popular and an ideal procedure. A transverse incision about 5 cm is made in the deltopectoral groove. The cephalic vein is isolated and the distal end of the vein is ligated so that venous blood does not leak. A nick is made in the vein, through which a sufficient sized cannula (infant feeding tube can be used) is introduced. A silk ligature is applied above, just tight enough to hold cannula in place. Free flow of venous blood in the cannula indicates that it is inside the vein. The cannula is advanced further for about 10–15 cm. It is connected to IV line containing fluid (Fig. 30.120).

Precautions

1. Neither air bubbles should be injected nor should they be present in the drip set, to avoid air embolism.

2. Upper ligature should not be tight. It may obstruct the flow of fluids.

3. Strict antiseptic principles must be followed to avoid septicaemia.

Other veins selected for cut down

- Basilic vein in arm
- Cubital vein at the elbow
- Long saphenous vein in the leg. Veins in the leg, as far as possible, should be avoided to prevent deep vein thrombosis.

7. Closure: Skin—interrupted silk

8. Postoperative management
- Care of wound by dressing
- To avoid air bubbles in the drip set

9. Postoperative complications
- Infection, chills, rigors and septicaemia
- Air embolism

10. Advice at discharge: Nil

Advantages of Cephalic Vein Cut Down

1. Reliable vein and easy to do.

2. If cannula is advanced into the right heart, CVP can be measured.

3. Mobility of the patient is not restricted.

4. Substances which cannot be given in a peripheral vein, such as 50% dextrose, lipids, amino acids, etc. can be given without risk of thrombosis of the vein, for hyperalimentation purposes.

Clinical Wisdom

Cannulate vein, not an artery for venesection. Thin-walled nonpulsatile blue structure is vein.

VASECTOMY

Division and removal of a part of the vas deferens is vasectomy (Fig. 30.121).

1. Indications
- Family planning
- To prevent epididymo-orchitis after prostatectomy (nowadays not routinely done).

2. Contraindications
- **Relative:** Tuberculosis epididymo-orchitis. The incision may result in a nonhealing sinus. Hence, control of tuberculosis is done first followed by vasectomy.

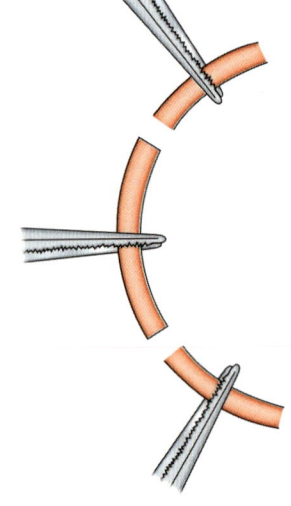

Fig. 30.121: Division of vas deferens by three-clamp method

- **Absolute:** Suspicion of testicular malignancy.

3. Position of the patient: Supine

4. Anaesthesia: Local anaesthesia using 3–5 ml of 2% lignocaine.

5. *Preparation of the parts*

- Savlon and spirit
- Iodine is better avoided

6. *Procedure*

Feeling the vas deferens: After cleaning and draping, the vas is felt, at the root of scrotum between the index finger and thumb. It feels like a cord. Lignocaine is infiltrated and wait for 1–2 minutes for lignocaine to act.

Incision: An incision of 2–4 cm is made in root of scrotum and it is deepened through layers of scrotum. An 'Allis forceps' is introduced within the incision and spermatic cord is held. During this step, fingers of the other hand help in guiding/locating/stabilising the cord. The coverings of the cord are incised.

Precautions

- Do not damage testicular vessels.
- Vas is separated. It is confirmed by its white colour, and it feels like a cord.
- Division of vas by three-clamp method (Fig. 30.121).
- Vas is cut in two places A and B so that a piece of vas is removed, which can be sent for histopathology to confirm that it is vas.
- Since a piece of vas is removed, reunion of the cut ends will not occur.
- The two cut ends of vas are doubly ligated by using silk.

7. *Closure*: The skin is closed by absorbable one or two sutures so that removal not required.

8. *Postoperative management*

- Rest for a few hours
- Antibiotics and analgesics.

> **Clinical Wisdom**
>
> The procedure is repeated on the other side.

9. *Postoperative complications*

- Injury to the vessels, resulting in a large haematoma.
- Infection
- Testicular atrophy can occur a few years later. It is due to immunological reaction rather than disuse atrophy.

10. *Advice at discharge*: To use other methods of family planning for two months while having sexual intercourse, as some sperms may be present in the distal end of the vas and seminal vesicle.

> **Clinical Wisdom**
>
> Vasectomy being a part of family planning project, every student should be familiar with this.

No Scalpel Vasectomy

- It is a novel technique to do vasectomy through one single puncture which does not require any suturing. It is less traumatic than conventional vasectomy and shortens recovery time.
- The procedure is done with LA.
- A special instrument is used to puncture the scrotum and grasp the vas deferens. Vas is then cut and through the same puncture, the other side is also operated.

TRACHEOSTOMY

An opening made in the trachea is tracheostomy.

1. *Indications*

a. Emergency

- Choking of the larynx due to dentures, foreign bodies, fish bones, etc.
- Stridor due to diphtheria, carcinoma larynx and bilateral recurrent laryngeal nerve paralysis after thyroidectomy.

b. Elective

- Coma
- Tetanus
- Barbiturate poisoning
- Head injuries
- Pulmonary insufficiency

2. *Contraindications*: Anaplastic carcinoma thyroid patients presenting with stridor due to infiltration of growth into trachea. It may not be possible to do a tracheostomy or an attempt to do tracheostomy may result in the growth fungating through the incision (which is best avoided). In such patients, **endotracheal intubation** is done, if possible. If not possible, no other intervention is done.

3. *Position of the patient*: Supine with extension of the neck and head by keeping a sandbag or a pillow under the shoulders.

4. *Anaesthesia*: Local infiltration anaesthesia.

5. *Preparation of the parts*: Iodine and spirit.

6. *Procedure*

- **Incision:** Transverse curved incision for about 3–4 cm is made at the level of 2nd tracheal ring.

- **Dissection:** Skin, subcutaneous tissue and deep fascia are incised. Isthmus of thyroid is separated.

- **Procedure:** A transverse cut is made in the 2nd tracheal cartilage, its edge is held with Allis forceps and a small cuff of cartilage is removed. 'Cricoid hook' can be used to stabilise the trachea (found more useful in children).

- A suitable-sized tracheostomy tube is introduced within.

- The cuff of tracheostomy tube is inflated by using 2–5 ml of air and is held in place by passing a tape around the neck.

- Confirm that the **tube** is in the **trachea**, not in the subcutaneous plane.

- Confirm **air entry** on both sides of lung.

7. *Closure*: A few interrupted skin sutures by the side of the tracheostomy tube and dressing is applied.

8. *Postoperative management*

- Suction of tracheostomy tube, regular dressing

- Humidification of air

- Check for air entry

9. *Postoperative complications*

- Wound infection

- Air leakage

- Improper air entry

- Cricoid stenosis (high tracheostomy).

Closure of tracheostomy

- Once patient improves and is able to take care of his own airway, the tracheostomy tube is blocked. Observe for 24–48 hours.

- If there is **no respiratory distress**, the cuff is deflated and the tube is removed. A few skin sutures can be put or dressing is applied. It closes automatically.

10. *Advice at discharge*

- Tracheostomy done after laryngectomy is permanent. Patients should learn to use metal tracheostomy, cleaning the tubes, etc.

- Inner tube should be removed, cleaned and replaced in cases of respiratory distress.

SUPRAPUBIC CYSTOSTOMY (SPC)

In this operation, urinary bladder is drained to the exterior by inserting a Malecot's catheter[1] into the bladder.

1. *Indication*: Retention of urine due to any cause where a catheter or a dilator cannot be passed through the urethra to empty the bladder. However, this operation is rarely done nowadays since suprapubic catheterisation with a trocar and cannula has simplified the procedure.

2. *Contraindication*: Carcinoma bladder

3. *Position of the patient*: Supine

4. *Anaesthesia*: SA or GA

5. *Preparation of the parts*: Iodine and spirit

6. *Procedure*

Incision (Fig. 30.122): A vertical incision of 6–8 cm is made below the umbilicus in the midline.

Layers opened

- Skin, subcutaneous tissue, and linea alba in the upper part of incision. (**Below the semilunar line, there is no linea alba.**)

- Rectus muscle is split in the midline (separated).

- Extraperitoneal tissue with fat is seen.

- With blunt dissection, fat and peritoneum are swept upwards so that anterior wall of the bladder is seen with its peritoneal covering. The bladder is identified by perivesical plexus of veins or aspirating the urine with syringe and needle.

- Two stay sutures are applied on the anterior bladder wall. The bladder is incised and urine drained out. The opening is enlarged and a

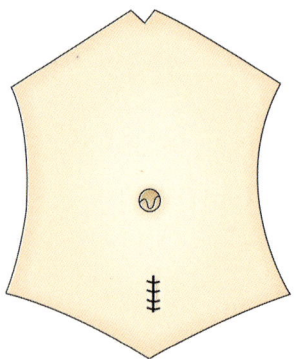

Fig. 30.122: Incision for SPC

---

[1]Malecot's catheter SPC is no longer done, trocar SPC is the choice today

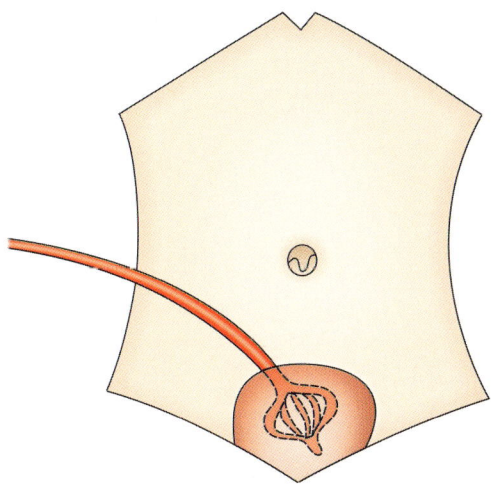

Fig. 30.123: Completion of SPC

Malecot's catheter is introduced within. It is brought outside from the upper part of the incision and connected to a closed bag (urosac) (Fig. 30.123).

- Urinary bladder is closed with absorbable 2–0 chromic catgut sutures.

- A corrugated drainage tube is kept in the prevesical space.

7. *Closure*

- Split rectus muscles are approximated by using catgut sutures.

- Anterior rectus sheath/linea alba—by nonabsorbable sutures.

- Subcutaneous tissue—chromic catgut

- Skin—silk

8. *Postoperative management*

- Antibiotics

- Analgesics

9. *Postoperative complications*

a. Wound infection

b. Haemorrhage: Bladder wash is given till the contents are clear. Rarely, it may need reexploration and control of the bleeding.

c. If urinary leakage occurs, it is usually minor.

10. *Advice at discharge*: Nil

THYROIDECTOMY

1. *Indications*: All goitres with symptoms—MNG, toxic goitre, colloid goitre and malignant goitre.

2. *Contraindications*: Asymptomatic goitre, Hashimoto's thyroiditis, anaplastic carcinoma thyroid.

3. *Position of the patient*

- Supine with extended neck by keeping a sandbag under the shoulders.

- Head end of the patient is elevated to about 30° to reduce venous congestion. This position is called **anti-Trendelenburg position**.

4. Anaesthesia: GA

5. *Preparation of the parts*: Iodine and spirit

6. *Procedure*

Incision (Fig. 30.124): 6–8 cm collar neck incision or crease incision.

Layers opened

- Skin, platysma, subcutaneous tissue in the line of incision.

- Deep fascia is incised vertically

- Strap muscles are separated (can be cut in very large goitres).

- Pretracheal fascia is incised

- Thyroid gland is mobilised by using blunt dissection.

- Assess the entire gland to know whether it is a solitary nodule or multinodular goitre.

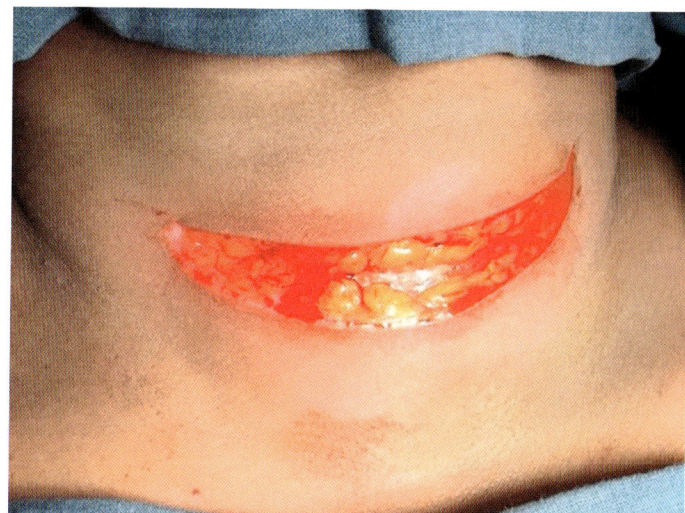

Fig. 30.124: Incision for thyroidectomy is given

- One of the lobes is mobilised by dividing middle thyroid vein (single, short, thin vein).
- Then, upper pole is dissected. This pedicle contains superior thyroid artery and veins. They are ligated and divided in between. **Please apply double ligature proximally.**

Clinical Wisdom

All major arteries should be ligated twice proximally. Example: Superior thyroid artery, facial artery, left gastric artery, cystic artery, renal artery.

- Upper pole should be ligated as close to the gland as possible to avoid damage to external laryngeal nerve.
- Inferior thyroid artery used to be ligated[1] well away from the gland. It has a horizontal course. It is thick and pulsatile. Then, the branches of inferior thyroid artery are ligated. This will avoid injury to recurrent laryngeal nerve and it will prevent hypoparathyroidism also. Multiple veins, present in the lower pole, are ligated and divided.
- Isthmus is separated from trachea, both above and below.
- In subtotal thyroidectomy, the entire isthmus, and parts of the right and left lobes are removed in flush with tracheal surface, leaving behind tissue in the tracheo-oesophageal groove to protect recurrent laryngeal nerve and parathyroid gland. Cut edges of thyroid gland are sutured by using Vicryl sutures (Fig. 30.125). In total thyroidectomy almost entire gland is removed (Fig. 30.126).

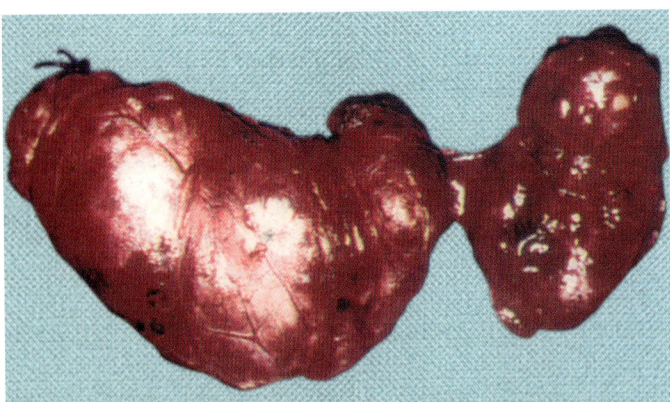

Fig. 30.125: Subtotal thyroidectomy for MNG

---

[1]Today, branches of inferior thyroid artery are ligated—not the main artery so as to preserve blood supply to parathyroid gland.

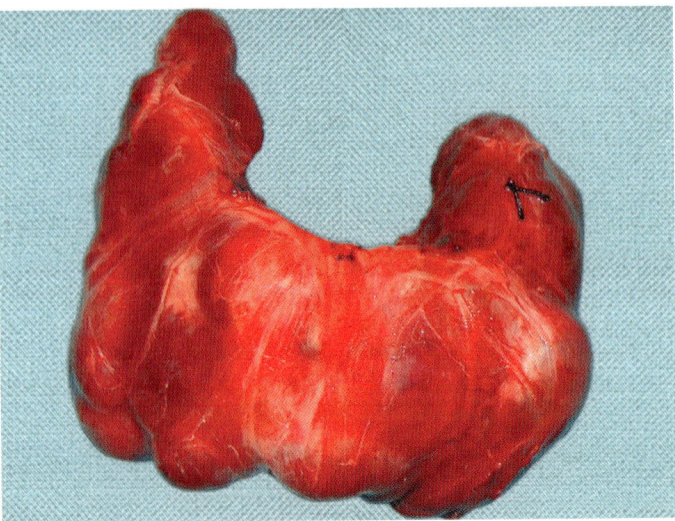

Fig. 30.126: Total thyroidectomy specimen for papillary carcinoma thyroid

Precautions

- Any structure directly entering the gland is unlikely to be RLN and hence, can safely be divided.
- Recurrent laryngeal nerve enters the thyrohyoid membrane, after running a vertical course, in the tracheo-oesophageal groove.

7. *Closure*

- A suction drain is kept in the thyroid bed.
- Deep fascia—continuous Vicryl
- Subcutaneous fat—Vicryl
- Skin—interrupted silk/subcuticular sutures
- A bandage is applied.

8. *Postoperative management*

- NPO for 6–8 hours followed by liquid diet
- Antibiotics are not necessary
- **Head end must be elevated** to reduce oedema of the wound.
- In toxic goitres, propranolol must be continued after surgery and slowly tapered over a week.
- Blood transfusion depending upon blood loss.
- Drain removal after 2–3 days (once it stops draining).
- Suture removal after 4–5 days.

9. *Postoperative complications*

A. **Haemorrhage: Tension haematoma.** Reactionary haemorrhage is due to slipping of ligature due to coughing, hypertension, etc. If it is alarming, deep fascial sutures have to be opened, haematoma drained and haemostasis has to be achieved.

B. **Thyrotoxic crisis** in patients with toxic goitre

C. **Tracheomalacia**—resulting in stridor

D. Recurrent laryngeal nerve paralysis

E. Hypothyroidism

F. Hypoparathyroidism

G. Wound infection

10. *Advice at discharge*: This depends on the type of indication for thyroid surgery, e.g. those who undergo subtotal thyroidectomy for thyrotoxicosis have to be closely followed for recurrent thyrotoxicosis or hypothyroidism. If calcium levels are low, it has to be supplemented.

Clinical Wisdom

Thyroidectomy is an operation which provides a surgeon to demonstrate his skills and capacity to be meticulous.

Different Types of Thyroidectomy (Table 30.2)

What is Zuckerkandl's Tubercle?

- **Zuckerkandl's tubercle** is a pyramidal extension of the thyroid gland, located at the most posterior side of each lobe.
- The structure is important in thyroid surgery as it is closely related to the recurrent laryngeal nerve, the inferior thyroid artery, Berry's ligament and the parathyroid glands.
- It is also important to remove this *in toto* while doing thyroidectomy for malignancies.

AMPUTATIONS

Definitions/Terminologies of Amputation

- **End bearing:** Weight is taken by the body.
- **Non-end bearing:** Here weight is taken by the joint.
- **Guillotine amputation:** Here no flaps are raised, all the tissues are divided at the same level and the stump is kept open.
- **Formal amputation:** In this case, depending upon the indications and the decisions taken by the surgeon, amputation is done with closure of the stump.

Table 30.2: Different types of thyroidectomy

Diseases	Before surgery	After surgery	Name of the operation
1. Solitary nodule (benign)			Hemithyroidectomy means removal of one lobe with isthmus
2. Multinodular goitre			Subtotal thyroidectomy
3. Toxic multinodular goitre			Subtotal thyroidectomy
4. Primary thyrotoxicosis			Subtotal thyroidectomy
5. Malignant neoplasm			Near total thyroidectomy
6. Malignant neoplasm— high-grade carcinoma			Total thyroidectomy

Indications

1. Vitality of the part is destroyed by injury or disease—*dead limb.*

2. Life of patient is threatened by spread of a local condition—*deadly limb.*

   Examples: Gas gangrene, extensive melanoma

3. Patient may be better served by an artificial limb because of deformity or paralysis—*deformed limb. In such cases, better to amputate and fit in an artificial limb.*

4. *Dying limb*—acutely ischaemic limb, late presentation.

Optimum Levels of Amputation

Level of amputation depends not only upon the extent of disease but also function desired in the remaining stump. This differs markedly in the upper and lower limbs.

Ideal Stump

* Should have ideal length for proper fitting of prosthesis. Examples: Below knee: 8 to 12 cm from tibial tuberosity; above knee: 23 cm from greater trochanter and, above and below elbow 20 cm stump.

* Should be conical and rounded

* Should not be tender

* Should have adequate muscle padding so that its movements are adequate.

* Should have adequate blood supply so that it heals with primary intention in the postoperative period.

* Should have a thin scar which should not interfere with prosthetic function.

* Should not have any redundant soft tissue hanging.

* Skin and scar should not be adhered to the underlying tissue.

Incisions

Depending upon the site of the level of amputation and keeping in mind the blood supply of the part, different types of incision are given. They are as follows:

* *Racquet incision:* This is used in amputation for digits or toes.

* *Elliptical or oval incision* is given for metatarsal amputations.

* *Circular incision* is given especially in *Guillotine* amputation.

* *U-shaped incisions:* These are given to raise flaps—anterior and posterior flaps as in below knee or above knee. By convention, equal flaps are used for above knee and a long posterior and short anterior flaps are used for below knee amputation. This is because vascularity of the posterior flap is good below the knee due to bulky muscles with good blood supply when compared to the thin, muscle less anterior flap (*see* Ten Commandments).

TEN COMMANDMENTS: GENERAL PRINCIPLES IN AMPUTATIONS

1. Should mark the incision

2. Should give prophylactic antibiotics

3. Should avoid **tourniquet** in arterial occlusive diseases.

4. Should ensure adequate blood supply to the flaps—if raised as in below knee and above knee amputations.

5. Should ligate the blood vessels securely to avoid haematoma and then infection in the postoperative period.

6. Should not clamp the nerves but they are pulled down and transected as high as possible so that nerve ends are not caught in the suture line.

7. Should saw the anterior part of the bone obliquely to give a smooth anterior bevel which prevents pressure necrosis of the flap.

8. Should excise the bulky muscles so as to give a good conical stump (Fig. 30.127). Example: Excise soleus muscle in below knee amputations.

9. Should use absorbable sutures to unite the muscle ends.

10. Should drain the cavity with a suction drain which is brought out through the skin clear of the wound.

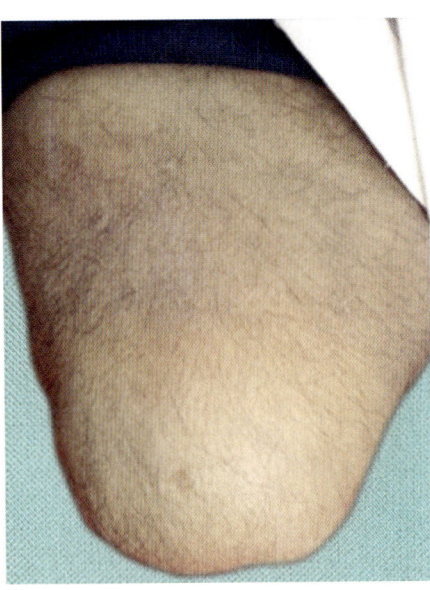

Fig. 30.127: Conical stump

AMPUTATIONS IN LEG

Skeleton of Foot

To have a better understanding of amputations kindly study Figs 30.128 and 30.129 first.

One of the common indications for lower limb amputations is diabetic ulcer/gangrene foot. Various types and various levels of amputations are done with the main aim to conserve as much as possible. However, when the limb is a useless limb, a below knee or an above knee amputation is done depending upon the seriousness of the problem.

1. *Ray amputation*: It is amputation of the toe with head of metatarsals.

2. *Transmetatarsal/amputation*: It is called Gilles' amputation. When multiple toes are involved with gangrene as in vasculitis syndromes or in diabetic patients, amputation is done through metatarsal bones—proximal to the neck, distal to the base. Long volar flap is created and sutured to the dorsal skin.

3. *Lisfranc's amputation (tarsometatarsal amputation)*: Tarsometatarsal articulations are called Lisfranc joint. The bones forming these are the first, second, and third cuneiforms, and the cuboid, which articulate with the bases of the metatarsal bones. The bones are connected by dorsal, plantar, and interosseous ligaments. These ligaments have to be divided. A long volar flap is used. Patient needs a surgical boot.

4. *Chopart's amputation*: Francis Chopart first described disarticulation through midtarsal joint. It is midtarsal amputation. Disarticulation of the foot is completed through talonavicular joint and through calcaneocuboid joint. Thus, Chopart amputation removes the forefoot and midfoot, saving talus and calcaneus. Tibialis anterior muscle is sutured to the drilled talus bone.

- **Contraindication:** Ischaemic feet as in atherosclerosis.
- **Disadvantages:** It is a very unstable amputation, because most of the tendons supporting the foot will be removed. Thus, it will go for equinus and

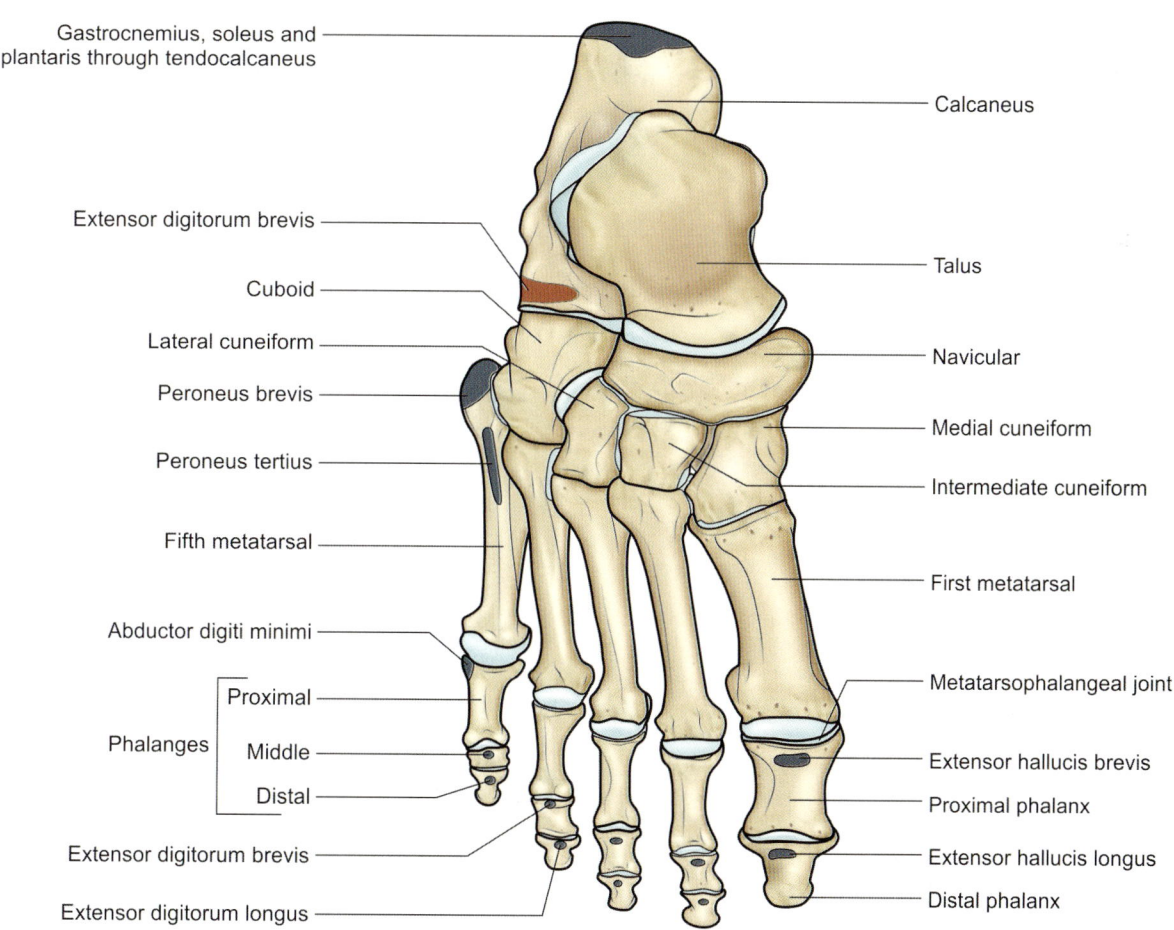

Fig. 30.128: Skeleton of the foot as seen from the dorsal aspect

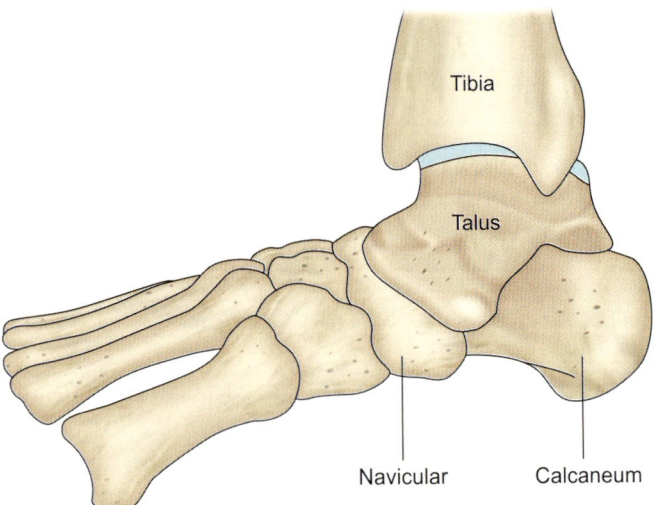

Fig. 30.129: Tarsal bones

must usually be fitted with a prosthesis that extends up to the patellar tendon level.

5. *Syme's amputation*: The tibia and fibula are divided at or immediately above the level of ankle joint and their ends are covered with a single flap obtained from heel.

- The end of the stump is at a height of about 6–8 cm from the ground.
- 50% of people will be able to walk on the stump without prosthesis.
- It is of value in patients who do not have access to modern artificial limbs.
- **Pirgroff's modification of Syme's amputation** retains a small portion of calcaneum in the flap obtained from heel.
- Heel flap is supplied by medial and lateral calcaneal vessels, both are branches of posterior tibial artery.
- Those who will not be able to walk after this amputation, can be fitted with elephant boot.

6. *Below knee amputation*
- It is the operation of choice when it is not possible to preserve the foot or heel.
- The ideal length of the tibial stump is 14 cm.
- Minimum length required to fit an artificial leg is 8 cm. Stump shorter than this tends to slip out of the socket of an artificial limb.
- The stump is covered by creating long posterior flap.
- This is the amputation commonly done in patients who are in severe sepsis involving the leg with uncontrolled diabetes and life is in danger.

- All the rules mentioned above in Ten Commandments are followed here such as division of the nerve, flap vascularity, reduction of bulky muscles and the anterior scar, thus prosthesis will not cause discomfort while walking.
- Advantages of below amputation include greater range of movements without limp and without support.
- This amputation is also called Burgess amputation.
- POP cast should be put to present contractures (Fig. 30.130).

7. *Amputations through thigh*
- Ideal length is 25–30 cm as measured from tip of trochanter.
- It is done when it is not possible to save at least 8 cm of tibia as in some cases of diabetes or spreading infections of the leg and when muscles involved are not bleeding at surgery.
- When this amputation is done in children, as much length as possible should be preserved (growing epiphysis of femur is at lower end).
- Unlike, below knee amputation, equal flaps are raised—anterior and posterior.
- Any length less than 10 cm of femur will not help. In such cases, hip disarticulation is done.
- In peripheral arterial occlusive disease, an attempt is made first by raising below knee flaps. If edges of the skin flaps do not bleed, it is better to go ahead with above knee flaps because vascularity of above knee flaps are better. Stump healing is better with above knee amputation than below knee.

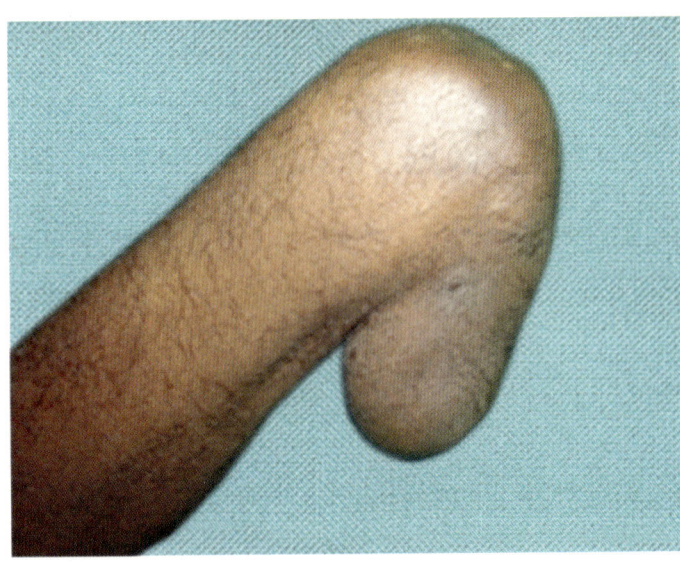

Fig. 30.130: Amputation contracture

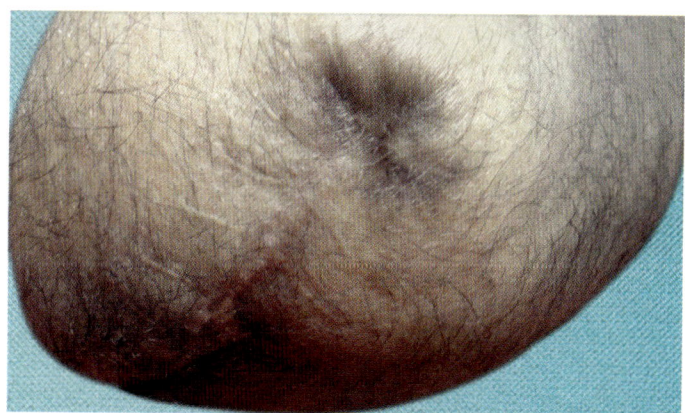

Fig. 30.131: Infected scar

- Disadvantages of this amputation are difficult rehabilitation (not easy), prosthesis fitting is not good, invariably patient needs one more support (Fig. 30.131).

8. *Hip disarticulation*

- When it is not possible to get minimum of 10 cm length of stump of the femur, hip disarticulation is done. This situation can occur in trauma or malignancies to get a wide clearance. Examples: Sarcomas or in cases of malignant melanomas.

- Usually, a single posterior flap is raised—Solcum's approach.

- Anterior approach can also be used (2nd option)—Boyd's approach.

9. *Hindquarter amputation*

- In this amputation—one side of pelvis with innominate bone, pubis, muscles and vessels are removed. Hence, it is called hemipelvectomy today.

- Indications are trauma and tumour (malignancy).

- In the original description, common iliac artery used to be ligated. However, now the branches of external and internal iliac artery are ligated.

- A large posterior flap based on superior gluteal artery is used.

- Variations in this amputation are: Extended hemipelvectomy with removal of posterior part of the sacrum.

- Limb preserving hemipelvectomy: It is called internal hemipelvectomy.

UPPER LIMB AMPUTATIONS

General Principles

- Conserve as much tissue as possible.

- Skin closure should not be under tension.

- Soft tissue cover over bony stump is desirable. Otherwise, painful adherent scar will result.

- Amputation through middle or terminal phalanx is preferred to disarticulation at interphalangeal joints since attachment of flexor tendons is thereby preserved.

- Every effort should be made to preserve as much of the thumb.

Amputation through Forearm and Upper Arm

- Ideal stump is 16–20 cm measured from olecranon.

- Stump less than 8 cm is useless for transmitting movement to an artificial elbow joint.

- A stump measuring 20 cm from acromion is ideal for fitting prosthesis.

Krukenberg's amputation: In this amputation, a gap is created between radius and ulna like a claw. It helps in holding objects.

Interscapulothoracic amputation (forequarter amputation)

- Indications are for malignancy involving axial skeleton such as sarcoma. Sepsis involving the upper limb is another indication such as gas gangrene.

- It is a very radical mutilating operation, hence all possible limb saving attempts should be done first.

- Entire upper limb with scapula and lateral 2/3rds of the clavicle with all the muscles attached to it are removed.

Complications Following Amputation

1. *Wound infection*: Especially it is common in amputations done for diabetic gangrene cases. Stitches may have to be opened to release pus followed by secondary suturing at a later date.

2. *Flap necrosis*: It is a common complication because of several reasons—important one being decreased blood supply to the limb either due to arterial occlusive disease or due to diabetes. Necrotic skin and subcutaneous tissues should be removed followed by secondary suturing at a later date. Hence, blood supply of the flap has to be kept in mind when raising the flaps.

3. *Stump ulcers* are common in the initial stages of wearing artificial limbs.

4. *Contracture*: If the artificial limb is not fitted, the stump will develop flexion contracture.

5. *Amputation neuroma*: This is an end neuroma. The cut end of the nerve is entrapped in the scar tissue and gives rise to pain. To avoid this, nerve end is pulled and cut so that after division of the nerve, the end gets retracted.

6. *Phantom limb*: A **phantom limb** is the sensation that a missing limb is attached to the body. Approximately 60 to 80% of individuals with an amputation experience phantom sensations in their amputated limb, and the majority of the sensations are painful. It is probably due to presence of a severe pain at the amputated site before surgery and the corresponding site in the brain has registered this sensation.

EXCISION OF SWELLINGS

Lipoma

1. *Indications*

- Large size (cosmesis/patient's wish)
- Recent rapid increase in size (sarcomatous change)
- Symptomatic naevo/neurolipomas
- Causing pressure symptoms based on site

2. *Contraindications*: Strictly speaking, there are no contraindications. However, asymptomatic lipomas in a difficult location need not be excised. However, small the surgery may be, safety is important principle to be kept in mind.

3. *Position of the patient*: Supine/lateral/prone depending upon the location.

4. *Anaesthesia*: If small, under LA. If large, regional anaesthesia or GA.

5. *Preparation of the parts*: Povidone-iodine and spirit.

6. *Surgical procedure*

- **Incision:** A linear incision over the summit of the swelling is placed and flaps raised on both sides of the incision.
- **Layers opened:** Skin and some part of the subcutaneous tissue till the capsule of the swelling is encountered.

- **Dissection:** Using an artery forceps or a mosquito forceps (if a small swelling), a plane is created between the raised flaps and the capsule of the swelling. Pressure is given at the base of the swelling to deliver out the lipoma. A small vessel may be encountered as the base is being dissected that should be identified and cauterised or ligated. The specimen should be sent for histopathological evaluation.

7. *Closure*: If a large cavity is created due to excision of swelling, the excised skin flaps can be refreshed and excess skin can be removed. A few interrupted Vicryl sutures can be placed to close subcutaneous layer. The skin is closed with 2–0 ethilon vertical mattress suture. Sometimes, a drain may have to be kept in the cavity.

8. *Postoperative management*: Rest to the part to prevent bleeding.

9. *Postoperative complications*

- Infection, bleeding
- Injury to vital structures around
- Seroma formation, if large cavity remains

10. *Advice at discharge*: Suture removal after 7–10 days.

Sebaceous Cyst

1. *Indications*

- Infection
- Complications such as **Cock's peculiar tumour**, horn and calcification
- Patient's wish (cosmesis).

2. *Contraindication*: No specific contraindication.

3. *Position of the patient*: Supine/lateral/prone depending upon the location.

4. *Anaesthesia*: Mostly LA. Multiple cysts over scalp and scrotum may require GA or regional anaesthesia.

5. *Preparation of the parts*: Povidone-iodine and spirit.

6. *Surgical procedure*

- **Incision: Elliptical incision** around the summit of the swelling encircling the punctum.
- **Layers opened**
  - Incision should be superficial. Care should be taken not to cut open the cyst wall.

– The principle is to **completely excise the cyst with its wall** and the overlying punctum and a bit of the surrounding skin around the punctum.

- **Dissection**
  - A plane is created between the skin and the cyst wall, carefully, preventing opening of the cyst wall.
  - An Allis forceps may be applied to the punctum and the elliptical skin to get a traction. Flaps need to be raised gradually on either sides of the incision and then deliver the cyst *in toto*.
  - If the cyst wall opens up, the sebum is removed completely and an effort to remove all the cyst wall, in piecemeal, is made.

7. *Closure*: Single layer closure of the skin.

8. *Postoperative management*: To keep the wound clean—proper hygiene.

9. *Postoperative complications*

- Flap necrosis, if too large a swelling and thin skin flaps.
- Infection
- Recurrence, if cyst wall is not completely removed.

10. *Advice at discharge*: Suture removal after 7–10 days.

Neurofibroma

1. *Indications*

- Cosmesis
- Symptoms of pain on pressure
- Pressure effects causing neurological deficits
- Sarcomatous changes

2. *Contraindication*: In von Recklinghausen's disease, only symptomatic neurofibromas should be removed.

3. Position of the patient: Supine/lateral/prone depending upon the location.

4. *Anaesthesia*: Mostly LA, sometimes GA

5. *Preparation of the parts*: Povidone-iodine and spirit.

6. *Surgical procedure*

- **Incision:** A linear incision over the summit of the swelling is placed and flaps raised on both sides of the incision.
- **Layers opened:** Skin and some part of the subcutaneous tissue till the capsule of the swelling is encountered.
- **Dissection:** Using an artery forceps or a mosquito forceps (if a small swelling), a plane is created between the raised flaps and the capsule of the swelling. Pressure is given at the base of the swelling to deliver out the neurofibroma. Care should be taken not to injure the underlying nerve while dissecting.

7. *Closure*: It can be closed in two layers, subcutaneous—Vicryl, interrupted and skin 2–0 ethilon vertical mattress.

8. *Postoperative management*: Rest to the affected part, to keep the wound clean.

9. *Postoperative complications*

- Infection
- Injury to the nerve causing weakness, loss of sensations of the affected part.
- If partially left behind, recurrence and chance of sarcomatous changes.

10. *Advice at discharge*: Suture removal after 7–10 days.

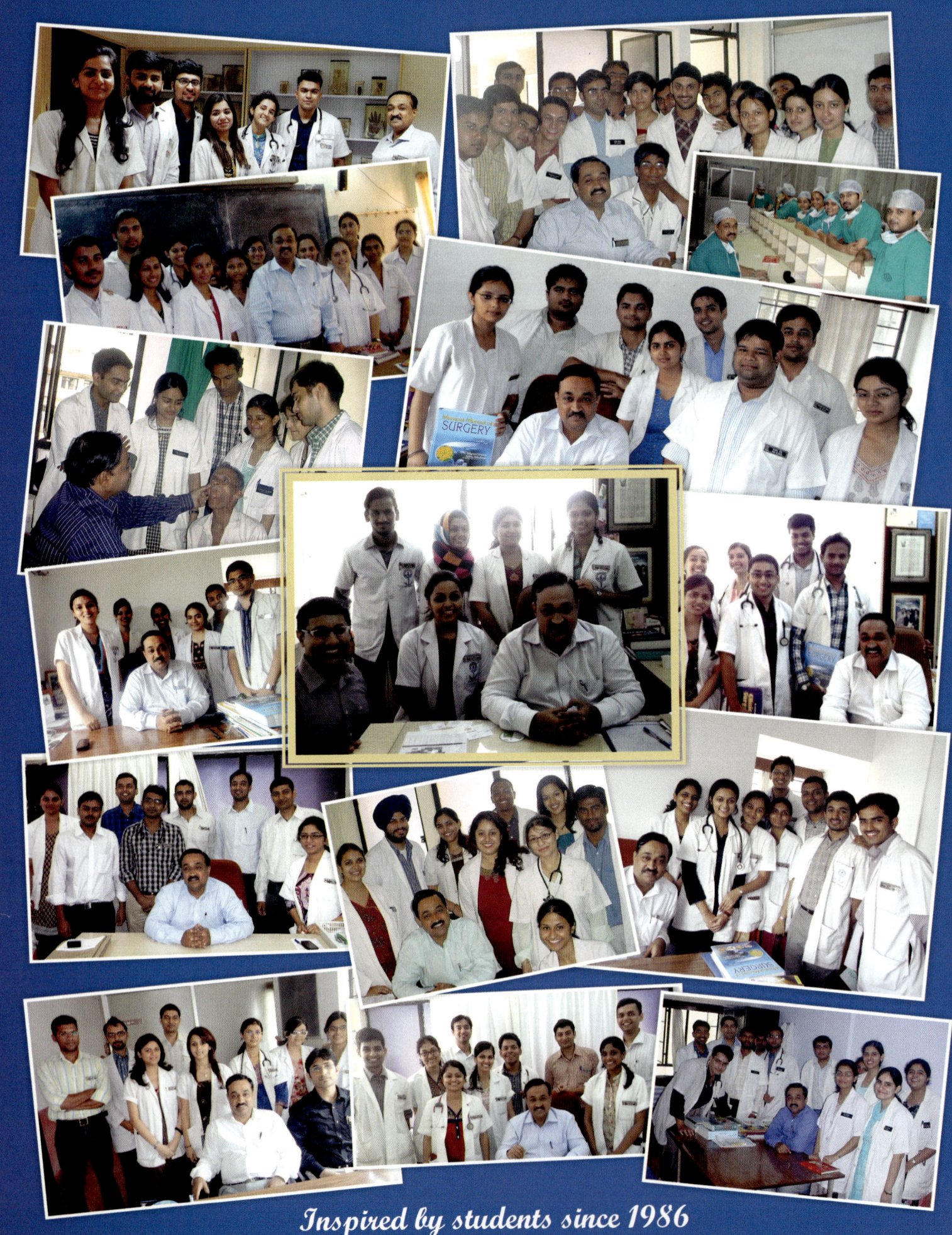

Inspired by students since 1986

Index